Prehospital Emergency Care & Crisis Intervention

FOURTH EDITION

Prehospital Emergency Care & Crisis Intervention

BRENT Q. HAFEN, Ph.D.
KEITH J. KARREN, Ph.D.

WITH WRITING ASSISTANCE FROM
Kathryn J. Frandsen
Lavina Fielding Anderson

MEDICAL CONSULTANT:
Keith R. Hooker, M.D., FACEP

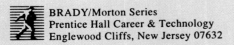
BRADY/Morton Series
Prentice Hall Career & Technology
Englewood Cliffs, New Jersey 07632

Library of Congress Cataloging-in-Publication Data

Hafen, Brent Q.
  Prehospital emergency care & crisis intervention / Brent Q. Hafen,
Keith J. Karren. -- 4th ed.
      p.   cm.
  "Brady Morton series."
  Includes bibliographical references and index.
  ISBN 0-89303-930-6
    1. Emergency medicine.   2. Disaster medicine.   3. Crisis
intervention (Psychiatry) I. Karren, Keith J.   II. Title.
III. Title: Prehospital emergency care and crisis intervention.
  [DNLM: 1. Crisis Intervention.   2. Emergencies.   3. Emergency
Medical Services.   WX 215 H138p]
RT86.7.H34   1992
616.02′5--dc20
DNLM/DLC
for Library of Congress   91-32195
                                                        CIP

ACQUISITION EDITOR: Natalie E. Anderson
PRODUCTION EDITOR: Ed Jones/Penelope Linskey
MARKETING MANAGER: Ann Elizabeth Hendrix
COPY EDITOR: Kathryn Beck
DESIGNER: Maureen Eide
COVER DESIGNER: Maureen Eide
PREPRESS BUYER: Ilene Levy
MANUFACTURING BUYER: Ed O'Dougherty
SUPPLEMENTS EDITOR: Judy Casillo
EDITORIAL ASSISTANT: Louise Fullum

COVER PHOTO: Linda Gheen

Notice: The author and the publisher of this book have taken care to make certain that the equipment, doses of drugs, and schedules of treatment are correct and compatible with the standards generally accepted at the time of publication. Nevertheless, as new information becomes available, changes in treatment and in the use of equipment and drugs become necessary. The reader is advised to carefully consult the instruction and information material included in the package insert of each drug or therapeutic agent, piece of equipment, or device before administration. This advice is especially important when using new or infrequently used drugs. Prehospital Care Providers are warned that use of any drugs or techniques must be authorized by their medical advisor, in accord with local laws and regulations. The publisher disclaims any liability, loss, injury, or damage incurred as a consequence, directly or indirectly, of the use and application of any of the contents of this book.

ISBN 0-89303-978-0

ISBN 0-89303-936-5 {INST. ED.}

Prentice-Hall International (UK) Limited, *London*
Prentice-Hall of Australia Pty. Limited, *Sydney*
Prentice-Hall Canada Inc., *Toronto*
Prentice-Hall Hispanoamericana, S. A., *Mexico*
Prentice-Hall of India Private Limited, *New Delhi*
Prentice-Hall of Japan, Inc., *Tokyo*
Simon & Schuster Asia Pte. Ltd., *Singapore*
Editora Prentice-Hall do Brasil, Ltda., *Rio de Janeiro*

contents

Introduction   x

chapter 1
Introduction to Emergency Medical Services   1

The Need for EMTs, 2
History of Emergency Medical Services, 2
The EMS System, 3
The Role and Responsibilities of the EMT, 4
Job Description, 6
Functions of the EMT, 7
Legal Problems and Emergency Care, 10
EMT Code of Ethics, 14
National Organizations, 15

chapter 2
Anatomy and Physiology of Body Systems   17

Anatomical Terminology, 18
Medical Terminology, 19
Anatomical Regions and Topography, 19
The Skeletal System (Bones and Joints), 21
Body Cavities, 28
The Muscular System, 28
The Circulatory System, 31
The Respiratory System, 34
The Digestive System, 36
The Urinary System, 38
The Endocrine System, 38
The Reproductive System, 39
The Nervous System, 39
The Skin, 44
The Eye, 45
The Ear, 46

chapter 3
Patient Assessment   47

The Ten-Step Sequence of Patient Assessment, 49
   1. Receiving the Call from the Emergency Medical Dispatcher, 49
   2. Arriving at the Scene, 49
   3. Establishing Rapport and Controlling the Scene, 50
   4. Conducting a Primary Survey, 52
   5. Identifying the Chief Complaint, 58
   6. Taking the Vital Signs, 58
   7. Spotting Medical Information Devices, 64
   8. Conducting a Neuro Examination, 65
   9. Taking a History, 68
   10. Conducting a Secondary Survey, 69
Considerations before You Transport the Patient, 78

chapter 4
Basic Life Support: Artificial Ventilation   79

Understanding the Respiratory System, 80
Respiratory Arrest, 83
Evaluation of Respiratory Status, 83
Basic Life Support, 86
Obstructed Airway Emergencies, 94
Common Medical Conditions that Cause Respiratory Emergencies, 101

chapter 5
Ventilation Equipment and Oxygen Therapy   104

The Use of Airway Adjuncts, 105
Suction Units, 107
Oxygen Equipment, 107
Oxygen Delivery Equipment, 112

chapter 6
Basic Life Support— Cardiopulmonary Resuscitation (CPR)   120

The Heart, 121
Location of the Heart and Associated Organs, 121
The Heart Action, 121
Cardiac Arrest, 123
How CPR Works, 123
Steps Preceding CPR, 124
Performing CPR, 126
Signs of Succesful CPR, 132
Errors in Performing CPR, 126
Complications Caused by CPR, 133

A Comment on ACLS, 133
CPR in Infants and Children, 133
Moving CPR, 136
When to Terminate CPR, 137
When to Withhold CPR, 137
CPR Retraining, 137
Supplementary Equipment, 138
Psychological Considerations in CPR, 138
Disease Transmission and CPR, 139

chapter 7
Control of Bleeding   140

Circulatory System, 141
Blood, 141
Blood Vessels, 141
Hemorrhage or Bleeding, 141
General Procedures for Controlling Bleeding, 144
Specific Methods of Controlling Bleeding, 147
Internal Bleeding, 152
Nosebleeds—Epistaxis, 154

chapter 8
Shock   156

The Physiology of Shock, 157
Causes of Shock, 158
Factors Influencing the Severity of Shock, 159
Types of Shock, 159
Stages of Shock, 161
Signs and Symptoms of Shock, 162
Patient Assessment, 166
Management of Shock, 167
Pneumatic Antishock Garment (PASG), 172

chapter 9
Mechanisms of Injury: The Kinetics of Trauma   176

Motion and the Interaction of Velocity and Mass, 177
Mechanisms of Injury, 179
Summary, 194

chapter 10
Soft-Tissue Injuries   195

What is a Soft-Tissue Injury?, 196
Closed Wounds, 196
Open Wounds, 196
Blunt Trauma, 203
General Emergency Care for Open Wounds, 203

chapter 11
Clamping and Penetrating Wounds   205

Clamping Objects, 206
Stab Wounds, 207
Gunshot Wounds, 207
Impaled Objects, 209

chapter 12
Bandaging   212

Dressings, 213
Bandages, 214
Special Types of Dressings and Bandages, 214
Principles of Dressing and Bandaging, 215
Applying Special Dressings and Bandages, 219

chapter 13
Musculoskeletal Injuries   220

Anatomy of the Musculoskeletal System, 221
Forces that Cause Musculoskeletal Injuries, 222
Patient Assessment, 222
Injuries to Muscles, 223
Dislocations of Joints, 225
Fractures, 227
Repositioning Fractured or Dislocated Limbs, 232
Types of Splints, 232

chapter 14
Fractures of the Upper and Lower Extremeties   236

Fractures of the Collarbone (clavicle), 237
Fractures of the Scapula, 237
Fractures of the Humerus, 238
Fractures of the Elbow, 238
Fractures of the Forearm and Wrist, 238
Fractures of the Hand and Fingers, 240
Fractures of the Pelvis, 241
Fractures of the Hip, 242
Fractures of the Femur, 242
Fractures of the Patella (Kneecap), 244
Fractures of the Lower Leg (Tibia, Fibula), 244
Fractures of the Ankle and Foot, 244

chapter 15
Head Injuries   249

The Nervous System, 250
Physiology of Brain Injury, 252

Obtaining a Patient History, 252
Physical Assessment, 253
Neurologic Assessment, 255
Skull Fracture, 258
Injuries to the Brain, 258
Emergency Care for Head Injury, 263

chapter 16
Injuries to the Spine 265

The Spinal Cord, 266
Mechanisms of Spinal Injury, 267
Assessment of Spinal Cord Injury, 268
Signs and Symptoms of Spinal Injury, 268
Emergency Care for Spinal Injury, 272
Helmet Removal, 285

chapter 17
Injuries to the Eye 289

Assessment of the Eyes, 290
Foreign Objects in the Eye, 290
Injury to the Orbits, 291
Lid Injuries, 291
Injuries to the Globe, 293
Chemical Burns of the Eye, 293
Impaled Objects in the Eye, 295
Extruded Eyeball, 295
Other Eye Injuries, 296
Basic Rules for Emergency Eye Care, 296
Removing Contact Lenses, 297

chapter 18
Injuries to the Face and Throat 299

Injuries to the Face, 300
Trauma to the Mouth and Jaw, 301
Fractures of the Face and Lower Jaw, 303
Injuries of the Nose, 305
Injuries of the Ear, 305
Injuries of the Throat, 306

chapter 19
Injuries to the Chest 310

Anatomy of the Chest, 311
Chest Injuries, 311
General Signs and Symptoms of Chest Injury, 311
General Principles for Treatment of Chest Injuries, 314
Flail Chest, 315
Pulmonary (Lung) Contusions, 316

Heart (Myocardial) Contusion, 317
Pericardial Tamponade, 317
Compression Injuries and Traumatic Asphyxia, 319
Broken Ribs, 319
Transection of the Great Vessels, 320
Hemothorax, 321
Tension Pneumothorax, 321
Pneumothorax, 322
Subcutaneous Emphysema, 322
Sucking Chest Wounds (Open Pneumothorax), 323

chapter 20
Injuries to the Abdomen and Genitalia 325

The Abdominal Cavity, 326
Abdominal Injuries, 326
Genitourinary System Injuries, 330

chapter 21
Farm, Rural, and Industrial Accidents 333

Why Farm and Rural Accidents Are So Serious, 334
Causes of Farm Accidents, 334
Operational Controls, 339
Equipment Shutdown, 339
Patient Assessment and Emergency Care, 340
Industrial Rescue, 340

chapter 22
Poisoning Emergencies 342

Ingested Poisons, 343
Inhaled Poisons, 348
Absorbed Poisons, 351
Poisonous Plants, 351
Food Poisoning, 353

chapter 23
Drug and Alcohol Emergencies 354

General Terminology, 357
How to Determine If an Emergency Is Drug/Alcohol/Related, 357
How to Determine If an Alcohol/Drug Emergency Is Life-Threatening, 358
Signs and Symptoms of Drug Abuse, 358
Observation and Assessment, 358
Alcohol Emergencies, 360
General Guidelines for Managing a Drug/Alcohol Crisis, 364

Managing the Violent Drug Patient, 365
Dealing with Hyperventilation Patients, 365
General Procedures for Overdoses, 365
Phencyclidine (PCP), 368
Cocaine, 368

chapter 24
Bites and Stings   370

Snakebite, 371
Insect Bites, 375
Insect Stings, 379
Marine Life Poisoning, 380

chapter 25
Respiratory Emergencies   384

Dyspnea (Shortness of Breath), 385
Chronic Obstructive Pulmonary Disease (COPD), 385
Pneumonia, 389
Pulmonary Embolism, 389
Acute Pulmonary Edema, 391
Hyperventilation, 392

chapter 26
Heart Attack and Other Cardiac Emergencies   394

Cardiac Anatomy and Physiology, 395
Coronary Artery Disease, 395
Cardiac Risk Factors, 396
Angina Pectoris, 397
Acute Myocardial Infarction (AMI), 398
Congestive Heart Failure, 403
Patient Assessment for Cardiac Emergencies, 405
General Emergency Care for Cardiac Patients, 406

chapter 27
Stroke   407

General Causes of Stroke, 408
Signs and Symptoms of Stroke, 410
Emergency Care, 412

chapter 28
Diabetic Emergencies   414

Causes of Diabetes, 415
Diabetic Coma (Ketoacidosis and Hyperglycemia), 415
Insulin Shock (Hypoglycemia), 417

chapter 29
Acute Abdominal Distress and Related Emergencies   422

Causes of Abdominal Pain, 423
Signs and Symptoms of Abdominal Distress, 423
Special Examination Procedures, 424
Emergency Care for Acute Abdominal Distress, 424
Ruptured Esophageal Varices, 425
Abdominal Aortic Aneurysm, 426
Vomiting, 427
Esophageal Reflux (Heartburn), 427
Diarrhea and Constipation, 428

chapter 30
Epilepsy, Dizziness, and Fainting   429

Seizures and Epilepsy, 430
Dizziness, Fainting, and Unconsciousness, 437

chapter 31
Infectious Disease Control   439

Bacteria, Viruses, and the Immune System, 440
Transmission of Infectious Diseases, 440
Identifying Patients with Infectious Diseases, 440
Diseases of Concern in the Emergency Setting, 441
Acquired Immunodeficiency Syndrome (AIDS), 441
Preventing Infection Spread During CPR, 446
Guidelines for Handwashing, 447
Guidelines for Protective Clothing, 447
Equipment Cleaning, Disinfecting, and Sterilization, 447
Disposing of Infectious Wastes, 448
Guidelines for Cleaning the Vehicle, 448
Recommended Immunizations for EMTs, 450
General Guidelines for Preventing the Spread of Infection, 450

chapter 32
Pediatric Emergencies   452

Dealing with Parents, 452
Dealing with the Child, 454
General Procedures, 456
Obtaining a Medical History, 456
Vital Signs for Children, 457
Neurological Assessment of Children, 458
Trauma, 459
Special Situations for Children, 460
Common Pediatric Emergencies, 461
Transporting the Child, 474
Take Care of Yourself, 476

chapter 33
Geriatric Emergencies   **477**

How Body Systems Change with Age, 478
Differing Signs and Symptoms in the Elderly, 480
Special Assessment Considerations, 480
Special Communication Considerations, 481
Special Examination Considerations, 481
Special Trauma Considerations, 481
Common Medical Problems in the Elderly, 482

chapter 34
Childbirth and Related Emergencies   **484**

Normal Pregnancy and Stages of Labor, 485
Managing an Obstetrics Call, 487
Emergency Home Delivery, 490
Newborn Care, 495
Evaluating the Newborn, 496
Other Emergency Deliveries, 497
Complications of Pregnancy, 498
Complications of Delivery, 504
Complications in Newborns, 506
Pregnancy and Trauma, 507

chapter 35
Burn Emergencies   **510**

Types of Burn Injuries, 511
Degree of the Burn, 512
Percentage of Body Burned: the Rules Of Nines, 514
Severity of the Burn, 514
Location of the Burn, 515
Accompanying Complications, 516
Age of the Patient, 516
Burn Management, 516
Inhalation Injuries, 519
Thermal and Radiant Burns, 521
Chemical Burns, 522
Electrical Burns, 525
Triage and Transportation of Burn Patients, 528

chapter 36
Hazardous Material Emergencies   **530**

Resources for Handling Hazardous Materials, 531
Identification, 532
General Procedures, 532
Radiation Emergencies, 540

chapter 37
Heat and Cold Emergencies   **546**

How the Body Adjusts, 547
Hyperthermia (Heat-Related Injury), 549
Hypothermia (Cold-Related Injury), 556

chapter 38
Water Emergencies   **568**

Drowning and Near-Drowning, 569
Diving Emergencies, 572

chapter 39
Psychological Emergencies and Special Communication Needs   **577**

Principles of Psychological Emergency Care, 578
Emotional Responses of Patients to Illness and Injury, 579
Responses of Family, Friends, or Bystanders, 580
Patient Assessment in Psychological Emergencies, 580
Physical Disorders that Resemble Psychological Emergencies, 581
General Guidelines for Management of Psychological Emergencies, 581
Communicating in Psychological Emergencies, 583
Helping Patients with Special Communciation Needs, 584
Stress Responses of EMTs, 587
Critical Incident Stress Debriefing, 591

chapter 40
Crisis Intervention   **593**

Anxiety Disorders and Phobias, 594
Depression, 594
Suicide, 595
Paranoia, 597
Rage, Hostility, and Violence, 598
Spouse Abuse, 601
Rape and Sexual Assault, 607
Death and Dying, 609

chapter 41
Patient Packaging, Moving, and Triage   **612**

When to Make an Emergency Move, 613
Emergency Moves, 614
Basic Guidelines for Moving Patients, 616
Understanding your Equipment, 618

The Mechanics of Lifting, 624
Lifts and Carries, 626
Moving a Cot, 633
Traversing Stairways, 633
Special Concerns in Moving Patients, 634
Triage, 636

chapter 42
Multiple-Casualty Incidents and Disaster Management 643

What is a Disaster?, 644
Phases of a Disaster, 644
Requirements of Effective Disaster Assistance, 644
General Procedures of a Disaster Plan, 644
Prewarning and Evacuation, 647
Setting up Communications, 648
Psychological Impact of Disasters, 648
General Guidelines for Disaster Rescuers, 649
Reducing Stress on Rescue Personnel, 651

chapter 43
Vehicle Stabilization and Patient Extrication 653

Importance of Protective Clothing, 654
Rescue Tools, 654
Principles of Extrication, 655
Other Extrication Situations, 671

chapter 44
Ambulance Operations 674

Driving Safety, 675
Ambulance Colors and Markings, 675
Laws, Regulations, Ordinances, 675
Factors Leading to Unsafe Driving, 677
Driving Excellence, 677
Controlling the Vehicle, 682

Warning Devices, 683
Ambulance Equipment, 684
Vehicle Maintenance, 686
Carbon Monoxide in Ambulances, 688
Phases of an Ambulance Run, 689
Air Ambulances, 693

chapter 45
Communications, Records, and Reports 697

Importance of Communications, 698
Basic Functions of Emergency Communications, 698
Components of an Emergency Communications System, 698
Permitted and Recommended Communications, 699
Relaying Information to the Physician, 699
Communications Control Center, 700
Patient Entry into the EMS System, 701
Dispatch, 701
Using Radio Communications Equipment, 702
Records and Reports, 704

Appendix 1: Advanced Airway Management 707

Appendix 2: Intravenous Fluid Therapy 719

Appendix 3: EMT-D Prehospital Defibrillation 733

Appendix 4: Maintaining a Healthy Lifestyle 745

Glossary 769

Index 789

Introduction

THE EFFECTIVE USE OF THIS TEXT

We have written and designed this text and the accompanying workbook with the needs of you — the EMT student —foremost in our planning. The design, text, photographs, and graphics are developed to allow you to use as many learning abilities and skills as possible and to enhance skill building and knowledge retention. The objectives and content of the text itself conform to the EMT National Standard Curriculum developed by the U.S. Department of Transportation.

The "Objectives" sections give you an overview of each chapter. Words that you should know stand out in a bold type in the text and are found in a glossary at the back of the book.

The accompanying workbook, which contains questions correlated to each chapter of the text, will help you to retain the new knowledge. The multiple-choice tests for each chapter will familiarize you with the types of questions that the majority of states use for EMT certification written tests and will help to prepare you for these tests.

The PARCER Method

Our goal is to help you experience success in this EMT course and to be a skilled, professional, certified emergency medical technician. One way of achieving that goal is to help you retain a high comprehension as you read and study this text through use of the **PARCER method.** This technique divides a chapter into its parts and allows you to discover the content relationships. The PARCER[1] process means:

- **Preview** the chapter (selection, etc.), noting title, objectives, major headings, subheadings, summaries, graphic materials, etc., to get a general idea of content and to understand organization and emphasis.
- **Ask** questions, based on each section heading, that should be answered in the reading. Start at the beginning of the chapter and do this for one short section at a time.
- **Read** each section, one section at a time, trying to find answers to the questions formulated in the

[1] Hansen, Dorothy M., Herlin, Wayne R., and Marrott, Janene, _Critical Reading_ (Provo, Utah; Brigham Young University Press, 1976), pp. 61–64).

"Ask" step. Be alert to any information not anticipated by the questions.

- **Check** your understanding of each section, one section at a time: (1) answer the question you asked, (2) note additional significant information not anticipated, (3) jot down key words and phrases that are important to remember (these are called check notes and are important if much detail is to be remembered), and (4) tie the current section to previous sections and anticipate its impact on subsequent sections. This section-by-section check should be done from memory _without looking at the book._
- **Evaluate** your understanding of the entire chapter by reciting the key points _from memory_ (do not use the book), or by filling in as much detail as possible while looking at the accumulated check notes prepared during the check step.
- **Relate** what you read to what you know from other sources (class lecture, previous reading, lab sessions, etc.). Criticize, verify, pose counter arguments, or make any applications that seem pertinent. This is the time to make the reading a part of yourself.

A few prior comments are helpful if you plan to try the PARCER study-reading system:

1. It takes about ten trials before the system smooths off to an efficient process. If you have learned how to speed up your reading, you can help yourself develop efficiency by pushing your reading speed during the "R" step. The time that you save by doing this can then be utilized for the other steps, and net study time will be no longer than your single reading used to be. But now you will deal with the content six times.

2. Your check notes should be as brief as possible. Never use a phrase when a word will do, and never use complete sentences. You should be able to understand your check notes, but no one else needs to understand them.

3. Note that the "Ask-Read-Check" steps are done section-by-section. In fact, the circular path implied by ARC should remind you of the circular repetition of these three steps. Take the sections in larger or smaller portions depending on the difficulty of the material and your purpose in reading. At the end of a section, you should be able to

recite *from memory* as much detail as your purpose for reading dictates. If you cannot recite from memory immediaely after reading, it is not likely that you will be able to do so the following week on a test; hence, the immediate check on yourself. If you do not know an answer, go back and re-read.

4. As you begin applying PARCER, you will notice that the last two steps, done after the entire chapter has been read, may be completed simultaneously and will have a mutual strengthening effect. Your self-evaluation becomes a part of relating your new knowledge to the old; and as you relate immediate content to your broader perspective, you also will evaluate your total understanding and power to apply that understanding. In fact, the "Evaluate" and "Relate" stages will often be so closely intertwined that you will feel as though you are involved in only one step that treats the question, "What use will this information have in my life as I view it now?" Don't be alarmed by that discovery. All the information you gain as an EMT takes on value only as you use it. Prepare well and you will be a successful EMT.

☐ ACKNOWLEDGMENTS

The authors wish to express special appreciation to the following individuals for their contributions to this book:

Kathryn J. Frandsen
Thom Dick
Lavina Fielding Anderson
Norman E. McSwain, Jr. M.D.
Mike Smith
Don Bloom
Ken Bouvier
Wayne Watson
Ray Andrews
Baxter Larmon
Twink Gorgen

Appreciation is also expressed to Valley Ambulance, Provo Fire Department, and Orem Fire Department for their assistance.

Photography and consultation was provided by Max Wilson with the assistance of the following individuals:

Ron Hammond
Mikki Abbate
Steve Hawks
Kevin Crawford
Judy Berryessa
Chuck Tandy
Gary Jolley
Joe McRae
Rick Nye
Max Wilson
Lynette Atwood
Andrew Goodman
Steve Russell
Eric Kapo'o
Laurel Turpen
Kent Boots

Appreciation is also expressed to the following for allowing us to use their color photographs — with special thanks to Blayne Hirsche, M.D.; James Clayton, M.D.; Spenco Medical Corp.; and Pennsylvania SIDS center. Companies and individuals that generously assisted with photographs are:

Linda Gheen
William F. Toon, NREMT-P

Dyna Med, Inc.
George D. Dodson
California Medical Products, Inc.
Lab Safety Supply, Inc.,
    Janesville, WI
David Clark Co.
REEL Research & Development
FERNO, a Division of FERNO-Washington, Inc.
Respironics, Inc.
Southern Ambulance Builders, Inc.
Wheeled Coach, Inc.
Minto Research
AMKUS Rescue Systems
Philip C. Anderson, M.D.
Cameron Bangs, M.D.
W. Henry Baughman, H.S.D.
Robert Biehn
John A. Boswick, Jr., M.D.
Jim Bryant
N. Branson Call, M.D.
Douglas C. Cox, Ph.D.
Bob Cross
Drug Intelligence Publications, Inc.
Corine A. Dwyer
Larry Ford
Michael D. Ellis
Bruce Halstead, M.D.
Niles W. Herrod, D.D.S.
Glen R. Hunt, M.D.
Renner Johnston, M.D.
Arthur K. Kahn, M.D.
Thomas Morton, M.D.
Pat Olsen
Eugene Robertson, M.D.
Rocky Mountain National Parks Service
Pat Sullivan
John Whitman
Lawrence Wolheim, M.D.
World Life Research Institute
Michael and Jacqueline Gelotte
Barry and Kathy Brewer
Michael Johnson
Mike Oaks
Mark and Sharlene Sumison
Julie White

Other individuals who participated in the development of this text are:

David Dodds
George E. Moerkirk
H. R. Seymour
Jerrell F. Gerdes
Kenneth Grassick
Cecil M. Castle, Sr.
Stanley E. Dempsey
Patricia Gaums
Nicholas Benson
Tom Ferrell
Mary "Posie" Mansfield

Gary Bilek
Judith Norberg
Clint Buchanan
Robert Aisenstat
Tod Stanford
Phillip W. Davis
John M. Landrum
Jessie Bailey
Brian J. Wilson
Marianne McBrien
Eileen Dean

Marilyn Bourne
Scott Bourne
John Lisle
Dr. Henry Baughman
Cynthia McCloud
Michael T. McEvoy
Robert Speser
Joe Desjardins
David S. Becker
Kathryn Hilgencamp
Robert Hawley

Don F. Black
Richard Bailey
William Hollis
Edward A. Wolfe
Bruce Maxwell
Stanley Batchelon
Steve R. Dargon
J. B. Tomassetti
Sharon A. Funderlich
Nancy Siekman
Clyde Tamboulian

Additional appreciation is expressed to Susan Strawn and Dennis Giddings and to Network Graphics for their artwork.

Credits

Chapter 1

Section on first responders from Harvey D. Grant et al., *Emergency Care,* 5th ed., p. 66.

Sections on patient rights — confidentiality and victims of crime from Harvey D. Grant et al., *Emergency Care,* 5th ed., p. 19.

Chapter 2

Figure 2-8, The skeletal system, Reprinted from Bledsoe, Porter, and Shade: *Paramedic Emergency Care,* Prentice-Hall, Englewood Cliffs, NJ (1991), p. 137.

Figure 2-14, The muscular system, Reprinted from Bledsoe, Porter, and Shade: *Paramedic Emergency Care,* Prentice-Hall, Englewood Cliffs, NJ (1991), p. 138.

Figure 2-15, Three types of muscle, Reprinted from Bledsoe, Porter, and Shade: *Paramedic Emergency Care,* Prentice-Hall, Englewood Cliffs, NJ (1991), p. 133.

Figure 2-17, The respiratory system, Reprinted from Bledsoe, Porter, and Shade: *Paramedic Emergency Care,* Prentice-Hall, Englewood Cliffs, NJ (1991), p. 143.

Figure 2-18, The digestive system, Reprinted from Bledsoe, Porter, and Shade: *Paramedic Emergency Care,* Prentice-Hall, Englewood Cliffs, NJ (1991), p. 144.

Figure 2-19, The urinary system, Reprinted from Bledsoe, Porter, and Shade: *Paramedic Emergency Care,* Prentice-Hall, Englewood Cliffs, NJ (1991), p. 145.

Figure 2-20, The reproductive system, Reprinted from Bledsoe, Porter, and Shade: *Paramedic Emergency Care,* Prentice-Hall, Englewood Cliffs, NJ (1991), p. 146.

Figure 2-21, The nervous system, Reprinted from Bledsoe, Porter, and Shade: *Paramedic Emergency Care,* Prentice-Hall, Englewood Cliffs, NJ (1991), p. 141.

Figure 2-22, The autonomic nervous system, Reprinted from Bledsoe, Porter, and Shade: *Paramedic Emergency Care,* Prentice-Hall, Englewood Cliffs, NJ (1991), p. 142.

Figure 2-23, Anatomy of the skin, Reprinted from Bledsoe, Porter, and Shade: *Paramedic Emergency Care,* Prentice-Hall, Englewood Cliffs, NJ (1991), p. 138.

Figure 2-24, Anatomy of the human eye, Reprinted from Bledsoe, Porter, and Shade: *Paramedic Emergency Care,* Prentice-Hall, Englewood Cliffs, NJ (1991), p. 135.

Figure 2-25, Anatomy of the human ear, Reprinted from Bledsoe, Porter, and Shade: *Paramedic Emergency Care,* Prentice-Hall, Englewood Cliffs, NJ (1991), p. 135.

Chapter 3

Section on assessing patient's level of consciousness from Harvey D. Grant et al., *Emergency Care,* 5th ed., p. 71.

Chapter 4

Figure 4-1, Anatomy of the upper airway, Reprinted from Bledsoe, Porter, and Shade: *Paramedic Emergency Care,* Prentice-Hall, Englewood Cliffs, NJ (1991), p. 201.

Chapter 5

Figure 5-21, The nasal cannula is comfortable and convenient, Reprinted from Bledsoe, Porter, and Shade: *Paramedic Emergency Care,* Prentice-Hall, Englewood Cliffs, NJ (1991), p. 259.

Figure 5-22, Simple mask, Reprinted from Bledsoe, Porter, and Shade: *Paramedic Emergency Care,* Prentice-Hall, Englewood Cliffs, NJ (1991), p. 260.

Figure 5-23, Nonbreather mask, Reprinted from Bledsoe, Porter, and Shade: *Paramedic Emergency Care,* Prentice-Hall, Englewood Cliffs, NJ (1991), p. 261.

Figure 5-28, Bag-valve-mask unit, Reprinted from Bledsoe, Porter, and Shade: *Paramedic Emergency Care,* Prentice-Hall, Englewood Cliffs, NJ (1991), p. 263.

Chapter 9

Chapter text provided by Twink Gorgen.

Figure 9-2, Vehicle collision, Reprinted from Bledsoe, Porter, and Shade: *Paramedic Emergency Care,* Prentice-Hall, Englewood Cliffs, NJ (1991), p. 379.

Figure 9-3, Body collision, Reprinted from Bledsoe, Porter, and Shade: *Paramedic Emergency Care,* Prentice-Hall, Englewood Cliffs, NJ (1991), p. 379.

Figure 9-4, Organ collision, Reprinted from Bledsoe, Porter, and Shade: *Paramedic Emergency Care,* Prentice-Hall, Englewood Cliffs, NJ (1991), p. 379.

Figure 9-5, Motor vehicle trauma based on type of impact, Reprinted from Bledsoe, Porter, and Shade: *Paramedic Emergency Care,* Prentice-Hall, Englewood Cliffs, NJ (1991), p. 381

Figure 9-7, Reprinted from Bledsoe, Porter, and Shade: *Paramedic Emergency Care,* Prentice-Hall, Englewood Cliffs, NJ (1991), p. 380.

Figure 9-8, Chest impacting the steering wheel, Reprinted from Bledsoe, Porter, and Shade: *Paramedic Emergency Care,* Prentice-Hall, Englewood Cliffs, NJ (1991), p. 383.

Figure 9-9, The "paper bag" syndrome, Reprinted from Bledsoe, Porter, and Shade: *Paramedic Emergency Care,* Prentice-Hall, Englewood Cliffs, NJ (1991), p. 382.

Figure 9-12, Injury mechanisms associated with frontal impact, Reprinted from Bledsoe, Porter, and Shade: *Paramedic Emergency Care,* Prentice-Hall, Englewood Cliffs, NJ (1991), p. 382.

Figure 9-13, Coup and contrecoup movement of the brain, Reprinted from Bledsoe, Porter, and Shade: *Paramedic Emergency Care,* Prentice-Hall, Englewood Cliffs, NJ (1991), p. 417.

Figure 9-15, Movement in the rear impact collision, Reprinted from Bledsoe, Porter, and Shade: *Paramedic Emergency Care,* Prentice-Hall, Englewood Cliffs, NJ (1991), p. 384.

Figure 9-17, Rotational impact, Reprinted from Bledsoe, Porter, and Shade: *Paramedic Emergency Care,* Prentice-Hall, Englewood Cliffs, NJ (1991), p. 385.

Figure 9-21, In falls, the energy is transmitted up the skeletal system, Reprinted from Bledsoe, Porter, and Shade: *Paramedic Emergency Care,* Prentice-Hall, Englewood Cliffs, NJ (1991), p. 391.

Figure 9-24, Severity of injury . . . , Reprinted from Bledsoe, Porter, and Shade: *Paramedic Emergency Care,* Prentice-Hall, Englewood Cliffs, NJ (1991), p. 396.

Figure 9-26, Blast injuries . . . , Reprinted from Bledsoe, Porter, and Shade: *Paramedic Emergency Care,* Prentice-Hall, Englewood Cliffs, NJ (1991), p. 393.

Chapter 10

Part of section on emergency care of amputations from J. David Bergeron, *First Responder,* 3rd ed., p. 230

Chapter 13

Figure 13-5, Closed and open fractures, Reprinted from Bledsoe, Porter, and Shade: *Paramedic Emergency Care,* Prentice-Hall, Englewood Cliffs, NJ (1991), p. 483.

Figure 13-6, Types of fractures, Reprinted from Bledsoe, Porter, and Shade: *Paramedic Emergency Care,* Prentice-Hall, Englewood Cliffs, NJ (1991), p. 482.

Chapter 14

Section on emergency care of patients with pelvic fractures from Harvey D. Grant et al., *Emergency Care,* 5th ed., p. 274.

Chapter 15

Chapter written in conjunction with Thom Dick.

Chapter 16

Chapter written in conjunction with Thom Dick.

Boxed photo page on spinal injuries/rigid collars from Harvey D. Grant et al., *Emergency Care,* 5th ed., p. 313.

Seven warnings for use of short spine board from Harvey D. Grant et al., *Emergency Care,* 5th ed., p. 321.

Captions for illustrations showing helmet removal methods from Harvey D. Grant et al., *Emergency Care,* 5th ed., p. 307 (Originally from Campbell et al., *BTLS Basic Prehospital Trauma Care,* The Brady Company, 1988).

Chapter 18

Section on transportation of a patient with facial injuries from Harvey D. Grant et al., *Emergency Care,* 5th ed., p. 332.

Chapter 21

Chapter written by Mike Smith, Director of the Paramedic Training Program, Tacoma Community College, and Ray Andrews, Emergency Rescue Technician Instructor and Chief, Pleasant Valley Fire Department.

Chapter 26

Boxed text on acute myocardial infarction (AMI) from Harvey D. Grant et al., *Emergency Care,* 5th ed., pp. 390–391.

Chapter 28

Summary of diabetic emergencies from Harvey D. Grant et al., *Emergency Care,* 5th ed., p. 405.

Chapter 30

Section on progression of a grand mal seizure from Bryan E. Bledsoe et al., *Paramedic Emergency Care,* p. 737.

Chapter 32

Section on pediatric infectious diseases from J. David Bergeron, *First Responder,* 3rd ed.

Chapter 34

Figure 34-1, Anatomy of the placenta, Reprinted from Bledsoe, Porter, and Shade: *Paramedic Emergency Care,* Prentice-Hall, Englewood Cliffs, NJ (1991), p. 927.

Figure 34-16, Normal delivery, Reprinted from Bledsoe, Porter, and Shade: *Paramedic Emergency Care,* Prentice-Hall, Englewood Cliffs, NJ (1991), p. 945.

Figure 34-17, Suctioning the mouth . . . , Reprinted from Bledsoe, Porter, and Shade: *Paramedic Emergency Care,* Prentice-Hall, Englewood Cliffs, NJ (1991), p. 947.

Figure 34-18, Encouraging the newborn to breathe, Reprinted from Bledsoe, Porter, and Shade: *Paramedic Emergency Care,* Prentice-Hall, Englewood Cliffs, NJ (1991), p. 947.

Figure 34-26, Prolapsed cord, Reprinted from Bledsoe, Porter, and Shade: *Paramedic Emergency Care,* Prentice-Hall, Englewood Cliffs, NJ (1991), p. 950.

Figure 34-27, Patient positioning for prolapsed cord, Reprinted from Bledsoe, Porter, and Shade: *Paramedic Emergency Care,* Prentice-Hall, Englewood Cliffs, NJ (1991), p. 951.

Figure 34-28, Provide and maintain an airway . . . , Reprinted from Bledsoe, Porter, and Shade: *Paramedic Emergency Care,* Prentice-Hall, Englewood Cliffs, NJ (1991), p. 949.

Chapter 38

Figure 38-4, Water Rescue—possible spinal injury, Reprinted from Bledsoe, Porter, and Shade: *Paramedic Emergency Care,* Prentice-Hall, Englewood Cliffs, NJ (1991), p. 840.

Chapter 41

This chapter was written in conjunction with Thom Dick.

Chapter 42

Figure 42-1, The incident command system . . . , Reprinted from Bledsoe, Porter, and Shade: *Paramedic Emergency Care,* Prentice-Hall, Englewood Cliffs, NJ (1991), p. 83.

Figure 42-2, Triage tagging . . . , Reprinted from Bledsoe, Porter, and Shade: *Paramedic Emergency Care,* Prentice-Hall, Englewood Cliffs, NJ (1991), p. 86.

Appendix 1

Figure A1-7, Lighted stylet/endotracheal tube in position, Reprinted from Bledsoe, Porter, and Shade: *Paramedic Emergency Care,* Prentice-Hall, Englewood Cliffs, NJ (1991), p. 247.

Figure A1-8, The properly positioned stylet . . . , Reprinted from Bledsoe, Porter, and Shade: *Paramedic Emergency Care,* Prentice-Hall, Englewood Cliffs, NJ (1991), p. 247.

CREDITS (continued on p. 801)

chapter 1

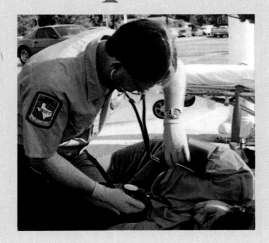

Introduction to Emergency Medical Services

✻ OBJECTIVES

- Identify the need for properly prepared emergency medical technicians.
- Become familiar with the history of emergency medical services.
- Identify the components of a functioning emergency medical services (EMS) system.
- Understand the job description, roles, responsibilities, training and functions of the emergency medical technician (EMT).
- Learn how to safeguard yourself while providing emergency care.
- Understand legal and ethical aspects of emergency medical care.
- Identify the major national emergency medical technician organizations.
- Become familiar with the PARCER method of comprehension in order to increase your understanding of this text.

It is recommended that EMTs wear protective gloves whenever there is a possibility of coming in contact with a patient's blood, body fluids, mucous membranes, traumatic wounds, or sores. See Chapter 31.

□ THE NEED FOR EMTS

One of the most critical and visible health problems in the United States today is the sudden loss of life and disability caused by catastrophic accidents and illnesses. While facts and figures are not essential in preparing emergency rescuers, they do paint a picture of the great need for properly prepared **emergency medical technicians (EMTs).**

You are joining a proud force of approximately one-half million EMTs who have saved millions of lives. Welcome to the health-care team!

* Over 70 million Americans receive hospital emergency care each year.
* Over 150,000 people die each year from **trauma** and 400,000 receive permanent injuries, making trauma the fourth largest cause of death in the United States.
* 1.4 million injuries occur on U.S. highways, including 51,900 traffic deaths and 150,000 permanent disabilities.
* Homicides and suicides each account for approximately 25,000 deaths per year.
* Each year there are 2 million burn accidents, 1.5 million heart attack victims (50 percent die within two hours), and 5 million poisonings (90 percent of them children).
* Each year, brain-spine injuries paralyze 80,000 victims.
* Another way to understand the scope of the injury problem in the United States is as "the three times rule": "Every second, we spend $3,000 on injury; this year, an injury will strike one in three people; and it will take one life every three minutes."[1]

For further statistics on the impact of trauma on the U.S. population, see Figure 1-1.

Each year more than 100,000 people die needlessly in the United States because of the lack of adequate and available emergency medical services. Most of the deaths occur from heart disease, accident injury, burns, poisoning, alcohol and drug overdose. The training offered in this book will enable you to give assistance in these cases.

□ HISTORY OF EMERGENCY MEDICAL SERVICES

Many improvements originated in the care of wounded soldiers during various wars. The **International Red Cross** was formed in Switzerland in 1863. American

[1] Committee on Trauma Research, *Injury in America: A Continuing Public Health Problem* (1985), as cited in Bud Hoekstra, "An Ounce of Prevention," *Emergency*, September 1989, p. 34.

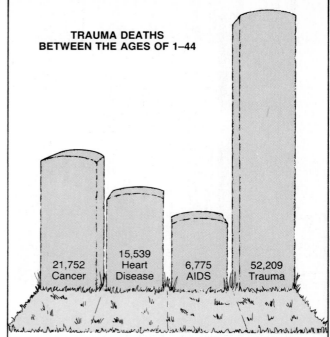

TRAUMA DEATHS BETWEEN THE AGES OF 1–44

21,752 Cancer

15,539 Heart Disease

6,775 AIDS

52,209 Trauma

Trauma can strike you at any minute of any day. Each year, more than 62 million people are injured. That's about one out of every five persons in the United States.

Trauma permanently disables more than 325,000 people each year. As former Surgeon General C. Everett Koop stated in his address to the U.S. Senate, "There are no one-time costs associated with injuries. There are only *lifetime* costs."

Trauma most often strikes at the prime of life. This means children and young adults. Each year, 19 million children under the age of 15 — one child in every four — are injured seriously enough to need to visit a doctor.

FIGURE 1-1
Source: American Trauma Society. 1988

Clara Barton, a nurse during the Civil War, headed the drive to bring the Red Cross to the United States in 1905. Since that time, the **American Red Cross** has trained hundreds of thousands of Americans in first aid and emergency care. Ambulance systems began to develop nationwide after World War II when fire departments also became more involved in providing emergency care.

Emergency medical services were really initiated in the 1950s when the older "load-and-go" methods began to be replaced with professional-level care at the scene before the patient was transported to the hospital.

In 1966, two important developments occurred:

1. The National Highway Safety Act charged the **Department of Transportation (DOT)** with developing an **Emergency Medical Services (EMS)** system and upgrading prehospital emergency care.

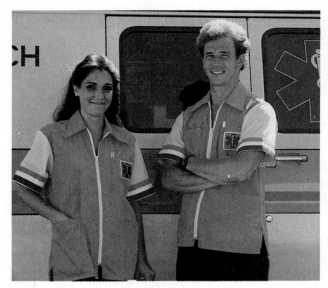

FIGURE 1-2 EMTs who look and act professional instill confidence in the patient.

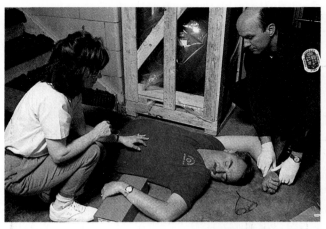

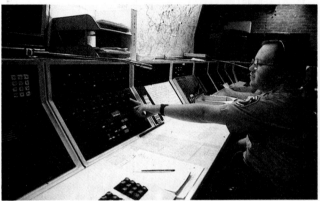

Out of this development emerged the emergency medical technician course, in which you are now involved.

2. The **American Heart Association (AHA)** began to publicly teach **cardiopulmonary resuscitation (CPR)** and **basic life support.** During this time, the National Academy of Sciences Research Council stressed professional training for prehospital emergency personnel.

Advances in emergency medical services and equipment and in the training of emergency medical technicians continue. The present-day EMS system and the EMT program extend a much-needed professional arm of the hospital emergency room out into the field to save many lives. You are joining that needed profession by becoming an emergency medical technician. Be the best one that you can be through study, practice, and keeping up with the advancements in emergency medical services (Figure 1-2).

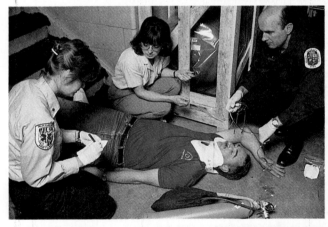

☐ THE EMS SYSTEM

As part of the EMS team, you join an elite group dedicated to helping people. The personnel in the emergency room are the foundation of the system. A vital extension from the emergency room out to the field and the patients is the EMT team, which works from a well-equipped emergency vehicle or ambulance. The most basic level is the first responder, who, if well trained, can successfully attend to immediate emergency-care needs until the ambulance team arrives (Figure 1-3).

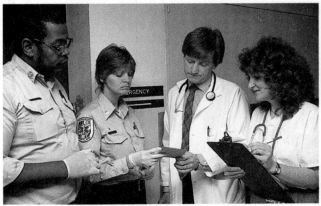

FIGURE 1-3

There are four basic emergency medical services:

1. Rescue operations.
2. Ambulance transportation.
3. Emergency department services.
4. Public education.

Such emergency services are required as the result of an unforeseen attack of illness or as the result of injury.

An EMS system should meet two objectives:

1. It should promptly identify and respond to a wide range of emergency situations.
2. It should use proper emergency medical-care measures and life-support systems to sustain and prolong life, both at the scene and during transportation of the patient to the appropriate medical facility, without further injuring the patient (Figure 1-4).

Star of Life — EMS Symbol

In 1973, DOT adopted the "Star of Life" emblem as a symbol of EMS. The use of the Star of Life symbol by both the private sector and the government has served to identify emergency medical services and contributed greatly to a realignment of objectives and commitment to improved emergency medical care. States and federal agencies have been authorized to assist in exercising supervisory control over the use of this symbol. In addition, steps are being taken to have the symbol appear on highway signs to help alert citizens about the EMS system and how to enter and use it.

FIGURE 1-4 EMTs in action at the scene.

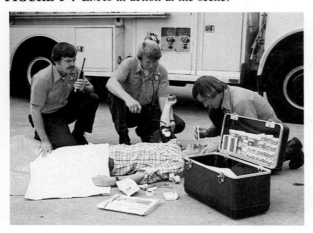

☐ THE ROLE AND RESPONSIBILITIES OF THE EMT

The Health-Care Professional

The EMT is a crucial member of the EMS team. As such, you are a health-care professional, a person who has special skills and knowledge in emergency medicine. You are concerned about other people's health and well-being, as well as your own.

Some EMTs are remunerated financially, while others volunteer their services. Professional standards in the EMT ranks are maintained by individuals pursuing quality continuing education.

EMTs are professionals. To some that may mean to "act educated, be credible, and instill confidence." Others understand professionalism as a quality that comes with hard work and dedication. Becknell gives the following advice regarding professionalism and self-improvement:

- Value yourself and what you do. Believe in your own worth as an EMT and in the worth of your work.
- Be *the best* for those you are called upon to help. Skills need to be sharp and knowledge must be fresh. Constantly improve emergency-care abilities.
- Continue to learn and grow as a human being. Work on improving relationships with others. This includes fellow EMS providers as well as patients.
- Develop a positive image of yourself. If you feel good about how you look, you feel better about what you do![2]

Although most EMTs now serve in the field, an increasing number are beginning to hold positions within hospital emergency departments. Some EMTs are training other emergency medical technicians, including those in administrative positions, for work as managers and supervisors. Some EMTs have become public educators; for example, some are certified instructors for the American Heart Association. As public educators, EMTs can help people learn how to call for emergency services efficiently and how to respond in a medical emergency when a police officer, firefighter, or EMT is not present. In addition, citizens are trained in such first-aid techniques as CPR, thus becoming "extenders" for EMTs.

[2] Becknell, John M., "Discover Professionalism in EMS," *JEMS*, December 1987, pp. 30-32.

Whatever the job, an EMT's professional responsibilities include:

- Maintaining a working understanding of the different components of the EMS system.
- Maintaining a professional level of ethics, technical skills, and appearance.
- Working cooperatively with other members of the EMS team.

As a health-care professional, the EMT is a vital member of the team. As such, you must understand the EMS system in which you work as well as your responsibility to the public before, during, and after a medical emergency.

Initial Role of the EMT

The major role of the EMT is to quickly respond to and assist an ill or trauma patient, then efficiently and quickly transport the patient to the nearest appropriate medical facility.

The initial care of a trauma patient includes:

- Airway management.
- Hemorrhage control.
- Treatment of shock.
- Stabilization of fractures.

The amount of patient stabilization performed by EMTs at the scene is based on the critical nature of the patient's injuries. A professional EMT should be trained to make these appropriate time judgments, giving the patient every medical opportunity without compromising the patient's chance of survival and full recovery by spending too much time stabilizing in the field.

Recent research on heart attacks and early defibrillation has identified CPR as a holding pattern (CPR at best can produce only 30 percent of normal cardiac output). The goal of emergency care is to restore circulation and oxygen supply to the brain, heart, and lungs with normal cardiac contractions. Many EMTs are now being trained in the use of automatic defibrillators to accomplish this goal. As you can see, the professional EMT has become a very important member of the emergency medical services team.

Levels of EMT Training

This text provides the material for the basic-level EMT, or EMT-A. However, there are other levels with which you should be familiar:

- EMT-A (emergency medical technician-ambulance) or EMT-1: a rating given to those who successfully complete the minimum DOT 110-hour course (some states require more hours) and who have been certified as EMTs by the state EMS division. The DOT course prepares the EMT to utilize major life-saving skills. These skills cover three areas:

1. Controlling life-threatening situations, including maintaining an open airway, keeping the lungs and heart working, controlling accessible bleeding, treating shock, and caring for poison cases.
2. Non-life-threatening conditions that require stabilization before transport, including dressing and bandaging wounds, splinting fractures and dislocations, delivering babies and caring for them, and dealing with the psychological stress of the patient, family members, neighbors, and, if necessary, colleagues.
3. Nonmedical requirements, which include using appropriate driving skills, maintaining supplies and equipment in proper order, using good communication skills, keeping good records, knowing proper extrication techniques, and coping with related legal issues.

All of these functions are described in this and other chapters.

- *EMT-I (intermediate)*: EMT-2, or A-EMT, these are the most common designations for advanced EMT levels, although the titles vary widely from state to state. These levels signify EMTs who have completed training in locally determined procedures in intermediate and advanced life support (e.g., IV training, use of field drugs, etc.). In some states, advanced training qualifies EMTs as cardiac technicians or cardiac rescue technicians.
- EMT-P: the paramedic level, assigned to EMTs who successfully complete state-certified paramedic training that is at least commensurate with the DOT.

First Responders

There will be times when the first person on the scene is someone with formal training in first aid, basic life support, or elementary emergency care. This person may be a police officer, a firefighter, or an industrial health officer. In some cases, this person may have advanced training, such as nursing. These individuals have traditionally been called first responders.

As an EMT, you will interact with first responders who have had American Red Cross training, American Heart Association basic cardiac life support training, or special industrial first responder training. Today, many police officers, firefighters, and industrial health personnel are trained to Department of Transportation guidelines and are certified First Responders. As a member of the EMS System, you should respect the work done by all of these individuals as they attempt to help the patient and you at the emergency scene.

First responders can provide valuable information about how the emergency came about, how the patient was acting when they arrived, what they found to be wrong with the patient, and what care procedures have been started. True, you will still have to do a patient assessment and you must evaluate the care already provided, but you should appreciate what the first responders have done before you arrived. Their assessment and care may often make a difference, improving or stabilizing the patient's condition. The information they give you, along with your own assessment may alert you to the fact that the patient is improving or deteriorating.

When you arrive at an emergency scene and find first responders providing care for a patient, tactfully assume responsibility for the patient. Remember to thank the first responders and to give them credit for any prompt and efficient care they provided for the patient. Allow first responders to help when you need assistance.

Most emergency scenes will not provide you with the time or privacy necessary to give on-the-scene training to the first responders. When practical, point out any errors made by first responders, but do so tactfully and in private. Should you notice a mistake in the assessment or care provided by the first responders, and they are members of the police department, fire department, or industrial squads, alert the appropriate training officer as soon after the run as possible. Do not act as though the training officer is at fault or the first responders lacked ability. Be a professional helping another professional to improve the quality of care.

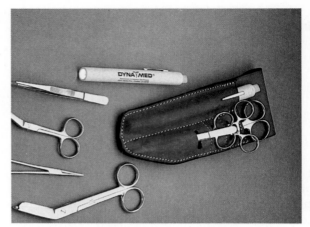

FIGURE 1-5 An EMT "holster" containing basic equipment.

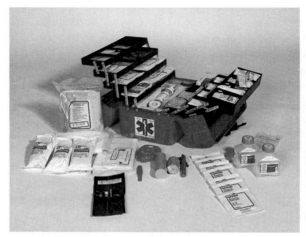

FIGURE 1-6 A basic EMT jump kit.

☐ JOB DESCRIPTION

Education, Training, and Experience

- A high-school education or its equivalent is recommended but not required.
- An EMT must be eighteen years of age or older.
- The minimum training is that prescribed in the basic training program for emergency medical technicians-ambulance (EMT-As) of the U.S. Department of Transportation.
- An EMT needs practical experience in the care and use of the emergency equipment commonly accepted and employed, such as suction machines, oxygen-delivery systems (installed and portable), spineboards, fracture kits, emergency medical-care kits, obstetrical kits, stretchers of various types, and light rescue tools (Figures 1-5 and 1-6).

- An EMT must understand sanitizing and disinfecting procedures.
- An EMT must know safety and security measures.
- An EMT must acquire, through critiques and conferences with emergency-department personnel, constructive criticism of care rendered and instruction about advances in patient care and new or improved equipment.
- An EMT must acquire a thorough knowledge of the territory within his or her service area and of the traffic ordinances and laws concerning the emergency care and transportation of the sick and injured. He or she must have necessary driver and professional licenses as required by law.

Physical Demands

An EMT must be able to meet the following requirements:

- Good physical health.

- Ability to lift and carry up to 100 pounds.
- Color vision (necessary for examining patients as well as for distinguishing traffic signs and lights).
- Good eyesight (necessary for driving and for examining the patient — correction by lenses is permitted).

Interests and Temperament

An EMT should possess the following characteristics:

- A pleasant personality. Much of your job will be to perform highly skilled and complex functions while at the same time speaking in a reassuring and calming voice to a patient who may be hysterical, in shock, and/or in a great deal of pain. Often, you must deal simultaneously with bystanders who are in an equally emotional state.
- Leadership ability. You should be able to assess a situation quickly, set action priorities, give directions clearly and simply, be persuasive enough to be obeyed, and carry through with what needs to be done. You must develop good judgment about handling difficult situations that involve human beings in crises.
- Neat appearance. Part of being professional is to be clean, well-groomed, and in proper uniform. You are a part of a *medical* team. Your appearance is part of the message that you are competent and can be trusted to make the right decisions.
- Good moral character. This chapter will discuss some of the legal constraints on your profession, but you have ethical obligations and a position of public trust that can never be wholly described by statute and case law.
- Emotional stability and psychological adaptability. Being an EMT is emotionally stressful. Exhaustion, frustration, anger, and grief are part of the package. Few people are initially prepared for the sights, smells, and sounds of intense human suffering. You will have to learn how to delay your response and how to express your response appropriately, but you should not try to deny it. If you do, you may burn out or become insensitive to the needs of your patients.

☐ FUNCTIONS OF THE EMT

Seniority and responsibility among the members of an EMT team should be determined by the EMS supervisor. All members of the team should be equally trained so that they may function interchangeably or independently in caring for multiple casualties.

First Response Duties

As a member of that team, your responsibilities are to:

1. **Respond to calls.**
   - After receiving the call from the dispatcher, drive your ambulance to the address or location given, using the safest route possible given traffic and weather conditions.
   - Observe traffic ordinances and regulations concerning emergency-vehicle operation.
   - At the scene of the accident or illness, park the ambulance in a safe location.
   - If police are present, receive a briefing and follow any necessary instructions that they may have about the situation. Avoid assuming the functions of police or other authorities when they are present, but do not permit their actions to compromise patient care.
   - Take over from the first responder, assess and express appreciation for the quality and care given, and ask for continued assistance if necessary.
   - If police are not present, enlist bystanders' help to create a safe traffic environment: place road flares, remove debris, and redirect traffic to protect both yourself and the injured persons.

2. **Assess the medical situation.**
   - Gain access to patients. In many cases, this will be easy; but in others you will need to deal with people entangled in automobile wreckage, in water or even under ice, under the debris of a caved-in house, and involved in a crime situation.
   - Recognize and evaluate problems. In some cases, you can see the situation at a glance. But even in obvious cases, ask bystanders (and the patient, if conscious) what happened and what's wrong as you begin your examination. This will help you reconstruct basically what happened and the probable injury (Figure 1-7).
   - Attend to life-threatening situations first: open and maintain the airway and stabilize the cervical spine, assure adequate ventilation, give CPR if indicated, control bleeding, treat shock.
   - Conduct a patient assessment.
   - Provide care before extricating/moving the patient, and continue care when extrication is delayed.
   - Avoid undue haste, carelessness, and mishandling while working as quickly as possible.
   - Respect the patient's dignity. Shield the patient from curious onlookers.

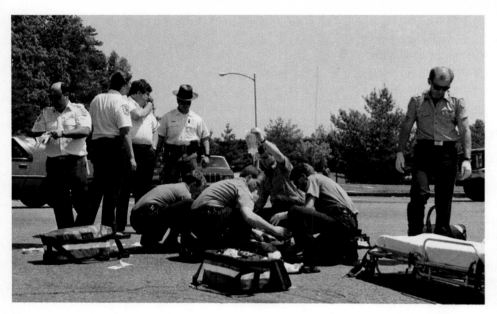

FIGURE 1-7 The EMT is an important component of the emergency medical services team and must interact with patients, bystanders, and other rescue personnel in a professional and efficient manner.

• Stay calm. Deal courteously and professionally with both patients and bystanders whose behavior has been altered by illness or anxiety.

3. **Extricate the patient and prepare him or her for transport.**

• Do not engage in extrication or rescue procedures when qualified rescue personnel are present.

• Stabilize life-threatening problems and immobilize injured parts before extrication.

• Contact the dispatcher for additional help or special rescue/utility services, fire personnel, etc., if needed. Do not attempt complicated extrication if the ambulance does not have the correct equipment and if the specialized unit is on the way.

• Extricate the patient in such a way as to minimize damage to the injured parts. Continue to administer essential care during the extrication.

• Evaluate the patient(s) after extrication to determine additional needed care and to prepare for transport.

• Lift the cot, place it in the ambulance, secure the stretcher and the patient, and continue emergency care. Protect the patient's valuables and transport them also.

• Determine which facility (poison center, children's hospital, etc.) will be most appropriate, given the patient's condition, the extent of the injuries, the relative locations, and the hospital staffing unless otherwise directed by the dispatcher or medical command.

4. **Provide proper care and appropriate communication en route.**

• Use the communications equipment in your ambulance effectively and correctly.

• To assure prompt medical care on delivery, contact the hospital emergency room and report the number of patients, the destination(s), and the nature and extent of the injuries. Alert the emergency department about high-priority patients and what will be needed immediately upon arrival.

• In some areas, you will be responsible for triage — deciding which hospital is best equipped to handle certain types of cases. In other areas, city-wide protocols make that determination. You will need to be aware of these rules.

• Ride in the compartment with the patient. Continually observe and protect the patient, administrating care as indicated.

• Report changes in the patient's condition. If necessary, ask for instructions from emergency room physicians for enroute care.

• Follow FCC regulations regarding communications equipment.

5. **Provide safe and efficient transport.**

• Drive in a way that will minimize further injury, maximize comfort, and prevent shock.

• Know and abide by laws and traffic regulations pertaining to ambulances. Exercise emergency privileges properly. Not all EMTs are required to be drivers; but if you certify as an EMT-A (meaning "ambulance"), you will, of course, have to have a valid driver's license, an acceptable driving record, certification as an ambulance driver, and a good working knowledge of the streets and roads within your working area.

- Proper use of lights and sirens is an important component of safe transport.
- Deliver the patient to the emergency department of a receiving hospital.

6. **Transfer the patient and patient information to the hospital emergency department in an orderly way.**

- Help remove the stretcher and carry it into the emergency department. Provide other assistance as needed.
- Maintain a courteous attitude toward emergency department personnel.
- Comply with hospital regulations.
- Deliver the patient's valuables or personal effects and obtain a receipt.
- Report verbally and in writing what injuries were identified and what patient care was administered both at the emergency scene and in transit. Keep one copy of the record for the official EMS record. (See "How to Document" later in this chapter.)
- Follow prescribed procedures for returning or exchanging equipment or supplies.

7. **Deal compassionately and reasonably (or honestly) with death.**

- If death is imminent either on the scene or in the ambulance during transport, be supportive and reassuring to the patient, but do not lie. If a patient asks, "I'm dying, aren't I?" respond with something like, "You have some very serious injuries, but I'm not giving up on you."
- If a patient requests that you pray with him or her, do so. Summon a priest or minister if there is time and if the patient makes such a request.
- If a patient dies, treat the body with dignity and follow local regulations. These may require you to leave the body at the scene of the accident to aid the police investigation. In this case, cover it and protect it from curious bystanders. Or, the regulations may require you to transport the body to the hospital where a physician will pronounce death. Notify the proper authorities.
- If a patient asks about others, particularly loved ones, involved in an accident, be as reassuring as possible without being dishonest. For example, if an injured parent asks about a child, also injured or possibly dead, respond with "Another member of my team is working with him (or

her) right now, doing everything possible. Now, let's concentrate for a minute on seeing if your legs seem okay." If possible, wait to inform a patient of a loved one's death or critical injury until psychological support (for example, a minister or emergency room personnel) is available.

8. **Maintain proper reports and records.**

- Maintain an up-to-date log of calls as described in Chapter 44.
- While treating the patient, collect information on circumstances by interviewing the patient, relatives, or bystanders.
- Enter the following medical information onto a permanent record and be prepared to share it with emergency department personnel: patient's name, type of accident or nature of illness, observed hazards (radiation, chemicals, hazardous gases, and so on); rescue measures before emergency care, care given at the scene and during transport, changes in vital signs, and any problems occurring en route.

9. **Care for the vehicle and equipment.**

- Properly maintain your vehicle and all medical, safety, and communications equipment. Routinely check the gas, all other fluid levels, and the tire pressure.
- Replenish supplies, linens, blankets, etc.
- Routinely sanitize and decontaminate the vehicle, supplies, and equipment. This is a must after exposure to infectious disease.
- Check all equipment. Keep the interior clean and tidy.
- Maintain familiarity with special equipment on the ambulance, such as oxygen equipment, extrication equipment, and so on.

Special Considerations

Some of the circumstances in which you will be required to provide emergency service will place extra demands on you. Some of those situations include the following:

1. Children and elderly people are particularly likely to panic if they are separated from other family members.

- It is best to have a familiar face near the patient during care and sometimes during transport. If you are clear, courteous, and specific about what you are doing, where the family member may stand, and what he or she may do, you will usually get excellent cooperation. For instance, say, "Please sit on the ground on her left side, ma'am, and hold her hand. Talk to her. Don't move her arm, and don't let her move her head. I'm going to be checking her hips and legs."

- Be extremely careful about what is said at the scene of an emergency. Verbal and other communication from the EMT to the patient can give great support and consequent physiological benefit, or go the other way and "cause untold harm." Resist the temptation to defuse a tense situation by making a joke if it can be misunderstood.

- Caring through touch as you attempt to win the patient's confidence is also a very important part of communication. Touch can often communicate what words cannot. A hand touch or arm around the shoulder, or a pat on the back are small gestures that tell the patient, "You're doing fine," or, "I care about you." Touch is a basic human need and can help a great deal in an emergency situation.

2. Some handicapped people have special communication needs. If you are caring for a blind patient, you will need to explain what has happened, who you are, what procedures you are taking, and what the person can expect. With a non-hearing or non-speaking victim, using eye contact, and giving reassuring nods, or gestures will facilitate treatment.

3. If a patient does not speak English and you do not have a second-language capability, you might consider having a sentence-book or phrase-book made up with basic medical information in it, explaining who you are, what you need to do, and where the patient will be taken.

4. Many religious people attach great significance to religious symbols. Unless it is necessary for treatment, do not remove crosses or amulets.

- Be aware that members of some ethnic groups may be highly emotional over apparently minor problems while those of other groups show little emotion even in the face of serious illness or injury. Other factors that can seriously influence patient responses include social and economic background, emotional dependence, level of maturity, fear of any authority figure including medical personnel, senility, mental disorders, alcoholism, drug addiction, effects of medication, malnutrition, and chronic disease.

Personal Safety

You must protect your own safety from a variety of hazards by doing the following:

- Avoid traffic accidents while going to the scene of an accident or to the hospital. Use a seat belt at all times unless you need to remove it to care for the patient.

- Wear reflective emblems or clothing at night; supply adequate light at an accident scene.

- Wear protective clothing (latex gloves, goggles, mask, etc.) for infectious disease prevention.

- Minimize personal injury from jagged metal or broken glass at a car accident site by wearing a firefighter's helmet or hard hat, turnout gear, goggles or face shield, and leather gloves.

- Remove yourself and your patient from such potentially hazardous sites as high-traffic areas, leaking gasoline or a burning car, chemical spillage, radiation leaks, etc.

- Do not enter an unstable accident before trained personnel have taken care of hazards such as poisonous gases, live electrical wires, fires, and hazardous materials.

- Do not enter a volatile crowd situation — a riot, a crime scene, or a hostage situation — until it has been controlled by the police.

- Take extra precautions (e.g., proceed cautiously, do not disturb possible evidence) when you have reason to suspect that a victim, relative, bystander, etc. is involved in a crime.

☐ LEGAL PROBLEMS AND EMERGENCY CARE

At a certain point, you may wonder whether an EMT can give a patient emergency care without being sued. This is a complex issue.

In facing potential medico-legal situations, Burton[3] suggests five tools that can be used to manage and reduce liability risks:

R: **Recording.** "If it isn't recorded, it wasn't done." (See Chapter 45.)

I: **Informing.** Inform physicians when a gray zone occurs and inform your insurance carrier when there is the possibility of a claim by a patient.

S: **Solving Problems.** When you recognize a problem, fix it.

K: **Keeping Up.** Continue your quest for updated knowledge and skills.

S: **Staying in communication with your patients.** Do this while you are giving emergency care and transporting.

---

[3] Burton, Richard M., M.D., "Risky Business," *Emergency*, April 1986, pp. 54–55.

The EMT's Legal Obligations

Legally, you are obligated to care for any patient requiring your services while you are on duty. However, when you are off duty, you have no more legal obligation than any other citizen. Let's say that you pass an automobile accident on your way home from work. You have three choices: (1) you can stop and help the accident victim at the scene; (2) you can pass the scene and telephone for an ambulance, the police, etc.; or (3) you can pass the scene and make no attempt to call for help.

However, if you stop, you (or any other citizen) are obligated to help as much as you can, and you may not legally leave the scene until another health-care professional with at least as much expertise as you takes over care or until the police order you from the scene. If you do, you may be charged with **abandonment.**

If you need to remove articles of clothing or jewelry, or if you pick up any personal property, such as a purse or wallet, you are legally responsible for them. You should turn them over to the team in the emergency room and obtain a signed receipt for them.

Many areas have **protocols** that provide guidelines for cooperation between police and EMT personnel. In their absence, be sure that there are clear understandings, worked out by periodic conferences. If you suspect that a crime has been committed at the scene of an emergency, you should immediately notify the dispatcher so that the police can be summoned. If the situation is safe, you should continue with appropriate emergency care. You may transport the patient to the hospital even before the police arrive.

However, you should be careful not to disturb the scene more than necessary. Make notes or drawings of the position of the patient, weapons, and other items. If you have reason to believe that potential evidence will disappear if you leave, take it with you, properly bagged and labeled. Be sure that your partner witnesses what you are doing. Include in your records pertinent details that you observe or are told about — dying statements, circumstances of death, statements by the patient or others — that may become part of an investigation.

Good Samaritan Laws

Most states have **Good Samaritan laws.** The first was passed by California in 1959 specifically to protect "persons licensed (such as a physician or surgeon) who in good faith render emergency care at the scene of the emergency" from liability "for civil damages as a result of any acts or omissions." Other states followed with laws of their own, some of which specifically cover prehospital-care providers.

Generally, these laws state that a person is not liable for acts performed in good faith unless they constitute gross negligence. Therefore, the person suing must prove that the care provided was markedly below the standard of care that the court could assume would have been provided to the same patient under the same circumstances by another EMT who had received the same training — the "reasonable person" test. Good Samaritan laws do not, therefore, protect you from being sued. They just make it more difficult for the suing patient to provide a legally persuasive case. You still may have to face large legal fees.

Most states have specific laws authorizing EMTs to perform prehospital emergency medical procedures without a medical license and also allow some form of immunity to nurses, physicians, supervisors, or other personnel who give directions to EMTs by phone or radio. The laws governing private and public providers may vary. Check your local laws.

What Happens if a Patient Files Suit?

If a patient files a suit, it will be a **tort** claim, a civil (not a criminal) suit, and will not involve a broken contract or failure to pay a debt. The court must determine whether the individual's natural rights were violated through negligence. **Negligence** is carelessness, inattention, disregard, inadvertence, or oversight that was accidental but avoidable.

To establish negligence, the court must decide that:

1. The EMT had a duty to act.
2. The patient was injured.
3. The EMT's actions violated the standard of care that a normal, prudent EMT with similar training under similar conditions would have given.
4. The EMT's actions or lack of action in violation of the standard of care caused or contributed to the injury.

The jury would then decide six critical issues:

1. Did the EMT act, or fail to act?
2. Did the patient sustain physical, psychological, or financial injury due to the EMTs actions?
3. Did the action or inaction of the EMT cause or contribute to that injury by violating the standard of care reasonably expected of an EMT with similar background and training?
4. Did the patient contribute to his or her own injury?
5. Did the EMT violate his or her duty to care for the patient?
6. If the patient proves his or her case, what damages should be awarded?

Your best defense for protection in a negligence suit, then, would be to display professional competence and a professional attitude, to provide a consistently high standard of care, and to correctly document that care.

Patient Consent

It is important that you receive consent to care for a patient. Touching the body or clothing of an individual without consent can constitute **battery.** The primary types of consent are:

1. **Express or actual consent.**
   - You need to say something like, "My name is Nick Prizzuti and I'm a trained emergency medical technician. I'm here to help you. Is that all right?" Oral consent, a nod, or an affirming gesture constitutes valid consent. Consider, however, the age and mental capacity of the person giving the consent. A child or mentally retarded patient should have a guardian give consent. The rule of **implied consent** may apply here.
   - **Informed consent** means that a patient has received, in terms that he or she understands, all of the information that would affect a reasonable person's decision to accept or refuse a treatment or procedure.

2. **Implied consent.** In a true emergency where the patient is unconscious or disoriented and there is a significant risk of death, disability, or deterioration of condition, the law assumes that the patient would give his consent. In some cases in which a person received treatment while comatose and then subsequently sued, the law affirmed that the medical technicians acted properly since the patient was not legally competent to refuse treatment.

3. **Minor's consent.** A parent or legal guardian needs to consent to treatment for a minor. A minor is considered to be any person under the age of eighteen or twenty-one, depending on state law. However, parental or guardian consent is *not* required for a person under legal age who is married, pregnant, a parent, a member of the armed forces, or financially independent and living away from home. If a minor needs emergency care and no guardian is present, implied consent usually takes effect.

Refusing Treatment

A competent adult has the right to refuse treatment to the extent permitted by law, either verbally, or by pulling away, shaking his or her head "no," gesturing you away, or pushing you away. "Competent" means that the person is lucid and capable of making an informed decision; people who are disoriented, in shock,

mentally ill, or under the influence of drugs or alcohol are not considered competent.

A parent may also refuse treatment on behalf of a child. The courts have made two exceptions to refusal: parents or spouses may not withhold consent for life-saving treatment, and a pregnant woman may not refuse treatment if the life of her unborn child is endangered.

If a competent adult refuses treatment, he or she needs to be informed in a calm, persuasive way of the medical consequences of this action. Sometimes the patient has not clearly understood what you need to do and why. However, if he or she still refuses, even after understanding the treatment and the possible consequences, you must ask the individual to sign an official release form acknowledging the refusal. Either the signing or a refusal to sign must become part of the official documentation of the case. Obtain written witnessed statements regarding "refusals to sign" and, if possible, regarding "refusals to care." Use direct quotes where possible. However, keep in mind that you must use common sense. Some victims may not be thinking rationally due to shock or mild hysteria.

Naturally, emergency conditions are not always ideal for obtaining informed consent; but if ideal circumstances existed, this is what you should do to provide a patient, especially one refusing treatment, with enough information:

1. Get the patient's undivided attention, even if it takes some time to calm him or her and get him or her to trust you.
2. Assess the patient's emotional, intellectual, and physical status to see if he or she is capable of absorbing the information. Document this assessment.
3. Communicate very clearly. Don't say things like, "Call us if you feel worse." Say, "Call us if you feel a burning pain in your stomach." Don't use technical terms.
4. Ask the patient direct questions. For example, ask "What did I tell you to do if you start seeing double?"
5. Give the patient a copy of the report and ask him or her to read aloud the section on possible risks of not receiving immediate treatment.

Patient Rights — Confidentiality

Many jurisdictions have yet to write specific laws about the confidentiality due a patient receiving emergency care from an EMT. Laws do exist that prevent the intentional invasion of a person's privacy. These may be applied to cases involving emergency care. In many states, the deliberate invasion of a patient's privacy by an EMT may lead to the loss of certification and could lead to legal actions being taken against you.

Individuals in emergency care usually feel very strongly about protecting the patient's right to privacy. You must not provide care for a patient and then speak to the press, your family, friends, or other members of the public about the details of the care. If you speak of the emergency, you must not relate specifics about what a patient may have said, who he or she was or was with, anything unusual about his or her behavior, or any descriptions of personal appearance. The same holds true if you receive this information from another member of the EMS System. Confidentiality applies not only to cases of physical injury, but also to cases involving possible infectious diseases, illnesses, and emotional and psychological emergencies. Grant, P.19.

Patient confidentiality however, does not apply if you are asked to provide information to the police or to testify in court. You may be asked to repeat what patients tell you, call out, or tell others while under your care. You should maintain notes about each incident to which you respond.

Victims of Crime

As in all aspects of emergency care, your first concern must be your own safety. If you arrive at the scene and a crime is in progress or the criminal is still active at the scene, *do not* attempt to provide care. Wait until the police arrive and they tell you that the scene is safe.

Your first priority at the controlled crime scene is to provide emergency care. While doing so, you must try to preserve the *chain of evidence* that will go from the crime scene to the courtroom. Touch only what you need to touch. Move only what must be moved to protect the patient and to provide proper care. Do not use the telephone unless the police tell you that you may do so. Unless you have police permission, move the patient only if he or she is in danger or if he or she must be moved to provide proper care (e.g., to a hard surface for CPR).

In cases in which you are called to the scene of a domestic dispute, wait for police assistance. Domestic disputes are dangerous calls because the people involved often act unpredictably. The call to have you respond was probably placed because someone has been beaten or injured by some act of violence. If the violent person is still on the scene, he may turn his aggression toward you. Sometimes, it is the victim of the aggressive act who will attack you because you are an outsider interfering with a family matter.

If the crime is rape, do not wash the patient nor allow the patient to wash. Ask the patient not to change clothing, use the bathroom, or take any liquids or food. To do so may destroy evidence. Obviously, you may not physically prevent anyone from doing these things, but you can explain why such activities may break the chain of evidence. The patient will probably cooperate and follow your requests. *Emotional support* is a must in

cases of rape. The privacy, comfort, and *dignity* of the patient must be considered from the beginning of care. The degree of future emotional problems faced by the rape victim may well depend on how the patient is initially treated by the professionals who respond to help.

Remember: As an EMT, you may have a legal duty to report any situation in which injury is a possible result of crime or was received in the commission of a crime. In most localities, you should not leave the crime scene until the police give you permission to do so.

How to Document

In a malpractice suit, documentation, as found in the written ambulance report (see Chapter 45) is your main line of defense. Review Chapter 45 and follow those procedures on each and every call.

Requirements to Report

Depending on the state, you may be required by law to report certain medically related conditions:

1. **Child abuse.** Many states require people to report suspected child abuse. Some states have very broad requirements (Utah, for instance, requires any adult who suspects child abuse to report it) while others require reporting from only a limited group, like physicians. Such statutes frequently grant immunity from liability for libel, slander, or defamation of character to the reporter if the report is made in good faith. Know what the statute in your state says.

2. **Felonies.** Many states require you to report an injury that may have resulted from a crime or to report certain injuries like gunshot or knife wounds or poisoning. Again, know what your state requires.

3. **Drug-related injuries.** Some states require you to report drug-related injuries; however, the U.S. Supreme Court has ruled that drug addiction (not drug possession) is an illness, and not a crime.

4. Other cases you may be required to report include rape, assault, attempted suicide, dog bites, and some communicable diseases.

Legal Requirements and the Dying Patient

An EMT has certain legal obligations when dealing with dying or terminally ill patients. It is important to be aware of these obligations as well as of the boundaries within which the EMT is required to work.

In many states, for example, only a doctor or coroner can pronounce a person dead. If a person is obviously dead (crushed, decapitated, rigor mortis setting in), you may be required to leave the body at the site so as not to hinder a police investigation. In other cases, you may be required to transport the body to a medical facility where death can be pronounced.

In some cases, you may be called to a home where a terminally ill patient has reportedly requested and the doctor has reportedly ordered no resuscitation measures if the heart and lungs cease to function. In the absence of written proof (a living will or a doctor's written instructions), you are obligated to begin resuscitation measures immediately.

The physician's instructions must be clear, concise, and unambiguous, typed or written in a clear hand on a letterhead form. Phrases like "no heroics" or "no extraordinary treatment" are not sufficiently clear. If your area doesn't have a standard form to express the patient's and/or doctor's treatment desires, press for the adoption of one.

And finally, even in the presence of signed and *witnessed* natural-death directives (living wills) and "do-not-resuscitate" orders, medico-legal experts agree that EMTs and paramedics must contact their base-station physician or supervisor before following or disregarding the order.

In some cases, information about terminally ill patients is registered at local rescue stations.

Malpractice Insurance

Although negligence suits against EMTs are comparatively rare, it may be a reasonable precaution for you to maintain malpractice insurance for the following reasons:

1. You are legally responsible for your own acts or malpractice, whether alone or working for a large organization. You are not immune from suit.

2. You will need the best legal defense available in case of a malpractice suit. Legal costs can be very expensive. Even if you win the case, you could be devastated financially.

☐ EMT CODE OF ETHICS

A code of ethics is a list of rules of ideal conduct. For a given group, a code of ethics is drawn up by responsible members of that group. The earliest known medical code of ethics is embodied in the oath of Hippocrates, dating to fourth century B.C., which, in modified form, many physicians still take. A Code of Ethics for Emergency Medical Technicians was issued by the National Association of Emergency Medical Technicians in January 1978. This code is as follows:

Professional status as an emergency medical technician is maintained and enriched by the willingness of the individual practitioner to accept and fulfill obligations to society, other medical professionals, and the profession of emergency medical technician. As an emergency medical technician, I solemnly pledge myself to the following code of ethics:

- *The fundamental responsibility of the emergency medical technician is to serve life, to alleviate suffering, and to promote health.*

- *The emergency medical technician provides services based on human need, with respect for human dignity, unrestricted by considerations of nationality, race, creed, color, or status.*

- *The emergency medical technician does not use professional knowledge and skill in any enterprise detrimental to the public good.*

- *The emergency medical technician respects and holds in confidence all information of a confidential nature obtained in the course of professional work unless required by law to divulge such information.*

- *The emergency medical technician as a citizen understands and upholds the laws and performs the duties of citizenship; as a professional person the emergency medical technician has particular responsibility to work with other citizens and health professionals in promoting efforts to meet health needs of the public.*

- *The emergency medical technician maintains professional competence and demonstrates concern for the competence of other members of the medical profession.*

- *The emergency medical technician assumes responsibility in defining and upholding standards of professional practice and education.*

- *The emergency medical technician assumes responsibility for individual professional actions and judgment, both in dependent and independent emergency functions, and knows and upholds the laws which affect the practice of the Emergency Medical Technician.*

- *The emergency medical technician has the responsibility to participate in study of and action on matters of legislation affecting Emergency Medical Technicians and emergency service to the public.*

- *The emergency medical technician adheres to standards of personal ethics which reflect credit upon the profession.*

- *The emergency medical technician may contribute to research in relation to a commercial product or service, but does not lend professional status to advertising, promotion, or sales.*

- *Emergency medical technicians, or groups of emergency medical technicians, who advertise professional services, do so in conformity with the dignity of the profession.*

- *The emergency medical technician has an obligation to protect the public by not delegating to a person less qualified any service which requires the professional competence of an emergency medical technician.*

- *The emergency medical technician works harmoniously with, and sustains confidence in, emergency medical technician associates, the nurse, the physician, and other members of the health team.*
- *The emergency medical technician refuses to participate in unethical procedures, and assumes the responsibility to expose incompetence or unethical conduct in others to the appropriate authority.*

Both the Code of Ethics for Emergency Medical Technicians and similar oaths (see Figure 1-8) express a very basic concept: concern for the welfare of others, from which all statutes of right and wrong ultimately arise. It is safe to say that if EMTs place the welfare of the patient above all else when providing medical care, they will rarely commit an unethical act.

☐ NATIONAL ORGANIZATIONS

The development of the emergency medical technician program in the United States has helped to create national organizations that provide support services to the EMT. One of the oldest is the **National Registry of Emergency Medical Technicians.** This organization is involved in developing educational programs for national certification, in determining qualifications for eligibility to certify, and in maintaining a directory of registered EMTs.

The National Registry provides certification at three levels: basic (EMT-ambulance and EMT-nonambulance), intermediate (EMT-intermediate), and advanced (EMT-paramedic). Its logo patch has been copyrighted.

The headquarters of this organization is:

The National Registry of Emergency Medical
  Technicians
6610 Busch Boulevard
P.O. Box 29233
Columbus, OH 43229

The **National Association of Emergency Medical Technicians (NAEMT)** is concerned primarily with maintaining and upgrading EMT knowledge and skills and with promoting the profession. It also helps to develop and upgrade EMS systems across the United States. Each state has a chapter of the NAEMT open to any nationally or state-certified EMT.

The address of the national office is:

The National Association of Emergency Medical
  Technicians
9140 Ward Parkway
Kansas City, MO 64114

The **National Council of State EMS Training Coordinators,** is a vehicle for communication among the state EMS training coordinators across the United

FIGURE 1-8

The EMT Oath

Be it pledged as an Emergency Medical Technician, I will honor the physical and judicial laws of God and man. I will follow that regimen which, according to my ability and judgment, I consider for the benefit of patients and abstain from whatever is deleterious and mischievous, nor shall I suggest any such counsel. Into whatever homes I enter, I will go into them for the benefit of only the sick and injured, never revealing what I see or hear in the lives of men unless required by law.

I shall also share my medical knowledge with those who may benefit from what I have learned. I will serve unselfishly and continuously in order to help make a better world for all mankind.

While I continue to keep this oath unviolated, may it be granted to me to enjoy life, and the practice of the art, respected by all men, in all times. Should I trespass or violate this oath, may the reverse be my lot. So help me God.

Adopted by The National Association of Emergency Medical Technicians, 1978

States. The national council works for reciprocity between the states, certification and recertification standards, and standardization of courses. Another important function is to upgrade and publicize the EMT and EMS systems in the various states. The address is:

The National Council of State EMT Training Coordinators and EMS Clearinghouse
P.O. Box 11910
Iron Works Pike
Lexington, KY 40578

Two other organizations that deal with emergency care of the critically injured are:

America Trauma Society
875 North Michigan Avenue
Chicago, IL 60611

National Association for Search and Rescue
P.O. Box 2123
La Jolla, CA 92038

chapter 2

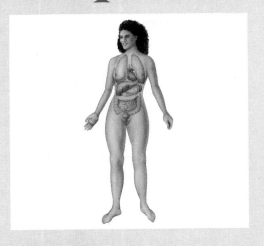

Anatomy and Physiology of Body Systems

✱ **OBJECTIVES**

- Define and locate the common anatomical and topographic terms of body position, location, direction, planes, regions, and cavities.
- Define and understand the common medical terms and abbreviations used by EMTs.
- Describe the common structures and functions of the major body systems.

It is recommended that EMTs wear protective gloves whenever there is a possibility of coming in contact with a patient's blood, body fluids, mucous membranes, traumatic wounds, or sores. See Chapter 31.

To effectively administer emergency care, you need to recognize disease states and injuries, and to do that successfully, you must have a basic knowledge of the structures and functions of the human body. **Anatomy** deals with the structure of the body and the relationship of its parts to each other; in other words, how the body is made. **Physiology** deals with the function of the living body and its parts; in other words, how the body works.

□ ANATOMICAL TERMINOLOGY

In the study of anatomy and physiology, you will encounter descriptive terms that you may not have used before. It is essential that you learn and use terms of position, direction, and location in reference to the body and its parts when describing illness or injury. Using correct terms will minimize confusion and enable you to communicate the exact extent of injury based on a careful visual examination of the patient.

Terms of Position

- **Anatomical position.** Unless otherwise indicated, all references made to the body will utilize the "anatomical position" — standing erect with the arms down at the sides, the palms facing you. This basic position is used as the point of reference when terms of direction and location are used. "Right" and "left" refer to the patient's right and left (Figure 2-1).
- **Supine position.** The patient is lying face-up (on the back) (Figure 2-2).
- **Prone position.** The patient is lying face-down (on the stomach) (Figure 2-3).
- **Lateral recumbent.** The patient is lying on the left or right side (Figures 2-4 and 2-5).

FIGURE 2-1 Anatomical regions of the human body.

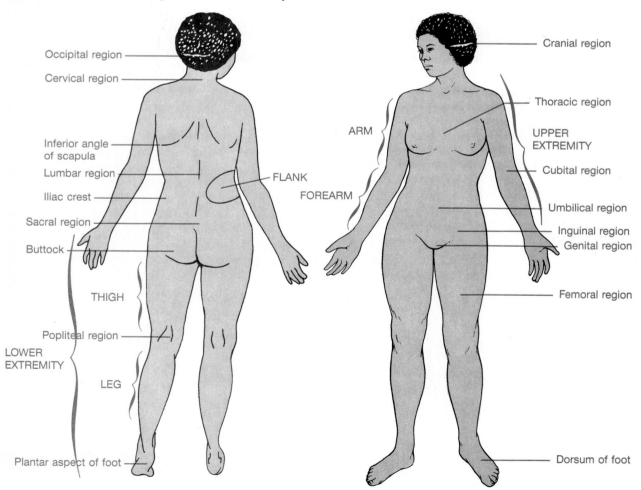

Occipital region
Cervical region
Inferior angle of scapula
Lumbar region
Iliac crest
Sacral region
Buttock
THIGH
Popliteal region
LOWER EXTREMITY
LEG
Plantar aspect of foot
FLANK
ARM
FOREARM
Cranial region
Thoracic region
UPPER EXTREMITY
Cubital region
Umbilical region
Inguinal region
Genital region
Femoral region
Dorsum of foot

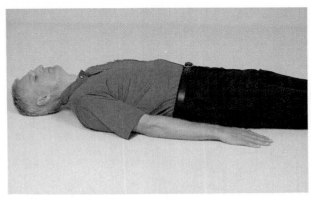

FIGURE 2-2 Supine position.

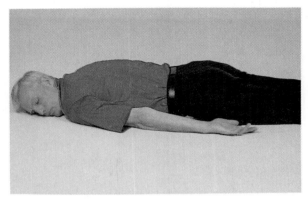

FIGURE 2-3 Prone position.

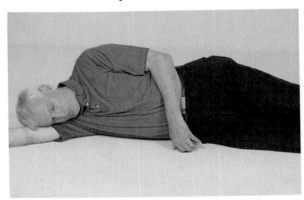

FIGURE 2-4 Right lateral recumbent position.

FIGURE 2-5 Left lateral recumbent position.

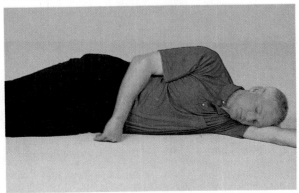

Terms of Direction and Location

- **Superior** — toward the head (**cranial**).
- **Inferior** — toward the feet (**caudal**).
- **Anterior** — toward the front (**ventral** — the belly side).
- **Posterior** — toward the back (**dorsal** — the backbone side).
- **Medial** — toward the midline or center of the body.
- **Lateral** — to the right or left of the midline or center of the body.
- **Proximal** — near the point of reference.
- **Distal** — far away from the point of reference.
- **Superficial** — near the surface.
- **Deep** — remote from the surface.
- **Internal** — inside
- **External** — outside.

Anatomical Planes

Imaginary straight-line divisions of the body are called planes. Medical illustrations and diagrams that indicate internal body structure relationships are labeled to indicate the plane divisions (see Figure 2-6).

☐ MEDICAL TERMINOLOGY

To understand most medical words, break the words into their parts and learn the meaning of these parts. Many medical words contain a stem or root to which is affixed either a prefix, a suffix, or both. A prefix is a group of letters combined with the beginning of a word to modify its meaning. A suffix is a group of letters added to the end of a word to modify its meaning. For example, the word "myocarditis" consists of the prefix "myo," the stem "card," and the suffix "itis." "Myo" means "muscle." "Card" means "cardiac" or "heart." "Itis" means inflammation." Thus, myocarditis means inflammation of muscles of the heart (Tables 2-1, 2-2, and 2-3). Also, become familiar with the abbreviations listed in Table 2-4.

☐ ANATOMICAL REGIONS AND TOPOGRAPHY

In evaluating a patient's condition, it is important to know certain external and internal landmarks; that is, the anatomical regions and systems of the body and their related parts. Reference to these landmarks makes the description of the patient's complaint or problem

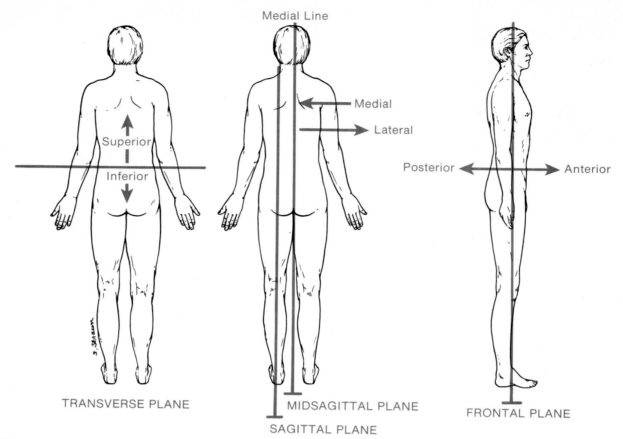

FIGURE 2-6 Anatomical planes.

TABLE 2-1
Common Stem Words

adeno	= gland
arthro	= joint
cardio	= heart
cephalo	= head
cysto	= bladder
cyto	= cell
dermo	= skin
entero	= intestine
gastro	= stomach
hemo	= blood
hepato	= liver
myelo	= spinal cord
	(or bone marrow)
myo	= muscle
nephro	= kidney
neuro	= nerve
oculo	= eye
osteo	= bone
oto	= ear
procto	= rectum
thoraco	= chest

TABLE 2-2
Common Prefixes

a– (or an–)	absence of, deficiency	in–, intra–	in, inside
ab–	away from	inter–	between
ad–	toward	leuko–	white
algia–	painful condition	macro–	large
ambi–	both	mal–	disordered, bad
angio–	tube or blood vessel	mamm–	breast
ante–	before, front	meno–	monthly, menstrual
anti–	against	micro–	small
arthro–	joint	myelo–	spinal cord, bone marrow
bi–	two	myo–	muscle
brady–	slow	nephro–	kidney
cardio–	heart	neuro–	nerve
cephalo–	head	ocul(o)–	eye
cerebro–	brain	olig–	little
chole–	bile	ophthal–	pertaining to eye
circum–	around	osteo–	bone
co–	with	oto–	ear
contra–	against	para–	beside
cost–	pertaining to rib	ped–	child, or foot
cyt–	sac	per–	through
derma–	skin	peri–	surrounding
di–	twice, double	pharyngo–	throat, pharynx
dys–	disordered, painful, difficult	pneumo–	air, lung
en–	in	poly–	many
endo–	inner, inside	post–	after
enter–	pertaining to the intestines	pre–	before
entero–	intestine	pro–	before, in front of, forward
epi–	upon, on the outside	pseudo–	false
erythro–	red	psych–	pertaining to the mind
ex–	out, away from	pulmo–	lung

TABLE 2-2 *(cont.)*
Common Prefixes

gastro–	stomach	pyelo–	kidney
glyco–	sugar	pyo–	pus
gynec–	pertaining to women	retro–	behind, backward
hem–, hema–	blood	rhino–	nose
hemi–	half	semi–	half
hepa–, hepato–	liver	sub–	under
hydro–	water	super–, supra–	above, greater
hyper–	above, excess	tachy–	fast
hypo–	below, deficient	thermo–	heat
hystero–	uterus	trans–	across

TABLE 2-3
Common Suffixes

–algia	pain	–paresis	weakness
–asthenia	weakness	–pathy	disease
–centesis	puncturing	–phasia	speech
–cyte	cell	–phobia	fear
–ectomy	surgical removal	–plasty	surgical repair
–emia	condition of the blood	–plegia	paralysis
–esthesia	feeling	–pnea	breathing
–genic	causing	–rhythmia	rhythm
–graph(y)	visualization machine	–rrhagia	bursting forth
–itis	inflammation	–scopy	see, looking into or through an instrument
–oma	tumor, swelling		
–omy	to cut	–stomy	surgical opening creating a hole
–osis	condition of		
–ostomy	opening	–tomy	surgical incision
–otomy	incision, to cut	–uria	urine

TABLE 2-4
Frequently Used Abbreviations

BP	–Blood Pressure	IV	–Intravenous (into a vein)
C.C.	–Chief Complaint	LOC	–Level of Consciousness
CO	–Carbon Monoxide	LLQ	–Left Lower Quadrant
CNS	–Central Nervous System	LUQ	–Left Upper Quadrant
COPD	–Chronic Obstructive Pulmonary Disease	MAST	–Military Antishock Trousers
CPR	–Cardiopulmonary Resuscitation	MI	–Myocardial Infarction
CVA	–Cerebrovascular Accident (stroke)	O_2	–Oxygen
DOA	–Dead on Arrival	OD	–Overdose
Dx	–Diagnosis	OR	–Operating Room
EEG	–Electroencephalogram	P	–Pulse
EKG	–Electrocardiogram	PASG	–Pneumatic Antishock Garment
EMT	–Emergency Medical Technician	PERL	–Pupils Equal and Reactive to Light
ER	–Emergency Room	R	–Respirations
Fx	–Fracture	RLQ	–Right Lower Quadrant
GI	–Gastrointestinal	RUQ	–Right Upper Quadrant
Hx	–History	Stat	–Immediately
ICU	–Intensive Care Unit	Sx	–Sign, symptom
IPPB	–Intermittent Positive Pressure Breathing		

more understandable to others, particularly when medical advice is sought by radio. Refer to Figures 2-1 and 2-7.

☐ THE SKELETAL SYSTEM (BONES AND JOINTS)

The human body is shaped by its bony framework. Without its bones, the body would collapse. Bone is composed of living cells and non-living, intercellular matter. The non-living material contains calcium compounds that help to make bone hard and rigid. The bony framework of the body is held together by ligaments that connect bone to bone; layers of muscles; tendons, which connect muscles to bone or other structures; and various connective tissue. Bones and their adjacent tissues help to move, support, and protect the vital organs.

The structural framework of the body, the **skeleton,** must be strong to provide support and protection, jointed to permit motion, and flexible to withstand stress.

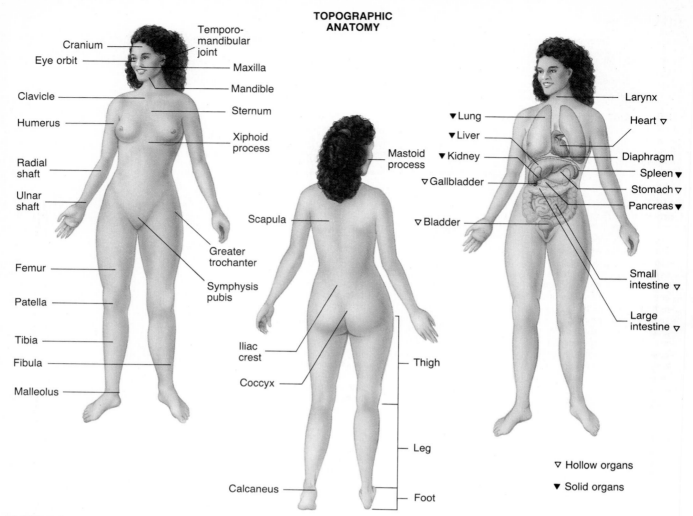

FIGURE 2-7

The adult skeleton has 206 bones that are classified by size and shape as long, short, flat, or irregular. These may be separated into two main divisions: (1) the **axial** skeleton and the (2) **appendicular** skeleton. The axial skeleton consists of the bones of the head, the neck, and the thorax. The appendicular skeleton consists of the bones of the extremities — the arms, shoulder girdle, and pelvic girdle (Figure 2-8).

The Axial Skeleton

Skull

The skull rests at the top of the spinal column. It contains the brain and the centers of special senses — sight, hearing, taste, and smell. The **brain** and the **spinal cord** (extending downward from the brain through the spinal column) constitute the **central nervous system.** **Cranial nerves** originate in the brain and pass through openings in the skull, thus differing from **spinal nerves,** which branch from the spinal cord.

The skull has two parts, the braincase **(cranium)** and the face. The eight interlocking bones of the cranium form a firm cover for the brain. Four of these bones — the occipital, two parietal, and the frontal — are typical flat bones. Their outer layer is thick and tough; the inner layer is thinner and more brittle. This arrangement gives maximum strength, lightness, and elasticity (Figure 2-8).

Although the skull is very tough, a blow may fracture it. Even if there is no fracture, a sudden impact may tear or **bruise** the brain and cause it to swell, as any **soft tissue** will swell following an injury or contusion. Because the skull cannot expand to accommodate brain swelling, injury to the brain is magnified by the contained pressure. Unconsciousness or even death may result from swelling **(edema),** a tearing wound **(laceration),** bleeding, or other damage to the brain.

The face, extending from the eyebrows to the chin, has fourteen bones, thirteen of which are immovable and interlocking. The immovable bones form the

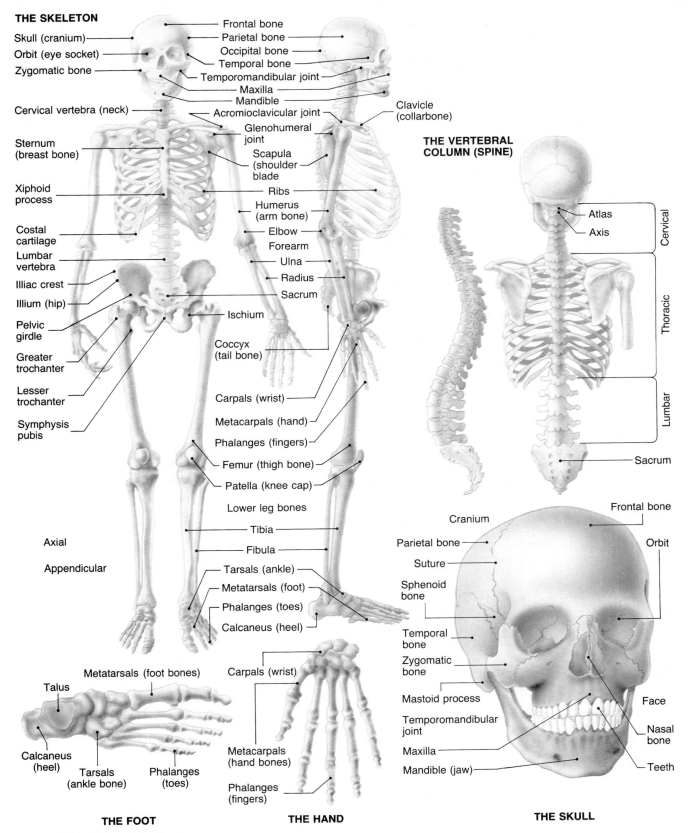

THE SKELETON

Skull (cranium)
Orbit (eye socket)
Zygomatic bone

Frontal bone
Parietal bone
Occipital bone
Temporal bone
Temporomandibular joint
Maxilla
Mandible

Cervical vertebra (neck)

Acromioclavicular joint
Glenohumeral joint
Scapula (shoulder blade)

Clavicle (collarbone)

Sternum (breast bone)

THE VERTEBRAL COLUMN (SPINE)

Xiphoid process

Ribs
Humerus (arm bone)
Elbow
Forearm
Ulna
Radius
Sacrum
Ischium

Atlas
Axis

Cervical

Costal cartilage
Lumbar vertebra
Illiac crest
Ilium (hip)
Pelvic girdle
Greater trochanter

Thoracic

Coccyx (tail bone)

Lumbar

Lesser trochanter
Symphysis pubis

Carpals (wrist)
Metacarpals (hand)
Phalanges (fingers)
Femur (thigh bone)
Patella (knee cap)
Lower leg bones

Sacrum

Axial

Appendicular

Tibia
Fibula
Tarsals (ankle)
Metatarsals (foot)
Phalanges (toes)
Calcaneus (heel)

Frontal bone

Cranium
Parietal bone
Suture
Sphenoid bone

Orbit

Metatarsals (foot bones)
Talus

Carpals (wrist)

Temporal bone
Zygomatic bone

Calcaneus (heel)
Tarsals (ankle bone)
Phalanges (toes)

Metacarpals (hand bones)
Phalanges (fingers)

Mastoid process
Temporomandibular joint
Maxilla
Mandible (jaw)

Face
Nasal bone
Teeth

THE FOOT

THE HAND

THE SKULL

FIGURE 2-8 The skeletal system.

bony settings of the eyes, nose, cheeks, and mouth. The fourteenth bone, the lower jaw **(mandible),** moves freely on hinge joints.

The upper jaw is formed by two **maxillary bones** that meet in the midline of the face. Together with the **palatine bones**, they form part of the **palate** or roof of the mouth, the floor of the eye sockets, and the floor and sides of the nasal cavities.

The lower jaw is shaped like a horseshoe. It is the largest and strongest bone of the face. The curved portion forms the chin. Two perpendicular portions form hinge joints with the **temporal bones** located on each side of the cranium just in front of the ears. Fractures and dislocations of the lower jaw are common.

Spinal Column

The **spinal column** is the principal support system of the body. Ribs spring from it much as the ribs of a ship spring from the keel. The rest of the skeleton is directly or indirectly attached to the spine.

The spinal column has a good deal of mobility. It is made up of irregularly shaped bones called **vertebrae** (the singular is "vertebra"). Lying one on top of the other to form a strong, flexible column, the vertebrae are bound firmly together by strong ligaments. Between each two vertebrae is a fluid-filled pad of tough elastic cartilage (the **intervertebral disc),** which acts as a shock absorber (Figure 2-9).

The spinal column may be damaged by disease or injury; the **cervical vertebrae** (the first seven) are mobile and delicate and are most prone to injury, while the sacrum, the lowest vertebrae, are least mobile and are seldom injured. If any of the vertebrae are crushed or displaced, the spinal cord at that point may be squeezed, stretched, torn, or severed. Movement of the disabled part by the injured person, or careless handling by well-

meaning but uninformed persons, may result in displacement of sections of the spinal column, causing further injury to the cord and possibly resulting in permanent paralysis. For this reason, *a person with a back or neck injury must be handled with extreme care.*

The spinal column, which lends support to the upper part of the body and the head and provides protection for the spinal cord, is composed of thirty-three vertebrae arranged in a column that is divided into five parts (Figure 2-8):

1. The **cervical vertebrae** are the first seven vertebrae — those that form the neck. The skull is attached to the top of this section of the spinal column. As mentioned, these are mobile and delicate and are most prone to injury.

2. The **thoracic vertebrae,** the twelve vertebrae directly following the cervical vertebrae, comprise the upper back. The twelve pairs of ribs are attached to these vertebrae and serve as a support to the vertebrae.

3. The **lumbar vertebrae,** the next five, form the lower back, one of the areas of the spine that is susceptible to injury. Since these vertebrae are the least mobile, however, they are the most seldom injured; many lower-back injuries involve musculature, not vertebrae.

4. The **sacrum,** composed of the next five vertebrae, are fused together to form the rigid part of the back side of the pelvis.

5. The **coccyx** (or **coccygeal spine),** the last four vertebrae, form the part of the spine most commonly referred to as the "tailbone." The four vertebrae of the coccyx are fused together and do not have the protrusions characteristic of the other vertebrae.

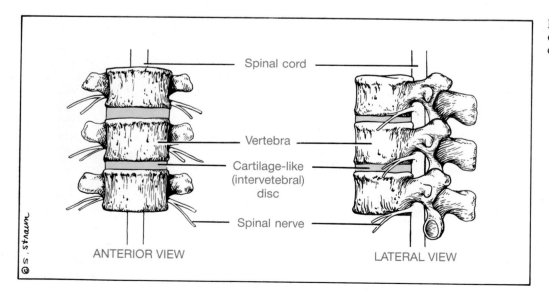

FIGURE 2-9 Anatomy of vertebrae of the spinal column.

Spinal cord

Vertebra

Cartilage-like (intervetebral) disc

Spinal nerve

ANTERIOR VIEW

LATERAL VIEW

© S. Strawn

These vertebrae are designated by letters and numbers. Those in the cervical spine are referred to by the letter "C" with numbers one through seven; those in the thoracic spine by the letter "T" with numbers one through twelve; and so on. In other words, if the third vertebra in the lumbar spine is injured, you report the injury as a "L-3."

The vertebrae, except for those in the coccyx and sacrum, are structured with a solid block of bone in their forward-facing part; this part bears the weight. The rear-facing (posterior) section is called the **vertebral arch,** and each arch has several bony protrusions. Some of these act as attachments for muscles or ligaments, and others form **joints.** In between the body (the solid block of bone) and the vertebral arch is a space; when all of the vertebrae are connected, these spaces combine to form the tunnel through which the spinal cord passes.

The vertebrae are connected by ligaments; lying between each vertebra is a disc or pad of tough cartilage that serves as a cushion and allows for movement of the spine. These discs are extremely susceptible to injury from twisting, grinding, or improper lifting of heavy objects. This can result in severe pain and sometimes total incapacitation.

Cylindrical in shape, about eighteen inches long, and weighing about one ounce, the spinal cord is a bundle of nerves that passes from the brain down through the spinal column. The protective outer covering of the spinal cord is rich with blood vessels and is composed of three membranes similar to the protective membranes of the brain. At different levels of the spine, pairs of nerves branch out between overlapping processes in the vertebrae and lead to various muscles and organs of the body.

Sternum (Breastbone) and Ribs

The **sternum** is a flat, narrow bone in the middle of the anterior wall of the chest. The **clavicles** and certain ribs are attached to the sternum (Figure 2-8).

The twenty-four **ribs** are semiflexible arches of bone. There are twelve on each side of the chest. The back end of the twelve pair of ribs are attached to the twelve thoracic vertebrae. Strong ligaments bind the posterior ends of the ribs to the backbone but allow slight gliding or tilting movements. The anterior ends of the top seven pairs of ribs are attached to the sternum by means of cartilage. They are the **true ribs.** The remaining five pairs are the **false ribs;** each of the upper three pairs is attached in front by cartilage to the pair of ribs above, and thus indirectly to the breastbone. The front ends of the last two pairs hang free; they are called **floating ribs.**

Fracture of the sternum or the ribs usually results from crushing or squeezing of the chest. A fall, blow, or penetration of the chest wall by a weapon may have the same effect. The chief danger from such injuries is that the lungs, heart, or blood vessels may be punctured by the sharp ends of broken ribs.

Appendicular Skeleton

The extremities contain no vital organs. A fracture or other injury to them is not likely to cause death except by a complication such as uncontrolled bleeding, **shock,** or **infection.** Permanent crippling can result from an injury to an **extremity.** However, this is less likely to happen today than in the days before effective surgery and rehabilitative education. Nonetheless, disfigurement and disability can result from improper handling of a patient. Emergency care, if correctly given, can minimize this possibility.

The upper and lower extremities are much alike. Each has one long, strong bone nearest to the trunk; two long bones parallel to each other; and several small bones forming the wrist and hand, or ankle and foot. However, ankles and feet, which are for locomotion, are not nearly as flexible as wrists and hands, which are for manipulation. Sturdy support for the body's weight, with a reasonable degree of mobility, is all that is required of the legs and feet.

Shoulder Girdle

Each clavicle (collarbone) and scapula (shoulder blade) form a **shoulder girdle.** With the muscles that extend from it to the arms, thorax, neck, and head, the shoulder girdle helps to attach the arms to the trunk.

Arms and Hands

The bone of the arm — the **humerus** — is the largest bone in the upper extremity. Its shaft is roughly cylindrical; its upper end (the head of the humerus) is round; its lower end, flat. The round head fits into a shallow cup in the shoulder blade, forming a **ball-and-socket joint.** This is the most freely movable joint in the body and is easily dislocated. **Dislocation** may tear the capsule of the joint (synovial membrane) and cause damage. Improper manipulation during attempts to **reduce** or "set" the dislocation may add to the damage. Therefore, it is well to treat dislocation of the shoulder with gentle care.

The bones of the forearm are the **ulna** and the **radius;** the end of the ulna forms most of the elbow joint. While the ulna can be palpated along its entire length, the upper two-thirds of the radius is sheathed in muscles and cannot be palpated; only the lower third of the radius, which enlarges to form most of the wrist joint, can be felt through the skin. The bony prominences on the ends of the ulna and radius that form the socket for the wrist joint are called the **styloid processes;** the **ulnar styloid** is on the little finger side of the wrist, and the **radial styloid** is on the thumb side of the wrist.

The wrist consists of eight bones called the **carpals;** a **metacarpal** bone lies at the base of each finger, and the metacarpal bones form the structural strength of the hands. The **phalanges** are the bones that make up the fingers and thumbs; each finger has three, and each thumb has two.

Pelvis

The two **ilia,** the sacrum, and the coccyx form the **pelvic girdle** (pelvis). Muscles help to attach the pelvic bones, the trunk, the thighs, and the legs together. The pelvis forms the floor of the **abdominal cavity.** The lower part of the cavity — sometimes called the **pelvic cavity** — holds the **bladder, rectum,** and internal parts of the reproductive organs. The pelvic cavity is extremely vascular, and a pelvic fracture may cause severe bleeding. The floor of the pelvic cavity helps to support the **intestines.**

Thighs and Knees

At the outer side of each hipbone (*os coxae*) is a deep socket into which the round head of the thighbone (**femur**) fits, forming a ball-and-socket joint called the **hip.** The head of the femur, not as easily dislocated as the less firmly fixed head of the humerus, is likely to be more difficult to put back into its socket (reduce). The lower end of the femur, like the humerus, is flat and has two knobs (**condyles**) that articulate with the shinbone (**tibia**) at the knee joint (Figure 2-8).

Although the femur is the longest and strongest bone in the skeleton, it is commonly fractured. Fracture of the femur is always serious because of the difficulty in getting a good position for union between the broken or splintered ends of this large, strong bone. Because of the force required to break the femur, laceration of the surrounding tissues, pain, and blood loss may be unusually extensive.

The knee joint is a strong **hinge joint** and, like the elbow, allows angular movement only. The joint is protected and stabilized in front by the kneecap (**patella**). The patella is a small, triangular-shaped bone in front of the large muscle of the front of the thigh. Because the patella usually receives the force of falls or blows upon the knee, it frequently is bruised and is sometimes fractured.

Legs

Anatomically speaking, the word "leg" is used only for that portion of the lower extremity between the knee and the ankle. Its two bones are the **tibia** (the weight-bearing bone) and **fibula.** The tibia is at the anterior and medial side of the leg. Its broad upper surface receives the condyles of the femur to form the knee joint. The lower end, much smaller than the upper end, forms the inner, rounded knob of the ankle. The fibula, more slender than the tibia, is at the outer side of the leg parallel to the shinbone. The fibula, not a part of the true knee joint, is attached at the top to the tibia. The fibula is more often fractred alone than is the tibia (Figure 2-8).

Ankle and Foot

The bony prominences at the ends of the tibia and fibula form the ankle joint socket; the **talus,** or ankle bone, fits inside the socket. The **calcaneus,** or heel bone, forms the prominence of the heel and fits against the undersurface of the talus. The talus, the calcaneus, and five other bones are referred to in a group as the **tarsal bones;** these make up the rear portion of the foot. Five **metatarsal bones** form the substance of the foot, and fourteen **phalanges** on each foot form the toes (two in the big toe, three in each other toe) (Figure 2-8).

Joint Movements

Different joints may be classified as immovable, slightly movable, and movable (see Figure 2-10 for examples). Movable joints allow change of position and motion. Examples of joint movement are:

- **Flexion** (bending).
- **Extension** (straightening).
- **Abduction** (movement away from the **midline.**
- **Adduction** (movement toward the midline).
- **Circumduction** (when a joint is capable of all four of the above motions).
- **Pronation** (turning the forearm so that the palm of the hand faces downward.
- **Supination** (turning the forearm so that the palm of the hand faces upward).

If the bone of a joint is capable of turning on its own long axis, the motion is called **rotation.** The motion of turning in toward the midline of the body is called inward or internal rotation, and the motion of turning outward is called outward or external rotation. (The humerus in the anatomical position is in external rotation.)

Attempts to force joints to move beyond their normal limitations can be disastrous. The structure of the joint determines the kind of movement that is possible, since the bone ends **articulate,** or fit into each other, at the joint. Examples of joint structure that permit certain kinds of joint movement include (Figure 2-11):

- Ball-and-socket joints, as in the shoulder and hip. These joints permit the widest range of motion — flexion, extension, abduction, adduction, and rotation.

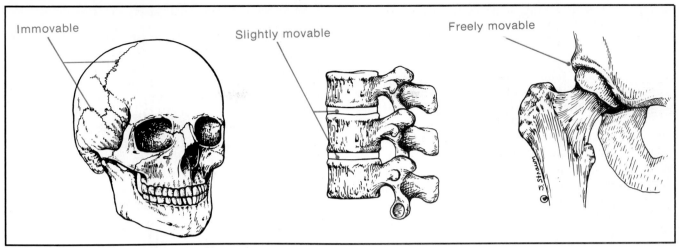

FIGURE 2-10 Anatomy of immovable, slightly movable, and freely movable joints.

- Hinge joints, as in the elbow, knee, and finger. Hinge joints permit flexion and extension. Elbow joints have forward movement — the **anterior** bone surfaces approach each other. Knee joints have backward movement — the **posterior** bone surfaces approach each other.

- **Pivot joints,** such as at the head and neck, at the first and second cervical vertebrae. The **distal** end of the **radius** and **ulna** also form a pivot joint for rotation of the wrist.

- The simplest movement between bones occurs in a **gliding joint,** where one bone slides part way

FIGURE 2-11 Types of freely movable joints.

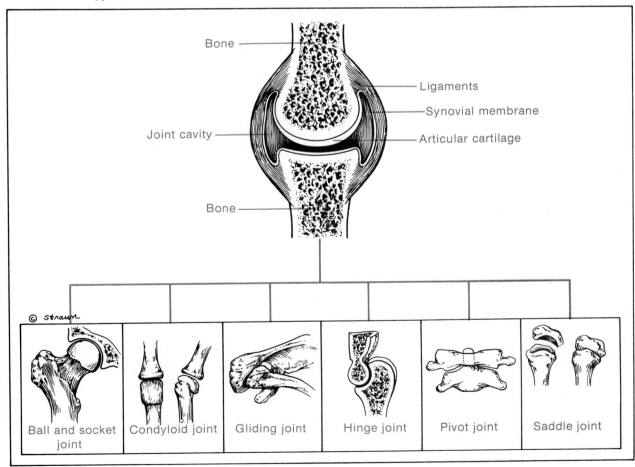

Bone

Ligaments

Synovial membrane

Joint cavity

Articular cartilage

Bone

Ball and socket joint   Condyloid joint   Gliding joint   Hinge joint   Pivot joint   Saddle joint

across another. Surrounding structures restrict the motion. Gliding joints connect small bones in the hands and feet, such as the carpals and metacarpals.

- The **saddle joint,** as in the ankle, is shaped to permit combinations of limited movements along perpendicular planes; hence, the ankle allows the foot to turn inward slightly as it swivels up and down. The carpo-metacarpal joint of the thumb is also an example of a saddle joint.
- The **condyloid joint** is a modified ball-and-socket joint that permits limited motion in two directions. In the wrist it permits the hand to move up and down and side to side but not to rotate completely.

□ BODY CAVITIES

The organs of the body are located in certain **cavities,** the major ones of which are the cranial, spinal, thoracic, abdominal, abdominopelvic and pelvic cavities (Figure 2-12).

FIGURE 2-12 Main body cavities.

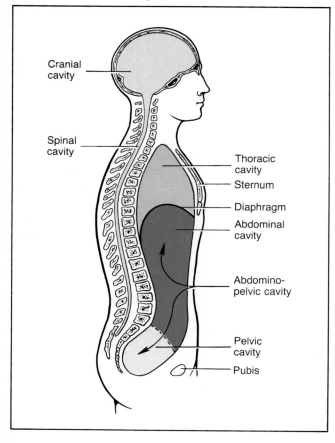

Anterior Abdominal Surface Area

The large anterior area of the **abdomino-pelvic cavity** is divided into four quadrants (Figure 2-13). The right upper quadrant (RUQ) contains the **liver, gallbladder,** and part of the colon; the left upper quadrant (LUQ) contains the **stomach, spleen,** and part of the colon. The right lower quadrant (RLQ) contains the ascending colon and the cecum, to which the appendix is attached; the left lower quadrant (LLQ) contains the **sigmoid** and descending portions of the colon. The initials of these quadrants are often used to indicate the approximate location of an organ, pain, wound, or surgical incision. In addition to identification by quadrants, the upper central abdominal region is referred to as **epigastric** (over the stomach), and the lower central region as **suprapubic** (above the pubis). The ribbed area is called **costal.**

□ THE MUSCULAR SYSTEM

Movements of the body are due to work performed by muscles Figure 2-14. Examples are walking, breathing, the beating of the heart, and the movements of the stomach and intestines. What enables muscle tissue to perform work is its ability to **contract** — to become shorter and thicker — when stimulated by a nerve impulse. The cells of a muscle, usually long and thread-like, are called **fibers.** Each muscle has countless bundles of closely packed, overlapping fibers bound together by connective tissue. Figure 2-15 illustrates the three different kinds of muscles:

1. **Striated** or skeletal **muscle** (voluntary).
2. **Smooth muscle** (involuntary) or visceral.
3. **Cardiac muscle** (heart).

They differ in appearance and in the specific jobs that they do.

Muscles can be injured in many ways. Overexerting a muscle may break fibers. Muscles subjected to trauma may be bruised, crushed, cut, torn, or otherwise injured, with or without breaking the skin. Muscles injured in any of these ways are likely to become swollen, tender, painful, or weak.

Skeletal Muscle

Skeletal muscles, under the control of a person's will, make possible all deliberate acts: walking, chewing, swallowing, smiling, frowning, talking, or moving the eyeballs. Most skeletal **(voluntary)** muscles are attached by one or both ends to the skeleton by **tendons.** However, some muscles are attached to skin, cartilage, and special organs such as the eyeball, or to other muscles, like the tongue.

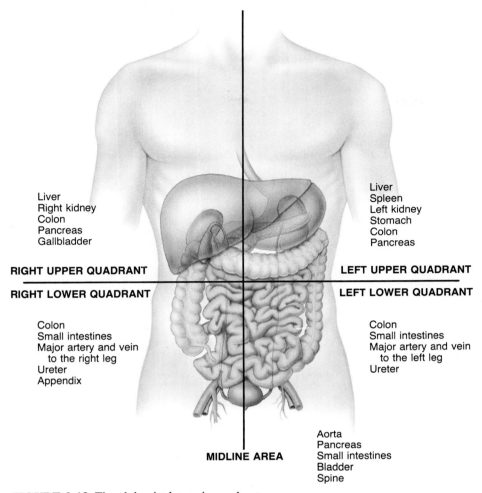

Liver
Right kidney
Colon
Pancreas
Gallbladder

RIGHT UPPER QUADRANT

RIGHT LOWER QUADRANT

Colon
Small intestines
Major artery and vein
   to the right leg
Ureter
Appendix

MIDLINE AREA

Liver
Spleen
Left kidney
Stomach
Colon
Pancreas

LEFT UPPER QUADRANT

LEFT LOWER QUADRANT

Colon
Small intestines
Major artery and vein
   to the left leg
Ureter

Aorta
Pancreas
Small intestines
Bladder
Spine

FIGURE 2-13 The abdominal area in quadrants.

Muscles help to shape the body and to form its walls. In the trunk they are broad, flat, and expanded to help form the walls of the cavities that they enclose — the abdomen and the chest. In the extremities, the skeletal muscles are long and much more rounded, somewhat resembling spindles. Most skeletal muscles end in tough, whitish cords (tendons or **leaders**) by which they are attached to the bones that they move. Tendons run through sleeves of dense, strong tissue **(fascia).** These are lined with a **synovial membrane** that secretes a lubricating substance, the **synovial fluid.** This makes it easier for the tendon to move when the muscle contracts or relaxes. If the synovial membrane becomes inflamed, stiffness and limitation of motion occur.

Smooth Muscle

Smooth muscles are made up of fibers that are larger than most striated fibers. A person has little or no con-

trol over these muscles and usually is not conscious of them. Smooth **(involuntary)** muscles are in the walls of tubelike organs, ducts, and blood vessels. In the intestines they form much of the walls. Some muscles are in two principal layers, circular and longitudinal. This arrangement strengthens the tubes and makes possible their rhythmic, wavelike movements. The **peristaltic waves** in the intestines propel food through the **alimentary canal.**

Cardiac Muscle

The walls of the heart have a special kind of muscle. **Cardiac muscle** is particularly suited for the work that the heart must do. It is smooth like involuntary muscle but is striated like voluntary (skeletal) muscle. Unlike either, it is made up of a cellular meshwork. Heart muscle is able to stimulate itself into contraction, even when disconnected from the central nervous system.

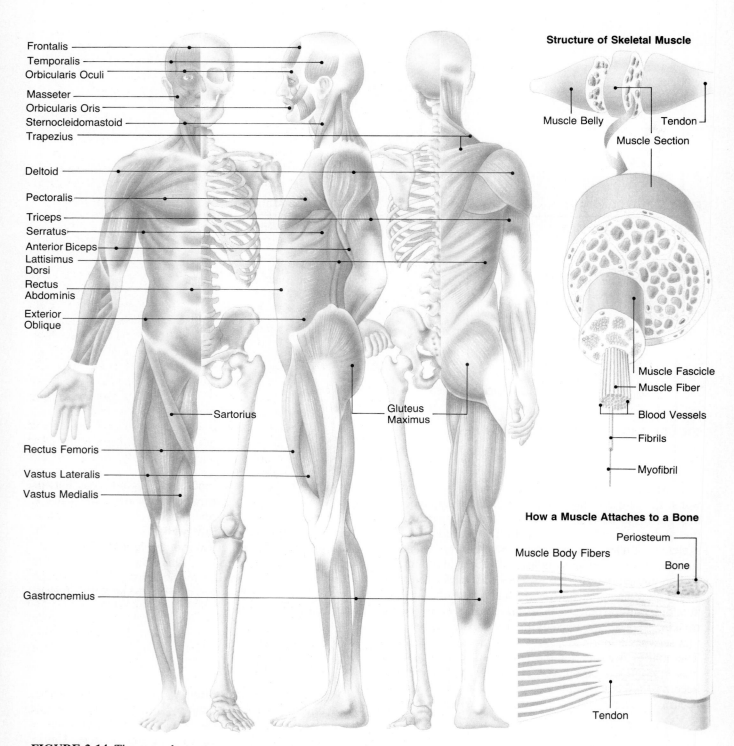

Structure of Skeletal Muscle

Frontalis
Temporalis
Orbicularis Oculi
Masseter
Orbicularis Oris
Sternocleidomastoid
Trapezius
Deltoid
Pectoralis
Triceps
Serratus
Anterior Biceps
Lattisimus Dorsi
Rectus Abdominis
Exterior Oblique
Sartorius
Rectus Femoris
Vastus Lateralis
Vastus Medialis
Gastrocnemius
Gluteus Maximus

Muscle Belly
Tendon
Muscle Section
Muscle Fascicle
Muscle Fiber
Blood Vessels
Fibrils
Myofibril

How a Muscle Attaches to a Bone

Muscle Body Fibers
Periosteum
Bone
Tendon

FIGURE 2-14 The muscular system.

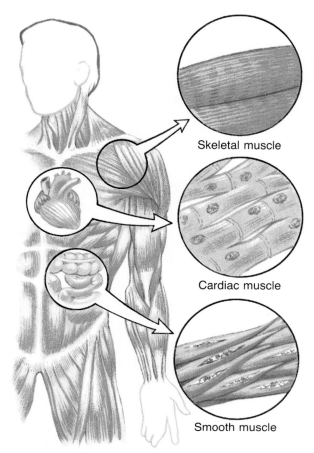

FIGURE 2-15 There are three types of muscle. Skeletal muscle, also called voluntary muscle, is found throughout the body. Cardiac muscle is limited to the heart. Smooth muscle, occasionally called involuntary muscle, is found in the intestines, arterioles, and bronchioles.

☐ THE CIRCULATORY SYSTEM

The **circulatory system** (Figure 2-16) has two major fluid transportation systems, the **cardiovascular** and the **lymphatic.** The cardiovascular system, which contains the heart, blood vessels, and blood, is a closed system, transporting blood to all parts of the body. Blood flowing through this circuit brings oxygen, food, and other chemical elements to tissue cells and removes **carbon dioxide** and other waste products resulting from cell activity. The **lymphatic system,** which provides drainage for tissue fluid, is an auxiliary part of the circulatory system, returning an important amount of tissue fluid **(lymph)** to the bloodstream through its own system of lymphatic vessels.

The Heart

The **heart,** designed to be a highly efficient pump, is a four-chambered, muscular organ lying within the chest.

About two-thirds of its mass is located to the left of the midline. It lies in the **mediastinal space** in the **thoracic cavity** between the two lungs. In size and shape, it resembles a man's closed first. Its lower point, the apex, lies just above the left **diaphragm.**

The **pericardium** is a double-walled sac enclosing the heart. The outer fibrous surface gives support, and the inner lining prevents friction as the heart moves within its protective jacket. The surfaces of the pericardial sac produce a small amount of fluid needed for lubrication to facilitate the normal movements of the heart.

The wall of the heart is made up of cardiac muscle called **myocardium.**

The heart has four chambers that are essentially the same size. The upper chambers, called the **atria,** are seemingly smaller than the lower chambers, the **ventricles.** The apparent difference in total size is due to the thickness of the myocardial layer. The right atrium communicates with the right ventricle; the left atrium communicates with the left ventricle. The **septum** (partition) that divides the interior of the heart into right and left sides prevents direct communication of blood flow from right to left chambers or left to right chambers. This is important, because the right side of the heart receives **unoxygenated** blood returning from the **systemic** (body) **circulation.** The left side of the heart receives **oxygenated** blood returning from the **pulmonary** (lung) **circulation.** The special structure of the heart keeps the blood flowing in its proper direction to and from the heart chambers.

The heart, then, is a hollow, muscular organ about the size of the fist. It rests on the diaphragm in the front part of the chest cavity, just underneath and to the left of the **sternum** (breastbone). It lies in front of the esophagus and the trachea (the tubes that lead to the stomach and the lungs), and it is protected by the bony **rib cage.**

Flow of Blood through the Heart

It is helpful to follow the flow of blood through the heart to understand the relationship of the heart structures (Figure 2-16). Remember — the heart is both the pump and the connection between the systemic circulation and the pulmonary circulation. Blood returning from the systemic circulation must flow through the pulmonary circulation for exchange of carbon dioxide for oxygen.

Blood from the upper part of the body enters the heart through a large vein, the **superior vena cava,** and from the lower part of the body via the **inferior vena cava.**

Blood from the superior vena cava and inferior vena cava enters the heart at the right atrium, which contracts, forcing blood through the open **tricuspid valve** into the relaxed right ventricle.

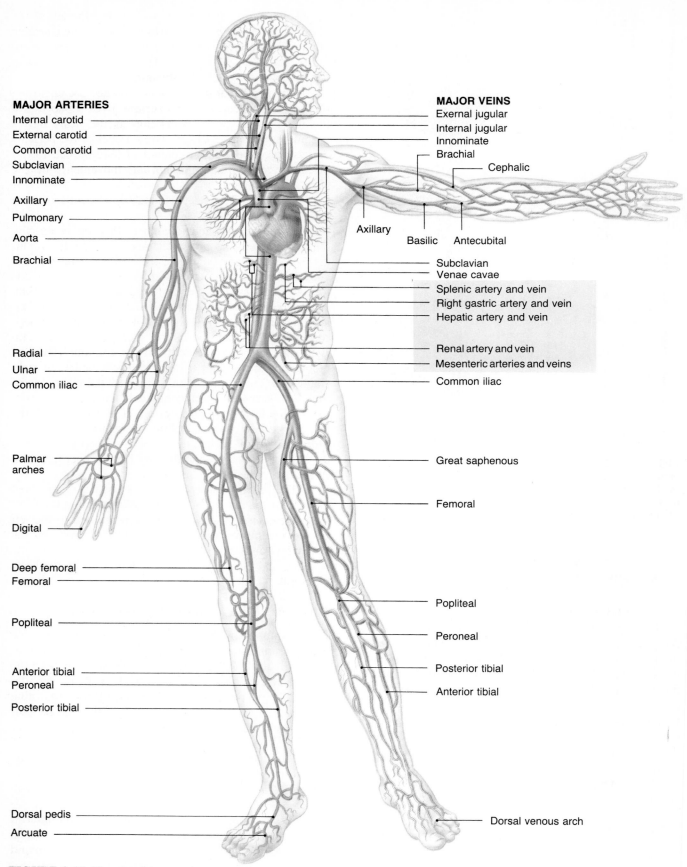

MAJOR ARTERIES

Internal carotid
External carotid
Common carotid
Subclavian
Innominate
Axillary
Pulmonary
Aorta
Brachial

Radial
Ulnar
Common iliac

Palmar
arches

Digital

Deep femoral
Femoral

Popliteal

Anterior tibial
Peroneal
Posterior tibial

Dorsal pedis
Arcuate

MAJOR VEINS

Exernal jugular
Internal jugular
Innominate
Brachial
Cephalic
Axillary
Basilic   Antecubital

Subclavian
Venae cavae
Splenic artery and vein
Right gastric artery and vein
Hepatic artery and vein

Renal artery and vein
Mesenteric arteries and veins

Common iliac

Great saphenous

Femoral

Popliteal

Peroneal

Posterior tibial

Anterior tibial

Dorsal venous arch

FIGURE 2-16 The circulatory system.

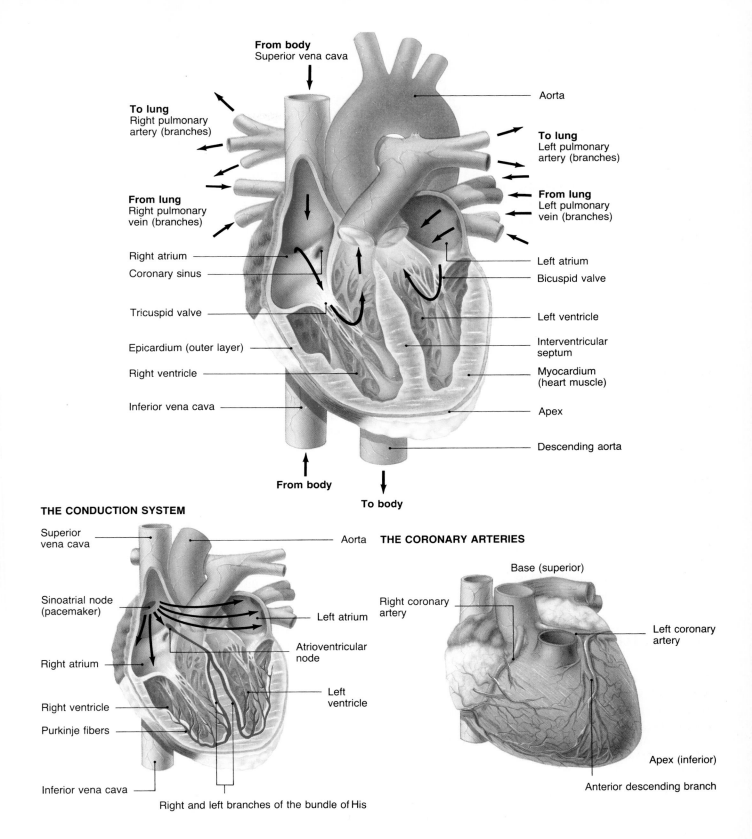

From body
Superior vena cava

Aorta

To lung
Right pulmonary
artery (branches)

To lung
Left pulmonary
artery (branches)

From lung
Right pulmonary
vein (branches)

From lung
Left pulmonary
vein (branches)

Right atrium

Left atrium

Coronary sinus

Bicuspid valve

Tricuspid valve

Left ventricle

Epicardium (outer layer)

Interventricular
septum

Right ventricle

Myocardium
(heart muscle)

Inferior vena cava

Apex

Descending aorta

From body

To body

THE CONDUCTION SYSTEM

Superior
vena cava

Aorta

THE CORONARY ARTERIES

Sinoatrial node
(pacemaker)

Left atrium

Base (superior)

Right coronary
artery

Atrioventricular
node

Left coronary
artery

Right atrium

Right ventricle

Left
ventricle

Purkinje fibers

Inferior vena cava

Right and left branches of the bundle of His

Apex (inferior)

Anterior descending branch

As the right ventricle contracts, the tricuspid valve closes, preventing backflow into the atrium. The **pulmonary semilunar valve** opens as a result of the force and movement of the blood, and the right ventricle pumps the blood into the **pulmonary artery.** While most arteries carry oxygenated blood away from the heart, the pulmonary artery carries unoxygenated blood from the heart to the lungs, where it can be oxygenated. (The oxygenated blood is returned to the heart through the pulmonary veins).

The blood is carried through the lung tissues, exchanging its carbon dioxide for oxygen in the **alveoli.** This oxygenated blood is collected from the main **pulmonary veins** and delivered back to the left atrium.

As the left atrium contracts, the oxygenated blood flows through the open **bicuspid (mitral) valve** into the left ventricle.

As the left ventricle contracts, the bicuspid valve closes. The **aortic semilunar valve** opens as a result of the force and movement of the blood, and the left ventricle pumps oxygenated blood through the aortic semilunar valve into the **aorta,** the main artery of the body. Oxygenated blood now starts its flow to all of the body cells and tissues. The systemic circulation starts from the left ventricle, the pulmonary circulation from the right ventricle.

Blood Vessels

The blood vessels are the closed system of tubes through which the blood flows. The **arteries** and **arterioles** are distributors, taking blood away from the heart. The **capillaries** are the vessels through which all exchange of fluid, oxygen, and carbon dioxide takes place between the blood and tissue cells. The **venules** and **veins** are collectors, carrying blood back to the heart. The capillaries are the smallest of these vessels but are functionally of the greatest importance.

□ THE RESPIRATORY SYSTEM

The body may store food to last for several weeks and water to last for several days, but it can store only enough oxygen for a few minutes. Ordinarily this does not matter, because we have only to inhale air to get the oxygen we need. If the oxygen supply of the body is cut off, as in drowning, choking, or smothering, death will come in about five minutes. Oxygen from air is made available to the blood through the **respiratory system** (Figure 2-17) and then to the body cells by the circulatory system.

Nasal Passages

Air normally enters the body through the nostrils. It is warmed, moistened, and filtered as it flows over the damp, sticky lining (**mucous membrane)** of the nose. When a person breathes through the mouth instead of the nose, there is less filtration and warming.

The nose is divided into two crooked passages by a wall (**septum)** of bone and cartilage. Each side of the nose has bones shaped like two inverted cones (**turbinates).** These protect the lungs from foreign body contamination, while warming and moistening the air. Air moving through the nasal passages enters the nasal portion of the **pharynx (naso pharynx)** (Figure 2-17).

Pharynx and Trachea

From the back of the nose or mouth, the air enters the throat (**pharynx).** The pharynx is a common passageway for food and air. At its lower end it divides into two passageways, one for food and the other for air. Food is routed by muscular control in the back of the throat to the food tube (**esophagus),** which leads to the stomach, and air is routed from the pharynx to the windpipe (**trachea),** which leads to the lungs.

The trachea and the esophagus are separated by a small flap of tissue (the **epiglottis),** which acts as a kind of valve that closes the trachea while food is being swallowed. At other times the trachea remains open to permit breathing. Usually this controlled diversion works automatically to keep food out of the trachea and air from going into the esophagus. However, when the epiglottis fails to close, food or liquids can enter the larynx instead of the esophagus, causing choking (Figure 2-17).

During unconsciousness, normal swallowing controls do not operate. *If liquid is poured into the mouth of an unconscious person to try to revive him, it may get into his windpipe and cause suffocation.* Foreign objects, such as false teeth or a piece of food, may lodge in the throat or windpipe and cut off the passage of air.

In the upper two inches of the trachea, just below the epiglottis, is the voice box (**larynx),** which contains the **vocal cords.** In the front of the throat, the larynx (**Adam's apple)** can be felt.

Lungs

The trachea branches into two main tubes (bronchial tubes or **bronchi),** one of each lung. Each bronchus divides and subdivides somewhat like the branches of a tree. Finally, the smallest ones end in thousands of tiny **alveolar pouches** (air sacs), just as the twigs of a tree end in leaves. Each air sac is enclosed in a network of capillaries (Figure 2-17).

The adjoining walls of the air sacs and the walls of the capillaries are very thin. Through these walls, the oxygen combines with **hemoglobin** in red blood cells to form **oxyhemoglobin,** which is carried to all parts of the body. Carbon dioxide and other waste gases in the blood move across the capillary walls into the air sacs

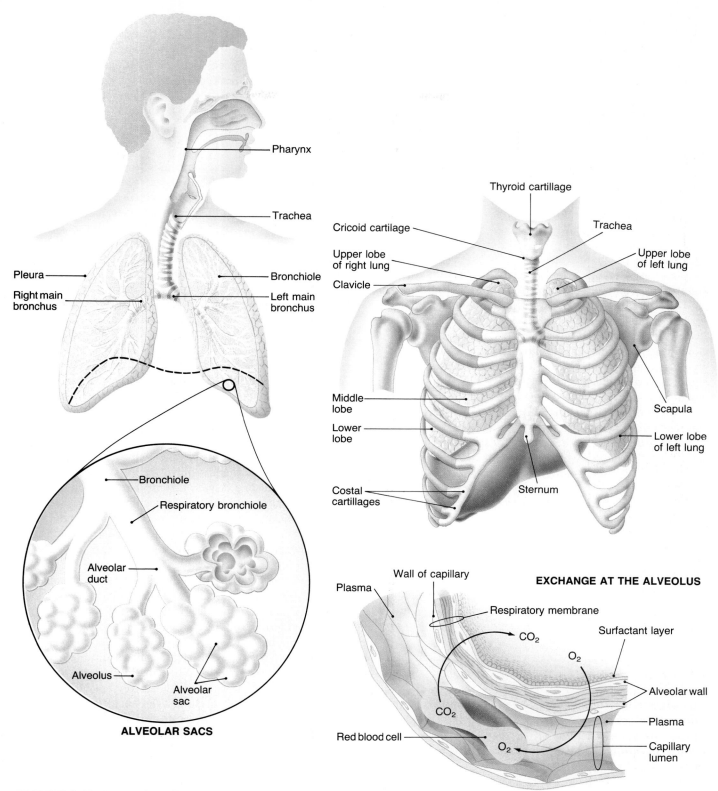

FIGURE 2-17 The respiratory system.

and are exhaled from the body. Tobacco smoke and other inhaled irritants cause the partitions between the air sacs to be destroyed, resulting in shortness of breath and eventually a disease called **chronic obstructive pulmonary disease.**

The respiratory system has two layers of connective tissue called **pleura.** The first layer, which is thin, covers the lungs. A thicker, more elastic layer covers the chest wall, between the two layers is the **intrapleural space,** a tiny space with negative pressure. If air from the outside enters the intrapleural space (as happens in some injuries), one or both lungs may collapse.

Mechanics of Breathing

The passage of air into and out of the lungs is called **respiration.** Breathing in is called **inspiration** or **inhalation;** breathing out is **expiration** or **exhalation.**

Respiration is a mechanical process brought about by alternately increasing and decreasing the size of the chest cavity. During inspiration, the diaphragm is drawn downward, and the vertical dimension of the chest cavity is increased. At the same time, muscles attached to the chest wall tighten and lift the ribs and sternum upward and outward, increasing the front-to-back and horizontal diameters of the chest. A relative vacuum in the respiratory system occurs.

By way of the nose, mouth, trachea, and bronchi, air enters the lungs, which expand to fill the enlarged chest cavity. Muscles can close the larynx to hold the breath.

During expiration, the muscles of the chest relax; the larynx opens to release the air trapped in the "pulmonary tree." Atmospheric pressure on the chest wall forces the ribs to fall, decreasing the size of the chest cavity. At the same time, the abdominal muscles contract and the abdominal contents press upward on the relaxed diaphragm, causing it to dome. This further decreases the size of the chest cavity, forcing out the same volume of air that was just taken in.

□ THE DIGESTIVE SYSTEM

The **digestive system** (Figure 2-18) is composed of the **alimentary tract** (food passageway) and the accessory organs. Its main functions are to ingest and carry food so that **digestion** and **absorption** can occur and to eliminate waste. The products of the accessory organs help to prepare food for its absorption and use (**metabolism**) by the tissues of the body.

Digestion consists of two processes, one mechanical and the other chemical. The mechanical part includes chewing, swallowing, **peristalsis** (the rhythmic movement of matter through the digestive tract), and defecation (the elimination of digestive wastes). The chemical part consists of breaking foodstuffs into simple components that can be absorbed and used by the body. In this process, foodstuffs are broken down by **enzymes,** or digestive juices, formed by digestive glands. **Carbohydrates** are broken into simple sugar (**glucose**), **fats** are changed into fatty acids, and **proteins** are converted to **amino acids.**

Abdominal Cavity

Except for the mouth and esophagus, the abdomen contains the major organs of the **gastrointestinal tract.** The abdominal cavity is protected above by the thorax, below by the heavy ring of pelvic bones, and on the sides and in the back by thick, tough muscles, the lower ribs, and the spinal column. It is protected in front by flat, muscular layers, which for greater strength run in different directions in the abdominal wall.

The major organs of the abdominal cavity are the **stomach, pancreas, liver, spleen, gallbladder,** and the **small** and **large intestines.** The stomach, a large hollow organ and the main organ of the digestive system, secretes gastric juices that begin converting ingested foods to a form that can be assimilated by the body. The pancreas, a flat solid organ that lies below and behind the stomach, secretes pancreatic juice to aid in the digestion of fats, starches, and proteins; the islets of Langerhans, located in the pancreas, produce the insulin that regulates the amount of sugar in the blood. The liver, the largest solid organ in the abdomen, lies immediately beneath the diaphragm in the right upper quadrant; it produces bile, which aids in the digestion of fat and stores sugars until they are needed by the body. The liver also produces components necessary for immune function, blood clotting, and the production of plasma. Toxic substances produced by digestion are rendered harmless in the liver.

The spleen, a solid organ located in the left upper quadrant just below the diaphragm, helps in the production and destruction of red blood cells. If it is injured or surgically removed, its function is assumed by the liver and the bone marrow. The gallbladder, a hollow pouch that is actually part of a bile duct leading from the liver, acts as a reservoir for bile. When food enters the small intestine, contractions are stimulated to empty the gallbladder into the small intestine. The small intestine — made up of the **duodenum, jejunum,** and **ileum** — receives food from the stomach and secretions from the pancreas and liver; digestion of the food occurs in the small intestine. In the large intestine, the water is absorbed from the waste products that remain to form the stool (Figures 2-7, 2-13, and 2-18).

Contraction of the abdominal muscles and the diaphragm puts pressure on the abdominal contents from the sides, front, and above. This pressure helps defecation, urination, and vomiting. Occasionally, the abdominal wall has weaknesses that may "give" under pres-

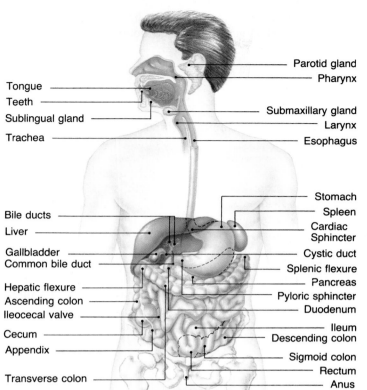

Parotid gland
Pharynx
Tongue
Teeth
Sublingual gland
Submaxillary gland
Larynx
Trachea
Esophagus

Bile ducts
Liver
Stomach
Spleen
Cardiac Sphincter
Gallbladder
Common bile duct
Cystic duct
Splenic flexure
Hepatic flexure
Pancreas
Ascending colon
Pyloric sphincter
Ileocecal valve
Duodenum
Ileum
Cecum
Descending colon
Appendix
Sigmoid colon
Rectum
Transverse colon
Anus

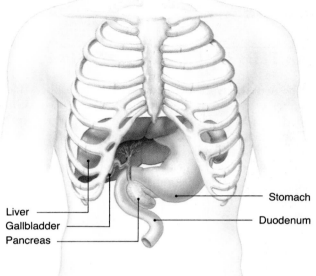

LIVER, STOMACH, AND PANCREAS

Stomach
Liver
Duodenum
Gallbladder
Pancreas

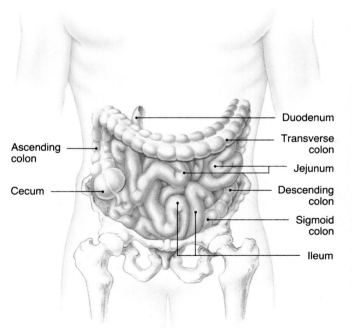

LARGE INTESTINE

SMALL INTESTINE

Esophagus

Duodenum
Diaphragm
Hepatic flexure
Stomach
Splenic flexure
Ascending colon
Transverse colon
Ileocecal valve
Descending colon
Cecum
Appendix
Sigmoid colon
Rectum
Anus

Ascending colon
Duodenum
Transverse colon
Jejunum
Cecum
Descending colon
Sigmoid colon
Ileum

FIGURE 2-18 The digestive system.

sure. These weaknesses are at points of some anatomical peculiarity, such as where two bundles of muscles cross at an angle to each other. Under sufficient pressure, the abdominal contents may bulge into or through the muscle wall but not through the skin. This is a **rupture (hernia).** Most hernias occur in the **groin (inguinal hernias).** A rupture at the navel **(umbilicus)** is called an **umbilical hernia.** Hernias also may occur in many other places, both **superficially** and deep in the abdominal cavity.

☐ THE URINARY SYSTEM

The **urinary system** (Figure 2-19), which filters and excretes wastes from the blood, consists of two **kidneys,** two **ureters,** one **urinary bladder,** and one **urethra.** The urinary system helps the body to maintain its delicate balance of water and various chemicals in the proportions needed for health and survival. During the process of urine formation, wastes are removed from circulating blood for elimination, and useful products are returned to the blood.

The kidneys are continually supplied with large quantities of blood and, when injured, bleed profusely and may leak urine into the abdominal cavity.

☐ THE ENDOCRINE SYSTEM

Endocrine (or **ductless**) **glands** (Figure 2-18—21) are the body's regulators. Secretions **(hormones)** of the glands are carried by the bloodstream to all parts of the body, affecting physical strength, mental ability, build, stature, reproduction, hair growth, voice pitch, and behavior. How people think, act, and feel depends largely on these minute secretions.

Endocrine glands, having no ducts, discharge their secretions directly into the bloodstream. Each gland produces one or more hormones, which are chemical substances that have a specific effect on the activity of certain organs. Good health depends on a well-balanced output of hormones. Endocrine imbalance yields profound changes in growth and serious changes in mental, emotional, physical, and sexual behavior.

FIGURE 2-19 The urinary system.
ORGANS OF THE URINARY SYSTEM

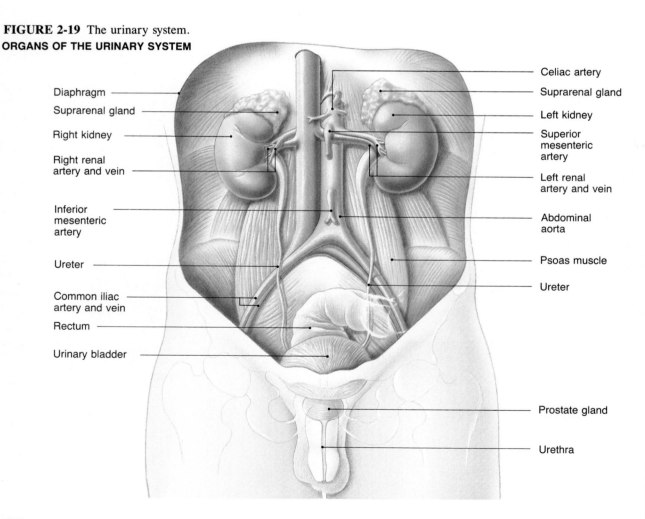

Diaphragm
Suprarenal gland
Right kidney
Right renal artery and vein
Inferior mesenteric artery
Ureter
Common iliac artery and vein
Rectum
Urinary bladder

Celiac artery
Suprarenal gland
Left kidney
Superior mesenteric artery
Left renal artery and vein
Abdominal aorta
Psoas muscle
Ureter
Prostate gland
Urethra

Some endocrine glands and their functions are as follows:

- The **thyroid gland** in the neck produces **thyroxine,** a hormone which regulates metabolism, growth and development, and activity of the nervous system.
- The **parathyroid glands,** back of the thyroid, produce **parahormone,** necessary for the metabolism of calcium and phosphorous in bones.
- The **adrenal glands** atop the kidneys produce hormones such as adrenalin that postpone muscular fatigue, increase the storing of **glycogen** (a sugar), control kidney function, and regulate the metabolism of salt and water.
- The **gonads (ovaries** and **testes)** produce the hormones governing reproduction and sex characteristics.
- The **islets of Langerhans** in the pancreas make **insulin** for sugar metabolism.
- The **pituitary gland** at the base of the brain behind the nose is the "master gland" because its various hormones regulate growth, the thyroid and parathyroid glands, pancreas, gonads, metabolism of fatty acids and some basic proteins, blood sugar reactions, and urinary excretion.

□ THE REPRODUCTIVE SYSTEM

The **reproductive systems** (Figure 2-20) in the male and female consist of complementary organs whose function is to accomplish reproduction and produce a new human being. The male, who provides the male germ cell (the **sperm),** and the female, who provides the female germ cell (the **ovum),** contribute the **genes** that determine the hereditary characteristics of the baby. Combination of a single sperm with a single ovum forms a fertilized ovum that can grow into an **embryo,** then into a **fetus,** and finally into a newborn baby.

The reproductive system of the male includes the two testes (singular, testis), a duct system, accessory glands, and the **penis.**

The female reproductive system consists of two **ovaries,** two uterine **(fallopian) tubes,** the **uterus,** the **vagina,** and the external **genitals.**

□ THE NERVOUS SYSTEM

The **nervous system** (Figure 2-21) has two major functions — communication and control. It enables the individual to be aware of and to react to his envioronment. It coordinates the responses of the body to **stimuli** and keeps body systems working together. (Stimuli are changes in environment that require the body to adjust.)

The nervous system consists of nerve centers and of nerves that branch off from the centers and lead to tissues and organs. Most nerve centers are in the brain and spinal cord. Nerves carry impulses from tissues and organs to nerve centers, and from these centers to tissues and organs. The **neurons** that carry impulses from the skin and other sensory organs to the central nervous system are **sensory neurons.** They make the body aware of its environment. The neurons that carry impulses from the central nervous system to muscles and

FIGURE 2-20 The reproductive system.

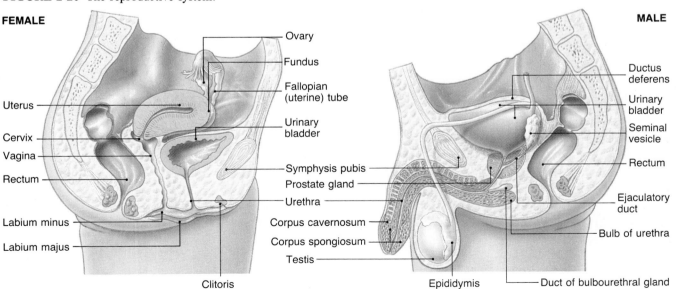

FEMALE

Uterus
Cervix
Vagina
Rectum
Labium minus
Labium majus

Clitoris

Ovary
Fundus
Fallopian (uterine) tube
Urinary bladder
Symphysis pubis
Prostate gland
Urethra
Corpus cavernosum
Corpus spongiosum
Testis

MALE

Ductus deferens
Urinary bladder
Seminal vesicle
Rectum
Ejaculatory duct
Bulb of urethra
Duct of bulbourethral gland

Epididymis

Labium minus (singular), Labia minora (plural)
Labium majus (singular), Labia majora (plural)

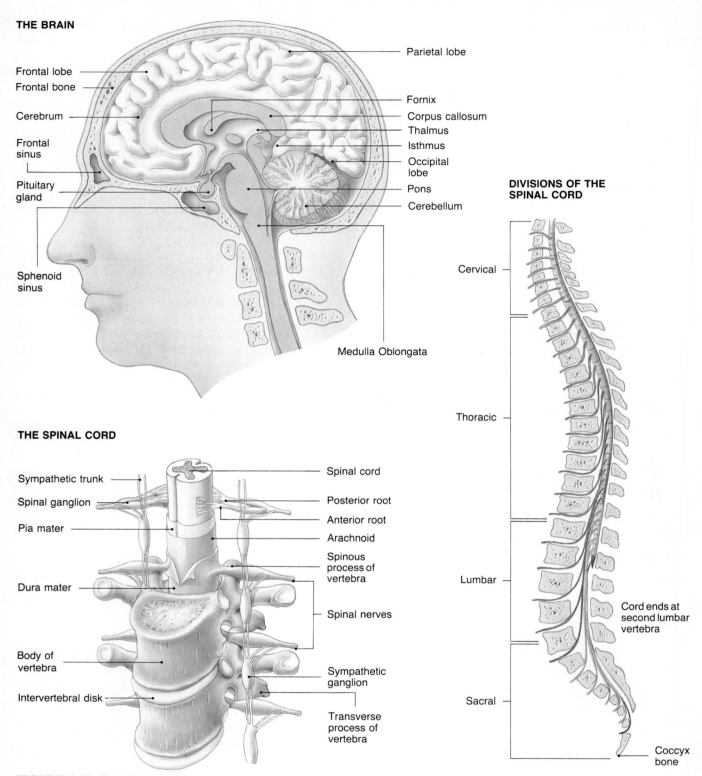

THE BRAIN

Frontal lobe
Frontal bone
Cerebrum
Frontal sinus
Pituitary gland
Sphenoid sinus

Parietal lobe
Fornix
Corpus callosum
Thalmus
Isthmus
Occipital lobe
Pons
Cerebellum
Medulla Oblongata

DIVISIONS OF THE SPINAL CORD

Cervical
Thoracic
Lumbar
Sacral
Cord ends at second lumbar vertebra
Coccyx bone

THE SPINAL CORD

Sympathetic trunk
Spinal ganglion
Pia mater
Dura mater
Body of vertebra
Intervertebral disk

Spinal cord
Posterior root
Anterior root
Arachnoid
Spinous process of vertebra
Spinal nerves
Sympathetic ganglion
Transverse process of vertebra

FIGURE 2-21 The nervous system.

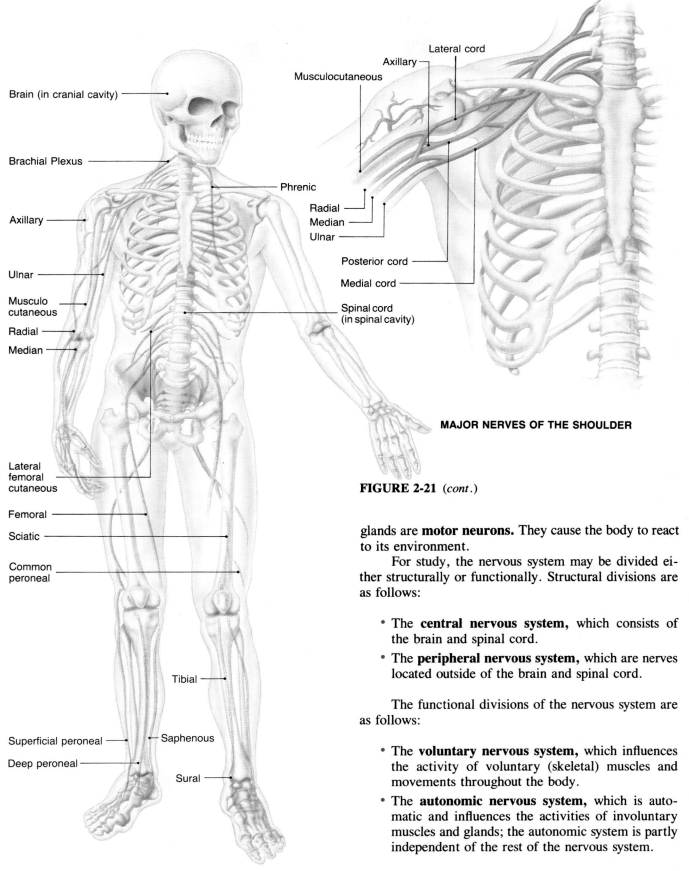

Brain (in cranial cavity)

Brachial Plexus

Axillary

Ulnar

Musculo cutaneous

Radial

Median

Lateral femoral cutaneous

Femoral

Sciatic

Common peroneal

Tibial

Superficial peroneal

Deep peroneal

Saphenous

Sural

Phrenic

Spinal cord (in spinal cavity)

Lateral cord

Axillary

Musculocutaneous

Radial

Median

Ulnar

Posterior cord

Medial cord

MAJOR NERVES OF THE SHOULDER

FIGURE 2-21 (*cont.*)

glands are **motor neurons.** They cause the body to react to its environment.

For study, the nervous system may be divided either structurally or functionally. Structural divisions are as follows:

- The **central nervous system,** which consists of the brain and spinal cord.
- The **peripheral nervous system,** which are nerves located outside of the brain and spinal cord.

The functional divisions of the nervous system are as follows:

- The **voluntary nervous system,** which influences the activity of voluntary (skeletal) muscles and movements throughout the body.
- The **autonomic nervous system,** which is automatic and influences the activities of involuntary muscles and glands; the autonomic system is partly independent of the rest of the nervous system.

The Central Nervous System

The central nervous system (CNS) consists of the brain and spinal cord. These are delicate structures that are protected by two coverings — bones and special membranes. The brain is encased by the skull; the spinal cord by the vertebrae. The three layers of protective membranes enclosing both brain and spinal cord are the **meninges.** The outer layer of strong, fibrous tissue is called the **dura mater.** The middle layer of delicate, cobwebby tissue is the **arachnoid.** The innermost layer, adherent to the outer surface of the brain and spinal cord, is the **pia mater.** Between the dura mater and arachnoid is the **subdural space,** and between the arachnoid and pia mater is the **subarachnoid space.**

In addition to protective bones and membranes, nature provides a cushion of fluid around and within the subarachnoid space, in the space within the brain called the ventricles, and in the central canal of the spinal cord. **Cerebrospinal fluid** filters out from networks of capillaries in the ventricles. It is formed and circulated constantly, and part of it is perpetually reabsorbed into the **venous blood** of the brain. Cerebrospinal fluid may drain from the nose and/or ears as a result of skull fracture or possible laceration of the dura (the outermost covering of the brain).

The Brain

The brain (Figure 2-21), which is the headquarters of the human nervous system, is probably the most highly specialized organ in the body. It weighs about three pounds in the average adult, is richly supplied with blood vessels, and requires considerable oxygen to perform effectively.

The brain has three main subdivisions: the **cerebrum** (large brain), which occupies nearly all of the cranial cavity; the **cerebellum** (small brain); and the **medulla oblongata** (brainstem). The cerebrum is divided into two hemispheres by a deep cleft. The outer surface of the cerebrum, about one-eighth inch thick, is composed mainly of cell bodies of nerve cells, called **gray matter** or the **cerebral cortex.** The inner mass of cerebral tissue, or **white matter,** has interconnecting nerve fibers intermixed with small sections of "gray matter" that form special **ganglia,** or control centers of nerve cells. These ganglia integrate and moderate the activities of nerve cells in the cortex.

Certain sections of the cerebrum control specific body functions, such as sensation, thought, and associative memory, which allow us to store, recall, and make use of past experiences. Also, the cerebrum initiates and manages motions that are said to be "under the control of the will."

The sight center of the brain is located in the back part called the **occipital lobe.** The **temporal lobe** at the side of the head deals with smell and hearing. The sensory and motor centers are separated by a **transverse** fissure at the middle of the top of the brain. Centers of touch, taste, smell, and speech, among others, have been recognized. An injury to any one center interferes with the specific function that it controls.

The cerebellum is located at the back of the cranium and below the cerebrum. Its main function is to coordinate muscular activity. Also it maintains balance in association with impulses from the eyes and the semicircular canals of the inner ears. Although the cerebellum cannot initiate a muscular contraction, it can hold muscles in a state of partial contraction, which keeps a person from collapsing.

A smaller subdivision of the brain, the **pons,** acts as a bridge that connects the cerebrum, cerebellum, and the medulla oblongata (brainstem). The medulla oblongata protrudes from the skull slightly where it joins the spinal cord. It controls the activity of the internal organs, such as the rate of respiration, heart action, muscular action of the walls of the digestive organs, and glandular secretions.

The Spinal Cord

The spinal cord (Figure 2-21), protected by meninges and vertebrae, is about eighteen inches in length. The cord is continuous with the medulla of the brain and terminates at a level between the first and second lumbar vertebrae.

The spinal cord has two major functions — **conduction** and connection. Many nerves enter and leave the spinal cord at different levels. These nerves all connect with nerve centers located within the spinal cord or the brain. Nerve centers within the cord form the gray matter of the cord's inner core. Surrounding the gray matter are columns of nerve fibers, forming the white matter.

The nerve fiber columns in the spinal cord are called **tracts;** these tracts connect the different levels of the nervous system. Ascending tracts, which transmit upward, are all sensory nerve fibers. Descending tracts, which transmit impulses downward, are all motor nerve fibers, controlling both voluntary and involuntary muscles. When the spinal cord is damaged, the extent of disability depends upon which nerve centers and tracts are injured.

The Peripheral Nervous System

The peripheral nervous system is composed of the nerves located outside the brain and spinal cord. **Cranial nerves** and their branches stem from the brain; **spinal nerves** and their branches stem from the spinal cord.

The twelve pair of cranial nerves arise from the undersurface of the brain and pass through openings in the skull to their destinations. The nerves are numbered and have names that describe their distribution or function. For example, the **vagus nerve** (a cranial nerve) is an important nerve in the autonomic nervous system, with both sensory and motor fibers distributed to organs in the thorax and abdomen.

The thirty-one pairs of spinal nerves arise from the spinal cord and pass through lateral openings between the vertebrae. Spinal nerves are numbered according to the level of the spinal column at which they emerge.

The Autonomic Nervous System

The autonomic nervous system (Figure 2-22) is an auxiliary network of nerve tissue that regulates unconscious, involuntary body functions that must continue day and night, regardless of our desires. It excites into action the smooth muscle of the walls of blood vessels, the gastrointestinal tract, and the lungs and heart, and it stimulates internal secretions. The system governs automatic functions to which we normally pay no attention — including vital functions like breathing and the heartbeat.

The autonomic nerves belong to a group that is not directly under control of the brain but that usually works in harmony with nerves that the brain controls.

The autonomic system is divided into the **sympathetic nervous system** and the **parasympathetic nervous system.** Both systems act in delicate balance.

Sympathetic Nervous System

The sympathetic nervous system helps to regulate heart action, arterial blood supply, secretions of ductless glands, smooth muscle action in the stomach and intestines, plus action of other internal organs. An important function of the system is to increase body activity to enable it to meet danger. When challenged to meet stress, body processes are stepped up by the discharge of stimulating secretions at nerve junctions. These secretions, plus **adrenalin,** released into the bloodstream, produce faster muscular action than could be obtained by hormonal releases from various glands. Heart and lung action increases, extra glucose is released from the liver for energy, and the body is prepared for "fight or flight."

Parasympathetic Nervous System

Ganglia of the parasympathetic nervous system are in the midportion of the brain, the medulla oblongata, and the sacral region of the spinal cord. This system opposes the sympathetic system. It prevents body processes from increasing to extremes. Secretions are discharged to slow the heartbeat, decrease lung action, and return body processes to normal after the threat of danger has been met.

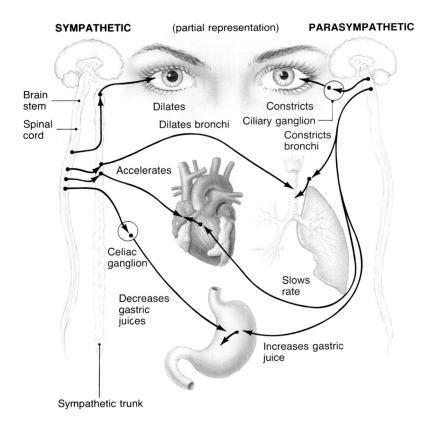

SYMPATHETIC   (partial representation)   **PARASYMPATHETIC**

Brain stem

Spinal cord

Dilates

Dilates bronchi

Constricts

Ciliary ganglion

Constricts bronchi

Accelerates

Celiac ganglion

Decreases gastric juices

Slows rate

Increases gastric juice

Sympathetic trunk

FIGURE 2-22 The autonomic nervous system.

One way to describe the nervous system is by function. There are two divisions: the voluntary (cerebrospinal) system, which for the most part sets up conscious, deliberate bodily actions under the control of the will — plus reflex actions which may or may not be conscious; and the involuntary (autonomic) system which is automatic and partly independent of the rest of the nervous system. The autonomic nervous system is subdivided into the sympathetic and the parasympathetic nervous systems.

☐ THE SKIN

The human body, composed of various tissues, organs, and systems, is separated from the outside world by the **skin (integument)** (Figure 2-23). The skin covers the whole body, protecting its deep tissues from injury, drying out, and from invasion by **bacteria** and other foreign bodies. The skin helps to regulate body temperature, aids in the elimination of water and various salts, and acts as the **receptor** organ for touch, pain, heat, and cold.

The four accessory structures of the skin are the nails, hair, sweat glands, and oil **(sebaceous glands).** The nails, the only external skeleton of the human body, are composed of a horny, elastic material that grows from a root and extends beyond the tips of the fingers and toes. Hair fibers are round, oval, or flat, thin or thick, and have a root and a shaft growing from a sac **(follicle).** Each hair is kept soft and pliable by two or more sebaceous glands that secrete varying amounts of a fatty substance **(sebum)** into the follicle near the surface of the skin. Between the hair follicles, coiled sweat glands open onto the surface of the skin.

Sweat or perspiration **glands** occur in nearly all parts of the skin. Sweat contains essentially the same minerals as blood **plasma** and urine but is more diluted.

Normally, only traces of the wastes excreted in urine are in sweat. But when sweating is profuse, or when the kidneys are diseased, the amounts of such wastes excreted in the sweat may be considerable. Several mineral salts are removed from the body in sweat. Chief among these in quantity is **sodium chloride** (common table salt).

The skin is the largest organ in the body. It gives protection against infection and foreign material for all of the other organs in the body.

The skin itself is composed of two separate layers. The **epidermis,** or outermost layer, has four layers of cells. Cells in the first two layers are dying and dead and are sloughed off as new cells replace them. The skin's pigmentation — the **melanin** — is located in the deepest layers of the epidermis.

The **dermis,** or second layer, is also composed of layers but is much thicker than the epidermis. In the thin, upper part of the dermis is the vast network of blood vessels that supply the skin; in the lower layers are the hair follicles, sweat and oil glands, blood vessels, and sensory nerves. Composed of dense connective tissue, the dermis is what gives the skin its elasticity and strength.

Just below the skin is a layer of fatty tissue called the **subcutaneous connective tissue;** it varies in thickness, depending on what part of the body it covers. Subcutaneous tissue of the eyelids, for instance, is ex-

THE SKIN

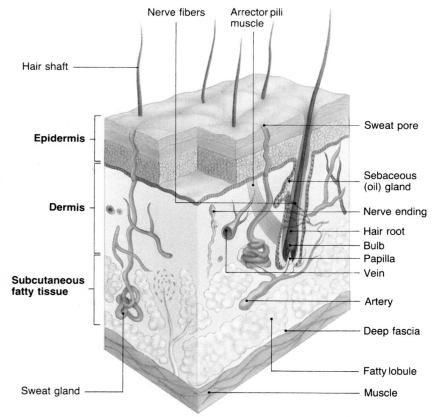

FIGURE 2-23 Anatomy of the skin.

The skin encloses the entire body and provides a watertight protection that is not penetrable by bacteria if it is in tact. It protects the deeper tissues from injury, drying out, and invasion from bacteria and other foreign bodies. The skin helps to regulate body temperature, aids in the elimination of water and various salts, and acts as a receptor organ for touch, pain, heat and cold. The outermost layer, the epidermis, contains cells with pigment granules. The dermis or second layer of skin contains many special structures as shown above.

The subcutaneous tissue is a layer of fatty tissue that is beneath the skin and serves as a body insulator.

tremely thin, while it is thick over the abdomen and **buttocks.** While the subcutaneous layer is not actually part of the skin, it can be involved in full-thickness (third-degree) burns and other soft tissue injuries.

□ THE EYE

The eye (Figure 2-24) is a sphere approximately one inch in diameter formed by a tough outer coat called the **sclera** and the clear front portion known as the **cornea.** Six muscles are attached to the sclera, and they work in various combinations to move the eye.

The cornea is the window through which light enters the eye. There are no blood vessels in the normal cornea, and it is extremely sensitive and especially susceptible to injury or infection. If **scarring** occurs from injury, the cornea loses its transparency at the site of the scar, which may markedly impair vision. The cornea has an extremely high concentration of nerve fibers which make it very sensitive. A superficial scratch, **abrasion,** or the smallest foreign object can cause extreme pain with reflex tearing and redness **(inflammation)** of the eye.

The back surface of the eyelids and the exposed portion of the white part of the eye (sclera) are lined with a paper-thin covering called the **conjunctiva;** it does not cover the cornea. The conjunctiva may become infected and produce a red eye with a variable amount of **pus, mucus,** or watery discharge. This infection is called **conjunctivitis.**

The internal portions of the eye are the **anterior chamber, iris, lens, vitreous body,** and **retina.** The anterior chamber, a space filled with watery fluid, called **aqueous humor,** lies between the cornea and the colored portion of the eye (iris). The iris is a pigmented muscular structure that opens and closes the pupil to allow more or less light to enter the eye, depending on the level of illumination. This works much the same as the iris diaphragm on a camera, which controls the amount of light that enters the camera.

Just behind the iris is a structure known as the lens, which can change shape to focus light rays on the back of the eye. When the lens becomes cloudy, it is called a **cataract.** In middle age the lens usually becomes somewhat less flexible, making it necessary to get reading glasses or bifocals. Behind the lens is the vitreous body, a cavity filled with a clear jelly known as the **vitreous humor.**

THE EYE

FIGURE 2-24 Anatomy of the human eye.

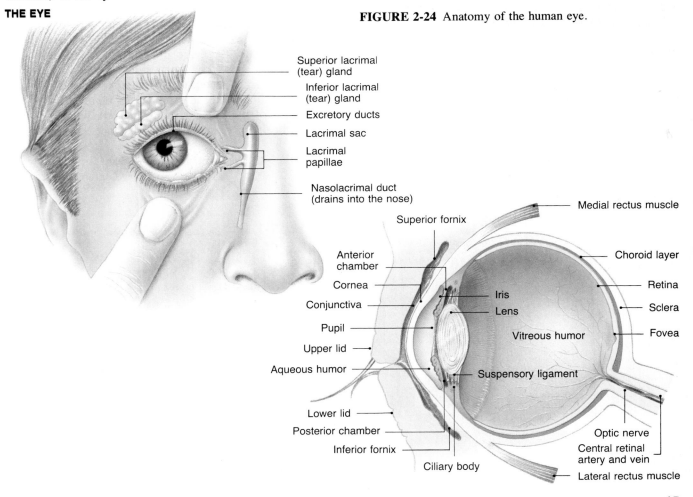

Superior lacrimal (tear) gland
Inferior lacrimal (tear) gland
Excretory ducts
Lacrimal sac
Lacrimal papillae
Nasolacrimal duct (drains into the nose)

Superior fornix
Anterior chamber
Cornea
Conjunctiva
Pupil
Upper lid
Aqueous humor
Lower lid
Posterior chamber
Inferior fornix
Ciliary body
Iris
Lens
Suspensory ligament
Vitreous humor
Medial rectus muscle
Choroid layer
Retina
Sclera
Fovea
Optic nerve
Central retinal artery and vein
Lateral rectus muscle

The innermost layer of the eye is the retina, with specialized nerve cells that are sensitive to light and color. The retina acts much the same as the film in a camera, except that the retina receives the light rays and converts them into nerve impulses that are transmitted to the brain by the **optic nerve.** In the brain, the nerve impulses are interpreted as sight.

A **lacrimal gland** (tear gland), located under the outer part of the upper lid, is constantly producing tears to keep the eye moist and lubricated so that the eyeball can glide smoothly under the eyelid. When the eye is irritated, tear production is increased to help wash away the irritant.

The eye is protected and cleansed by the **eyelids.** They spread the tears over the front of the eye and tend to wipe away dust and other foreign particles. Along the edges of the eyelids are openings of many small oil glands which help prevent the tears from evaporating too rapidly. The lashes and eyebrows help to prevent foreign material from entering the eye.

□ THE EAR

The ear (Figure 2-25) is concerned with the functions of hearing and **equilibrium.** There are three divisions of the ear: the **outer ear, middle ear,** and **inner ear.**

The outer ear is comprised of the **auricle (pinna),** a skin-covered, cartilaginous framework that projects from the head, and the **external auditory canal.** This canal, lined with hairs and glands that secrete **earwax (cerumen),** is S-shaped, about one inch long, and extends to the middle ear.

The **eardrum (tympanic membrane** or tympa-

num) separates the external auditory canal from the middle ear. In the middle ear, three tiny movable bones (the **ossicles)** modify and conduct sound vibrations from the eardrum to the inner ear.

The eardrum and the ossicles are so delicate that violent vibrations of the air, like those caused by the explosion of a bomb or the firing of a heavy gun, may injure them. The three ossicles of each ear are called the **malleus, incus,** and **stapes,** and in the order named, resemble a minature hammer, anvil, and stirrup.

Air is let into or out of the middle ear through the **eustachian tube** (internal auditory canal), which leads to the upper part of the throat. The eustachian tube allows air pressure in the middle ear to equal that of air entering the external ear canal. A nose or throat infection can spread to the middle ear by way of the eustachian tube. Blowing the nose may force infected material into the middle ear. An infection of the middle ear may **abscess** (form pus) resulting in a discharge from the ear. Sometimes infection may extend from the middle ear to the **mastoid cells** in the temporal bone and cause **mastoiditis.** When this happens, a brain abscess or permanent deafness may result.

Vibrations of the eardrum caused by sound waves are carried by the ossicles to the inner ear, which is a series of fluid-filled chambers hollowed out of bone. The fluids in the inner ear then vibrate, stimulating various nerve endings which send impulses to the auditory center in the brain; these are interpreted as sound. When the head and body change positions, the fluid moves; the inner ear has receptors that react to the motion and help the brain make adjustments to maintain balance. Infections of the inner ear can interfere with these receptors, causing dizziness and imbalance.

FIGURE 2-25 Anatomy of the human ear.

THE EAR

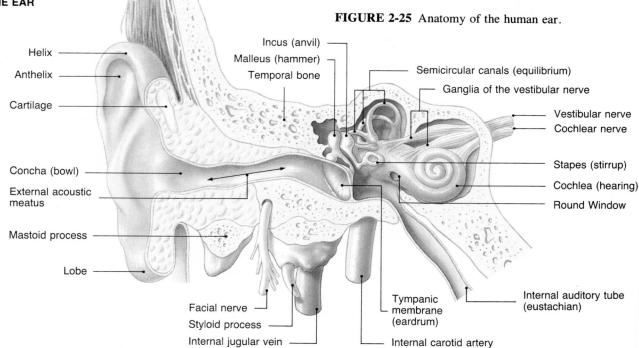

Helix
Anthelix
Cartilage
Concha (bowl)
External acoustic meatus
Mastoid process
Lobe
Facial nerve
Styloid process
Internal jugular vein

Incus (anvil)
Malleus (hammer)
Temporal bone
Semicircular canals (equilibrium)
Ganglia of the vestibular nerve
Vestibular nerve
Cochlear nerve
Stapes (stirrup)
Cochlea (hearing)
Round Window
Internal auditory tube (eustachian)
Tympanic membrane (eardrum)
Internal carotid artery

chapter 3

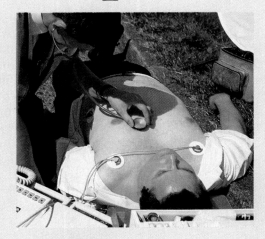

Patient Assessment

✱ OBJECTIVES

- ■ Discuss the importance of learning standard routines and standard medical terminology.
- ■ List the ten-step sequence of patient assessment.
- ■ Demonstrate how to establish rapport with the patient and how to control the scene.
- ■ Describe how to determine the mechanism of injury and make possible predictions of injury as a result.
- ■ Describe how to conduct a primary survey, doing the ABCDE evaluation for life-threatening problems, identifying the chief complaint, taking the vital signs, spotting medical information devices, conducting a neuro examination, and taking a history.
- ■ List the sequence of and practically apply the secondary survey.
- ■ Discuss psychological and convenience factors in transporting a patient.
- ■ Describe the special nature and care demands of trauma patients.

It is recommended that EMTs wear protective gloves whenever there is a possiblity of coming in contact with a patient's blood, body fluids, mucous membranes, traumatic wounds, or sores. See Chapter 31.

The Importance of Learning Standard Routines

As an EMT, you need to be an expert in the medical functions that fall within your responsibility: patient assessment and history taking, primary care, and transport. To administer proper field treatment, you must understand how to assess correctly. This chapter will teach you a routine that will cover all of the important points in an order that has been refined by the experience of many EMTs. If you follow this order, you will not overlook important areas and you will be able to establish priorities for treatment.

Having a well-practiced routine will also keep you professional during tense and disorienting situations (multiple, grotesque, or hemorrhaging injuries) when you could become "rattled."

You will also need to learn how to take a history in a certain order, covering the same points, and asking questions that omit no vital points. Patient assessment and history taking have three main purposes:

1. To win the patient's confidence and thereby alleviate some of the anxiety contributing to his or her discomfort.

2. To rapidly identify the patient's problem(s) and establish which one(s) require immediate care in the field.

3. To obtain information about the patient that may not be readily available later in the hospital (e.g., observations about the environment in which the patient was found).

Another reason for learning standard routines and practicing them in the proper sequence until they become habitual is that you will need to communicate information by radio to the hospital or care facility if the situation warrants on-the-scene instructions from a physician. You will also need to transfer information along with the patient when you reach the care facility at the other end. (See Chapter 45 for procedures on dispatch and radio reporting, and Chapter 41 for procedures on transferring the patient.)

The Importance of Learning Medical Terms

There are many technical medical terms in this chapter, all of them defined in the glossary. It is important for you to know them and be able to use them comfortably for two reasons:

1. They save time and are more precise. You can say "upper left quadrant" faster than you can say "over on the left side of the abdomen just below the ribs."

2. They are common language among medical personnel. That is the team that you are on. You can neither report information nor receive instructions accurately unless you can speak the same language.

For example, here are two terms that you will need to know: **signs** and **symptoms**. The terms are often used interchangeably by emergency medical personnel. They should *not* be. A **sign** (Figure 3-1) is something that the EMT observes or sees about a patient, such as a deep arm laceration or a leg deformed by a fracture. A **symptom** (Figure 3-2) is something that the patient feels and

FIGURE 3-1 A patient exhibiting a sign, such as a deformed wrist.

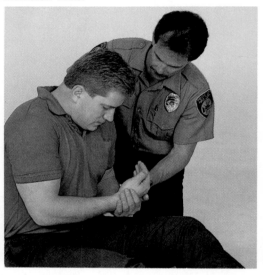

FIGURE 3-2 A patient describing a symptom, such as a stomach pain.

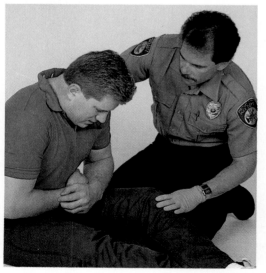

describes to the EMT, such as pain in the abdomen or head, or a feeling of **nausea** or dizziness.

☐ THE TEN-STEP SEQUENCE OF PATIENT ASSESSMENT

This chapter organizes the discussion on patient assessment in the order listed below: Remember — experience and local protocol will tell you when to adopt or change this sequence.

1. Receiving the call from the emergency medical dispatcher.
2. Arriving at the scene.
3. Establishing rapport and controlling the scene.
4. Conducting a primary survey.
5. Identifying the chief complaint.
6. Checking vital signs.
7. Spotting medical information devices.
8. Conducting a neuro exam.
9. Taking a history.
10. Conducting a secondary survey.

☐ 1. RECEIVING THE CALL FROM THE EMERGENCY MEDICAL DISPATCHER

However, not all dispatchers are trained in emergency medical dispatching. You will have to adapt accordingly.) The first assessment of a patient is usually performed by the emergency medical dispatcher (**EMD**) who receives the call (Figure 3-3). The EMD is trained

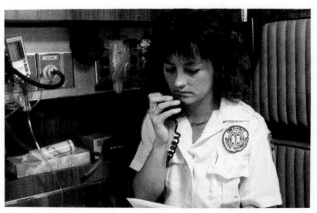

FIGURE 3-3 The EMS dispatcher communicates important information to the EMT in the field.

to gain specific patient information that is passed on to the EMTs who will respond to the call. This information helps the EMTs to prepare both physically and mentally as they respond to the call. The part that the EMD plays on the EMS team is vital and is discussed in detail in Chapter 45.

☐ 2. ARRIVING AT THE SCENE

Gain as much information about the illness or accident as possible before and en route to the scene. As you arrive at the scene, quickly assess the environment and/or the patient(s) before getting out of the ambulance (if possible).

The accident or illness situation may indicate potential problems (e.g., the presence of police cars may be indicative of trauma or violence). Are there any environmental dangers (e.g., dangling power lines, icy roads, fuel spills, etc.)? Are the police present and in control of the traffic? Is the mechanism of injury observable (how the person was injured)? (See Figure 3-4.)

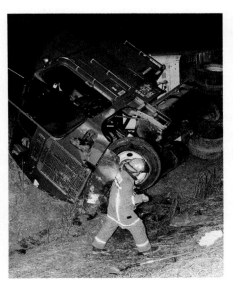

FIGURE 3-4 The initial survey of the scene can provide a great deal of information about the emergency.

Take all appropriate safety precautions to protect yourself, bystanders, and patients at the scene.

Park safely and carefully. As you leave the emergency vehicles (**jump kit** in hand), walk — don't run — to the patient.

☐ 3. ESTABLISHING RAPPORT AND CONTROLLING THE SCENE

When you arrive on a call, you may find the people at the scene hurt, frightened, anxious, and possibly angry and in shock. These are all high-intensity emotions. You will need to establish scene control by utilizing the three "C"s: competence, confidence, and compassion. If you convey these qualities, you will get better cooperation and have to deal with few irrational responses.

These three "C"s will be exhibited through your personal appearance and professional manner. If the patient is alert and no obvious life-threatening conditions are present, it may be appropriate to be briefed by the first responder, whether that person is a police officer, a relative, or someone who has given first aid. This need not take more than a minute. Look directly at the person (take off your sunglasses if you are wearing them) and say, "I'm John Brady and this is my partner, Susan Kelchow. We're certified emergency medical technicians, trained to provide emergency care." Remember that not everyone knows what "EMT" stands for. "Can you tell me what's happened here and what emergency care has been given?" Comment positively on the aid already given (for example, "You've done a good job of immobilizing the head"). However, if the patient is unconscious and life-threatening injuries are observed, go directly to the patient and ask bystanders questions while you give emergency care. (See also Chapter 1, p. 7.)

After the briefing, go directly to the patient. Observe any clues at the scene that may help you in assessment, such as:

- Possible mechanism of injury.
- The patient's position.
- Pills or food in the environment.
- Warmth of the environment.
- Anything else that may help you better assess the patient's condition.

Introduce yourself to the patient in much the same way and ask for the patient's name. With older people, err on the side of formality — "Mrs. Lubeck" or "Mr. Perez" — since they may consider it disrespectful for a stranger to address them by their first names. If you have time and are in doubt, simply ask, "What would you like me to call you?"

Be sure to also say "I'm going to help you. Is that all right?" This is the important matter of receiving consent for treatment discussed in Chapter 1. Continue to address the patient by name throughout the examination.

Don't be surprised if a patient says, "No!" or "I'm okay!" Usually he or she will be responding out of denial because he or she is simply frightened or confused. Keep talking quietly, saying something like, "Looks like an accident happened here. I can see there's something wrong with your shoulder. Does it hurt?" or "Your husband called us because he's worried about you. Would it be all right if we talked about it for a minute or two?"

Maintain eye contact during these important first few seconds (Figure 3-5). Speak calmly and deliberately. People who are under stress or in medical shock process information more slowly. Speak distinctly. Raise your voice only if the person is hard of hearing or disoriented. Otherwise, try to give orders quietly. People follow emotions, and emotions can escalate quickly in tense situations. Smooth movements rather than jerky movements also communicate competence and control.

Place yourself at a comfortable level in relation to the patient. If your eye level is above that of the patient, you are in a dominant position, denoting authority and control. If the eye levels are equal, so is the authority. Since you usually want the patient to remain immobile,

FIGURE 3-5 Establish rapport with the conscious patient by using eye contact, giving a warm smile, and introducing yourself, identifying yourself as an emergency medical technician.

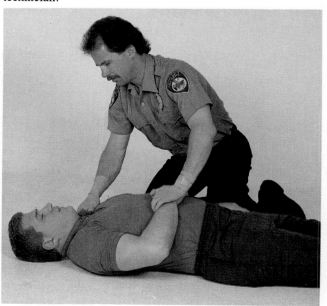

position yourself so that he or she is not tempted to twist his or her neck or tip his or her head.

Be courteous. Patients and bystanders are often emotionally unstable. Explaining what you are doing, giving them choices when possible, and apologizing for necessary discomfort are a way of acknowledging their control in the situation.

Be sensitive to the power of touch. In American culture generally, intimate space starts at about eighteen inches from the body. Eye contact is a way of allowing you into that space so that when you need to touch the person, it is not perceived as encroachment. Touching is an almost instinctive form of comforting another person, and it can be welcome, even from a stranger. Take a hand, pat a shoulder, smile reassuringly, or lay your hand on a forearm. Remember that you have to be comfortable doing it, too, and not just trying it as a gimmick.

As quickly as you can, bring order into the environment. If the television or radio is blaring, ask someone, "Will you please turn off the TV? I'll need to ask some questions." Or do it yourself with the same explanation. If pets, especially dogs, are in the room, ask to have them taken to another room. If children are present with no apparent supervision, ask the police or first responder to take care of them.

If a doctor is present or if fire-rescue personnel or police are also on the scene, an orderly transfer of authority must occur so that you do not become engaged in a dispute and try to care for the patient simultaneously. Sometimes just asking a clear question like, "We're emergency medical technicians. Is there anything we need to know before we give emergency care?" will let rescue and police personnel brief you quickly and allow you to begin your job. If a doctor is present, say, "We're certified EMTs, Doctor. How can we help?" In any situation, the EMT must be the advocate for good patient care and not allow secondary issues to interfere with good and proper patient care. All requests from any person that may impact the care being rendered must be carefully considered and adjusted to provide the best care for the patient.

Patient assessment must be systematic; a hasty, shotgun approach always leads to omissions. Learn to perform a patient assessment and take a history in a specific order so that no important information is missed. Let the urgency of the situation determine the detail of your questions.

The remainder of this chapter will focus on steps 4–10 of the sequence of patient assessment: 4. Conducting a **primary survey,** 5. Identifying the chief complaint, 6. Taking **vital signs,** 7. Spotting medical information devices, 8. Conducting a neuro exam, 9. Taking a history, and 10. Conducting a secondary survey. *In the field, the order will be dictated by circumstances.* You must always deal first with life-threatening emer-

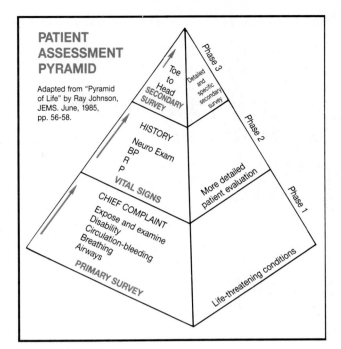

FIGURE 3-6

gencies like obstructed airways, cardiac arrest, and severe bleeding (Figure 3-6).

In the critical patient, life-threatening conditions determine priority. You may not have time to progress beyond the primary survey. In most trauma patients, however, there is time to conduct thorough primary and secondary surveys. Critical patients need rapid evaluation and early transport to a hospital emergency department. Efficient prehospital management is still essential — it just needs to be performed faster, more efficiently, and in some cases during transport to the hospital.

Some of the survey steps can be done simultaneously. You can take a pulse, notice skin color and temperature, and ask, "What happened?" all in the same few seconds. You may want to take the history while taking vital signs, conducting the secondary survey, or giving emergency care. Let judgment and experience dictate the best order of approach.

Be systematic but flexible. Remember — your patient's condition, or a change in that condition, warrants rearranging usual priorities. As you work through the evaluation, remember that your major concerns are:

1. To protect yourself from harm and injury, which includes wearing proper safety apparel such as a face mask, eye goggles, and gloves.

2. To identify and correct any life-threatening problems.

3. To render proper emergency care to correct other patient problems.

4. To stabilize and prepare the patient for transportation, then transport properly while continuing to monitor the patient's vital signs and provide needed emergency care.

☐ 4. CONDUCTING A PRIMARY SURVEY

The major goal of the primary survey is to detect life-threatening problems. With a conscious patient begin with a systemic scan:

- Ask, "What happened?" as you kneel beside the patient. The patient's response will tell you the airway status, the adequacy of **ventilations,** and the level of consciousness. You may also find out the **mechanism of injury** and information about other victims.

- Then ask, "Where do you hurt?" while you check for capillary refill. This question will identify the most likely points of injury.

- Visually scan the patient for general appearance, cyanosis (blueness from lack of oxygen), and sweating (Figure 3-9).

This scan should take less than sixty seconds and then you can begin immediately on the "ABCDE" procedure described below. If the patient is unconscious, begin immediately on the ABCDE procedure while asking bystanders, "Can you tell me what happened?" *Always assume possible spinal damage with an unconscious patient and do nothing that could aggravate a possible injury.*

You now have a very quick idea of your patient's overall **systemic** condition. The rest of the primary survey consists of identifying conditions that may become life-threatening. Remember the five steps of the primary survey alphabetically — A, B, C, D, E:[1]

1. **A**irway and cervical spine.
2. **B**reathing.
3. **C**irculation — bleeding.
4. **D**isability.
5. **E**xposure for examination.

You should be able to conduct this survey in *sixty seconds,* unless there are life-threatening problems that must be treated immediately.

[1] As suggested by *Pre-Hospital Trauma Life Support 1986 — Emergency Training,* p. 27.

Airway and Cervical Spine

- **Airway.** Is it open? Are blood, secretions, etc. making it hard for the patient to breathe? Chapter 4 describes two methods for clearing the airways: (1) the **head tilt/chin lift** (Figure 3-7) and (2) the **modified jaw thrust** (Figure 3-8).

- **Cervical Spine.** The way in which the airway is opened will be determined by the potential for a

FIGURE 3-7 Estabilsh an open airway, then check for adequate breathing by the Look-Listen-Feel technique. Assure an adequate open airway by the head-tilt/chin-lift method.

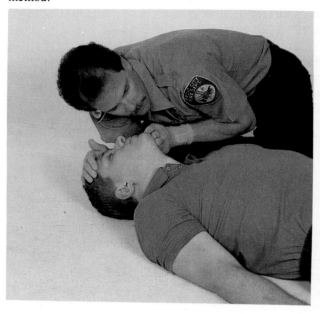

FIGURE 3-8 If a cervical spine injury is suspected, use a modified jaw thrust to open the patient's airway.

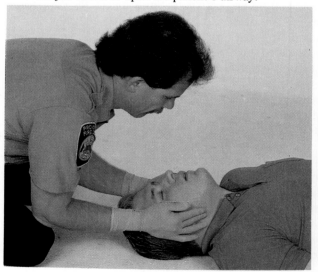

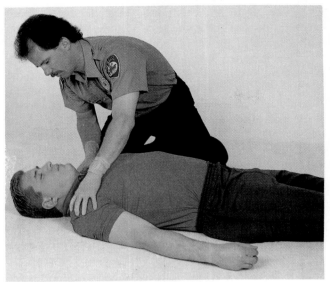

FIGURE 3-9 As you make contact with your patient, perform a systematic body scan.

cervical spine injury. Movement of a fractured spine to establish an airway can cause **neurological** damage. Pay attention to the mechanism of injury, what the patient tells you, and any deformity. If there is a potential cervical spine injury, the modified jaw thrust is used, and the patient's neck should be immobilized with the most efficient method available (Figures 3-10 and 3-11).

Breathing

Is the patient breathing? How well? Is breathing absent or adequate? Check approximate rate, depth, regularity, and ease. *Look* and listen at the chest for open wounds (**sucking chest wounds**), and at the diaphragm for nor-

FIGURE 3-10 Use in-line support to keep the head and neck in alignment as the cervical collar is applied.

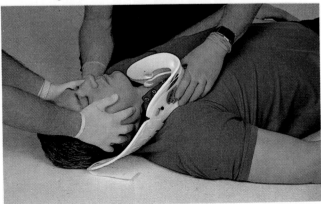

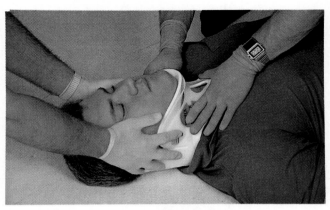

FIGURE 3-11 A cervical collar in place.

mal breathing movements. *Listen* for breathing sounds at the mouth and nose, and *feel* whether air is passing in and out of the nose and/or mouth (Figure 3-12). Note the skin color. Is there any cyanosis? If you suspect any chest injuries that may complicate breathing, give the proper emergency care.

If the patient is not breathing spontaneously, or is breathing too rapidly or too slowly, begin **artificial ventilation** immediately and continue until spontaneous breathing recurs or until you are relieved by trained personnel (see Chapter 4). If the patient is breathing adequately through an open airway, estimate the adequacy of the ventilatory rate and continue the primary survey.

FIGURE 3-12

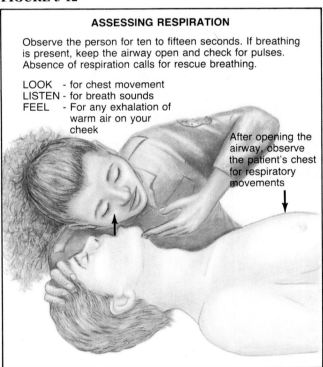

ASSESSING RESPIRATION

Observe the person for ten to fifteen seconds. If breathing is present, keep the airway open and check for pulses. Absence of respiration calls for rescue breathing.

LOOK - for chest movement
LISTEN - for breath sounds
FEEL - For any exhalation of warm air on your cheek

After opening the airway, observe the patient's chest for respiratory movements

Circulation — Bleeding

Now determine if there is heart action and blood circulation by palpating the **radial pulse** at the wrist (Figure 3-13) or, if the patient is unconscious and the radial pulse is absent, palpate the **carotid pulse** (Figure 3-14) in the neck. (The carotid pulse is usually the last pulse to disappear if the patient goes into shock.) Is the pulse absent or adequate? Be sure the patient is lying or sitting

FIGURE 3-13 Palpate the radial pulse at the wrist.

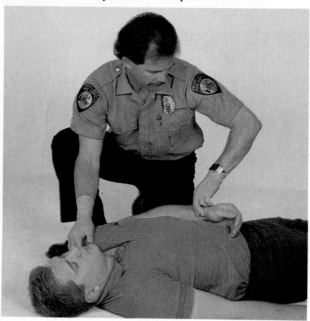

FIGURE 3-14 If the radial pulse is absent, palpate the carotid pulse in the neck.

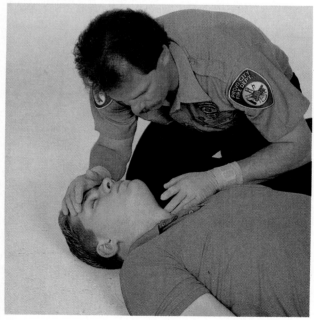

when you try to find this pulse. Never try to feel both carotid pulses at the same time. Excessive pressure on both arteries might cut off circulation to the brain.

Maintain an open airway by keeping one hand on the patient's forehead. With your other hand, place the tips of your index and middle fingers on the patient's Adam's apple, then slide your fingertips into the groove at the side of the patient's neck closest to you for five to ten seconds. Pay attention to the regularity and strength of the pulse (Figure 3-15). If in an emergency situation a **BP** cuff and stethoscope were not available, you could quickly establish an idea of the approximate blood pressure by palpating the different pulses and using the following rule of thumb:

- If the radial pulse is palpable, the blood pressure is at least 80 **systolic.**
- If the **brachial pulse** is palpable, the blood pressure is at least 70 systolic.
- If the **femoral pulse** is palpable, the blood pressure is at least 70 systolic.
- If the **carotid pulse** is palpable, the blood pressure is at least 60 systolic.

If the patient is pulseless, breathless, and not responsive, perform cardiopulmonary resuscitation (see Chapter 6). If there is a pulse, but no breathing, continue artificial ventilation and periodically check the

FIGURE 3-15

EVALUATING PULSES

Evaluate the circulatory status by palpating the carotid pulse with two fingers between the thyroid cartilage, anterior surface of the sternocleidomastoid muscle, and mandible.

If you feel no pulse, remember to quickly try the opposite side.

If pulses are palpable, continue rescue breathing until spontaneous ventilation resumes (or until help arrives with equipment to undertake more definitive airway management). If you cannot detect pulses, begin full CPR.

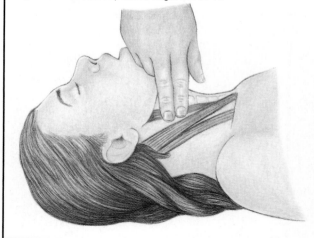

carotid pulse. If both breathing and a pulse are present, continue with the primary survey.

Now check for serious or profuse bleeding. Put on a pair of latex or surgical gloves to protect yourself against any contamination and gently but thoroughly and quickly run your hands over and under the head and neck, upper extremities, chest and abdomen, pelvis and buttocks, and lower extremities. Use extreme care in case a spinal injury may have occurred. Check your hands often for blood. Cut clothing away quickly to see a bleeding site clearly. (Figure 3-16). See Chapter 7 for the necessary emergency care in controlling bleeding.

Bleeding wounds can be misleading in that they sometimes are not as serious as they look; but during the primary survey, deal only with bleeding that requires immediate action, such as hemorrhage that is spurting or flowing freely.

Check the capillary refilling time by pressing down with your thumb and finger on the nail beds (Figure 3-17), on the fleshy part of the palm along the ulnar margin or on the forehead or cheeks. As you release pressure, the blanched area should disappear within one to two seconds. If refilling of the capillary bed takes longer, circulation is not adequate. Monitor the heart action closely.

Disability

After the airway, breathing, and circulation have been assessed, note any signs and/or symptoms that make you suspect damage to the central nervous system.

If the brain does not receive enough oxygen or glucose, it will not be able to control thought, speech, and skills. Changes in mental states may reveal a potential medical problem.

Assess the patient's level of consciousness (LOC) and reposition the patient if necessary. (See "Conduct-

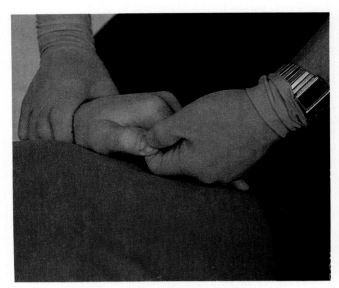

FIGURE 3-17 Assess the circulation by observing the capillary refill.

ing a Neuro Exam" later in this chapter for a more detailed discussion.)

1. Check for responsiveness (LOC). A conscious patient indicates breathing and circulation. Breathing may not be adequate and you may have to clear the airway, but the patient is breathing. Keep in mind that consciousness may be lost quickly, breathing may change, and circulation may stop. To check for responsiveness, *gently* tap the patient's shoulder and say: "Are you okay?"

2. Reposition the patient if necessary. You will find it difficult to determine if an unconscious patient in the prone position has an open airway and adequate breathing. Even though you have not surveyed the patient for possible spinal and other serious injuries, you will have to place him in a supine position. If the patient is not breathing, or you cannot tell if he or she is breathing, use a simple **log-roll** maneuver to move the patient from a prone to a supine position. (See Figures 3-18 through 3-22.) Kneel at the patient's side, leaving enough room so that the patient will not roll into your lap. Gently straighten the legs and position the arm that is closest to you above the head. Place one of your hands so that it cradles the head and neck from behind. Place your other hand under the patient's distant shoulder, at the armpit. Move the patient as a unit onto the side and then onto the back. You must move the head, neck, and torso as a unit to reduce the chances of aggravation to spinal injuries.

FIGURE 3-16 Perform a quick body sweep for bleeding and check your hands often for blood.

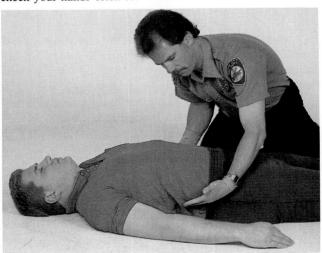

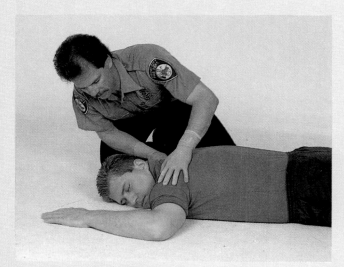

FIGURE 3-18 Reposition the patient *only* if necessary. Use a simple log-roll maneuver.

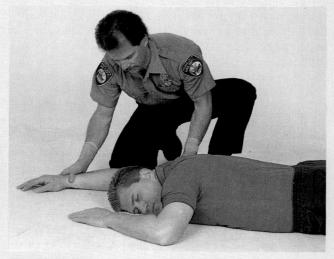

FIGURE 3-19

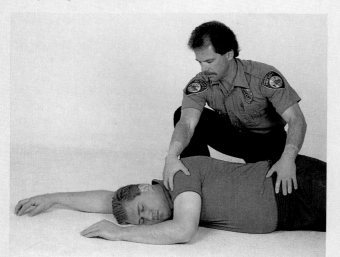

FIGURE 3-20

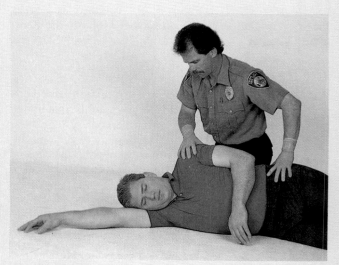

FIGURE 3-21

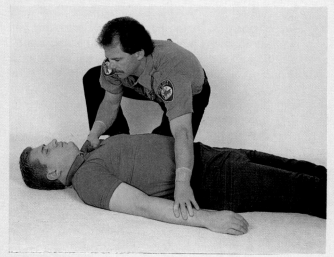

FIGURE 3-22

Note that this log roll is best done by two or more rescuers. One rescuer must be responsible for stabilizing the head and neck. This person directs the actual repositioning of the patient. The one-rescuer log roll is to be used only when basic life support may be needed and adequate personnel are not immediately on hand to assist.

As you assess the patient's LOC and responsiveness, the patient's LOC or "mental state" can be described using the following memory device — *AVPU:*

- ☐ **A** = Alert.
- ☐ **V** = Voice commands bring responses.
- ☐ **P** = Painful stimuli bring responses.
- ☐ **U** = Unresponsive.

Your patient is alert or **oriented** to person, place, and date if he or she can focus on you and answer the following questions. If not, the patient is **disoriented.** Ask:

- What's your name?
- What's happened to you?
- Where were you going, or where are you?
- Can you tell me the date (day of the week, year, etc.)?

Document and record the patient's condition precisely, e.g., "disoriented to time." Do not ask yes-no questions, do not ask questions for which you do not know the answer, and if your patient cannot answer a specific question, get more general.

Your patient is **responsive** if he or she seems to be unconscious but will:

- Open his or her eyes if you speak to the patient or try to answer a question.
- Respond to a light touch on the hand.

If your patient fails to respond and *if you have checked for possible head, back, and neck injuries,* then gently shake the patient by the shoulder while saying his or her name, pinch the earlobe or shoulder skin, or apply gentle pressure to the nailbed of a patient's finger, increasing the pressure as needed to get a response. If the patient makes a sound or movement of protest, he or she is responsive. Or, if you need to determine the level of consciousness earlier in the exam, immobilize the patient's head with one hand while you shake him or her gently, calling his or her name.

A patient with a spinal injury may not feel sensation in the hands or be unable to respond because of pain, a fracture, or another localized injury. The earlobe pinch avoids these problems and is suitable even in the case of very high spinal injuries (Figure 3-23).

Again, be sure to document and report the level of response, e.g., "unconscious but responds to verbal stimuli by opening eyes."

If you even suspect a head or neck injury, tell the patient to lie very still (**ground splint**), immobilize the neck with a rigid **cervical collar** or similar device, be

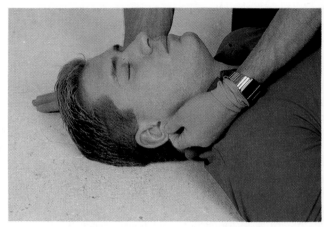

FIGURE 3-23 Check the patient's response by pinching the earlobe.

prepared to administer high-flow oxygen, and transport the patient as soon as possible. Keep the head and neck in alignment at all times. Another EMT can guard the stability of the spine. (See "Neuro Examination" under "Secondary Survey" to learn how to check for neurological damage.) (page 65)

Exposure for Examination

Expose as much of the body as necessary to examine for injuries and bleeding. Completely expose any bleeding sites so that you can examine and give emergency care to the whole wound. Clothing can hide injuries, so do not be afraid to remove clothing as necessary (Figure 3-24). It is a good idea to tell a conscious patient or concerned bystanders (family members, etc.) what you are doing and why you are doing it. Be cognizant of modesty, but do not compromise quality emergency care.

FIGURE 3-24 Completely expose any bleeding sites.

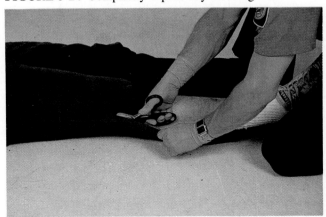

☐ 5. IDENTIFYING THE CHIEF COMPLAINT

Up to this point, you have looked for signs of immediate injury or illness to check the ABCs of emergency care. You were more concerned with the quality of the response when you asked the patient, "Are you okay?" Now it is time to ask specific questions and listen carefully to the patient's symptoms.

The answer you receive from the patient when you ask, "Can you tell me where you are hurt?" is the **chief complaint,** or the reason for the call. In many instances, this will be obvious, such as the patient who lies bleeding in the street after being struck by an automobile. Even in this circumstance, however, it is useful to determine what is bothering the patient most, for the report may lead you to unexpected findings. For example, the patient who is struck by a car may have a dramatically obvious **open fracture** of the leg, yet his chief complaint may be, "I can't breathe," leading you to discover an unsuspected chest injury. If the patient has two or more complaints ("I think I'm going to throw up and my back — something's wrong with my back"), ask: "Which is bothering you the most?" Most chief complaints are characterized by pain, abnormal function, some change from a normal state, or an observation made by the patient.

If the patient seems confused or gives an irrational answer, like "Everything's fine," ask more specific questions: "Are your legs okay?" If he or she gives a too-general answer (for example, "My legs hurt"), ask more specific questions: "Do you feel any numbness in your legs? A burning sensation? Some tingling?" All of these are symptoms of damage to the spinal cord.

If the patient is not conscious, ask a nearby relative or other bystander, "Can you tell me what happened?" The answer will usually be the chief complaint.

Later, when you are filling out the ambulance report form, record the chief complaint and who gave it — the patient or other person.

☐ 6. TAKING THE VITAL SIGNS

After you have investigated the chief complaint, assess the patient's vital signs:

1. Pulse
2. Respirations
3. Blood pressure
4. Skin temperature
5. Skin color.

If you are working as a team, one of you may take the vital signs while the other EMT can take a history of the illness or injury (also referred to as the **subjective interview**).

Knowing how to read and interpret these signs correctly determines how successful your prehospital emergency care will be. Vital signs should be repeated at two-to-five-minute intervals. Changes in vital signs reflect not only alterations in patient condition, but also how effectively you are managing the illness or injury.

You can monitor all of these vital signs, except for blood pressure, with your senses (look, listen, feel, smell). It is best, however, if you routinely carry the proper equipment:

- A **sphygmomanometer** (blood pressure cuff) to take blood pressure.
- A **stethoscope** to take blood pressure and listen to respiration and pulse rates.
- A wristwatch that counts seconds to measure pulses and respiratory rates.
- A penlight to examine pupils, mouth, ears, and nose.
- A pair of heavy-duty bandage scissors for cutting away clothing.
- A pen and a pocket notebook for entering vital signs, other findings, and emergency care given.
- Your own protective equipment, such as latex gloves, goggles, face mask, and mouth shields for artificial respiration.

Pulse

Each time the heart beats, the arteries expand and contract with the blood that rushes into them. The pulse is the pressure wave generated by the heartbeat. It directly reflects the rhythm, rate, and relative strength of the contraction of the heart. It can be felt at any point where an artery crosses over a bone or lies near the skin. When you take a pulse, you should note the following:

- Its rate — slow or fast. This important reading is expressed in beats per minute. Normal resting rates are 60 to 80 beats per minute for an adult and 80 to 150 beats per minute for a child (See Table 3-1).
- Its strength — a normal pulse is full and strong. A **thready pulse** is weak and rapid. A **bounding pulse** is unusually strong.
- Its rhythm — an **irregular pulse** is one that is irregularly spaced. A normal pulse is regular. Irregularity of beats usually signifies cardiac disease.

As an example, you might express the pulse of a

TABLE 3-1
Normal and Abnormal Pulse Rates per Minute, at Rest

AGE OF PATIENT	PULSE RATE	DESCRIPTION
Adult		
	60 to 80	Normal
	100+	Rapid (**tachycardia**)
	Below 60	Slow (**bradycardia**)
Infant		
	120 to 150	Normal
	Above 150	Rapid
	Below 120	Slow
Child (1–5 years)		
	80 to 150	Normal
	Above 150	Rapid
	Below 80	Slow
Child (5–12 years)		
	60 to 120	Normal
	Above 120	Rapid
	Below 60	Slow
Adolescent		
	55 to 105	Normal
	Above 105	Rapid
	Below 55	Slow

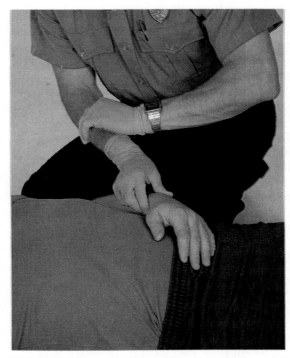

FIGURE 3-25 Palpate the radial pulse for 15 seconds, then multiply by 4.

patient as "72, strong and regular." The rate, strength, and regularity of the pulse are relative indicators of cardiac function. They tell what the heart is doing at any given time. When taken in conjunction with other vital signs and observations of a patient's overall appearance, the pulse can help a good EMT to determine the *effectiveness* of circulation.

EMTs most commonly take the pulse at the wrist where the radial artery crosses the **distal** end of the radius. This is the larger of the two major arteries that supply the hand. The other, not as easy to palpate, is the ulnar artery, also named for the bone associated with it. To take the radial pulse (see Figure 3-25):

- The patient should usually be lying down or sitting.
- Use the tips of two or three fingers, and examine the pulse gently by touch.
- You can count the number of beats for fifteen seconds and multiply by four to obtain the number of beats per minute.
- Always write down the pulse and any other vital signs immediately after taking them. Do not rely on your memory.
- Avoid using your thumb to take pulses, as the thumb has a prominent pulse of its own that may be palpated by mistake.

Other areas where a pulse may be taken include the carotid arteries (see Figure 3-14) in the neck (especially for unconscious patients), the femoral artery in the groin, the dorsalis pedis on top of the foot, and the posterior tibial artery above the ankle. The latter two pulse points may be difficult to obtain and are used primarily to check adequacy of circulation.

Another method is to take the **apical pulse.** Place a stethoscope under the patient's left breast and count each complete "dub-lub" heard as one beat.

A pulse rate should be taken as early as possible. Changes in rate and intensity are important, so also take the pulse frequently. You can gauge what is happening to the patient by the pulse (See Table 3-2). A rapid pulse may indicate shock; a rapid, bounding pulse

TABLE 3-2
Pulse Types and Related Problems

PULSE	POSSIBLE PROBLEM
Rapid, regular, and full	Exertion, fright, fever, high blood pressure, or first stages of blood loss.
Rapid, regular, and thready	Reliable sign of shock, often evident in later stage of blood loss.
Slow	Head injury, barbiturate/narcotic use, some poisons, possible cardiac problems.
No pulse	Cardiac arrest leading to death.

can occur with fright. Absence of a pulse indicates that an artery has been blocked or injured, that the blood pressure is very low, or that the heart has stopped beating. A change in the pulse can mean changes in the heart (due to injury, alarm, or death), in the amount of blood circulating through the vessels, in the blood vessels themselves, or even in the effectiveness of respiration.

The absence of a pulse in a single extremity may indicate obstruction to an artery. Numbness, weakness, and tingling follow the pain. The skin gradually turns mottled, blue, and cold. Always assess pulses in several areas to determine how well the entire circulatory system is functioning as well as appraising circulation to the extremities.

Respirations

The number of times per minute that a person breathes in and out can be a telltale sign of injury or illness. A respiration consists of one inhalation plus one exhalation. The normal number of respiration per minute varies with the sex and age of the patient, on the average twelve to twenty times per minute. Normal respirations are easy and occur without pain or effort.

The depth of a patient's respirations gives a clue as to the *volume* of air that is being exchanged in a given amount of time; say, a minute. You can gauge depth of respiration by placing your hand on the patient's chest and feeling for chest movement. If the patient appears to be an **abdominal breather** (the chest does not seem to move, but the abdomen does), simply feel the abdomen instead. Either way, you should note at least one inch of expansion in a forward direction (Figure 3-26).

How difficult does breathing seems to be for the patient? You can tell this in several ways. Normally, the work required by breathing is very small; we do not

FIGURE 3-26 Gauge the depth of respirations by placing your hand on the chest or abdomen.

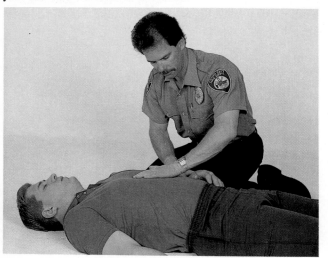

even think about it. But it does require some effort to inhale and almost none to exhale. For this reason, normal inspiration takes slightly longer than normal exhalation. If exhalation takes as long or longer than inhalation, we note this as a *prolonged expiratory phase* of breathing. Prolonged expiration is frequently seen in patients with **chronic, obstructive pulmonary disease (COPD)** such as emphysema. Prolonged inspiration indicates an upper airway obstruction. Cardinal signs of respiratory distress include flaring of the nostrils, contracting of the trachea, and the use of accessory muscles in the neck and abdomen (Figure 3-27).

Although a patient's respiration may be influenced by fear, age, gender, size, and physical conditioning, abnormal ranges that require a physician's care immediately are:

- Adults: Below ten and above twenty-eight breaths per minute.
- Infants: Below thirty-five and above sixty breaths per minute.
- Children below age five: Below twenty-five and above forty-four breaths per minute.
- Children between ages five and twelve: Below twelve and above thirty-six breaths per minute.

Also check for:

1. Rhythm: Is it regular or irregular?
2. Depth: Is it deep or shallow? This is a somewhat subjective judgment, but use your own experience.

As soon as you have determined the pulse rate, start counting respirations, still keeping your hand on the patient's wrist. (Many people's breathing rates change if they know someone is watching them breathe.) Watch the patient's chest or diaphragm for movement, count the number of breaths taken in thirty seconds and multiply by two. Note rhythm, depth, ease, and sounds associated with respiration, and record the assessment ("Respirations 16, regular and normal") with the time of the assessment.

Abnormal respiratory conditions of which you should be aware include:

- **Cheyne-stokes breathing,** common in disturbances of the central nervous system. In this pattern, periods of rapid, irregular breaths — starting shallowly, becoming deeper, then becoming shallower — alternate with periods of **apnea** (cessation of breathing). The cycle repeats every thirty seconds to two minutes, with five- to thirty-second periods of apnea.
- **Bradypnea** is an abnormally slow rate of breathing — less than eight respirations a minute. **Dys-**

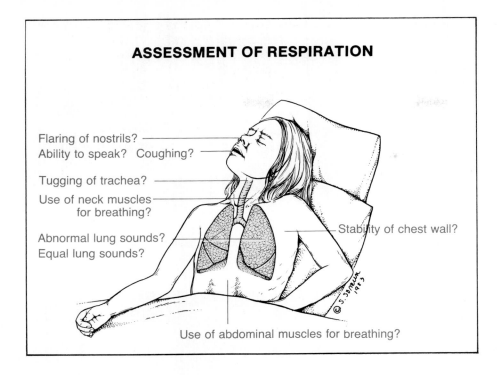

ASSESSMENT OF RESPIRATION

Flaring of nostrils?

Ability to speak? Coughing?

Tugging of trachea?

Use of neck muscles for breathing?

Abnormal lung sounds?

Equal lung sounds?

Stability of chest wall?

Use of abdominal muscles for breathing?

FIGURE 3-27

pnea is a shortness of breath or a difficulty in breathing that may be caused by cardiac problems, strenuous anxiety, or anxiety.

- **Neurogenic hyperventilation** is often a grave sign. It is characterized by very deep, rapid respirations. Abnormally deep respirations are called **hyperpnea;** abnormally rapid respirations, more than twenty-five per minute, are called **tachypnea.**

A too great of volume of air per minute can constitute **hyperventilation.** Other causes of hyperventilation are head trauma and complications of **diabetic coma.** Too little volume per minute can indicate **agonal respirations** or the respirations of death. They are inadequate, whatever their rate, and require vigorous intervention.

Blood Pressure

Blood pressure can fall drastically due to severe bleeding, heart attack, or shock. Low blood pressure means that there is insufficient pressure in the arterial system to keep the organs supplied adequately. The organ may be severely damaged, and death could result. You should promptly identify and treat bleeding that is causing low blood pressure.

High blood pressure can be equally dangerous because it may rupture or damage vessels in the arterial circuit; but the causes are more complex and usually require hospitalization.

The sphygmomanometer is the instrument used to measure blood pressure (Figure 3-28). Blood pressure normally varies with the age, sex, and medical history of an individual. The result of the contraction of the heart which forces blood through the arteries is called **systolic pressure.** The result of relaxation of the heart between contractions is called **diastolic pressure.**

With most diseases or injuries, these two pressures either rise or fall together. However, there are two exceptions. Head injuries sometimes cause a rise in the systolic pressure accompanied by a stable or falling diastolic pressure. In **cardiac tamponade** (the sac

FIGURE 3-28 Equipment for taking a blood pressure — stethoscope and sphygmomanometer.

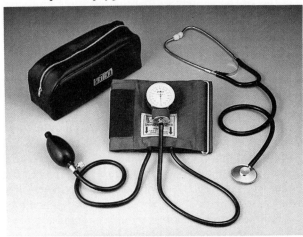

around the heart fills with blood; see p. 317), the diastolic pressure will rise while the systolic pressure falls.

The usual guide for systolic pressure in the male is 100 plus the individual's age, up to 140 to 150 mmHg. Normal diastolic pressure in the male is 65 to 90 mmHg. Both the systolic and diastolic pressures are 8 to 10 mmHg lower in the female than in the male. Blood pressure is reported as $\frac{systolic}{diastolic}$ as in $\frac{120}{80}$ **mmHg (millimeters of mercury).**

Remember that these figures are derived from averages in a large group of healthy adults. Age, diet, physical conditioning, and other factors can produce higher or lower "normal" readings.

Blood pressure is considered "very serious" in the following cases:

1. When an adult's systolic reading is above 180 or below 90 mmHg.
2. When an adult's diastolic reading is above 104 or below 60 mmHg.
3. When a child, age five or younger, has a systolic reading above 120 or below 70 mmHg.
4. When a child, age five or younger, has a diastolic reading above 76 or below 50 mmHg.
5. When a child between age five and twelve has a systolic reading above 150 or below 90.
6. When a child between age five and twelve has a diastolic reading above 86 or below 60.

All EMTs are taught how to take blood pressures, but many do not realize that it is not unusual for a "shocky" or anxious patient's blood pressure to vary from 24 to 34 mmHg (both diastolic and systolic) between the first reading at the accident scene and the reading at the hospital emergency room. The blood pressure may actually change as a result of medication, but the problem may be the sphygmomanometer, the EMT, or both! Blood pressure readings may also fluctuate from the right to the left arm. Record the pressure at the site accurately so that the receiving physician can tell how much it has changed since you first saw the patient.

To take a blood pressure (Figures 3-29–3-31):

1. Choose the proper size of sphygmomanometer cuff. The cuff should completely encircle the patient's arm about one inch above the elbow crease, without overlapping, and its bladder should cover half of the arm circumference. If it covers less, it will not compress the blood vessels properly. If it covers more, it will suppress the pulse too quickly. The cuff thus fits snugly, the lower edge at least an inch above the **antecubital space** (the "hollow" of the front of the elbow), and the bladder centered over the brachial artery.

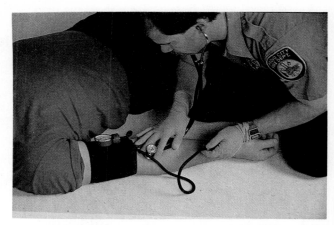

FIGURE 3-29 Proper positioning of the blood pressure cuff and stethoscope.

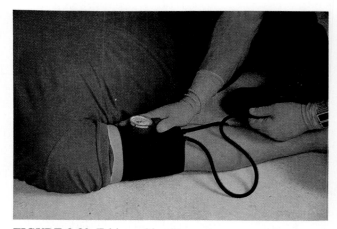

FIGURE 3-30 Taking a blood pressure.

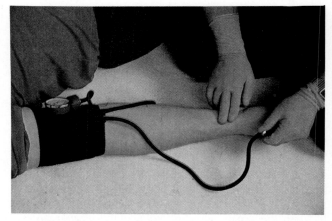

FIGURE 3-31 Palpate the radial pulse until it cannot be felt.

Some cuffs have markers for overlap placement, but they are not always in the correct location. The American Heart Association states that the only accurate method is finding the bladder center. Know your equipment well enough to know whether you can trust its markings, the tubes entering the bladder, or your own ability to find the center. The cuff should not be too tight. You should be able to place one finger easily under its bottom edge.

2. Now inflate the cuff rapidly with the rubber bulb while palpating the radial pulse until it cannot be felt. Make a mental note of the reading (as this may be the only BP recorded — this records as $\frac{120}{P}$;

This is known as palpated blood pressure. Without stopping, continue to inflate the cuff to 30 mm above the level where the pulse was obliterated (cannot be felt).

3. Apply the stethoscope. Place the diaphragm of the stethoscope over the brachial artery just above the hollow of the elbow (artery on the medial anterior surface). The diaphragm may be held with the thumb.

4. Deflate the cuff at approximately 2 mm per second (faster if skill permits), watching the mercury column of needle indicator drop.

5. As soon as you hear two or more consecutive beats (clear tapping sounds of increasing intensity), record the pressure. This is the systolic pressure.

6. Continue releasing air from the bulb. At the point where you hear the last sound, record the diastolic pressure. Continue to deflate slowly for at least 10 mm. Remember that slow pulses require slower-than-normal rates of inflation. With children and some adults, you may hear sounds all the way to zero. In such cases, record the pressure when the sound changes from clear tapping to soft, muffled tapping.

After you have measured the blood pressure, leave the cuff deflated but in place. Take several BP readings during the time of your care and transport. Watch for changes in BP that are diagnostically significant. Carefully record the BP each time you measure it, with the time when it was taken. Remember — during shock, the pulse can change much more rapidly than the BP!

With all the variables that may occur, it is essential that you have the proper equipment and expertise for accurate readings. The standards for blood pressure readings are published by the American Heart Association and should be studied thoroughly.

Recognizing and combatting the more than twenty potential mistakes that can occur in taking blood pressure is also essential. The most critical of these possible errors include:

- Using a too-wide bladder. This error will give you a false-low reading.
- Using a too-wide cuff. If the width of the cuff is more than 20 percent of the circumference of the arm, use a narrower cuff. A cuff should cover one-half to one-third of the upper arm. If the cuff is too wide, you will get a false-low reading. If it is too narrow, you will get a false-high reading.
- Improperly placing the stethoscope ear pieces. If the ear pieces do not bend downward and forward, you will probably record a false-low systolic and a false-high diastolic pressure.
- Inflating the cuff too fast. If you do, you will get a false-low systolic and a false-high diastolic reading.
- Not palpating the systolic pressure at the highest level.
- Not hearing properly due to noise, a head cold, or other distraction. If you cannot hear clearly, you will get a false-low systolic and a false-high diastolic reading.
- Improper conditions. Remember that you must measure blood pressure when the person is seated or lying down. The cuff should be at heart level for best results. If the patient is sitting up, prop his or her arm on a table or support it during the procedure. Use caution when moving a patient or the patient's arm lest you aggravate other injuries.

Hemorrhage

Hemorrhage and its corresponding changes in blood pressure come in four grades:

1. Grade 1, 15 percent blood loss. This corresponds to 1.5 pints for a 150-pound patient. Signs: slight increase in heart rate, dizziness when standing, usually normal blood pressure and capillary refill.

2. Grade 2, 15–30 percent blood loss. This corresponds to 1.5 to 3 pints for a 150-pound patient. Signs: Tachycardia, pallor, delayed capillary refill, thirst, increased respiratory rate, and a narrowed pulse pressure (mathematical difference between the systolic and diastolic blood pressure reading). The systolic blood pressure may be normal or slightly decreased. Blood pressure usually falls if the patient sits or stands up.

3. Grade 3, 30–40 percent blood loss. This corresponds to 3 to 4 pints in a 150-pound patient. Signs: same as above, plus a decreased blood pressure. As long as brain is perfused with blood, the patient will remain responsive.

4. Grade 4, more than 40 percent blood loss. This corresponds to a loss of 4 pints or more in a 150 pound patient. Signs: the patient is unresponsive, pulses are usually not palpable, and the patient seems dead.

Skin Temperature

The most common temperature taken by EMTs in the field is **relative skin temperature,** accomplished by touching the patient's skin with the back of the hand (Figure 3-32). It is useful as an indicator of abnormally low and high temperatures.

Normally, skin temperature rises as blood vessels near the skin **dilate,** and it falls as blood vessels **constrict. Fever** and high environmental temperatures cause vessels to dilate, while shock causes vessels to constrict under most circumstances. Normal skin is fairly dry. Stimulation of the sympathetic nervous system — as in shock — normally results in perspiration, **pallor,** and cool skin. Depression of the sympathetic nervous system — as may occur in cervical, thoracic, or lumbar spine injuries — can cause the skin in the affected areas to be abnormally dry and cool. Placing the back of your hand against the patient's forehead will give you some idea of skin temperature.

Changes in temperature can alert you to certain injuries and illnesses. A patient whose temperature is low may be suffering from shock, **heat exhaustion,** or exposure to cold; a high temperature can result from fever in illness or **heat stroke.**

The body temperature can change over a period of time or be different in various areas of the body. Circulatory problems may result in a cold **appendage,** while an isolated "hot" area may indicate a localized infection and/or inflammation. Be alert to changes and record them along with times at which you notice changes.

FIGURE 3-32 For relative skin temperature, touch the patient's skin with the back of your hand.

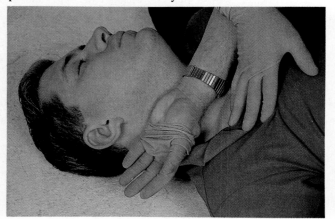

Skin Color

A related sign that can communicate a great deal is skin color. It is a good indicator of heart and lung function and can also alert you to other problems:

- Pallor may be caused by shock, heart attack, fright, anemia, simply fainting, or emotional distress.
- Redness may be caused by high blood pressure, stroke, heart attack, carbon monoxide poisoning, alcohol abuse, sunburn, heat stroke, fever, infectious disease, or blushing.
- Blueness (cyanosis) results from poor oxygen levels in the circulating blood, making the blood very dark. It appears first in the fingertips and around the mouth. It may be caused by suffocation, lack of oxygen, heart attack, or poisoning and is always a serious problem.
- Yellowish color may be a symptom of liver disease.
- Black-and-blue mottling shows a seepage of blood under the surface of the skin, most usually as the result of a blow.

If your patient has dark skin, check for color changes on the lips, nailbeds, palms, ear lobes, whites of the eye, inner surface of the lower eyelid, gums, or tongue.

☐ 7. SPOTTING MEDICAL INFORMATION DEVICES

While taking vital signs, be on the lookout for a **medic alert** tag, necklace, anklet, or bracelet (Figure 3-33). Over a million Americans wear these life-saving infor-

FIGURE 3-33 Medic Alert necklace.

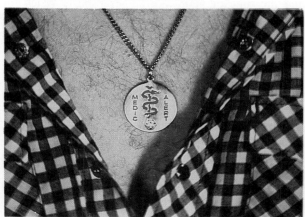

mation devices. This medical identification may give important information about the patient.

The Medic Alert system was directly credited with saving 2,000 lives during a recent twelve-month period. Medic Alert is a nonprofit, charitable, tax-exempt organization that provides a twenty-four-hour emergency information system for the one out of five people who have a hidden medical condition, such as a heart problem, **diabetes, epilepsy,** or allergies to **penicillin** and other medications. In case the patient is unable to speak or communicate due to an accident or sudden illness, the emblem on the tag can alert EMTs to the possible problem.

The **Vial of Life Program** is a similar emergency medical information system being used extensively. The system uses a small prescription-type bottle or vial that contains a medical information form filled out in advance by the patient. This vial is usually kept in the home refrigerator. Stickers near or on the front entrance of the patient's home and on the refrigerator tell EMTs that the vial is present.

□ 8. CONDUCTING A NEURO EXAMINATION

Conduct this examination any time you suspect possible central nervous system injury. Local protocol may place it normally during the primary or secondary exam. This exam checks three areas:

1. Level of consciousness (orientation and responsiveness).
2. Motor functions, such as voluntary movement and response to pain.
3. Sensory functions — what can the patient feel? Can he or she identify the stimulus? How does he or she respond to pain?

Level of Consciousness

See the discussion on p. 52 on level of consciousness. Talk to the patient to determine whether he or she is alert or confused.

- Is the patient oriented to time (time of day, day of week, date), to place, and to person?
- Note the patient's speech. Progressive slurring of words or vagueness in answering questions, especially when the patient formerly spoke clearly and coherently, indicates a decreasing level of consciousness. Garbled words may indicate a **stroke.** (Identify whether a patient may be intoxicated. An alcohol effect may duplicate or cover up signs and symptoms of another medical problem.)

- If the patient cannot speak, try to discover whether he or she can understand by giving a simple command (such as "squeeze my hand").
- Estimate the alertness of young children or infants by observing their interest in their surroundings and their voluntary movements.

Motor and Sensory Functions

- With unconscious or sleeping patients, determine how easily they can be aroused. If they cannot be aroused by verbal stimuli, can they be aroused by a pain stimulus like a pinch?
- If the patient moves in response to a given stimulus, observe the nature of the movement. Is it purposeful — that is, does the patient try to move away from the painful stimulus or try to remove the annoying stimulation?
- In all areas of palpation, ask about pain and feeling. Does the patient move both sides equally well? Do his or her hands grip with equal strength (Figure 3-34)? Can the patient wiggle his or her toes?
- With unconscious patients, stimulate both arms and legs simultaneously to test for equality of responses on both sides. Does the patient show abnormal, jerky movements?
- Is the patient restless, irritable, or combative? Restlessness can indicate general discomfort, a full bladder, a reaction to restraints, etc. However, restlessness is also one of the earliest signs of lack of oxygen in the blood, internal bleeding, or poisoning.
- Discover the level of consciousness as soon as possible, and check it often for changes.

FIGURE 3-34 Test for grip strength (possible nervous system damage) by having the patient squeeze your fingers.

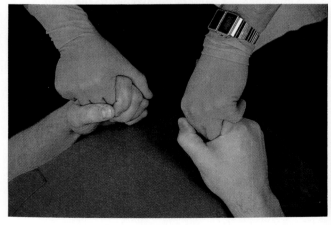

- Describe the patient's status by reaction to special stimuli or responses to specific inquiries. For example, "the patient responds purposefully to deep pain but not to verbal stimuli," or, "the patient knew his name and address but could not remember the date." This type of report provides information that can be rechecked very precisely to determine whether a genuine change has occurred in the patient's status.

Generally, the damage is in direct proportion to the amount of stimuli required to rouse the patient. Damage to one side of the brain stem does not usually produce unconsciousness, but **bilateral** damage may produce deep **coma.**

A great deal of neurological damage is caused by trauma. An understanding of trauma and trauma scores will aid the EMT in assessing neurological damage.

Trauma Assessment

Trauma kills more than 140,000 people per year and kills more Americans between ages one and thirty-four than all disease combined. Trauma is the leading cause of death for people under forty-four. Every six months, accidents kill far more Americans than died in Vietnam. Injuries permanently disable more than 300,000 Americans. The National Safety Council estimates the direct and indirect costs of trauma at a minimum of $75 to $100 billion annually. Trauma victims die from **hypoxemia** (inadequate oxygen), shock, central nervous system damage, and hemorrhage. They drown, suffocate, are burned, or are crushed.

Some services use a simple four-step procedure for determining the trauma patient's status: CUPS.

1. Critical: cardiac arrest, respiratory arrest, or respiratory assistance required.
2. Unstable: patients with severe injuries to upper airway, serious chest trauma, shock from hidden or uncontrollable hemorrhage, rising intracranial pressure, or penetrating wound to the head, neck, chest, abdomen, or pelvis.
3. Potentially unstable: patients with early signs of shock, possible hidden injuries, major isolated injuries.
4. Stable: patient with minor injuries or injuries to limbs; may have sustained neurovascular damage.

Much of the prehospital emergency care in which EMTs are involved is trauma-related. It has been suggested by some that prehospital care is a major area of inadequacy in trauma care. What is the role of the EMT in trauma management?

Cardiologists have set a standard of scene stabilization; surgeons are calling for speedy transport. The key is to combine the best that speed and stabilization can offer. The paramount importance is to get the patient to the hospital with the greatest opportunity for survival. In trauma management, the need is to rapidly assess and move traumatized patients. It may help to use an assessment that can rapidly identify the trauma patient or patients who are candidates for trauma surgery and so need to be transported quickly to the hospital trauma center. In prehospital trauma care the two important assessments are:

1. Evaluate the mechanism of injury as soon as you arrive; this will trigger proper concern.
2. Formulate a **trauma score.** A trauma score is not an end unto itself, but it is helpful in indicating the condition of the trauma victim.

Then put these two assessments together. The trauma score and mechanism of injury seem to be the best and quickest ways to identify patients who are surgical candidates. These patients will need quick but efficient:

- Airway care.
- Cervical spine protection.
- Control of external hemorrhage.
- Transport to the proper medical facility.

A trauma score is a numerical way to identify trauma severity. A good trauma score should be simple to use and should accurately identify patients who must be transported speedily to a trauma facility or other suitable medical facility. An example is the revised trauma score. The Trauma Score (Champion et al.), includes the **Glasgow Coma Scale** (Table 3-3).

Revised Trauma Score

The revised trauma score, endorsed by the American Trauma Society, assigns a number to each finding. The total score, between one and twelve, identified the severity of the trauma. The lower the number, the greater the severity. The trauma score examines:

- The respiratory rate (RR).
- Systolic blood pressure (SBP).
- Glasgow Coma Scale (GCS).

Patients with a GCS less than 13 or SBP less than 90 or RR greater than 29 or less than 10 should be triaged to a trauma center.

TABLE 3-3
Trauma Score

BRIEF NEUROLOGICAL EVALUATION

A — **Alert**
V — Responds to **Vocal** stimuli

P — Responds to **Painful** stimuli
U — **Unresponsive**

REVISED TRAUMA INDEX

TRAUMA SCORE OPERATIONAL DEFINITIONS

Respiratory Rate

Number of respirations in 15 seconds; multiply by 4

Systolic Blood Pressure

Systolic cuff pressure; either arm
— auscultate or palpate
No pulse — no carotid pulse

Best Verbal Response

Arouse patient with voice or painful stimulus

Best Motor Response

Response to command or painful stimulus

Project estimate of survival for each value of the Trauma Score based on results from 1,509 patients with blunt or penetrating injury.[2]

TRAUMA SCORE	PERCENTAGE SURVIVAL
12	99
11	97
10	88
9	77
8	67
7	64
6	63
5	46
4	33
3	33
2	29
1	25
0	4

REVISED TRAUMA SCORE

The Trauma Score is a numerical grading system for estimating the severity of injury.[1] The score is composed of the Glasgow Coma Scale (reduced to approximately one-third total value) and measurements of cardiopulmonary function. Each parameter is given a number (high for normal and low for impaired function) Severity of injury is estimated by summing the numbers. The lowest score is 1, and the highest score is 12.

Respiratory Rate	10-29/min	4
	29/min	3
	6-9/min	2
	1-5/min	1
	None (0)/min	0
Systolic Blood Pressure	>89 mmHg	4
	76 mmHg	3
	50-75 mmHg	2
	1-49 mmHg	1
	No Pulse or 0 SBP (Systolic Blood Pressure)	0

Trauma Scale Total

GLASGOW COMA SCALE

Eye Opening	Spontaneous	4	**Total Glasgow Coma Scale Points**
	To Voice	3	
	To Pain	2	13-15 = 4
	None	1	9-12 = 3
Verbal Response	Oriented	5	6-8 = 2
	Confused	4	4-5 = 1
	Inappropriate Words	3	<3 = 0
	Incomprehensive Words	2	
	None	1	
Motor Response	Obeys Command	6	
	Localized Pain	5	
	Withdraw Pain	4	
	Flexion (pain)	3	
	Extension (pain)	2	
	None	1	

Glasgow Coma Scale Total

Total Trauma Score
Trauma Scale + GCS   1-12

Source: "A Revision of the Trauma Score," *The Journal of Trauma.* 29(5): 1989, pp. 623–29.

[1] Champion, H. R., Sacco, W. J., Carnazzo, A. J., et al. "Trauma Score," *Crit Care Med.* 9(9): 1981, pp. 672–76.

[2] Endorsed by the American Trauma Society.

Guidelines for Reporting a Patient's Condition

When reporting a patient's condition for trauma assessment, remember that it is better to report the patient's actual response than the score itself. In other words, instead of saying, "Eyes, 2," report, "Patient opens eyes in response to pain." Also, for information purposes, the approximate level of injury can be estimated by testing for sensation of touch, starting at the feet and moving upward. As a rough guide, the navel is approximately at the level of the tenth thoracic nerve distribution (T10), the nipple line is around T4 to T5, and the shoulder blades are at about the third cervical nerve distribution (C3). As an example, if sensation is absent all the way up to the ribs, but is present at the nipple line, the injury is likely to be somewhere between the fifth and tenth thoracic vertebrae (T5 to T10).

☐ 9. TAKING A HISTORY

Taking a history begins with scene assessment. If the patient is home, how does it look? Is it clean and well-maintained or disorderly and dirty? Are any medications visible? Do empty glasses or bottles suggest alcohol consumption? Check for bracelets or necklaces, refrigerator stickers, etc., that may describe a **chronic** medical condition.

What is the patient's position? Do the placement of the patient and any objects at the scene give clues about how the injury occurred?

Generally, it is best to talk to the patient, if he or she is able to communicate. If time permits and you need to question others, do so one at a time, or have your partner take a family member into another room for the history while you question the patient.

Depending on the urgency of the situation, either ask yes-or-no questions ("Have you eaten today?" "Does it hurt when you move your arm?") or open-ended questions ("When does the pain come on?" "Tell me about your last meal"). It is preferable to ask open-ended questions (if this is possible) so that you do not suggest answers to the patient. You might also get additional information that you did not think to ask about.

If you are questioning the patient during the exam, ask questions about an area or organ *before* you examine it. If you ask afterwards, the patient will probably assume that you found something wrong.

If the patient is unconscious or experiencing a life-threatening condition, the history, of course, can wait. The most effective way to collect this history is for your partner to fill out the patient information form while you talk to the patient and conduct first the primary, then the secondary, examination.

You probably asked your patient's name within the first minute or so. Also estimate your patient's age.

If the information is required in your areas for reports and transmission to the hospital, ask for it directly. Children expect to be asked their ages. You'll need to ask an adolescent his or her age to determine if he or she is a minor. If an adult is reluctant to disclose his or her age, explain matter-of-factly, "We need to know this for our records."

If your patient is a child or teenager away from the family setting, ask, "How can we contact your parents?" Reassure young patients that someone will stay with them, that you'll find their parents as quickly as possible, and that you'll be helping them all the time.

It is important for you to know about and record any major medical problems and medical procedures that may affect the patient. This information can be obtained by using two memory devices. The first word is "SAMPLE."

S: Symptoms. What is the patient feeling? When and where did the first symptoms occur? What was the patient doing at the time?

A: Allergies. Does the patient have any allergies to drugs, foods, or foreign proteins? Does the patient regularly see a certain doctor?

M: Medications. Does the patient take any medications regularly? If so, what are they? Were they taken today? When? How much? If the patient's medications are available, gather all the containers or ask a family member to do so and transport them with the patient. Such information may be critical to the hospital staff, especially if the patient becomes unconscious. Remember to say "medication," not "drugs," since the second word may connote illegal activity to your patient. If you have the feeling that your patient or a bystander you are interviewing is holding back information because the patient was involved in drug abuse, say, "I'm an EMT, not a police officer. I need all the information you can give me so that I can give you proper care. Let's work on helping you right now."

P: Previous Illnesses. Does the patient have any underlying medical problems (e.g., **cardiac, renal,** epilepsy, respiratory, etc.)? Is he or she a **diabetic?** Is the patient under a doctor's care for any serious condition?

L: Last Meal. What did the patient eat? When?

E: Events Prior to Emergency. What occurred before the patient became ill or had the accident? Where there any unusual circumstances? Did the patient have any peculiar feelings or experiences?

These questions will help you to obtain pertinent information about the patient's past medical history *that relate to the current problem.* You need to know which conditions are directly related to the present problem or could adversely affect the outcome of the present problem. When caring for a burn victim, for example, it is important to know whether there are underlying cardiac or respiratory problems that might impair breathing. It is not relevant to learn whether the patient went under a hernia operation five years earlier or had **measles** as a child. It is relevant, however, to find out if the patient had a similar episode, and if so, when. What was the cause? Was the patient hospitalized?

One of the common complaints of an emergency-care patient is pain. Knowing the nature and extent of the pain can help you to understand what emergency care your patient needs. The questions relating to "PAIN" can be remembered by using this second word as the acronym:

P: **Period of the Pain.** What started it? How long ago?

A: **Area.** Where does it hurt the most? Does the pain travel (**radiate**) from one area to another or stay in the same place?

I: **Intensity.** How intense is the pain? Dull? Throbbing? Sharp? Crushing? Stabbing? Does the pain change in intensity or remain constant?

N: **Nullify.** What alleviates or reduces the pain? Changing body position? Rest? Medications?

Remember that patients suffering from hysteria, violent shock, or drug or alcohol abuse may feel no pain from an injury for several hours and may continue to try to use the injured limb. Be sure to ask open-ended questions if possible, and wait for the patient's response, unless he or she is unable to do so. Also, through observation and questioning, try to identify the mechanism of injury in a trauma situation (cars colliding, patient falling off a roof, etc.). Then write all pertinent findings of the history on the patient's record.

☐ 10. CONDUCTING A SECONDARY SURVEY

Once you have completed the quick primary survey, have attended to life-threatening problems, and have taken vital signs, and the medical history, take a closer look at the patient and systematically examine him or her from head to toe for less obvious injuries or medical problems. This examination, called the **secondary survey,** consists of conducting a full body assessment with your hands, checking for swelling, depression, deformity, bleeding, etc. (Figure 3-35). (If the patient has life-threatening injuries or illness, you will probably begin immediate resuscitation and transport. In that case, the secondary examination must be postponed.)

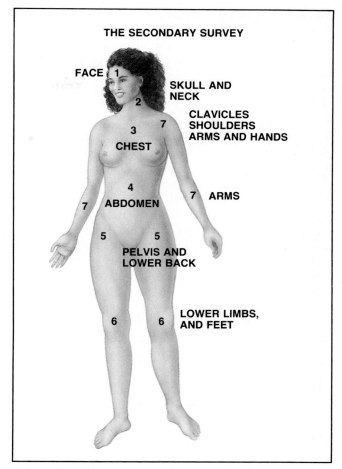

FIGURE 3-35

Use a common sense approach and perform the head-to-toe survey where possible. Before you begin, warn the patient that the survey may cause some pain and discomfort, but explain that you will be as careful as possible.

Use a "Look, Listen, Feel, Smell" approach by:

- **Look for:** deformities, wounds, bleeding, discolorations, penetrations, openings in the neck, and any unusual chest movements.

- **Listen for:** any unusual breathing sounds, gurgling, or crepitus (a noise like sandpaper rubbing together and made by broken bone ends rubbing against each other). Do *not* ask the patient to move so you may listen for these sounds!

- **Feel for:** unusual masses, swelling or hardness, softness or mushiness, muscle-spasms, pulsations, tenderness, deformities, and temperature.

- **Smell for:** Any unusual odors on the patient's breath, body, or clothing.

Any clothing that interferes with your ability to examine the patient properly should be cut on the anterior part and allowed to fall away. Be as modest as possible, and try to insure the patient's privacy.

While you conduct the secondary exam, keep talking calmly to the patient, even if there is no apparent response. Don't frighten the patient by describing wounds or injuries but rather describe what you are doing to help. For example, instead of saying, "There seems to be a lot of blood soaking your shirt on this side," say, "I'm going to pull up your shirt on this side so I can examine your abdomen." Keep glancing at the patient's face, both to maintain rapport and to catch nonverbal responses, like a grimace in response to pain.

Be very careful not to move the patient unnecessarily until you are sure that there are no neck or spinal injuries. Keep the head and neck in alignment. The examination itself may cause the patient some discomfort, but it helps if you explain what you are going to do. Be very systematic in your approach; it will keep patient discomfort to a minimum.

Use common sense in your examination. *Do not* remove **wound dressings** (unless there is an important reason to check on the nature of the wound) or probe wounds. *Do not* pull on clothing attached to a wound. Explain to the patient what you are doing to his or her clothing and why. Be modest and professional in your demeanor. If there is any question about the patient's condition, assume the worst and work from there.

Begin the head-to-toe survey by kneeling at the side of the patent's head. If you have a partner or a responsible bystander, have him kneel behind the patient and apply slight traction to the head to immobilize the head and neck until you are sure there is no spinal injury. If the trauma patient is seated or in an unusual situation, have your partner stabilize the head with slight traction before you begin the survey. If you are by yourself, use one hand on the patient's chin to stabilize the head and use your other hand for the inspection. Then proceed in the following order, checking the facial features first.

Check the Facial Features

Run your fingers over the forehead, eye orbits, and facial structure to feel for any abnormalities. Gently press on the patient's cheekbones, then on the jawbone, checking for fractures. Omit this step if there is obvious facial damage.

Check the ears and nose for fluid, the mouth for internal lacerations, and the eyes for **pupillary** response and injuries. The face should be symmetrical and the teeth should align well. There should be no fluids coming from the ears, nose, or throat. The eyes should track a moving object smoothly and together into all four quadrants of their normal range of motion (Figures 3-36–3-43).

If the pupils are dilated or unresponsive to light, the patient may be suffering from cardiac arrest or drugs

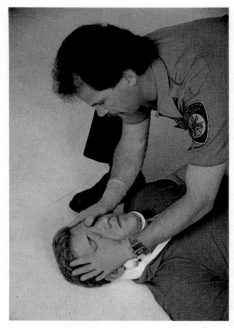

FIGURE 3-36 Run your fingers over the forehead, orbits of the eyes, and facial structure.

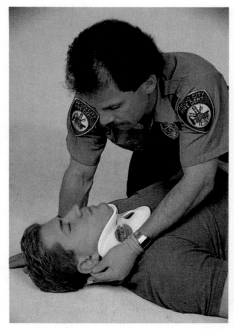

FIGURE 3-37 Check the nose and ears for blood or clear fluid (cerebrospinal fluid).

such as LSD or amphetamines. If the patient is unconscious, the pupils will not respond to light. If the pupils are constricted and unresponsive, the patient may be suffering from a disease of the central nervous system or the influence of such narcotics as heroin, morphine, or codeine. Unequal size of pupils may indicate a stroke or head injury.

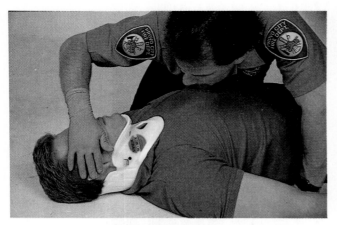

FIGURE 3-38 Check behind the ears for discoloration or bruising.

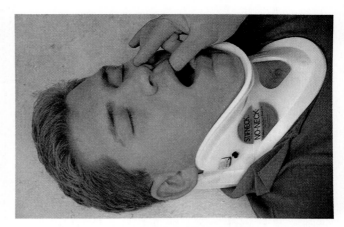

FIGURE 3-41 Open the mouth using the scissors technique.

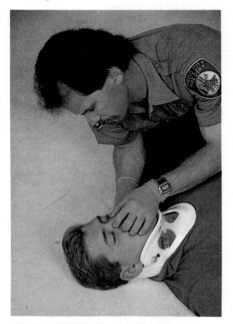

FIGURE 3-39 Gently check the nose for any possible injury.

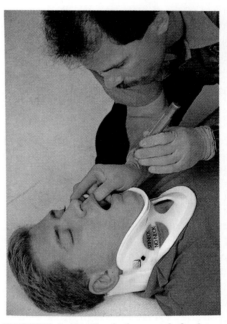

FIGURE 3-42 Check the mouth for lacerations or obstructions. Is any unusual breath odor present?

FIGURE 3-40 Check the eyes for reactive pupils and for possible damage.

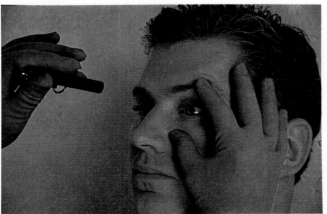

It may be necessary to remove contact lenses in an unconscious patient. Place the contacts in a safe place in a container and make sure that they are transported with the patient. Do not try to remove **foreign objects** embedded in the eye.

If the patient has burns, cuts, or any injuries to the eyelids, assume that there is damage to the eye. Do not attempt to open the eyelids. Do not apply any pressure on the eye.

In some cases you can locate a problem by smelling the breath; for example, you may be able to tell if a patient has been drinking alcohol. Also, some conditions related to diabetes cause a sweet, fruity breath odor. Be wary of deciding that a patient is "just drunk"

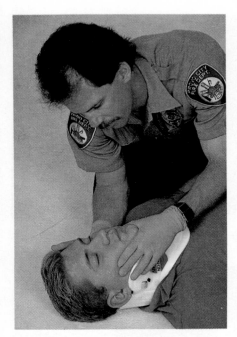

FIGURE 3-43 Check the face for symmetry and the teeth for alignment.

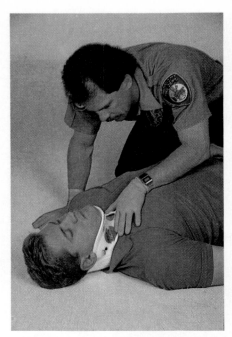

FIGURE 3-44 Observe the neck for abnormal signs.

if you smell alcohol. Another more serious problem may be occurring simultaneously. Be sure to note *any* unusual breath odor.

Feel the Skull and Neck

Check for depressions and bruises that may indicate skull **fracture** or dislocation of cervical vertebrae. The trachea should be in the midline of the neck (Figure 3-44). The neck veins should not be distended if the patient is sitting upright, except perhaps near the end of exhalation. If the patient's neck veins remain distended when he or she is sitting, it may be a sign of cardiac or thoracic problems.

The carotid pulses should be equal in intensity. The patient should be able to swallow without discomfort. The voice should not be hoarse, unless this is normal for the patient. Any tenderness in the posterior neck should be regarded as an indicator of cervical fracture until the patient has been examined *for that possibility* by a physician. Anterior neck pain may indicate an injury that might **occlude** the airway or circulation to the brain.

If you find midline deformities of the cervical spine, point tenderness (a painful response) when you apply gentle finger pressure, or muscle spasms, suspect cervical spine injury. Examine the anterior neck and sides, then *stop the survey* until you can immobilize the head and neck. Use a rigid cervical or extrication collar or a blanket roll in the absence of an extrication collar. (See Chapter 41 for detailed procedures.) This procedure will take two trained people, and one EMT will need to immobilize the neck and head during the rest of the examination. If the patient is unconscious, *assume* that there has been spinal injury and proceed accordingly.

Check the anterior neck for signs of injury, deviations of **larynx** (voice box) or **trachea** (windpipe) from the midline of the neck, bruises, deformity, or a **stoma** (permanent surgical opening at the base of the throat with a metal or plastic tube in it to keep it open. The patient breathes through this opening. Approximately 25,000 people in the United States have them).

In checking the scalp, be very careful not to move the patient's head. Run your fingers through the patient's hair, feeling for wounds. If hair is matted with blood over a possible injury site, do not attempt to part the hair. Check the hidden part of the scalp by *very gently* running your fingers up through the scalp (Figure 3-45). Do not perform this test until after the patient's neck has been immobilized, if you suspect spine injuries. Take great care not to drive bone fragments or dirt into a scalp wound.

If the patient is wearing a hairpiece or wig, do not attempt to remove it. It may be held in place with permanent adhesive or tape. Feel gently through the netting to check for bleeding, swellings, or deformities. Do not reach under the wig.

If cervical spine mechanism of injury, neck pain, or neurological deficit are *not* present, continue the survey. If they are, have a second rescuer maintain neutral or in-line immobilization and apply a cervical collar.

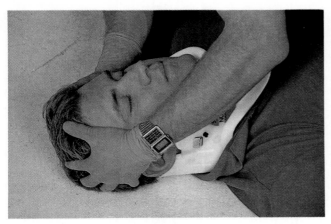

FIGURE 3-45 Run your fingers gently over the patient's scalp.

Check the Chest

The chest should be checked again even if you noted injuries during the earlier exam (Figure 3-46). In addition to the examination of the chest administered during the primary survey, watch for respiratory disturbances:

Listen to the patient's speech. A spinal cord injury in the neck at or just below C4 may paralyze the chest muscles so that the patient can breathe only with his diaphragm. Because of this, the patient can speak only a few words at a time. A patient with severe shortness of breath from any cause may also speak in short phrases.

Feel the chest to confirm the findings of the inspection. Check for symmetry of respirations by placing the tips of your thumbs on the **xiphoid process** (the lower tip of the breastbone) and spreading your hands over the lower rib cage (Figure 3-47). Both hands should move an equal distance with each breath. In injury patients, also feel for tenderness and instability over the ribs and for air crackling beneath the skin (**subcutaneous emphysema**).

FIGURE 3-46 Cut away clothing if necessary to inspect visually the chest and abdomen.

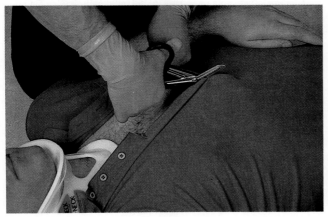

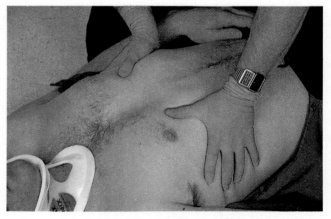

FIGURE 3-47 Check for symmetry of respirations. Both hands should move an equal distance with each breath.

Place the ulnar edge of one hand or both hands on the sternum, one on top of the other, and push down gently (rib spring), and check for any pain (Figure 3-48). If the patient is already complaining about chest pain, do not apply pressure to the ribs or sternum.

If your patient is a child, remember that his or her flexible rib cage may transmit more impact to the organs underneath. He or she may develop breathing or heart problems up to twenty-four hours after an injury.

When checking breath sounds (auscultation) with a stethoscope, it is best to listen to the front and back sides in at least four sections if possible, comparing left and right sides at each level. In trauma, *do not* move the patient. Listen to inspiration and expiration (Figure 3-49).

Listen to the chest to be certain that breath sounds are present and are equal on both sides. Absent, diminished breath sounds on one side may indicate bronchial obstruction, pneumothorax, or **hemothorax** (discussed in Chapter 19)? When listening for abnormal sounds, recall that fluid transmits sound better than air. Most

FIGURE 3-48 Gently press on the sternum for possible chest injury.

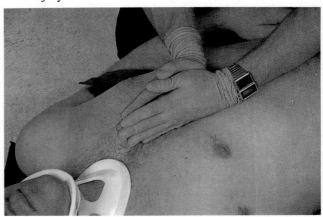

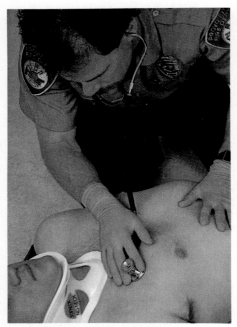

FIGURE 3-49 Listen to breath sounds at the front and back of the chest.

abnormal sounds in the lungs are caused by fluid in the form of pus, abnormal quantities of mucus, or fluid due to swelling.

Another abnormal sound produced by obstruction of the upper airway that can usually be heard without a stethoscope is **stridor.** Stridor is a harsh, high-pitched sound, sometimes resembling a bark. It indicates a narrowing of the upper airway, usually caused by foreign material, spasm, or swelling. It usually occurs on inspiration.

Coughing is a response to bronchial irritation. Simple chemical irritation from inhaled material or smoke may cause a cough. A nonproductive cough indicates that the cause is irritation only or that the cough is ineffective in clearing the airways. If a cough produces **sputum,** note the color, consistency, amount, and odor. Mucus is white or clear; a **purulent** (infected) sputum is usually yellow or green. Coughing up blood may indicate cardiac or pulmonary disease. Frothy or foamlike sputum may be caused by an injury to the chest. You should note the volume, color, and other characteristics of any sputum that is produced.

Check the Abdominal Region

Look first for obvious injury: cuts, bruises, penetrations, impaled objects, open wounds with protruding organs, rashes, or burns.

Usually it is best to have the patient lying down. Keep him or her warm, and be sure that your hands are warm. Shivering will make the abdominal muscles tense. Be gentle. Sudden pokes will also make the muscles tense.

If you see signs of swelling, ask the patient if his or her abdomen seems larger than usual. It may be **bloated** (filled with gas), **edematous** (engorged with water due to heart failure), or **distended** by blood. Is the swelling **generalized** or **localized?** Are there bruises over the **flank** (between the ribs and pelvis on the sides) or around the navel? If there are, the patient may be bleeding internally.

Then gently palpate the four quadrants of the abdomen separately, using the pads of your fingers and holding your hands almost parallel to the patient's abdomen (Figures 3-50 and 3-51). If you suspect injury in any area, check that region last. Gently feel for the presence of any abnormal masses. A vigorously pulsating mass in the abdomen may be a weakened bulge in the aorta that needs immediate attention.

Do not press or palpate if there is an obvious injury. If the patient complains of abdominal pain and is also spitting or vomiting blood, the stomach may be injured. Bright red blood may be from a damaged esophagus. Whole blood irritates body tissues and therefore

FIGURE 3-50 Palpating the upper quadrant of the abdomen.

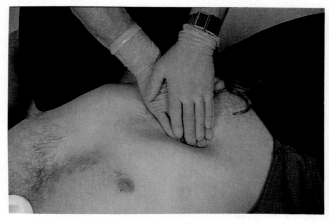

FIGURE 3-51 Palpating the lower quadrant of the abdomen.

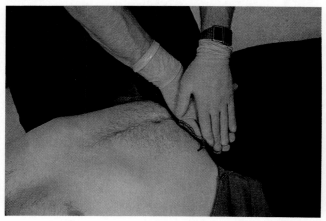

results in pain, guarding, and abdominal rigidity. If digestive organs are lacerated, they may release toxins and infectious microorganisms which can cause bloating.

The liver is in the upper right quadrant of the abdomen but extends behind the notch at the base of the rib cage. Injury to the liver is extremely serious because of the high probability of serious internal bleeding and shock. The stomach is in the upper left quadrant of the abdomen, partially protected by the rib cage. The spleen, again an organ which can produce serious internal bleeding, is to the left of the stomach.

The appendix is in the lower right quadrant. Pain in that location and a rigid abdomen are classic symptoms of appendicitis, but not all cases show these symptoms. Blood in urine usually means kidney damage. Dark blood in feces is usually a symptom of intestinal bleeding, while bright blood in feces is probably from hemorrhoids. Incontinence of bowel or bladder may be caused by head or spinal injury.

If your patient has clear signs of internal bleeding or injury, do not palpate. You will only cause further suffering.

If the patient instinctively **guards** his or her abdomen by protecting or by tightening his muscles, it may indicate the presence of blood, urine, gastric contents, or feces — all of the irritation agents — in the abdominal cavity. You can test by distracting the patient with conversation. Voluntary guarding will stop. If the abdomen still feels rigid (wooden or boardlike) it is a sign of **peritonitis** or serious internal injury. Taking a deep breath will also hurt, so the patient usually breathes shallowly. In such cases, do not put pressure on the tender area during palpation.

If the patient has had a **colostomy** or **ileostomy** (surgical removal of the colon or intestine), you will see a surgical opening in the abdominal wall and a bag to hold excretions from the digestive tract. Leave the bag in place and make every effort to keep it covered from view to save the patient from possible embarrassment.

Check the Pelvic Region and Lower Back for Tenderness

Damage to the pelvis can cause great pain, so be gentle. Tell the patient what you are doing and prevent embarrassment. First put your hands on each side of the hips and compress inward, checking for tenderness, **crepitus,** and instability (Figure 3-52). Put the base of your hands on the **pubic bones** with your hands covering the **iliac crest** (wings) and hip bones. Compress gently, then more firmly (Figure 3-53). Note any tenderness. Visually note any possible loss of bladder control, bleeding, or an erection in a male patient (a possible CNS injury). Check the strength of the femoral pulses. Remember that a pelvic fracture can bleed *vigorously*.

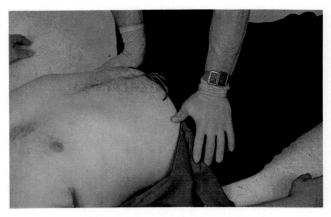

FIGURE 3-52 Apply gentle, then firmer compression to check for pelvic fractures.

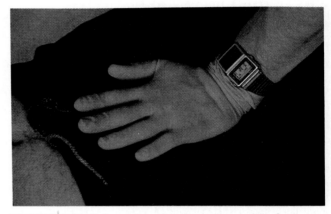

FIGURE 3-53 Palpate the pubic bone for possible fracture.

If a male patient has a persistent erection of the penis (**priapism**), consider this a symptom of spinal injury or possible sickle-cell crisis. Do not touch a patient's genitals except to stop dangerous bleeding.

Without moving the patient, slip your hand beneath his or her back and feel for possible fractures, dislocations, or deformities.

If you need better access to the back, and if you have already ruled out possible spine damage, gently lift the patient's arm on the side that you are examining across his or her chest with his or her hand toward the opposite shoulder (Figure 3-54). This will let you slip your hand down the full length of the spine. Do not lift more than is absolutely necessary. Ask the patient to tell you if there is any tenderness at any point. If there is, keep the patient immobile (and secure him or her on a backboard before transporting). Check simultaneously, with little or no spine movement, for any bleeding in this area.

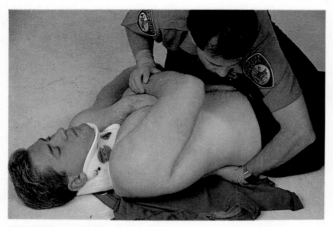

FIGURE 3-54 Check the back for point tenderness and deformity. Keep the head and neck in alignment, and be very careful of movement.

Check the Lower Limbs and Feet

Inspect each lower limb, one at a time, from hip to foot. Look for possible bruises, fractures, dislocations, or swelling. Check for abnormal positions of the legs. Signs of a fractured hip are a leg that is turned away, shortened, and/or rotated. Palpate the entire limb for protrusions, depressions, abnormal movement, and tenderness (Figures 3-55—3-57).

Follow the instructions on pages 58 through 63 under "Vital Signs" for checking skin temperature, pulse, etc.

If you suspect an injury to the legs or feet, cut pant legs along the seam and fold the clothing back.

FIGURE 3-55 Check the upper leg for pain and deformity.

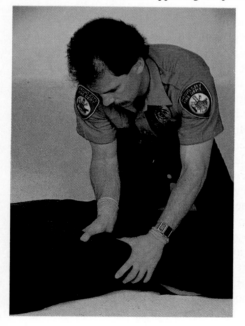

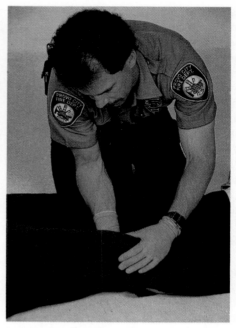

FIGURE 3-56 Palpate the knees and feel the patella (kneecap) for any pain or deformity.

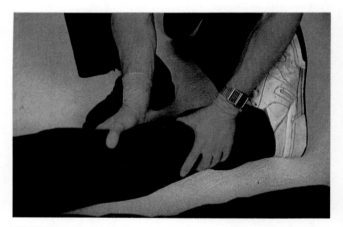

FIGURE 3-57 Feel the lower legs; palpate the tibia, ankles, and feet.

Follow local protocol on whether to remove shoes. You can take a distal pulse without removing a pair of low-cut shoes. If the patient is wearing gym shoes, high-top dress shoes, or boots, you may need to cut the laces or cut away the footwear if unlacing and pulling the footwear off might aggravate an injury. Do not attempt to remove ski boots unless you have been specifically trained in that procedure.

Do not move or lift the patient's legs. Do not change the position of the legs or feet during the examination.

If the patient reports extreme pain in a leg but has no skin sensation, it may be the result of occlusion (blockage) of the main artery to that limb. Usually the pulse in that limb is absent. A similar situation may exist in an arm as well.

In all patients with spinal injury or suspected stroke, check strength and sensation. Spinal injuries more commonly result in **paraplegia** (**paralysis** of both legs) or **quadriplegia** (paralysis of arms and legs), while stroke patients are more likely to have **hemiplegia** (paralysis of an arm and a leg on the same side of the body). Usually the patient will not be able to move the limb and will not be able to feel a pinch or touch (Figures 3-58–3-60).

Be aware, however, that some spine-injured patients can still move and the patient may complain only of tingling or numbness in the extremities. If these symptoms are present, treat the patient for spinal injury.

Immobilization is the most important action to take in the field, since accurate diagnosis can be done only in the hospital.

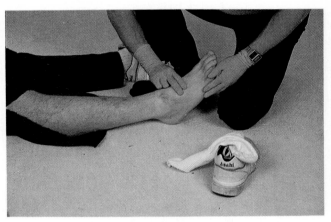

FIGURE 3-60 Inspect the bare foot; then check for a distal pulse in each foot.

Squeeze the calves of the legs looking for tenderness. Be gentle and do not repeat the test if the patient reports pain, since clots may be present which you could dislodge. If they reach the lungs, they could be fatal.

Check for the distal pulse in each foot either behind the medial ankle or on the anterior surface of the foot straight up from the big toe. The second pulse, on top of the foot, is more reliable than the ankle pulse. If there is no pulse, suspect that a major artery has been pinched or severed, usually by a broken or displaced bone end or a blood clot. If you cannot find a pulse, check skin color and test capillary refill.

Check the Upper Extremities

Gently palpate the clavicles and shoulders to check for pain and deformity (Figure 3-61). Gently run your hands over the patient's arms, checking for fractures and/or dislocations at the joints (Figure 3-62). Have him or her grip your hands to see if he or she has equal

FIGURE 3-58 Check strength and sensation by having the patient pull up against your hand.

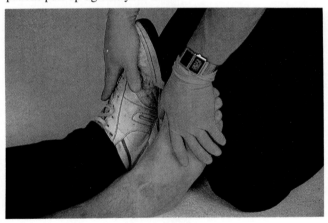

FIGURE 3-59 Then have the patient push his or her foot against your hand.

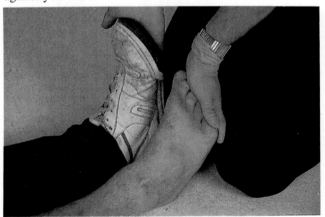

FIGURE 3-61 Gently, palpate the clavicles and shoulders.

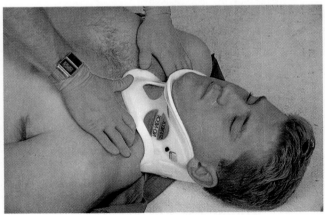

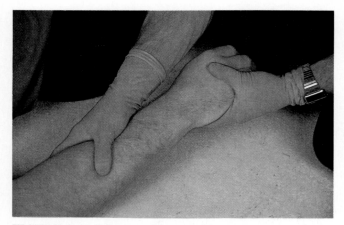

FIGURE 3-62 Palpate each arm and hand.

strength in both hands. Check both radial pulses for equal strength.

If the patient is conscious and there are no obvious injuries to the arm or hand, have him or her identify which finger you are touching, wave the hand, and grasp your hand. If he or she cannot, assume spinal injury. Also, be on the alert for the sudden onset of difficult breathing or respiratory arrest. Monitor the patient's breathing constantly.

If the patient is unconscious, assume possible spine injury. Gently hold his or her arm near the wrist and pinch the skin on top of the hand, noting any reaction to the pain. This may be a fairly unreliable test. If the patient shows some reaction to the pain, you still cannot rule out spinal injury. Furthermore, if the patient is deeply unconscious, he or she will not react to pain.

□ CONSIDERATIONS BEFORE YOU TRANSPORT THE PATIENT

When you are getting ready to transport, take a minute or two to clean up. Are all of your bandage wraps cleaned up? If someone needs to accompany the patient to the hospital, can a bystander escort that person to the ambulance and be sure that the seatbelt is fastened?

If the patient is elderly, does she have a wheel-chair, cane, crutches, walker, dentures, hearing aid, or eyeglasses that need to go too? The isolation and inconvenience that can result from not having these familiar aids can be serious. If you take along the patient's regular medications, be sure to give them to the hospital staff.

Try to have family members keep the patient's valuables. If the case is not a crisis, taking a minute to be sure that children, pets, etc., are cared for may ease unnecessary worries. See Chapters 44 and 45 for transporting the patient and reporting by radio.

When you arrive in the emergency department or write your report, it is important to present information in an orderly, concise fashion (Figure 3-63). Make a careful recording of all findings and emergency care given. Document any repeat assessments. Record vital signs and neurological status. A clear, complete report will provide better communication with the emergency department staff, safeguard you against omitting important details, and create a permanent record that may be used in court. Remember — "If it isn't written down, you didn't do it."

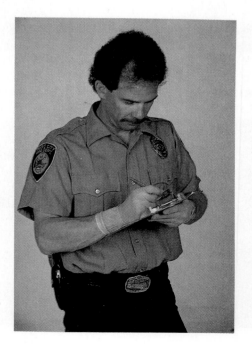

FIGURE 3-63 Write your report in orderly, concise fashion.

chapter 4

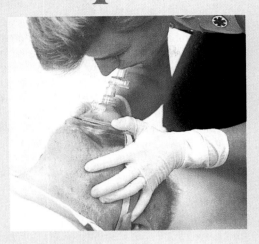

Basic Life Support: Artificial Ventilation

✳ OBJECTIVES

- Describe the respiratory system and the role of the airways and lungs, the exchange of oxygen and carbon dioxide, and the significance of oxygen to body tissue.
- Discuss the physiology of respiratory arrest.
- Demonstrate how to assess respiratory status by taking a history and by the "Look, Listen, and Feel" assessment method.
- List the initial steps of basic life support, including assessment, patient positioning, opening the airway, and restoring breathing through artificial ventilation.
- Identify an obstructed airway and demonstrate the techniques for dislodging foreign objects that are obstructing the airway.
- Explain how to adapt ventilation support procedures to infants and children.
- Discuss the common medical conditions that cause airway problems.

It is recommended that EMTs wear protective gloves whenever there is a possibility of coming in contact with a patient's blood, body fluids, mucous membranes, traumatic wounds, or sores. See Chapter 31.

The first priority in any emergency is to establish and maintain an adequate airway. Because breathing is vital, your quick and efficient care will spell the difference between life and death for many of your patients. In some instances, airway obstruction itself may be the emergency: a swimmer stays underwater too long and inhales water, a business executive at a banquet begins to choke on a piece of steak, or a woman carrying a bag of groceries trips on the curb and is knocked unconscious and quits breathing. Such instances cause 3,900 avoidable deaths per year. By understanding the physiological process of breathing and the methods of care, you will be able to quickly initiate and maintain an adequate airway in cases of emergency.

□ UNDERSTANDING THE RESPIRATORY SYSTEM

The respiratory system consists of all of the body structures involved in breathing (or **respiration**). The parts include (1) **airways,** consisting of the nose, mouth, throat, larynx, trachea, and bronchi, (2) the **lungs** (where oxygen-carbon dioxide exchange occurs), and (3) muscles that permit respiration (the **diaphragm,** the muscles of the chest wall, and accessory muscles). The air passages begin in the head and pass through the throat into the **thorax,** which is protected by the rib cage, the **clavicles,** and the diaphragm. **Oxygen** is essential to all life. Oxygen enters the body through respiration, the breathing process. Any interference with breathing produces oxygen depletion (**hypoxia**) throughout the entire body, and carbon dioxide levels rise in the blood and tissues. At the same time, respiratory **acidosis** (an accumulation of acid) occurs. If this situation is not reversed, the patient will die. Partial airway obstruction may also have the same end result due to a lack of oxygen (**anoxia**), but it will take longer for the patient to die.

During respiration, air is taken into the lungs (inhalation) and allowed to pass out (exhalation). It passes through the nose, throat (**pharynx**), and trachea (**windpipe**). Air is warmed, moistened, and filtered by the **cilia** (hairs) and mucous membrane.

The pharynx is a continuation of the nose and mouth. At its lower end are two openings, one anterior to the other. The anterior opening is called the trachea, and it leads to the lungs. The one posterior is called the esophagus, which leads to the stomach (Figure 4-1).

At the top of the trachea is a flap, the epiglottis, which closes over the trachea during swallowing to keep food or liquid from entering it. When a person is unconscious, the flap may fail to respond. This is why you never give solids or liquids to an unconscious person by mouth, since the risk of **aspiration,** or foreign matter inhaled into the lungs, is serious and may be fatal. The

tongue of an unconscious person, especially if he or she is lying on his or her back, is apt to collapse against the back of the throat and interfere with air reaching the lungs. In some cases, it may block the throat entirely (Figure 4-2).

The throat, or pharynx, is the passageway for both food and air. The larynx connects the pharynx with the trachea. The **voice box** is found in the larynx, the organ of voice. The outside view is often referred to as the Adam's apple.

The trachea extends into the chest cavity, where it divides into two bronchial tubes (bronchi), one going to each lung. Within the lungs, the tubes branch out like limbs of a tree, until they become very small (Figure 4-3).

After subdividing into very small branches, the bronchial tubes end in a group of air cells or sacs (alveoli) resembling a very small bunch of hollow grapes. Around each of the air cells with its very thin walls is a fine network of small blood vessels, or capillaries. The blood in these capillaries releases carbon dioxide and other waste matter — the byproducts of tissue activity from all over the body — through the thin cell wall and, in exchange, takes on a supply of oxygen from the air breathed into the alveoli cells.

As the blood returns to the heart in veins, it collects in the right atrium of the heart and is pumped into the lungs by the right ventricle. In the lungs, it passes through a fine network of pulmonary capillaries, which form a mesh among the alveoli. Healthy lungs contain about 700 million alveoli. The blood gives up carbon dioxide to these air sacs and absorbs new oxygen from them. This reoxygenated blood leaves the lungs, collects in the left atrium, and is pumped into the aorta from the left ventricle. Then it circulates throughout the body again while the wastes and carbon dioxide are exhaled.

The lungs are two cone-shaped bodies that are soft, spongy, and elastic. Each lung is covered by a layer of smooth tissue called pleura; another layer of pleura lines the inside of the chest cavity. These two layers are called **parietal** pleura (lining the chest wall) and **visceral** pleura (covering the lungs). A small potential space filled with a small amount of lubricant is between the pleura. The inside of the lungs communicates freely with the outside air through the windpipe.

Breathing consists of two separate acts: inhalation and exhalation. During inhalation, an active act, the chest muscles raise the ribs, and the arch of the diaphragm falls and flattens, expanding the chest cavity so that the air pressure within becomes less than that outside. Air rushes to fill the vacuum, inflating the lungs. In exhalation, a relatively passive act performed with slight muscular action, the ribs fall to their normal position, the arch of the diaphragm rises, decreasing the capacity of the chest cavity, and air is forced out (Figure 4-4).

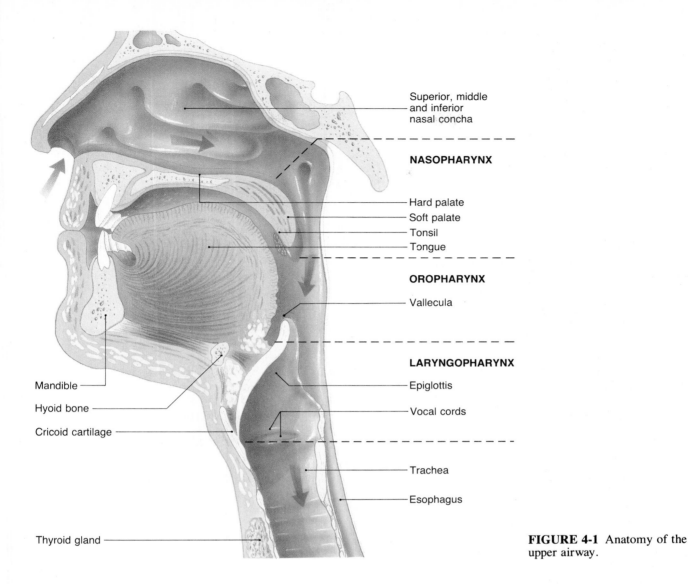

Superior, middle and inferior nasal concha

NASOPHARYNX

Hard palate

Soft palate

Tonsil

Tongue

OROPHARYNX

Vallecula

LARYNGOPHARYNX

Epiglottis

Vocal cords

Mandible

Hyoid bone

Cricoid cartilage

Trachea

Esophagus

Thyroid gland

FIGURE 4-1 Anatomy of the upper airway.

FIGURE 4-2 Relaxed tongue blocking the airway.

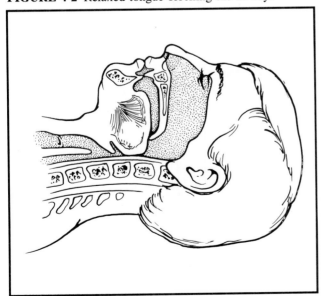

If any air gets through the chest wall, or if the lung is punctured so that air from the outside can fill the **pleural space,** the lungs will not fill. This is because the air pressure is equal outside and inside the chest cavity. Thus, no negative pressure is created and the patient cannot inhale.

Breathing is usually automatic, and a person generally exerts only a limited degree of control over the process. The brain continually monitors oxygen and carbon dioxide levels in all parts of the body. If these levels become abnormal, the brain signals the respiratory system to correct the abnormality.

Carbon dioxide diffuses through the alveolar membrane about twenty times faster than oxygen. As a result, the body is extremely sensitive to carbon-dioxide levels. An increase of 5 percent of carbon dioxide in the air will double a person's rate and depth of breathing.

The amount of air breathed and frequency of breathing vary according to whether the person is at rest or engaged in work or exercise. At rest, a healthy adult

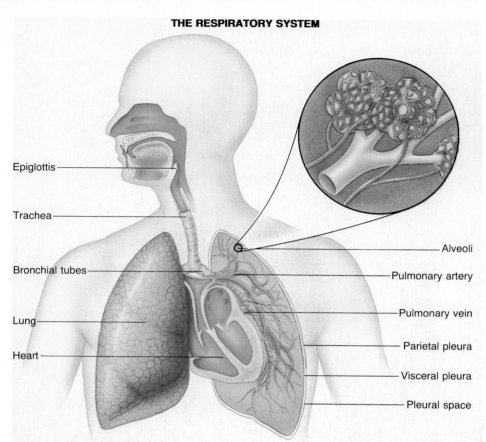

Epiglottis

Trachea

Bronchial tubes

Lung

Heart

Alveoli

Pulmonary artery

Pulmonary vein

Parietal pleura

Visceral pleura

Pleural space

FIGURE 4-3

FIGURE 4-4

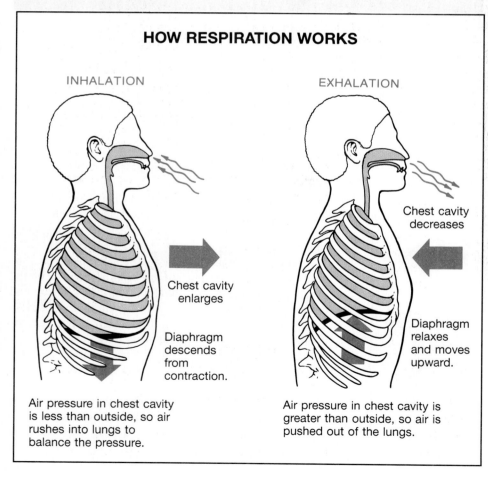

HOW RESPIRATION WORKS

INHALATION

EXHALATION

Chest cavity
enlarges

Diaphragm
descends
from
contraction.

Air pressure in chest cavity
is less than outside, so air
rushes into lungs to
balance the pressure.

Chest cavity
decreases

Diaphragm
relaxes
and moves
upward.

Air pressure in chest cavity is
greater than outside, so air is
pushed out of the lungs.

breathes between twelve and twenty times a minute. During strenuous work, the breathing rate and amount inhaled may be increased several times.

For additional information on the anatomy and physiology of the respiratory system, see Chapter 2.

☐ RESPIRATORY ARREST

Breathing may stop as a result of a variety of medical disorders or serious accidents. The most common causes of **respiratory arrest** are electric shock, drowning, suffocation, inhalation of poisonous gases, head injuries, airway closure, stroke, drug overdose, heart problems, and allergy reactions.

When oxygen is cut off to the lung, hence to the brain and heart, the heart will continue to pump. Oxygen stored in the lungs and blood will continue to circulate to the brain and other vital organs. But the heart will gradually become weaker as the brain cells that send signals to the heart begin to die from lack of oxygen. When the heart muscle or myocardium experiences hypoxia, the heart falters and stops, resulting in **cardiac arrest.**

When respiration and heart action cease, the patient is classified as **clinically dead,** because the two essential systems that continue life have been shut down. However, cells have a residual oxygen supply and can survive for a short time. The brain cells, which use approximately 20 percent of the oxygen in the circulatory system, are the first to begin to die — usually four to six minutes after being deprived of oxygenated blood. This irreversible brain damage is called **biological death** (Figure 4-5). The period between clinical and biological death is short, which means that the EMT must act quickly to **reoxygenate** the blood through artificial ventilation and get it to flow to the brain. Proper emergency care can keep the brain cells alive and hence save the patient from biological death. The key is knowing *immediately* the status of the respiratory and circulatory systems.

☐ EVALUATION OF RESPIRATORY STATUS

You must learn to evaluate a patient's respiratory status by looking at, listening to, and touching him or her. Educated eyes, ears, and hands can give you valuable information.

Taking a History

Assuming that your patient is conscious and does not require immediate emergency measures, get as much information as possible about the chief complaint. In most

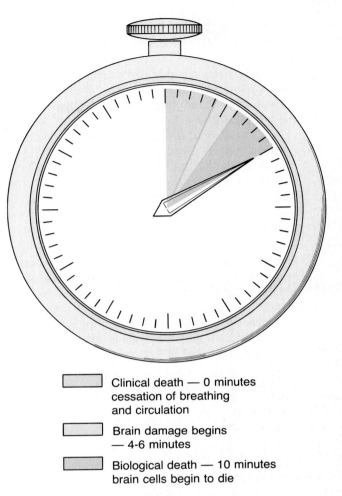

☐ Clinical death — 0 minutes cessation of breathing and circulation

☐ Brain damage begins — 4-6 minutes

☐ Biological death — 10 minutes brain cells begin to die

FIGURE 4-5 Clinical and biological death.

instances, this will be **dyspnea** (difficulty in breathing or shortness of breath). (Patients may have serious respiratory problems without dyspnea, as when their breathing has been depressed by **drugs** or **trauma.**) Assuming that the chief complaint is dyspnea, ask:

1. **How long have you felt like this?** Is this a chronic situation, as in the patient with chronic obstructive pulmonary disease; or as it of recent origin, as in pneumothorax (the presence of air within the chest cavity in the pleural space but outside the lung)?

2. **Was the onset gradual or abrupt?** The dyspnea associated with asthma or **congestive heart failure** may develop gradually over several hours, while that associated with pulmonary **embolism** (a blood clot in a pulmonary vessel) or pneumothorax may come on suddenly.

3. **Is the dyspnea made better or worse by any particular position?** Dyspnea that gets worse when the patient lies down is often related to congestive heart failure, for the horizontal position fa-

vors pooling of blood in the lungs. Most patients with dyspnea caused by disease feel more comfortable sitting.

4. **Have you been coughing?** Patients with chronic obstructive pulmonary disease often have a chronic cough and thick, white sputum. When these patients develop problems, their sputum changes in amount and character and may become purulent (yellow-green, thick). Purulent sputum is also associated with pneumonia. The patient with pulmonary edema often produces a foamy, blood-tinged sputum. Coughing up bright, clear blood may be associated with a variety of conditions, including **heart disease, tuberculosis,** and trauma to the lungs.

5. **Is there any associated pain?** If so, what is the nature of the pain? Abrupt dyspnea occurring with sudden, sharp chest pain may indicate a spontaneous pneumothorax or pulmonary embolism. Dyspnea occurring with heavy, squeezing chest pain underneath the breastbone is one of the symptoms of **myocardial infarction** (heart attack).

6. **Has this happened before?** The patient with congestive heart failure may have a long history of cardiac problems or high blood pressure. The asthmatic often will have had a prior attack and may report that previous episodes were relieved by epinephrine injected in the emergency room. The patient with chronic obstructive pulmonary disease will often give a history of heavy smoking and chronic cough. Find out which medications the patient takes regularly. Certain medications and inhalants suggest **obstructive airway disease.**

7. **Are you taking any medication for it?** The medication **digitalis** indicates that the patient is under care for an underlying cardiac problem. The patient taking "blood thinners" (**anticoagulants,** such as **coumadin**) may have had a previous episode of pulmonary embolism.

Visual Assessment

By the time you complete the history, you will already have some important information about the patient's physical signs. Does the patient appear anxious, uncomfortable, in distress? Does the dyspnea cause the patient difficulty in speaking? Does he or she have to stop to catch his breath? Or did your questions easily distract him or her from the symptoms? Was the patient lying down or sitting very upright, straining to breathe? Were the answers appropriate and coherent, or were they confused and disoriented?

Such observations assess the patient's general appearance and mental status. The patient in severe respiratory distress is frightened and intensely uncomfort-

able, is usually sitting upright, and may be gasping, laboring to breathe, confused, or disoriented.

After completing your primary survey, take the patient's vital signs. Pay particular attention to the breathing.

Are the respirations abnormally rapid (tachypnea) or unusually deep (hyperpnea)?

Injury often causes the patient to breathe up to twice the normal rate (twenty to forty times per minute). If an injured patient is breathing under the normal rate, he most likely has a problem in the airway, diaphragm, lungs, chest wall, and/or central nervous system.

Is the respiratory pattern abnormal? Cheyne-Stokes respirations, consisting of rhythmic waxing and waning of the depth of breathing with periods of absent breathing, suggest a disorder in the central nervous system. An irregular respiratory pattern may be associated with severe head injuries.

Signs of Respiratory Distress

Look for signs of respiratory distress (Figure 4-6):

- Diminishing of speech, or whispering and grunting.
- Restlessness and anxiety.
- Nasal flaring — the nostrils open wide during inhalation.
- Tracheal tugging — the Adam's apple is pulled upward on inhalation.
- Retraction of intercostal muscles (those between the ribs) during inhalation.
- Use of the diaphragm and neck muscles to assist in inhalation.
- Use of the abdominal muscles during exhalation.
- Cyanosis (bluish discoloration of the skin and mucous membranes). This symptom is a late sign.

Look also at the chest wall. A "barrel chest" suggests chronic obstructive pulmonary disease. A deformed chest in a trauma patient is a sign of damage to the chest wall and internal structures. Does the chest move symmetrically during respiration? Does any area bulge or flair during expiration? Is the trachea in the midline, or does it deviate toward one side?

Listening Assessment

When you have completed your visual inspection, the next step is auscultation (listening) as the patient breathes. Listen first with the unaided ear, then apply the diaphragm of your stethoscope firmly to the patient's chest at the nipple level in the mid-axillary line and listen to at least one full inhalation and exhalation

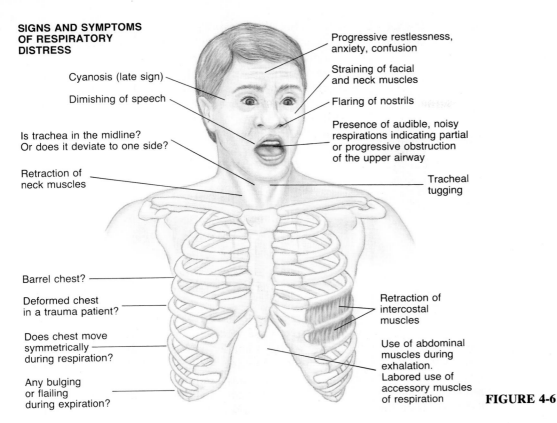

Cyanosis (late sign)

Dimishing of speech

Is trachea in the midline?
Or does it deviate to one side?

Retraction of
neck muscles

Progressive restlessness,
anxiety, confusion

Straining of facial
and neck muscles

Flaring of nostrils

Presence of audible, noisy
respirations indicating partial
or progressive obstruction
of the upper airway

Tracheal
tugging

Barrel chest?

Deformed chest
in a trauma patient?

Does chest move
symmetrically
during respiration?

Any bulging
or flailing
during expiration?

Retraction of
intercostal
muscles

Use of abdominal
muscles during
exhalation.
Labored use of
accessory muscles
of respiration

FIGURE 4-6

of each lung apex. Different respiratory problems have characteristic sounds.

- **Snoring** occurs when the upper airway (mouth, nose, larynx, main bronchus) is partially obstructed by the base of the tongue. Snoring, and the obstruction that it signals, can be corrected by the head tilt-chin lift maneuver, which lifts the base of the tongue away from the back of the throat, or by use of the **modified jaw thrust** if a neck injury is suspected.

- **Crowing** is a sound like a cawing crow that occurs when the muscles around the larynx (voice box) begin to **spasm.**

- **Gurgling,** a sound like gargling, usually indicates the presence of foreign matter in the airway, such as a liquid.

- **Stridor** (low wheeze) is a harsh, high-pitched sound heard on inspiration. It is characteristic of tight upper airway obstruction, as in swelling of the larynx. If you have ever heard the "seal bark" of a child with **croup,** you have some idea of how alarming this sound can be.

- **Wheezing** is a whistling sound heard diffusely all over the chest area in asthma, in some cases of pulmonary embolism, and in congestive heart failure. It is caused when **bronchospasm** (constriction), edema (swelling), or foreign materials nar-

row the airways. Wheezes can also be heard when a foreign body is obstructing the trachea or a bronchus, as in the child who aspirates a peanut. Wheezing due to the presence of foreign bodies may be quite localized to the obstructed area, so you need to listen carefully over all **lung fields.**

- **Rhonchi** are rattling noises in the throat or bronchi and are commonly due to partial obstruction of the larger airways by mucus.

- **Rales** or crackles, are usually fine, moist sounds, sometimes crackling or bubbling in quality. They are associated with fluid in the smaller airways (e.g., pulmonary edema, pneumonia). Auscultate the bases of the lungs posteriorly, for it is here where the rales of pulmonary edema are usually first heard in cases of congestive heart failure.

You must also determine whether the breath sounds are equal on both sides of the chest. Diminished or absent breath sounds on one side of the chest mean that the lung is not being adequately ventilated because of obstruction, collapse, or other causes.

Palpating the Chest

After auscultation comes palpation (examination by touch). Feel the chest wall of the trauma patient for tenderness and instability over the ribs. Feel for subcuta-

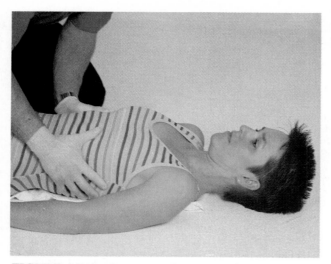

FIGURE 4-7 Apply compression to the rib cage to discover any rib cage damage. At the same time, visually inspect the chest for deformities, wounds, and equal chest expansion.

neous emphysema (air in the fatty tissues just underneath the skin). The skin in such cases will make a crackling sensation under the fingertips. Trauma to the chest may produce subcutaneous emphysema if air invades the chest wall from the neck or directly from the lungs.

Assess **symmetry** of breathing by placing your thumbs on the xiphoid (tip of the breastbone) and spreading your hands over the front of the chest wall. If the patient is breathing normally, your hands should move symmetrically with each breath (Figure 4-7).

☐ BASIC LIFE SUPPORT

The first crucial step in basic life support is assessment. All too often in CPR training the complete assessment phase is overlooked. The American Heart Association has stated: "The assessment phases of basic life support are crucial. No victim should undergo any one of the more intrusive procedures of cardiopulmonary resuscitation (i.e., positioning, opening the airway, rescue breathing, and external chest compression) until the need for it has been established by the appropriate assessment."

The instructions in this chapter assume that there are no injuries to the neck or spine. If you suspect such injuries, you must quickly open the airway using spinal precautions, collar early, then deal with the respiratory emergency, since the risk of paralysis of the respiratory system is very high, and is irreversible.

Assume cervical spine injury if the patient has suffered injuries to the head or face; or has an altered level of consciousness. Mechanism of injury alone frequently warrants assumption of a cervical spine injury. Maintain the head and neck in a neutral position, with the shoul-

ders in line, then use the jaw thrust to open the airway. This manuever is safe if the head and neck are being maintained in neutral alignment. Using a **nasopharyngeal** or **oral airway** will leave the head and neck in a neutral position. A **bag-valve-mask** breathing apparatus, when used properly, leaves the head and neck in a position of neutral alignment. All of these devices are discussed in Chapter 5.

Patient Assessment

The initial steps in patient assessment are:

1. Determine unresponsiveness.
2. Activate the EMS system (911), if necessary.
3. Achieve control of the cervical spine.
4. Open the airway with the appropriate maneuver, either the head-tilt/chin-lift or jaw-thrust.

First assess the level of consciousness. (If the patient is responsive, your procedures will differ.) Tap the patient gently on the shoulder and ask loudly, "Are you OK?" You are not looking for an answer to the question as much as you are any kind of response — fluttering eyelids, muscle movement, turning from the noise, etc. If there is no response, activate the EMS system (911). If you suspect or observe trauma to the head and neck, move the patient only if absolutely necessary.

Positioning the Patient

To perform CPR, the patient must lie supine (on the back) on a firm, flat surface. If the patient is lying on his side or face down, position your hands so that you can roll him as a unit with head, neck, and torso moving simultaneously. Do not allow the head to roll, twist, or tilt backward or forward. Place the arms along the side of the body. Kneel at shoulder level. (See Figure 4-8.)

Plan the move, perform it carefully, and move the patient only once if possible. Position the patient as the condition warrants it, *not* as an automatic basic life support step.

If your patient is unresponsive, follow the A-B-C procedure: Airway, Breathing, and Circulation (see p. 124). You need to implement basic life support within four minutes.

Open the Airway

Next open the airway. When unconsciousness causes the tongue to relax, it will frequently fall back and block the airway (see Figure 4-2). The epiglottis can also relax and obstruct the larynx. Efforts to breathe will create negative pressure which may draw the tongue, epiglottis, or both into the airway to block the trachea.

Open the mouth with the **crossed-finger technique.** (See Figure 4-9.)

☐ Repositioning the Patient for Basic Life Support

WARNING: This maneuver is used to initiate basic cardiac life support when you must act alone. For all other repositionings, use the four-rescuer log roll. (Chapter 11)

1

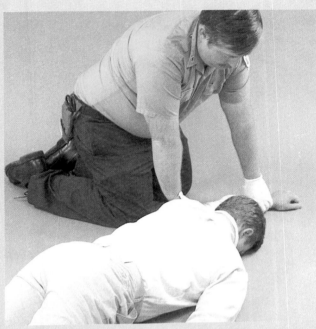

Straighten the legs and position the closest arm above the head.

2

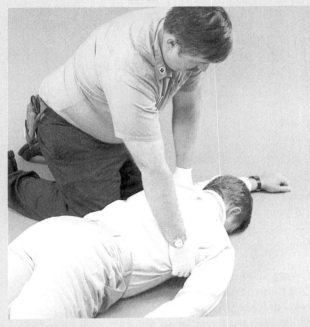

Cradle the head and neck. Grasp under the distant armpit.

3

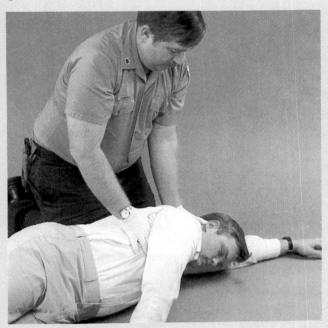

Move the patient as a unit onto his side.

4

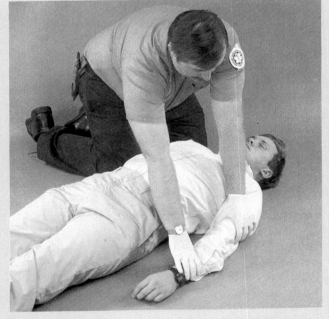

Move the patient onto his back and reposition the extended arm.

FIGURE 4-8

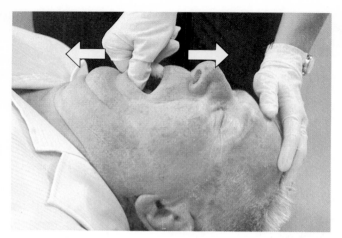

FIGURE 4-9

1. Kneel above and behind your patient.
2. Cross the thumb and forefinger of one hand.
3. Place the thumb on the patient's lower incisors and your forefinger on the upper incisors.
4. Use a scissors motion or finger-snapping motion to open the mouth.

If you can see liquids like vomitus or blood clots inside, suction the patient. If you do not have suction equipment, quickly wipe the fluids away with your index and middle fingers, wrapped in cloth. If you can see solid foreign objects, such as food, broken teeth, or dentures, hook them out with your index finger. Do this quickly. Guard against the patient biting you, gagging, or vomiting.

Use one of the two methods described below to open the airway. Note that the general method is the head-tilt/chin-lift maneuver, unless a cervical spine injury is suspected, then use the jaw–thrust maneuver.

Take special precautions with children. Hyperextending the head and neck can cause a child's supple trachea to collapse more easily than that of an adult. Never tilt an infant's head beyond neutral position. In older children, tilt it only slightly more than the **sniffing position.** A rolled towel under the shoulders may adjust the position enough.

Head-Tilt/Chin-Lift Maneuver

The American Heart Association recommends the head-tilt/chin-lift maneuver if there is no evidence of head or neck trauma. (Figure 4-10).

1. Place the tips of the fingers of one hand underneath the lower jaw on the bony part near the chin. Put the other hand on the patient's forehead, and apply firm backward pressure.
2. Bring the chin forward, supporting the jaw and tilting the head backward as far as possible. *Do not*

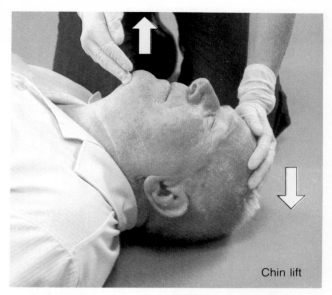

Chin lift

FIGURE 4-10 The head-tilt/chin-lift maneuver.

compress the soft tissues underneath the chin; they might obstruct the airway.

3. Continue to press the other hand on the patient's forehead to keep the head tilted backward.
4. Lift the chin so that the teeth are nearly brought together. (If necessary, you can use your thumb to depress the lower lip; this will keep the patient's mouth slightly open.)
5. If the patient has loose dentures, hold them in position, making obstruction by the lips less likely. If rescue breathing is needed, the mouth-to-mouth seal is easier when dentures are in place. But if the dentures are hard to manage in place, remove them.

Jaw-Thrust Maneuver

If the head-tilt/chin-lift is unsuccessful, or if you suspect a cervical spine injury, forward displacement of the jaw may be necessary. To do this (Figure 4-11):

1. Kneel at the top of the patient's head. Place your elbows on the surface on which the patient is lying, putting your hands at the side of the patient's head.
2. Grasp the patient's lower jaw on both sides where it angles up toward the patient's ears. Move the jaw forward and simultaneously tilt the head backward.
3. Retract the lower lip with your thumb if the lips close.

If you suspect a neck injury, *first* perform the jaw–thrust maneuver *without* the head-tilt/chin-lift. After you have displaced the jawbone forward, support the

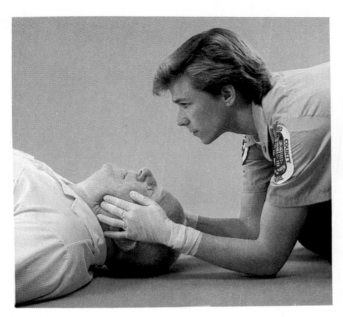

FIGURE 4-11 The jaw thrust.

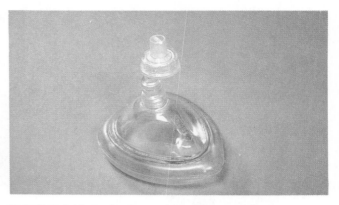

FIGURE 4-12 Pocket face mask with one-way valve.

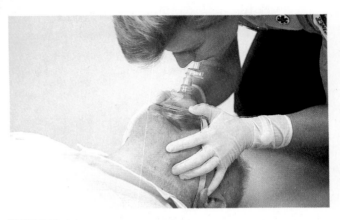

FIGURE 4-13 Providing breaths with a pocket face mask.

head carefully without tilting it backward or turning it from side to side.

If you need to perform ventilation, you will need to keep the head and neck stable with both hands while you are delivering the ventilations.

Breathing

Now that the airway is opened, check to see if the patient is breathing. While maintaining an open airway, place your ear close to the patient's mouth and nose for three to five seconds, and:

- ☐ **LOOK** for the chest rising and falling.
- ☐ **LISTEN** for air escaping during exhalation.
- ☐ **FEEL** for air flow against your cheek.

Be aware that though the patient may make respiratory efforts, the airway may still be obstructed and opening the airway may be the only emergency care needed. Possible reflex gasping respiratory efforts (agonal respirations) also may occur early in the course of primary cardiac arrest and should not be mistaken for adequate breathing.

Provide Rescue Breathing

You do not need any equipment to start rescue breathing — and you should not waste time waiting for supplies or devices. To minimize the risk of contracting an infectious disease, however, use a pocket face-mask with a one-way valve (see instructions on p. 116) or bag-valve-mask unit, and wear gloves, if they are available (see Figures 4-12 and 4-13). Deliver artificial ventilation, and do it at the pace of about twelve breaths per minute (faster for infants and children). The most efficient method is **mouth-to-mouth** or **mouth-to-mask ventilation.** If breathing seems obstructed, repeat the airway-opening maneuver and the two rescue breaths. If signs of effective ventilation are still lacking, assume the patient has upper airway obstruction and proceed to the airway-obstruction maneuvers.

Mouth-to-Mouth or Mouth-to-Mask Ventilation

The atmosphere that we breathe in contains about 21 percent oxygen. Of this 21 percent, only 5 percent is used by the body, and the remaining 16 percent is exhaled. Because the exhaled breath contains about 16 percent oxygen, a patient can be oxygenated using only the EMT's breath.

Use the hand engaged in the head tilt (forehead) to pinch together the patient's nostrils.

Follow these basic procedures for mouth-to-mouth or mouth-to-mask ventilation (Figures 4-14–4-22) and see also section on mouth-to-mask ventilation:

1. Open your mouth wide, take in a deep breath, and cover the patient's entire mouth with your mouth or place your mouth on the mask's chimney, forming a tight seal; then give two initial ventilations at 1.5 to 2 seconds per ventilation. Allow for full exhalations between ventilations and for completely refilling your own lungs after each breath. Use

Basic Life Support: Artificial Ventilation **89**

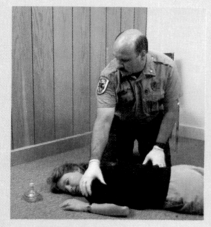

FIGURE 4-14 Position a patient who is not suspected of having a spinal injury on his or her back.

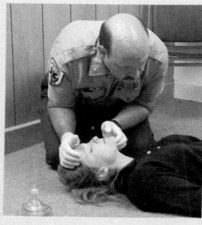

FIGURE 4-15 Open the airway by the head-tilt/chin-lift maneuver. Use two fingers just under the mandible, not on the soft part under the chin.

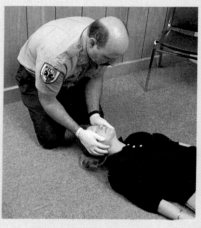

FIGURE 4-16 Open the airway by the jaw–thrust maneuver, if you suspect spinal injury.

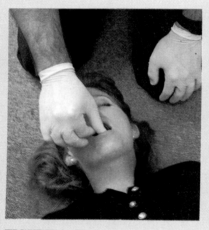

FIGURE 4-17 If the patient's mouth remains closed, open it with the cross-finger technique.

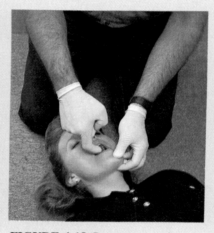

FIGURE 4-18 Remove any obstructions from the mouth if they are visible.

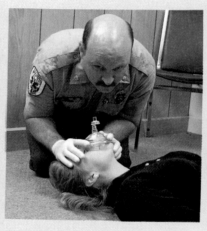

FIGURE 4-19 Establish breathlessness with the Look-Listen-Feel method, 3 to 5 seconds.

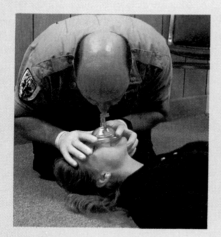

FIGURE 4-20 Perform mouth-to-mouth (mouth-to-mask) ventilation. Give two successive full breaths of air.

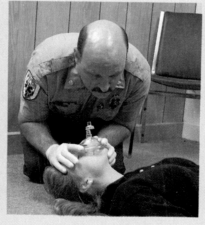

FIGURE 4-21 Observe passive exhalation by the patient.

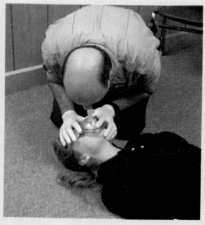

FIGURE 4-22 Or provide mouth-to-nose ventilation.

full, slow breaths. If you hurry or blow too hard, you will blow air into the stomach, which may cause a condition called **gastric distention,** which will almost certainly cause vomiting and the risk of aspiration (sucking vomitus into the lungs).

2. Remove your mouth and turn your head toward the patient's chest each time you take a breath. With your peripheral vision, watch the patient's chest rise, and with your head turned you can watch it fall.

3. Give these first ventilations in succession, allowing for deflation between ventilations. Remove your mouth, look at the patient's chest and abdomen, and let him or her exhale passively. Feel for exhaled breath on your cheek.

4. If you must use the jaw thrust, continue to hold the lower lip down with your thumb and forefinger; press your cheek against the patient's nostrils to seal them off. Form a tight seal over the mouth while you hold the lip down.

5. If you cannot blow air into the lungs, reposition the patient's airway and try again. The most common cause of difficulty with ventilation is improper positioning of the head and chin. If the second try also fails, assume that the airway is blocked by a foreign object and follow the instructions under "Emergency Care for Obstruction by a Foreign Object," pp. 94–95.

6. After the first successful ventilations, give one breath every five seconds, or approximately twelve per minute.

7. To assess whether breathing has recurred spontaneously, put your ear about an inch above the patient's mouth and nose and listen carefully, watching the patient's chest and abdomen for movement at the same time. Hearing the movement of air or feeling a breath against your ear is more reliable than body movement. A patient's chest and abdomen could rise and fall considerably in the struggle to breathe but it is possible that no air will be exchanged. Furthermore, a patient can breathe with relatively little perceptible chest movement.

8. The most common problems with the mouth-to-mouth technique are: (1) failure to form a tight seal over the patient's mouth; often, you are pushing too hard; (2) failure to pinch the nose completely closed; (3) failure to keep an open airway because the patient's head is not positioned correctly; (4) failure to have the patient's mouth open wide enough to receive ventilations adequately; and (5) failure to clear the upper airway of obstructions.

Mouth-to-Nose Ventilation

Use **mouth-to-nose ventilation** when the patient's mouth cannot be opened, when it is seriously injured, or when you cannot achieve a tight mouth-to-mouth seal.

1. Place one hand on the forehead, and tilt the patient's head backward. With your other hand, lift the lower jaw forward to seal the lips.

2. Take a deep breath, and place your mouth over the patient's nostrils, forming a tight seal.

3. Breath slowly into the nostrils for 1.5 to 2 seconds until you feel the lungs expand or see the patient's chest rise.

4. Remove your mouth and make sure that air is escaping through the patient's nostrils; the chest should fall as exhalation occurs. If the patient is not exhaling enough, open the mouth to let air escape.

5. If you use the jaw thrust, keep the jaw in place with your hand, and seal the mouth with your cheek.

Ventilating Infants and Children

The technique for ventilating infants and children varies only slightly. If the patient is an infant or a small child:

1. Gently open the airway. Tilt the head to the neutral + position or only as much as necessary since you can actually obstruct (kink) a child's airway (Figure 4-23).

2. Cover the patient's nose and mouth with a tight seal during inhalation (Figure 4-24).

3. Deliver only small breaths or puffs of air — just enough to make the chest rise.

4. The breathing rate for infants (one month to one year) is once every three seconds; for a child (one to eight years), once every three seconds; and for a child above eight years, once every five seconds, the same as for an adult.

A child's smaller air passages provide a greater resistance to airflow; therefore, your blowing pressure will probably be greater than you would assume.

Mouth-to-Stoma Ventilation

Some people have all or part of their larynx removed through surgery (**laryngectomy**). A patient who has had a laryngectomy has a permanent opening (**stoma**) in the neck and breathes through the stoma. The stoma is usually in the center, in front, and at the base of the neck.

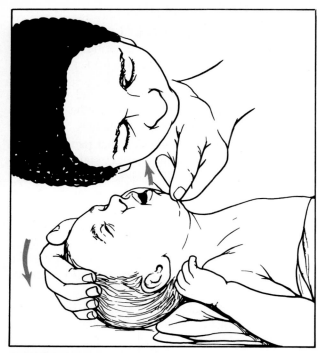

FIGURE 4-23 Head-tilt/chin-lift.

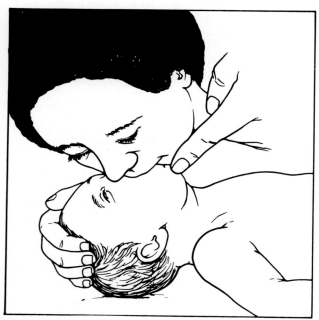

FIGURE 4-24 Mouth-to-mouth and nose seal.

Sometimes there will be other openings in the neck, depending on the kind of surgery done on the patient, but the stoma is the only one pertinent to artificial ventilation and is almost always the only one on the midline (see Figure 4-25). To perform artificial ventilation (Figure 4-26):

1. Remove all coverings (i.e., scarves, ties, etc.) from the stoma area.

2. Clear the stoma of any foreign matter. Do not remove the tube. Clean the neck opening of mucous or foreign matter with a gauze pad or a handkerchief, not tissue. Pass a sterile suction catheter tube through the stoma and into the trachea no more than three to five inches and suction enough to partially open the airway. It is not necessary to open the tube completely to begin ventilation.

3. You will not need to perform a head tilt on a patient with a stoma. Keep the patient's head straight and the shoulders slightly elevated. Place your pocket face-mask over the stoma or breathe directly into the stoma, forming a seal with your mouth. (Mouth-to-stoma ventilation is bacteriologically cleaner than mouth-to-mouth ventilation, but you may still be exposed to infectious diseases.) Or, breathe through the **tracheostomy tube** in the stoma if there is one. Blow slowly through the stoma for 1.5 to 2 seconds, using just enough force to cause the patient's chest to rise.

4. Watch for the patient's chest to fall, and feel to make sure that the air is escaping back through the stoma during the exhalation.

5. If the chest does not rise, suspect a **partial neck breather.** Seal the nose and mouth with one hand so that air will not leak out the mouth or nose, and repeat the process. Pinch off the nose between the third and fourth fingers; seal the lips with the palm of the hand; place the thumb under the chin, and press upward and backward. Repeat ventilations.

Mouth-to-Mask Ventilation

In most parts of the country, EMT protocols require the use of pocket face-masks, usually with one-way valves and sometimes with an additional inlet for supplemental oxygen. These masks are made of soft materials and fit easily in a pocket. You supply ventilation by breathing through a chimney on the mask.

Advantages of the mouth-to-mask ventilation are:

1. It cuts down on the risk of contracting an infectious disease by preventing direct contact with the patient's saliva, mucous, vomitus, and blood.

2. It reduces the effort required to keep an airway open. You can use both hands to maintain the proper head-tilt while keeping a good seal between the mask and the patient's face.

3. Because the mask is transparent, you can see the color of the patient's lips, whether there is any vomiting, and whether the patient has resumed breathing.

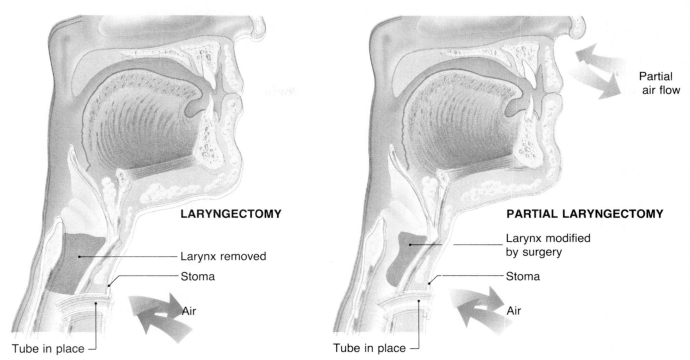

LARYNGECTOMY

Larynx removed

Stoma

Air

Tube in place

PARTIAL LARYNGECTOMY

Partial air flow

Larynx modified by surgery

Stoma

Air

Tube in place

FIGURE 4-25 The neck breather's airway has been changed by surgery.

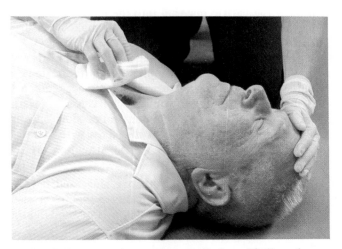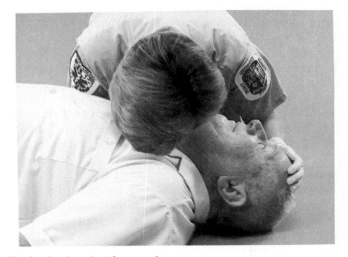

FIGURE 4-26 Mouth-to-stoma ventilations. If allowed, use a pediatric-sized pocket face mask.

Some masks are designed to be used one way on an adult and inverted for use on a child; however, some manufacturers no longer recommend this method. Know the manufacturer's specifications for the mask you are using. Be aware that masks are also available in infant sizes as well; serious communicable diseases are not limited to adults.

Follow the procedure already described:

1. Determine if the patient is unconscious.

2. Activate the EMS system, if necessary.

3. Position the patient properly.

4. Open an airway, and, if necessary, clean it.

5. If ventilation is necessary, kneel at the top of the patient's head and position the mask on the patient's face so that the upper tip of the triangle extends to the bridge of the patient's nose while the base is settled between the lower lip and the chin.

6. Hold the mask in place firmly and simultaneously maintain the proper head-tilt. Please both thumbs at the dome of the mask over the chin. Apply pressure to both sides of the mask.

7. Use your index, third, and fourth fingers to grasp the patient's lower jaw between the earlobe and

Basic Life Support: Artificial Ventilation **93**

the angle of the jaw. Lift it forward. With your palms or the heels of your hand, apply pressure to the patient's temples to keep the head tilted back.

8. Breathe into the mask, then lift your head and check for passive exhalation. Follow the directions already given for rates of respiration.

9. If you are doing both mouth-to-mask breathing and chest compressions, strap the mask to the patient's face and work from the side of the head.

Car Accident Victims

There are special problems if you need to provide ventilation for the victims of automobile accidents who are still in their vehicles. Artificial ventilation works best, as we have said, when the patient is lying down; but a patient who is not breathing requires immediate assistance.

If you suspect spine or neck injuries and if the patient is lying down, use the jaw-thrust maneuver and mouth-to-mask or mouth-to-nose techniques already described. Use your cheek to seal either the mouth or nose. You should tilt the head very slightly, if and only if the airway will not open and if you feel strong resistance to your efforts to ventilate.

If you suspect spine or neck injuries and the patient is slumped forward or has been thrown backward, do not try to reseat him or her. If you are alone, cradle the patient's head by wrapping one arm around the top of the head and hold the chin in your hand while you slide the patient to his or her back. If you have help, one of you should hold the patient's head and neck in line with both your hands and forearms. Be aware that these maneuvers will not and cannot fully protect the spine; but if the patient is not breathing, death is certain.

If the patient is seated and you do not suspect spinal or neck injuries, lay the patient flat or, if this is not possible, cradle the patient with his or her neck on your upper arm, letting the head tilt back slightly. If the patient is lodged in the front seat in a way that prevents easy access, go to the rear seat and deliver mouth-to-mask or mouth-to-mouth ventilation from this location.

Gastric Distention

During artificial ventilation, it is common for air to get into the esophagus and therefore into the stomach. Gastric distention (inflation) happens most often in children and in airway-obstructed patients when you have exerted excessive pressure while blowing air into the patient's mouth or nose. If the distention is slight, you can safely ignore it. However, a larger quantity is dangerous because it can make the patient vomit and can force up the diaphragm, limiting the amount of air that the lungs can hold.

You can minimize gastric distention by avoiding the common mistakes in administering ventilation:

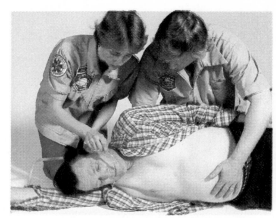

FIGURE 4-27 Relieving gastric distention and suctioning the patient.

- Ventilating the patient too forcefully. Stop when the chest rises, thus not blowing forcefully enough to open the esophagus.
- Not keeping the head tilted, when appropriate.
- Not allowing deflation between the first two ventilations.

If you hear any gurgling or bubbling while you are ventilating a patient, stop resuscitation immediately or you will blow the gastric material into the lungs.

Reposition the head and neck to make sure that the airway is open.

The American Heart Association recommends *not* relieving gastric distention by pressing on the abdomen because of the danger of aspirating stomach contents into the lungs. Aspirated vomitus can cause a severe chemical pneumonia. Attempt **decompression** only if the distention is so great that it interferes with ventilation. Procedures for relieving gastric distention are as follows:

1. Turn the patient's body to one side, and have a suction device at hand, if readily available, in case the patient vomits and begins to aspirate (Figure 4-27).

2. Use the flat of your hand to exert moderate pressure on the patient's abdomen between the navel and rib cage.

3. After the vomiting has occurred, quickly wipe the mouth out with 4 × 4 gauze pads, suction any remaining vomitus out of the airway, wipe off the face, and return to resuscitation.

□ OBSTRUCTED AIRWAY EMERGENCIES

Any agent that causes upper airway obstruction blocks either the nasal passages, the **oropharynx,** or the **laryngopharynx.** Lower airway obstruction can be

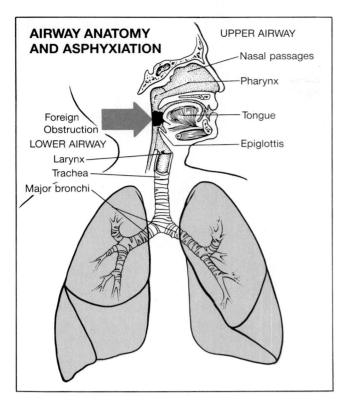

AIRWAY ANATOMY AND ASPHYXIATION

UPPER AIRWAY
Nasal passages
Pharynx
Tongue
Epiglottis

Foreign Obstruction
LOWER AIRWAY
Larynx
Trachea
Major bronchi

FIGURE 4-28 The structure most commonly responsible for upper airway obstruction is the tongue. The type of foreign object that most frequently causes lower airway obstruction is food. Another common cause of obstruction is acute epiglottitis, which is more frequently seen in children than in adults. Do not overlook nasal obstruction as a cause of upper airway obstruction in infants who are nasal breathers rather than mouth breathers.

caused by breathing in foreign materials or by a severe bronchospasm (Figure 4-28). In any case, the airway will need to be cleared so that the patient can breathe efficiently.

Causes of Airway Obstruction

If your patient is unresponsive, try ventilating the lungs first. If a foreign object is present, it will become evident when your efforts to ventilate the lungs fail. The most common source of upper airway obstruction is the tongue.

Foreign bodies may also obstruct the lower airway. According to the National Safety Council, an annual estimated 3,900 people choked on a foreign object and died in 1989.

You should strongly suspect food choking if the patient had been eating or had anything in his or her mouth prior to collapsing. Elderly people are at particular risk for food choking because they have a slower gag reflex and are more frequently misdiagnosed as having coronary disease if they collapse. The typical victim of the so-called **cafe coronary** is middle-aged or elderly and is commonly a denture wearer. He has usually had a few drinks, which both **depress** his protective reflexes and adversely affect his judgment about the size of bites he is taking. When the piece of solid food, often a chunk of meat, lodges in the airway, the patient becomes completely **aphonic** (unable to talk, breathe, groan, cough, or cry out). He may try to get up and walk from the table or may pitch forward, all in complete silence, and is usually cyanotic (blue).

Other causes of upper airway obstruction include **blood clots** that are the result of trauma or surgery, cancerous conditions of the mouth or throat, **tonsil** enlargement, injury to the face or jaw, acute **epiglottitis,** aspirated vomitus, and broken dental bridges. Nasal passage obstruction may be a cause of upper airway obstruction in infants who can breath only through their noses.

When possible, educate people to prevent choking by following these steps:

- Avoid excessive intake of alcohol before and during meals.
- Cut food into small bite-size pieces.
- Chew slowly and thoroughly; this precaution is especially important for denture wearers.
- Avoid talking and laughing during chewing and swallowing.
- Teach children not to put foreign objects in their mouths.
- Do not allow children to run about when they are eating.

□ Emergency Care for Obstruction by a Foreign Object

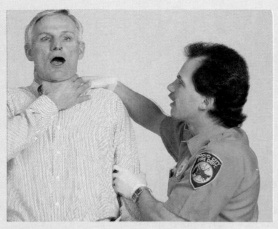

FIGURE 4-29 The universal sign of choking. Ask the patient, "Are you choking?"

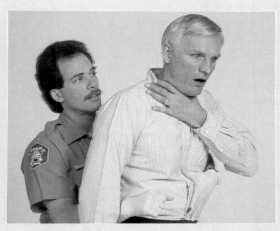

FIGURE 4-30 Positioning of the fist, thumb side in, for the abdominal thrust.

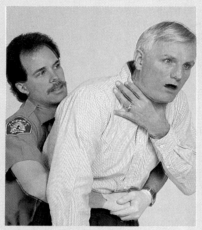

FIGURE 4-31 Administering the abdominal thrust on a standing patient.

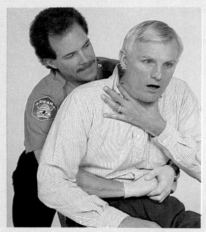

FIGURE 4-32 Administering the abdominal thrust to a sitting patient.

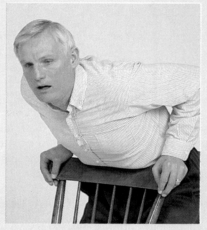

FIGURE 4-33 The choking victim performing an abdominal thrust on self.

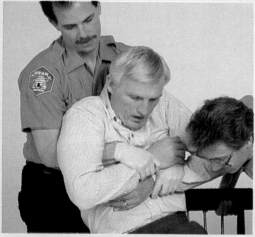

FIGURE 4-34 Remove an unconscious, sitting patient from the chair and lay him or her face-up on the floor.

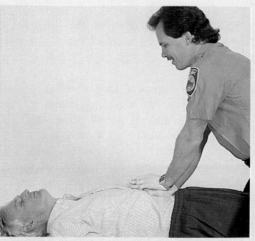

FIGURE 4-35 Performing abdominal thrusts on an unconscious patient.

Signs and Symptoms of Airway Obstruction

Sudden respiratory failure can be caused by conditions other than choking; for instance, fainting, stroke, heart attack, epilepsy, an obstructing **tumor, laryngeal edema,** or drug overdose; but these emergencies are managed differently. It is important to recognize foreign-body airway obstruction quickly. The following signs will help you.

- Audible, noisy breathing, or no breath sounds. If the patient is conscious, you can ask, "Are you choking?" A patient with airway obstruction will be able to nod but unable to speak or cough. A person having a heart attack will usually be able to speak or whisper.
- Labored use of muscles required in breathing; nostrils are flared; neck and facial muscles are strained.
- Progressive restlessness, anxiety, and confusion.
- Cyanosis: lips and skin turn blue from lack of oxygen.
- Patient becomes unresponsive.

Emergency Care for Partial Obstruction

The most common source of upper airway obstruction is the tongue. (If it partially blocks the airway, your patient will make snoring sounds while breathing.) Reposition the head and neck with the head-tilt/chin-lift maneuver or jaw–thrust maneuver and attempt to ventilate.

A foreign body may cause a partial or complete airway obstruction. If the obstruction is partial, the patient may get some air exchange. If the patient can cough forcefully, air exchange is occurring. Allow the patient time to remove the obstruction himself.

Encourage the patient to cough. Do not interfere with his or her attempts to expel the foreign object, but do *not* leave the patient. Monitor him or her closely, looking for signs of reduced air passage: a weak, ineffective cough, a high-pitched wheeze during inhalation, increased strain in breathing, clutching the throat, and the beginning of cyanosis.

Abdominal thrusts (the Heimlich maneuver) are usually ineffective in dislodging the partially obstructing object and may lodge it further down in the airway. Open the airway if necessary by the head-tilt/chin-lift or jaw–thrust maneuvers, and administer 100 percent oxygen. Transport the patient promptly to a medical facility where the partial obstruction can be removed.

Emergency Care for Complete Obstruction

If the Patient is Conscious

1. Recognize the obstruction, either from your observations or, if you have just arrived, by asking the patient, "Are you choking?" If the patient cannot make a sound, and has one or two hands over his throat, the airway may be blocked (Figure 4-29). If the patient is having a heart attack or another problem, he or she will be able to speak or whisper.

2. Use the **Heimlich maneuver** to clear the airway. (See Figure 4-36.) When this maneuver thrusts the diaphragm quickly upward, it can force enough air from the lungs to create an artificial cough that can dislodge and expel the foreign object (Figures 4-30–4-32).

3. If the patient is standing or sitting, stand behind him or her and wrap your arms around the waist. Keep your elbows out, away from the patient's ribs. Make a fist with one hand, and place the thumb side on the midline of the abdomen slightly above the navel and well below the xiphoid process (Figure 4-30).

FIGURE 4-36 The function of abdominal thrusts for a complete airway obstruction victim.

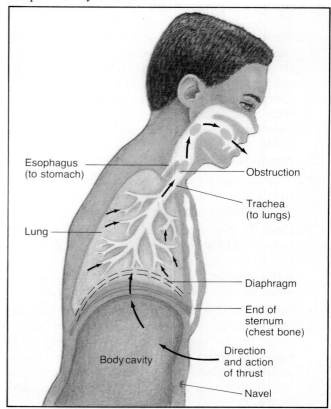

4. Grasp your fist with your other hand, thumbs toward the patient. Press your fist into your patient's abdomen with a quick, inward and upward thrust. If you need to repeat this movement, make each thrust separate and distinct. Continue with up to five thrusts, then reassess airway. Repeat this cycle until the object is released or the patient becomes unconscious.

5. See Figure 4-33 for performing an abdominal thrust on yourself.

6. It may take six to ten thrusts to succeed, but persist. It may take several thrusts to be sure you are delivering the correct pressure. Success often comes later because increasing hypoxia will cause more muscle relaxation in the patient. This may cause the obstructed airway to become only partially obstructed, thereby making the foreign object easier to remove.

7. Be aware of these dangers: (1) If you are improperly positioned or perform the thrusts too rapidly and too forcefully, you may lose your balance and fall into the patient; (2) if your hands are too high (on the lower edges of the rib cage), you can cause internal ruptures or lacerations; and (3) the maneuver will often cause vomiting. Correct hand placement and the correct amount of force can help minimize this danger.

If the Patient Is Unconscious or Becomes Unconscious

1. Place the patient on his or her back, face up, if the patient was unconscious when you arrived, and go through the assessment and breathing steps of rescue breathing (p. 90). Perform a finger sweep by using the tongue jaw lift to open the mouth and, with your index finger, sweep deeply into the mouth to remove a foreign body (see Figure 4-37). Attempt ventilations. If unsuccessful, prepare to perform abdominal thrusts.

2. Straddle the patients thighs or close to the patient's hips. If the patient is very large or you are small, straddle one leg only.

3. Place the heel of one hand on the midline of the patient's abdomen, between the xiphoid process and umbilicus (navel.) Put your second hand directly over the first. Spread and lift your fingers to avoid applying too much pressure to the ribs.

4. Lock your elbows and, exerting pressure from the shoulders, press downward and forward with a quick thrust (Figure 4-35). Your body weight will make the thrust more energetic. (Take care to avoid the xiphoid process. Putting pressure on it may lacerate vital organs.) Perform five abdominal thrusts.

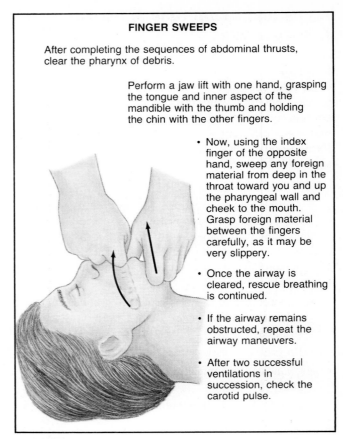

FINGER SWEEPS

After completing the sequences of abdominal thrusts, clear the pharynx of debris.

Perform a jaw lift with one hand, grasping the tongue and inner aspect of the mandible with the thumb and holding the chin with the other fingers.

- Now, using the index finger of the opposite hand, sweep any foreign material from deep in the throat toward you and up the pharyngeal wall and cheek to the mouth. Grasp foreign material between the fingers carefully, as it may be very slippery.

- Once the airway is cleared, rescue breathing is continued.

- If the airway remains obstructed, repeat the airway maneuvers.

- After two successful ventilations in succession, check the carotid pulse.

FIGURE 4-37

5. If this action does not dislodge the foreign body, open the patient's mouth by gripping the tongue and lower jaw between the thumb and fingers of one hand and shift the jawbone forward. This will draw the tongue away from the back of the throat and may partially relieve the obstruction.

6. Perform finger sweeps (Figure 4-37). Insert the index finger of your other hand along the cheek and deep into the throat to the base of the tongue with a slow, careful hooking motion. Use this maneuver only on an unconscious patient. A conscious patient will gag. Never use it on a baby, since the foreign body may be pushed farther back in the throat and cause further obstruction.

7. Be careful not to force the object deeper into the airway. You may have to push the object against the opposite side of the throat to dislodge it. Hook it up into the mouth where you can remove it. Remove dentures if they are present and are causing difficulties.

8. If the foreign object is still not expelled, open the airway and perform mouth-to-mouth resuscitation. If you cannot succeed in providing ventilation, repeat the cycle of abdominal thrusts, the finger sweep, and resuscitation again.

If the Patient Is Pregnant or Obese and Conscious

1. In the advanced stages of pregnancy, or in a particularly obese patient, there is no room between the rib cage and the expanding uterus or the abdomen to perform the Heimlich maneuver.
2. With the patient standing or sitting, stand behind him or her with your arms directly under the armpits. Wrap your arms around the chest.
3. Position the thumb side of your fist on the middle of the breastbone. If you are near the margins of the rib cage, you are too low.
4. Seize your fist firmly with your other hand and thrust backward sharply.
5. Repeat until the object is expelled or the patient becomes unresponsive. (See Figures 4-38–4-41.)

□ A Pregnant or Obese Choking Victim

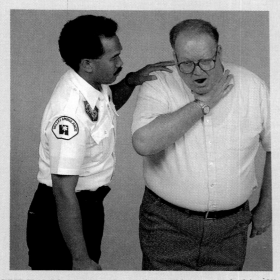

FIGURE 4-38 Asking the patient, "Are you choking?"

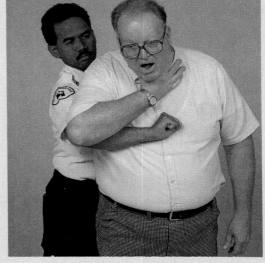

FIGURE 4-39 Position the thumb side of your fist on the middle of the patient's breastbone or sternum.

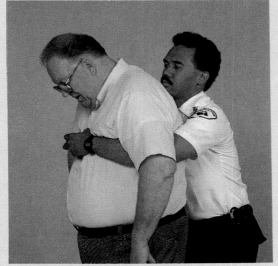

FIGURE 4-40 Seize your fist firmly with your other hand and thrust backward sharply.

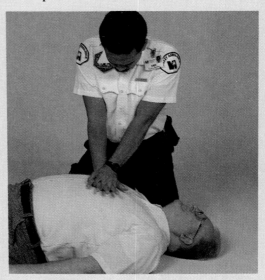

FIGURE 4-41 If the patient becomes unconscious, lie him or her on his or her back and perform chest thrusts.

If the patient is or becomes unresponsive:

1. Place the patient on his or her back and kneel beside or straddle him or her.

2. Place the heel of your hand directly over the *lower* one-half of the breastbone.

3. Give distinct, separate thrusts downward and forward (Figure 4-42).

After the foreign object is removed, transport the patient to the emergency room. The airway may close again from edema. The patient should also be routinely evaluated for a fractured rib or sternum, or a ruptured liver or spleen. All of these complications are possible results of the Heimlich maneuver.

Obstructed Airway in Children and Infants

More than 90 percent of the **pediatric** fatalities resulting from foreign bodies occur in children under the age of five. Sixty-five percent occur in infants.

Remember that, compared to an adult, an infant has a proportionately larger tongue, a larger and stiffer glottis, and concave vocal cords. Infants under the age of eight months breathe only through their noses.

FIGURE 4-42

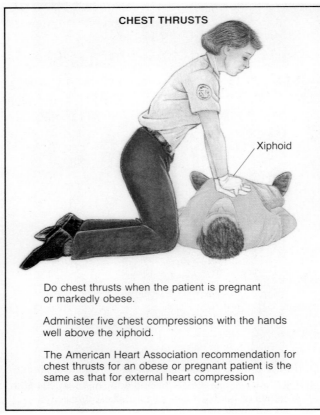

CHEST THRUSTS

Xiphoid

Do chest thrusts when the patient is pregnant or markedly obese.

Administer five chest compressions with the hands well above the xiphoid.

The American Heart Association recommendation for chest thrusts for an obese or pregnant patient is the same as that for external heart compression

In a great majority of cases, cardiopulmonary arrest in childen results from respiratory arrest, while cardiac arrest usually occurs first in adults. You will need to ventilate children in many of these emergencies: aspirating foreign objects (toys, food, and other items); poisoning, drug overdose, airway infections, near-drowning, and sudden infant death syndrome (SIDS). For the purpose of CPR, an infant is a child under the age of twelve months. A child above eight years of age can usually be resuscitated using the same techniques as for adults.

The narrowest part of a child's airway is not at the level of the vocal cords, but the **cricoid cartilage** below the cords. This is true of children up to age twelve. Below the vocal cords, the airway is lined with a loose mucous membrane that can be easily inflamed or bruised, with resultant swelling.

Overextending a child's neck can occlude the trachea more easily than in an adult. Tilt an infant's head to neutral position or neutral + (until breaths go in easily). In older children, tilt it only slightly more than sniffing position.

For partial obstruction — and assuming no cervical or spinal injuries — place the child on his or her right side so that secretions, blood, and vomit can drain out to the mouth. The jaw will also fall forward, bringing the tongue and epiglottis away from the airway.

For the conscious, choking infant under twelve months:

1. Assess the airway. Perform the following procedures only if the obstruction is a foreign body. If obstruction is caused by airway swelling from infection or disease, transport the patient immediately to a medical facility. Also transport if the patient is still conscious but having breathing difficulties. *If the infant is choking and coughing but still breathing, let him or her try to expel the foreign object before taking the following steps.*

2. Straddle the infant over one arm with the face down and the head lower than the trunk at about a sixty-degree angle. With the heel of your other hand, deliver five **back blows** rapidly (within three to five seconds) between the shoulder blades. The blows should be forceful, but remember that this is an infant (Figure 4-43). The reason for doing back blows first is that there is some risk of injuring an infant's liver with chest thrusts.

3. While supporting the infant's head, sandwich the body between your hands and turn the patient on his or her ·back, with the head lower than the trunk. Lay the infant on your thigh or over your lap with the head supported. Deliver five slow, firm thrusts in the midsternal region in the same manner as for external chest compressions (Figure 4-44).

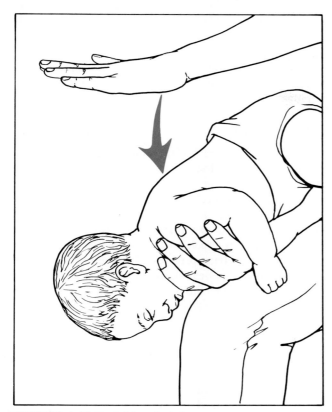

FIGURE 4-43 Back blow in infant.

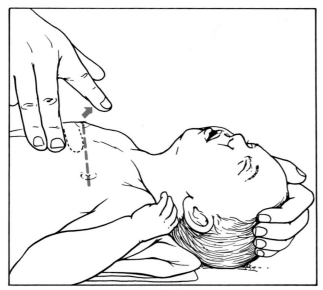

FIGURE 4-44 Locating the finger position for chest thrusts in infant.

4. Repeat steps 2 and 3 until the obstruction is expelled or the infant becomes unconscious.

Do not use blind finger sweeps and probes with infants and children. You must see the obstruction before trying to grasp it with your fingers. For infants and small children, use your little finger.

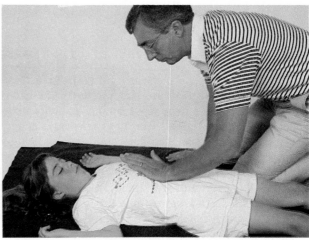

FIGURE 4-45 Performing abdominal thrusts on a child lying down. For a larger child, place other hand on top of first hand, as in an adult.

For the unresponsive nonbreathing infant:

1. Open the airway.
2. Attempt ventilation. If unsuccessful, reposition the head and try again.
3. Deliver five back blows within three to five seconds.
4. Deliver five chest thrusts within three to five seconds.
5. Perform a jaw-thrust maneuver to check for a foreign body. Do *not* perform a blind finger sweep. Remove the foreign body only if visible.
6. Reattempt ventilation and repeat steps 2 to 5 as necessary.

In a child over one year, use the same techniques as for an adult with the following modifications:

1. Kneel beside, not astride, a child lying down. Use one hand, rather than both hands (Figure 4-45).
2. Be sure to direct the thrusts at the midline of the abdomen, and not to either side. (See Chapter 31 for more information on pediatric breathing difficulties).

□ COMMON MEDICAL CONDITIONS THAT CAUSE RESPIRATORY EMERGENCIES

Although this chapter has focused on the kinds of accidents and trauma that cause respiratory emergencies and require airway management, you should also be familiar with the five most common medical conditions that can also result in airway failure.

Asthma

More than 9 million Americans suffer from asthma. About 50 percent of them are children under the age of ten, with a 52 percent increase among patients under eighteen during the 1980s. Twice as many boys as girls are afflicted, with urban and black children also being at higher risk. The fatality rate for children under fourteen doubled between 1977 and 1983. After the age of thirty, the gender ratios are approximately equal. The overall rate of death from asthma grew 23 percent between 1980 and 1985, most probably as a result of increased environmental pollution.

Symptoms include dyspnea, difficulty in breathing, and chest tightness. The patient will often wheeze audibly while expiring and have a very long exhalation phase. The patient may be extremely fatigued, able to speak only a word or two at a time, be dehydrated from the increase in respiration rate, and be coughing up a white, sticky sputum.

Procedure:

1. Assuming that it is not a life-threatening emergency, obtain a medical history. Pay particular attention to the patient's medications.
2. Auscultate the breath sounds. A patient with chronic asthma who has a silent chest is on the verge of respiratory arrest.
3. Check the skin for cyanosis, although this is not so reliable a sign as respiratory status.
4. Administer humidified oxygen with a bag-valve-mask or nonrebreathing mask to increase arterial oxygen saturation.

Chronic Bronchitis

More than 17 million Americans suffer from chronic bronchitis, often in association with emphysema. It is nearly always caused by cigarette smoking and afflicts more men than women. It is most common in adults between forty-five and sixty-five. The irritated brochial tubes overproduce mucous, and the cilia that sweep the bronchial tubes are damaged. As a result, the small airways are swollen, the patient chronically retains carbon dioxide and suffers persistently from mild oxygen shortage and cyanosis. Such patients are extremely susceptible to respiratory infection and, in acute emergency cases, are candidates for **septic shock.**

The treatment of choice is supplemental high-flow oxygen during transport. Also be prepared to use a bag-valve-mask (see Chapter 5). Depending on local protocols, you may also need to apply a heart monitor and start an IV as well.

Because the rate and depth of respiration are controlled primarily by carbon dioxide levels in the blood and secondarily by oxygen levels, some texts warn against "erasing" the respiratory drive by supplemental oxygen. Always give supplemental oxygen and be prepared to ventilate.

Emphysema

Emphysema is caused by irreversible destruction of the alveoli, which characteristically assume a rounded shape, rather than the normal "cauliflower" look. This condition causes decreased flexibility, collapsed alveoli, and a lower surface available for oxygen–carbon-dioxide exchange. To keep the collapsed alvioli inflated, the chronic emphysemic patient purses his lips during exhalation to create a back pressure. The patient seldom has a cyanotic look, but develops a barrel chest as a result of constantly using the intracostal muscles for breathing. The treatment is the same as for chronic bronchitis.

Pneumonia

Pneumonia is still the fifth-leading cause of death for Americans, even though it can usually be treated successfully. It results from an infection or inflammation of the lung tissue caused by infection, fungi, chemicals, and aspiration.

The symptoms of bacterial pneumonia include a shaking chill, a persistent temperature above 102°, a hacking cough that produces sputum, and pleuritic chest pain. The patient has often had a recent upper respiratory infection.

Viral pneumonia can accompany influenza and immunosuppression treatments (as for organ transplant or cancer therapy) or AIDS. Alcoholism, cancer (especially lung cancer), and sickle-cell anemia increase the risk of pneumonia. A leading cause of death in trauma patients is aspiration pneumonia.

You should treat pneumonia cases conservatively with oxygen. Since pneumonia patients can become septic quickly, however, you should monitor them closely.

Pulmonary Embolism

Pulmonary embolism affects an estimated 6 million Americans, and 40,000 die from it annually. Since it quickly causes respiratory collapse, it is often mistaken for cardiac arrest. Prime candidates are women who both smoke and take oral contraceptives.

Sometimes the symptoms are a deceptively mild dyspnea. Other potential symptoms (often not all present or not all present simultaneously) are pleuritic chest pain, **hemoptysis,** and dyspnea in about 25 percent of the patients. Because the emboli form in the feet or legs about 75 percent of the time, phlebitis is a common cause. In these cases, flexing the ankle causes calf pain.

The treatment should include high-flow oxygen and EKG-monitoring, if possible, during transport.

Hyperventilation

The symptoms of **hyperventilation** overlap with those of pulmonary embolism, so take them seriously. Furthermore, hyperventilation is also commonly caused by diabetic ketoacidosis. Until you have ruled out this possible problem, do not use the common treatment of breathing into a paper bag.

Rebreathing carbon dioxide reduces oxygen to the brain, causes **vasodilation** around the respiratory center, removes the excess carbon dioxide from the center, and slows the breathing.

chapter 5

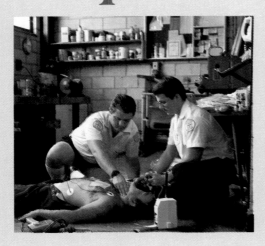

Ventilation Equipment and Oxygen Therapy

✱ OBJECTIVES

- Define hypoxia and the need for supplemental oxygen by some patients.
- Demonstrate how to insert oropharyngeal and nasopharyngeal airways correctly.
- Correctly use both portable and fixed suction units.
- Describe the need for supplemental oxygen and demonstrate how to properly and safely deliver it with oxygen equipment, including cannulae and masks.
- Identify the hazards of supplemental oxygen.

It is recommended that EMTs wear protective gloves whenever there is a possibility of coming in contact with a patient's blood, body fluids, mucous membranes, traumatic wounds, or sores. See Chapter 31.

Hypoxia develops when the body is underoxygenated, and is nearly always a danger when the patient needs assisted ventilations and cardiac compression. Even though the amount of oxygen entering the body is theoretically sufficient, external chest compression at best produces only 25 to 30 percent of the normal heart activity, so the oxygen delivered to the vital organs is inadequate. You should always deliver 100 percent concentrations of oxygen to any patient who has had a cardiopulmonary arrest.

Causes of hypoxia include:

1. Respiratory insufficiency, a condition in which the the alveoli receive too little oxygen.
2. Circulatory insufficiency, a condition in which the blood flow is dangerously reduced.
3. Hemoglobin insufficiency, a condition in which the red blood cells do not carry sufficient hemoglobin.
4. Cellular exchange problems. Poisons like cyanide prevent oxygen exchange between the bloodstream and the cells. Drug and alcohol abuse have the same effect.

Although basic life support needs no mechanical ventilatory aids, such aids may provide the EMT with valuable advantages. The use of supplementary oxygen may make a big difference in the saving of a life.

☐ THE USE OF AIRWAY ADJUNCTS

Airway and oxygen equipment can be excellent tools for well-trained EMTs in certain situations. It is important, however, to:

- Not wait for airway and oxygen equipment to arrive before beginning emergency care.
- Not depend on mechanical devices entirely, for they may fail.

There are two types of artificial airways: oropharyngeal, which pass through the mouth, or nasopharyngeal, which pass through the nose. The airways extend down to but do not pass through the larynx. Keep in mind that:

- The equipment must be clean and in good operational use.
- The proper equipment and correct size must be selected.
- These devices can be used only on an unconscious patient.

- The patient must be monitored continually and carefully. If the patient begins to regain consciousness, gags, or vomits, remove the equipment immediately.

Oropharyngeal Airway

The **oropharyngeal airway** (Figure 5-1), a semicircular device made of hard plastic or rubber helps prevent the tongue or jaw from falling backward and allows sufficient drainage or suction of secretions in the deeply unconscious patient. The oropharyngeal airway may be used initially when working on an unresponsive patient. Do not use this device on responsive or semiconscious patients, because it may cause vomiting or spasm of the vocal cords.

If you choose the wrong length or put it in the wrong way, you could cause vomiting or even force the tongue back into the pharynx.

The airway set should consist of multiple infant, child, and adult sizes. This type of airway is easy to insert with minimal friction and is usually rigid enough to hold the base of the tongue in a forward position.

The procedures for inserting the airway are as follows (Figure 5-2):

1. Select the proper size. The airway should extend from the center of the patient's mouth to the angle of the lower jaw. Before you insert the airway, hold it next to the patient's lower face to check for proper size. *Do not* use an airway of incorrect size. If you select an airway that is too long, you can force air into the esophagus, causing hypoventilation or laryngospasm of the trachea.
2. Ventilate the patient for thirty seconds.

FIGURE 5-1 The oropharyngeal airway helps prevent the jaw or tongue from obstructing breathing. These airways have a reinforced bite block and permit access of a suction catheter.

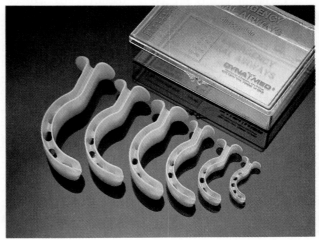

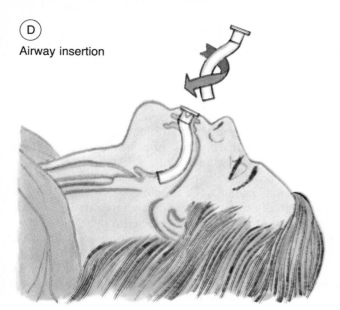

Ⓓ
Airway insertion

FIGURE 5-2 The oropharyngeal airway.
Step A:
Open mouth with cross-finger technique.
Step B:
Insert airway in a backward position as it enters the mouth.
Step C:
Rotate airway into proper position.
Step D:
Airway in position.

3. Open the patient's mouth by using the cross-finger technique (see Chapter 4).

4. Insert the airway with the tip facing upward, or toward the roof of the patient's mouth.

5. When the airway contacts the **soft palate,** gently continue to insert the airway while rotating it 180 degrees. Continue inserting until the flange rests on the patient's lips. The curve of the airway follows the patient's tongue.

Performing this procedure requires practice, because it is done primarily by feel as well as by vision.

Note: If the tongue gets in the way during insertion of the airway, use the jaw thrust maneuver. This will move the tongue forward and allow correct insertion of the airway.

Once the airway is in place, position the nontrauma patient on his or her side to decrease the possibility of aspiration if vomiting occurs. If you suspect any spinal injuries, leave the patient in the supine position.

Remove the airway when the patient can swallow, regains consciousness, or tries to dislodge it. Remove the airway by gently pulling it out and down. Follow the mouth's natural curvature.

Nasopharyngeal Airway

Nasopharyngeal airways (Figure 5-3) are curved hollow tubes made of soft rubber or plastic with a flare at the top end. Their use is increasing because they are less likely to stimulate vomiting and may be used on a responsive patient who cannot maintain an open airway.

Due to the risk of infection, do not use this device if the patient is bleeding from the nose or cerebrospinal fluid is draining nasally.

FIGURE 5-3 Inserting lubricated nasopharyngeal airway.

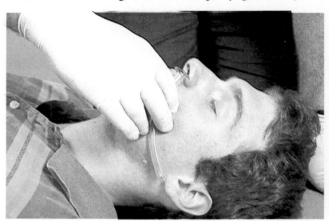

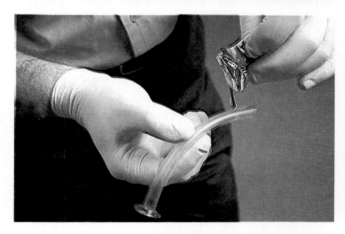

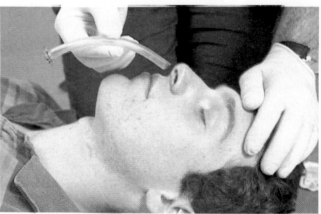

The procedures for inserting this airway are as follows:

1. Select the proper size. The length of the tube should approximate the distance from the tip of the patient's nose to the earlobe. Sizes are measured by internal diameter, like endotracheal tubes. Typically, they range from 5 mm to 9 mm with lengths to match.

2. Lubricate the airway with a sterile, water-based lubricant, preferably one with a topical **anesthetic,** or with water if you have no lubricant. *Do not* use petroleum jelly. It may damage the tissue lining of the nasal cavity and pharynx.

3. Insert the tube through the larger nostril, and gently slide the tube into the nose until the flange lies against the flare of the nostril. Insert it along the floor of the nasal cavity straight back to the posterior pharynx, *not* upwards. A gentle back-and-forth rotation may help it slip in easier. When the flared end is about an inch from the nostril, the airway will usually stop because it has encountered the back of the tongue. Simply lift the jaw and let the airway pass behind the tongue. If you meet resistance when inserting the tube, *do not* force it. Pull the tube out and try the other nostril.

4. Rotate the tube fifteen or thirty degrees until you can hear the maximal airflow. Then, as the patient breathes in, advance the tube quickly and gently. The flange should lie against the flare of the nostril.

5. If the patient is responsive, have him exhale with his mouth closed.

6. The tube is in place if you feel air coming through it.

☐ SUCTION UNITS

The purpose of a **suction unit** (Figure 5-4) is to remove blood, vomitus, and other liquids from the airway.

The fixed or installed suction system should be a part of the required equipment on any ambulance. A fixed system can be powered by an electric vacuum pump or by the vacuum produced by the engine manifold.

Portable suction units can be oxygen- or air-powered. Whatever the suction source, the portable unit should:

- Have a wide-bore, thick-walled, non-kinking tubing and semi-rigid or rigid suction tips.

- Have several sterile, disposable suction **catheters** of various sizes for suctioning the mouth, the pharynx of children, and stomas. Rigid pharyn-

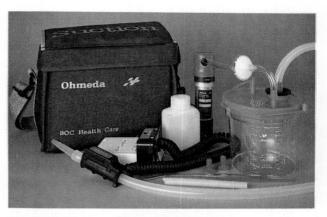

FIGURE 5-4 A portable suction unit.

geal suction tips (**tonsil suction tips**) are best for suctioning the pharynx.

- Have an unbreakable collection bottle and a supply of water for rinsing tubes and catheters.

- Have enough vacuum pressure and flow for pharyngeal suction.

Though there are many variations in suctioning procedures, the following technique is an effective one (Figure 5-5–5-10):

1. Inspect the unit to make sure that all the parts are assembled and are in proper working order. Measure the suction catheter to be sure it is the proper length.

2. Switch on the suction.

3. Position yourself beside the patient's head, and open the mouth with the cross-finger technique.

4. Insert the rigid tonsil suction tip into the mouth with the **convex** (bulging) side along the roof of the mouth. Insert the tip to the beginning of the throat, *not* into the throat or the larynx.

5. After the catheter or rigid tip is in place, suction for no more than fifteen seconds in the breathing patient.

6. No suction unit will handle food particles. Wipe out the patient's mouth with a 4 × 4 gauze pad or part of the patient's clothing, if nothing else is available.

☐ OXYGEN EQUIPMENT

Oxygen is a colorless, odorless gas normally present in the atmosphere in a concentration of approximately 21 percent. Pure or 100 percent oxygen is obtained commercially by fractional **distillation,** a process in which air is **liquefied** and the gases other than oxygen (primarily **nitrogen**) are boiled off. Liquid oxygen is then con-

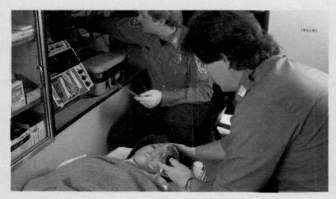

FIGURE 5-5 Position yourself at the patient's head and turn the patient to the side.

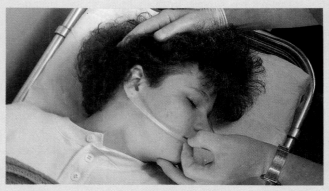

FIGURE 5-6 Measure suction catheter: the distance between the patient's earlobe and the corner of the mouth, or center of the mouth to the angle of the jaw.

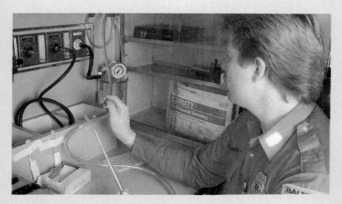

FIGURE 5-7 Turn unit on and test for suction.

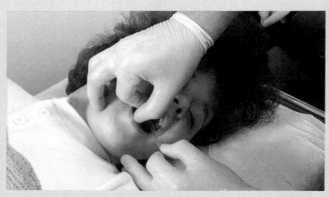

FIGURE 5-8 Open the patient's mouth by the crossed-finger technique and clear mouth.

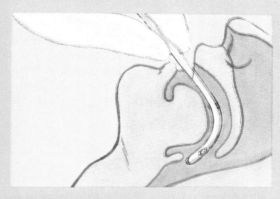

FIGURE 5-9 Place the rigid pharyngeal tip so that the convex (bulging out) side is against the roof of the patient's mouth. Insert the tip to the beginning of the throat. *Do not* push the tip down into the throat or into the larynx.

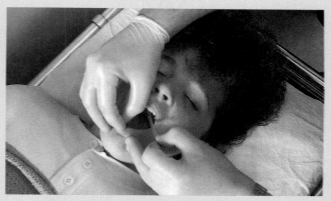

FIGURE 5-10 Apply suction *only* after the tip of the catheter or the rigid tip is in place.

verted under high pressure to a gas and stored in steel cylinders under pressure of about 2,000 pounds per square inch (**psi**) (Figure 5-11).

These cylinders are given letter designations according to their size. For example, the three most common used in emergency medical care are D, E and M cylinders. An E cylinder is 4.5 inches by 30 inches and contains 625 liters of oxygen, while an M cylinder is larger and contains 3,000 liters of oxygen.

Gas flow from an oxygen cylinder is controlled by regulators that reduce the high pressure in the cylinder to a safe range (around 50 psi) and control the flow from 1 to 15 liters per minute (Figure 5-12). These regulators attach to the cylinder by a yoke; each yoke is designed so that its pins will fit only the cylinders for one type of gas (e.g., oxygen, **helium**). In addition, all gas cylinders are color-coded according to their contents. Oxygen cylinders in the United States are generally steel-green or aluminum gray.

Two types of regulators may be attached to an oxygen cylinder — **high-pressure regulators** and **therapy regulators.** The high-pressure regulator can provide 50 psi to power a **demand-valve** resuscitator or a suction device. It has only one gauge (registering cylinder contents) and a threaded outlet. It cannot be used interchangeably with the therapy regulator because it has no mechanism for adjusting flow rate and is designed specifically for use with other equipment. To use the high-pressure regulator, attach the equipment supply line to the threaded outlet and open the cylinder valve fully; then turn it back one-half turn for safety.

The therapy regulator can administer oxygen up to 15 **lpm** (liters per minute). It has two gauges: one shows cylinder contents, the other allows you to provide a metered flow of oxygen to the patient. The cylinder is "full" when the pressure is 2,000 psi or greater, and this pressure drops directly proportional to the contents (1,000 psi is half full). Adjust the flow meter to provide oxygen appropriate to the device used and the condition of the patient.

FIGURE 5-11 A basic portable resuscitator.

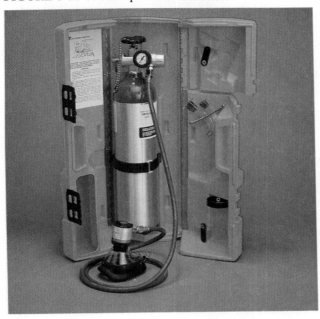

FIGURE 5-12 An oxygen regulator with calibrated flow control. High-flow outlet capacity is 25 lpm with outlet pressure at 40 to 60 psi.

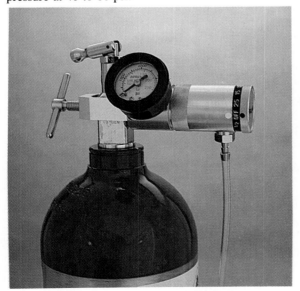

Safety Precautions

Observe these safety precautions in handling oxygen cylinders:

- Never allow combustible materials, such as oil or grease, to touch the cylinder, regulator, fittings, valves, or hoses. Oil and oxygen under pressure will explode if they come in contact. This includes petroleum-based adhesive (adhesive tape) or lubricating a delivering system with petroleum jelly.

- Never smoke or allow others to smoke in any area where oxygen cylinders are in use or on standby. Because oxygen makes fire burn more rapidly, it greatly increases the risk of fire, not only from the tube but in towels, sheets, and clothing in which the oxygen has been in contact.

- Store the cylinders below 125° Fahrenheit.

- Never use an oxygen cylinder without a safe, properly fitting regulator valve. Never use a valve that has been modified from another gas.

- Keep all valves closed when the oxygen cylinder is not in use, even if the tank is empty.

- Keep oxygen cylinders secured to prevent toppling

□ Preparing the O₂ Delivery System

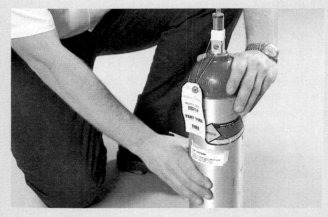

FIGURE 5-13 Place the cylinder in an upright position and stand to one side.

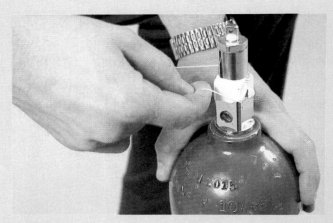

FIGURE 5-14 Remove the plastic wrapper or cap protecting the cylinder outlet.

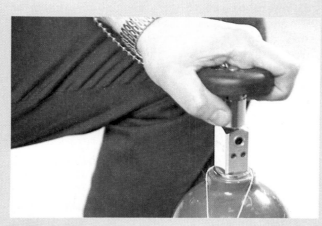

FIGURE 5-15 "Crack" the main valve for one second.

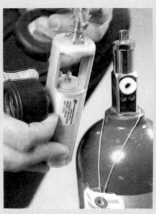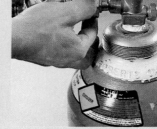

FIGURE 5-16 Select the correct pressure regulator and flowmeter.

over. In transit, they should be in a carrier rack or be strapped to the stretcher with the patient.

- When you are working with an oxygen cylinder, never place any part of your body over the cylinder valve. A full cylinder usually has 2,000 or 2,200 psi. If the tank is punctured or if a valve breaks off, a supply tank can accelerate with enough force to penetrate concrete walls. A loosely fitting regulator can be blown off the cylinder with sufficient force to amputate a head or demolish any other object in its path. Never stand an oxygen tank upright by the patient. If the tank is not in a commercial pack, lay it on its side by the patient.

Oxygen Administration

To administer oxygen:

1. Prepare the tank if it is not used every day (Figure 5-13—5-19):
   a. Place the cylinder securely upright, and position yourself to the side.
   b. "Crack" the tank with the wrench supplied; i.e., slowly open and rapidly close the cylinder valve to clean it of debris.
   c. Inspect the regulator valve to be certain that it is the right type for an oxygen cylinder and that it has an intact washer.

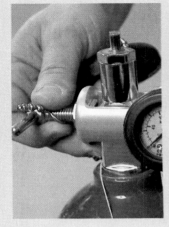
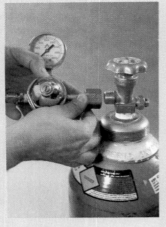

FIGURE 5-17 Align pins, for DISS, thread by hand.

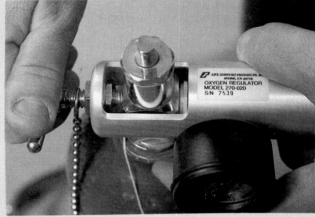

FIGURE 5-18 Tighten T-screw for pin-index, and tighten with a wrench for DISS.

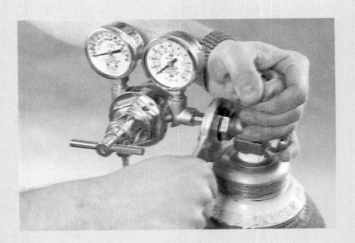

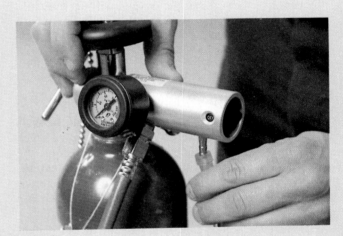

FIGURE 5-19 Attach tubing and delivery device.

d. Apply the regulator valve and tighten securely.

2. Regulate the oxygen flow:

   a. Open the main cylinder valve slowly about one-half turn beyond the point where the regulator valve becomes pressurized. Read the gauge to be sure that the tank has an adequate amount of oxygen (follow local protocol here; the usual residual pressure is 200 psi).

   b. Open the control valve to the desired liter flow.

   c. When you are ready to terminate oxygen administration, detach the mask from the patient and shut off the control valve until the liter flow is at zero.

d. Shut off the main cylinder valve.

e. Bleed the valves by opening the control valve and leaving it open until the needle or ball indicator returns to zero flow.

f. Shut the control valve on all tanks carried on ambulances. It should be part of your daily routine to open the main cylinder valve on the oxygen tank carried in your vehicle and to check the pressure remaining in the cylinder. It is extraordinarily discouraging, not to mention negligent, to arrive at the scene of an accident with lights and sirens and other fanfare only to discover that you have an empty oxygen cylinder. Always replace a cylinder when the pressure is low (e.g., 200 psi or less). Carry backup portable oxygen cylinders in the vehicle.

□ OXYGEN DELIVERY EQUIPMENT

Using an Oxygen Mask

1. Select a mask with the oxygen supply tube pre-attached; the other end attaches to the humidifier nipple or oxygen source. Turn on the oxygen, at first with a higher flow than prescribed (10 to 15 liters per minute) to quickly flush the mask. Then set the flow at the prescribed level. If the mask has a reservoir bag, make sure that the bag is filled before using it.

2. Gently place the mask over the patient's face. Slip the loosened elastic strap over the head so that it is positioned below or above the ears.

3. Pull the ends of the elastic until the mask fits the patient's face so that the oxygen will not leak into the eyes. If any gaps remain, plug them with gauze pads. Place 4 × 4-inch pads under any irritation areas.

General Guidelines for Using Masks and Oxygen

Often the plastic face mask or nonrebreathing mask is preferred in the field because it can deliver high oxygen concentrations. Some patients, however, tolerate the masks poorly and complain of feelings of **suffocation.** In such situations, the nasal cannula is a better alternative, may be adequate, and is more comfortable than a mask.

Whatever device you use, explain to the patient what it is and why you are using it. Forewarn the patient that the mask may feel confining but that it is nonetheless providing the proper amount of oxygen will help considerably.

Warning: A rare complication that EMTs may encounter as they administer oxygen is respiratory depression in a chronic obstructive pulmonary disease (COPD) patient. The drive to breathe may come from the lack of oxygen (hypoxic drive). Very high oxygen levels may eliminate the COPD patient's hypoxic drive in isolated cases. Monitor the patient carefully.

The control of the rate and depth of breathing rests primarily in the brainstem. The brainstem measures carbon dioxide (CO_2) and pH levels in the blood. This is used as an indicator for the correct respiratory rate to blow off the proper amount of carbon dioxide

and provide the right amount of oxygen. Some COPD patients are unable to eliminate carbon dioxide normally, so their respiratory centers become accustomed to high carbon-dioxide levels and low O_2 levels. These patients are stimulated to breathe by receptors located in the aorta and carotid arteries, which are sensitive to decreases in oxygen levels. Therefore, oxygen administration may supply high enough oxygen levels to discontinue the body's messages to breathe.

Take a good medical history before beginning oxygen therapy. If your patient suffers from chronic obstructive pulmonary disease, closely monitor his breathing as you give oxygen.

With any hypoxic patient, think in terms of percentages of oxygen before the liter flow is set. The following are reasons to initiate O_2 therapy:

1. An adequate past medical history.
2. Present ventilatory status.
3. The degree of hypoxia present.

Remember — oxygen is a vital drug and can be beneficial in field care. Proper concentrations and observant patient monitoring will generally prevent problems.

Oxygen Delivery Devices

A variety of devices are available to provide supplemental oxygen to the victim of cardiopulmonary arrest and other breathing problems. Proper training for the use of these devices is essential (Follow state and local protocol) (See Table 5-1.) They include:

* Nasal cannula.
* Simple plastic face masks.
* Partial rebreathing masks.
* Non-rebreathing masks.
* Venturi masks.

These devices are all used on patients who are breathing spontaneously. If the patient is not breathing spontaneously and requires resuscitation, the following devices can be used in the field:

* Pocket masks.
* Bag-valve-masks.
* Demand-valve resuscitators.
* Intermittent positive-pressure breathing (IPPB) resuscitators.

Nasal Cannula

One of the most common oxygen devices is the nasal cannula, two soft plastic tips that are inserted a short

TABLE 5-1
Oxygen Delivery Devices and Their Characteristics

DEVICE	FLOW RATE USED	PERCENTAGE OF OXYGEN DELIVERED	COMMENT
Nasal cannula	4–6 liters/min	24–44%	Usually well tolerated.
Plastic face mask	8–12 liters/min	35–60%	Preferred on trauma patients with no shock developing.
Partial rebreathing masks	6–10 liters/min	35–60%	For trauma patients
Non-rebreathing masks	10–15 liters/min	80–95%	Permits administration of high O_2 concentration.
Venturi masks			Useful in long-term treatment of patients with COPD. Limited usefulness in the field.
24%	4 liters/min	24%	
28%	4 liters/min	28%	
35%	8 liters/min	35%	
40%	8 liters/min	40%	

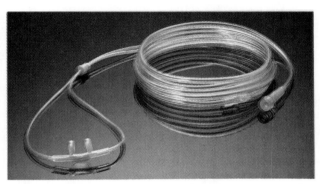

FIGURE 5-20 The nasal cannula is used for low (1 to 6 liter, 24 to 44 percent) oxygen concentration. This type is an over-the-ear placement.

distance into the nostrils and that are attached to the oxygen source with thin tubing (Figures 5-20 and 5-21). The nasal cannula provides safe, comfortable, "low-flow" oxygen in concentrations up to 40 percent with a two- to six-liter flow. It should be used at flow rates of under six liters per minute. Higher flows cause drying of nasal **mucosa,** and possible nosebleeds. The cannula is most widely used in oxygen therapy for the emphysema or chronic lung disease patient.

To use a nasal cannula:

1. Set the liter flow to the desired rate. Make sure that you can feel oxygen flowing from the prongs.
2. Insert the two prongs of the cannula downward

FIGURE 5-21 The nasal cannula is comfortable and convenient.

Ambient air containing 21% oxygen

100%

100% oxygen

24 to 36% oxygen concentration delivered

113

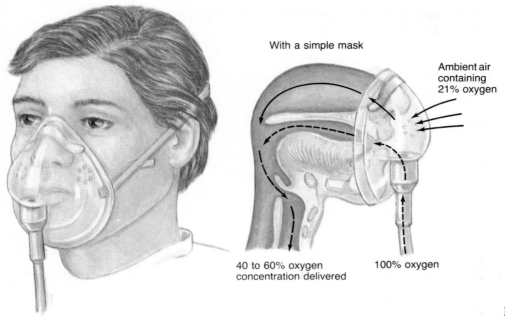

With a simple mask

Ambient air containing 21% oxygen

40 to 60% oxygen concentration delivered

100% oxygen

FIGURE 5-22 Simple mask.

into the patient's nostrils, with the tab facing down. Make sure that the prongs curve downward.

3. Position the tubing over and behind each ear. Gently secure it by sliding the adjuster underneath the chin. Do not adjust the tubing too tightly. If an elastic strap is used, adjust it so that it is secure, yet comfortable.

4. If the tubing causes irritation, pad the cheeks and behind the ears with 2 × 2-inch gauze pads.

5. Use a sterile, packaged humidifier with a patient who has respiratory burns, asthma, or croup. These patients are generally given O₂ by mask, however.

6. Check often. The cannula can be dislodged easily.

Simple Plastic Face Masks

Simple plastic face masks (Figure 5-22) can deliver up to 60 percent oxygen, depending on the oxygen flow rate and the patient's **tidal volume** (amount inhaled and exhaled during one full breath). Exhaled air exits through holes on each side of the mask. At low oxygen flow rates and high tidal volumes, the patient may draw more room air in through the side holes, thus diluting the oxygen concentration received. In general, a flow rate between 8 and 12 liters per minute should ensure adequate oxygen delivery.

Partial Rebreathing Masks

Partial rebreathing masks (Figures 5-23 and 5-24) look similar to plastic face masks but are equipped with reservoir bags that permit the patient to rebreathe about one-third of his or her expired air. Since this air is prin-

cipally from the patient's **deadspace** (i.e., from areas of the respiratory tract where gas exchange does not take place), it contains mostly oxygen inspired during the previous inhalation. At flow rates of 6 to 10 liters per minute, partial rebreathing masks can provide an oxygen concentration of 35 to 60 percent.

Non-Rebreathing Masks

Non-rebreathing masks (Figure 5-25) also have an oxygen reservoir, but they are equipped with a one-way valve that permits inhalation of oxygen from the reservoir bag and exhalation through the valve. Adjust the oxygen flow to prevent the bag from collapsing during inspiration — usually about 10 to 12 liters per minute. If the mask is fitted tightly to the face, it can deliver oxygen concentrations approaching 100 percent and thus is ideally suited to situations involving severe hypoxemia. Remember — the flow rate must be adequate to keep the bag inflated.

FIGURE 5-23 Partial rebreathing oxygen mask. Fill the reservoir for this mask to function properly. At flow rates of 6 to 10 lpm, it delivers 35 to 60 percent oxygen.

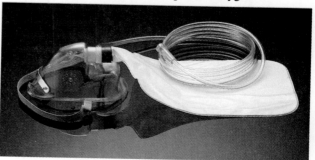

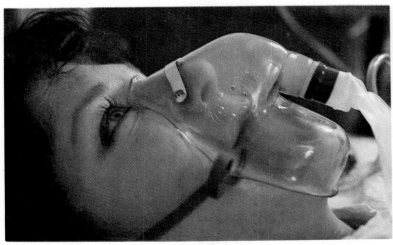

FIGURE 5-24 A partial rebreathing oxygen mask in position.

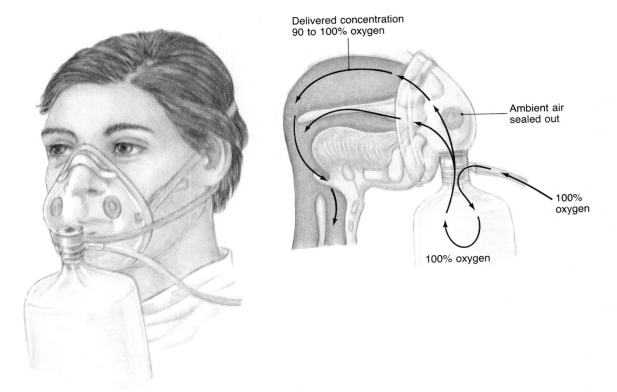

Delivered concentration 90 to 100% oxygen

Ambient air sealed out

100% oxygen

100% oxygen

FIGURE 5-25 Nonrebreather mask.

Venturi Masks

The Venturi mask is a low-flow oxygen system that provides different concentrations of oxygen through a delivery tube that is connected to a standard face mask. The mask contains diluter jets that can be dial-turned, or changed, to alter the oxygen concentration. It can be used to deliver humidity and does not dry the mucous membranes. However, the mask is hot and confining and may irritate the skin. Complications (e.g., kinked tubing) can lower the oxygen delivery. The Venturi mask is used with patients who have chronic obstructive pulmonary disease.

Pocket Masks

The **pocket mask** (Figure 5-26) is the preferred device for delivering artificial ventilation in the field. Its oxygen inlet valve helps to supply oxygen to supplement rescue breathing and eliminates direct contact with the patient's nose and mouth. It will deliver up to 90 per-

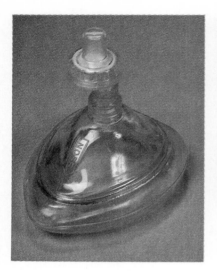
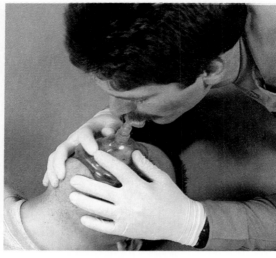

FIGURE 5-26 Pocket face masks. Note the chimney with one-way valve for mouth-to-mask ventilations.

cent oxygen at a flow rate of 10 liters per minute and delivers a higher tidal volume than the bag-valve-mask.

It has these important advantages:

- Because you can carry it in your pocket, it is instantly available.
- It minimizes patient contact and reduces the risk of infectious exposure.
- You will not need to switch to another device once an oxygen supply arrives.
- If the patient begins breathing spontaneously, you can simply strap the mask to his or her face and use it to deliver 40 to 60 percent oxygen.
- You can use both hands to hold it in place and simultaneously maintain a maximum airway by tilting the head back and moving the jaw forward. Both of these maneuvers are hard with the bag-valve-mask, which requires you to use one hand on the bag. As a result, you can ventilate the lungs in larger amounts and risk less gastric distention.
- Through the mask, you can feel lung resistance, just as you can in mouth-to-mouth ventilation.

To apply the pocket mask:

1. Connect the oxygen line to the inlet valve on the mask.
2. Perform a modified jaw thrust maneuver. Position the rim of the pocket mask between the patient's lower lip and chin to retract the lip downward and hold the mouth open.
3. Clamp the remainder of the mask to the patient's face, keeping both of your thumbs along the sides of the mask.
4. With your fingers, grasp the patient's jaw just be-

neath the jaw angles and pull upward, maintaining a backward tilt of the head. Do not perform this tilt if you suspect spine damage.

5. Blow into the mask, forcing your breath, plus the supplementary oxygen, into the patient's lungs. Watch for the chest to rise.
6. Remove your mouth, but do not disturb the mask, because you need to allow for exhalation.
7. For placement of a pocket mask on an infant's face, see Figure 5-27.

FIGURE 5-27 Ventilating infants and small children: watch for chest to rise.

Establish an adequate airway
(do not overextend neck)

Provide adequate breaths

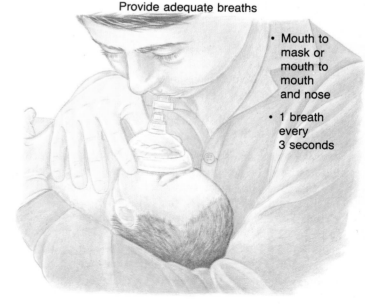

- Mouth to mask or mouth to mouth and nose
- 1 breath every 3 seconds

116   *Chapter 5*

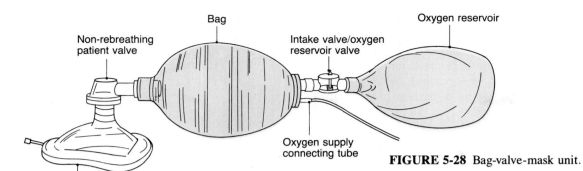

Non-rebreathing patient valve | Bag | Intake valve/oxygen reservoir valve | Oxygen reservoir | Oxygen supply connecting tube | Face mask

FIGURE 5-28 Bag-valve-mask unit.

Bag-Valve-Masks

Bag-valve-mask devices (Figure 5-28) are self-inflating, manual resuscitators; and when used without supplemental oxygen, deliver room air (21 percent oxygen) to the patient. If a source of oxygen at a flow rate of twelve liters per minute is attached to the bag-valve-mask device, the delivered oxygen concentration can be increased to 40 to 60 percent. Adding an oxygen reservoir to the bag can further increase the oxygen concentration to almost 100 percent.

The mask used with a bag-valve device should be transparent so that you can see vomitus or secretions around the patient's mouth. The mask should fit snugly over the patient's chin, beneath the lower lip, and over the bridge of his nose.

To operate the device (see Figures 5-29 and 5-30):

1. Place your thumb and index finger on the mask, the thumb above and the index finger below the valve connection.

2. Use your other fingers to grip the mandible and hold a tight seal.

3. Tilt the patient's head backward to open the airway, and compress the bag with your other hand. Do not perform this head tilt if you suspect injuries to the spine.

4. Keep checking whether the chest rises and falls to be certain that ventilation is occurring. An oropharyngeal airway is often desirable to keep the airway **patent** (open).

A new approach in the operation of a bag-valve-mask is the FATS approach[1], which stands for face and thigh squeeze. Place your thighs on either side of the patient's face, put the mask on the patient's face in the normal position, then place the heel of your hand on top of the mask or valve. Grasp the patient's jaw with your middle fingers. A head-tilt/chin-lift is then performed, and the knees are squeezed together to keep the patient's head hyperextended.

---

[1] Pumpin, Douglas Austin, Jr., and Judith Reid Graves, *JEMS*, September 1988, pp. 62–65.

FIGURE 5-29 Fill the reservoir bag and fit the mask over the patient's chin, beneath the lower lip, and over the bridge of the nose.

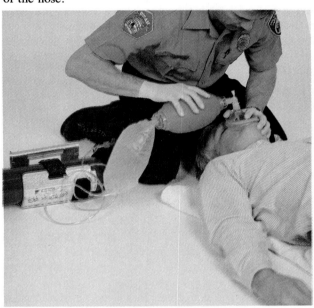

FIGURE 5-30 Create a good mask seal by placing the thumb above and the index finger below the valve connection. Grip the patient's mandible with the other fingers.

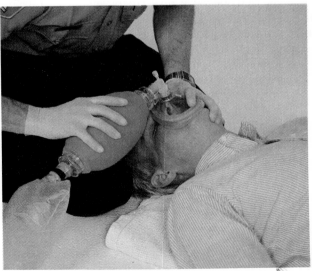

The principal advantages of the bag-valve-mask device over mouth-to-mouth ventilation are convenience to the EMT and the ability to deliver enriched oxygen mixtures. However, the bag-valve-mask rarely generates the tidal volumes that are possible with mouth-to-mouth ventilation, and gastric distention remains a problem with both techniques.

However, you should be aware that the bag is harder to use than it looks and is fatiguing to operate. One researcher summarized, "The BVM requires extraordinary coordination, dexterity, and practice to simultaneously seal the mask, hold the head in position, and empty the bag."[2] It is best if two people can administer oxygen with the bag-valve-mask, but this is not always practical. Also be aware that it takes frequent practice to maintain high skills. Rural volunteer services may not be able to maintain these levels. In such cases, the pocket mask may have advantages over the bag-valve-mask.

Demand-Valve Resuscitators

The demand-valve ventilation device (Figure 5-31) is designed to assist or control ventilation. If the mask has a good seal, the demand valve will deliver 100 percent oxygen to the patient's lungs. The valve is automatic in that when inspiration occurs (demand), the device will deliver oxygen, then shut off the oxygen supply when an expiration begins. In this way, a conscious breathing patient can have his or her oxygen supply augmented but not interfered with. These devices should not be used in emergency field conditions unless they deliver a flow rate of at least 1 liter per second.

They may be connected to a mask, **endotracheal tube,** or **esophageal obturator airway;** but they are most effectively used to assist ventilation in the spontaneously breathing patient. It is the preferred method for delivering oxygen to a conscious patient in pulmonary edema.

The demand-valve resuscitator should also have a manual control so that the EMT can activate the valve and ventilate the patient. To use the demand valve successfully:

1. Apply the face mask (if the mask has a collar, make sure that it is blown up), assuring an airtight fit between the patient's face and mask.

2. Begin pressure initially at 8 to 15 mmHg. Increase as necessary during use.

3. Ventilate the patient by periodically depressing the valve button. Do *not* over-inflate the lungs!

4. Carefully monitor the valve control at all times, looking for signs that the patient is being oxy-

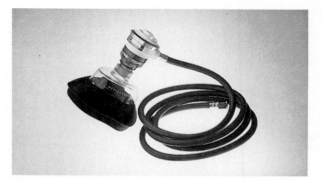

FIGURE 5-31 A demand-valve resuscitator with a manual trigger.

genated (chest rising, coloring of skin, etc.). If you suspect that mechanical resuscitation is not working, switch to mouth-to-mouth resuscitation.

5. An oxygen powered breathing device with a mask may cause severe gastric distention on an apneic patient if used improperly.

6. Do not use the device at all on patients under twelve years of age, except under very special circumstances (i.e., airway obstruction due to croup or epiglottitis). *Bag-valve masks provide finer control of ventilation and better assessment of the patient's lung compliance.*

> **NOTE: Pressure-cycled automatic resuscitators should not be used for artificial ventilation, especially while performing CPR. External chest compressions will prematurely trigger the termination of the inflation cycle and cause inadequate ventilation.**

Intermittent Positive-Pressure Breathing (IPPB) Resuscitator

A positive-pressure resuscitator without a demand valve has a manual control button on top of the valve unit to which the face mask is also connected. To operate this device:

1. Make a tight seal with the face mask around the patient's face and nose. Have a position on the manual control so that both of your hands can remain on the mask to provide an airtight seal while supporting and tilting the patient's head and keeping the jaw elevated. It is critical that an air-tight fit continues between the patient's face and the mask.

2. Depress the control button; this allows oxygen to flow into the face mask at a rate of up to 150 liters per minute. The patient's lungs inflate until the manual control button is released or until a preset back pressure is reached (approximately 40 mmHg).

---

[2] Lahaie, Ulysses David, "The Bag-Valve Mask: Do Not Resuscitate!" *Emergency Prehospital Medicine,* April 1990, p. 14.

3. You must remain constantly alert for gastric (stomach) distention during positive-pressure resuscitation.

4. Although **positive-pressure ventilators** can deliver large volumes of 100 percent oxygen, they prevent you from feeling when respiratory resistance is developing. With a bag-valve-mask, you can feel the bag becoming harder to squeeze when respiratory resistance occurs. This does not occur with ventilators. Also, because of the high volumes made possible with ventilators, you risk pressure injury to the lungs, esophagus, and stomach.

Oxygen Delivery Devices and Children

Most of the techniques and devices discussed can be applied to children with only modification for sizes. Be aware, however, of the danger of overinflating a child's lungs. Also, delivering too much volume can result in gastric distention or possibly pneumothorax. Check the chest movement carefully during respiration.

Suggested rates of respiration are: newborn, forty breaths per minute; infant, twenty to thirty breaths per minute; child, sixteen to twenty breaths per minute.

Medical Hazards of Oxygen

Although oxygen is a life-saving substance, there are some medical hazards associated with its use. They are not serious considerations for EMTs because they re-quire longer exposure and higher concentrations of oxygen than you will be delivering in field conditions. However, they include:

1. Oxygen toxicity, or the destruction of lung tissue due to high concentrations for a long period of time. This is *not* a consideration in EMT-level emergency care.

2. Alveolar collapse, or the constriction of the air sacs in the lungs, due to a too-rich oxygen concentration. This condition is sometimes permanent. In severe cases, whole sections of the lung collapse. Again, this is *not* a concern in prehospital emergency care.

3. Infant eye damage, or the formation of scar tissue behind the lens of the eye in infants, especially premature infants. This condition can cause permanent eye damage or even blindness, but is caused by oxygen levels in the bloodstream, not by oxygen touching the eyeball. Again, this does *not* occur in emergency field conditions.

Intubation

Intubating a patient with an **endotracheal tube** or an **esophageal obturator** airway for establishing and maintaining a clear airway are advanced procedures. Proper training is essential and is most often beyond the scope of practice of the basic EMT. Only patients for whom the simpler airway management techniques just described are not effective will require these advanced airway techniques. See Appendix 1.

chapter 6

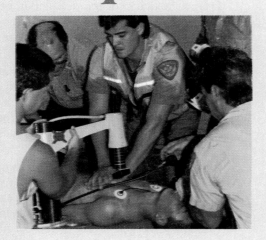

Basic Life Support — Cardiopulmonary Resuscitation (CPR)

✱ OBJECTIVES

- List and discuss the components and function of the circulatory system.
- Describe the specific signs of cardiac arrest.
- Define cardiac arrest and identify its major cause.
- Understand and practice cardiopulmonary resuscitation (CPR), as appropriate, on adults, children, and infants.
- List possible complications of CPR and know when to terminate CPR.
- Discuss CPR and disease transmission.

It is recommended that EMTs wear protective gloves whenever there is a possibility of coming in contact with a patient's blood, body fluids, mucous membranes, traumatic wounds, or sores. See Chapter 31.

Heart attacks and associated heart disease are America's number-one killer. Fortunately, hospitals have perfected a number of techniques that help to reverse cardiac disease and its crippling effects. Still, life-saving techniques exercised in the field by EMTs are critical keys in saving lives.

Coronary artery disease takes the lives of approximately 600,000 Americans each year. This killer does not just occur in the older population, but also incapacitates people in their thirties and forties. Ten percent of all heart attack patients could be saved by immediate, efficient prehospital emergency care.

Other situations besides heart attacks that require CPR include near-drownings, electric shocks, crushing chest injuries, drug overdoses, and toxic gas inhalation.

□ THE HEART

The heart is a hollow, muscular organ about the size of a fist. It lies in the lower central region of the chest cavity, commonly referred to as the **mediastinum.** The heart is surrounded by the **pericardial sac** or pericardium.

The heart contains four chambers. The two upper chambers are the left and right atria, and the two lower chambers are the left and right ventricles. The septum divides the right side of the heart from the left side. The heart also contains several one-way valves that keep blood flowing in the correct direction.

□ LOCATION OF THE HEART AND ASSOCIATED ORGANS

The heart is located in the chest cavity under the sternum and between the lobes of the lungs. Two blood receptacles are located just below the heart — the liver to the right and center, and the spleen to the left (Figure 6-1). It is important to know the location of these organs to each other, because improper **cardiac compressions** may cause a fractured sternum or ribs. A piece of splintered or jagged bone could lacerate the lungs or liver which could prove fatal to the patient.

□ THE HEART ACTION

By the heart's pumping action, blood is kept under pressure and in constant circulation throughout the body. In a healthy adult at rest, the heart contracts between sixty and eighty times per minute; in a child, eighty to one hundred times per minute.

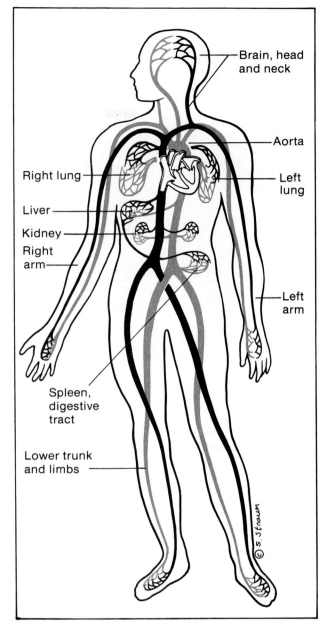

FIGURE 6-1 The heart pumps blood through the pulmonary and systemic circulation.

The average adult has approximately six liters of blood in the system. Children have two to three liters, depending on their size, while infants have only about 300 ml. Thus, blood loss that would be insignificant for an adult may be fatal in an infant.

The heart may be likened to a four-cylinder pump, except that the "cylinders" of the heart do not discharge into a common outlet. The left side of the heart receives oxygenated blood from the lungs and pumps it to all parts of the body. The right side of the heart receives blood from all parts of the body and pumps it to the

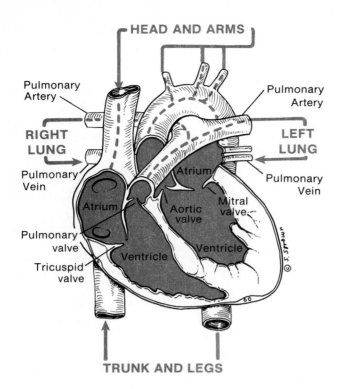

RIGHT HEART:
receives blood from
the body and pumps it
through the pulmonary
artery to the lungs where
it picks up fresh oxygen.

FIGURE 6-2

LEFT HEART:
Receives oxygen-full
blood from the lungs
and pumps it through
the aorta to the body.

lungs to be reoxygenated (Figure 6-2). The effect of these contractions can be noted by means of the pulse — the pressure exerted against the arterial wall during each contraction. Each time the heart pumps, a pulse can be felt throughout the **arterial system.** The pulse can most easily be felt where a large artery is close to the skin surface, such as:

• The radial pulse in the wrist.
• The carotid pulse in the neck.
• The femoral pulse at the upper thigh.

The pulse is most easily felt over the carotid artery on either side of the neck, or on the thumb side of the inner surface of the wrist (radial).

A heart attack occurs when there is a complete blockage of blood so that the heart can't get the oxygen and nutrients it needs. Most often, this occurs when a blood clot forms in an artery narrowed by fatty plaques and blocks the flow of blood. This form of heart attack is a coronary thrombosis, coronary occlusion, or **myocardial infarction.**

Cardiac arrest occurs when the heart is not generating an effective and perceptible flow of blood. Arrest can occur even while there is still movement and muscular activity. The dying part of the heart may trigger electrical activity that causes uncoordinated twitching, instead of smooth contractions. This twitching is called **ventricular fibrillation.**

Three vital organs of the body — the heart, the lungs, and the brain — have a close relationship in sustaining life within the body because they are closely intertwined in function. When one of the organs cannot perform properly, the other two are handicapped in performing their functions (Figure 6-3). For example, a motorcycle accident victim is thrown against the motorcycle bars, crushing his trachea. This results in respiratory arrest. As the seconds tick by, the blood becomes deprived of oxygen because the oxygen in the lungs has been depleted. Therefore, the blood carries less and less oxygen to the brain, seriously impairing brain function. The cardiac control centers stop sending signals to the heart, which begins beating improperly, then stops beating (cardiac arrest). Within four to six minutes, the brain cells begin to die. The smooth functioning of each organ is crucial to the other two, and ultimately to the whole system. If one organ fails, the other two will follow.

FIGURE 6-3

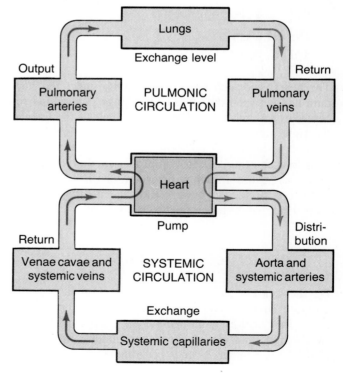

□ CARDIAC ARREST

Cardiac arrest refers to the heart "stopping" because the heart muscle (**myocardium**) is not getting the blood (hence, nutrients and oxygen) that it needs to work efficiently. The disease process called **atherosclerosis** is the main cause.

A heart that is not being adequately circulated with blood will result in the victim experiencing one or more of the following signs and symptoms:

1. Chest pain that may radiate to the shoulders and jaws.
2. Nausea and/or vomiting.
3. Cool, pale, moist skin.
4. Weakness, and a feeling of being sick.
5. A fluctuating pulse (faster or slower than normal).
6. **Diaphoresis** (perspiring).
7. **Dyspnea** (difficulty in breathing).

A heart attack may result in cardiac and respiratory arrest. Immediate, effective CPR and Advanced Cardiac Life Support (ACLS) is then needed to attempt to save a life. A more complete discussion on heart attack and other cardiac emergencies is found in Chapter 26, beginning on p. 394. See Chapter 4 for signs and emergency care of respiratory arrest.

The key principles of CPR are to oxygenate and circulate the blood of the cardiopulmonary arrest victim until definitive corrective measures (advanced cardiac life support) can be given. Any delays in initiation of CPR increase the possibility of neurological impairment and reduce the patient's chance of survival. Survival rates improve with shorter time intervals between the onset of the cardiopulmonary arrest and the delivery of **defibrillation** and other ACLS measures (such as **endotracheal intubation** to secure the airway, monitoring and diagnosing of cardiac rhythm disturbance, defibrillation, and delivering of **intravenous** medication). ACLS is administered by EMT-Paramedics and physicians, although EMTs in many states are being trained to defibrillate and are successful in that function. Statistics show that the most successful program includes rapid inception of basic life support by EMTs with possible defibrillation, followed by ACLS performed by EMT-Paramedics within seven minutes of the cardiac arrest.

□ HOW CPR WORKS

You should immediately assess all unconscious patients for airway, breathing, and circulation. Assume that an unconscious person has experienced respiratory or cardiac arrest or both (**cardiopulmonary arrest**) until proven otherwise. Obvious cases where assistance is needed include trauma accidents, electric shock, suffocation, and near-drowning.

It is important to closely monitor an unconscious person who is breathing because respiratory arrest can occur at any time. The heart muscle, being incapable of storing oxygen, is severely affected by hypoxia (lack of oxygen) and loses its ability to contract forcefully.

Proper emergency care involves airway management, efficient artificial ventilation, and correct artificial circulation by cardiac compressions (Figure 6-4). Cardiopulmonary resuscitation consists of opening and maintaining a patent airway, providing artificial ventilation through rescue breathing, and providing artificial circulation by means of external cardiac compression.

It was formerly thought that cardiac compressions work because the blood is pumped out of the heart as the heart is squeezed between the sternum and backbone. Newer evidence indicates that **closed-chest compression** produces a generalized rise in **intrathoracic** (inside the chest cavity) pressure. The pressure in the chest cavity is transferred to the blood vessels outside the chest. Due to thicker muscular walls in arteries, the pressure is greater there than in veins. This difference in pressure and the resistance created by one-way flow valves in the veins probably forces the blood to flow from the arteries into the capillaries. This allows oxygenated blood to reach the brain and other vital organs. Support for this position comes from the fact that forceful coughing *alone* can sustain blood pressure and flow for up to thirty seconds after the heart has stopped beating.

During the compression phase of CPR, blood is forced out of the right ventricle and into the lungs while blood in the left ventricle is sent out to the body. When you release pressure on the sternum, the chest wall "rebounds," allowing the sternum to return to its normal position. This release of pressure in the chest creates a sucking action that probably draws blood from the body into the right side of the heart and blood from the lungs into the left side of the heart. In other words, compressing the chest makes the blood circulate; releasing compression lets the heart fill with blood.

Because chest compressions are only 25 to 33 percent as effective as normal heart action, you should give the patient supplemental oxygen at 90 percent or higher as soon as possible.

The key to the survival of a cardiac arrest patient is:

- Early access to the patient by rescuers (including first responders trained in CPR).
- Early CPR.
- Early oxygen and defibrillation (see Appendix 3).

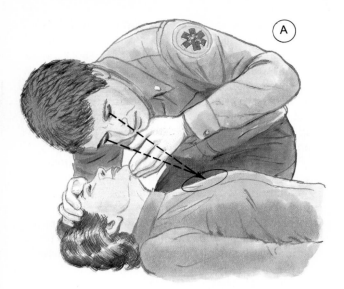

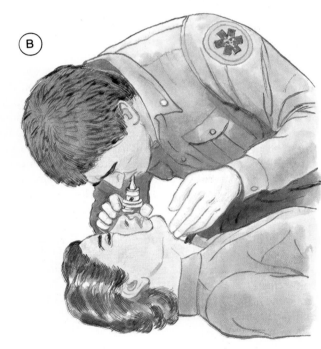

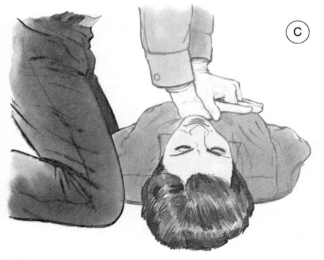

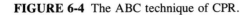

FIGURE 6-4 The ABC technique of CPR.

☐ STEPS PRECEDING CPR

A victim of cardiac arrest will be unconscious, will have no pulse, or a pulse so slow, weak, or irregular that it is not circulating the blood effectively. He or she will not breathe, and will have a deathlike appearance (grayish-blue skin and dilated or midpoint and non-reactive pupils). The major factor, however, is the absent pulse.

The sequence of basic life support steps preceding CPR are:

1. **Establish unresponsiveness.**

    Try to rouse the patient by tapping him gently on the shoulder and loudly asking him, "Are you okay? Are you okay?"

    * If he or she does not respond to touch, your voice, or pain, the patient is unresponsive. This evaluation should take no more than ten seconds.

2. **Activate the EMS (911).**

    Unless you are responding as a member of an ambulance or other rescue crew, you should activate the EMS system by calling an ambulance or the emergency number 911. Go to a phone yourself if you are alone, or send someone else. You should not leave the patient for more than thirty seconds. The person who makes the call should be prepared to give the following information as calmly as possible:

    * Exact location, including cross street names and numbers.
    * Phone number of the telephone from which you are calling.
    * Description of what happened, such as auto accident or heart attack.
    * Number of patients who need help.
    * Condition of the patients.
    * Description of emergency care being given to patients.
    * Any other information requested.

    Hang up the phone only after dispatcher has all the information required.

3. **Position the patient on his or her back (supine position) on a hard, flat surface** (floor, sidewalk, etc.). If the patient is on the side or stomach, roll him or her as a unit into the supine position. A patient with a suspected neck injury must have the neck stabilized during the roll onto the back (see Chapter 4). The nonbreathing patient should be supine with arms alongside the body.

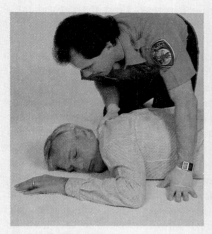

FIGURE 6-5 Establish unresponsiveness and call for help.

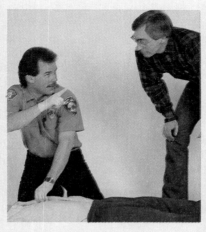

FIGURE 6-6 If you are NOT a rescue team, send someone to activate the Emergency Medical Services System (e.g., 911).

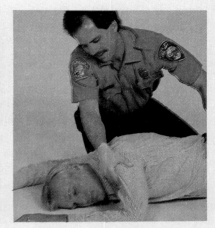

FIGURE 6-7 Position the patient on his or her back on a hard, flat surface.

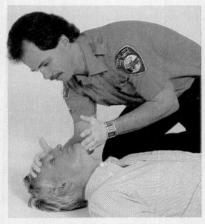

FIGURE 6-8 Open the airway with the head-tilt/chin-lift maneuver.

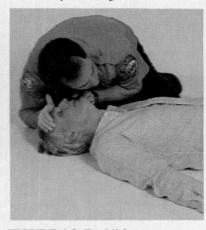

FIGURE 6-9 Establish breathlessness with the Look-Listen-Feel method.

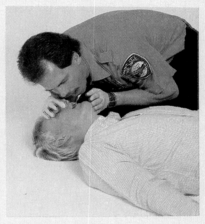

FIGURE 6-10 Perform mouth-to-mouth or mouth-to-mask ventilation. Give two full breaths of air within five seconds.

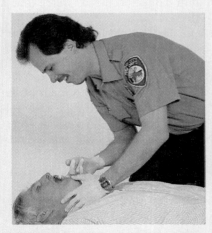

FIGURE 6-11 Clear an obstructed airway.

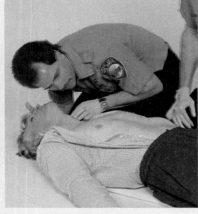

FIGURE 6-12 Establish pulselessness by palpating the carotid artery.

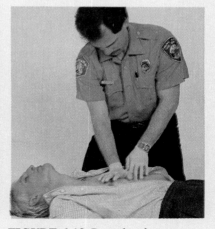

FIGURE 6-13 Bare the chest, landmark properly, and perform cardiopulmonary resuscitation.

4. **Position yourself at the patient's side.**

5. **Perform the ABCs of CPR.** Assess airway, breathing, and circulation.

   - **Open the patient's airway and establish breathlessness** by the head-tilt/chin-lift or modified jaw thrust. Take three to five seconds to look, listen, and feel for breathing.

   - **Give two full breaths.** If the patient is not breathing, deliver two slow successive breaths by mouth-to-mouth or mouth-to-mask ventilation at 1.5 to 2 seconds per ventilation.

   - **Clear an obstructed airway.** If the patient's chest does not rise and fall with the ventilations, open his mouth and check for foreign matter. If you see nothing, reposition the head for an open airway. If that is unsuccessful, take the necessary steps to clear the obstructed airway. Then reattempt rescue breathing (see Chapter 4).

   - **Establish pulselessness.** Find the carotid pulse by placing two fingers on the larynx (Adam's apple), then slide distally into the groove between the larynx and the **sternocleidomastoid** muscle (large muscle in the neck). Then palpate the pulse (Figure 6-14). Keep your thumb out of the way, and *do not* rest your hand across the trachea. This step should take five to ten seconds. If you feel no pulse, quickly try the opposite side. *If a patient has a pulse, even a weak or irregular one, do not begin chest compressions.* You could cause serious complications by doing so. Continue rescue breathing until spontaneous ventilation resumes or until paramedics take over to perform more definitive airway management. If you cannot detect a pulse, begin CPR.

   - If the patient's heart is not beating, continue CPR. Effective CPR is essential if the patient is to survive.

   If in doubt about the assessment of cardiorespiratory arrest, assume that an arrest has occurred, and begin resuscitative procedures immediately.

FIGURE 6-14 After you have completed ventilation, check the carotid pulse. Palpate the thyroid cartilage in the midline with your index and middle fingers. Slide your fingers laterally to the groove between the trachea and the sternocleidomastoid muscle, and gently feel for the carotid pulse. If you do not feel a pulse, immediately try the opposite side. If you feel no pulse, begin compressions.

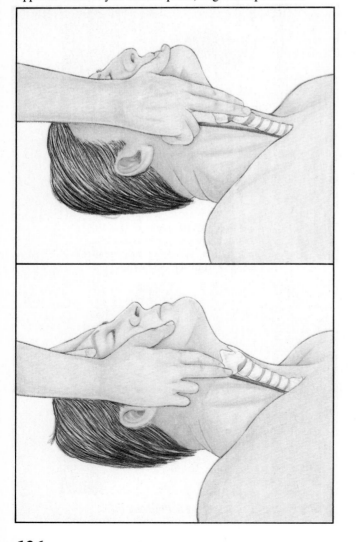

□ PERFORMING CPR

Cardiopulmonary resuscitation combines rescue breaths and chest compressions. When you perform CPR by yourself, deliver fifteen consecutive chest compressions at a rate of 80 to 100 compressions per minute, then two rescue breaths (allowing 1.5 to 2 seconds per inspiration). This cycle is continued.

If you have a partner, you may perform two-rescuer CPR. One EMT delivers compressions at the same rate of 80 to 100 per minute, but a 1.5–2-second pause is made after every fifth compression to allow a single breath to be delivered by the second rescuer. This same pattern is continued until fatigue occurs, at which time a switch is made.

A critical part of CPR is performing the chest compressions. It is essential that you pay as much attention to the duration of the chest compression as you do to the rate of closed-chest compression.

Compression should last at least 50 percent of the cycle. While study continues, you should rigorously follow the current CPR protocol of the American Heart Association described here and stay current on new CPR developments.

One-Person CPR

As you read this section, refer to the photo series "One-Person CPR," Figures 6-15–6-20.

1. The patient should already be lying horizontally on his or her back on a firm surface, preferably the

☐ One-Person CPR

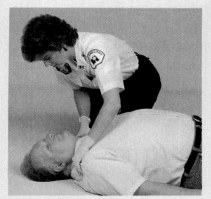

FIGURE 6-15 Establish unresponsiveness. Activate the EMS system.

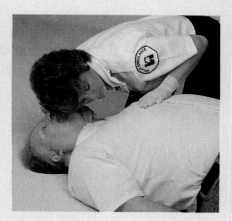

FIGURE 6-16 Open the airway with the head-tilt/chin-lift maneuver, then establish breathlessness with the Look-Listen-Feel method.

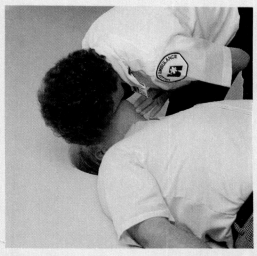

FIGURE 6-17 Give two breaths of air within five seconds.

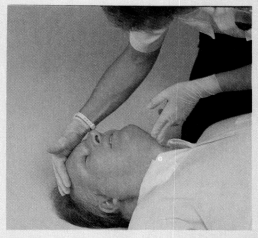

FIGURE 6-18 Establish pulselessness by palpating the carotid artery in the neck.

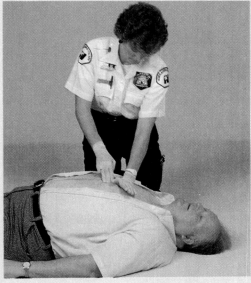

FIGURE 6-19 If you detect no pulse, locate the xiphoid process, or sternal notch, and measure two finger-widths above it.

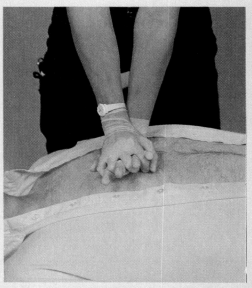

FIGURE 6-20 Compress one and one-half to two inches on an adult at the rate of 80 to 100 per minute.

ground, the floor, or a **spineboard** on a wheeled **litter.** The patient's legs should be elevated.

2. Remove the patient's shirt or blouse. (Do not waste time unbuttoning it — rip it open or pull it up.) Cut a woman's bra in two or slip it up to her neck.

3. Kneel on the firm surface *close* to the side of the patient's shoulders. Have your knees about as wide as your shoulders.

4. Locate the lower tip (xiphoid process) of the patient's breastbone (sternum) by feeling the lower margin of his rib cage on the side nearest you with the middle and index fingers of the hand closest to the patient's feet. Then run your fingers along the patient's rib cage to the notch where the ribs meet the sternum in the center of the lower chest (**substernal notch**) (Figure 6-21).

5. Place one finger on that notch, and put your other finger on the lower end of the patient's sternum.

6. Now place the heel of the hand closest to the patient's head *above* the two fingers. When you apply pressure at that point with the heel of your hand, the sternum is flexible enough to be compressed. (If you do not position your hand prop-

FIGURE 6-21

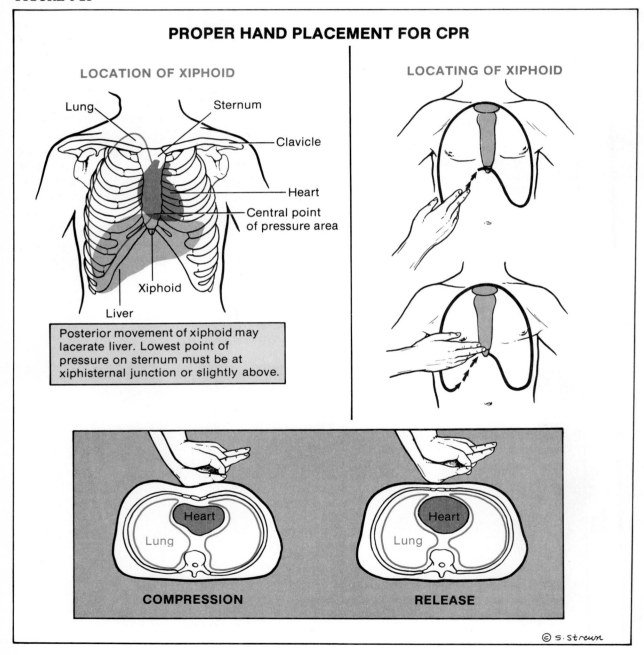

PROPER HAND PLACEMENT FOR CPR

LOCATION OF XIPHOID

Lung · Sternum · Clavicle · Heart · Central point of pressure area · Xiphoid · Liver

Posterior movement of xiphoid may lacerate liver. Lowest point of pressure on sternum must be at xiphisternal junction or slightly above.

LOCATING OF XIPHOID

Heart · Lung

COMPRESSION   RELEASE

© S. Streun

erly, compression can fracture the sternum or the ribs, lacerating the heart, the lungs, and/or the liver. See Figure 6-22.)

7. Place your second hand on top of your first, bringing your shoulders directly over the patient's sternum.

8. Interlace your fingers. The fingers should be held off the chest wall.

9. Keeping your arms straight and your elbows locked, thrust from the shoulders and apply firm, heavy pressure so that you depress the sternum about one and one-half to two inches (four to five centimeters) on an adult. Do not make sudden, jerking movements. Even this amount of effective compression provides only one-fourth to one-third

of normal blood flow, so anything less is ineffective. Your compressions should be regular, smooth, and uninterrupted, with compressions and relaxation time being about equal. Jabs make the blood spurt but do not increase the volume of flow, and they enhance the risk of injury. Make sure you administer pressure directly from above, not from the side. Use the weight of your upper body as you lean down over the patient to deliver the compressions. If necessary, add additional weight with your shoulders, but never with your arms — the force is too great, and you may fracture the sternum. Compression duration should occupy 50 percent of the pumping cycle (Figure 6-23).

* An acceptable alternative for those who have hand or wrist problems is to grasp the wrist of the hand lying on the chest with the hand that has been locating the lower end of the sternum. Pull your *fingers* upward, off the chest. If your fingers stay on the chest, the pressure from your compressions increases the possibility of fracture or rib-joint separation.

10. After each compression, completely relax the pressure so that the sternum returns to its normal position, but do not remove your hands from the patient's chest or you will lose the proper positioning. The heel of your bottom hand should continue to touch the chest even during relaxation.

11. Count as you administer compressions. It should take a little less than two seconds from the time

FIGURE 6-22 Improper positioning of the hands during CPR can damage the rib cage and underlying organs.

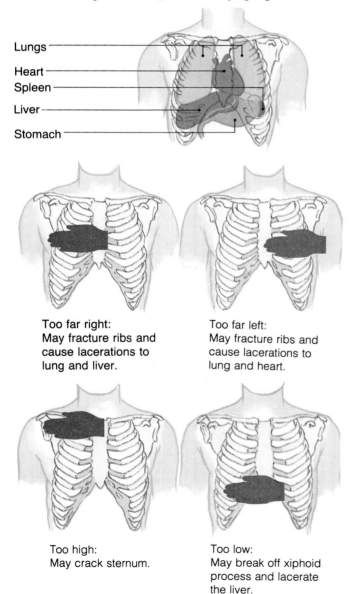

Lungs

Heart

Spleen

Liver

Stomach

Too far right:
May fracture ribs and cause lacerations to lung and liver.

Too far left:
May fracture ribs and cause lacerations to lung and heart.

Too high:
May crack sternum.

Too low:
May break off xiphoid process and lacerate the liver.

FIGURE 6-23 Proper positioning of the EMT to perform chest compressions.

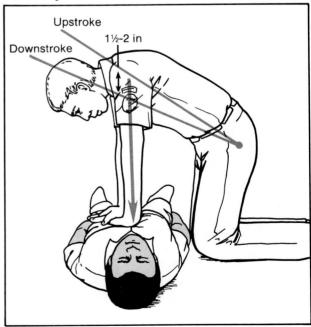

Upstroke

Downstroke

1½–2 in

you say "one" and compress the first time until you say "two" and compress the second time. This will enable you to administer eighty compressions per minute. Time yourself. Fifteen compressions should take between nine and eleven seconds.

☐ **One** — push down
☐ **and** — let up
☐ **two** — push down
☐ **and** — let up, etc.

12. Deliver compressions at the rate of 80 to 100 per minute for an adult or child, and at least 100 per minute for an infant.

13. Give the two lung inflations within five seconds (1 to 1.5 seconds per lung inflation).

14. After the first minute (four cycles of fifteen compressions and two ventilations) of CPR, and periodically thereafter, palpate the carotid artery (within five seconds) to check for the return of a spontaneous, effective heartbeat. Do this pulse check regularly in four- to five-minute intervals, or every few minutes thereafter, but do not interrupt CPR for more than a few seconds (Figure 6-24).

Periodically, pause for a pulse and breathing check (one minute after beginning CPR and every few minutes thereafter.) After you do this check, resume chest compressions followed by the breath.

You may interrupt CPR for no more than seven seconds to check for pulse and breathing, to reposition yourself and the patient, and to change positions with another EMT in two-person CPR. The first recommended interruption comes after one minute when you check for pulse and breathing. You should continue to check for these vital signs every few minutes. You should also be able to move the patient to a stretcher within seven seconds.

Other permissible interruptions are:

- Moving the patient downstairs (30 seconds at a time).
- Getting help (30-second maximum after 1 minute of CPR).
- Allowing advanced cardiac life-support measures (usually no more than 15–30 seconds per interruption).
- Suctioning to clear an obstructed airway.

Two-Person CPR

As you read this section, refer to the photo series "Two-Person CPR," Figures 6-25–6-33.

1. If two EMTs are present, you should kneel at the patient's side and perform cardiac compressions while the other EMT kneels on the *opposite side* near the patient's head and delivers artificial ventilation.

2. In this case, ventilation should be delivered during a pause after every fifth cardiac compression so that ventilation is at the rate of twelve per minute.

FIGURE 6-24

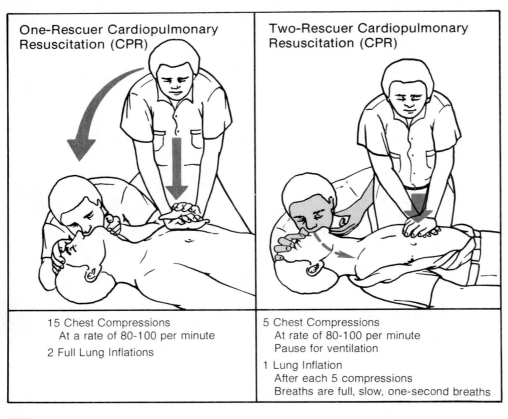

One-Rescuer Cardiopulmonary Resuscitation (CPR)	Two-Rescuer Cardiopulmonary Resuscitation (CPR)

15 Chest Compressions
   At a rate of 80-100 per minute
2 Full Lung Inflations
	5 Chest Compressions
	   At rate of 80-100 per minute
	   Pause for ventilation
	1 Lung Inflation
	   After each 5 compressions
	   Breaths are full, slow, one-second breaths

☐ Two-Person CPR

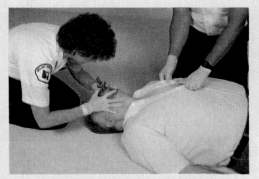

FIGURE 6-25 After establishing breathlessness, one rescuer gives two breaths while the other rescuer bares the chest and gets into position to perform chest compressions.

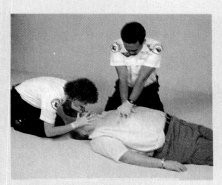

FIGURE 6-26 After establishing pulselessness, one rescuer gives a ventilation. The other rescuer then begins chest compressions.

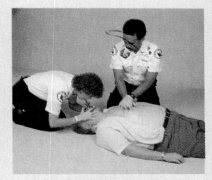

FIGURE 6-27 CPR continues at a ratio of five compressions to one ventilation, during which the rescuer performing the compressions pauses.

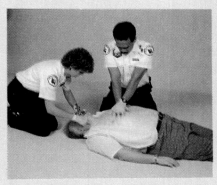

FIGURE 6-28 Stop CPR to assess the carotid pulse after the first minute, and every few minutes thereafter.

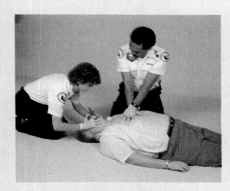

FIGURE 6-29 The tired compressor requests a switch.

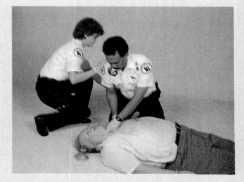

FIGURE 6-30 Changing positions in two-rescuer CPR. The EMT ventilating delivers a breath as usual, then moves into position to assume cardiac compressions while the other EMT checks the carotid pulse and gets into position to ventilate.

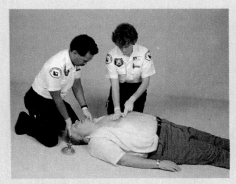

FIGURE 6-31 The EMT performing the compressions quickly moves to the patient's head and opens the airway while the other EMT landmarks the patient's chest.

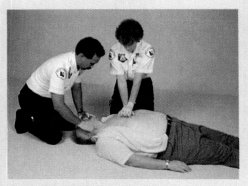

FIGURE 6-32 The rescuer at the patient's head checks the carotid pulse and breathing for five seconds. The other EMT readies for compressions.

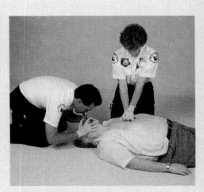

FIGURE 6-33 Completing the change. If no pulse is found, the EMTs continue CPR.

3. Use an audible count of "one and two and three and four and five and pause," so that you achieve five compressions every three to five seconds.

4. The compression EMT counts the sequence aloud. Compressions occur on each number (one, two, etc.).

5. The ventilation EMT takes a deep breath on "three and," positions himself to ventilate on "four and," and begins breathing into the patient after "five." The compressor pauses for 1.5 to 2 seconds so that the patient receives a full breath.

6. Always stop CPR to assess the carotid pulse (five to ten seconds) after the first minute, and every few minutes thereafter.

7. The ventilator should occasionally check the carotid pulse *during* the chest compression to be sure that a regular pulse is there. This indicates that blood is being moved from the heart satisfactorily.

Changing Positions in Two-Person CPR

When the EMT performing cardiac compressions gets tired, he or she should switch with the one who is performing ventilations. Here is the seven-second method:

1. The EMT doing compressions calls for a switch at the end of the compression cycle by substituting "change" for "one." The audible count remains the same for the remaining four compressions. (Any mnemonic that satisfactorily accomplishes the change is acceptable. Another popular technique uses as the count, "Change, on, the, next, breath.") A similar phrase can also be used to "call" for the move of the patient, or to "call" for a pulse check. It simply involves substituting:

   "1-and   2-and   3-and   etc."
   "CHANGE-and   2-and   3-and   etc."

2. After the fifth compression, the EMT performing the ventilations gives the full breath, then moves to the chest, locates the landmark notch, and gets into position for compressions.

3. The EMT performing the compressions moves quickly to the patient's head after the fifth compression and checks the carotid pulse and breathing for a maximum of five seconds.

4. If no pulse is found, the EMT at the head gives a breath and announces, "No pulse; continue CPR."

5. The EMT at the chest is in position and begins compressions.

6. If the compressor becomes short of breath and cannot give the full count out loud, at least say the "four and, five and," count so that the ventilator will know when to breathe.

Even when the patient lives and spontaneous circulation occurs, there is irreversible damage in 20 to 40 percent of the patients.

If one EMT is performing CPR and a second EMT or other rescuer becomes available, follow this procedure:

1. He should identify himself as qualified in CPR.

2. The first EMT nods as compressions are continued and he completes the cycle of fifteen compressions and two ventilations.

3. At the end of the cycle (15-2), the first EMT checks the carotid pulse for five seconds, then gives one ventilation. The second rescuer gets into position and becomes the compressor.

4. Compressions resume. A ventilation should be given during a pause after each fifth chest compression.

5. Continue CPR until pulses resume or until ACLS (Advanced Cardiac Life Support) can be initiated.

6. Because the ventilator has only 1.5 to 2 seconds to interpose a breath, a number of circumstances — including resistance from the patient's airways and personnel fatigue — may make it impossible to deliver a full breath to the patient. In this case, do *not* wait another five compressions but try to interpose the missed ventilation before the next set of compressions.

☐ SIGNS OF SUCCESSFUL CPR

- Each time that the sternum is compressed, you should feel a pulse (it will feel like a flutter) in the carotid artery.
- The lungs should expand.
- The pupils *may* react, or appear normal.
- A normal heartbeat *may* return.
- A spontaneous gasp of breathing *may* occur.
- The patient's skin color *may* improve or return to normal.
- The patient *may* move his arms or legs on his own.
- The patient *may* try to swallow.

Remember that "successful" CPR does not mean that the patient lives. "Successful" means that you performed it correctly. Very few patients will survive, despite the best CPR, if they do not receive advanced life support, defibrillation, oxygen, and drug therapy. The goal of CPR is to prevent biological death in a clinically dead person for a few crucial moments in hopes that advanced life support will reach him quickly.

☐ ERRORS IN PERFORMING CPR

The most common ventilation mistakes are:
- Failing to tip the head back far enough and thereby not giving adequate ventilations.
- Failing to maintain an adequate head tilt.
- Failing to pinch the nose or maintain the pinched nose during ventilations, allowing air to escape, not covering the mouth *and* nose during infant ventilations.
- Not giving full breaths.
- Completing a cycle in fewer than five seconds.
- Failing to watch and listen for exhalation.
- Failing to maintain an adequate seal around the patient's mouth, nose, or mask during ventilation. (The seal should be released when the patient exhales.)

Some common chest compression mistakes:
- The patient is not on a hard surface.
- Elbows bent instead of straight.
- Shoulders not directly above sternum of the patient.
- Heel of bottom hand not in line with the sternum, or too low; not depressing the chest (sternum) one-half to two inches.
- Fingers touching the patient's chest.
- Pivoting at knees instead of at hips.
- Incorrect compression rate.
- Compressions given in jerky movements rather than smoothly.
- Hand not remaining on patient's chest between compressions.

☐ COMPLICATIONS CAUSED BY CPR

Even properly performed, CPR may cause rib fractures in some patients. Other complications that may occur with properly performed CPR include fracture of the sternum, **costochondral** separation, pneumothorax, hemothorax, lung **contusions,** lacerations of the liver, and fat emboli. You can minimize these complications by giving careful attention to performance — but remember, effective cardiopulmonary resuscitation is necessary even if it results in complications, since the alternative is death.

The rib cartilage in elderly patients will often separate easily. You will hear it crunch as you compress. Be sure that your hand is positioned correctly and that you are compressing to the correct depth, but do not stop.

☐ A COMMENT ON ACLS

Although you are not able to perform Advanced Cardiac Life Support as a basic EMT, an understanding of the procedures performed by the EMT-Paramedic is helpful.

As soon as possible after CPR is initiated, the following ACLS steps should be administered by qualified paramedics:

1. Electrical defibrillation is attempted (and repeated twice if unsuccessful).
2. If necessary after defibrillation, CPR should be continued.
3. Endotracheal intubation is performed.
4. Ventilation with 100 percent oxygen is begun.
5. An intravenous line is placed.
6. Intravenous epinephrine is administered every five minutes during CPR, along with other possible medications.
7. The patient is transferred to the hospital while emergency care continues.

☐ CPR IN INFANTS AND CHILDREN

Cardiac arrest in children is rarely caused by heart problems. The heart nearly always stops beating because of oxygen deprivation due to injuries, suffocation, smoke inhalation, **sudden infant death syndrome (SIDS),** or infections. See the discussion on pediatric respiratory arrest in Chapter 4 and Chapter 32, "Pediatric Emergencies," for a more detailed discussion.

Infants (up to one year) and children (one to eight years) require slightly different procedures for evaluation and performance of CPR. The best time to activate the EMS system is also different. After unresponsiveness is established in an infant or child, provide one minute of CPR or rescue breathing. Then activate the EMS system.

As you read this section, refer to the photo series "Infant and Child CPR," Figures 6-34–6-42.

Establishing Unresponsiveness or Respiratory Difficulty

- No brachial pulse.
- No chest movements.
- No audible heart sounds.
- Blue or pale skin.

☐ Infant and Child CPR

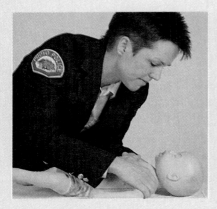

FIGURE 6-34 Determine unresponsiveness in the infant by a GENTLE "Shake and shout" method. You may also try flicking the soles of the baby's feet.

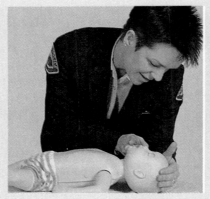

FIGURE 6-35 Gently open the airway using the head-tilt/chin-lift maneuver. Do NOT tilt the head back very far.

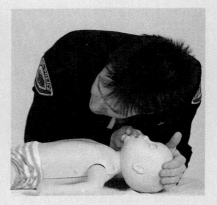

FIGURE 6-36 Establish breathlessness by the Look-Listen-Feel method.

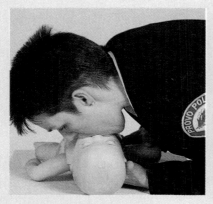

FIGURE 6-37 Infant mouth-to-mouth and nose ventilation. The rescuer covers the baby's mouth and nose with a good seal, then gives two ventilations.

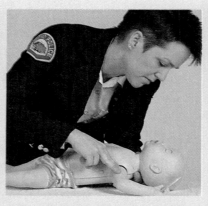

FIGURE 6-38 Check the infant for pulselessness by gently palpating the brachial artery.

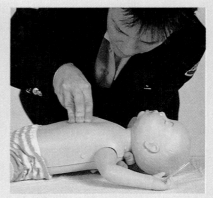

FIGURE 6-39 Perform cardiac compressions in an infant by placing the middle and ring fingers in the midline, one finger's breadth below the intermammary line.

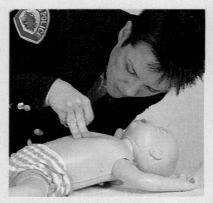

FIGURE 6-40 The lower sternum is depressed one-half to one inch at a minimum compression rate of 100 per minute.

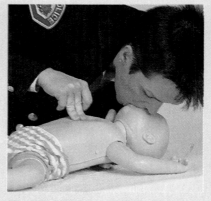

FIGURE 6-41 A gentle puff of air is given after each fifth compression. Perform CPR for one minute, then activate the EMS system.

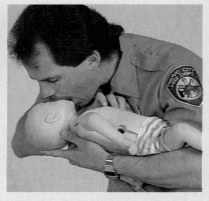

FIGURE 6-42 Performing infant CPR while carrying the baby.

- No response when shaken or gently tapped.
- Gasps, muscular contractions, and seizure-like convulsive activity.

An infant or child with breathing difficulty but who is not blue probably has an adequate airway and should be immediately transported to an advanced life-support facility.

Opening the Airway

1. Tilt the head.
   - **Infant.** When performing the head-tilt/chin-lift technique, apply a *slight* tilt. Tilting the head aggressively may injure the infant's neck or kink the trachea and close off the airway. Support the infant's head and watch for the chest to rise during ventilations.
   - **Child.** Open the airway of a larger child by the standard head-tilt/chin-lift or jaw-thrust techniques.

Breathing

Often, an infant or child will resume breathing when the airway is open. If the child gasps or struggles to catch his breath after the airway is open, let him breathe on his own if the lips are pink. Transport immediately. If the lips are blue (cyanotic), the patient is not getting adequate oxygen.

1. If the patient does not breathe, begin ventilations by giving two gentle breaths at 1 to 1.5 seconds per ventilation. Allow deflation between breaths.
2. Force and volume used should be that of a puff from the cheeks. Do not overinflate. Use only enough air to make the chest rise.
3. Watch the motion of the chest wall with each breath to be sure that air is getting in and out.
4. Use oxygen if it is available.

Establishing a Pulse

After you are successful in delivering the two consecutive breaths, *check the carotid pulse in a child,* but *check the brachial pulse in the infant.*

- **Infant.** The brachial pulse can be felt when compressing the brachial artery of the upper arm. You can find the brachial pulse by:
  1. Locating the point halfway between the infant's elbow and shoulder.
  2. Placing your thumb on the lateral side of the upper arm at this midway point.
  3. Placing the tips of your index and middle

fingers at the midway point on the medial surface of the infant's upper arm. You will feel a groove in the muscle at this location.
  4. Pressing your index and middle fingers in toward the bone, taking care not to exert too much pressure. To do so may collapse the artery, stopping circulation to the lower arm and perhaps causing you to miss feeling the pulse.
  5. Take 5 to 10 seconds to determine pulselessness.
- **Child.** Check for circulation in a child by palpating the carotid pulse, the same as you would in an adult.

Cardiopulmonary Resuscitation

If there is no pulse, begin performing ventilations and chest compressions. Make sure that the patient is lying on a firm surface.

- **Infant.**
  1. The correct area of compression in the infant is one finger width below an imaginary line between the nipples, and where that bone intersects the sternum (lower half of sternum).
  2. Use the flat part of your middle and ring fingers to compress the infant's sternum one-half to one inch.
  3. The compression rate for infants is at least 100 times per minute.
- **Child.**
  1. Locate the lower margin of the child's rib cage on the side next to you, with the middle and index fingers — while the hand nearest the child's head maintains head tilt.
  2. The margin of the rib cage is followed with the middle finger to the notch where the ribs and breastbone meet.
  3. With the middle finger on this notch, the index finger is placed next to the middle finger (Figure 6-43).
  4. While looking at the position of the index finger, lift that hand and place the heel of that hand next to where the index finger was (lower half of sternum), with the long axis of the heel parallel to that of the sternum. (See Figure 6-44.)
  5. The chest is compressed with one hand to a depth of 1 to 1.5 inches at a rate of 80 to 100 compressions per minute. Keep the fingers off the ribs.
  6. Use smooth, compressions; the chest should be allowed to return to its resting position after

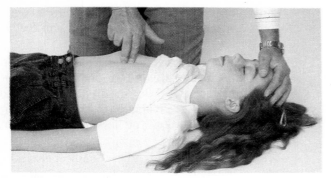

FIGURE 6-43 Proper finger position on a child.

each compression, but the hand should not be lifted off the chest. Each compression and relaxation phase should be equal in time.

7. If the child is large or above the age of approximately 8 years, the method described for adults should be used.

* The ratio of compressions to respirations is five to one in both infants and children.
* In one-person CPR, breathe once for the patient after each fifth compression.
* With two-person CPR on a child, ventilate during a pause after each fifth compression. Count compressions at this rhythm:

Infant — one, two, three, four, five, breathe.
Child — one and two and three and four and five and breathe.

* Periodically pause for a pulse and breathing check (one minute after beginning CPR and every few minutes thereafter). After you do this check, resume chest compressions followed by the breath.

See Summary for pediatric CPR in Figure 6-44.

□ MOVING CPR

Use the following guidelines for moving CPR:

* The best number of EMTs on a CPR call is three. Two should perform CPR while the third organizes help, has a bystander get the ambulance cot, radios for additional assistance, prepares to replace one of the workers, etc.
* Never interrupt CPR for more than seven seconds. The only exceptions are for transportation in which the interruption may last fifteen to thirty seconds.
* If you are transferring a patient from the ground to the ambulance cot, the leader tells the compressor to "call for the move." The third EMT places a

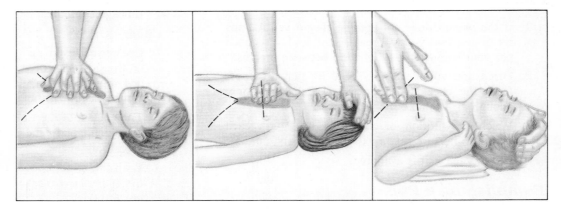

	ADULT	**CHILD** (1 to 8 yrs)	**INFANT** (less than 1 year)
HAND POSITION	Two hands on lower half of sternum.	One hand on lower half of sternum.	Two fingers on lower half of sternum (one finger width below nipple line).
COMPRESS	Approximately 1½ to 2 inches.	Approximately 1½ to 2 inches.	Approximately ½ to 1 inch.
BREATHE	Slowly until chest gently rises (about 1.5 to 2 seconds per breath).	Slowly until chest gently rises (about 1 to 5 seconds per breath).	Slowly until chest gently rises (about 1 to 5 seconds per breath).
CYCLE	15 compressions. 2 breaths.	5 compressions. 1 breath (pause for ventilation).	5 compressions. 1 breath (pause for ventilation).
RATE	15 compressions in about 10 seconds or 80–100 per minute.	5 compressions in about 3 seconds or 100 per minute.	5 compressions in about 3 seconds or at least 100 per minute.

FIGURE 6-44 The technique for chest compressions differs for adults, children, and infants.

CPR board or short backboard on the cot. The compressor counts: "Move, and, two, and, etc.," then after "five, pause," shifts his or her hands to lift under the patient's back. The ventilator picks up the head and shoulders, while the leader already has the feet and legs. They quickly move the patient to the cot, the ventilator gives two full ventilations, and the compressions continue in rhythm.

* If you are moving a patient downstairs, do a full cycle of CPR at the head of the stairs with the compressor giving a similar call to move one cycle ahead. Then move the patient quickly to the next level area, give two full ventilations, and continue CPR through another full cycle before calling for the next necessary move.

* As you carry the cot and load it, always step frontward or sideways (step with the forward foot and bring the back foot to it). Never cross your feet or you might be off-balance.

* When the patient is on the cot, do not straddle the patient or kneel on the cot while it is moving. If the cot is low, stand at the side.

* It is nearly impossible to maintain a tight seal around the patient's nose and mouth while moving him or her if you are using a bag-mask or demand-valve resuscitator. It is best to return to mouth-to-mouth ventilations or use a pocket mask for this step.

* Always load the cot into the ambulance head first, lifting from the sides.

* If possible, have three EMTs in the patient compartment to rotate for greater efficiency. (This may be difficult, especially in rural areas and depending on the cabin design.) The third EMT can sit on the squad bench behind the compressor and hold the patient by the hips to help brace him or her as the ambulance moves.

* The driver should warn the EMTs of turns, rough roads, proximity to the hospital, or any other factors that may affect their performance. This is not a time for "heroic" driving. The driver should turn slowly around corners and curves so that compressions and ventilations are not interrupted.

□ WHEN TO TERMINATE CPR

EMTs, as they recognize cardiac arrest, must administer CPR to the best of their ability and knowledge and should not be held liable for failure to initiate CPR if that decision is consistent with current American Heart Association standards. They should continue resuscitation efforts until one of the following occurs:

* Effective spontaneous ventilation and circulation have been restored.
* Another responsible or professional person assumes responsibility for life support.
* A physician, physician-directed individual, or physician-directed team assumes responsibility for life support.
* The patient is transferred to an appropriate emergency medical service facility.
* The rescuer is exhausted and unable to continue life support.
* The patient is declared dead by a physician.

□ WHEN TO WITHHOLD CPR

You are legally required to begin CPR on any patient who needs it for whom "there is no legal or medical reason to withhold it," according to the 1986 American Medical Association guidelines. For all practical purposes, there is no way you can tell if such a legal or medical reason exists, and you should simply initiate CPR under all reasonable conditions.

The medical reasons for not beginning CPR are "irreversible cessation of all functions of the entire brain, including the brain stem." You, of course, have no way of determining whether the condition is irreversible until you try to reverse it. Only in the presence of **rigor mortis, decapitation,** obviously **mortal** wounds, severe crushing of the chest and/or head, or established **lividity** (signs of death) could you be absolutely sure that resuscitation would not be possible.

You should not try to resuscitate a stillborn infant. This child died before birth, and the symptoms may include blisters on the skin, a very soft head, and strong, disagreeable odor.

As a practical matter, however, long-term survival decreases dramatically if the patient has not been resuscitated after thirty minutes (exceptions are drowning and hypothermia cases). Also, children and infants may tolerate longer periods of cardiac arrest than adults.

□ CPR RETRAINING

Several studies have shown that CPR technical skills deteriorate rapidly without frequent practice and retraining. Retraining in CPR skills should occur quarterly, and recertification should occur every one to two years.

□ SUPPLEMENTARY EQUIPMENT

CPR does not require adjunctive equipment, but it can be used, when available, by specialized personnel who have had adequate training. *You should never delay basic life support while you are waiting for equipment,* nor should the arrival of equipment divert your attention from your basic life-support efforts. If your team is trained to use specialized adjunctive equipment, and you are equipped with it, test it periodically for satisfactory performance. Maintain accurate records of these tests.

Mechanical CPR Devices

Mechanical chest compression devices are designed to imitate the appropriate manual techniques for chest compression.

To operate most of these devices, you should position the patient on the back support to which the compressor is attached. This molded board automatically tilts the patient's head up to maintain the airway. Then position the compressor carefully on the lower third of the patient's sternum. The compressor, when activated, automatically compresses the chest 1–1.5 to 2 inches approximately once per second. Generally, such units also come with automated ventilation support.

One advantage of mechanical compressors is that they do not get tired. They will deliver consistent compressions of unvarying speed and depth of compression for an indefinite period of time. They will also maintain the compression for the recommended 50 percent of the cycle. The compactness of the unit is also an advantage in crowded conditions when there is less room for two or three crew members to surround the patient. Furthermore, the compression cycle need not be interrupted for monitoring pulse and defibrillation, moving the patient, or during transport to the hospital.

It is important that the compression piston remain positioned exactly over the sternum. If the pad moves sideways out of position, a gauze pad underneath the pad will help keep the piston in the proper place.

Defibrillation

The 1985 CPR national conference strongly recommended that EMTs be trained in the use of defibrillators, since early defibrillation (within ten to twelve minutes after arrest) is the best predictor of patient recovery. Fibrillation occurs when the muscle fibers of the heart (usually of the ventricle) contract rapidly and irregularly. The standard treatment is a shock of ordinary DC electrical current which interrupts the irregular pattern and gives the regular pattern a chance to resume control. This treatment is called defibrillation.

Training and managing an EMT defibrillation program requires the close supervision and involvement of a physician. Training on manual defibrillators requires approximately ten hours, followed by quarterly reviews of two or three hours. Training on automatic defibrillators requires approximately four hours, followed by biannual reviews of two hours.

Follow local protocol in the use and standards of defibrillation techniques. (See Appendix 3.)

Oxygen

Supplemental oxygen should be administered as soon as it becomes available. Exhaled-air ventilation (used in emergency breathing) delivers about 16 percent oxygen to the patient — a concentration that, under normal circumstances, would produce an acceptable level. But because external cardiac compression is usually associated with low cardiac output, an acceptable level of oxygen may not be reached. A usual result is hypoxemia (or lack of oxygen), a condition that often impairs patient recovery. Supplemental oxygen should always accompany bag-valve-mask systems. See Chapter 5 for details on these systems and how to use them.

□ PSYCHOLOGICAL CONSIDERATIONS IN CPR

Because a life is literally on the line in a CPR call and because every second counts, CPR calls are emotionally challenging. The necessity for speed and precise techniques increases the natural tension. Keep these considerations in mind:

- This is not the time to be a hero. Share the responsibility of resuscitation as a team. Call for changes as needed. A tired chest compressor is frequently an ineffective one.

- If someone criticizes you, do not argue. Obey your leader's instructions or use your best judgment, but do not stop in the middle of resuscitation to justify what you are doing.

- If you need to criticize a fellow worker, do it quietly and tactfully as a suggestion. Certainly do not announce mistakes in front of the distraught family.

- Take time after the call to debrief with your team, express appreciation for crucial support, discuss what went well, and talk about areas for improvement. Share feelings about the call as well. Do not try to suppress feelings. Just delay their expression to an appropriate time.

□ DISEASE TRANSMISSION AND CPR

What about the risks of catching a cold, tuberculosis, **mononucleosis, hepatitis B, herpes,** or even **AIDS** while performing CPR? Use the following guidelines to reduce your risk:

- Clear, plastic face masks with one-way valves to divert the patient's exhalations away from you are available. Using these masks may be a local option in your area, and some experts recommend the routine use of a pocket mask after you have been correctly trained in their use. The American Medical Association observes, "The need for and effectiveness of this adjunct in preventing transmission of an infectious disease during mouth-to-mouth ventilation are unknown." They should be used only during two-person CPR, where the ventilator provides breaths until he becomes fatigued. Masks are not practical for one-person CPR because one person performs both the ventilations and compressions and therefore does not have time to adjust the mask each time he resumes ventilations.

- The AMA suggests the use of latex gloves to prevent transmitting blood or saliva that may carry the AIDS virus to your hands. It also suggests the use of disposable airway equipment.

- Thorough and scrupulous **decontamination** of resuscitation equipment and devices contaminated with blood or other bodily fluids should be standard operating procedure.

- If you have a cut, laceration, or needle stick, or your eye or mouth have been splashed by a patient's bodily fluids, rinse copiously with clear water, inform your supervisor, and consult a physician.

- During training, every effort should be made to follow the manufacturer's instructions on decontaminating practice mannequins.

- You should not participate in practice sessions if you have a known infection or have been exposed to one.

- Maintain proper hygiene during training sessions

(wash hands, do not eat or chew gum, etc.) to minimize unnecessary contamination.

- During two-person CPR practice, there is obviously no time to decontaminate the mannequin while switching positions. The American Red Cross, the American Heart Association, and the American Medical Association recommend that the second student only simulate ventilation in the correct rhythm, rather than blow into the mannequin.

- Use a decontaminated mannequin to practice finger sweeps in the obstructed airway procedure or only simulate the sweep. Between students, scrub out the mannequin's airway with a gauze pad that is wet with (a) a sodium hypochlorite solution — at least one-fourth cup of liquid household bleach per gallon of water, or (b) a 70 percent alcohol solution. Then wipe the surface vigorously with a clean gauze pad. The chlorite solution has a strong odor, but alcohol is less effective against a broad range of bacteria.

- Use individual face shields during practice.

- After use, scrub the mannequins with warm, soapy water, rinse with a sodium hypochlorite solution, then rinse with clear water. Both the AIDS and hepatitis type B viruses are relatively delicate and will die in less than ten minutes at room temperature if treated by soap-and-water scrubbing plus either the sodium hypochlorite or alcohol solution.

Current research indicates consistently that there is no evidence that AIDS is transmitted by casual personal contact, by indirect contact with an inanimate surface, or by air. Thus, only direct mouth-to-mouth or mouth-to-nose contact with a directly contaminated individual or mannequin would place you at risk for contracting AIDS. Furthermore, although approximately 150 million individuals worldwide have learned mouth-to-mouth ventilation on mannequins in the last twenty-five years, there has never been a documented case of a bacterial, fungal, or viral disease being transmitted by a mannequin. Likewise, there is no documented case of transmission of hepatitis B virus infection from mouth-to-mouth ventilation, either on a person or on a mannequin.

chapter 7

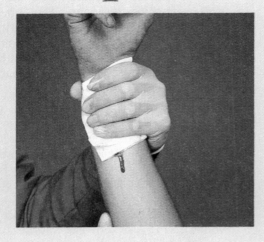

Control of Bleeding

✳ OBJECTIVES

■ Describe the significance of bleeding and how it affects various aspects of the circulatory system.

■ Describe and demonstrate how to control external bleeding using direct pressure, elevation, pressure points, splints, air splints, pneumatic counterpressure devices, tourniquets, and cryotherapy.

■ Identify the most common sites and signs and symptoms of internal bleeding.

■ Describe and demonstrate the general procedures for controlling internal bleeding.

It is recommended that EMTs wear protective gloves whenever there is a possibility of coming in contact with a patient's blood, body fluids, mucous membranes, traumatic wounds, or sores. See Chapter 31.

□ CIRCULATORY SYSTEM

The life processes depend on an adequate and uninterrupted blood supply. An understanding of what blood is and how it is circulated will help explain why and how blood loss must be stopped quickly and effectively.

In order to function, a person's body must receive a constant supply of nourishment (such as oxygen), which is distributed by the blood. If the supply of blood is cut off, the tissues in the body will die for want of nourishment.

The circulatory system, by which blood is carried to and from all parts of the body, consists of the heart and blood vessels. Through the blood vessels, blood is circulated to and from all parts of the body under pressure supplied by the pumping action of the heart.

□ BLOOD

Blood is composed of **serum** or plasma, **red cells, white cells,** and **platelets.** Plasma is a fluid that carries the blood cells and transports nutrients to all tissues. It also transports waste products resulting from tissue metabolism to the organs of excretion. Red cells give color to the blood and carry oxygen. White cells aid in defending the body against infection. Platelets are essential to the formation of blood clots, which are necessary to stop bleeding. Clotting normally takes six to seven minutes.

The process whereby body cells receive oxygen and other nutrients and wastes are removed is called **perfusion.** An organ is perfused if blood is entering through the arteries and leaving through the veins.

One-twelfth to one-fifteenth of the body weight is blood. A person weighing 150 pounds will have approximately ten to twelve pints of blood. If the blood supply is cut off from the tissues, they will die from lack of oxygen. The loss of two pints, 8 to 10 percent of the body's blood, by an adult, usually is serious, and the loss of three pints may be fatal if it occurs over a short time, such as one to two hours. At certain points in the body, fatal hemorrhages may occur in a very short time. The cutting of the principal blood vessels in the neck, in the arm, or in the thigh may cause hemorrhage that will prove fatal in one to three minutes or less if uncontrolled. Rupture of the main blood vessels of the chest and abdomen may cause fatal hemorrhage in less than thirty seconds.

The loss of blood causes a state of physical **shock.** This occurs because there is insufficient blood flowing through the tissues of the body to provide food and oxygen. All processes of the body are affected. When a person is in shock, vital bodily functions slow down. If the conditions causing shock are not reversed, death will result.

□ BLOOD VESSELS

Oxygenated blood is carried from the heart by a large artery called the aorta. Smaller arteries branch off from this large artery, and those arteries in turn branch off into still smaller arteries. These arteries divide and subdivide until they become very small, ending in threadlike vessels known as capillaries, which extend into all the organs and tissues. Through the very thin capillary walls, oxygen, carbon dioxide, and other substances are exchanged between body cells and the circulatory system.

After the blood has furnished the necessary nourishment and oxygen to the tissues and organs of the body, it takes on waste products, particularly carbon dioxide. The blood returns to the heart by means of a different system of blood vessels known as **veins.** The veins are connected with the arteries through the capillaries. Veins collect deoxygenated blood from the capillaries and carry it back to the heart.

Very small veins join, forming larger veins, which, in turn, join until the very largest veins return the blood to the heart. Before the blood is returned to the heart, it passes through the kidneys, where certain waste products are removed. When the blood from the body reaches the heart, carbon dioxide and other waste products contained in the blood but not removed by the kidneys must be eliminated, and the oxygen used by the body replaced. The heart pumps the blood delivered to it by the veins into the lungs, where it flows through another network of capillaries. There, the carbon dioxide and other waste products are exchanged for oxygen through the delicate walls of air cells, called alveoli. Thus, the blood is oxygenated and ready to return to the heart, which recirculates it throughout the body. The time taken for the blood to make one complete circulation of the body through miles and miles of blood vessels is approximately seventy-five seconds in an adult at rest.

□ HEMORRHAGE OR BLEEDING

Severity of Bleeding

Generally, hemorrhage is considered more severe as the breathing rate increases, the pulse quickens, the blood pressure drops, and the level of consciousness falls (Figure 7-1). The severity of hemorrhage depends on a number of factors:

- How fast the blood is flowing from the vessel (the size of the vessel).
- Whether the bleeding is arterial or venous (arterial bleeding is more rapid and profuse).

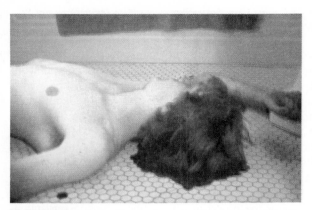

FIGURE 7-1 Detecting and controlling profuse bleeding are part of the primary survey.

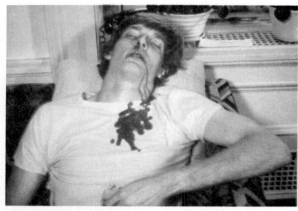

FIGURE 7-2 Bleeding from the mouth and/or nose in an unconscious patient can be a serious threat to respiration if proper precautions are not taken for drainage.

- Whether blood is flowing freely or into an enclosed body cavity (the most dangerous bleeding is into a confined space, such as the skull or the pericardial sac surrounding the heart).
- Where the bleeding originated.
- How much blood has already been lost.
- The patient's age and weight.
- The patient's general physical condition.
- Whether bleeding is a threat to respiration (Figure 7-2).

There are four general stages of hemorrhage, and they are based on the amount of blood lost (Figure 7-3). It is difficult to estimate the amount of blood lost by looking at it, but relying on signs and symptoms can give you a pretty clear indication of how much blood has been lost. The signs and symptoms caused by hemorrhage depend on these classifications, which can be very useful in the field.

Effects of Hemorrhage

Hemorrhage causes the following effects:

- The loss of red blood cells causes a lack of oxygen to the body systems.
- A decrease in **blood volume** causes a decrease in blood pressure.
- The heart's pumping rate increases to compensate for reduced blood pressure.
- The force of the heartbeat is reduced, since there is less blood to pump.

If hemorrhage goes uncontrolled, it will lead to the following signs:

- Moderate shock (follows loss of 15 percent of blood volume, or two pints in the average male).
- Severe or fatal shock (follows loss of 30 percent or more of blood volume, or four pints in the average male).

How the Body Controls Hemorrhage

The body reacts to various hormonal, metabolic, and sympathetic nervous system changes that occur during bleeding to begin the processes that help to control hemorrhage. Specific physical reactions that occur include:

- The blood vessel spasms and contracts (vasoconstriction), partially shutting off the flow of blood; arteries seal more efficiently than veins.
- Platelets adhere to the vessel wall, forming a sticky plug.
- A network of **fibrin** threads forms in the vessel; platelets and other blood components stick to the threads, forming a clot.
- When completely severed, an artery can sometimes constrict and seal itself off.

Normal clotting can be compromised by a number of factors and disease conditions, including head injury, and acidosis (a metabolic result of shock).

Bleeding from an Artery

When bright red blood spurts from a wound, an artery has been cut. The blood in arteries comes directly from the heart and spurts with each heart contraction. Because the blood has a fresh supply of oxygen, it is bright red in color (Figure 7-4). Blood loss from an artery is often rapid and profuse. Unless the artery is very small, blood in an artery usually will not clot, because the flow

THE FOUR STAGES OF HEMORRHAGE

CLASS 1 Up to 15% blood loss*	CLASS 2 Up to 30% blood loss	CLASS 3 Up to 40% blood loss*	CLASS 4 More than 40% blood loss*
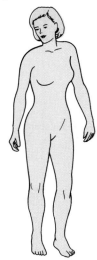	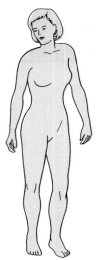	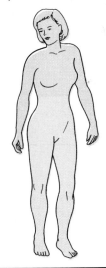	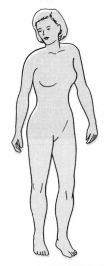

HOW THE BODY RESPONDS

Compensatory mechanisms (essentially sympathetic nervous system responses such as vasoconstriction) maintain homeostasis.

EFFECT ON PATIENT

- Patient remains alert.
- Blood pressure stays within normal limits.
- Pulse stays within normal limits or increases slightly; pulse quality remains strong.
- Respiratory rate and depth, skin color and temperature all remain normal

*The average adult has 5 liters (1 liter = approximately 1 quart) of circulating blood; 15% is 750 ml (or about 3 cups). With internal bleeding, 750 ml will occupy enough space in a limb to cause swelling and pain. With bleeding into the body cavities, however, the blood will spread throughout the cavity, causing little, if any. initial discomfort.

- Vasoconstriction continues to maintain adequate blood pressure, but with some difficulty now.
- Blood flow is shunted to vital organs, with decreased flow to intestines, kidneys, and skin.

EFFECT ON PATIENT

- Patient may become confused and restless.
- Skin turn pale, cool, and dry because of shunting of blood to vital organs.
- Diastolic pressure may rise or fall. It's more likely to rise (because of vasoconstriction) or stay the same in otherwise healthy patients with no underlying cardiovascular problems.
- Pulse pressure (difference between systolic and diastolic pressures) narrows.
- Sympathetic responses also cause rapid heart rate (over 100 beats per minute). Pulse quality weakens.
- Respiratory rate increases because of sympathetic stimulation.
- Delayed capillary refill

- Compensatory mechanisms become overtaxed. Vaso-constriction, for example, can no longer sustain blood perssure, which now begins to fall.
- Cardiac output and tissue perfusion continue to decrease, becoming potentially life threatening. (Even at this stage, however, the patient can still recover with prompt treatment.

EFFECT ON PATIENT

- Patient becomes more confused, restless, and anxious.
- Classic signs of shock appear—rapid heart rate, decreased blood pressure, rapid respiration and cool, clammy extremities.

- Compensatory vasoconstriction now becomes a complicating factor in itself, further impairing tissue perfusion and cellular oxygenation.

EFFECT ON PATIENT

- Patient becomes lethargic, drowsy, or stuporous.
- Signs of shock become more pronounced. Blood pressure continues to fall.
- Lack of blood flow to the brain and other vital organs ultimately leads to organ failure and death.

FIGURE 7-3

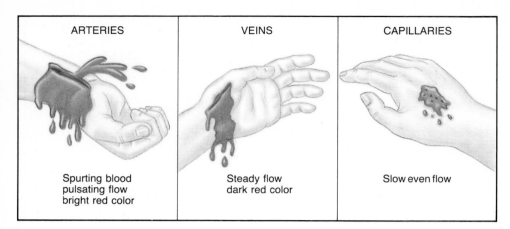

ARTERIES	VEINS	CAPILLARIES
Spurting blood pulsating flow bright red color	Steady flow dark red color	Slow even flow

FIGURE 7-4 Bleeding characteristics.

is too rapid; even if a clot forms, it can be forced out by the pressure of the blood flow. As mentioned, a completely severed artery can constrict and seal itself off, as often happens in cases of traumatic **amputation.**

Bleeding from a Vein

When dark bluish-red blood flows from a wound in a steady stream, a vein has been cut (Figure 7-4). The blood in veins, on its way back to the heart, flows more slowly than arterial blood. Having given up its oxygen and received carbon dioxide and waste products in return, the blood is dark in color. While bleeding from a vein can be profuse, it is usually easier to control than bleeding from an artery. Veins have a tendency to collapse when cut, which helps to control bleeding.

Bleeding from Capillaries

When dark red blood oozes slowly from a wound, capillaries have been cut (Figure 7-4). There is usually no danger from the bleeding, since little blood can be lost. Blood drips steadily from the wound until clotting occurs; direct pressure with a **compress** applied over the wound is usually enough to cause clotting. Bleeding from capillaries often clots spontaneously, without any treatment. When a large skin surface is involved, the threat of infection is of much greater concern than the loss of blood.

"Bleeders"

Hemophiliacs, sometimes called "**bleeders,**" are people whose blood will not clot due to congenital abnormalities in the clotting mechanisms. Even a slight wound that cuts a blood vessel can cause a hemophiliac to bleed to death. In addition to aggressive measures to control bleeding through direct pressure, you should administer oxygen and transport a wounded hemophiliac to the hospital as quickly as possible, as you would any patient with significant bleeding.

☐ GENERAL PROCEDURES FOR CONTROLLING BLEEDING

If bleeding is severe enough to threaten life, you must act rapidly to control it. The control of life-threatening bleeding takes priority over almost everything else, such as positioning the victim or taking a history. You may even have to control bleeding simultaneously with efforts to maintain an airway and provide ventilation.

The following are *general* procedures for control of bleeding (see Figure 7-5):

- Before handling the patient, put on a pair of latex gloves to protect yourself from the AIDS virus or other blood-borne contaminants.
- Conduct a quick assessment to determine the cause and source of bleeding and the general condition of the patient.
- Control the bleeding with direct pressure or use of pressure points.
- Maintain an open airway and administer oxygen. Be cautious when administering oxygen to victims of chronic obstructive pulmonary disease; oxygen hunger is often the only thing that keeps them breathing.
- While preparing the patient, obtain a brief history of the injury to determine the possibility of internal bleeding.
- Place the patient in a position in which he or she will be least affected by the loss of blood. If possible, have the patient lie down with the legs elevated in a semi-flexed position (to prevent aggravation of spinal injury and breathing impairment).
- Keep the patient at rest to prevent increased heart action, which interferes with clot formation and causes the blood to flow faster.

SUMMARY — CONTROL OF EXTERNAL BLEEDING

Type & Nature of Bleeding

CAPILLARY Oozing, most common type of external hemorrhage. This type of bleeding is expected in all minor cuts, scratches, and abrasions. Dark red color.

VENOUS Slow, even blood flow. Occurs when a vein is punctured or severed. Venous blood is dark in color. Danger in venous bleeding from neck wound is that an air bubble may be sucked into the wound.

ARTERIAL Occurs when an artery is punctured or severed. Less common than venous bleeding because arteries are located deep in the body and are protected by bones. Arterial bleeding is characterized by spurting of bright red blood. Common arteries injured in accidents: carotid, brachial, radial, femoral.

Emergency Care

External bleeding is bleeding that can be seen coming from a wound. Excessive external bleeding can create a crisis situation; the platelets, which usually help the blood clot, aren't effective in cases of severe bleeding or when the blood vessels have been damaged.

Serious blood loss is defined as one liter in an adult and half a liter in a child. If the bleeding remains uncontrolled, shock and death may result.

Elevate Extremity

Direct Pressure

1. Apply direct pressure against the bleeding site.

2. Use a dressing; if necessary, even your gloved hand. If dressing soaks through do not remove it — put another on top and continue applying pressure.

3. Maintain firm pressure until the bleeding stops or until the patient reaches the hospital.

4. If the wound is on an extremity, elevate it while you apply direct pressure.

Pressure Points

The most important arteries used in pressure point control include:

Brachial Artery Along the inside of the upper arm midway between the elbow and the shoulder; compression will stop or control bleeding below the pressure point.

Femoral Artery In the groin, slows bleeding in the leg on the appropriate side. See Figure 7-9.

Splints & Counterpressure Devices

In cases of open fractures, splintered bone ends can damage tissue and cause external bleeding. Properly applied splints can immobilize the fracture and lessen the chance of further injury. Air splints can aid in controlling bleeding, particularly in the upper extremities.

Pneumatic counterpressure devices, used to control and reverse shock, can also be effective in controlling bleeding of the lower extremities, abdomen, and vagina.

Tourniquet

Use of a tourniquet is rarely warranted, because control of external bleeding can almost always be achieved by using some other means. Tourniquets should be used as a *last resort only,* and only after trying all other methods of control.

FIGURE 7-5

- Prevent the loss of body heat by putting blankets over and underneath the patient; do not overheat.

- Take vital signs every five minutes; repeat patient assessment every fifteen minutes. When the body loses its ability to compensate for blood loss, the patient can suddenly and rapidly deteriorate.

- Stabilize any fractures; fractures, especially those of the pelvis or femur, can be a hidden cause of hemorrhage. Unless contraindicated, inflate a PASG on the affected part to both stabilize the fracture and control bleeding.

- Remain alert for complications of blood loss.

□ SPECIFIC METHODS OF CONTROLLING BLEEDING

Direct Pressure

The best method of controlling bleeding — and the one that should be tried first — is applying pressure directly to the wound. Direct pressure is best applied by placing **sterile** gauze or the cleanest material available (such as a handkerchief, sanitary napkin, or bed sheet) against the bleeding point and pressing firmly with the heel of your hand until a **bandage** can be applied. (A dressing is a sterile covering for a wound, while a bandage holds the dressing in place.) Check the dressing every few minutes; if it soaks through with blood, do not remove it — simply place another dressing on top of it and resume pressure (Figures 7-6–7-9 and 7-13–7-15).

To bandage, wrap the dressing firmly with a self-adherent **roller bandage;** cover the area both above and below the dressing. Tie the bandage knot over the wound unless otherwise indicated. Do not remove the bandage or the dressing once they have been applied; bleeding may restart if the bandage is disturbed.

When **air splints** or **pressure bandages** are available, they can be used over dressings to supply direct pressure. See the section on air splints later in this chapter.

A blood pressure cuff can also be used to create a pressure bandage; use only slight pressure, and monitor it frequently to avoid damage from too much pressure (Figure 7-10).

To make a pressure dressing, use several layers of gauze (Figure 7-15) topped by a bulky dressing, firmly wrapped with a self-adhering roller bandage to hold the dressing in place. Pressure dressings must remain undisturbed for at least ten minutes; earlier removal can disrupt the clot and cause bleeding to start again. If bleeding continues after the pressure bandage has been applied, it is not tight enough; either tighten the bandage or apply more pressure with the heel of your hand.

Without removing the original bandage, apply more pads or more bandages.

In cases of severe hemorrhage, do not waste time trying to find gauze or some other material; use your gloved hand (Figure 7-13) to apply direct pressure.

Elevation

Elevation of the injured limb should be used in conjunction with direct pressure to stop bleeding. Elevating the bleeding part above heart level slows the flow of blood and speeds clotting (Figure 7-16).

Do not elevate an injured limb if you suspect that a fracture, dislocation, impaled object, or spinal injury has occurred.

Pressure Points

Arterial bleeding can be controlled by digital thumb or finger pressure applied at **pressure points.** Pressure points are places where an artery is close to a bony structure and also near the skin surface; pressing the artery against the underlying bone can control the flow of blood to the injury (Figure 7-11). Use of pressure points requires skill and a knowledge of the exact location of each point.

In severe bleeding that is not being controlled by direct pressure and elevation, digital pressure can be used. Do not substitute indirect pressure for direct pressure — both kinds of pressure should be used simultaneously. The wound is probably supplied by more than one major blood vessel, so using the presure point alone is rarely enough to control severe bleeding. Hold the pressure point only as long as necessary to stop the bleeding; reapply indirect pressure if bleeding recurs.

Pressure points on the arms (brachial pressure points) and in the groin (femoral pressure points) are the ones most often used (Figure 7-12). The location of these pressure points should be thoroughly identified and the method to occlude them practiced until the technique can be applied quickly and effectively.

Brachial Artery

Pressure on the brachial artery (Figure 7-12 and 7-17) is used to control severe bleeding from an open wound on the upper extremities. This pressure point is located in a groove on the inside of the arm between the armpit and the elbow. To apply pressure to the brachial artery:

1. Grasp the middle of the patient's arm with the thumb on the outside of the arm and the fingers on the inside.
2. Press the fingers toward the thumb.
3. Use the flat, inside surface of the fingers, not the fingertips. This inward pressure closes the artery by pressing it against the humerus.

□ Control of Bleeding from Lacerated Wound

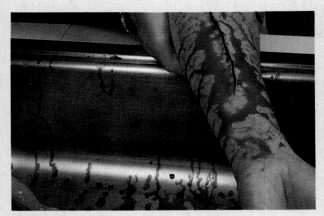

FIGURE 7-6 Bleeding from a lacerated wound on the forearm.

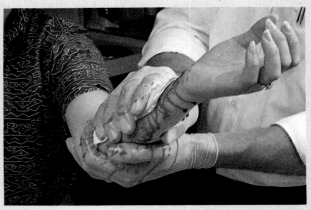

FIGURE 7-7 Control bleeding with direct pressure and elavation; if necessary, use your gloved hand.

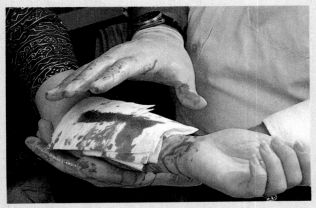

FIGURE 7-8 If bleeding soaks through the dressing, do not remove the original dressing.

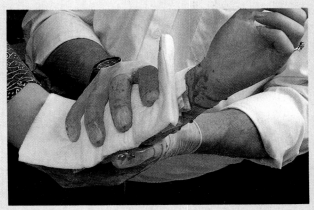

FIGURE 7-9 Add a new dressing on top of the original and continue with direct pressure and elevation. After bleeding is under control, bandage the dressing in place.

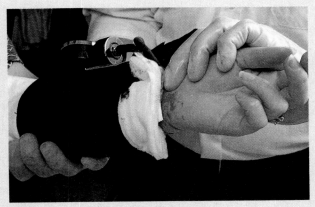

FIGURE 7-10 A blood pressure cuff can be used to apply pressure and control bleeding in an extremity.

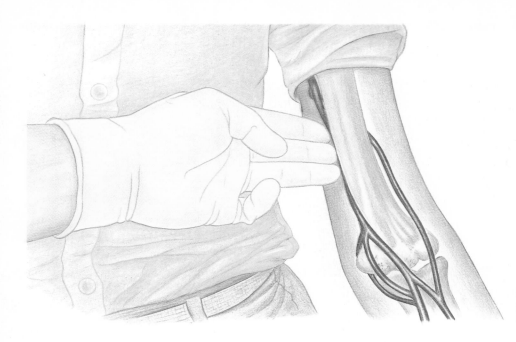

FIGURE 7-11 Using pressure points can stop profuse bleeding from an arm or leg.

FIGURE 7-12

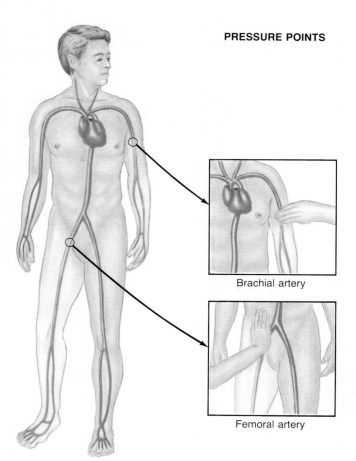

PRESSURE POINTS

Brachial artery

Femoral artery

Femoral Artery

The femoral artery (Figure 7-12 and 7-18) is used to control severe bleeding from a wound on the lower extremity. The pressure point is located on the front center part of the crease in the groin area. This is where the artery crosses the pelvic basin on the way into the lower extremity. The femoral artery needs more pressure than the brachial artery because of the number and size of muscles in the thigh and the fat content of the thigh. To apply pressure:

1. Position the patient flat on his or her back, if possible.
2. Kneeling on the opposite side from the wounded limb, place the heel of one hand directly on the pressure point, and lean forward to apply the small amount of pressure needed to close the artery.
3. If bleeding is not controlled, it may be necessary to press directly over the artery with the flat surface of the fingertips and apply additional pressure on the fingertips with the heel of the other hand.

Splints

Significant bleeding may accompany fractures, since the jagged bone end may lacerate skin, muscle, and underlying tissue, causing bleeding. Left unsplinted, the bone ends can continue to irritate surrounding tissue, with continued bleeding. In cases of fracture, splinting the bone can help control bleeding. Specific instructions on splinting are given in Chapter 13.

☐ Summary of Methods for Controlling External Bleeding

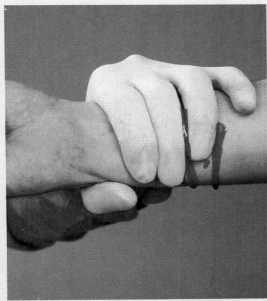

FIGURE 7-13 In cases of profuse bleeding, do not waste time hunting for a dressing.

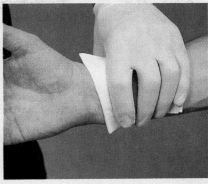

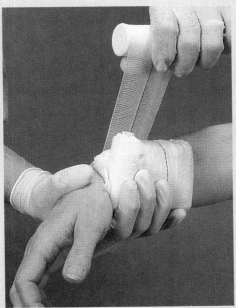

FIGURE 7-14 A Apply direct pressure with a dressing. **B** Apply additional dressing if necessary. **C** Bandage wound.

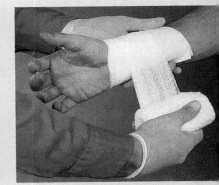

FIGURE 7-15 A B Applying a pressure dressing.

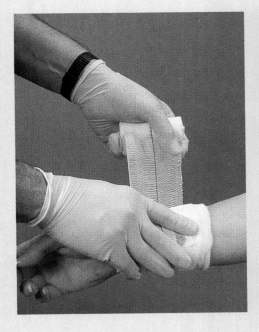

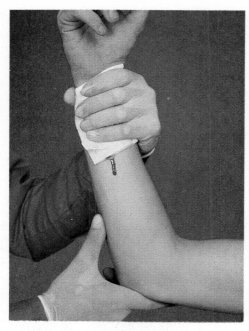

FIGURE 7-16 Combine elevation and direct pressure.

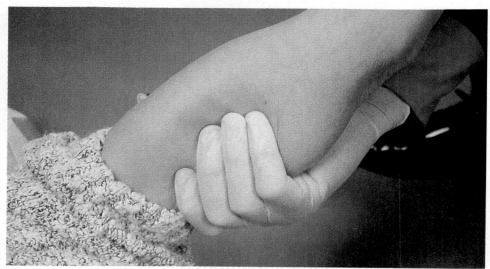

FIGURE 7-17 Apply pressure to the brachial artery pressure point to control bleeding from the arm.

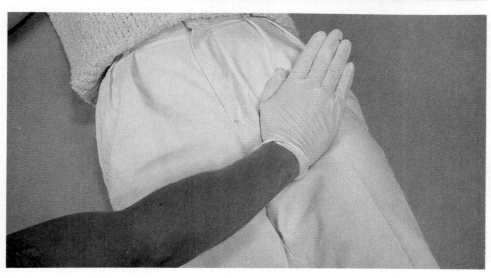

FIGURE 7-18 Apply pressure to femoral artery pressure point to control bleeding from the leg.

Air Splints

If air splints are available, they can be used to create a pressure dressing and control bleeding in an extremity (Figure 7-19).

To use an air splint:

1. Cover the wound with a thick sterile dressing; use several layers of thick sterile gauze, a sanitary napkin, or some other thick material.
2. Slip the splint over the dressing, without moving the dressing.
3. Inflate the splint until bleeding is controlled.

Pneumatic Counterpressure Devices

When significant external hemorrhage occurs in the lower extremities, a pneumatic counterpressure device, often referred to as PASG (pneumatic antishock garment) or MAST (military antishock trousers) can provide an excellent means of control through circumferential counterpressure (Figure 7-20). Actually a form of direct pressure, the pneumatic counterpressure device can be applied to the entire extremity and has the added benefit of stabilizing fractures. See Chapter 8 for application procedures. *Follow local protocol.* Do not exert too much pressure, and do not deflate the device until a physician is present. Notify the base physician when the garment was applied and monitor the patient continually. Follow specific guidelines given by the base physician.

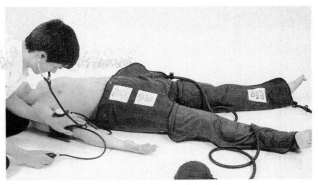

FIGURE 7-20 A pneumatic counter-pressure (PASG) device can be used to control bleeding in the lower extremities.

Tourniquet

A **tourniquet** is a device used to control severe bleeding. It is used *only as a last resort* after all other methods of control have failed and is used only on the extremities. Before you use a tourniquet, you should thoroughly understand the dangers and limitations of its use. Improper use by inexperienced, untrained persons can cause severe tissue injury or loss of a limb. The tourniquet may halt venous — but not arterial — blood flow, actually increasing blood loss. It may completely shut off the blood supply to a limb, killing all tissue below the tourniquet. The pressure from a tourniquet can crush underlying tissue, causing permanent damage to skin, nerves, and muscles. And, finally, when the tourniquet is finally removed, it may flood the central circulation with blood that is extremely acidic and hypoxic (lacking in oxygen). As a general rule, consider a tourniquet only when a large artery has been severed, when a limb has been partially or totally severed, and when bleeding is uncontrollable by any other means. Use a tourniquet only for a wound of an extremity.

With some cautions, you can use a blood pressure cuff as a tourniquet. Secure it well so that the Velcro does not pop open as a result of the pressure. Continually monitor the pressure so that it does not drop; the pressure should be maintained in the 150 mmHg range for as long as the tourniquet is in place. A blood pressure cuff used as a tourniquet can be safely left inflated for up to thirty minutes; do not release pressure until a physician is present.

The procedures for applying a tourniquet are shown in Figure 7-21.

Once the tourniquet is tightened, it should not be loosened except by or on the advice of a physician. *Never* remove a tourniquet unless you are assisted by a physician. The loosening or removal of a tourniquet may dislodge clots and result in sufficient loss of blood to cause severe shock and death.

FIGURE 7-19 Air splints can be used to apply pressure and control bleeding from an extremity.

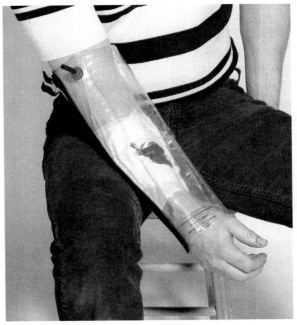

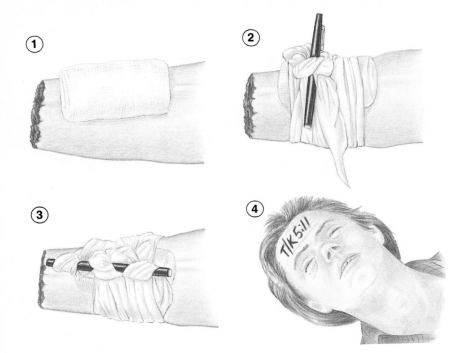

FIGURE 7-21 Apply a tourniquet as a last resort. 1. Apply pad. 2. Tighten tourniquet. 3. Fix in place. 4. Record time.

Cryotherapy

Cryotherapy, the use of cold packs to reduce bleeding, is not effective on its own but can be effective when used in combination with direct pressure and/or elevation. In addition to slowing the flow of blood, cold packs relieve pain and reduce swelling.

When using cold packs, never let the ice or cold pack come into direct contact with the patient's skin; guard against **frostbite** by placing a layer of gauze or other suitable material between the cold pack and the skin. Never use a cold pack for longer than twenty minutes at a time. If prolonged treatment is needed, use the cold pack for twenty minutes, wait ten minutes, then use it again for twenty minutes.

☐ INTERNAL BLEEDING

Internal bleeding generally results from blunt trauma, a deficiency of the body's clotting mechanism (sometimes due to medication), the spontaneous rupture of a blood vessel, or certain fractures (such as pelvic fracture). Although internal bleeding is not visible, it can be very serious — even fatal. A victim of internal bleeding can develop life-threatening shock before you even realize that he or she is bleeding. And assessment is not easy: many times you will need to assume that a victim has internal bleeding based on the mechanism of injury (such as a fall, a deceleration injury, severe blunt trauma, and so on) and on signs and symptoms. Internal bleeding can accompany external bleeding (and is often more severe), or can occur in the absence of external bleeding.

How rapidly internal bleeding progresses depends on the patient's overall condition, age, pre-existing disease, and the source of bleeding (whether blood loss is from a vein or an artery). Internal bleeding is especially severe if it seems from an internal organ that is richly supplied with blood, such as the spleen, liver, or kidney.

Assume that a patient has internal bleeding if he has a bone fracture (especially of the hip or pelvis), a rib fracture, or a penetrating wound of the skull, chest, or abdomen.

Signs and symptoms of internal bleeding include the following:

- Bruises or contusions.
- Pain, tenderness, swelling, or discoloration at the site of suspected injury.
- Bleeding from the mouth, rectum, or other body openings; blood or bloody fluid in the nose or ears.
- Nonmenstrual bleeding from the vagina.
- Dizziness in the absence of other symptoms (dizziness when going from lying to standing may be the only early sign of internal bleeding).
- Cold and clammy skin, shock-like signs and symptoms.
- Profuse sweating.
- Dull eyes, clouded vision, dilated pupils that are slow to respond to light.
- Severe respiratory distress.
- Restlessness, combativeness, and anxiety.
- Feeling of impending doom.

- Weak, rapid pulse.
- Nausea and vomiting.
- Abdominal bruising, pain, rebound tenderness, rigidity, spasms, or distention.
- Lower back pain.
- Blood in urine or decreased urinary output.
- Shallow, rapid breathing.
- Thirst.
- Weak, helpless feeling.
- Dropping blood pressure (late sign).
- Altered levels of consciousness.

Don't wait for symptoms to develop if the mechanism of injury suggests that there is probable internal bleeding. Early on, there may be no symptoms — and by the time they develop, it may be too late to render life-saving care.

Serious internal bleeding can result from fractures (Figure 7-22). As an example, a fractured shaft of the femur (thigh bone) can lacerate the femoral artery and result in an internal loss of one liter of blood. One of the most serious causes of internal blood loss is pelvic fracture.

The patient with a history of gastrointestinal **ulcer** or one who reports having vomited blood or passed blood by the rectum may have lost a significant amount of blood internally. Vomited blood can be bright red, dark red, or blackened, with the appearance of coffee grounds.

The highest priorities in terms of treatment are internal bleeding into the chest cavity and into the abdominal cavity.

To treat patients of internal bleeding:

1. The goal of treatment is to maintain adequate oxygen perfusion to all cells. Secure and maintain an open airway; administer high concentrations of humidified, high-flow oxygen.

2. Check for fractures; splint if appropriate.

3. Keep the patient quiet; position and treat for shock. Loosen restrictive clothing at the neck and waist. Unless you suspect spinal injuries, elevate the feet six to twelve inches.

4. Monitor vital signs every five minutes.

5. Anticipate vomiting; if you do not suspect spinal injuries, position the patient on his or her side with the face pointing downward, and have suc-

FIGURE 7-22 Internal bleeding.

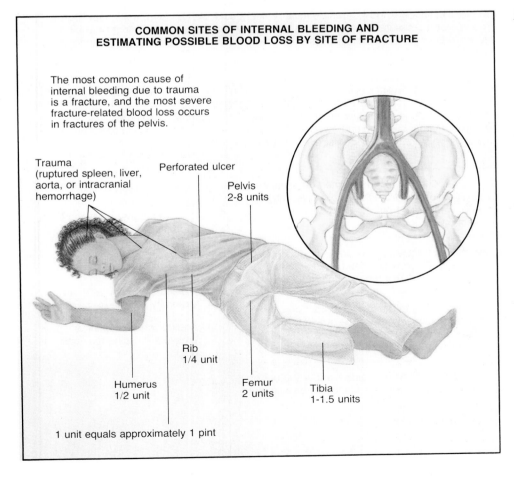

COMMON SITES OF INTERNAL BLEEDING AND
ESTIMATING POSSIBLE BLOOD LOSS BY SITE OF FRACTURE

The most common cause of internal bleeding due to trauma is a fracture, and the most severe fracture-related blood loss occurs in fractures of the pelvis.

Trauma
(ruptured spleen, liver, aorta, or intracranial hemorrhage)

Perforated ulcer

Pelvis
2-8 units

Rib
1/4 unit

Humerus
1/2 unit

Femur
2 units

Tibia
1-1.5 units

1 unit equals approximately 1 pint

tion ready. Give the patient nothing to eat or drink; he or she may need surgery at the hospital.

6. Transport the patient to a medical facility as quickly and safely as possible.

If the internal bleeding is into an extremity, use a pressure bandage or air splint to apply pressure; pressure will tend to close off the ends of the bleeding vessels. Elevate the limb after it has been immobilized. If you suspect a fracture, use extreme caution in applying any kind of pressure bandage — application directly over the fracture could further injure tissue or complicate the fracture.

If the internal bleeding is in the abdomen or lower extremities, consider use of a pneumatic counterpressure device. Thoroughly assess the patient before applying a pneumatic counterpressure device, and do not use

it with a patient who has heart failure or pulmonary edema. Deflate a pneumatic counterpressure device only on the "order" and in the presence of a physician.

For a general summary of emergency care for internal bleeding, see Figure 7-23.

☐ NOSEBLEEDS—EPISTAXIS

Nosebleeds are a relatively common source of bleeding and can result from an injury, disease, activity, the environment, or other causes. Generally, they are more annoying than serious, but enough blood may be lost to cause shock.

If a fractured skull is suspected as the cause of the nosebleed, *do not* attempt to stop the bleeding — to do so might increase pressure on the brain. Cover the nasal

FIGURE 7-23

SUMMARY — EMERGENCY CARE FOR INTERNAL BLEEDING

Internal bleeding is an extremely serious condition. It is just as dangerous as external bleeding and, when uncontrolled, can lead to death due to shock. It may be caused by a tearing or bruising force that actually ruptures or tears apart one of the internal organs or tissues. Pressure on nerves from internal bleeding can cause great pain or paralysis. The most common cause of internal bleeding due to trauma is a fracture. The most severe blood loss occurs in fracture of the pelvis. Extensive swelling can cut off blood circulation to a limb. Internal bleeding is often hard to assess and can prove rapidly fatal. The signs of internal bleeding are similar to those of shock — look for restlessness, anxiety, cold, clammy skin, weak, rapid pulse, rapid breathing, and, ultimately, a drop in blood pressure. In addition, the victim may cough up or vomit bright red blood, vomit dark blood (the color of coffee grounds), pass dark stools, pass bright red blood, or have a tender, rigid abdomen that enlarges.

Common Causes	Signs and Symptoms	Emergency Care
Hard blow to any part of the body will cause contusions and/or rupturing of internal organs.	A fractured bone, hard blow, or other force may cause internal bleeding and swelling. A closed fracture may cause loss of blood internally.	Internal bleeding usually requires surgical correction.
Fractured ribs, causing puncture of lungs. Fractured sternum from too vigorous CPR.	Bright red frothy blood coughed up usually means bleeding from the lungs. Pale, moist skin; weak, rapid pulse; shallow, rapid respiration.	1. Activate the EMS system immediately. 2. Secure an open airway; administer high concentrations of oxygen if properly trained to do so and allowed by local protocol. See pages 443-454.
Bleeding ulcer. Ingestion of a sharp object, i.e., glass.	Vomiting bright red blood may indicate stomach bleeding. Blood which has been in stomach a longer time will resemble coffee grounds.	
Disease corroding intestines, tapeworms, blow to abdominal area, appendicitis.	Slow bleeding in the intestinal tract above the sigmoid colon will cause the stools to be jet black (tar color). Hardness or spasm of abdominal muscles accompanies.	3. If bleeding originates in an extremity, elevate it. 4. Application of a splint or pressure dressing may also help.
Blockage of urethra may result in rupture of bladder, causing internal bleeding; multiple trauma may cause fractured pelvis, which may puncture kidneys.	Blood in urine may indicate bladder rupture or injury to the urinary tract. Urine may be a smoky color.	

opening loosely with a dry, sterile dressing to absorb blood; do not apply pressure. Treat the patient for skull fracture as outlined in Chapter 12.

Nosebleed from other suspected causes may be treated as follows:

1. Keep the patient quiet and in a sitting position, leaning forward to prevent aspiration of blood (Figure 7-24). If a sitting position is made impossible because of other injuries, have the patient lie down with head and shoulders elevated.

2. If there is no nasal fracture, apply pressure by pinching the nostrils together (Figure 7-25) or by placing rolled gauze between the patient's upper lip and gum; press with your fingers if necessary.

3. Apply cold compresses to the nose and face.

4. If this does not control the bleeding, insert a small clean pad of gauze into one or both nostrils and apply pressure again, pinching the nostrils. Make sure that a free end of gauze extends outside the nostril to facilitate removal later.

5. If the patient is conscious, apply pressure beneath the nostril above the upper lip.

6. Instruct the patient to avoid blowing his nose for several hours, as this could dislodge the clot.

7. If bleeding continues, transport.

FIGURE 7-24 For a nosebleed patient, keep the patient quiet and leaning forward in a sitting position.

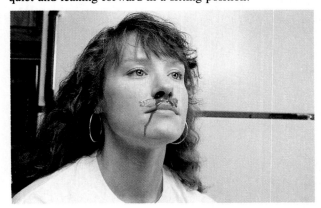

FIGURE 7-25 Apply pressure by pinching the nostrils and, if necessary, apply cold compresses to the nose and face.

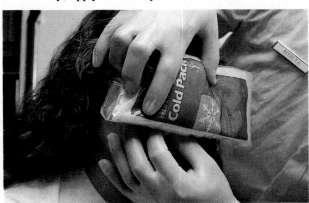

chapter 8

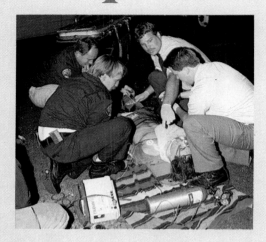

Shock

✳ OBJECTIVES

- Describe the basic causes and physiology of shock.
- Outline the factors that may influence the severity of shock.
- List the various types of shock.
- Identify the signs/symptoms and stages of shock.
- Describe and demonstrate the management of shock.
- Describe and demonstrate how to apply pneumatic antishock garments.

It is recommended that EMTs wear protective gloves whenever there is a possibility of coming in contact with a patient's blood, body fluids, mucous membranes, traumatic wounds, or sores. See Chapter 31.

In 1852, shock was defined as "a rude unhinging of the machinery of life." Probably no better definition exists to describe the devastating effects of this process on a patient, but a more recent definition calls shock "the collapse and progressive failure of the cardiovascular system." Shock, left untreated, may be fatal — and it may well be the EMT's worst enemy. In the field, shock must be recognized and treated immediately, or the patient may die. If shock can be prevented or arrested, on the other hand, the chances for survival will be greatly enhanced.

The definition of shock does not involve low blood pressure, rapid pulse, or cool clammy skin — these are merely the signs. Simply stated, shock results from inadequate **perfusion** of the body's cells with oxygenated blood.

Shock is a step-by-step process that may be either gradual or rapid in onset; often, there is enough warning that you can anticipate shock and begin to stabilize the patient. Throughout the development of shock, the patient's condition is constantly changing — and it is critical that his or her condition be constantly monitored.

To understand the abnormal condition of shock, you need to know what is happening and how the body responds to protect itself from these changes.

☐ THE PHYSIOLOGY OF SHOCK

Every cell in the body requires oxygen to function. Oxygen is delivered to the cells through the bloodstream, is taken in by the cells, and undergoes a complicated physiologic process (metabolism) that produces energy and waste by-products. Simply stated, oxygen and glucose produce energy and waste products such as carbon dioxide. Long-term survival requires delivery of nutrients and oxygen to body cells. The cells most sensitive to a lack of oxygen are those in the heart, brain, and lungs; they can be irreparably damaged in just four to six minutes without oxygen and glucose.

In order to prevent death, **oxygenation** of the red blood cells — which includes having an adequate airway and proper ventilation — is one of the most critical parts of the shock resuscitation process. (The majority of all blood cells are red blood cells, which carry oxygen to the body's cells.) Proper airway and ventilation procedures are covered in detail in Chapters 4 and 5.

The other critical aspect of shock prevention and treatment is the adequate perfusion of body cells.

The cardiovascular system consists of the heart, the blood vessels, and the blood that circulates throughout the system. If any one of the three components malfunctions, adequate amounts of blood (and the nutrients it carries) will not be delivered to individual cells.

The heart, with its set of paired pumps, collects blood from the veins, circulates it through the lungs (where it dumps carbon dioxide and picks up oxygen), returns it to the heart, circulates it through the body, and then starts the cycle all over again. The effectiveness of the heart as a pump depends on its ability to change the rate and force of its contractions as needed.

In order for blood to be circulated through the system, two things are required: enough blood, and enough pressure to move the blood. Two factors help to maintain the necessary blood pressure:

1. The amount of blood pumped out of the heart per minute (cardiac output).
2. The pressure created by constriction of the arteries, which creates resistance (**peripheral vascular resistance**). When the arteries constrict, the passageway through which the blood travels becomes narrower, and pressure increases. When the arteries dilate, the passageway opens up, and pressure decreases. The central nervous system constantly regulates the blood pressure by signaling the arteries to constrict or relax.

The volume of blood pumped out by each contraction (stroke) is called the **stroke volume.** A small stroke volume can occur under any of the following conditions:

* The heart fails to pump enough blood or fails to pump at all.
* The heart cannot enlarge enough to receive the required amount of blood.
* There is not enough blood to fill the heart chambers. (Blood vessels are cut or burst open.)
* The heart is not strong enough to empty completely.

When blood flow is compromised, the body uses the following method to compensate: Smooth muscles in the blood vessels contract, causing blood to flow away from the extremities and abdomen and to the chest and brain. Blood vessels in some parts of the body then become deprived of nutrients. Eventually, the affected blood vessels become smaller and allow capillaries to develop small holes through which plasma leaks. As a result, fluid accumulates in the space between the cells and the blood vessels, making transport of oxygen even more difficult.

The heart is then forced to work under three conditions, which eventually decrease its efficiency:

1. Increased resistance to blood flow in the muscle and capillary beds makes the heart work harder to force blood through the vessels.

2. The oxygen supply is decreased, yet the heart needs more oxygen in order to work harder.

3. There is not enough blood to adequately fill the chambers of the heart; with the heart only half-full, it has to contract more often to pump less blood.

The body responds to shock with the following defenses (Figure 8-1):

- When the blood supply is inadequate, the blood vessels constrict.
- Cardiac output increases through stronger and more rapid contractions.
- The adrenal glands release epinephrine.
- The body tries to rid itself of wastes by making respirations faster.
- As shock progresses, the brain decreases its functioning as perfusion and oxygenation drop. The victim first develops anxiety and belligerent behavior, then slowing of the thought processes, and, finally, slowing of the motor and sensory functions of the body.

□ CAUSES OF SHOCK

There are four primary ways in which inadequate perfusion might occur, i.e., there are four basic causes of shock (Figure 8-2):

1. Fluid is lost from the circulatory system (hypovolemic shock). This loss usually results from injury that causes hemorrhage, from burns (which lead to loss of plasma), or through **dehydration** (which is the loss of fluids). In response, the brain releases signals and hormones that cause increased cardiac output and that cause the vessels to increase their resistance. A person can lose 25 percent of his total blood volume and be in moderate shock; if he loses 30 to 35 percent of his total volume, he is considered to be in serious shock.

2. The heart fails to pump enough blood (cardiogenic shock). Shock is a vicious cycle: the heart fails to pump enough blood, which makes the blood flow diminish. This, in turn, lowers the blood pressure, which weakens the heart — and a weakened heart fails to pump enough blood.

FIGURE 8-1

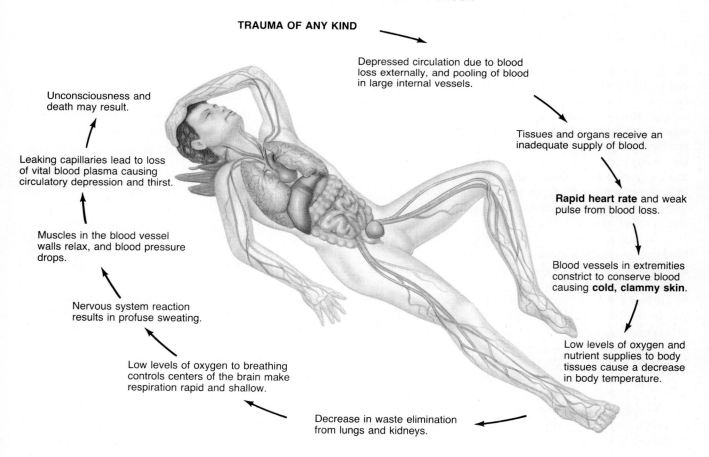

CONTINUOUS CYCLE OF TRAUMATIC SHOCK*

TRAUMA OF ANY KIND

Depressed circulation due to blood loss externally, and pooling of blood in large internal vessels.

Tissues and organs receive an inadequate supply of blood.

Unconsciousness and death may result.

Leaking capillaries lead to loss of vital blood plasma causing circulatory depression and thirst.

Rapid heart rate and weak pulse from blood loss.

Muscles in the blood vessel walls relax, and blood pressure drops.

Blood vessels in extremities constrict to conserve blood causing **cold, clammy skin.**

Nervous system reaction results in profuse sweating.

Low levels of oxygen and nutrient supplies to body tissues cause a decrease in body temperature.

Low levels of oxygen to breathing controls centers of the brain make respiration rapid and shallow.

Decrease in waste elimination from lungs and kidneys.

CAUSES AND RESULTS OF SHOCK

Some of the major causes of shock are as follows:

- Allergic reactions
- Bites or stings of poisonous snakes or insects
- Poisons
- Exposure to extremes of heat and cold
- Emotional stress
- Myocardial infarction
- Spinal injuries

- Severe trauma
- Severe pain
- Loss of blood
- Severe burns
- Electrical shock
- Gas poisoning
- Certain illnesses

Resulting in one or more of:

- Failure of heart to pump sufficient blood

- Severe blood or fluid loss so that there is insufficient blood in the system

- Enlargement: dilation of blood vessels so that there is insufficient blood to fill them

- Breathing problems result in insufficient oxygen traveling through the system

RESULT: No matter what the reason, the result is the same: all normal bodily processes are affected. There is insufficient blood flow (perfusion) to provide nourishment and oxygen to all parts of the body. The key to managing shock is adequate ventilation and oxygenation.

FIGURE 8-2

3. The blood vessels dilate or constrict, causing blood to pool away from vital areas (peripheral shock, which includes septic and neurogenic shock). There can be many reasons for this, including head injury.

4. Inadequate oxygen.

☐ FACTORS INFLUENCING THE SEVERITY OF SHOCK

Some degree of shock occurs from all injuries; its severity depends on factors such as the stability of the patient's central nervous system, his or her age, his or her state of health, the presence of any existing disease, and so on. What might cause a mild case of shock in one person could cause a severe case in another.

☐ TYPES OF SHOCK

Shock may be caused by conditions that affect fluid volume, peripheral vascular resistance, or cardiac output. Within those three categories, there are seven types of shock (see Figure 8-3).

Hemorrhagic Shock

Simply stated, **hemorrhagic shock** (Figure 8-4) results from the loss of blood in the circulatory system, usually as a result of internal or external bleeding associated with injury or the loss of plasma associated with serious

SUMMARY — TYPES OF SHOCK	
TYPE	**DESCRIPTION AND CAUSE**
Hemorrhagic	Loss of blood resulting in not enough blood going to tisues, i.e., wounds, internal bleeding. Possible causes — multiple trauma and severe burns. There is insufficient blood in the system to provide adequate circulation to all body parts.
Neurogenic	Spinal or head injury resulting in loss of nerve control and thus **integrity** of blood vessels. The nervous system loses control over the vascular system — blood vessels dilate and there is insufficient blood to fill them.
Psychogenic	Something psychological affects the patient, i.e., the sight of blood, loved one injuried, etc.; blood drains from the head and pools in the abdomen, person faints due to lack of blood in the brain because of a temporary dilation of blood vessels.
Cardiogenic	Cardiac muscle not pumping effectively due to injury or previous heart attack. The heart muscle no longer imparts sufficient pressure to circulate the blood through the system.
Metabolic	Loss of body fluids with a change in biochemical equilibrium. Example: insulin shock or diabetic coma, vomiting, diarrhea.
Septic	Severe infection. Toxins cause pooling of blood in capillaries with dilation of blood vessels; not enough blood to tissues. Bacteria attack small blood vessel walls so that they lose blood and plasma and can no longer constrict.
Anaphylactic	Severe allergic reaction of the body to sensitization by a foreign protein, such as insect sting, foods, medicine, ingested, inhaled or injected substances. It can occur in minutes or even seconds following contact with the substance to which the patient is allergic.

FIGURE 8-3

HEMORRHAGIC SHOCK

Watch for shock in all trauma patients; they can lose fluids not only externally, through hemorrhage, vomiting, or burns, but also internally, through crush injuries or punctures of organs.

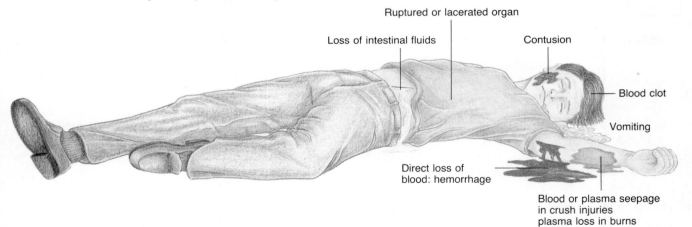

Ruptured or lacerated organ

Loss of intestinal fluids

Contusion

Blood clot

Vomiting

Direct loss of blood: hemorrhage

Blood or plasma seepage in crush injuries plasma loss in burns

FIGURE 8-4

burns. In hemorrhagic shock, there is not enough blood in circulation to supply all of the body's organs.

Metabolic Shock

Metabolic shock results when injury or untreated illness leads to profound fluid loss. Examples are severe burns (in which plasma is lost) or by serious illness that causes

dehydration (following diarrhea, vomiting, or excessive urination).

Septic Shock

Septic Shock develops when a severe infection (usually bacterial) creates poisonous **toxins** that cause blood to pool in the extremities, or toxins cause the blood vessels to dilate. While the culprit is usually a bacterial infection, septic shock can also stem from a viral, fungal, or **rickettsial** infection. Simply stated, the toxins produced by the infection damage the blood vessels, causing them to leak; in addition, damaged vessels lose muscle tone and are no longer able to constrict to create pressure. Septic shock can follow a prolonged illness, an injury that leads to infection, or a surgical procedure. Half of all those who develop septic shock die as a result.

Neurogenic Shock

Usually following spinal or head injury, **neurogenic shock** develops when the autonomic nervous control of the blood vessels fails; it can be caused by spinal cord injury, diabetes, pulmonary embolism, cirrhosis, or gastric distention, to name a few causes. Normally, the nervous system instructs the blood vessels to constrict or dilate and thus controls blood pressure. In neurogenic shock (usually because of injury) that control is lost; the blood vessels dilate, and blood pools in the peripheral areas of the body, away from vital organs. Blood vessels then lack the pressure required to adequately circulate the blood throughout the body. Simply stated, there is enough blood volume, but the blood vessels are enlarged; blood pressure drops significantly. Remember that other central nervous system controls are also lost — body temperature, for example, usually drops rapidly in neurogenic shock.

Psychogenic Shock (Fainting)

When a patient is affected psychologically (such as by fear, the sight of blood, bad news, or the death/injury of a loved one), a sudden, rapid, temporary dilation of the blood vessels occurs. As a result, blood pools in the abdomen and extremities, leaving the brain with inadequate blood circulation. At that point, the patient faints (temporarily loses consciousness). **Psychogenic shock** is self-correcting: when the patient faints (collapses), his or her head assumes a lower position; blood then returns to the brain, and the patient regains consciousness. Because an isolated episode of fainting is generally not serious, your greatest concern is to treat any injuries sustained in the fall.

Anaphylactic Shock ("Allergy Shock")

Anaphylactic shock results from a severe allergic reaction of the body to a foreign protein, such as an insect sting, food, medicine, pollen, or some other inhaled, ingested, or injected substance. The most common causes of anaphylactic shock are bee stings and drugs; at least 1 percent of the general population is at risk for developing anaphylactic shock from bee stings alone. The reaction can occur within minutes — or even seconds — following a sting or other exposure, and immediate treatment is required to prevent death.

Anaphylactic shock should be considered a grave medical emergency. The severity of the reaction is inversely related to the time elapsing between exposure and the onset of symptoms: the shorter the time before symptoms appear, the greater the risk of a fatal reaction.

Cardiogenic Shock

Cardiogenic shock occurs when the heart itself is damaged or injured; 10 to 15 percent of all patients suffering myocardial infarction develop cardiogenic shock. Other conditions that can cause cardiogenic shock include **coronary artery disease, valvular heart disease,** left **ventricular failure, pulmonary embolism, cardiac tamponade, tension pneumothorax,** or a mechanical obstruction to the blood flow to the heart. Simply stated, the heart muscle does not pump efficiently due to injury or myocardial infarction, so not enough pressure is exerted to circulate blood through the system.

Cardiogenic shock is progressive and very difficult to reverse; treatment is effective only if started *very* early. Only 5 percent of those who develop cardiogenic shock following myocardial infarction survive; overall, 80 to 100 percent die as a result of cardiogenic shock, regardless of the condition that caused it.

□ STAGES OF SHOCK

Shock is progressive — it passes through three stages and, if left untreated, may end in death. The three basic stages of shock include the following (Figure 8-5):

Compensatory Shock

In **compensatory shock,** the first stage, the body uses its normal defense mechanisms to try to maintain normal function. There are minimal signs and symptoms at this stage. As the patient's blood pressure begins to drop, the heart rate increases and the blood vessels constrict in an attempt to restore normal blood pressure. If no further complications occur, the body corrects the condition within twenty-four hours. Signs and symptoms of compensatory shock include pale skin, tachycardia, and normal blood pressure.

Progressive Shock

When bleeding is uncontrolled, the body's mechanisms can compensate only so much. Then the patient progresses to the second stage, or **progressive shock.** In an attempt to keep the vital organs perfused with oxygenated blood, the body shunts blood away from the extremities and the abdomen and toward the heart, brain, and lungs. As a result, the tissues in the extremities and the abdomen produce toxic by-products. At this stage, the body cannot correct the shock itself; without medical intervention, further decline occurs. Signs and

Shock is inadequate perfusion of bodily tissues. It is not a disease in itself but occurs secondary to trauma or illness. Shock may develop when serious injury causes significant blood loss, pump (heart) damage, spinal cord injury, or pulmonary injury, or when serious illness causes peripheral vasodilation or severe dehydration. Remember — in order for blood to circulate properly there must be adequate blood volume, a good working pump, and a intact vascular system.

When the cells of the body are not adequatelly oxygenated and/or nourished, a sequence of events may occur that, if left uncorrected, will result in death. The body will set in motion a series of complex mechanisms in an attempt to achieve homeostasis and compensate for shock. If the state of shock is severe or prolonged, it may become irreversible. If this occurs, no intervention will save the patient. Recognizing the signs and symptoms of each stage of shock will help you classify the patient's condition according to its severity so you can intervene appropriately.

COMPENSATORY STAGE

- Restlessness, anxiety, irritability, apprehension
- Slightly increased heart rate
- Normal blood pressure or sligthly elevated systolic pressure or sligthly decreased diastolic pressure
- Pale and cool skin in hypovolemic shock, warm and flushed skin in septic, anaphylactic, and neurogenic shock
- Slightly increased respiratory rate
- Slightly decreased body temperature (except fever in septic shock)

PROGRESSIVE (UNCOMPENSATED) STAGE

- Listlessness, apathy, confusion, slowed speech
- Rapid heart rate
- Slowed, irregular, weak, thready pulse
- Decreased blood pressure
- Cold, clammy, cyanotic skin
- Rapid breathing
- Severely decreased body temperature
- Confusion and incoherent, slurred speech, possibly unconsciousness
- Depressed or absent reflexes
- Decreased blood pressure with diastolic pressure reaching zero
- Dilated pupils slow to react
- Slow, shallow, irregular respirations

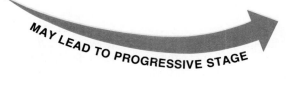

MAY LEAD TO PROGRESSIVE STAGE

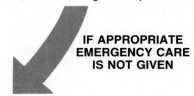

IF APPROPRIATE EMERGENCY CARE IS NOT GIVEN

IRREVERSIBLE SHOCK AND DEATH

FIGURE 8-5

symptoms include cyanotic or mottled skin, decreased blood pressure, and major changes in level of consciousness.

Irreversible Shock

There are no clear immediate signs and symptoms of **irreversible shock,** which is the final stage. Damage usually begins to manifest itself several days later, when organs die and stop functioning. In this last stage, blood is shunted away from the liver and kidneys to the heart and brain; the liver and kidneys then die. Blood vessels are no longer able to sustain the pressure needed to feed the heart and brain; blood begins to pool away from the vital organs, and death occurs.

Even with treatment, damage to the vital organs is permanent; untreated, this stage of shock leads to death.

☐ SIGNS AND SYMPTOMS OF SHOCK

Remember — the most obvious changes in vital signs occur late in the shock process. If you are "fooled" by normal early vital signs and wait to begin treatment until vital signs start to deteriorate, you may reduce the overall effectiveness of the emergency care rendered. It is vital to know that low blood pressure is a late and very serious sign of shock. A person can be in serious shock and still have near-normal blood pressure!

The signs and symptoms of shock should not be studied merely as a means of identifying shock, but are of tremendous value in helping to determine what will be required in treating the condition. The clinical picture of shock depends on what is occurring in the body. Decreased blood flow to the skin causes it to become pale, clammy, and cyanotic. When cardiac output decreases, the pulse will be more rapid as the heart tries to compensate. As blood pressure drops, the pulse will become shallow. Inadequate perfusion of the brain will cause anxiety, confusion, apathy, and loss of consciousness. Inadequate perfusion to the stomach will cause nausea and/or vomiting.

Signs and Symptoms Common to All but Anaphylactic Shock

All the signs and symptoms of shock do not occur at one time; they don't occur in any specific pattern or order, either. Generally, the patient's condition deteriorates — sometimes rapidly — over time, and signs and symp-toms tend to change constantly. Signs and symptoms *that are common to all but anaphylactic shock* include the following (Figure 8-6):

- Weakness (may be the most significant symptom).
- Restlessness, anxiety, fear, disorientation, mental confusion, and an anxious or dull expression.
- Feeling of impending doom.
- Cold, clammy, moist skin (except in septic shock).
- **diaphoresis** (profuse sweating).
- Extreme thirst.
- Nausea and/or vomiting.
- Initial dull, chalklike appearance to the skin; later cyanosis at the lips, tongue, or ear lobes.
- Shallow, irregular breathing; may also be labored, rapid, or gasping.
- Dizziness.
- Loss of consciousness or altered levels of consciousness.
- Closed or partially closed eyelids; dilated pupils; dull, lusterless eyes.

FIGURE 8-6

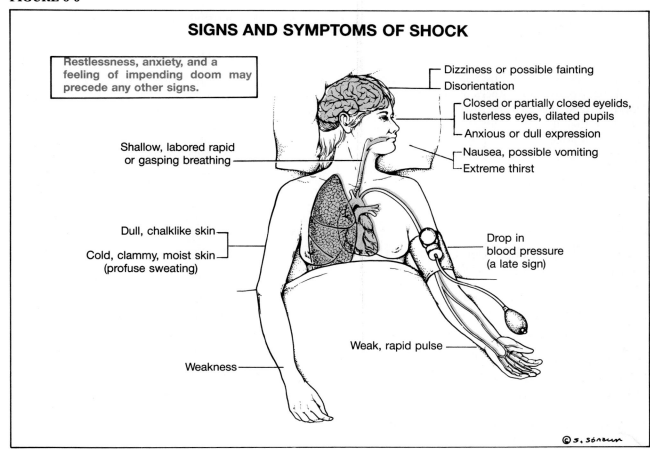

SIGNS AND SYMPTOMS OF SHOCK

Restlessness, anxiety, and a feeling of impending doom may precede any other signs.

Dizziness or possible fainting
Disorientation
Closed or partially closed eyelids, lusterless eyes, dilated pupils
Anxious or dull expression
Nausea, possible vomiting
Extreme thirst

Shallow, labored rapid or gasping breathing

Dull, chalklike skin
Cold, clammy, moist skin (profuse sweating)

Drop in blood pressure (a late sign)

Weak, rapid pulse

Weakness

- Weak, rapid pulse.
- Rarely, shaking and trembling of the arms and legs, as if chilled, or trembling of the entire body.
- Delayed capillary refill.
- Late sign: **hypotension** — gradual and steady drop in blood pressure (to 90/60 or lower), and eventually unobtainable blood pressure. A marked drop in blood pressure in a short period of time when no trauma or external bleeding is apparent is often an indication of internal bleeding.
- Eventual cardiac arrest, respiratory arrest, and death.

In assessing the signs and symptoms of shock, watch for a general pattern that indicates that the body is trying to compensate for circulatory problems. At first, pulse will increase and respiratory rate will increase. The victim will become restless. Then changes start to occur, sometimes rapidly: pulse gets weak and rapid. The patient's level of alertness starts to fail. Finally, respiratory arrest and cardiac arrest lead to death.

Signs and Symptoms of Specific Types of Shock

In addition to the above, you may note some or all of the following specific signs and symptoms.

Psychogenic Shock

The greatest signs and symptoms of psychogenic shock are a sudden drop in blood pressure and a feeling of faintness. This feeling is generally relieved if the patient sits with his head between his knees or lays on the floor.

Don't assume that because psychogenic shock is self-correcting that it is also not serious. The patient may have been injured in the fall, the patient may need strong emotional support, and the fainting may be a sign of a serious underlying condition (such as heart disease, undetected diabetes, brain disorders, or serious inner ear problems).

Septic Shock

This type of shock is not often seen in the field. Look for the following specific signs and symptoms:

- Confusion (generally the earliest sign).
- A greater-than-normal cardiac output.
- Warm, flushed skin.
- Low blood pressure (a very late sign).
- Increased pulse (a very late sign).
- Increased respiration (a very late sign).

The high mortality rate from septic shock (as high as 50 percent) is probably due to the fact that many cases are not recognized and therefore not adequately treated.

Cardiogenic Shock

Look for the following specific signs and symptoms:

- Chest pain.
- Shortness of breath.
- Rapid, thready (irregular) pulse.
- Peripheral cyanosis.
- Anxiety, confusion, lethargy, unresponsiveness.
- Decreased or absent peripheral pulse.
- Cool, clammy mottled skin.

In cardiogenic shock, watch for progressive changes instead of relying on isolated signs or symptoms to aid in assessment.

Hemorrhagic Shock

In trauma that has caused bleeding, watch for:

- Rapid pulse.
- Rapid, shallow respirations.
- Delayed or absent capillary refill.
- Low blood pressure (this is a very late sign, especially among children and adolescents).

Anaphylactic Shock

Anaphylactic shock is a severe allergic reaction that can occur when the body comes into contact with an allergen. Common causes of anaphylactic shock are insect bites or stings, foods (especially seafood or shellfish), spices, food additives or preservatives (especially sulfite), medications (especially antibiotics), chemicals, and inhaled substances. The signs and symptoms of anaphylactic shock are acute, generalized, and violent — they can develop within a few seconds of exposure, and rarely take more than a few minutes to develop.

The signs and symptoms of anaphylactic shock can occur in any combination of the following (Figure 8-7):

1. **Signs and symptoms involving the skin:**
   - Itching and burning of the skin with flushing, especially around the face and chest.
   - Blueness (cyanosis) around the lips.
   - Raised, hivelike patches with severe itching.
   - Swelling of the face and tongue.
   - Paleness.
   - Swelling of the blood vessels just underneath the skin.

ANAPHYLACTIC SHOCK

Anaphylactic shock is a severe allergic reaction of the body to sensitization by a foreign protein, such as insect sting; foods; medicine; ingested, inhaled, or injected substances. It can occur in minutes or even seconds following contact with the substance to which the patient is allergic. This is a grave medical emergency.

Rapidity of onset

As a rule, anaphylactic reactions occur more frequently and rapidly when the antigen is injected (seconds to minutes). By the oral route, they may be delayed (up to hours), although immediate, catastrophic progression is also a possibility with oral ingestion.

Common early symptoms and signs

Flushing, itching

Sneezing, watery eyes and nose

Skin rash, airway swelling

'Tickle' or 'lump' in the throat which cannot be cleared, cough

Gastrointestinal complaints

These signs and symptoms may swiftly lead to:

and/or

Acute respiratory obstruction

Circulatory collapse

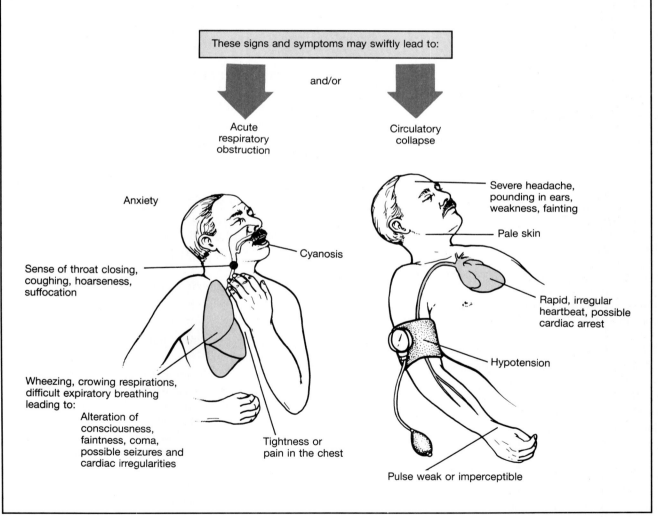

Anxiety

Cyanosis

Sense of throat closing, coughing, hoarseness, suffocation

Wheezing, crowing respirations, difficult expiratory breathing leading to:
Alteration of consciousness, faintness, coma, possible seizures and cardiac irregularities

Tightness or pain in the chest

Severe headache, pounding in ears, weakness, fainting

Pale skin

Rapid, irregular heartbeat, possible cardiac arrest

Hypotension

Pulse weak or imperceptible

FIGURE 8-7

2. **Signs and symptoms involving the heart and circulation:**
   - Weak, rapid pulse; pulse may be undetectable.
   - Low blood pressure.
   - Dizziness.
   - Restlessness.
   - Diminished stroke volume and cardiac output.

3. **Signs and symptoms involving the respiratory tract:**
   - Spasm of the bronchioles.
   - A painful, squeezing sensation in the chest.
   - Difficulty in breathing.
   - Coughing; bronchial obstruction.
   - Swelling of the lungs.
   - Swelling of the larynx.
   - Swelling of the epiglottis.
   - Respiratory wheezes.

4. **Signs and symptoms involving the gastrointestinal tract:**
   - Nausea.
   - Vomiting.
   - Abdominal cramps.
   - Diarrhea.

5. **Signs and symptoms involving the level of consciousness:**
   - Restlessness.
   - Faintness.
   - Convulsions.
   - Loss of consciousness (occurs very early in anaphylactic shock).

Shock in a Child

Shock in a child can present a somewhat different picture: it develops early, and it progresses extremely rapidly. Sometimes a child will show no symptoms at all, or only very subtle ones, until very late in the shock process; the only visible clues may be pallor or an altered sensorium. *Because of that, always begin shock treatment very early for a child; never wait to see if symptoms develop.*

Sometimes the best clues to shock in a child are general physical appearance and the presence of lethargy: always worry about a lethargic child who will let you do anything to him.

Vital signs are often a very late sign of shock in a child. The lower limit of normal systolic blood pressure is 70 in infants and children under six; in children six to fourteen, the normal measurement should be above 80 to 90. A child's pulse also gives an indication: under the age of two, less than 110 beats per minute is serious;

from two to six, under 80 is serious; and from six to fourteen years of age, a pulse of less than 60 indicates a serious problem.

☐ PATIENT ASSESSMENT

Never wait for the symptoms of shock to develop — by the time shock symptoms are obvious, it is often too late to really help the patient. If the history of the injury or illness suggests that shock may occur, *immediately* suspect shock and begin treating it. You will never hurt a patient who does *not* have shock by treating for shock.

Assessment for shock is similar to assessment for any other trauma: you should follow the basic ABCs (airway, breathing, and circulation). Your rapid initial assessment should determine whether major to moderate bleeding has occurred, whether the patient has a strong or weak pulse, and whether the level of consciousness has been altered.

During the primary survey, rapidly assess all conditions to isolate those that might be causing problems. During the secondary survey, do a complete, in-depth assessment of each body region or system.

Primary Survey

1. Visually assess the situation.
   - Look at how the patient is lying.
   - Note the patient's skin color.
   - Note the patient's level of consciousness.
   - Note whether there is blood on the ground.
   - Find out what caused the emergency.

2. Check airway viability. If the patient's skin is a normal color and respirations are full and at a rate of twelve to twenty per minute, the airway is functional.

3. Check the patient's carotid or radial pulse.
   - If there is a radial pulse, systolic blood pressure is at least 80 mmHg.
   - If there is a carotid pulse, systolic blood pressure is at least 60.
   - As you ask the patient what happened, check the skin color and capillary refill. To test capillary refill, squeeze a spot on the patient's forehead until it blanches (goes white); let go, and see how long it takes for color to return. If capillary refill is good, color should return within two seconds.
   - Note whether the airway is open and whether the patient is responsive and can move.
   - Life-threatening conditions are indicated by an absence of the carotid or radial pulse. Capillary

refill of longer than two seconds, and pale or cyanotic skin may also be an indication of inadequate circulation.

4. Check for adequate perfusion.
   - The first sign of *inadequate* perfusion is a change in the level of consciousness; anxiety and belligerence are early manifestations.
   - Exaggerated air hunger and the patient's attempts to remove the oxygen mask are other signs of inadequate perfusion.
   - The pulse should be palpable, strong, and normal in rate.
   - Danger signs are a pulse that is weak or unobtainable, thready, rapid, or extremely slow.

5. Do a more detailed check of the level of consciousness. Unless there is head injury, the level of consciousness is a good measure of circulation to the brain. Significant changes in consciousness indicate problems with circulation and perfusion.

6. Check the patient's skin color (Figure 8-8).

FIGURE 8-8 A healthy person with dark skin will usually have a red undertone and show a healthy pink color in the nailbeds, lips, mucous membranes of the mouth, and tongue. However, a black patient in shock from a lack of oxygen does not exhibit the marked skin color changes. Rather, the skin around the nose and mouth will have a grayish cast, the mucous membranes of the mouth and tongue will be blue (cyanotic), and the lips and nailbeds will have a blue tinge. If shock is due to bleeding, the mucous membranes in the mouth and tongue will not look blue but will have a pale, graying, waxy pallor. Other landmarks include the tips of the ears, which may be red during fever.

DETERMINING SHOCK IN A DARK-SKINNED PERSON

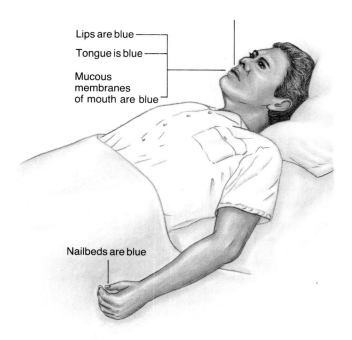

Lips are blue

Tongue is blue

Mucous membranes of mouth are blue

Nailbeds are blue

- Cyanosis indicates lack of adequate oxygen in the lungs and unoxygenated blood; less commonly, it is caused by poor blood circulation.
- Pale-colored skin can be caused by constriction of the blood vessels, a decreased number of red blood cells, or interruption of the blood flow to that part of the body.
- Compare the skin color of one part of the body to the skin color in other parts of the body.

7. Note the skin temperature. Skin that is cool to the touch for reasons other than cold weather may indicate that blood is being shunted to the vital organs — a possible sign of shock.

After completing the primary survey, perform any treatment suggested by your findings. Then move on to perform a secondary survey.

Secondary Survey

As time and the patient's condition permit, go back over the points covered in the primary survey and study each in greater detail. If it is possible to transport the patient early, you might complete parts of the secondary survey in the ambulance en route to the hospital. Get exact measurements of vital signs, survey for associated injuries, check the moisture and color of the skin, and examine the cardiac system in greater detail. Modify your treatment if necessary based on what you find in the secondary survey.

□ MANAGEMENT OF SHOCK

General Principles

Management of shock begins during the resuscitation phase of the primary survey and does not end until all bodily tissues are being properly perfused (this sometimes does not occur until the patient is at the hospital).

The top priority in shock management is to keep the vital organs functioning, and the primary goal is to halt the progression of shock. To accomplish these objectives, the EMT must administer high-flow oxygen. Unless you improve the delivery of oxygenated blood to the body's cells, the patient will not improve; rather, the patient will continue to deteriorate rapidly until he or she dies.

You cannot reverse shock, but rapid treatment can prevent shock from getting worse. If a victim is in shock, he should be transported immediately; treat and stabilize en route. The following steps should be taken to manage shock in the field:

1. Secure an open airway. (Give extra attention to patients with an obvious airway compromise, with

respiratory rates over twenty per minute, with noisy respiration, or to those not breathing.)

2. Control any obvious bleeding; use direct pressure, pressure points, elevation, an air splint, a blood pressure cuff, a pneumatic antishock garment, or a tourniquet if indicated. Early use of the pneumatic antishock garment can help control bleeding in the abdomen or lower extremities.

3. Administer oxygen in as high a concentration as possible. *Every patient in shock should immediately receive 100 percent oxygen at high-flow rates.*

4. Place the patient on his or her back with the legs and feet elevated approximately eight to twelve inches (Figure 8-9). If patient has serious injuries to the extremities, put flat on his or her back in supine position (Figure 8-10). *Follow local protocol.* Do *not* place the patient in the Trendelenburg position (a thirty-degree, head-down tilt), since it increases the work of the heart in circulating the blood.

5. Apply the pneumatic antishock garment (PASG) if the patient is suffering from hypovolemic shock and if use of the PASG is not contraindicated. Follow local protocol.

6. Splint any fractures. This can help reduce shock by slowing bleeding and helping to relieve pain.

7. Maintain the patient's normal body temperature. If he or she is too hot, sponge with tepid water. If the patient is too cool, keep warm by conserving body heat.

8. Keep the patient quiet and still; shock is aggravated by rough and/or excessive handling.

9. Give the patient nothing by mouth because of the possible need for surgery, because of possible injury to the digestive system, and because it may cause vomiting. If the patient complains of intense thirst, it may help to wet his or her lips with a wet towel.

10. Transport the patient rapidly to the nearest facility capable of handling the patient's injuries or condition.

    • The recommended transport position is for the patient to be on his or her back with the feet and legs elevated approximately twelve inches (Figure 8-11). However, this position should not be used if the patient has sustained suspected head injuries, chest injuries, abdominal injuries, neck/spinal injuries, pelvic fracture, or hip fracture/dislocation.

    • If the patient has severe extremity injuries, transport in a supine position.

    • If the patient has cardiac problems, respiratory problems, or difficulty breathing, transport in a semi-sitting position (Figure 8-12); do not use the semi-sitting position if the patient is hemorrhaging heavily. If there are possible spinal injuries, keep the patient in a supine position.

The general principles of management of shock are also illustrated in the photo series that includes Figures 8-13–8-21.

Management of Shock in Pregnant Women

Pregnancy presents an especially difficult situation for a patient in shock: trauma is now the number-one nonobstetrical killer of pregnant women, and shock compromises the lives of both the mother and the fetus, which is dependent on a rich supply of oxygenated blood. The lack of adequate perfusion to the uterus, in fact, can be serious enough to kill the fetus without causing evident signs or symptoms in the mother. You must be extremely wary of shock in any injured or ill pregnant woman and should act rapidly to provide corrective treatment, even in the absence of the traditional signs and symptoms.

To manage a pregnant woman in shock, follow these guidelines:

1. Secure an open airway.

2. Administer 100 percent high-flow oxygen.

3. Control any obvious bleeding.

4. Because the woman's stomach is displaced upward, remain constantly alert to the possibility of vomiting.

5. Place the woman in a left lateral recumbent position; put a pillow or folded blanket under the patient's left hip, and let her flex her right hip until it is comfortable. This position is critical: it prevents the heavy uterus from pressing against the inferior **vena cava** and slowing blood supply to the heart.

6. Apply the PASG if you suspect that the patient may go into shock, even if you do not see specific signs or symptoms. Apply only the leg sections; do not apply or inflate the abdominal section. Follow local protocol regarding application of the PASG for pregnant women.

7. Splint any existing fractures.

8. Keep the patient warm, and avoid rough or excessive handling.

9. Transport the patient rapidly in a left lateral recumbent position, monitoring vital signs and continuing ventilation during transport.

☐ Positioning the Shock Patient

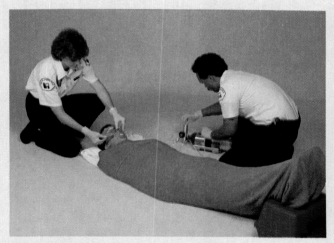

FIGURE 8-9 Shock patient with lower extremities elevated.

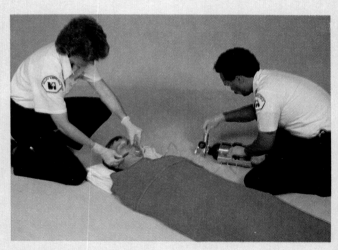

FIGURE 8-10 Shock patient in supine position.

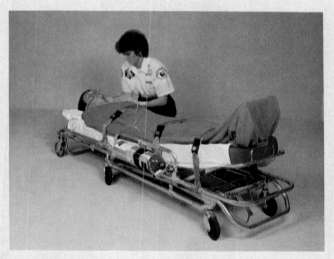

FIGURE 8-11 Shock patient ready for transport with lower extremities elevated.

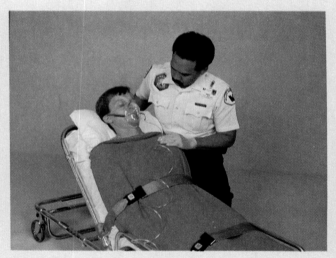

FIGURE 8-12 Shock patient ready for transport in semi-sitting postion.

Management of Anaphylactic Shock

Anaphylactic shock is a true life-threatening emergency: death can occur rapidly, and treatment must be aggressive.

1. The first priority is to secure an open airway.
2. Administer 100 percent high-flow oxygen; use a bag-valve-mask if necessary. Begin CPR if needed.
3. Radio your dispatcher and ask that the receiving facility be informed of the patient's condition.
4. *If state and local protocol allow it,* help the patient administer his medication (usually epinephrine and/or **antihistamines**).
5. Transport the patient rapidly for life-saving medical treatment.

□ Management of Shock

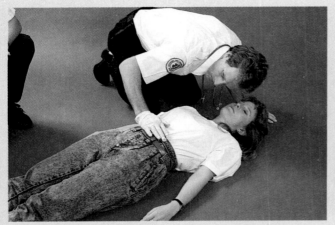

FIGURE 8-13 As with any emergency patient, assess the ABC's first.

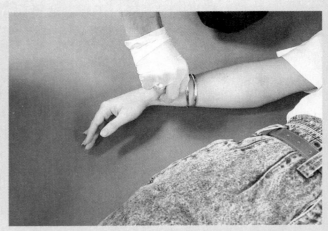

FIGURE 8-14 The presence and character of the pulse is a good indicator of the status of the patient's circulatory system

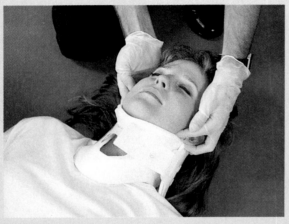

FIGURE 8-15 The airway in the shock patient should be assessed and maintained. If cervical spine injury is suspected, use the jaw-thrust maneuver.

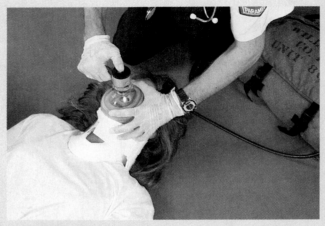

FIGURE 8-16 If necessary, assist or provide respirations and oxygenation.

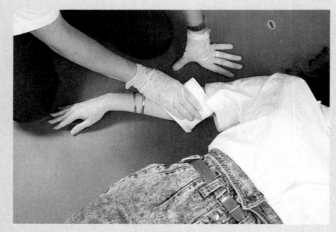

FIGURE 8-17 Control any obvious bleeding.

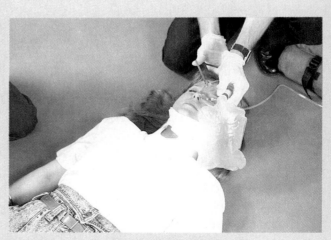

FIGURE 8-18 Provide high-flow oxygen.

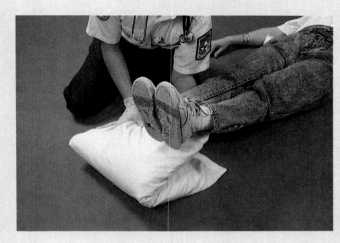

FIGURE 8-19 Elevate the feet if a head injury is not suspected.

FIGURE 8-20 Always maintain the patient's body temperature.

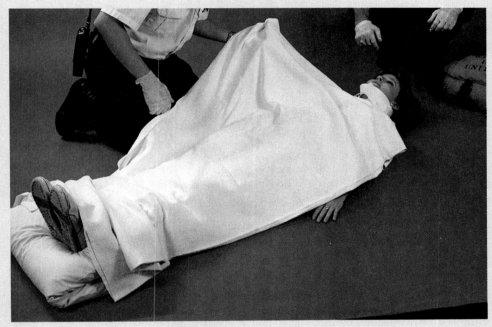

FIGURE 8-21 If shock is present the patient should be transported immediately with stabilization attempted en route.

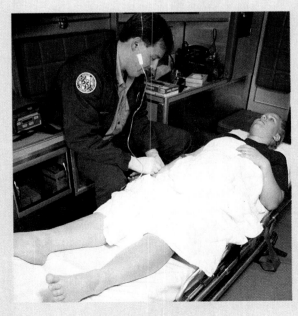

Preventing Shock

The preventive measures illustrated in Figure 8-22 should be carried out in all cases of impending shock except those in which the specific measure would be against the best interests of the patient.

□ PNEUMATIC ANTISHOCK GARMENT (PASG)

First used at the turn of the century by Dr. George Crile for maintenance of blood pressure in the operating room, the pneumatic antishock garment underwent a variety of changes before becoming widely used during the 1970s. At first it was called "pneumatic rubber suit," but it was not widely accepted because technology could not produce a suit that did not leak. For years it was called the "Curity suit," and it resembled a large balloon that compressed the patient from the waist down. Because too many were unfamiliar with how to use it and because blood transfusions became widely accepted, interest in the PASG declined.

During World War II, the garment — then called a "G-suit" — gained popular use as a way to keep high-performance diving pilots from blacking out during maneuvers. During the 1950s and 1960s, researchers experimented with the suit as a way of improving blood pressure. Initially tested in Vietnam, it was later used by the Miami Fire Paramedic Service as a way to support blood pressure and improve survival so that severely injured patients could be transported to the hospital for definitive care.

Today, it is used by most ambulance systems in the United States (Figure 8-23). However, recently their lifesaving benefits have been questioned by a few researchers. Until the controversy has been settled, the following indications are appropriate. Always follow local protocol.

The three main reasons for using the PASG are:

1. **Control of bleeding.** The PASG will control both

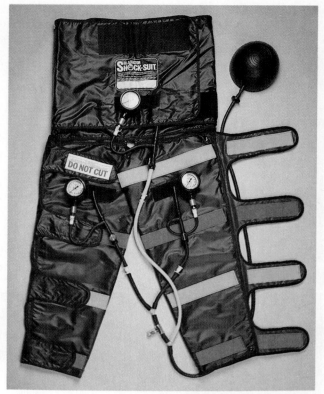

FIGURE 8-23 One type of pneumatic antishock garment. There are different types of PASG, with or without gauges or pop-offs. Some apply circumferential pressure around the entire leg; some only apply pressure to the bottom side. Some work at low pressure; some at high pressure. Follow local protocol in purchase and use of PASG.

external and internal bleeding in the area it covers; it is especially valuable for controlling the bleeding from a fractured pelvis, or injuries to the kidneys, bladder, or uterus.

2. **Stabilization of leg or pelvic fractures.** If possible, apply a traction splint to the leg before applying the PASG.

3. **Increasing the amount of blood available to the heart, lungs, and brain by reducing flow to the**

FIGURE 8-22

Assure adequate breathing

Loosen restrictive clothing

Maintain body heat

Administer high-flow oxygen

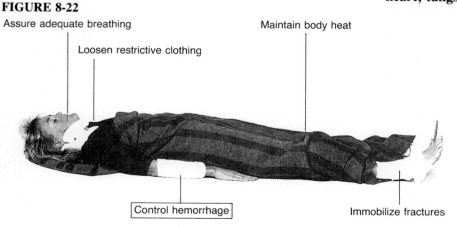
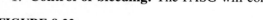

Control hemorrhage

Immobilize fractures

Reassure patient

Position patient

Relieve pain

extremities. Authorities now believe that the amount of blood actually *moved* by the PASG may be very low; instead, the valuable effect of the PASG may be due to the fact that it increases the resistance of the peripheral blood vessels.

Indications for PASG Use

Unless contraindicated, use the PASG for the following:

- Hemorrhagic shock (especially when signalled by increased heart rate and delayed capillary refill).
- Anaphylactic shock.
- Septic shock.
- Neurogenic shock.
- Suspected fracture of the lower extremities or pelvis.
- Suspected internal abdominal hemorrhage.
- Multiple trauma with shock.

Many studies have demonstrated an improved short-term survival with use of the PASG in patients with severe correctable hemorrhage, such as an **abdominal aortic aneurysm, hepatic** injuries, or **venacaval** injuries — especially if transport time is delayed or the patient is subjected to delays at the hospital while a room is being prepared.

Contraindications

If you believe that the patient will die without the use of PASG, use it, regardless of the patient's underlying conditions. Always follow local protocol. If the patient will not die without use of the PASG, you should probably *not* use it if the following conditions exist:

- Heart failure with pulmonary edema.
- Significant head injuries.
- Severe hemorrhage on the upper body, above the line where the PASG is against the body.
- Bleeding into the chest cavity (the PASG can cause increased bleeding).

If any of the above conditions exist, check with a physician by radio before using the PASG. *The PASG should never be used to treat patients with cardiogenic shock; the PASG results in decreased cardiac output, which worsens cardiogenic shock and can lead to death.*

In the following situations, use of the PASG should be altered as indicated:

- **Pregnancy.** Unless uterine bleeding is the cause of hemorrhagic shock, inflate the legs only for a patient in third-trimester pregnancy.
- **Impaled object in abdomen.** Leave the **impaled**

object in place; stabilize it with bulky bandages; inflate the leg sections only of the PASG. Check local protocol.

- **Impaled object in leg.** Leave the impaled object in place; stabilize it with bulky dressings and bandages; apply and inflate one side only of the PASG leg section on the uninjured leg.

Application of the PASG

Remember that you can apply a PASG during transport; you should *never* delay a patient's arrival at a hospital for PASG application. Remember, too, that the PASG is a temporary means of stabilizing the patient until he or she is able to get definitive care at the hospital.

When applying a PASG, *you should always follow local protocol.* Some areas require an EMT to obtain permission before inflating a PASG. In general, apply the PASG as quickly as possible and without delay if you suspect shock. You should be able to apply the suit within sixty seconds from start to finish. Follow these general guidelines *in conjunction with local protocol* (Figures 8-24–8-32):

1. Open and establish a viable airway, finish the primary survey, take the patient's vital signs, and administer oxygen. Once these are accomplished, apply — *but do not inflate* — the PASG in the following steps:
2. Remove the patient's outer clothing that would lie beneath the PASG; leave only the underwear on where possible. If you cannot remove clothing because of injuries, at least remove the patient's belt, empty pockets, and get rid of any sharp objects that could perforate the suit. Then cut away the clothing that will be under the suit. Do a final examination of the area to be covered by the garment to make sure that you have not overlooked any injuries or wounds.
3. Open the PASG completely and place it on a stretcher, a long backboard, or a gurney. Attach the foot pump, and open the valves.
4. Place the patient face-up directly on the PASG. If you suspect that the patient may have spinal injuries, log-roll the patient onto the PASG, taking extreme care to keep the head, neck, and back in alignment. Position the patient so that the top of the PASG is just below the patient's lowest rib.
5. Fold the PASG across the patient. First wrap the left leg of the garment around the patient's left leg; fasten the Velcro strips. Repeat with the right leg. Then wrap the abdominal section of the PASG around the patient's abdomen; fasten the velcro straps. Check to make sure that all straps are firmly fastened.

☐ Application of Antishock Garment

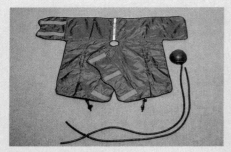

FIGURE 8-24 Unfold PASG on a firm surface and open stop-cock valves.

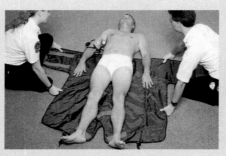

FIGURE 8-25 Unfolding PASG on a long spineboard or lifting apparatus is preferred. Then place or log roll the patient onto PASG so that it will be just below the patient's last rib.

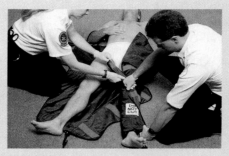

FIGURE 8-26 Wrap the left leg of PASG around the patient's left leg and secure with velcro strips.

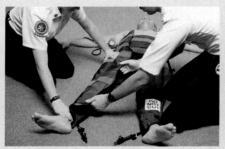

FIGURE 8-27 Wrap the right leg of PASG around the patient's right leg and secure with velcro strips.

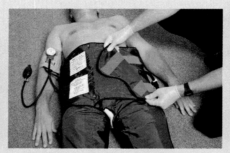

FIGURE 8-28 Wrap the abdominal portion of PASG around the patient's abdomen and secure with velcro strips.

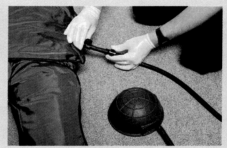

FIGURE 8-29 Check tubes leading to pump and PASG, and make sure stop-cocks are open.

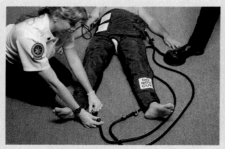

FIGURE 8-30 Inflate with foot pump until systolic blood pressure stabilizes at 100 or until "pop-off" valves release.

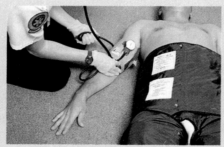

FIGURE 8-31 Check patient's blood pressure.

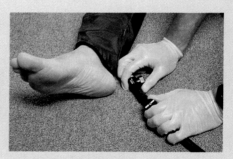

FIGURE 8-32 Close stop-cock valve.

6. Take the patient's vital signs again. *Wait for a physician's orders before you inflate the PASG.*

7. When you receive the physician's go-ahead, inflate the PASG with the foot pump; inflate the legs before you inflate the abdominal section. Begin with inflation of approximately 30 mm Hg, and continue inflating until the patient's systolic blood pressure is 100 mm Hg or until the Velcro makes a crackling noise or until air exhausts through relief valves. Close the stopcock valves.

8. Monitor the patient's blood pressure continuously throughout the use of the PASG.

9. Discontinue inflation, recheck vital signs, and continue transport to the hospital. Check inflation frequently during transport; changes in temperature can cause significant changes in the suit's pressure. If you are transporting by air, differences in atmospheric pressure as you change altitude can cause a sudden increase in the garment's pressure.

10. *Transport the patient rapidly;* he or she needs immediate hospital care.

Deflation of the PASG

Improper deflation of the PASG accounts for almost all complications associated with its use. Remember: deflation of the PASG is equivalent to losing two units of blood within a few seconds.

The PASG should seldom, if ever, be deflated in the field. *It is critical that you follow local protocol for deflation of a pneumatic antishock garment;* some areas do not allow for any deflation by prehospital personnel *at all, even in a hospital setting.* You should never deflate a PASG in the field unless extreme extenuating circumstances occur. Even then, you should have strict medical control of the situation. A PASG should be deflated and removed only under a physician's orders and with a physician present. Normally, a physician will okay deflation only when the patient is stable, two good IV infusions are running to replace lost fluids, any necessary x-rays have been taken, and an operating room is ready to receive the patient. *The PASG should never be deflated until there is an adequate amount of cross-matched blood available for transfusion.*

chapter 9

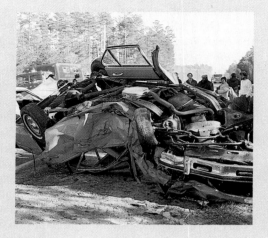

Mechanisms of Injury: The Kinetics of Trauma[1]

✴ OBJECTIVES

- Explain motion and the interaction of velocity and mass.
- Discuss mechanisms of injury and their effects upon the human body.
- List the five types of motor vehicle accidents.
- Describe the types of body trauma caused by falls.
- Explain the kinetics of penetrating trauma, including stabbings and bullet wounds.
- Discuss the effects of blast injuries.

[1] Chapter written by Twink Gorgen, R.N., REMT–P,
Paramedic Nurse Coordinator, Omaha Fire Dept.,
Omaha, NE.

It is recommended that EMTs wear protective gloves whenever there is a possibility of coming in contact with a patient's blood, body fluids, mucous membranes, traumatic wounds, or sores. See Chapter 31.

Since the early 1970s, trauma has been recognized as the leading cause of death for those between the ages of 14 and 40. Trauma is the third leading cause of death overall, only after cardiovascular disease and cancer. Trauma, or traumatic injury, makes up a significant percent of the calls to which prehospital personnel respond (Figure 9-1).

With any trauma victim, determining the extent of injury is important for determining treatment and decision making. The obvious injuries are usually the ones treated, but the hidden injuries usually are not. Hidden injuries that are not recognized — and thus not treated — may be fatal. In trauma, it is not sufficient merely to have good patient assessment skills; one must also develop a high index of suspicion.

Mechanism of injury refers to *how* a person was injured. The mechanism may be a fall, motor vehicle accident, gunshot wound, and so on. The science of analyzing the mechanism of injury, sometimes called **kinetics** of trauma or kinematics of injury, helps the EMT determine the most likely injuries sustained as well as develop a "high index of suspicion" for probable injury. Together, the mechanism of injury and index of suspicion will help the EMT determine whether to stabilize the patient at the scene or to provide rapid transport to the hospital. In the absence of acute physical injury, the decision to transport the patient to a trauma center is usually based on the mechanism of injury.

The process of analyzing the mechanism of injury is based on physical laws. Basically, the laws state that:

1. A mass in motion contains energy.
2. Energy is influenced by the interaction of velocity and mass.
3. Energy travels in a straight line.
4. Energy is neither created nor destroyed, only changed in form.

☐ MOTION AND THE INTERACTION OF VELOCITY AND MASS

The interaction of velocity and mass results in energy or force. This interaction can be explained in terms of the total amount of energy contained by an object in motion and by the energy created when the velocity accelerates or decelerates.

The term "kinetic" energy refers to the total amount of energy contained by an object in motion. The relationship is clearly illustrated by the formula:

$$\text{Kinetic Energy} = \frac{\text{Mass (WEIGHT)} \times \text{Velocity}^2}{2}$$

The mass is expressed in pounds, the velocity in feet per second. Therefore, kinetic energy is the amount of energy it takes to move one pound, one foot. The higher the velocity, the more energy is available to move a given mass a given distance.

This formula illustrates that as the weight of an object is doubled, the energy of its motion is also doubled. It would be twice as damaging to be hit by a two-pound baseball as to be hit by a one-pound ball. It would be three times as damaging to be hit by a three-pound ball, and so on. Velocity, or speed, is a much more significant factor in the kinetic energy produced than the weight of the object.

While velocity is a key factor in determining the kinetic energy of a body in motion, acceleration and deceleration also play key roles.

$$\text{Force} = \text{Mass} \times \text{Acceleration (or Deceleration)}$$

This formula points out the importance of the rate at

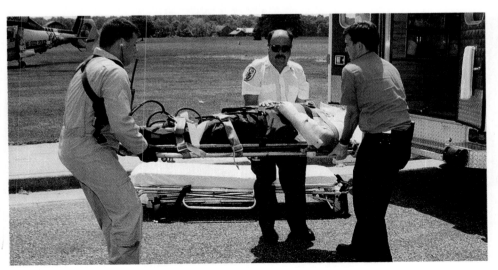

FIGURE 9-1 Victims of severe trauma have enhanced chances of survival if they can be delivered to the operating room within one hour after their accident (the "Golden Hour").

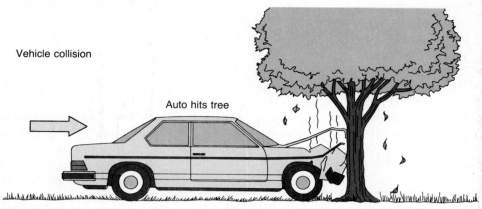

FIGURE 9-2 Step 1 — Vehicle collision. The vehicle strikes an object.

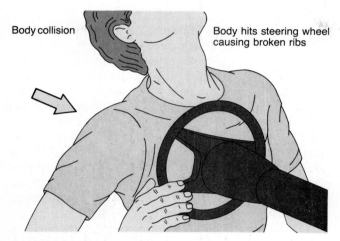

FIGURE 9-3 Step 2 — Body collision. The occupant continues forward and strikes the inside of the automobile.

FIGURE 9-4 Step 3 — Organ collision. The organs continue to move forward and strike the inside of the chest or other organs.

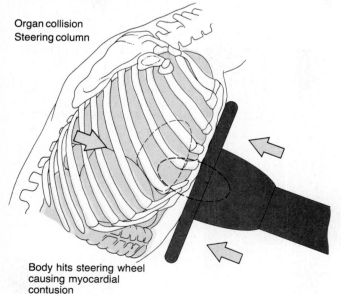

which an object *changes* speed. The faster the change of speed, the more force is exerted. This formula helps explain why the faster one is traveling, the longer it takes to stop when the brakes are applied.

These principles can be illustrated in the case of a person (mass) being struck by a car. The car causes the person (mass) to gain velocity or speed. A given amount of kinetic energy from the moving car is transferred to the person, putting him or her into motion. This same person, with a given amount of kinetic energy from motion, or velocity, now lands on the pavement, suddenly losing motion or decelerating. The process of gaining and losing velocity has occurred with each impact. Each impact, with the associated energy involved, had the potential to cause injury.

In most collisions, there are three impacts. For example, in the case above, the impacts began with the impact of the car against the person's body. The second impact was that of the body against the pavement, and the third impact was that of the internal organs against the body compartments. The number of impacts is the same with occupants in a vehicle. The vehicle impacts an object, the body impacts the inside of the vehicle, and the organs impact the compartments inside the body (Figures 9-2–9-4).

The number of impacts may change slightly with falls. In general, the body impacts the ground; then the organs impact surfaces inside the body. (This will be further explained in the section on falls.)

Occasionally, there may be more impacts, such as the case of a motorcycle rider who hits a car and is thrown. The motorcycle impacts the car, the cyclist impacts the handlebars of the motorcycle, impacts the hood of the car, and finally impacts the ground. With the impact of the car and the ground, the internal organs also impact the body compartments. There are six potential impacts, each of which produces energy.

When comparing the number of impacts, it is easier to understand why a person in or on a moving vehicle who gets thrown has a much greater chance for in-

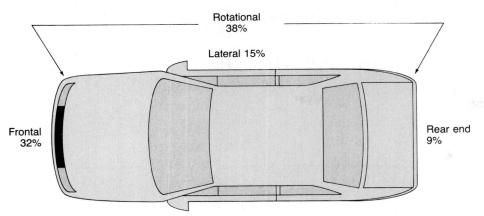

Rotational
38%

Lateral 15%

Frontal
32%

Rear end
9%

FIGURE 9-5 Motor vehicle trauma based on the type of impact.

jury. It is equally easier to understand why the faster a vehicle is traveling, the greater the kinetic energy produced and thus the greater the potential for injury.

The amount of kinetic energy that reaches the body is affected by how much energy is absorbed by other objects and material prior to reaching the body. For example, if a falling body strikes freshly plowed dirt, a major portion of the energy produced is absorbed by the soft dirt. On the other hand, if the falling body strikes concrete, the energy will be absorbed by the body, creating greater injury. The same principle is applied to vehicles. This is one reason why automobile manufacturers are now making vehicles out of materials that absorb energy more easily. These materials are more compressible, thus absorbing more energy. This results in greater structural damage to the vehicle, but less damage (injury) to the occupant.

Effect of Energy

Energy travels in a straight line. If energy, transmitted to a human body, continues to travel in a straight line without interruption, injury may not occur. However, energy traveling through the human body is frequently interrupted. The interruption may be because there is a curve in the bone, or an organ or tissue is caught between two hard surfaces (crushing or compression force) or pulled against a fixed point (shearing or deceleration force). In both instances, energy is forced to change form because it can no longer travel in a straight line. This results in injury. The injury is either blunt or penetrating.

In adults, the incidence of blunt and penetrating trauma is about equal, but varies by location. In children, however, over 90 percent of trauma is blunt. Blunt trauma is much more insidious and hidden. Penetrating trauma is usually obvious and may be very distracting. The index of suspicion is based on the mechanism of injury and how it may result in varying patterns of blunt and penetrating trauma to the body, especially to the internal organs.

□ MECHANISMS OF INJURY

The most common mechanism of injury is a fall, accounting for over half of all trauma incidents. Other common mechanisms include vehicular accidents; burns; penetrating wounds, such as gun shots and stabbings; and explosions.

Of all the mechanisms of injury, the most lethal is the motor vehicle accident. Over one-third of all deaths due to trauma occur from vehicular accidents. Many of those deaths occur because the occupants were not wearing seat belts. Seat belts prevent the occupant from impacting the inside of the vehicle and prevent ejection. The following discussion is based on the majority of the population who do not wear seat belts.

Motor Vehicle Accidents — Auto

There are five basic types of motor vehicle accidents. They are the head-on or frontal impact, rear impact, lateral or side impact, rotational impact, and the rollover (Figure 9-5). Each type has a predictable pattern of injury, and therefore, an index of suspicion.

The Head-On Impact

The head-on impact occurs in approximately 32 percent of the auto accidents in an urban area (Figure 9-6). It is estimated that there is probably a greater percentage that occur in rural areas. This impact results when a vehicle, traveling in a forward motion, suddenly loses velocity without deviating from its forward motion. Usually the loss of velocity is due to an immovable object — that is, a tree, wall, or another vehicle. The greater the velocity, the greater the energy produced.

A vehicle and its occupants travel at the same speed. When a collision occurs, the vehicle stops but the unrestrained occupants inside the vehicle continue their forward motion, at that same speed (Figure 9-7). The motion takes one or both of the following pathways:

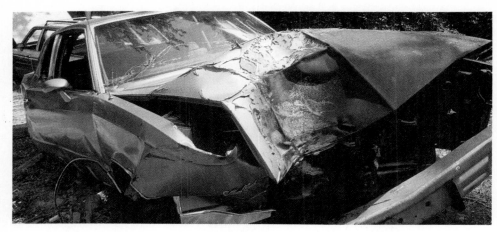

FIGURE 9-6 Frontal impact.

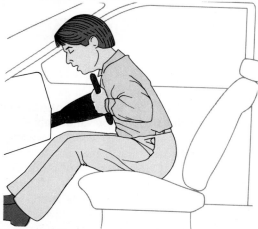

FIGURE 9-7

down and under, or up and over. Each pathway has a distinctive pattern of injury.

DOWN AND UNDER   The body slides down and under the steering wheel. The knees strike the dash, dissipating energy there first. Classic signs are dents in the dash. Remaining energy travels down the femur to the hip. Energy may dissipate mid-thigh, at the natural curve, causing a fractured femur. If the energy continues to travel down the femur, the hip socket is the last place for energy to dissipate. Posterior dislocations of the hip and/or a fractured pelvis can also result, as can secondary impacts as the body continues to travel forward with the abdomen and chest striking the steering wheel. (See Figure 9-12 on page 183.)

UP AND OVER   In addition to the down-and-under pathway, the torso may be thrown up and over the steering wheel. The chest and abdomen impact the steering wheel, and the face, head, and neck may impact the windshield.

• **Abdomen:** Observing the condition of the steering wheel can be a valuable index for suspicion. As the abdomen impacts the steering wheel, the liver,

spleen, and hollow organs of the abdomen are compressed between the anterior abdominal wall and the posterior abdominal wall, including the spine. The hollow organs are more easily displaced, leaving the liver and spleen to bear the brunt of the compressing force.

In addition to the compression force, the liver may be cut in half as it is forced against the ligament which holds it in place. In either case, lacerations may occur.

The spleen is attached to the body by a stalk-like structure that contains large blood vessels. In addition to the compression force, causing lacerations, the shearing force of the impact may tear the spleen from its attachment. Heavy bleeding may result from either the lacerations or tearing of vessels.

• **Chest:** As the chest impacts the steering wheel (Figure 9-8), bones and soft tissue are both affected. The bones of the chest, ribs, and sternum may break. As the sternum impacts the steering wheel, the sternum may break, and the cartilage connecting the ribs to the sternum may separate. The ribs are curved and as the sternum and spine are forced together, the ribs are forced to bend. This may result in rib fractures or flail chest.

The heart and lungs are the major soft-tissue organs affected. The heart suffers the effect of two forces, compression and shear. The compression force occurs when the heart is caught between the sternum and the spine. This may result in a bruise to the heart muscle (cardiac contusion). Ineffective pumping action of the heart and/or a pulse that is irregular or too fast or too slow may occur.

The heart is suspended by the aorta which is attached at the arch by a ligament. The shear force tends to pull the aorta at the ligament. This may

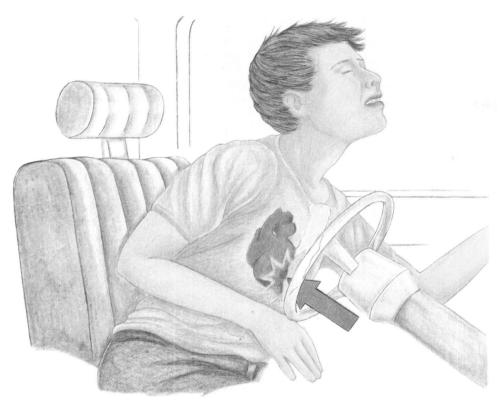

FIGURE 9-8 The chest impacting the steering wheel.

cause a traumatic aortic tear resulting in an aneurysm or dissection of the aorta.

The lungs may also be affected. Air, trapped in the lungs by a glottic spasm, is caught in a compression force between the ribs and spine. Air is forced into limited areas of the lung, expanding only that area affected to accomodate the compression. This may result in a bruise to the lung tissue (pulmonary contusion) or a ruptured lung. This is a pneumothorax and can occur in the absence of a rib fracture (Figure 9-9).

• Face, Head, Neck: The face, head, and neck are next to impact the windshield and/or dashboard.

The head may impact the rearview mirror and/or the windshield. The rearview mirror may be broken or have hair, tissue, or blood on it. The classic sign of impact to the windshield is the "bulls eye" pattern of broken glass. Occasionally the windshield will not be fully broken, but will bulge outward.

The face, depending on the impact point and amount of glass, may have extensive soft-tissue damage. Because of the vast blood supply of the face, what appears to be extensive bleeding may not be as serious as it looks (Figures 9-10 and 9-11).

FIGURE 9-9 The "paper bag" syndrome results from compression of the chest against the steering column.

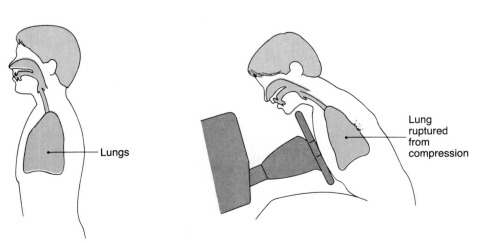

Lungs

Lung ruptured from compression

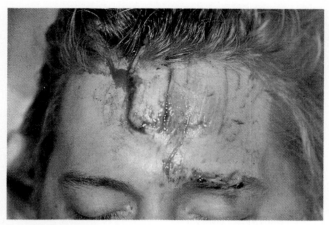

FIGURE 9-10

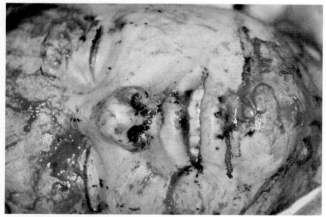

FIGURE 9-11

Head injuries from these impacts usually result in soft-tissue injury. Sometimes a skull fracture may occur. Depending on the force involved, penetrating bone shards or a depressed skull fracture may result, and both lacerate brain tissue. However, in the absence of outward bone injury, the force of the impact may cause damage to the brain itself, which may be more serious.

The brain is encased in a close-fitting box of bone surrounded by a thin layer of tissue (meninges) and fluid (cerebrospinal fluid). There is little room for movement. Therefore, when energy is transmitted through the skull, the energy proceeds through the brain tissue to the opposite side. Because the brain tissue itself is compressible, it will move. Two things may happen. First, the floor of the skull is very rough, with many sharp points that normally serve as sites for attachment. When the brain moves across these points, it can become lacerated or bruised. Second, as the brain moves,

it tends to move in a straight line. This may cause it to rebound against the opposite side of the skull from the original impact point. As the brain hits the wall of the skull it may again become bruised. This pattern of opposite bruising sites is termed a "coup-contre coup" injury or "brain whiplash" (Figure 9-13).

Because force tends to travel in a straight line, energy not dissipated by the face or head will continue down the neck causing a potential for cerebral spine injury. Depending on the impact site on the head and face, the line of energy may dissipate at differing points in the spine. If the impact point is at the top of the forehead, the neck may be forced in a **hyperflexion position.** If the impact point is the nose and mouth, the neck may be forced in a hyperextension position. If the impact point is on the top of the head, the entire C-spine may be involved with energy dissipating at any point, including the C_7–T_1 (Cervical 7–Thoracic 1) junction, causing compression fractures and/or dislocations.

If the driver or passenger is thrown forward at such an angle that the neck is either caught by the steering wheel or the dashboard, the trachea is in direct danger of cartilage ring separation. The key sign is a single dent in the top of the steering wheel or in the dashboard. The mark on the neck may be as simple as a small red mark. When the cartilage rings separate in the neck, air escapes into the soft tissue of the neck, putting pressure on surrounding structures and decreasing the effectiveness of ventilation.

The Rear Impact

The rear impact occurs in approximately 9 percent of the vehicular accidents in an urban area. This impact occurs when a vehicle with less speed is struck from behind by a vehicle traveling at a greater speed (Figure 9-14 on page 184). The vehicle that is struck suddenly accelerates at a greater speed. This sudden acceleration causes the body of the occupant to move out from under the head. The head rest is made to prevent hyperextension of the head in such cases. If the head rest is down or not present, sudden hyperextension can result in soft-tissue tears in the neck as well as cervical cord compression, whether or not vertebral fractures have occurred (Figure 9-15).

If the driver of the vehicle struck slams on the brakes, the occupant(s) will be thrown forward and suffer the same consequences of the "down-and-under/up-and-over" pathways discussed above.

DASHBOARD INJURIES

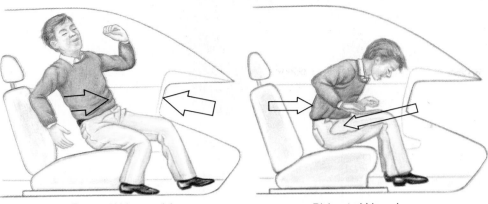

Fractured hip or pelvis

Dislocated hip or knee

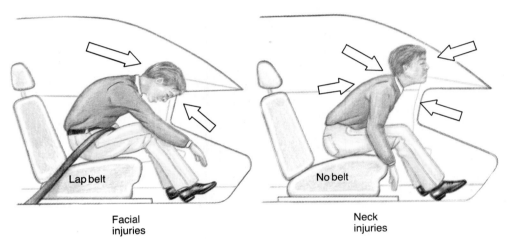

Lap belt

Facial injuries

No belt

Neck injuries

FIGURE 9-12 Examples of injury mechanisms associated with frontal impact.

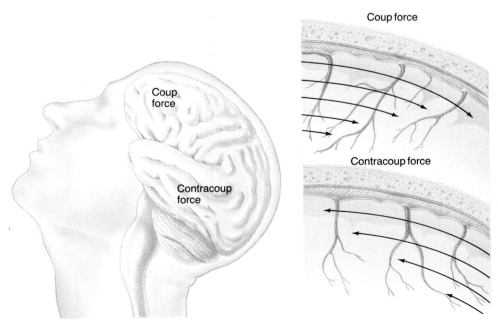

Coup force

Coup force

Contracoup force

Contracoup force

FIGURE 9-13 Coup and contrecoup movement of the brain.

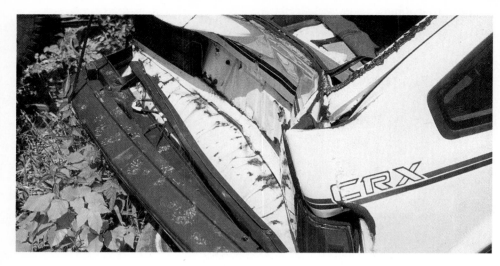

FIGURE 9-14 Rear impact.

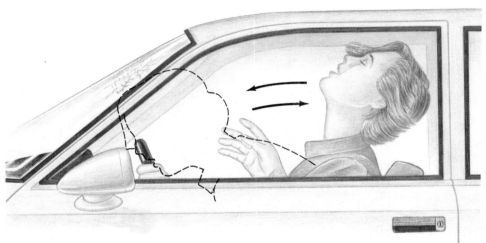

FIGURE 9-15 Movement in rear-impact collision.

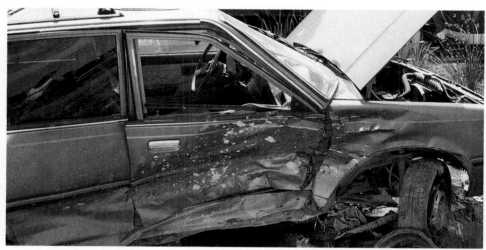

FIGURE 9-16 Lateral impact.

The Lateral Impact

A lateral impact occurs approximately 15 percent of the time in urban-area vehicular accidents. It occurs when the vehicle is struck from the side (Figure 9-16). These are sometimes termed "T-bone" impacts, or "broadside" collisions. In these cases, the person on the side of the impact absorbs a greater amount of energy than a person on the opposite side. However, both occupants may be injured with slightly different patterns of injury.

As the energy of the impact is absorbed by the person on that side, the body is pushed laterally, out from under the head. This causes the head to move in the opposite direction. Injuries occur to the head and neck, chest, and pelvis.

HEAD AND NECK   As the head moves in the opposite direction, it often impacts the door post causing injury to the parietal and temporal areas. The structures in the lateral areas of the neck are not as strong as in the anterior/posterior portion of the neck, thus resulting in more frequent muscle tears and ligamentous injuries. The vertebrae are not designed for extreme lateral movement, and vertebral fractures are common.

CHEST   Injuries to the chest occur when the door impacts on the chest wall. If the impact is on the shoulder, the energy traveling in a straight line may dissipate at the curve in the clavicle, resulting in a fracture. If the arm is caught between the door and chest, or if the door impacts the chest wall itself, fractured ribs and flail segments are possible. If the fractures occur low in the rib cage, the liver or spleen may be affected.

PELVIS   The impact of the vehicle door to the chest wall also causes a lateral impact to the pelvis. Fractures of the pelvis and upper femur usually complete this pattern.

The person opposite the impact site is also prone to injury. The body is shoved out from under the head, resulting in a similar neck injury. The head, lagging behind the rest of the body, often rebounds back, only to strike the door post on the opposite side. If there is more than one person sitting on the seat, heads will frequently collide causing head injuries.

The Rotational Impact

A rotational impact occurs in approximately 38 percent of the accidents in an urban area. It is an impact that occurs off-center. For the energy to dissipate, the vehicle will often rotate around the object struck until the energy has exhausted itself or another object is hit (Figure 9-17). Both head-on and lateral injury patterns occur. Steering wheels, the dashboard, door posts, and windows are the sturdiest structures, and often cause the most significant injury.

THE ROLLOVER   During a rollover (Figure 9-18), the occupant changes direction every time the vehicle does. Every protruding fixture in the vehicle becomes a potentially lethal object. A specific pattern of injury is impossible to predict, though there are a few characteristics. Multiple systems injury is common, and ejection is frequent with the unrestrained occupant. Ejection greatly increases the possibility of a crushing injury resulting from the vehicle rolling over the occupant.

Ejection

As stated above, ejection is frequent in rollover accidents when restraints are not used. Partial ejection is also possible. Partial ejection refers to only a portion of the body ejected from the vehicle. An example would be only the head protruding through the windshield. Severe soft-tissue injuries, including avulsions and crushing injuries, often result. The chance of sustaining a mortal injury is increased by 300 percent when the occupant is ejected. The chance of a cervical-spine injury is increased by 1,300 percent. Ejection and other trauma is prevented by the use of seat belts and other restraints, as noted below.

Restraints

As stated previously, the above discussion is based on the unrestrained driver. While the majority of the injuries discussed can be either prevented or their severity reduced by the use of seat belts, restraints are not without their own injury patterns.

There are several types of restraints: lap belts, lap

FIGURE 9-17 Rotational impact.

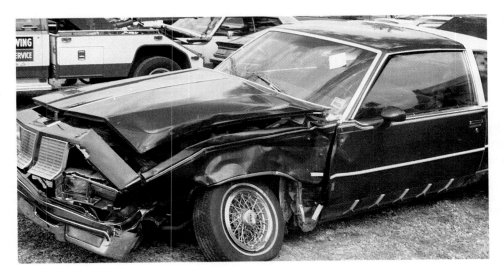

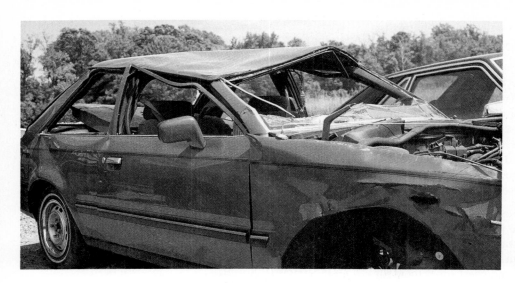

FIGURE 9-18 Rollover.

and shoulder belts, air bags, and car seats for infants and toddlers.

LAP BELTS Lap belts, when worn properly, distribute force across the iliac crests of the pelvis. This device prevents the occupant from being ejected, but does not prevent the chest from striking the steering wheel or the head and neck from striking the dashboard or steering wheel. Compression fractures of the lumbar spine occur as the torso is forceably flexed forward. This type of fracture of the spine is relatively mild compared to the potential for fractures of the C-spine.

Improperly worn lap belts can also cause injury to the internal organs. Compression between the seat belt and the posterior abdominal wall and spine may injure the spleen, liver, or pancreas. Compression may increase intra-abdominal pressure enough to herniate the diaphragm, forcing abdominal contents into the thoracic cavity.

LAP AND SHOULDER BELTS Properly positioned lap and shoulder belts will cause the force of the impact to be more evenly distributed and absorbed by the chest and pelvis. This reduces the force of the impact and the severity of injuries. One relatively minor injury that may occur is a fractured clavicle from the restraining shoulder strap.

Properly applied lap belts and shoulder straps do not, however, prevent the head and neck from moving laterally or forward and back. Properly positioned head rests will prevent excessive backward movement. It is impractical to restrict the forward movement of the head and neck. Fortunately, this pattern of movement is more easily tolerated.

AIR BAGS These devices are triggered to inflate from the steering wheel when a collision occurs. Air bags cushion the forward motion of the occupant by absorbing the energy from the collision and slowing the stopping rate of the occupant. The bag deflates immediately after the impact. Thus, air bags work best in the first collision of a head-on impact (65 to 70 percent of all collisions are head-on). They do not work well in multiple collision events nor in rear-end, lateral, or rollover collisions. For maximum effect, seat belts should be worn.

CAR SEATS Car seats are designed to protect an infant or toddler from becoming a missile during a collision. The properly secured car seat restrains the child at three or four points: the mid-pelvis, using one or two points, and at both shoulders. During a collision, the part or parts of the body that are not restrained continue forward at the same speed the vehicle was traveling prior to the impact. This includes the head and all four extremities. Of these, the head has a much greater body mass. Because of its greater mass, it tends to have greater kinetic energy and snap forward with more force. This literally stretches the neck against the resistance of the infant seat's shoulder restraints. The result is cord injury in the absence of vertebral injury. Even if facing backward, the same type of injury can happen if the car seat is rotated into a reclining position. To prevent head snapping, the proper position for the car seat is to face backwards, in the upright position. In this position and with proper restraints, injury is much less likely.

Motor Vehicle Accidents — Motorcycle

Motorcycle accidents account for a significant number of motor vehicle accidents that occur on and off our nation's highways. Morbidity and mortality is greatly affected by the presence or absence of a helmet (Figure 9-19).

There are three main types of impacts: head-on, angular, and ejection. Ejection is most often associated with the head-on impact. An evasive action known as

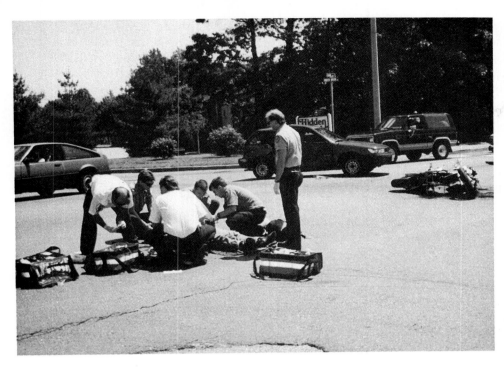

FIGURE 9-19 Motorcycle accidents can result in many types of trauma due to lack of protection of the rider.

"laying the bike down" is an associated mechanism that will also be discussed.

Head-On Impact

When a head-on impact occurs, the rider continues forward at the same speed the bike was traveling prior to the abrupt stop. The motorcycle tends to tip forward, due to the location of the center of gravity of the motorcycle. This causes the rider to travel into the handlebars at the same speed the bike was traveling. Depending on what part of his or her anatomy strikes the handlebars, a variety of injuries will occur. If the feet remain fixed or are caught on the pegs, the handle bars will impact at mid-thigh. This may result in bilateral femur fractures. If the pelvis does not clear the handle bars, pelvic fractures may also occur.

Angular Impact

In angular impacts, the rider strikes an object, usually a protruding object, at an angle. The object impacts whatever body part it comes into contact with, usually breaking or collapsing in on the rider. Examples include the edges of signs, outside mirrors on motor vehicles, or fence posts. The result can be severe avulsion injuries or even traumatic amputations.

Ejection

After any collision, if the rider clears the handlebars, ejection occurs. Ejection continues until a body part impacts with the object of the collision, or the ground, or both. There is the potential for six impacts to occur.

With each impact, energy changes form and is converted to body injury.

For protection, riders often wear boots, leather clothing, and helmets. The boots and leather clothing help protect against soft-tissue damage. The helmet is the best protection against head and facial injuries. If the rider is not wearing a helmet, the incidence for severe head injury and death increases 300 percent, the same as that for auto ejections.

"Laying the Bike Down"

This evasive action is designed to prevent ejection and separate the driver from the bike in an impending accident. The bike is turned sideways and "layed down" with the driver's inside leg dragging on the pavement or ground. The driver tends to lose speed faster than the bike, thus moving the bike out from under the driver. If the maneuver is successful, the driver clears the bike and slides along the ground, avoiding being trapped between the bike and the object it hits. There are two injury patterns from this evasive action: abrasions and burns.

ABRASIONS These are relatively minor injuries compared to the injuries sustained from ejection. However, they can be extensive and very painful. Abrasions are classed according to the the depth of the wound in a similar manner to burns. Superficial abrasions involve the epidermis, and partial thickness abrasions extend through the dermis. Full-thickness abrasions extend through the subcutaneous tissue and, in severe cases, to the periosteum or covering over the bone. Often the abrasions are complicated by particles embedded in the tissue — for example, dirt, grass, asphalt, sand and gravel, and so on. Embedded asphalt that is not completely scrubbed out of the tissue can result in "tattooing," a permanent discoloration of the skin at the site.

BURNS Burns are most often sustained when the inside leg does not clear the bike. The leg becomes caught between the exhaust pipe and the ground. The bike is often so heavy that the victim, regardless of his or her physical state, cannot move the bike off the leg. The longer the contact with the hot pipe, the worse the burn.

Recreational Vehicles Accidents

Traumatic incidents involving recreational vehicles has increased. Two of the most common vehicles involved are snowmobiles and all-terrain vehicles (ATVs) (Figure 9-20). Both have very similar patterns of injury to the motorcycle, with some differences due to the areas in which they are used. These vehicles are most commonly used in fields, hilly terrain, and sometimes areas inaccessible to cars or trucks. Therefore, detecting, gaining access to, and often extricating victims may be very difficult.

Snowmobiles

Snowmobiles are designed to be driven over snow, which may hide irregularities in the ground surface. Therefore, crush injuries and rollovers are common. Because snow tends to hide rocks and other obstructions, glancing blows may cause crush injuries to extremities.

Snowmobiles are also frequently operated at high speed. Inexperienced snowmobilers may be subject to severe head and neck damage when collisions with other vehicles or trees occur, which are exacerbated by the high speeds of the vehicle.

One of the most dangerous injuries can occur with either a snowmobile or an ATV when the vehicle and rider run into an unseen wire fence. Documented cases of lacerated vessels in the neck and severed tracheas are in the literature. Decapitation may even occur.

ATVs

There are two types of ATVs, the three-wheel and four-wheel type (Figure 9-20). The three-wheel ATV is very unstable and prone to rollovers even when turning. The injury pattern with rollovers include crush injuries and head injuries. Both types of vehicles are also prone to collision with other vehicles, resulting in head, neck, and extremity injury. Unfortunately, the majority of those who ride ATVs are children with lesser body weight. This factor also contributes to the instability of the vehicles.

Falls

Falls are the most common mechanism of injury causing trauma. The severity of the trauma depends upon the distance, surface, and the body part that impacted first. Associated factors that also affect the severity of injury are those that interrupt the fall prior to landing.

DISTANCE Increased height increases the velocity. In general, the greater the distance of the fall, the

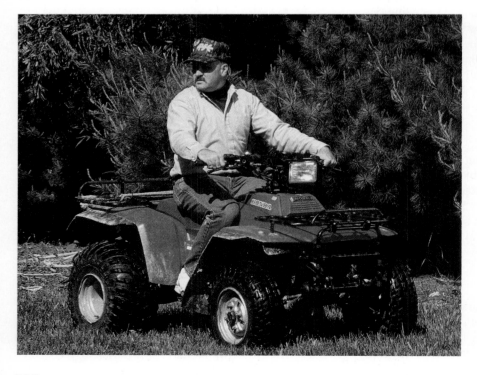

FIGURE 9-20 All-terrain vehicles (ATVs) can cause a multitude of injuries due to their speed and instability.

more severe the injury. This generality is only true when the surface is taken into account.

SURFACE   Some experts feel that the surface is more of a determining factor of injury than the height. Diving into deep water from a fifteen-meter height is done recreationally. However, diving that same distance onto a concrete sidewalk can hardly be called recreational.

BODY PART   The pattern of trauma seen is dependent on the body parts that impact first. Energy travels in a straight line until it is forced to curve. At that point or points, energy changes form to dissipate and injury occurs.

A fall of fifteen feet onto an unyielding surface is considered severe. Internal organ damage is very frequent, and attention should be directed toward a high index of suspicion regardless of the initial presentation of the patient.

Feet-First Fall

A feet-first landing causes energy to travel up the skeletal system. The heels (calcaneious bones) and ankles are the first points of impact. Possible fractures of the heels and/or fractures and dislocations of the ankles are common (Figure 9-21).

If the knees are flexed at the time of impact, the majority of energy will be dissipated and preserve the

FIGURE 9-21 In falls, the energy is transmitted up the skeletal system.

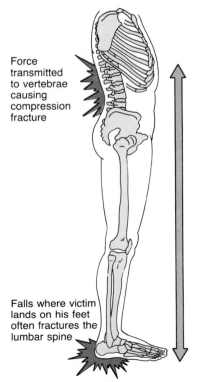

Force transmitted to vertebrae causing compression fracture

Falls where victim lands on his feet often fractures the lumbar spine

rest of the skeletal system. However, if the person lands flat-footed, energy will be transmitted up through the femurs to the hips and pelvis. Because the femur has a natural curve at mid-thigh, fractured femurs may also occur. The next energy dissipation points are the hips. Energy may dissipate at the socket, forcing the ball of the femur up through the acetabulum, fracturing the hip socket. If energy remains, the spine will absorb the force at every curve. The natural curves are at the lumbar, mid-thoracic, and the cervical spine.

In falls of fifteen feet or greater, the internal organs are more likely to be subjected to the same deceleration forces. The liver may be forced against the ligamentum teres and be literally sliced in two. The spleen may be torn from its stalk-like attachment. The heart may be torn from the aorta, and the ligament attaching the aorta at its arch may be ripped, causing traumatic aortic tears. As the body continues its downward motion, it is thrown either forward or backward.

Extending the arms to break the fall is natural during the forward motion. The first point of dissipation of energy is at the wrist. Colles' fractures (impacted bones at the wrist) are very common. The elbow and shoulder are the next points of potential injury with dislocations of the elbow being less common than dislocations and fractures of the shoulder and fractures of the clavicle. Again, forces are transmitted to the internal organs as the trunk of the body strikes the ground.

A backward motion leads more commonly to head, back, and pelvic injury.

Head-First Fall

In head-first falls, the pattern of injury begins with the arms and extends up to the shoulders, with head and spine injury very common. The extent of injury is similar to the forward motion of the feet-first fall. The head may be forceably hyperextended, hyperflexed, or compressed (axial loading), all of which can cause extensive damage to the C-spine. Again, as the body continues its downward motion, the torso and legs are thrown either forward or backward. Chest, lower spine, and pelvic injuries are common.

Penetrating Trauma

Between 30,000 and 35,000 people are killed each year by firearms. It is estimated by some experts that 300,000 to 500,000 are injured. The high incidence of injury and death due to firearms is second only to motor vehicle accidents. Firearms, however, are not the only cause of penetrating injury. Penetrating trauma results when any object penetrates the surface of the body. Objects may include darts, nails, bullets, knives, and so on.

The amount of damage that results depends on the amount of kinetic energy transferred to the tissue and the area of the body it penetrates. Of these two factors, the amount of kinetic energy that is transferred to the tissue is the greatest indicator of potential damage.

The amount of kinetic energy transferred to the tissue by a given mass is more a factor of velocity than the mass. A high-velocity bullet of small mass has the potential to cause more damage than a knife of larger mass. The kinetic energy formula explains why:

$$\text{Kinetic Energy} = \frac{\text{Mass} \times \text{Velocity}^2}{2}$$

As stated earlier, kinetic energy is more affected by a change in velocity than a change in the mass of an object. The ability of kinetic energy to be transferred to body tissue explains tissue injury. Energy changes form, and when it does, in relation to the human body, tissue damage may occur. Kinetic energy produced by an object is transferred to the tissues when that object enters the body. Energy impacting the tissues may result in compression, tearing, expansion, or fragmentation of body parts. If the object is a knife, the low kinetic energy limits the damage to the immediate impact site. On the other hand, if the object is a bullet, the higher kinetic energy results in tissue damage relatively far from the impact site. If the kinetic energy produced by the bullet is totally absorbed by the body tissues, the bullet will not exit. If, however, kinetic energy remains with the bullet, an exit wound will occur.

There are various categories of projectile injury depending on the types of weapons used. They are: low velocity, medium velocity, and high velocity. For the purposes of this text, the term "low velocity" is reserved for those projectiles that are manually powered, such as knives or arrows. Medium- and high-velocity projectiles are terms referring to those projectiles powered by an augmented force, such as gunpowder or other propellant. Typically these are the various types of handguns and rifles.

Low Velocity

Objects such as a knife, arrow, or other object impaled in the body exert damage to the immediate area of impact. Occasionally, knives will have a double edge, thus cutting with both edges. Sometimes the attacker will move the object while it is inside the body, increasing the potential for severe damage.

There are some guidelines to follow when dealing with stabbing victims. They include:

1. Never assume the perpetrator is absent from the scene until the police tell you the perpetrator is in custody.
2. Never assume there is just one wound.

3. Factors that help determine what organs may be affected include:
   a. The sex of the offender.
   b. The position the person was in when stabbed.
   c. The length of the knife or object used in the stabbing.

Enough cannot be said concerning the importance of assuring scene safety prior to the EMT entering the area of a shooting or stabbing. Most systems have definite protocols to follow when responding to such a scene. These procedures must be strictly adhered to in order to maintain the safety of all those who are responding.

With any assault, especially those victims of shootings and stabbings, the "expose" step of assessment is particularly important. A thorough examination of the victim is necessary to find all open wounds. Taking note of the location of the open wounds will help determine the most likely organ system affected. In the case of stabbings, the immediate organs under the area of impact are the ones most likely damaged.

The sex of the offender and the position the person was in when stabbed, may help determine the path of trajectory. Due to lesser upper-body musculature, women tend to stab overhand, or down, while men, with greater upper-body musculature, tend to stab up with an outward or crosswise stroke. Body position must also be taken into account. For instance, if a man in a standing position was stabbed in the right side by a woman, the most likely sites of injury would be the liver, kidney, and intestine. If, however, he was stabbed by a man, while in the same position, the potential injury sites would include the lungs.

If a person is trying to defend himself or herself against an attack, defense wounds may occur. These are slash marks noted in the hands and upper arms. This occurs when the victim puts up either or both arms, to ward off the attacker, or tries to grab the knife itself.

The length of the object used is also valuable information. For instance, a person sitting in a chair, stabbed in the anterior left chest from behind, may suffer vastly different injuries depending on the length of the blade. If the wound is from a short paring knife (approximately 3- to 3 1/2-inch blade), the victim may suffer a pneumothorax. On the other hand, if the same person were stabbed in the same place with a boning knife (approximately 7- to 8-inch blade), the injuries may include lacerated pulmonary veins, lacerated aorta, cardiac tamponade, and even a laceration to the heart muscle itself.

A thorough assessment and repeated evaluations of the patient's status, in addition to the factors listed, will help the EMT deliver the best care possible to the victim. Maintaining a high index of suspicion will keep the EMT from being caught unprepared when the unexpected happens.

Medium and High Velocity

Medium- and high-velocity projectiles are bullets (Figure 9-22). Generally shotgun pellets, or handgun bullets such as .22 gauge and .45 gauge, are considered medium velocity. Generally, this implies a muzzle velocity of less than 2,000 feet per second (f/s). True ballistics experts further divide them into low-velocity cartridges (less than 1,100 f/s) and medium-velocity cartridges (between 1,100 and 2,000 f/s). High-power, high-speed rifles, such as an M-16 or 30-30 Winchester, are considered high-velocity weapons. These weapons have a muzzle velocity of 2,000 f/s or greater.

Two other aspects of ballistics — trajectory and the dissipation of energy — need to be discussed.

- **Trajectory:** Trajectory is the path or motion of a projectile during its travel. Normally a bullet, once fired, follows a curved trajectory or path. However, the faster the bullet, the flatter the curve of the trajectory, and the straighter the path of the bullet.
- **Dissipation of Energy:** Dissipation of energy is affected by drag, profile, and cavitation.

DRAG "Drag" refers to the factor(s) that slow a bullet down. A bullet, fired into the air, experiences wind resistance, or drag. The greater the speed of the bullet, the more effect from wind resistance, and the greater the drag or slowing effect. This explains why a bullet fired from close range does more damage than the same bullet fired from a distance.

PROFILE This refers to the impact point of the bullet. The greater the size of the impact point, the more energy is transferred. This occurs in four ways: diameter of the projectile, modification of the "point" or bullet tip, tumble, and fragmentation.

- In addition, there are bullets designed to fragment upon impact. Soft-nose bullets, hollow-nose bullets, and bullets with vertical cuts in the nose all have a tendency to fragment upon impact. The total mass of fragments presents a larger surface area and thus causes more tissue damage. Soft-nose, high-velocity bullets are especially destructive, causing a cavitation ten to thirty times the diameter of the bullet. The zone of permanent injury can be up to ten times the bullet diameter.

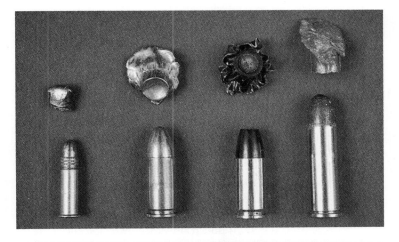

FIGURE 9-22 The profile of a bullet will vary based on its design.

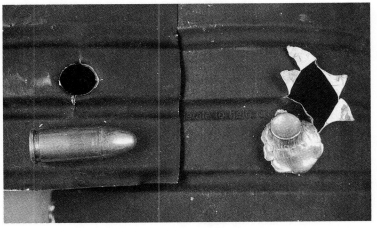

FIGURE 9-23 Destructive effect of .32 caliber handgun.

CAVITATION **Cavitation,** or pathway expansion, is formed by a pressure wave caused from the kinetic energy of the bullet traveling through body tissue. Cavitation greatly extends the tissue damage beyond the initial bullet pathway (Figure 9-24). The process of cavitation also pulls clothing, gunpowder, bacteria, and other small pieces of surrounding foreign material into the tissues, complicating the injury.

Shotgun Wounds

Shotgun wounds may differ significantly from gunshot wounds. Shotguns have multiple pellets that spray in a pattern. The multiple pellets increase the surface area and thus increase the amount of energy transferred to the tissues. Close-range shotgun wounds can cause devastating tissue damage, while long-range wounds may cause no more than relatively minor surface wounds (Figure 9-25).

Specific Pathologies

Of fatal wounds that occur due to firearms, 49 percent of them occur to the torso, 42 percent to the head, and 9 percent below the waist. These are specific body areas where trauma from this mechanism presents with certain characteristics that should be emphasized. The head, chest, abdomen, and extremities are included.

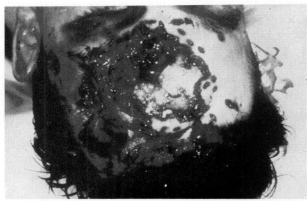

FIGURE 9-25 Wound resulting from close-range shotgun blast. Note the tattooing of the skin from the gunpowder.

Head

There are two regions that bear mentioning here: the skull and the face. The skull is a fixed space with little to no room for expansion. When a missile penetrates the skull and energy begins to dissipate, more injury than is usual results because of the cavitation within a fixed space. Brain tissue is naturally severely compressed. With no room to expand, brain tissue is sometimes forced out the entrance wound. If the force is severe enough, the skull may shatter into pieces.

Occasionally, a medium-velocity bullet, entering at an angle, may follow the curvature of the interior or exterior of the skull. The amount of damage is due to the location. If the bullet penetrates the skull and follows the interior curve, severe injury may occur with little outside evidence. Bleeding from the entrance wound may be minimal. If, however, the bullet does not penetrate the skull and follows the exterior curvature of the skull, the victim typically looks too good for the mechanism of injury.

The face is composed of soft tissues as well as bone. Gunshot wounds to the face typically result in major soft-tissue injuries that immediately threaten the airway. Attempted suicides where the weapon is held under the chin often result in fractures to the mandible, maxilla, nasal bones, and the frontal sinuses, with damage to the major contours of the face and the frontal lobe of the brain. Damage to the frontal lobe usually does not result in the death of the victim from the blast. However, the airway problem is major. There is no way to get a good seal to ventilate the patient with the lack of facial contours. Bleeding is extensive and the airway is difficult to manage.

FIGURE 9-24 The severity of injury associated with penetrating trauma is, in many ways, related to the velocity of the penetrating object.

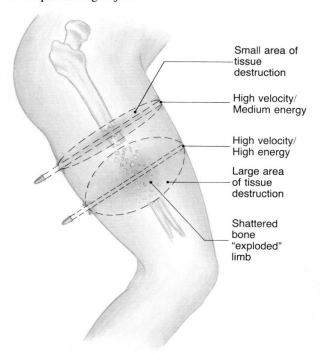

Small area of tissue destruction

High velocity/ Medium energy

High velocity/ High energy

Large area of tissue destruction

Shattered bone "exploded" limb

Chest

The chest is a relatively large target and often hit by projectiles. The full implications of chest wounds can be appreciated by considering the anatomy of the thorax. There are three thoracic cavities; the right and left thoracic cavities and the mediastinum. There are also three main types of tissue: pulmonary, vascular, and cardiac. Each thoracic cavity contains pulmonary and vascular tissue, while the mediastinum contains the major structures of all three.

Pulmonary, or lung, tissue is more tolerant of the cavitation formed by projectiles. The numerous air-filled alveoli form a spongy mass that is easily movable. Projectiles striking the ribs, however, often form other projectiles of bone. This multiplies the potential for injury. Common injuries to the pulmonary tissue include a pneumothorax, hemopneumothorax, and a tension pneumothorax. Associated injuries include rib fractures and possibly a sucking chest wound. There are three facts to note with sucking chest wounds:

1. Not all chest wounds need to be sealed *if positive pressure ventilations are being done for the victim.*
2. When the lung is completely collapsed, the wound will not manifest the characteristic "slurping" sound nor the bubbling of secretions.
3. If a tension pneumothorax is suspected in the presence of a penetrating wound to the chest, manipulation of the wound may relieve enough pressure to reduce the tension.

Vascular and cardiac tissue are not as tolerant of projectiles as lung tissue. However, the outer covering of the pulmonary vessels, aorta, and heart (pericardial sac), are tough and elastic. This characteristic allows for a "self-sealing" effect with small-caliber projectiles. Consequences include cardiac tamponade, traumatic aortic aneurysm, and vessel occlusion by the bullet. High-velocity projectiles tear the organ structure leading to rapid exsanguination.

The lower boundary of the thoracic cavity is formed by the diaphragm. With each cycle of respiration, the diaphragm moves, altering the size of the thoracic cavity and position of the abdominal organs immediately inferior to it. If a projectile strikes the lower half of the thoracic cavity during expiration, when the thoracic cavity is deflated, the projectile is more likely to cause an abdominal wound. On the other hand, if the projectile strikes the upper abdomen during inhalation, when the thoracic cavity is at its largest, the projectile is more likely to cause a thoracic wound. A good rule of thumb to follow is to suspect *both* a thoracic and abdominal wound when the entrance wound is between the nipple line and the waist.

Abdomen

The abdominal cavity is very large and contains structures that are fluid-filled, air-filled, solid, and bony. The abdomen is often secondarily injured when the thorax is injured. The major portion of the abdomen contains air-filled structures than are more tolerant of cavitation than are the solid organs. This implies that the majority of abdominal wounds due to projectiles are not rapidly fatal. However, 70 to 80 percent of medium-velocity injuries (such as those produced by a handgun) require surgical repair.

Extremities

The major structures include bone, muscle, vessels, and nerves. Bony injury due to projectiles results in bony fragments becoming secondary missiles, lacerating surrounding vessels, muscle, and nerves. Muscle expands due to the cavitation, resulting in capillary tears (leading to bleeding) and swelling. Vessels can be severed, ripped, buckled, and/or obstructed. As a result, circulation to the distal extremity may be completely blocked.

Blast Injuries

Blast injuries are not uncommon in prehospital care. Explosions can occur with natural gas, gasoline, fireworks, and even in grain elevators. No matter what the cause, each explosion has three phases: primary, secondary, and tertiary. Each has its own specific patterns of injury that are typical for that phase (Figure 9-26).

PRIMARY PHASE Injuries that occur during this phase are due to the pressure wave of the blast. These injuries primarily affect the gas-containing organs, such as the lungs, stomach, and intestines. Unsuspected gas-containing organs that are also affected include the inner ears and the sinuses.

Primary phase injuries include pneumothorax, pulmonary emboli, and perforation of the stomach and intestines. External bleeding from the nose and ears and internal bleeding from the pressure waves rupturing small vessels and organ membranes may be severe. Severe damage and death, without any external sign, may occur from this phase.

SECONDARY PHASE Injuries in this phase are due to flying debris from the force of the blast. Contrary to the injuries in the primary phase, the injuries of this phase are obvious. Lacerations, impaled objects, fractures, and burns are most common.

TERTIARY PHASE Injuries from this phase occur when the victim is thrown away from the source of the blast. Injuries are much the same as would be expected from ejection from a vehicle. The pattern is dependent upon the distance thrown and the point of impact.

Injuries sustained in the secondary and tertiary

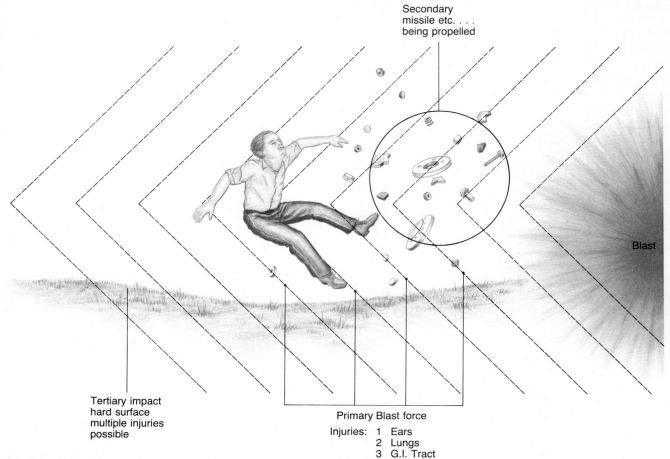

Secondary
missile etc. . . .
being propelled

Blast

Tertiary impact
hard surface
multiple injuries
possible

Primary Blast force
Injuries: 1 Ears
         2 Lungs
         3 G.I. Tract

FIGURE 9-26 Blast injuries can cause injury with the initial blast, when the victim is struck by debris, or by the victim being blown away from the site of the blast.

phases are the most obvious and more easily assessed and treated. Injuries of the primary phase are most often ignored or unsuspected and thus go untreated. Unfortunately, injuries of the primary phase are just as severe, if not more severe, than injuries obtained during the other phases. A thorough assessment and repeated observations must be done to ensure the best avenue of treatment for the victim. The index of suspicion on all blast-injury victims *must* remain high, regardless of the initial presentation.

☐ SUMMARY

Mechanisms of injury are an important part of the scene assessment, indicating the most likely areas of injury and what body systems should be repeatedly reassessed.

With any traumatic incident, it is important to discover and document the following:

1. The body position at the time of the impact.
2. The part of the body impacted.
3. What object/surface impacted.
4. The distance (if any) involved.

In cases of assault, where a stabbing may have occured, the sex of the offender and the length of the knife, if known, are also valuable pieces of information that should be noted and documented.

Above all, it is most important for the EMT to maintain a high index of suspicion with any patient involved in a traumatic injury.

chapter 10

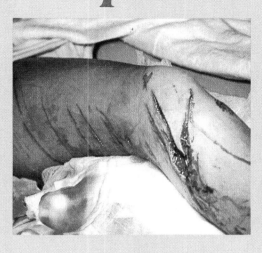

Soft-Tissue Injuries

✳ **OBJECTIVES**

■ Describe the various types of open and closed wounds, including contusions, abrasions, incisions, lacerations, punctures, and avulsions and the emergency care of each.

■ Describe the special precautions necessary for treating bites and amputations.

■ Describe how to properly care for amputated body parts.

■ Describe the general emergency care for open wounds.

It is recommended that EMTs wear protective gloves whenever there is a possibility of coming in contact with a patient's blood, body fluids, mucous membranes, traumatic wounds, or sores. See Chapter 31.

□ WHAT IS A SOFT-TISSUE INJURY?

In the injured patient, the skin not only reflects blood circulation but may itself (as well as underlying structures) be the site of damage. The entire surface of the body must therefore be inspected for soft-tissue injuries. Although this type of injury may be the most obvious and dramatic, it is seldom the most serious unless it compromises the airway or is associated with massive hemorrhage. Thus, the EMT must search systematically and thoroughly for other injuries or life-threatening conditions before treating the soft-tissue trauma.

Soft-tissue injuries involve the skin and underlying **musculature.** An injury to these tissues is commonly referred to as a wound. More specifically, a wound is a traumatically caused injury to the body that disrupts the normal **continuity** of the tissue, organ, or bone affected.

Wounds may be generally classified as **closed** or **open,** single or multiple. They are also classified according to anatomical location (position on the body). These include head wounds (subdivided into skull, face, and jaw wounds); abdominal wounds; chest wounds; wounds of the limbs (arms and legs); wounds of the joints; and spinal and pelvic wounds. The part of the body most severely injured determines the subclassification of multiple wounds.

Note: Always take appropriate infection-control measures before handling any patient, especially if blood is present. At a minimum, wear latex gloves; if there is likely to be splashing of blood or other body fluids, wear protective eyewear. For detailed infection-control procedures, see Chapter 31, "Infectious Disease Control."

□ CLOSED WOUNDS

In a closed injury, such as a bruise, or contusion, soft tissues beneath the skin are damaged but the skin is not broken (Figure 10-1). Contusions are marked by local pain and swelling. If small blood vessels beneath the skin have been broken, the patient will also exhibit ecchymosis (black and blue discoloration); blood and fluid will leak into the damaged tissue. If large vessels have been torn beneath the bruised area, a **hematoma** — a collection of blood beneath the skin — will be evident as a lump with bluish discoloration. Generally, closed wounds are characterized by pain at the injury site, ecchymosis, and swelling.

Small bruises generally require no treatment. Larger bruises, however, can signify serious internal injury and blood loss: a deep bruise the size of the patient's fist represents a 10 percent blood loss. Blood

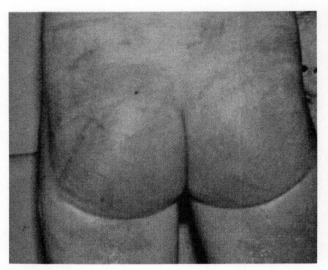

FIGURE 10-1 Contusions.

from a deep bruise can actually separate tissue and pool in a pocket, forming a hematoma.

In a closed injury, treat for internal bleeding if you are in doubt. If large bruised areas are present, assess carefully for fracture, especially if any swelling or deformity is present.

□ OPEN WOUNDS

In an open wound, the skin is broken and the patient is susceptible to external hemorrhage and wound **contamination.** An open wound may be the only surface evidence of a more serious injury, such as a fracture. Open wounds include **abrasions, incisions, lacerations, punctures, avulsions, bites,** and **amputations** (Figure 10-2).

Abrasions

An abrasion is a superficial wound caused by rubbing or scraping (friction) in which part of the skin layer — usually the epidermis and part of the dermis — has been lost (Figure 10-3). Blood may ooze from the abrasion, but bleeding is usually not severe. All abrasions, regardless of size, are extremely painful because of the nerve endings involved. Abrasions can pose a threat if large areas of skin are involved (as can happen in a motorcycle accident when the rider is thrown against the road). The most serious threat from abrasions is that of contamination and infection.

Emergency Care

Provide the following care for abrasions:

1. Cover the abrasion with a sterile dressing of nonadherent material and bandage in place.

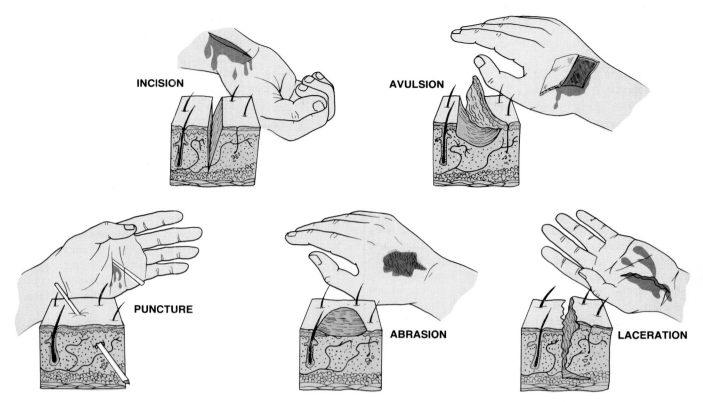

FIGURE 10-2 Classification of open wounds.

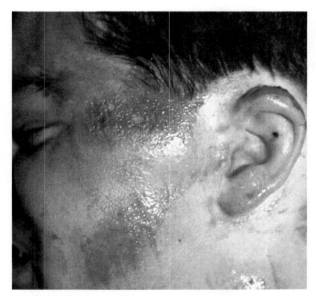

FIGURE 10-3 Abrasions.

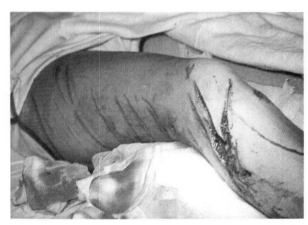

FIGURE 10-4 Incision and lacerations.

2. You should leave the cleaning of embedded debris to a physician. If you cannot transport the patient, however, bathe the abrasion with a normal **saline** solution and gently remove debris from around the wound. Loosely cover with a sterile dressing and bandage in place. *Follow local protocol*.

Incisions

Incisions are sharp, even cuts with smooth edges that tend to bleed freely because the blood vessels and tissue have been severed (Figure 10-4). Incisions are caused by any sharp, cutting object, such as a knife, razor blade, or broken glass. The greatest dangers with incisions are severe (often profuse) bleeding and damage to tendons and nerves. Incisions usually heal better than lacerations because the edges of the wound are smooth and straight.

Emergency Care

Provide the following care for incisions:

1. The first priority is to control bleeding by direct pressure.
2. Apply a sterile pressure dressing.
3. Give emergency care for shock.
4. Transport the patient.

Lacerations

A laceration is a tear inflicted by a sharp, uneven instrument (such as a broken glass bottle) that produces a ragged incision through the skin surface and underlying tissues (Figures 10-5 and 10-6). A laceration can also result from blunt trauma to tissue overlying a bone.

Lacerations can cause significant bleeding if the sharp instrument also cuts the wall of a blood vessel, especially an artery. This is especially true in areas where major arteries lie close to the skin surface, such as in the wrist. Because the edges of the wound are jagged, healing is not as good as in incisions; skin and tissue may be partly or completely torn away, and the laceration may contain foreign matter that can lead to infection.

FIGURE 10-5 Laceration of the forehead and scalp.

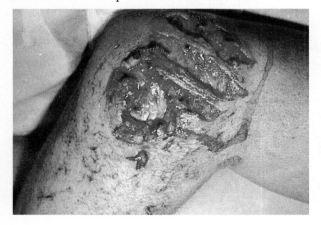

FIGURE 10-6 Deep abrasions and lacerations.

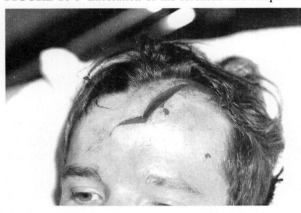

Emergency Care

Provide the following care for lacerations:

1. Control bleeding with direct pressure and elevation; if possible, use sterile gauze over the wound.
2. Cover with a sterile dressing.
3. Elevate the affected part to help control pain and bleeding.
4. Give emergency care for shock.
5. Transport.

Punctures

A puncture wound is caused by the penetration of a sharp object (such as a nail) through the skin and underlying structures (Figure 10-7). Even though the opening in the skin may appear very small, the puncture wound may be extremely deep, posing a serious threat of infection.

Internal organs may also be damaged by punctures. In some cases, the object that causes the injury remains embedded in the wound.

In a puncture wound, always assess for an exit wound as well. (See pages 207–209 for discussion of stab and gunshot wounds.)

Emergency Care

Provide the following care for a puncture wound:

1. Control bleeding with direct pressure. If an object remains impaled in the wound, spread your fingers out around the object; avoid putting any pressure on the object or the tissue around its edges.

FIGURE 10-7 Puncture wound of the foot.

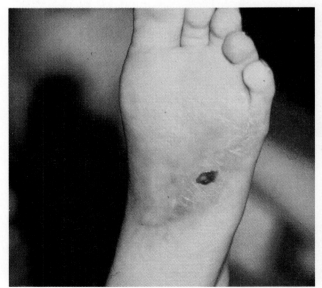

2. Cover the wound with a light sterile dressing.

3. Give the patient emergency care for shock.

4. Transport the patient with the injured part immobilized in a comfortable position.

If there is an impaled object in the wound, do *not* remove it: efforts to do so can cause underlying tissue damage and severe hemorrhage. See Chapter 11.

Avulsions

An avulsion is the tearing loose of a flap of skin, which may either remain hanging or be torn off altogether (Figures 10-8 and 10-9). Scarring is often extensive, and avulsions usually bleed extensively. In some cases, however, blood vessels might seal themselves and retreat into surrounding tissue, limiting the amount of blood loss — but limited blood loss does not signify a less serious injury. If the avulsed tissue is still attached by a flap of skin and is folded back, circulation to the flap can be severely compromised. The seriousness of an avulsion depends on how disrupted circulation is to the flap. Always make sure that the flap is lying flat and that it is aligned in its normal position.

FIGURE 10-8 Forearm avulsion.

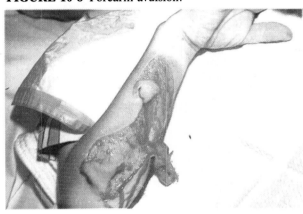

FIGURE 10-9 Ring avulsion.

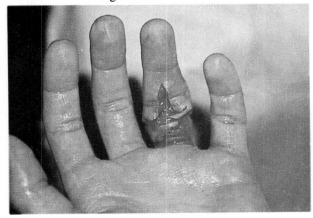

The most commonly avulsed skin on the body is that on the fingers and toes, hands, forearms, legs, feet, ears, nose, and penis. Most often, the patient with an avulsion works with machinery — home accidents involving lawnmowers and power tools are especially increasing in number. Avulsions also commonly occur in automobile or motorcycle accidents.

Emergency Care

To care for an avulsion:

1. Fold the skin flap back into normal position.

2. Control bleeding by direct pressure.

3. Apply a bulky, dry, sterile or compression dressing once the bleeding has been controlled.

4. Give the patient emergency care for shock.

5. Transport.
   - If the avulsion is complete, transport all avulsed parts.
   - Rinse the part with saline to remove gross debris. Follow local protocol.
   - Wrap the part in dry sterile gauze, seal it in a plastic bag, and transport it on ice in another container. Do not use dry ice.
   - Prevent freezing of the tissue; never submerge the plastic bag in the ice.

Bites

More than two million domestic animal bites and more than two thousand snakebites occur in the United States each year. The number of human bites is not recorded but would probably be staggering if known. Nine out of ten animal bites are inflicted by dogs; 10 percent require suturing; and 1 percent require hospitalization (Figure 10-10). Complications can include infection (greatest in those under the age of four or over fifty), **cellulitis, tetanus, septicemia,** and hepatitis.

FIGURE 10-10 Dog bite.

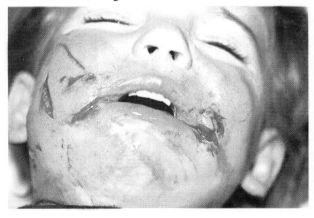

Of all domestic animal bites, dog bites are the most common (Figure 10-11). Most bites are inflicted by family pets or familiar dogs, with stray dogs inflicting only 6 percent of the bites. The most common victims are young children, with two times as many boys as girls being bitten. Most dog bites occur in the afternoon and early evening on cool summer or warm winter days. Among victims of all ages, 30 percent of the bites occur on the hands and arms, 30 to 50 percent on the legs, 10 percent on the torso, and 10 percent on the head and neck; children under the age of twelve are most frequently bitten on the face.

See Table 10-1 for breeds of dogs most associated with dog-attack fatalities. The worst dog bites are those that leave puncture wounds and those that occur in low vascular areas. A bite wound is actually a combination of a penetrating injury and a crushing wound (which can involve soft tissues, internal organs, and bones, and which may include rupturing of tissues or organs). The power of a dog's jaws can cause a severe crushing injury: a large breed can bite with the estimated force of 400 pounds per square inch.

Emergency Care

When you encounter a patient with a dog bite:

1. If the neck or face are involved, manage the airway to ensure adequate breathing.

FIGURE 10-11

DOG BITES

Over 1 million people suffer dog bites in the United States annually. The typical victim is male, under 20 years of age, and bitten by his own pet or some "familiar" large dog between 1 and 9 PM during summer. Facial wounds occur predominantly in young children and teenagers.

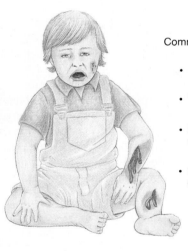

Commonly bitten areas:

- Face 11%
- Trunk 7%
- Upper extremities 28%
- Lower extremities 31%

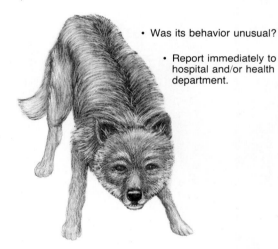

If possible, ascertain where the dog can be located: If an address is not possible, obtain a description of the dog, where it was encountered, and if the attack was provoked.

- Was its behavior unusual?
- Report immediately to hospital and/or health department.

EMERGENCY CARE

- In bites of the head, neck and face be sure airway is clear and position for drainage or suctioning.
- Cover wound with a thick dressing and apply gentle firm pressure.
- If wound is deep leave original dressing in place and add more gauze and then bandage in place.
- Immobilize injured part.
- The patient is usually frightened — calm him/her by talking to him while you are giving necessary care.
- If wounds are severe, monitor for shock, and maintain body heat.
- Always have a dog bite patient transported to a hospital.

2. Control hemorrhage with direct pressure.

3. Apply a dry sterile dressing and bandage in place.

4. Transport the patient with the limb elevated.

The bites of other animals should be cared for in the same manner as dog bites. Care for snakebite is more specific and is discussed in Chapter 13.

The most difficult bite is the human bite because of the high infection rate associated with it. Human bites usually involve the ears, nose, and fingers. They are inflicted most frequently by children involved in play or fights, or by people of all ages confined in mental institutions or involved in sexual assault and fights. Self-inflicted bites can result from ill-fitting dentures, broken teeth, the rough edges of decayed teeth, or seizures. Police may be bitten while breaking up disturbances or trying to apprehend suspects.

Human bites should be considered serious. Even though the wound may look minor, the tissue may be badly lacerated. More serious than the tissue damage, however, is the threat of infection. The human mouth harbors millions of bacteria, in a greater variety than found in the mouths of animals, and massive contamination may result. Human bites on fingers have sometimes resulted in loss of the fingers involved and, in some cases, the entire hand.

To treat a human bite:

1. Apply a sterile dressing.

2. Transport the patient as soon as possible to a hospital, where the wound can be cleaned in a sterile, controlled atmosphere, where unhealthy tissue can be removed, and where a **culture** can be taken.

TABLE 10-1
Breeds of Dogs Responsible for Fatal Single-Dog Attacks Over a Fourteen-Year Period

(Other Breeds Involved in Fatal Pack Attacks Include Boxers, Collies, Rottweilers, Labrador Retrievers, and Yorkshire Terriers)

German shepherd	10
Husky	8
St. Bernard	7
Bullterrier (pit bull)	4
Great Dane	4
Malamute	5
Golden retriever	2
Dachshund	2
Doberman pinscher	2
Basenji	1
Chow chow	1
Mixed breed	5
Unknown breed	4

Reprinted with permission from N. L. McGaffey, *Family Practice Recertification*, MRA Publications.

Traumatic Amputations

The ripping, tearing force of industrial and automobile accidents is great enough to tear away or crush limbs from the body (See Figures 10-12–10-14). The patients are usually young males, and the effects can be tragic.

FIGURE 10-12 Finger amputation.

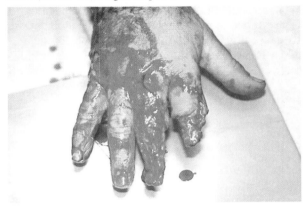

FIGURE 10-13

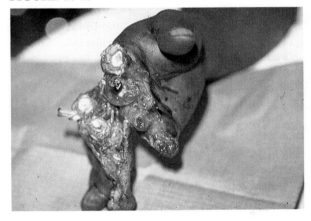

FIGURE 10-14 Toe amputation.

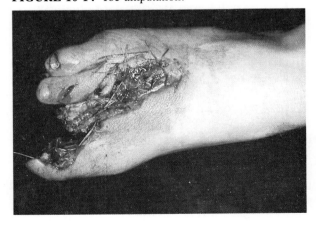

Therefore, the initial emergency management of the patient and of the dismembered limb is critical. New techniques in micro-reconstructive surgery make it possible to save many amputated limbs or digits, so care of the amputated part has become almost as crucial as care of the patient. A surgeon's ability to replant amputated tissue depends on the amount of time the tissue was without blood and oxygen.

Because blood vessels are elastic, they tend to spasm and retract into surrounding tissue in cases of complete amputation; therefore, complete amputations usually cause less bleeding than partial or degloving amputations, in which lacerated arteries continue to bleed profusely.

Emergency Care

Proper sequence of care for the amputation patient is as follows:

1. Establish and maintain the patient's vital functions (the ABCs of emergency care). Remember that trauma great enough to cause an amputation may also cause other bodily injury.

2. The limb, if crushed, may not bleed a great deal. Any hemorrhage should be controlled by direct pressure and elevation; use a tourniquet *only* as a lifesaving last resort. *Never* clamp blood vessels in an attempt to control bleeding; preserve the injured blood vessels as much as you can in case the amputated part can be reconstructed. If necessary, use a blood pressure cuff or antishock garment to help control bleeding.

3. After bleeding has been controlled, apply a dressing to the stump, and wrap the end of the stump with an elastic bandage to replace hand pressure.

4. If the amputation is incomplete, splint and elevate the extremity.

5. Treat the patient for shock. If the patient is conscious and alert, protect him or her from seeing the amputation by draping the area with a sheet.

6. Transport as rapidly as possible to minimize the amount of time the tissue is without blood and oxygen; use a helicopter or aircraft if necessary.

Do *not* waste time in the field searching for amputated parts (*follow local protocol*), and do not neglect patient care in search of amputated parts. If you cannot locate the part, assign someone to find it and bring to the hospital later. If you can quickly find the amputated parts, or if someone you assign to the task can find them, handle them in the following manner (Figure 10-15):

Save the part by wrapping it in a dry *sterile* gauze dressing secured in place by self-adherent roller bandage and placing the wrapped part in a plastic bag, plas-

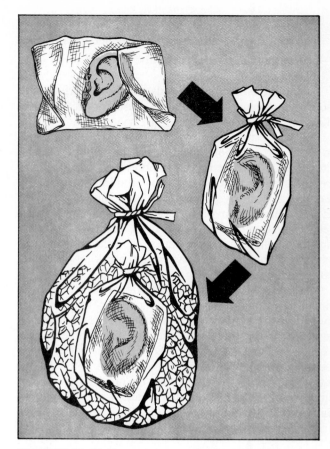

FIGURE 10-15 Emergency care for amputated parts consists of the following: (1) Wrap part completely in dry, sterile gauge or towel; (2) Place in plastic bag and seal shut; (3) Place bagged part on top of a cold back or sealed bag of ice.

tic wrap, or aluminum foil, in accordance with local protocol. If none of these items is available at the scene, wrap the part in a lint-free, sterile dressing. Make certain that you label the wrapped part as to what it is and the patient's name, date, and time the part was wrapped and bagged. Your records should show the approximate time of the amputation.

The part should be kept as cool as possible, without freezing. Place the wrapped and bagged part in a cooler or any other available container so that it is on top of a cold pack or a *sealed* bag of ice (do not use dry ice). *Do not* immerse the part in ice, cooled water, or saline. Label the container the same as the label used for the saved part.

Note: The care of amputated tissues is directed by local protocols, often written to match the reimplantation procedures of the hospitals in your EMS region. Some EMS systems prefer that the dressing used to wrap the part be moistened with normal sterile saline (sterile distilled water is not recommended).

Occasionally, you may find a patient whose limb has been severely lacerated or mangled but not completely amputated. The limb may be attached by a few strands of soft tissue and a small piece of skin. *Do not complete the amputation.* An important consideration in amputation is to preserve as much as possible of the original length of the limb. Even if a limb has been severely mangled and will eventually require amputation, the flap of skin holding the limb together may be used by the surgeon to cover the end of the stump, thereby allowing him or her to preserve a significant amount of limb length. In addition, the strands of soft tissue connecting the limb might contain nerves or blood vessels that, with proper surgical management, might allow the limb to survive.

Care for the open wound as previously described. Make sure that the skin bridge is not twisted or constricted by the pressure dressing.

☐ BLUNT TRAUMA

Blunt trauma is caused by a sudden blow or force that has a crushing impact. This type of injury is treacherous, because the crushing force can result in serious internal injuries that initially display few, if any, external signs. A victim of an accident or other injury can look fine when first examined by EMTs, providing a false sense of security. The patient may then quickly decompensate, resulting in deep shock and/or death. For this reason, always suspect hidden internal damage in patients with injuries involving force.

☐ GENERAL EMERGENCY CARE FOR OPEN WOUNDS

Immediate care for open wounds focuses on maintaining an airway, controlling severe blood loss, and managing any severe injuries that are part of soft-tissue injury (Figure 10-16). Before any other treatment takes place, assess the patient carefully to make sure that the airway is not compromised by bleeding or foreign object aspiration.

Assess the patient thoroughly and carefully, examining all parts of the body. Don't stop with the immediately obvious wound; you may miss others that can become life-threatening.

All open wounds are contaminated to some extent; proper care can reduce the chances for further contamination and enhance the prospect for complete healing.

1. Completely expose and assess the wound; tear or cut away clothing so that you can see the entire wound. Clear the wound and the area around it with sterile gauze so you can see what you're dealing with.

FIGURE 10-16

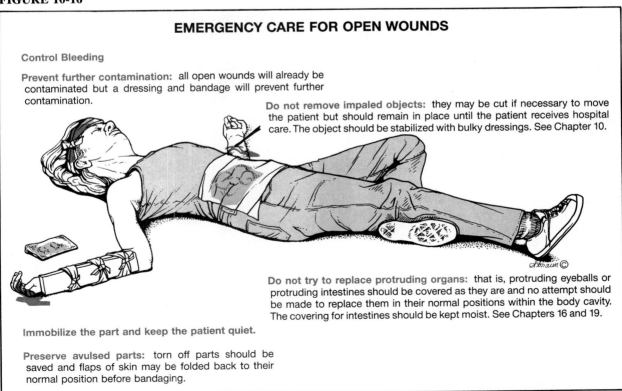

EMERGENCY CARE FOR OPEN WOUNDS

Control Bleeding

Prevent further contamination: all open wounds will already be contaminated but a dressing and bandage will prevent further contamination.

Do not remove impaled objects: they may be cut if necessary to move the patient but should remain in place until the patient receives hospital care. The object should be stabilized with bulky dressings. See Chapter 10.

Do not try to replace protruding organs: that is, protruding eyeballs or protruding intestines should be covered as they are and no attempt should be made to replace them in their normal positions within the body cavity. The covering for intestines should be kept moist. See Chapters 16 and 19.

Immobilize the part and keep the patient quiet.

Preserve avulsed parts: torn off parts should be saved and flaps of skin may be folded back to their normal position before bandaging.

2. If there is severe bleeding from an artery, always control it by direct pressure using your gloved hand or a dry, sterile compression dressing. A roller bandage can provide further pressure, and elevation of the affected limb can also help to control hemorrhage. Use a pressure point only if necessary. Use a tourniquet *only* as a last resort, lifesaving measure.

3. Shock usually follows open wounds, especially if a considerable amount of blood was lost. Give emergency care promptly, and administer 100 percent oxygen (Figure 10-17).

4. If loose foreign particles are present around the wound, wipe them away with sterile gauze or other clean material. Always wipe away from the wound, not toward it. *Never* pick out particles or debris that are embedded in the wound itself.

5. Do not attempt to remove a foreign object that is embedded in the wound; stabilize it with a bulky dressing and transport.

6. Keep the wound as clean as possible. Do not touch the wound with your hands, clothing, or anything that is not clean if possible.

7. Immobilize the injured part to the body or with a rigid splint; immobilization aids in the clotting process, helps prevent further bleeding, helps relieve pain, and helps reduce swelling. Do *not* use an elastic bandage to immobilize — it can cut off circulation.

8. Keep the patient lying still, if possible, since activity increases blood circulation and aggravates bleeding.

9. Place a bandage compress or dressing over the wound, and tie or tape it in place.

10. The bandage should be securely tied or fastened in place so that it will not move. Monitor the area distal to the bandage frequently to ensure adequate distal pulse, circulation, capillary refill, skin temperature, and skin color. If venous circulation is restricted, pain and edema increase.

11. Preserve all avulsed parts.

12. Calm and reassure the patient.

FIGURE 10-17 Treat for shock and adminster oxygen.

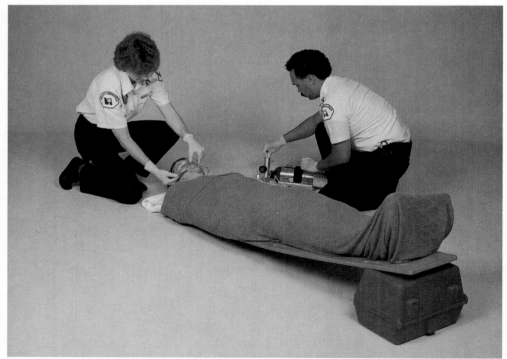

chapter 11

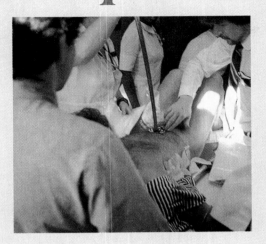

Clamping and Penetrating Injuries

✳ OBJECTIVES

- Outline the special concerns and precautions necessary for treating clamping injuries and stab and gunshot wounds.

- Describe the appropriate emergency care necessary for treating clamping injuries and stab and gunshot wounds.

- Describe the special concerns, precautions, and emergency care necessary for treating impaled object wounds.

It is recommended that EMTs wear protective gloves whenever there is a possibility of coming in contact with a patient's blood, body fluids, mucous membranes, traumatic wounds, or sores. See Chapter 31.

A number of soft-tissue injuries involve foreign objects. Broken glass, sheet metal, knives, bullets, and power tools cause the worst and most extensive damage. To care for such injuries, use common sense, and inspect each wound to determine the following:

- How did the injury occur?
- What object caused the injury?
- How much force was involved?
- What kind of underlying tissue damage might have resulted?
- What are the possibilities of contamination?
- Could a foreign object (or part of one) be left behind in the wound?

Foreign bodies damage soft body tissues in four ways:

1. By clamping onto or around skin.
2. By penetrating skin.
3. By becoming embedded in skin.
4. By penetrating the skin on one end and protruding from the other.

☐ CLAMPING OBJECTS

Most **clamping injuries** involved the hand (Figure 11-1) — more specifically, a finger, which can be strangled when it is stuck into a hole and cannot be pulled out. Try to free the finger as quickly as possible. The longer the finger is stuck, the harder it will be to remove, because the swelling will become more severe by the minute.

Emergency Care

Give the following emergency care:

1. Apply a lubricant such as green soap, and slowly but firmly wiggle the finger until it is loose.
2. If possible, elevate the hand above the patient's head while you remove the finger from the object.
3. If you are unable to loosen the finger, and the object that is clamping is movable and small enough transport the patient and object immediately. When possible keep the hand elevated above the patient's head during transport.

Another kind of **strangling injury** occurs when a ring (or some other constricting object) strangles the finger or other body part due to severe constriction caused by inflammation from an injury. Remove the ring from the finger immediately, and record the exact

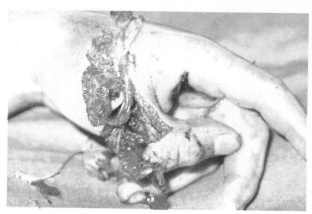

FIGURE 11-1 Clamping injury.

circumstances of removal. A ring cutter should be available in every jump kit. If you are unable to remove the ring, bend it so that the blood supply to the finger will resume. Transport the patient immediately.

A third kind of strangling injury occurs when an object is wound around a body part, cutting off circulation. Swelling is sometimes so bad that you will not be able to easily detect what is causing it (a rubber band, string, or hair).

Give the following care:

1. Examine the area closely. Find the cause of the swelling, and remove it promptly.
2. Elevate the body part to help reduce swelling.
3. Apply a cold pack.
4. Transport the patient immediately.

Use your judgment in deciding if you should care for the clamping injury at the site of the accident or first transport the patient to the hospital. Usually, life-saving measures must be taken in the field prior to transport because time is essential. However, a clamping injury that involves only skin and fat just underneath the skin (and no major blood vessels or nerves) is less serious, and the patient can be transported first. Emergency room personnel can then separate the patient from the clamping mechanism.

If you decide to care for the injury in the field, observe and assess the injury carefully. If the clamp is restricting blood flow, it is best to attempt removal even if some additional damage is inflicted — you may save an entire limb. During transport:

1. Apply a cold pack.
2. Elevate the injured area as high as possible.
3. Keep it well supported.
4. Never cool the injured area for longer than fifteen to thirty minutes at one time.
5. Treat for shock.
6. Administer oxygen.

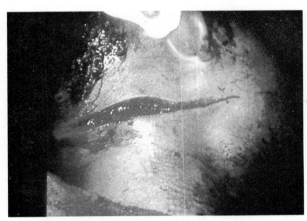

FIGURE 11-2 Knife wound of the neck.

☐ STAB WOUNDS

Knife and stab wounds are dangerous — and oftentimes fatal — and you must develop an efficient method of evaluation and emergency care. Because knife wounds are easier to detect than internal wounds, EMTs too frequently concentrate only on the superficial wound to the skin. Remember — the superficial skin wound is almost never fatal. The fatalities all relate to the injured organs that lie beneath the skin wound (Figure 11-2).

Emergency Care

1. Use local pressure to control external bleeding. Do not use tourniquets unless bleeding cannot be controlled in any other way.

2. Maintain an adequate airway. Poor respiratory exchange and failure to maintain an adequate airway are the leading causes of death from stab wounds to the head, face, and neck.

3. Cover all open wounds with a sterile dressing.

4. Shock is usually caused by hemorrhage and breathing problems. Check for sucking chest wounds. Administer oxygen.

5. Stabilize (with bulky dressings), and leave impaled knives in place during transport.

6. Immobilize extremities that have been injured, including the neck (fractures may have occurred).

7. Transport the patient immediately. Survival is directly related to the length of time that elapses between injury and surgery. Continuously monitor pulse and blood pressure.

☐ GUNSHOT WOUNDS

Gunshot wounds may cause both entrance and exit wounds (Figures 11-3–11-8). The entrance wound is generally much smaller and may be surrounded by pow-der burns if the victim was shot at close range, while the exit wound is generally two to three times larger and tends to bleed heavily. Assess this victim carefully — many have multiple gunshot wounds. Examine regions that may disguise a wound, such as pubic hair or rectal areas.

Ensure your own safety first. If the police are not present and you judge the scene to be unstable, leave until the police have arrived and secured the scene. *Do not enter the scene of a gunshot incident until the area has been secured by the police.* If the scene deteriorates after you enter it, exit quickly. Follow local protocol for reporting gunshot wounds (names, addresses, license numbers, and so on) to police. To protect your own safety and that of your patient, try to determine the location of the weapon and the person with the weapon before arriving on the scene.

Emergency Care

In the assessment of a gunshot-wound victim, it is critical that you quickly determine the damages done in the shooting. Remove all possible clothing and examine closely for wounds and bleeding. Examine all extremities, even if the bullet wound was not to the extremity itself: an arm or leg can be compromised by a bullet wound elsewhere.

The goal of emergency care for gunshot wounds is *rapid transport* — do not take unnecessary time in the field assessing and treating the patient. The secondary survey and all routine stabilization should be done during transport.

To treat the victim of a gunshot wound:

1. Make sure that the patient has an open airway, and assess for breathing.

2. If the patient is not breathing, administer artificial ventilation. If the wound is to the head, neck, chest, or abdomen, suspect cervical spine damage and immobilize as appropriate; ventilate using the modified jaw-thrust technique.

3. Check the patient's pulse. If there is no pulse, commence CPR.

4. Look for both entrance and exit wounds, and remember that the exit wound probably will *not* be in a direct line with the entrance wound. Apply pressure or compression dressings to control external bleeding.

5. Treat all life-threatening injuries. Gunshot wounds to the chest commonly result in pericardial tamponade, sucking chest wounds, or tension pneumothorax.

6. Immobilize injured extremities. If you suspect neck or spinal damage, place the patient on a backboard and apply a rigid cervical collar.

☐ Gunshot Wounds

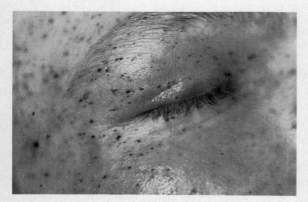

FIGURE 11-3 Powder burns from gunshot.

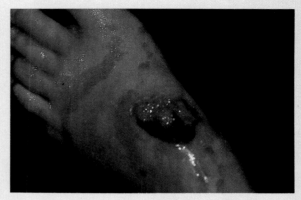

FIGURE 11-4 Gunshot wound to foot.

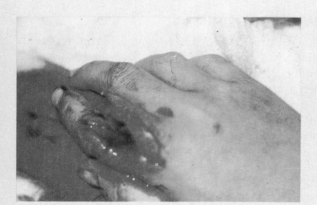

FIGURE 11-5 Gunshot wound to finger.

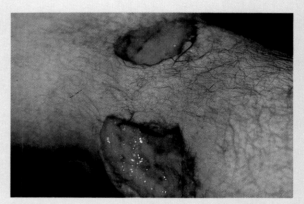

FIGURE 11-6 Gunshot entrance and exit wound to lower leg.

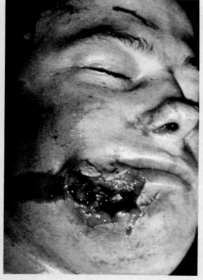

FIGURE 11-7 Gunshot wound to chin.

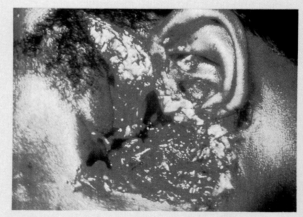

FIGURE 11-8 Gunshot wound to side of head.

7. Treat for shock; elevate the legs and keep warm. Administer oxygen to all victims of gunshot wound.

8. Apply, but do not inflate, a PASG. Before applying the PASG, carefully inspect the area it will cover to make sure there are no additional wounds. Inflate the PASG only if directed to do so by medical control.

9. Keep the patient as quite as possible, and allow nothing by mouth (food or drink can aggravate internal injuries, and the patient will also likely need anesthesia when he reaches the hospital).

10. Transport immediately and rapidly; most gunshot wound victims need surgical intervention. Monitor vital signs continuously throughout transport.

11. If you suspect that a crime has been committed, take care not to disturb potential crime scene evidence; contact the police.

□ IMPALED OBJECTS

Impaled objects occur when there is penetration of a body part by a rigid object, almost always with great force. Objects that both penetrate and protrude are said to be impaled (Figure 11-9). The object may be a stick, glass, arrow, knife, steel rod, or other similar object that penetrates any part of the body. The severity of the resulting wound depends on the body part that is impaled, the size and shape of the object, and the velocity with which it penetrated the body. The damage is not limited to the actual penetration, but also includes blunt trauma. Bleeding can be external or internal.

This type of injury requires careful immobilization of the patient and the injured part. Impaled objects need surgical removal; if impaled objects are removed in the field, the patient can rapidly bleed to death. (An exception is the removal of an impaled object in the cheek. See below.) Any motion of the impaled object can cause additional damage to the surface wound, and particularly the underlying tissues.

Emergency Care

The only time an impaled object should be removed in the field is when it is impaled in the cheek. Follow local protocol (Figure 11-10). To remove an object impaled in the cheek:

1. Assess and maintain the patient's airway; suction out any blood. Ventilate if necessary. Airway obstruction is the leading cause of death among facial trauma victims.

2. Palpate inside the patient's mouth to determine whether the object has penetrated completely.

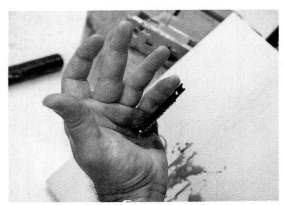
FIGURE 11-9 Penetrating injury with retained foreign body. (Courtesy of Scotland White Hospital and Clinic)

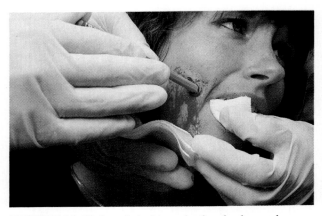
FIGURE 11-10 Impaled objects in the cheek may be removed. Dress outside of wound and put dressing on inside wound between cheek and teeth. Hold in place if necessary.

3. Control bleeding on the cheek, and dress the wound.

4. If the object penetrated completely, pack the inside of the cheek (between the cheek wall and the teeth) with sterile gauze to control bleeding.

5. Radio ahead and transport immediately.

If you encounter too much resistance in trying to remove the object from the cheek, maintain the airway and transport immediately. Stabilize the penetrating object prior to transport.

In cases of other impaled objects, provide the following emergency care (Figures 11-11–11-13):

1. Assess and maintain the airway; use suction to keep the airway clear, and ventilate if necessary. If the head, neck, or back is involved, immobilize immediately, using manual immobilization if necessary.

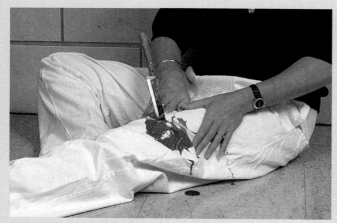

FIGURE 11-11 Impaled object injury.

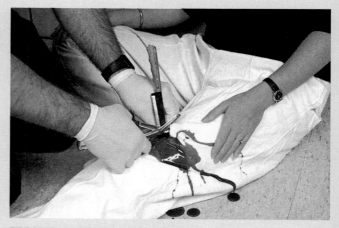

FIGURE 11-12 Cut away clothing.

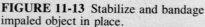

FIGURE 11-13 Stabilize and bandage impaled object in place.

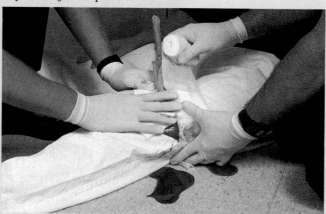

2. Remove clothing so the wound is exposed; cut it away without disturbing the impaled object. Do not move or remove the impaled object; to do so may cause added bleeding and damage to underlying tissues (muscles, nerves, blood vessels, bones, organs, and so on).

3. Control bleeding with direct pressure, but do not exert any pressure on the impaled object or on the tissue margins around the cutting edge of the object.

4. Stabilize the impaled object with bulky dressings and bandage in place. The impaled object itself must be completely surrounded by bulky dressings; the objective is to pack dressings around the object and tape them securely in place so that motion is reduced to a minimum. If possible, at least three-fourths of the object must be covered by

dressings. The use of a "doughnut"-type ring pad may also help in stabilization (Figure 11-14).

5. Calm and reassure the patient as you monitor for shock.

6. Keep the patient at rest, and administer oxygen.

7. Do not attempt to cut off, break off, or shorten an impaled object unless transportation is not possible with it in place. If the object must be cut off, stabilize it securely before cutting. Remember — any motion is transmitted to the patient and can cause additional tissue damage and shock.

8. Promptly but carefully transport the patient to the hospital, avoiding as much movement as possible. Notify the receiving facility of the nature of the injury so that appropriate arrangements can be made.

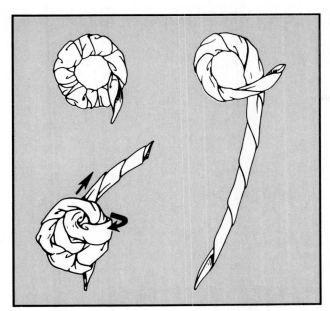

FIGURE 11-14 The penetrating object can be encircled and immobilized with a ring pad that can be improvised from a cravat, handkerchief, stocking, or even a small towel. Bandage in place.

chapter 12

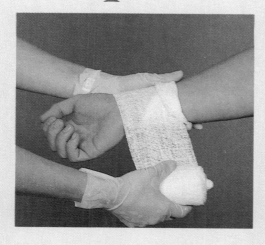

Bandaging

✱ **OBJECTIVES**

- Identify the various types of dressings and bandages.
- Demonstrate how to apply bandages to different parts of the body.
- Demonstrate the use of a sling and a pressure dressing.
- Describe the basic principles of dressing and bandaging wounds.

It is recommended that EMTs wear protective gloves whenever there is a possibility of coming in contact with a patient's blood, body fluids, mucous membranes, traumatic wounds, or sores. See Chapter 31.

Once heavy hemorrhaging from a wound has been controlled, the wound should be dressed and bandaged to manage further bleeding. Proper wound care enhances healing, adds to the comfort of the patient, and promotes more rapid recovery. Improper wound care can delay healing, cause infection, cause severe discomfort to the patient, and — in rare cases — result in the loss of a limb.

The basic purposes of dressing and bandaging are to:

- Control bleeding.
- Prevent further contamination of the wound.
- Protect the wound from further damage.
- Keep the wound dry.
- Immobilize the wound site.

□ DRESSINGS

A dressing is a sterile covering for a wound that controls bleeding and prevents further contamination of the wound. It should be **sterile** (meaning that all microorganisms and spores have been killed) and **aseptic** (meaning that it is free of bacteria). Commercial dressings are usually gauze pads that are individually wrapped and sealed to prevent contamination. **Bulky dressings** are thick dressings that are large enough to cover significant wounds. They are used to control bleedings and stabilize impaled objects.

The ideal dressing is layered and consists of coarse-mesh **gauze** and self-adhering roller material (such as **kling** or **kerlix**). It should be bulky enough to immobilize the tissues and to protect the wound; such protection cuts down on renewed bleeding and wound contamination. In an emergency, you can use *clean* handkerchiefs, towels, sheets, cloth, or sanitary napkins as dressings; never use elastic bandages (they have a tourniquet effect) or paper towels, toilet tissues, or other material that could shred and cling to the wound.

Type of wound dressings include (Figures 12-1–12-3):

- Aseptic (a sterile dressing free from bacteria).
- Wet (a moist dressing that may not be sterile).
- Dry sterile (a sterile dressing free from moisture).

□ Dressings

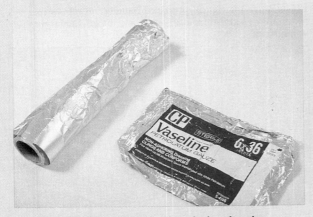

FIGURE 12-1 Petroleum and occlusive dressings.

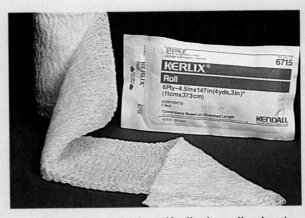

FIGURE 12-2 Nonelastic, self-adhering roller dressing and bandage.

FIGURE 12-3 Multi-trauma dressing.

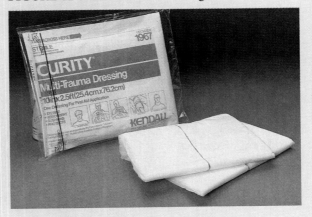

- Petrolatum gauze (sterile gauze saturated with petrolatum to prevent the dressing from sticking to an open wound).
- **Occlusive** (plastic wrap, aluminum foil, petroleum gauze, or other dressings that form an airtight seal).
- Compress (a bulky, usually sterile, dressing intended to stop and control bleeding).
- **Universal** (made from a nine-by thirty-six-inch piece of thick, absorbent material).

☐ BANDAGES

A bandage holds a dressing in place over a wound, creates pressure over a bleeding wound for control of hemorrhage, secures a splint to an injured part of the body, and provides support for an injured part. Properly applied, bandages promote healing, prevent severe complications, and help the patient remain comfortable during transport.

A bandage should not normally contact a wound; it should be used only to hold the dressing in place. A bandage should be applied firmly and fastened securely. It should not be applied so tightly that it stops circulation, or so loosely that it allows the dressing to slip. If bandages work themselves loose or become unfastened, wounds may bleed or become infected, and broken bones may become further displaced. It is essential, therefore, that bandages be properly applied and well secured.

Self-adhesive, highly comforming roller bandages do not stick to the skin, but the bandage surfaces adhere to each other to make bandaging easier.

Before you bandage a wound on the arm or hand, remove rings from the fingers and other jewelry that could restrict circulation as a result of swelling. Rings or hidden tape can cause pressure that may restrict circulation and could lead to **gangrene.**

If the bandaged part of the body is mobile, apply the bandage snugly to counter stretching. Make sure that the bandage is not too tight; loosen it slightly if signs of restriction occur. Signs that indicate an overtight bandage include:

- The skin around the bandage becomes pale or cyanotic (bluish).
- The patient complains of pain usually only a few minutes after you have applied the bandage.
- The skin is cold distally.
- The skin is tingling or numb distally.

If the pain or discomfort disappears after several hours, severe damage may have already occurred. Permanent muscle paralysis may result. Improper bandaging can be defined in a court of law as negligence.

☐ SPECIAL TYPES OF DRESSINGS AND BANDAGES

Bandage Compress

A **bandage compress** is a special dressing to cover open wounds (Figure 12-4). It consists of a pad made of several thicknesses of gauze attached to the middle of a strip of bandaging material. Pad sizes range from one to four inches. Bandage compresses usually come folded so that the gauze pad can be applied directly to the open wound with virtually no exposure to the air or fingers.

The strip of gauze at either side of the pad is folded back so that it can be opened up and the bandage compress tied in place with no disturbance of the sterile pad. The dressing portion of a bandage compress may be extended to twice its normal size by continued unfolding.

Unless otherwise specified, all bandage compresses and all gauze dressings should be covered with open triangular, cravat, or roller bandages.

FIGURE 12-4 Ready-prepared bandage compresses, available in individual packages, are useful for larger wounds.

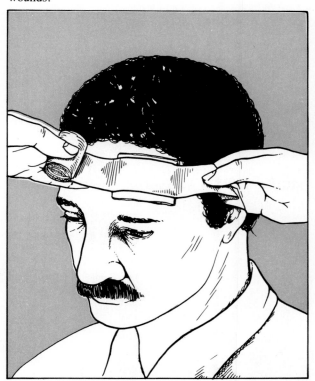

Gauze Pads

Gauze is used several ways in applying dressings; plain gauze may be used in place of a bandage compress to cover large wounds. Plain gauze of various sizes is supplied in packets. Care should be taken not to touch the portion of the gauze that is to contact the wound.

Sterile gauze pads, two-by-twos, four-by fours, and four-by-eights, are the most popular dressings that come individually wrapped. In cases of major multiple trauma, nonsterile bulk packages of four-by-four dressings are often used.

Special Pads

Large, thick-layered, bulky pads (some with water-proofed outer surfaces) are available in several sizes for quick application to an extremity or to a large area of the trunk (see Figure 12-3). They are used where bulk is required in cases of profuse bleeding. They are also useful for stabilizing embedded objects. These special pads are referred to as **multitrauma dressings, trauma packs, general purpose dressings, burn pads,** or **ABD dressings.**

Because of their absorbent properties, sanitary napkins are well suited for emergency care work. If purchased in individual wrappers, they have the added advantage of cleanliness.

Occlusive Dressing

An occlusive dressing is used to close an open wound that has penetrated a body cavity. Usually made of plastic, an occlusive dressing creates an airtight, moisture-proof seal. In an emergency, you can use a plastic bag.

Triangular Bandage

A standard triangular bandage is made from a piece of cloth approximately forty inches square by folding the square diagonally and cutting along the fold. It is easily applied and can be handled so that the part to be applied over the wound or burn dressing will not be soiled. A triangular bandage does not tend to slip off once it is correctly applied. It is usually made from unbleached cotton cloth, although any kind of cloth will do. In emergencies, a triangular bandage can be improvised from a clean handkerchief or clean piece of shirt.

The triangular bandage is used to make improvised tourniquets, to support fractures and dislocations, to apply splints, and to form slings. If a regular-size bandage is found to be too short when a dressing is applied, it can be lengthened by tying a piece of another bandage to one end.

Roller Bandages

The self-adhering (nonelastic), form-fitting roller bandage is the most popular and easy to use (Figures 12-5–12-16). It eliminates the need for much of the complex bandaging techniques required with regular gauze roller bandages or **cravats.**

This type of roller bandage is applied to hold a dressing securely in place over a wound. For this reason, it should be applied snugly, but not tightly enough to interfere with circulation. Fingers and toes should be checked periodically for coldness, swelling, cyanosis, and numbness. If symptoms occur, the bandage should be loosened immediately.

Self-adhering roller bandages are easily secured with several overlapping wraps and can then be cut and tied or taped in place. Commercial examples are Kerlix and Kling. Roller bandages of the head can be used to either hold a large dressing on a head wound or to encompass the complete cranial area. (See Figures 12-6 and 12-7.)

Roller bandages of the cheek, shoulder, elbow, arm, thigh, and knee can also be applied as illustrated in Figures 12-8–12-14 and 12-17–12-19.

□ PRINCIPLES OF DRESSING AND BANDAGING

There are no hard-and-fast rules for dressing and bandaging wounds: often, adaptability and creativity are far more important ingredients of rescue than even the best-intentioned rules. In dressing and bandaging, use the materials you have on hand and the methods to which you can best adapt, as long as the following conditions are generally met:

- Material used for dressings should be as clean as possible (sterile, if you can obtain sterile materials).
- Bleeding is controlled. Generally, you should not bandage a dressing into place until bleeding has stopped; the exception, of course, is a pressure bandage designed to stop bleeding.
- The dressing is opened carefully and handled in an aseptic manner; in other words, dirt and debris are kept off the dressing material.
- The original dressing is not removed. If blood soaks through, add another dressing on top of the original instead of removing it.
- The dressing adequately covers the entire wound (Figure 12-20).
- Wounds are bandaged snugly, but not too tightly, and bandage application should proceed from distal to proximal.
- Tips of the fingers and toes are left exposed when arms and legs are bandaged so that you can check for circulation impairment.

□ Self-Adhering Roller Bandages

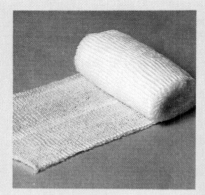

FIGURE 12-5 Self-adhering roller bandage.

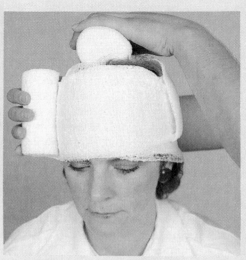

FIGURE 12-6 Head bandage.

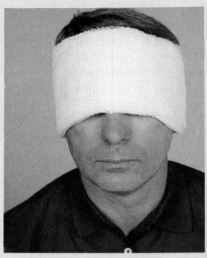

FIGURE 12-7 Head and/or eye bandage.

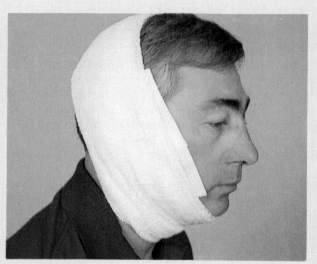

FIGURE 12-8 Cheek bandage (make sure the mouth will open).

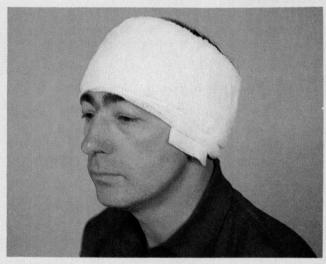

FIGURE 12-9 Head and/or ear bandage.

FIGURE 12-10 Shoulder bandage.

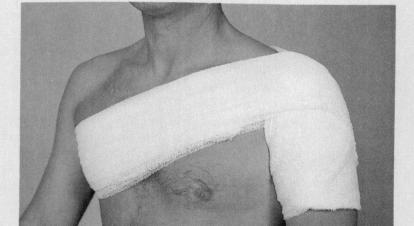

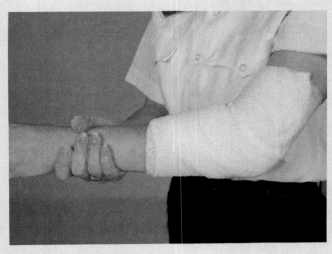

FIGURE 12-11 Elbow bandage.

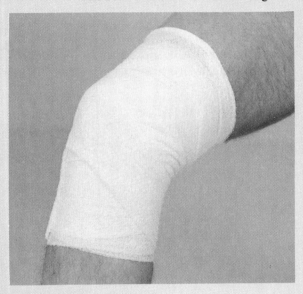

FIGURE 12-12 Lower arm bandage.

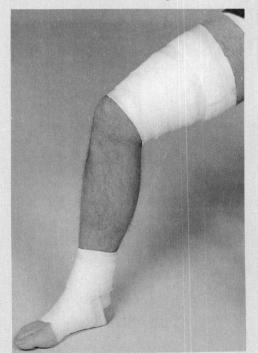

FIGURE 12-14 Knee bandage.

FIGURE 12-13 Thigh and ankle bandage.

FIGURE 12-16 Foot and/or ankle bandage.

FIGURE 12-15 Hand bandage.

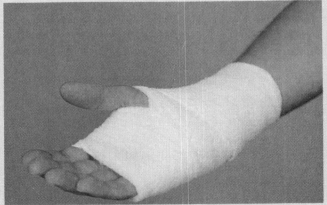

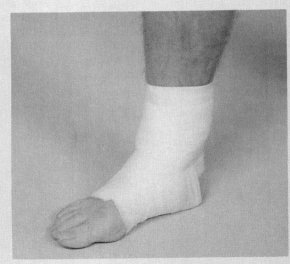

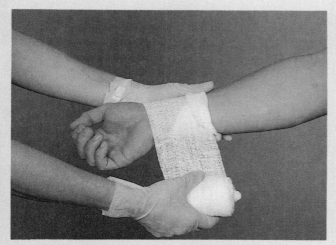

FIGURE 12-17 Secure with several overlying wraps.

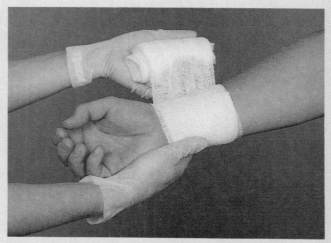

FIGURE 12-18 Overlap the bandage, keeping it snug.

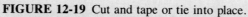
FIGURE 12-19 Cut and tape or tie into place.

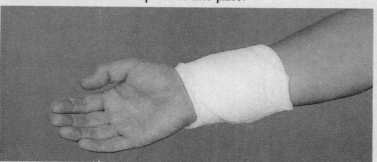

FIGURE 12-20 Dressings should adequately cover wounds, and bandages on extremities should cover a larger area than the wound.

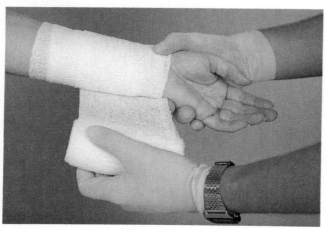

- If you are bandaging a small wound on an extremity, cover a larger area with the bandage to avoid creating a pressure point and to distribute pressure more uniformly (Figure 12-20).

- On an extremity, start bandaging at the distal end and work toward the heart — this pattern is much less likely to impair circulation.

- Always place the body part to be bandaged in the position in which it is to remain. You can bandage across a joint, but do not try bending a joint *after* the bandage has been applied to it.

- Question the patient regarding how the bandage feels. If he complains that it is too tight, loosen it and make it comfortable, but snug.

☐ APPLYING SPECIAL DRESSINGS AND BANDAGES

Pressure Dressing

Apply a pressure dressing in the following way:

1. Cover the wound with a bulky, sterile dressing.
2. Apply hand pressure over the wound until the dressing is in place.
3. Apply a firm roller bandage, preferably the self-adhering type; use an elastic bandage only in cases of profuse or difficult-to-control bleeding, and monitor constantly for signs of overtightness. An air splint or blood pressure cuff may also be used to hold a pressure dressing in place. See Chapter 7.
4. If blood soaks through the original dressing and bandage, do not remove them — leave them in place and apply another dressing, securing it in place with another roller bandage.

Slings

Slings are used to support injuries of the shoulder, upper extremities, or ribs. In an emergency, they may be improvised from belts, neckties, scarves, or similar articles. Triangular bandages should be used if available.

Tie a triangular bandage sling as follows (Figure 12-21):

1. Place one end of the base of an open triangular bandage over the shoulder of the injured side.
2. Allow the bandage to hang down in front of the chest so that its **apex** will be behind the elbow of the injured arm.
3. Bend the arm at the elbow with the hand slightly elevated (four to five inches).
4. Bring the forearm across the chest and over the bandage.
5. Carry the lower end of the bandage over the shoulder of the uninjured side, and tie a square knot (12-22) at the uninjured side of the neck, being sure that the knot is at the side of the neck.
6. Twist the apex of the bandage, and tuck it in at the elbow.

The hand should be supported with the fingertips exposed, whenever possible, to permit detection of impaired circulation.

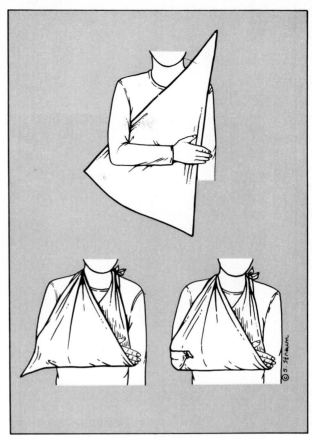

FIGURE 12-21 Triangular bandage as an arm sling.

FIGURE 12-22 Tying a square knot.

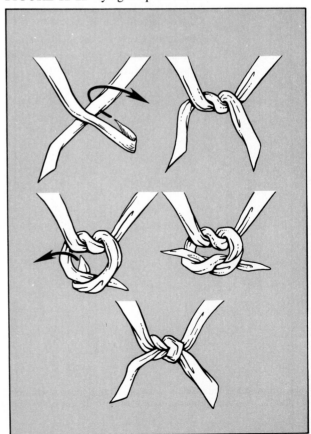

chapter 13

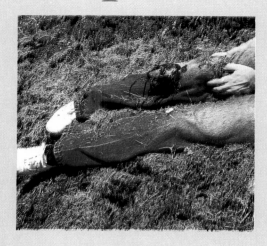

Musculo-skeletal Injuries

✳ OBJECTIVES

- Discuss the anatomy and physiology of the musculoskeletal system, including the major muscles and bones.
- Describe the types and causes of musculoskeletal injuries.
- Demonstrate a patient assessment at the scene of an accident or injury.
- Demonstrate emergency care for sprains, strains, and dislocations.
- Demonstrate how to assess for a fracture.
- Describe the two classifications and five types of fractures.
- Demonstrate the proper techniques of emergency care for fractures, including the various techniques of splinting.

It is recommended that EMTs wear protective gloves whenever there is a possibility of coming in contact with a patient's blood, body fluids, mucous membranes, traumatic wounds, or sores. See Chapter 31.

Injuries to muscles, joints, and bones are some of the most common situations encountered by EMTs. These injuries can range from the simple and non-life-threatening (such as a broken finger or sprained ankle) to the critical and life-threatening (such as a fracture of the femur or spine). Whether the injury is mild or severe, your ability to provide emergency care efficiently and quickly may prevent further painful and damaging injury and may even keep the patient from suffering permanent disability or death.

Emergency care of fractures, dislocations, and soft-tissue injuries during the first hours following injury is critical in preventing permanent disabilities. An immediate, systematic evaluation of the patient is essential so that concealed injury is not overlooked.[1]

□ ANATOMY OF THE MUSCULOSKELETAL SYSTEM

A major discussion and diagramming of the **musculoskeletal system** is presented in Chapter 2. While musculoskeletal injuries are common, they do not have to be difficult to care for and are generally not a threat to life.

The two main parts of the system are the muscles and the skeleton. **Tendons** and **ligaments** connect muscles to bones, and bones to bones, respectively (Figure 13-1):

Muscle

Muscle is a special type of tissue that contracts, or shortens, when stimulated. The three major types of muscles are:

- Involuntary (smooth) muscles, which are not under conscious control. They handle the work of the internal organs with the exception of the heart.
- Voluntary (skeletal) muscles, which are under conscious control. Voluntary muscles include muscles that make up the arms, the legs, the upper back, and the hips, and they cover the ribs and the abdomen. Skeletal muscles are attached to the bones either directly or by tendons (tough, fibrous, connective tissue). When the voluntary muscle contracts through stimulation, it shortens and pulls on a part of the skeletal system, causing movement.
- Cardiac, or heart muscle, also known as myocardium.

---

[1] For specialized information on how to treat fractures in children, see Chapter 32, "Pediatric Emergencies." See Chapter 14 for a more specific discussion of "Fractures of the Upper and Lower Extremities." For rib fractures, see Chapter 19, "Injuries to the Chest."

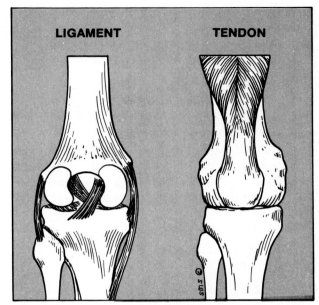

FIGURE 13-1 Ligaments connect bone to bone, while tendons attach muscles to bone.

Tendons

Tendons are highly specialized **connective tissue** composed of **collagen** and elastic fibers. They allow for maximum strength because they are oriented in the direction of muscle pull (Figure 13-1). Tendons form a shiny white band that attaches to the muscles and, through a network of tiny fibers, connects with a bone.

If sharp, sudden force is applied, the tendon may pull loose from the bone and may even pull a small piece of bone away with it. The skin over the injured area will remain intact, but local swelling and tenderness usually occur. Apply a splint as you would for a suspected fracture.

Ligaments

Ligaments connect bone to bone (Figure 13-1). When a ligament is injured, the individual parts give way at different places along the entire ligament length. Skin lacerations are rarely involved.

Torn ligament ends resemble a mop head. As the ligament heals, **scar tissue** forms throughout much of the ligament, affecting its ability to stretch. A ligament that is completely torn can never return to its previous stability and stretching ability.

Most bodily joints have ligaments at their sides located farthest from the center plane of motion. These are called **collateral ligaments.** More complex joints (like the knee) feature ligaments that are attached to the **joint capsule.** The ligament is often injured simultaneously with the joint, causing early joint swelling due to internal bleeding.

The Skeletal System

The skeletal system (Figure 13-2) has four major functions:

- It gives shape or form to the body.
- It supports the body, allowing it to stand erect.
- It provides the basic for **locomotion,** or movement, by giving muscles a place to attach and contains joints that allow movement.
- It protects major body organs, such as the brain (skull), the heart and lungs (rib cage), the pelvic organs, and the spinal cord (vertebrae).

The major parts of the skeletal system are discussed in Chapter 2.

FIGURE 13-2 The skeletal system.

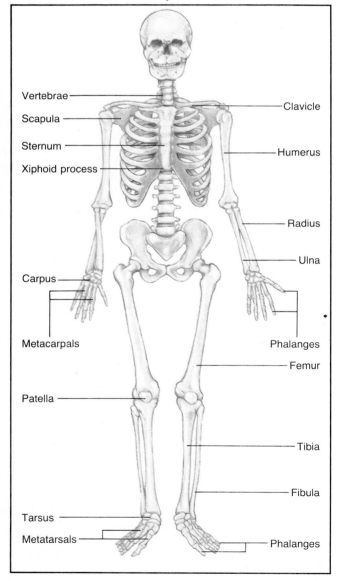

Vertebrae
Scapula
Sternum
Xiphoid process
Carpus
Metacarpals
Patella
Tarsus
Metatarsals

Clavicle
Humerus
Radius
Ulna
Phalanges
Femur
Tibia
Fibula
Phalanges

☐ FORCES THAT CAUSE MUSCULOSKELETAL INJURIES

Your EMT experience will most likely involve the recognition and emergency care of musculoskeletal injuries because they occur so frequently. Musculoskeletal injuries are usually associated with external forces, though some may occur through disease (e.g., bone degeneration).

The force applied to the body may cause injuries to the surrounding soft tissues (e.g., nerves and arteries), and even to body areas distant from the fracture site. This is why it is essential for you to complete efficient primary and secondary patient assessments so that more serious injuries may not be overlooked.

As you approach the accident scene and talk with the patient, bystanders, etc., try to imagine the forces that the patient's body experienced and the direction in which those forces propelled the body. Different types of forces (Figure 13-3) may cause differing types of injuries, such as:

- Direct blows — the fracture from a direct blow occurs at the point of impact (e.g., a patella hitting an automobile dashboard and being fractured).
- Indirect forces — the force impacts on one end of a limb, causing injury to the limb some distance away from the point of impact (e.g., a person thrown from a horse lands on two outstretched hands; one arm sustains a fractured wrist, and at the proximal end of the other arm, a clavicle is fractured).
- Twisting forces — one part of the **appendage** (e.g., the foot) remains stationary while the rest of the appendage (lower leg) twists.

☐ PATIENT ASSESSMENT

When you arrive on the scene of an accident or injury, do the following:

1. Conduct a primary survey of the airway, breathing, major bleeding, and circulation.
2. Conduct a secondary evaluation to identify other less serious injuries.
3. Obtain the history of the injury and observe the scene carefully so that you can determine the mechanism of injury.
4. If the patient cannot remember what happened, or felt dizzy or nauseated, check on the possibility of heart attack, seizure drug reaction, or chemical

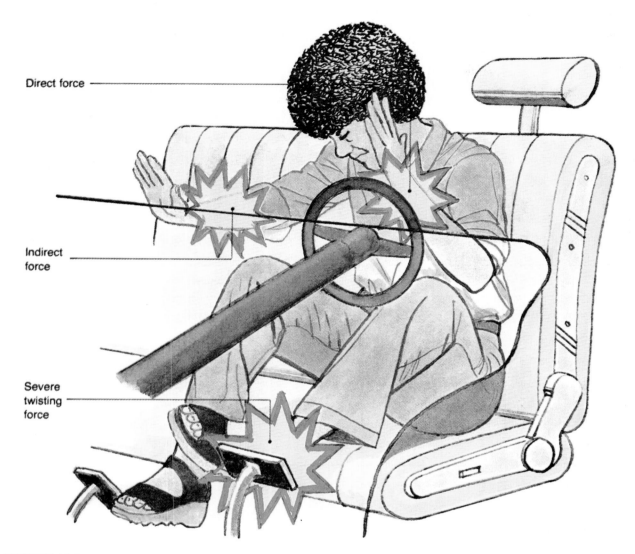

Direct force

Indirect force

Severe twisting force

FIGURE 13-3

imbalance. Do not overlook the possibility of physical abuse.

5. Treat all unconscious patients as if they had neck injuries.

☐ INJURIES TO MUSCLES

Two major types of muscle injuries are:

- **sprains.**
- **strains.**

Other muscle injuries are lacerations or punctures (discussed in Chapter 10, "Soft Tissue Injuries") and contusions. If severe enough to care, contusions may also indicate damage to underlying bones or nerves.

Sprains

Sprains are injuries in which ligaments are stretched and/or torn, usually due to sudden twisting of a joint beyond its normal range of motion. Sprains most commonly affect the knees and ankles and are characterized by pain, immediate swelling, inability to use the joint, and discoloration over the injured area (Figure 13-4).

Emergency Care

In most cases it is best to care for the sprain as if it were a fracture and immobilize it accordingly. In the case of a sprained ankle, assume that the injury is a fracture since, without an x-ray, a sprain cannot be differentiated from a fracture. Most sprains (about 80 percent) will occur because the ankle turns outward, toward the outside of the body, with a popping or ripping sound.

SIGNS AND SYMPTOMS OF COMMON ORTHOPEDIC INJURIES			
Sprain	**Strain**	**Fracture**	**Dislocation**
Pain on movement	Immediate, burning pain	Pain, tenderness	Pain
Tenderness	Little swelling	Deformity	Deformity
Painful movement, swelling	Little discoloration	Loss of use, swelling	Loss of movement
Redness		Bruising	
		Crepitus (grating)	
		Possible exposed bone ends	

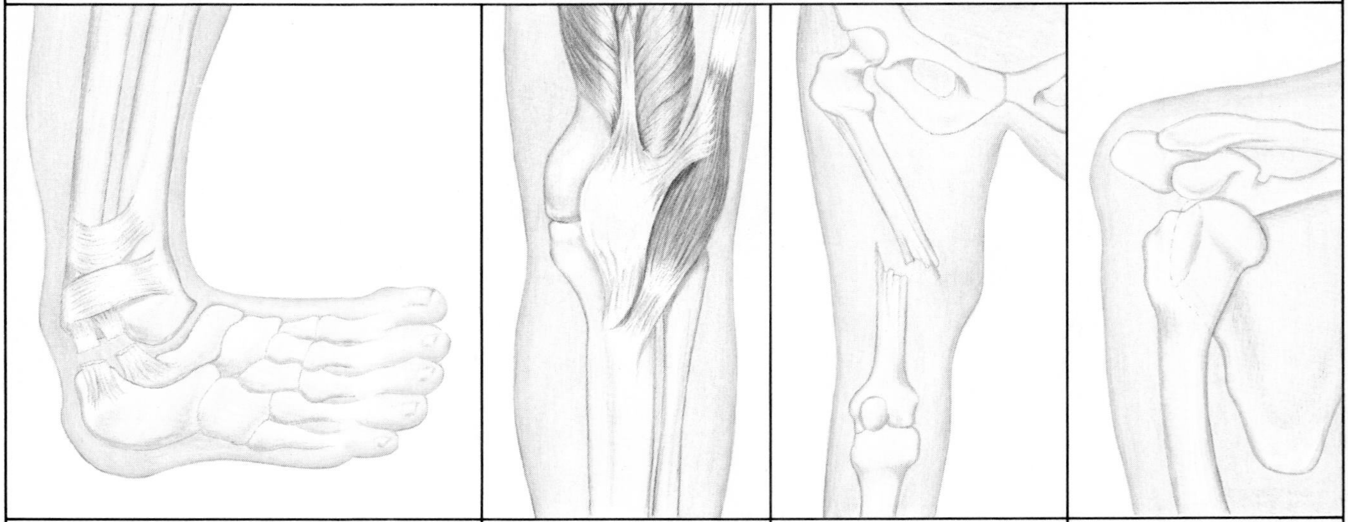

FIGURE 13-4

Do not allow the patient to walk or stand on a sprained knee or ankle. Loosen the shoelaces and remove the shoe as needed.

Before transport, provide care based on the acronym RICE.[2]

R: Rest
I: Ice
C: Compression
E: Elevation

1. **Rest.** A severely sprained ankle may have torn tissues and even a fracture. If you suspect major tissue damage, give the sprained joint complete rest by splinting it. Do not allow the patient to walk on it. Make sure that the sprain is evaluated by a physician.

2. **Ice.** Cold reduces pain, bleeding, swelling, and muscle spasms in injured muscles. Put cold packs, crushed ice, frozen gel, or cold towels on the injured area, or immerse it in ice water. Protect against frostbite by putting a towel or a single layer of elastic wraps next to the skin and by applying the cold pack for fifteen to thirty minutes. (Gel is colder than ice.)

3. **Compression.** In a long transport situation, a compression bandage will limit internal bleeding and may also squeeze some fluid and debris out of the injury site. Wrap the injured area with an elastic bandage, apply a cold pack, then wrap the pack to the sprained part with another layer of elastic bandage. Leave fingers and toes exposed so that you can check for color change or swelling that would indicate the bandage is too tight. Ask about pain, numbness, and tingling.

4. **Elevation.** Raise the injured area, propped and supported with pillows, to about heart level, if possible. This will reduce circulation to the area and thus help to control internal bleeding.

---

[2] Thygerson, Alton L., "Muscle Injuries," *Emergency*, July 1985, pp. 50–51; Levin, Susanna, "Sprains Are a Pain," *Walking Magazine*, June/July 1987, p. 75.

Apply an appropriate splint, then transport. (See "Types of Splints" later in this chapter.)

For maximum benefit, begin the RICE treatment as soon as possible but not later than sixty minutes after the injury has occurred.

Strains

Strains are caused by soft-tissue injuries or muscle spasms that occur around a joint and anywhere in the musculature (Figure 13-4). They are characterized by pain on active movement. No deformity or swelling is usually associated with a strain, and slow, gentle movement will cause little, if any, pain. The muscle fibers involved are stretched and may be partially torn due to overexertion. The most common strain injuries occur in the back and are usually caused by lifting an object that is too heavy or lifting it improperly.

Signs and symptoms include:

- Acute tearing pain at the time of injury. In the case of a back strain, pain may radiate downward to the leg muscles. The patient may have heard or felt a snap at the time of injury.
- Pain when moving the affected part.
- Spasm in the area of the strain.
- Disfigurement — either an indentation where tissues have separated or a swelling indicating contracted tissue.
- Severe weakness and loss of function.

Emergency Care

Strains are best cared for by having the patient avoid stress on the injured area. In most cases, assume that a fracture may be involved and immobilize accordingly. If the exact nature of the injury is in question, immobilize the extremity pending evaluation in the emergency department. To care for the patient:

1. Place the patient in a comfortable position, such as reclining with the knees drawn up to take pressure off the back muscles.
2. Immobilize the area by splinting if needed.
3. Transport for diagnosis.

□ DISLOCATIONS OF JOINTS

Bones that come together without a bony union form a joint. The body contains **immovable joints, joints with limited motion,** and **freely movable joints.** A dislocation is the displacement of a bone end from a joint. In a dislocation, the ligaments holding the bones in proper position are often stretched and sometimes are torn loose (Figure 13-4).

Dislocations cause serious pain because the joint surfaces are rich in nerves. Unstable joints or muscle spasms cause movement of the joint surfaces that are extremely irritating to these nerves. Although joint surfaces are not sharp, they can injure adjacent structures by contusion, compression, and vascular obstruction.

The general signs and symptoms of dislocations are:

- Rigidity (stiffness) and loss of function.
- Deformity or irregularity of the affected joint.
- Pain at the joint.
- Moderate or severe swelling around the joint.

The principle symptom of dislocation is pain or a feeling of pressure over the involved joint, as well as loss of motion of the joint. The principle sign of dislocation is deformity. If the dislocated bone end is pressing on a nerve, numbness or paralysis may also occur below the dislocation. If a blood vessel is being compressed, loss of pulse may occur below the dislocation. The absence of pulses means that the extremity is not receiving adequate blood. Transport the patient promptly but prudently, advising the hospital of the circulatory impairment.

Throughout these procedures, check distal pulses and sensation after every immobilization and splinting.

1. To check distal pulses:
   - Palpate the pulse on the side of the injury away from the heart.
   - You may also check capillary refill by pressing a fingernail or toenail and observing how quickly color returns to the area. Normal refill time is two seconds or less.
   - Absence of pulses or a prolonged refill time means that either the injury itself or your splinting procedures are reducing circulation to the area. You must correct this situation immediately by straightening the fractured limb or loosening the splint.

2. To check distal motion and sensations:
   - Ask the patient to wiggle his or her fingers and toes.
   - Touch a finger or toe and ask the patient if he or she can feel it.
   - If the patient is unconscious, gently probe or pinch the skin and note any reactions to this mild pain.

Emergency Care

Since dislocations involve the joints and are often accompanied by fractures, emergency care is to immobilize all suspected dislocations *in the position found.*

1. Do not try to straighten, or reduce, a dislocation unless specifically ordered to do so by a physician.
2. Splint above and below the dislocated joint to maintain stability.
3. Apply cold packs during transport.

If more than one hour elapses from the time of the patient's injury to arrival at the medical facility, contact a physician for instructions. He or she may request that you try to gently reduce the dislocation. For instructions on reducing a dislocation of the knee, see the section "Dislocation of the Knee" later in this chapter.

Dislocation of the Shoulder

The ball-and-socket shoulder joint is relatively unstable. Many forces — blows, falls, throwing a football — can cause dislocation of the shoulder. In 96 percent of all shoulder dislocations, the head of the humerus (upper arm) is forced forward. It is common for fractures of the shoulder girdle or upper arm to accompany a dislocated shoulder.

Nerves and blood vessels are often injured in a shoulder dislocation. The patient becomes immobilized, usually falls to the ground, and may faint due to the excruciating pain. To prevent further injury from falling or fainting, gently help the patient to sit or lie down. Shoulder pain is sometimes difficult to diagnose, and the cause may be irritation of a neck nerve or a problem involving an organ like the heart, lungs, gallbladder, or spleen. If there was no accident or obvious mechanism of injury, ask:

1. If the pain developed gradually, what seemed to be the cause? How long has the pain lasted? How intense is it? Where is the pain located? (Have the patient point with one finger to the painful area.)
2. Are there cold and warm areas on the skin? (Coldness can indicate circulation difficulties, while a heated area may indicate inflammation.)
3. Are any areas of skin numb? Is the joint tender?
4. How freely does the arm move compared to the other shoulder? (Also compare the painful side with the other side to see if the shoulders are even, if the arm needs to be supported, etc.)
5. Is there any weakness?

Emergency Care

Provide the following emergency care for a dislocated shoulder:

1. Examine the patient for other injuries. Check for distal pulse.
2. Give the patient care for shock, and keep him or her quiet and warm. The patient is often most comfortable sitting forward.
3. Do not let the patient eat or drink, because he or she may require general **anesthesia** at the hospital.
4. Let the patient hold the injured arm in a position most comfortable for him, but have him or her grasp the injured arm firmly with the hand of his or her unaffected arm to prevent any shoulder movement.
5. If it is necessary to move the patient at any time, let him or her move himself if he can. If he or she cannot move, help by giving gentle, firm support to the arm and by holding the arm only at the elbow and wrist.
6. Immobilization can be achieved by applying a roller bandage or sling and swathe.

Dislocation of the Elbow

Dislocations of the elbow usually occur when a patient falls forward and breaks the fall with his outstretched hand. This injury is often accompanied by dislocation or fracture of the wrist and fracture of the arm. The elbow usually is grossly deformed, and it is hard to tell the difference between dislocation and fracture.

Emergency Care

Provide the following emergency care:

1. Examine for other injuries and check distal pulses.
2. Examine the patient closely to determine whether the wrist or one of the bones in the arm has been fractured.
3. Immobilize the arm with an appropriate splint, such as a **ladder splint.**
4. Immobilize the distal and proximal joints by attaching the injured extremity to the body.
5. Transport the patient as soon as possible.

Dislocation of the Wrist

Dislocations of the wrist rarely occur without a fracture of either the wrist or arm bones. Do not straighten either a fractured or a dislocated wrist unless circulation is compromised.

Emergency Care

To prepare the patient for transport to the hospital:

1. Gently immobilize the arm with an appropriate splint.

2. Immobilize the joints distal and proximal to the location.

Dislocation of the Hip

There are two types of hip dislocations:

- With an anterior dislocation, the thigh is stretched out from the side of the body, lies flat, and is externally rotated away from the body.
- With a posterior dislocation, the knee is usually drawn up and the thigh is rotated inward toward the body.

Emergency Care

It is very difficult to splint a dislocated hip. Provide the following emergency care:

1. Adequate immobilization may be achieved by using a scoop stretcher to place the patient on a firm surface, like a full spine board, and using pillows or blankets tied with long straps to support the extremity in its abnormal position.
2. Sometimes the hip will relocate by itself during transport or during efforts to remove the patient from an automobile. If this happens, transport the patient to the hospital, advising the receiving physician of the possible dislocation with spontaneous reduction.
3. If you suspect a fractured femur and the patient will not tolerate straightening of the flexed knee, suspect a hip dislocation. *Do not use a traction splint.* Some protocols allow the use of PASG for splinting hip fractures (see pp. 242).

Dislocation of the Knee

Dislocations of the knee are severe injuries because blood vessel and nerve damage frequently occurs. It is sometimes difficult to tell whether the knee has been dislocated or broken.

Emergency Care

Provide the following emergency care:

1. If the patella, or kneecap, has been dislocated sideways, gently try to straighten the knee *once,* and only if it does not cause additional pain. Sometimes merely straightening the knee will help the kneecap relocate itself. If the pain increases, follow the procedures below for immobilizing a leg for transport.
2. Check for pulses at the ankle. Dislocations particularly threaten the popliteal artery just below the knee at the back of the leg. If you cannot find a

pulse, try moving the leg gently into a straighter position. Do not force it. Stop if pain increases or if you sense resistance on the leg. *Try only once* (local protocol may vary).
3. If the pulse is present, splint the injured leg in its current position to immobilize the knee.

Dislocation of the Ankle

Dislocations of the ankle are commonly complicated by fractures of the tibia and fibula. In many situations, deformity will not be present, but there will be swelling.

Emergency Care

Give the following emergency care:

- Immobilize with a pillow, full-leg air splint or other optional splint, making sure that you immobilize the joints proximal and distal to the injury.

☐ FRACTURES

Types of Fractures

A fracture is a break in the continuity of a bone. It may be either closed, in which the overlying skin is intact, or open, in which the skin over the fracture site has been broken (Figure 13-5). Bone may or may not protrude through the wound. Open fractures are more serious than closed fractures because the risks of contamination and infection are greater.

Fractures are further classified according to their appearance on x-rays.

A fracture may be produced by the direct application of force to the bone, which causes the bone to break. It may also be caused by the indirect application of force to the bone, such as a fall with weight on an outstretched hand which fractures the distal end of the radius. Many diseases, such as **osteoporosis,** and bone tumors, can gradually weaken a bone until only slight stress can cause it to fracture.

Fractures may also be classified according to the position, number, and shape of the bone fragments (Figure 13-6).

- In a **transverse fracture,** the fracture line is more or less at right angles to the long axis of the bone. It is usually produced by an angulation force.
- In a **longitudinal fracture,** the fracture line splits the bone lengthwise.
- An **oblique fracture** is one in which the fracture line extends obliquely across the bone, and fragments of the bone tend to slip by each other. It is usually produced by a twisting force.
- In a **spiral fracture,** the fracture line is spiral or

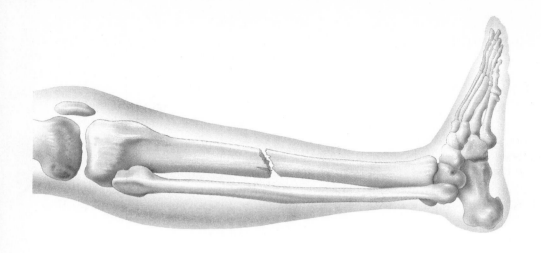

OPEN
Bone is protuding or has
protuded through the skin

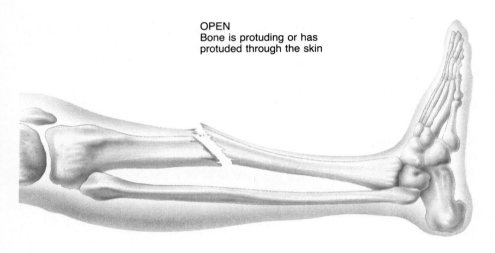

FIGURE 13-5 Closed and open fractures.

FIGURE 13-6 Types of fractures.

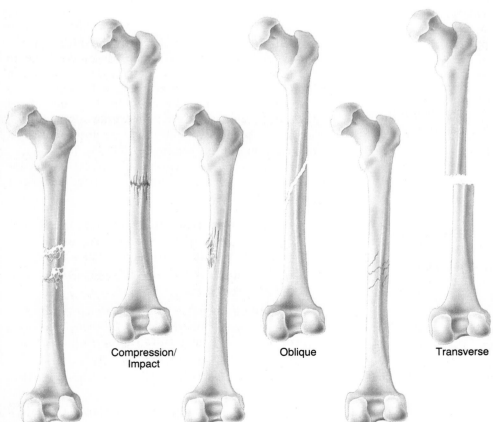

Comminuted

Compression/
Impact

Greenstick

Oblique

Spiral

Transverse

S-shaped. These fractures are produced by twisting injuries of the type seen among skiers or by torsion produced by muscular contraction.

- In an **impacted fracture,** the broken ends are violently jammed together so that they more or less telescope into each other.
- In a **comminuted fracture,** which is produced by severe, direct violence, there are three or more fragments. Reduction is difficult to maintain in this type of fracture, and associated soft tissue injuries are frequently severe.
- A **greenstick fracture** is an incomplete fracture caused by a compression force in the long axis of the bone. Usually the convex surface breaks, while the concave surface remains intact. This type of fracture is most common among children, whose bones are more elastic than those of adults.
- In **depressed fractures,** a fragment is driven below the surface of the bone. This type of fracture occurs in flat bones, such as the skull.
- A **compression fracture** damages the bones with force from both ends. For example, one or more of the vertebrae of the spinal column may be compressed as a result of a blow or **acceleration-deceleration** accidents.

Mechanisms of Injury

Injury to bones may result from a variety of mechanisms:

- Direct force — the bone breaks at the point of impact with a solid object, such as a dashboard or automobile bumper.
- Indirect force — this type of injury involves fracture or dislocation at some distance along the bone from the point of impact, such as a hip fracture caused by the knees forcefully striking the dashboard.
- Twisting force — this type of injury commonly occurs in football or skiing and results in fractures, sprains, and dislocations. Typically, the lower end of the limb remains fixed, such as when cleats or a ski hold the foot to the ground, while torsion develops in the upper end of the limb. The resulting forces causes shearing and fracture.
- Powerful muscle contractions — this type of injury, which occurs in seizures or tetanus, may tear muscle from bone or actually break away a piece of bone.
- Fatigue fractures — these are caused by repeated stress and most commonly occur in the feet after prolonged walking ("**march** or **stress fractures**").
- Pathological fractures — these are seen in pa-

tients with diseases that weaken areas of bone and may occur with minimal force. The elderly also have weaker bones and are thus more prone to fracture, especially of the hip.

History

Ask specific questions, such as:

- When did the injury occur?
- What happened?
- Where does it hurt?
- What did you feel?

Most patients with significant musculoskeletal injury will complain of pain localized to the area of injury. The patient may also report feeling or hearing something snap.

Signs of Fractures

The primary signs of fractures are (Figure 13-7):

- Swelling and bruising (discoloration). Blood leaks from ruptured vessels in and about the fractured ends of bones.
- Deformity and/or shortening. Compare the injured extremity to the normal extremity. Is it in an unnatural position? Is its motion false or unnatural? Is there a difference in size or shape? In the case of the skull or rib cage, does any portion apper caved in?
- Point tenderness to touch. Press gently along the length of the bone to locate the area of the injury.
- Grating, or crepitus. Broken fragments of bone grind against each other with a grating noise. *Do*

FIGURE 13-7

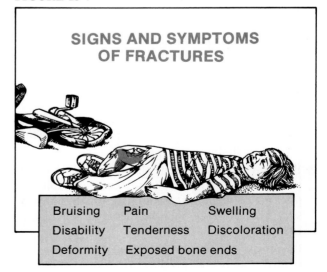

SIGNS AND SYMPTOMS OF FRACTURES

Bruising	Pain	Swelling
Disability	Tenderness	Discoloration
Deformity	Exposed bone ends	

not attempt to cause crepitus or ask the patient to move so you can hear it. You will only cause additional injury and pain.

- Guarding and disability. The patient with a fracture will try to hold the injured area in a comfortable position and will avoid moving it. The patient with a dislocation will be unable to move the dislocated extremity.
- Exposed bone ends.

Physical Examination

With rare exceptions, fractures and other **orthopedic** (bone) injuries are not life-threatening. In the multiple-injury patient, fractures may be the most obvious and dramatic injuries but may not necessarily be the most serious. Therefore, complete the primary survey and manage any life-threatening conditions first.

1. Establish an airway, protect the C-spine, and control moderate to severe hemorrhage.
2. When life-threatening conditions have been dealt with, identify and immobilize all fractures in preparation for transport.
3. Priorities for treating fractures are:
   - Spinal fractures (protect the C-spine).
   - Fractures of the head and rib cage.
   - Pelvic fractures.
   - Fractures of the lower limbs.
   - Fractures of the upper limbs.

   Remember, if there was enough force to damage the pelvis or cause severe head and facial injuries, assume that there are also injuries to the spine.

   Although life-threatening injuries must be dealt with first, you must take time to examine the extremities for fractures. Use the sings of fracture previously listed to conduct your assessment.

   Your examination of the patient should also assess nerve and circulatory status. Consider the five "**P**"s (Figure 13-8):

- **Pain.** Determine the area of pain and look for possible causes.
- **Pulse.** Carefully assess the pulses of an injured extremity. Evaluate circulation and nerve function every fifteen minutes.
- **Paresthesia.** The patient should be asked to describe the sensation in the involved extremity. A pricking or tingling sensation is **paresthesia.** Sensory changes may indicate nerve or circulatory changes.
- **Paralysis.** Assess the patient's ability to move the hand or foot of the involved extremity. Inability to

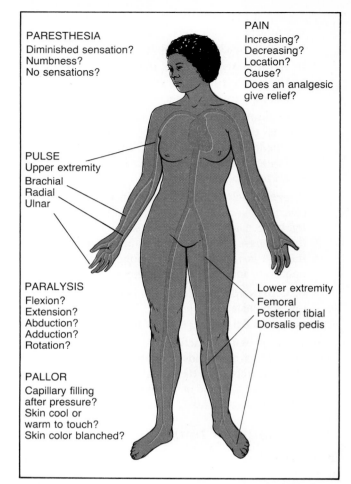

FIGURE 13-8 Assessing for nerve function and circulation after fracture.

move the injured extremities or paralysis may indicate peripheral nerve injury or circulatory impairment. For an upper extremity, ask the patient to make a fist, undo the fist, spread his or her fingers, then make a hitchhiking sign with the thumb (motor assessment). Nerves in the upper extremities are intact if the patient can perform all of these tasks. To test the lower extremities, ask the patient to tighten the kneecap, then to alternately move his or her foot up and down (as if he or she were pumping an automobile accelerator pedal). Nerves in the lower extremities are intact if the patient can perform this movement.

- **Pallor** (paleness). Carefully note the color and temperature of the fractured extremity. Feel the skin, and note how quickly color returns to the nailbed after you press it.

Emergency Care

The most important emergency care is immobilization for suspected fracture or extensive soft-tissue injury

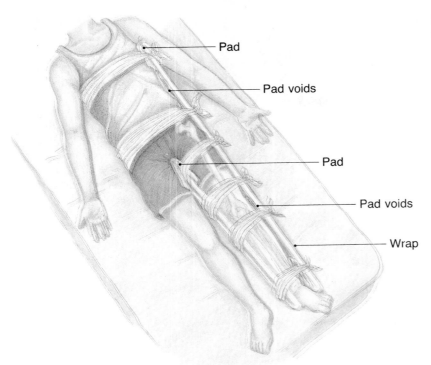

FIGURE 13-9 Splinting immobilizes fractures and dislocations.

Pad

Pad voids

Pad

Pad voids

Wrap

(Figure 13-9). The following are important reasons for immobilizing:

- To minimize damage to soft tissue, muscle, or **periosteum** (bone sheathing) which may become wedged between the fracture fragments.
- To prevent conversion of a closed fracture into an open one.
- To prevent more damage to surrounding nerves, blood vessels, and other tissues from the broken bone ends.
- To minimize bleeding and swelling.
- To diminish pain; this may help to control shock.

General principles for immobilizing fractures are as follows:

1. Remove clothing and jewelry around the injury site. Cut the clothing away with a pair of bandage scissors so that you will not move the fractured bone ends and increase the patient's pain. Give any of the patient's jewelry to a confirmed family member or bag it and put it with the patient so that it can be transported with the patient and turned over to the hospital staff with a receipt from the hospital.

2. Check the distal pulse of the suspected fracture site and control bleeding. (See Figures 13-10 and 13-11.)

3. With a few exceptions, never attempt to straighten

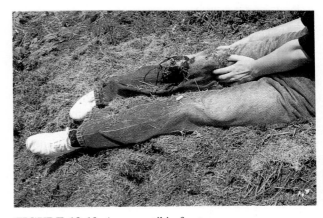

FIGURE 13-10 An open tibia fracture.

FIGURE 13-11 Support the limb, control bleeding, apply traction, locate a distal pulse, and splint. Brace the fracture with your hand under the fracture site.

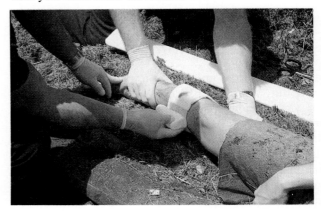

Musculoskeletal Injuries **231**

fractures of the spine, shoulder, elbow, wrist, or knee. Fractures involving joints should be splinted in the position in which they are found.

4. Cover all wounds, including open fractures, with sterile dressing. Then gently bandage. Do not attempt to push the bone ends back underneath the skin. Avoid excessive pressure on the wound. Brace the fracture with your hand under the fracture site.

5. Immobilize the joints above and below the fracture. (If the radius is fractured, for instance, immobilize the wrist and elbow.)

6. Wrap from the distal end of the splint to the proximal end. Splint firmly but not tightly enough to stop circulation. Check pulses below the splint (or at its lower end) after your splint is in place to be certain that circulation is still adequate. If a pulse is absent, loosen your splint until you can again feel the pulse. Check and recheck splints to make certain that they are not compromising circulation.

□ REPOSITIONING FRACTURED OR DISLOCATED LIMBS

A number of complications may accompany the attempt to reposition fractured or dislocated limbs. Unnecessary manipulation, for instance, may create additional pain or injury. Sharp bone ends can cause trauma to ligaments or tendons; allow contamination of the fracture site; and damage arteries, veins, the periosteum, and/or muscles. As a general rule, never straighten a wrist, elbow, knee, or shoulder. The major nerves and arteries near these joints mean that you would run a very high risk of causing further damage. Except for the wrist and shoulder, *make one attempt to straighten closed angulated fractures if no distal pulse is found.* If pain, resistance, or crepitus increase, stop. Joints, however, should not be manipulated unless circulation is compromised. *Follow local protocol.*

□ TYPES OF SPLINTS

Any device used to immobilize a fracture or dislocation is a **splint.** A splint may be soft or rigid improvised from virtually any object that can provide stability; or it may be one of the several commercially available splints, such as wooden, inflatable, and traction splints (Figure 13-12). Some splints are more suitable to certain types of cases than others, but many are interchangeable (Figure 13-13). Follow local protocol in such cases.

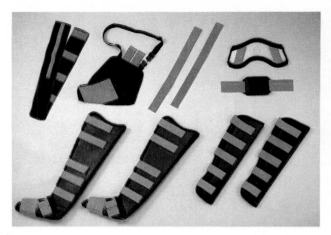

FIGURE 13-12 A set of commercial splints.

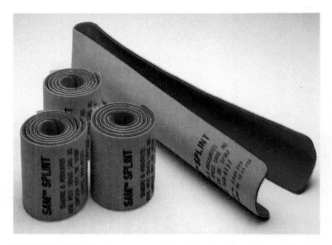

FIGURE 13-13 A commercial splint that can be molded to fit any appendage.

Remember — after every splinting, monitor distal pulses, swelling, and sensation.

Improvised Splints

EMTs will generally have access to commercial splints in an emergency, but should still be familiar with improvising; therefore, it is important to know how to make and apply improvised splints. An effective improvised splint must be:

- Light in weight but firm and rigid.
- Long enough to extend past the joints and prevent movement on either side of the fracture (two splints may be tied together to reach the necessary length).
- As wide as the thickest part of the fractured limb.
- If cardboard, board, etc., is used, pad well so that the inner surfaces are not in contact with the skin. Pad hollows of the limbs well.

Improvised splints have been made from a cardboard box, a cane, an ironing board, or a rolled-up newspaper or magazine, umbrella, broom handle, a catcher's shin guard, etc.

Self-Splint

A simple emergency splinting technique is to tie the patient's injured leg to the uninjured one, or secure the injured arm to his chest if the elbow is bent or to his side if the elbow is straight. Always put padding between the legs and underneath the arm if possible.

Fixation Splint

A fixation splint is a nonflexible device attached to a limb to maintain stability. It may be a padded board, a piece of heavy cardboard, or an aluminum splint molded to fit the extremity (Figures 13-14 and 13-15). Whatever the construction, it must be long enough to be secured well above and below the fracture site.

FIGURE 13-14 Cardboard splint of the lower arm.

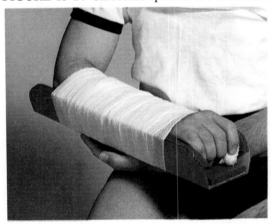

FIGURE 13-15 You must know how to make emergency splints.

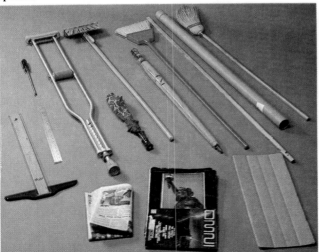

Be sure that the splint is adequately padded to assure even pressure along the extremity. While your assistant maintains stabilization, wrap the limb to the splint with self-adhering (Kling or Kerlix) bandages, tightly enough to hold the splint firmly to the extremity but not so tight as to cut off circulation.

Air Splint

Air splints are useful primarily for immobilizing fractures of the lower leg or forearm (Figure 13-16). Like all conforming splints, they are generally more comfortable for the patient and usually permit more uniform contact with the limb that is being splinted. However, they can sometimes impair circulation, even when properly inflated. Follow local protocol in their use.

To apply an air splint:

1. Remove clothing and jewelry from the splint area.
2. If the air splint is not equipped with a zipper, gather the splint on your arm so that the bottom edge is just above your wrist.
3. Grasp the patient's hand or foot while your assistant holds traction above the fracture. Slide the air splint over your hand onto the patient's arm or leg. The hand or foot of the injured limb should always be included in the splint.
4. The air splint should be positioned free of wrinkles.

FIGURE 13-16 Examples of inflatable air splints.

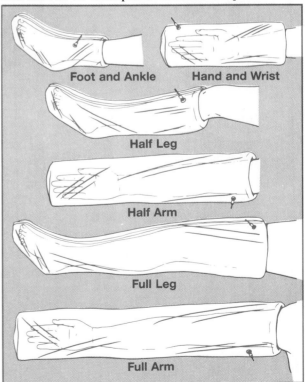

5. While you maintain traction, your assistant inflates the splint by mouth.

6. If the air splint has a zipper, position it over the injured area while your assistant maintins traction above and below the splint. Zip up the splint, and inflate it (Figure 13-17).

7. In either instance, the splint should be inflated just to the point at which your finger will make a slight dent against the splint.

FIGURE 13-17 Grasp the patient's hand or foot while your assistant holds traction above the fracture. Slide the air splint over the hand onto the patient's arm or leg. While you maintain traction, have your assistant inflate the splint by mouth. If the splint has a zipper, apply it to the injured area. Zip up the splint and inflate it just to the point at which your finger makes a slight dent against it.

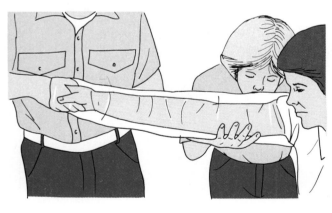

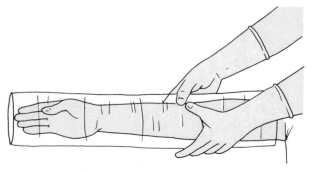

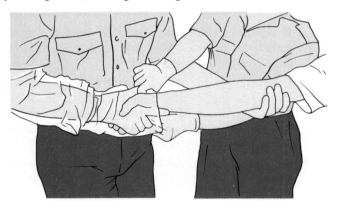

Air splints must be carefully monitored to be certain that they do not lose pressure or become overinflated. Overinflation is particularly apt to occur when the splint is applied in a cold area and the patient is moved to a warmer area. The air in the splint will then expand. Temperature, as well as surrounding air pressure, can cause detrimental changes.

Another problem is that many air splints completely enclose the hand or foot, making it difficult to palpate for circulation.

Sling and Swathe

The sling and swathe are particularly useful in stabilizing clavicular and scapular fractures (Figure 13-18).

To apply a sling and swathe:

1. Place a triangular bandage (about 40 by 40 by 55 inches) over the patient's chest, with the long edge parallel to the uninjured side. (An option is to first place a pillow between the arm and chest.)

2. Place the arm on the injured side in a flexed position on the bandage so that the point of the triangle extends beyond the injured elbow.

3. Fold the lower edge of the triangle up over the bent arm, and tie it to the other end of the bandage at the side of the neck (not over the spine.)

4. Bring the point of the bandage forward over the elbow, and pin it securely to the sling front, or twist the point end until it is snug, and tie a single knot to hold it in place.

5. Position the bandage so that the fingers remain slightly exposed. Check them often for signs of restricted circulation.

6. Slide a wide cravat under the small of the patient's back. Raise the cravat to the chest, and tie it securely to the uninjured side.

7. Continue to monitor during transport.

FIGURE 13-18 Immobilizing a fractured collarbone or humerus.

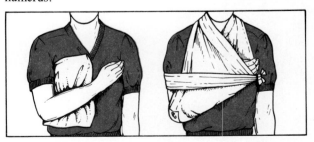

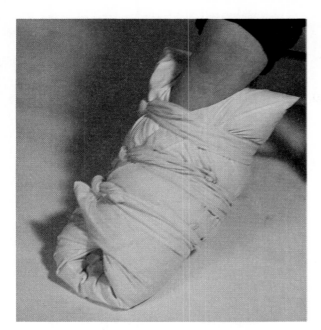

FIGURE 13-19 Pillow splint for a crushed foot or fractured ankle.

Pillow Splint (Soft Splint)

A pillow splint is an effective means to immobilize an injured foot or ankle. Wrap an ordinary pillow around the foot in a comfortable position and secure it with several cravats (folded triangular bandages) (Figure 13-19).

chapter 14

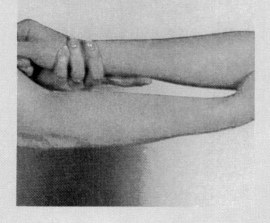

Fractures of the Upper and Lower Extremities

✳ ## OBJECTIVES

■ Identify fractures at various body sites.

■ Demonstrate how to choose the proper splint.

■ Demonstrate how to splint injuries to the following areas:

— Clavicle.	— Pelvis.
— Scapula.	— Hip.
— Humerus.	— Femur.
— Elbow.	— Patella.
— Forearm and wrist.	— Tibia and fibula.
— Hands and fingers.	— Ankle and foot.

Note: A discussion of fracture assessment and splinting principles is found in Chapter 13.

It is recommended that EMTs wear protective gloves whenever there is a possibility of coming in contact with a patient's blood, body fluids, mucous membranes, traumatic wounds, or sores. See Chapter 31.

Fractures to the upper extremities are very common. When a person falls, he or she automatically stretches out his or her hands to break the fall. The hands receive the full weight of the body, which can result in fractures anywhere between the hand and the clavicle.

The bones of the pelvis and lower extremities are very strong because they must bear considerable weight. Therefore, these bones are typically fractured from severe trauma due to heavy blows, falls, and automobile accidents.

When dealing with a fracture victim, first conduct a primary assessment and take the patient's history to identify and provide emergency care for life-threatening problems (fractures are seldom life-threatening). Then immobilize the fracture site by splinting. After splinting and during transport, evaluate and monitor distal **neurovascular** function (Figure 14-1).

□ FRACTURES OF THE COLLARBONE (CLAVICLE)

Fractures of the collarbone often occur when a person falls with the hand outstretched or sustains a blow to the shoulder. Signs and symptoms of collarbone fractures include:

- The arm on the injured side is partially or completely immobile.

- The shoulder on the injured side is lower and droops forward.
- The patient tilts his or her head in the direction of the injury with the chin turned in the opposite direction.
- The collarbone may appear crooked or deformed.

Emergency Care

Emergency care for a fractured collarbone involves:

1. Giving support to the arm and shoulder blade with a sling and swathe (Figure 14-2). The sling supports the weight of the arm, and the swathe binds the arm to the chest wall to prevent it from swinging freely.
2. Treat for shock if necessary.

□ FRACTURES OF THE SCAPULA

Fracture of the scapula is not a common injury. When a scapula fracture occurs, it is usually the result of a direct blow. Signs and symptoms are:

- Pain and swelling in the injured area.
- The patient is unable to swing his or her arm backward or forward from the shoulder.

FIGURE 14-1

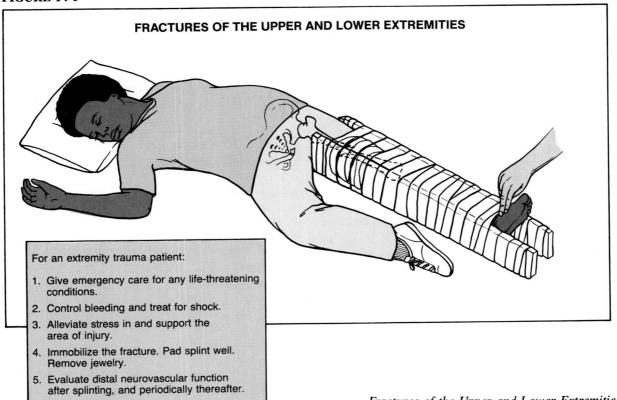

FRACTURES OF THE UPPER AND LOWER EXTREMITIES

For an extremity trauma patient:

1. Give emergency care for any life-threatening conditions.
2. Control bleeding and treat for shock.
3. Alleviate stress in and support the area of injury.
4. Immobilize the fracture. Pad splint well. Remove jewelry.
5. Evaluate distal neurovascular function after splinting, and periodically thereafter.

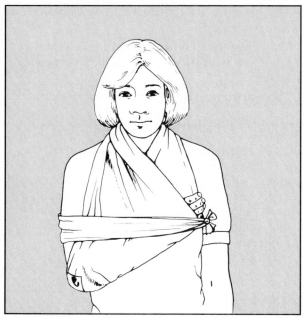

FIGURE 14-2 Immobilizing a fractured collarbone or clavicle.

Emergency Care

Emergency care for a fractured scapula is as follows:

> Splint the fracture with a sling and swathe.
> Continually check for respiratory inefficiency and transport.

☐ FRACTURES OF THE HUMERUS

Fractures of the humerus may be hard to detect because a bone break close to the shoulder causes less pain and disability than a break at the mid-shaft. This type of injury is also difficult to immobilize. A patient may sustain a fracture *anywhere* along the humerus, however, and other fracture sites along the humerus are not difficult to detect. If the mechanism of injury suggests a possible fracture and the patient has pain, treat as a fracture.

Emergency Care

Emergency care for fractures of the humerus is as follows (Figures 14-3–14-6):

1. If the arm is angulated, grasp the injured arm at the elbow and provide steady, gentle pressure. At the same time, grasp the wrist and move the lower arm across the abdomen in preparation for putting on a sling.

2. Check the distal pulse, sensation, and motor function. The risk of vessel and nerve damage from fractures of the humerus is high. Therefore, use great caution to prevent any unnecessary movement of the fractured bone ends.

3. Apply the splint:
   • The first EMT applies and maintains stabilization while the second EMT prepares the necessary splinting material.
   • Apply a sling and swathe without moving the fracture site.
   • A **fixation splint** may also be applied successfully (Figure 14-7).

4. Check distal pulse at the radial artery. Check motor ability by asking the patient to move his fingers. Check sensory ability by touching a finger and asking which digit was touched.

5. Monitor the fractured extremity frequently.

☐ FRACTURES OF THE ELBOW

Emergency Care

The type of emergency care required for a fractured elbow depends upon the position of the elbow at the time of the injury. Immobilize in the position found, using an appropriate splint. (See Figure 14-8.)

☐ FRACTURES OF THE FOREARM AND WRIST

Emergency Care

For a forearm fracture (Figure 14-9–14-12, page 240):

1. Remove all clothing and jewelry from or near the injury site.
2. Apply stabilization; hold until the splint is on.
3. Apply a rigid splint.
4. Check distal pulse and distal sensation.
5. Support with a sling.

☐ Open Fracture of the Humerus

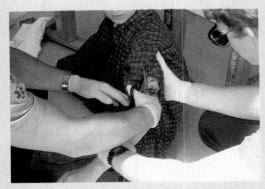

FIGURE 14-3 Cut away clothing to expose wound.

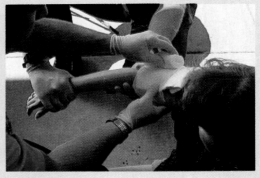

FIGURE 14-4 One EMT supports limb while the other EMT controls bleeding and dresses the exposed bone.

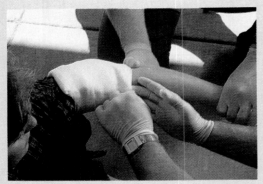

FIGURE 14-5 Wound is securely bandaged.

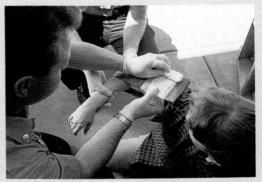

FIGURE 14-6 Limb is splinted in the most efficient way possible.

FIGURE 14-7 Fixed splints for a fractured humerus.

FIGURE 14-8 Immobilizing fracture of the elbow.

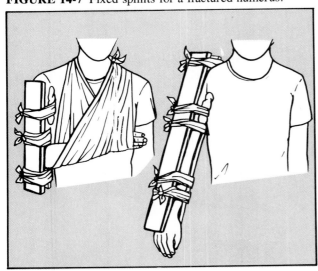

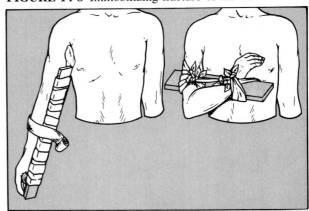

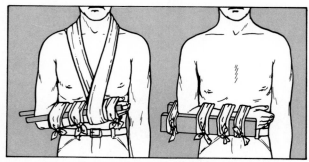

FIGURE 14-9 Immobilizing fractures of the forearm, wrist, and hand. Pad the splints well.

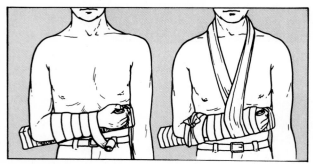

FIGURE 14-10 Immobilizing fractures of the forearm, wrist, and hand. Place the hand in position of function. Place a roller bandage in the hand.

If the fracture is in the wrist:

1. Apply a pillow or well-padded splint that supports the hand, wrist, and forearm and that prevents all movement in the wrist or elbow (Figure 14-13).
2. Elevate the injured arm.

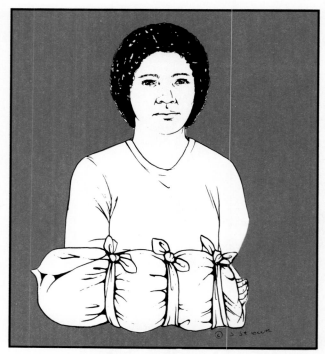

FIGURE 14-13 Pillow splint for fractures of the forearm, wrist, and hand.

□ FRACTURES OF THE HAND AND FINGERS

Emergency Care

If the break is a closed fracture of a single finger (Figure 14-14):

1. Place the injured finger in a comfortable position, usually slightly bent.

□ Splinting a Fractured Forearm

FIGURE 14-11 A fractured, angulated forearm may be straightened by gently pulling in opposite directions on the long axis of the arm.

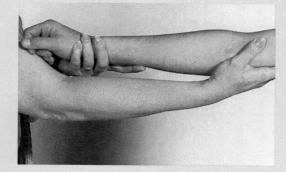

FIGURE 14-12 Splint should extend beyond both joints and support the hand. Splint is securely bandaged into place.

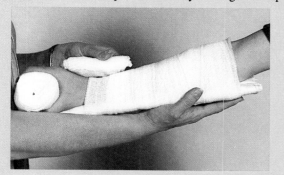

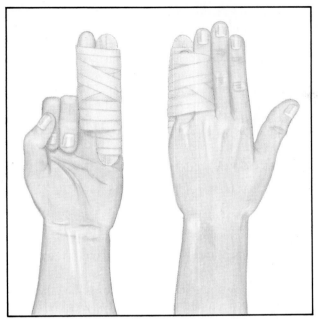

FIGURE 14-14 Fractured finger splinted with a tongue depressor.

2. Apply a padded splint to prevent movement. Fractures of the fingers can be splinted with a tongue depressor, a commercial aluminum splint, or even an adjacent finger (but not the thumb)!

3. Elevate the hand.

If the hand has been severely crushed:

1. Do not cleanse the wound.

2. Place a ball of gauze or padded cloth in the patient's hand so that the fingers can curve around the ball (position of function). Cover the entire hand with sterile 4 by 4s.

3. Apply splints.

4. Keep the hand elevated at all times to reduce swelling and prevent further damage.

☐ FRACTURES OF THE PELVIS

The pelvic girdle is formed by the sacrum (lowest five fused vertebrae) and the pelvic bone. It also contains the sockets of the hip joint into which the head of the femur fits (Figure 14-15). Fractures of the pelvis usually result from compression of the hips or from a direct blow and may puncture the enclosed organs.

Pelvic fractures may result in serious blood loss. Large blood vessels near the pelvis can be easily torn or lacerated at the time of the fracture. Even if there is only minimal swelling at the site, be alert for the possibility of hypovolemic shock. The body cavities can hold several liters of blood, making it possible for the patient to actually die of blood loss without any external bleeding.

Signs and symptoms of a pelvic fracture include:

• Marked pain at the fracture site.
• Severe shock.

FIGURE 14-15

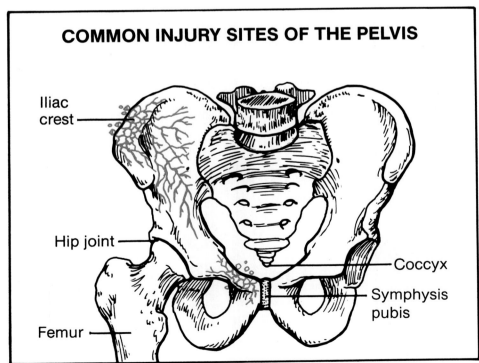

COMMON INJURY SITES OF THE PELVIS

Iliac crest

Hip joint

Femur

Coccyx

Symphysis pubis

Emergency Care

Every injury causing severe pelvic pain should be cared for like a spinal fracture.

1. Care for shock, providing a high concentration of oxygen.
2. Move the patient as little as possible. Any moves should be done so that the patient moves as a unit. Never lift the patient with the pelvis unsupported.
3. Determine the status of circulation and nerve function distal to the injury site.
4. Straighten the patient's lower limbs into the anatomical position if there are no serious injuries to the hip joints and lower limbs and if it is possible to do without meeting resistance or causing excessive pain.
5. Prevent additional injury to the pelvis by stabilizing the lower limbs. Place a folded blanket between the patient's legs, from the groin to the feet and bind them together with wide cravats.
6. Assume that there are spinal injuries and immobilize the patient on a long spine board (See Figure 14-16). When securing the patient, avoid placing the straps or ties over top of the pelvic area.
7. Reassess distal circulation and nerve function.
8. Transport the patient as soon as possible.
9. Monitor vital signs.

☐ FRACTURES OF THE HIP

A hip fracture is a break in the proximal or upper end of the femur (thighbone) or a fracture of the socket (when the bone is forced into it). Hip fractures are common among elderly patients who fall while standing or walking. In this case, the fracture is caused by the twisting force exerted on the femur during the fall.

Other patients, such as those involved in automobile accidents, sustain hip fractures from the force that pushes the thighbone into the socket. The patient will usually lie with the affected leg turned outward, and the leg may appear to be shortened. Blood loss can be severe, and shock is common.

Emergency Care

To care for hip fractures:

1. Watch the patient for signs and symptoms of shock and give emergency care accordingly.
2. Immobilize the pelvic girdle in a comfortable position.
3. Place pillows, a folded blanket, or some other soft object between and underneath the legs.
4. With the patient's knees bent, strap the legs together with belts, bandages, or straps.
5. Transport the patient on a rigid stretcher (Figure 14-17), backboard, or scoop.

☐ FRACTURES OF THE FEMUR

A fractured femur usually causes the following (Figure 14-18):

* Marked deformity may or may not be evident.
* Pain and swelling.
* Circulation impairment in the foot.
* Possibility of open fracture. Such fractures commonly result from automobile accidents.

FIGURE 14-16 Immobilizing a patient with pelvic injuries on a long spine board.

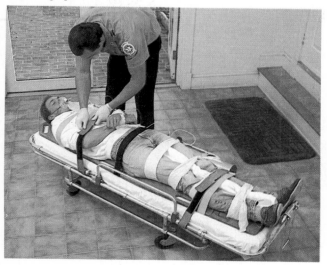

FIGURE 14-17 Immobilizing a fracture or dislocation of the hip or pelvis.

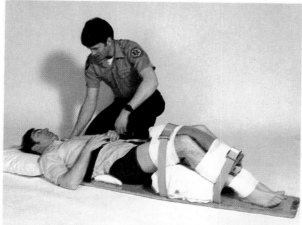

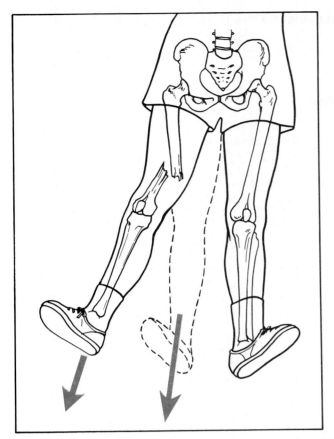

FIGURE 14-18 Fracture of the shaft of the right femur with angulation, shortening, and rotation of the limb below the fracture site. Apply gentle traction parallel to the normal axis of the fractured leg.

- Possible major blood loss; be alert for signs of shock.
- Limb shortening due to muscle contractures.

Emergency Care

The care for a fracture of the femur calls for splinting to immobilize the limb and to reduce pain and blood loss.

Traction splints are used exclusively on femur fractures, usually mid-shaft fractures. The PASG may also be used to splint a femur. You may also use board splints. You will need two, both padded.

1. The outside board should be long enough to reach from the patient's armpit to below his heel. The inner splint should be long enough to reach from the groin to below the heel.
2. Slide the cravat bandages underneath the patient at the ankle, knee, and lower back.
3. Position the padded splints, and add extra padding at the knee and ankle.
4. Tie the cravat bandages snugly around the chest, flank, groin, knee, and ankle (Figure 14-19).

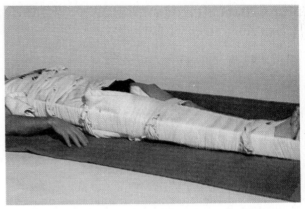

FIGURE 14-19 Immobilizing a high femur fracture with a fixation splint.

Traction Splints

Fractures of the femur and some fractures below the knee can be treated with the traction splint. *Never use a traction splint if the fracture is within one to two inches of the knee or ankle. Traction splints are not generally used for hip fractures, but may be acceptable under certain circumstances. Follow local protocol.*

A traction splint provides a counterpull, and it alleviates the pain, reduces blood loss, and minimizes further injury. It is not intended to reduce the fracture, but simply to *immobilize the bone ends and prevent further injury.*

Several types of traction splints are available. Basic traction splints are discussed, but learn to use the traction equipment available in your area, and learn how to use new equipment when it becomes available. Do not use traction splints on femur fractures when the break is close to the knee or there is any significant injury to the knee or a possible dislocated hip. Without x-rays, it is impossible to distinguish joint injuries from breaks, and traction could cause joint damage. Also, do not use a traction splint when there is a suspected break at or near the ankle, a fractured pelvis, a hip injury with gross displacement, or fractures to the lower third of the leg.

Applying a Traction Splint

To apply a traction splint:

1. The first EMT removes or cuts away clothing to completely expose the fracture site and controls any bleeding. (Make sure that a possible hemorrhaging wound on the back of the thigh does not go unexposed.) Dress and bandage open wounds.
2. The second EMT checks and records circulation and neurological status distal to the injury, then stabilizes the limb.

Fractures of the Upper and Lower Extremities **243**

3. The second EMT applies manual traction to the injured leg by grasping the lower part of the heel with one hand and placing the other hand under the slightly bent knee. He then exerts a strong, steady pull until the patient feels relief. The leg should be elevated sufficiently for the splint to be properly applied by the first EMT. The second EMT should maintain traction of the leg until traction is applied with the splint.

4. The first EMT should simultaneously adjust the splint for length and make all other necessary preparations to apply the splint. In doing so, remember that movements of the injured leg must be kept at an absolute minimum.

5. Apply the traction splint as shown in "Applying a Traction Splint" (Figures 14-20–14-28). This splint can be applied over the PASG if needed.

The **Sager splint** (Figures 14-29–14-31) used widely in some areas, can be applied quickly. It has a padded arch support designed to fit into the patient's crotch on one end and an ankle harness on the other end with an internal spring pulley-and-cable apparatus. The metal tubes of the splint can be adjusted to any length and locked into position. It fastens with Velcro tapes and will not interfere with applying and using the PASG. In fact, the PASG can be applied first. Do not use the Sager splint when the patient also has pelvic fractures.

☐ FRACTURES OF THE PATELLA (KNEECAP)

Fractures of the patella often result from a direct blow or from muscle pull on the cap when control of the knee is lost. Pain and swelling occur and there may be deformity and/or impaired circulation of the foot.

Emergency Care

Apply one of the following splints:

1. Pillow or blanket splint (Figure 14-32 on page 246).

2. A padded splint that extends from the buttocks to below the heel on the back of the leg.

☐ FRACTURES OF THE LOWER LEG (TIBIA, FIBULA)

Open fractures of the lower leg are common because of the thin layers of skin and tissue surrounding these bones. Fractures of the fibula may not be apparent, be-

cause this bone does not support any body weight and is splinted naturally by the tibia. Impaired circulation in the foot may occur.

Emergency Care

Emergency care consists of immobilizing the injury:

1. Gently straighten the leg. Grasp the extremity, one hand above and one hand below the fracture site. Provide two to five pounds of gentle counterpressure until the extremity returns to its normal anatomical position. If you meet any resistance in the leg, stop and immobilize it in the position found.

2. Check the distal pulse by palpating either the dorsalis pedis artery on the anterior surface of the foot or the posterior tibial artery on the medial side of the ankle and posterior to the tibia. Check distal movement and sensation by asking the patient to wiggle his or her toes, and ask if he or she can feel you touch each toe. If the patient is unconscious, gently palpate the foot for injuries.

3. Remove clothing and shoes so that you can observe the injured extremity for changes and prevent soft tissue injury from pressure caused by swelling. Cut the seam of the pant leg or skirt, and remove the shoe and sock or hose. Maintain traction during this process.

4. Apply the splint.
   • The first EMT applies and maintains adequate alignment of the limb, while the second EMT prepares the splint material.
   • Immobilize the leg with a padded, rigid long leg splint.
   • Alternate splinting includes an air splint that extends from the foot to the upper thigh, or even a traction splint.

5. Check the distal circulation by capillary refill. Check distal sensation at the same time by asking the patient to wiggle his or her toes or asking if he or she can feel your touch through the splint.

6. In an emergency, with no other equipment available, place blankets between the patient's legs, and tie the legs together, or use padded boards (Figures 14-33 and 14-34).

☐ FRACTURES OF THE ANKLE AND FOOT

Ankle fractures are most commonly caused by direct blows from heavy, crushing objects, by twisting, and by jumps and falls. Toes are frequently broken by blows or stubbing.

□ Applying a Traction Splint

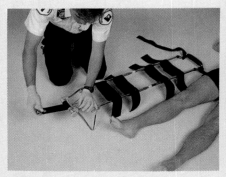

FIGURE 14-20 Expose, dress, and bandage any wound. Adjust splint for length: (1) Unlock splint and fold down heel stand. Slide up the splint until aligned with ankle. (2) Adjust to desired length; tighten sleeves. (3) Position opened leg support straps.

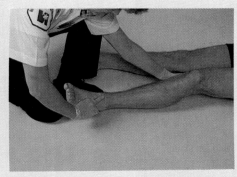

FIGURE 14-21 Palpate the distal pulse to check circulation.

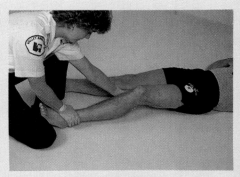

FIGURE 14-22 Stabilize the fractured limb by pulling along the long axis.

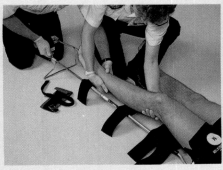

FIGURE 14-23 Move adjusted splint to injured leg and make final adjustments. Brace the fracture with your hand under the fracture site or as close as possible to it.

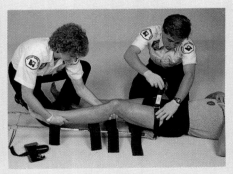

FIGURE 14-24 EMT 1 positions splint and attaches ischial strap; EMT 2 continues traction.

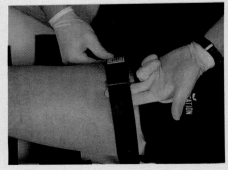

FIGURE 14-25 Make sure ischial strap is snug but not so tight as to cut off circulation.

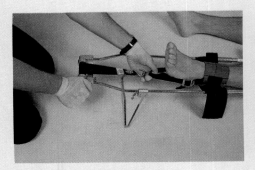

FIGURE 14-26 Apply the ankle hitch and insert S-ring into the D-rings. EMT 1 applies mechanical traction.

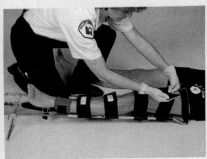

FIGURE 14-27 Leg support straps are fastened in place.

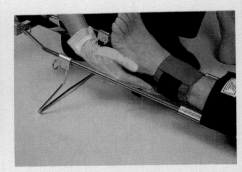

FIGURE 14-28 EMT monitors distal pulse. Adjust location of heel stand when patient is on the gurney.

Fractures of the Upper and Lower Extremities **245**

☐ The Sager Traction Splint

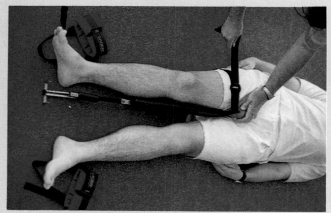

FIGURE 14-29 A Sager bilateral splint shown in "position."

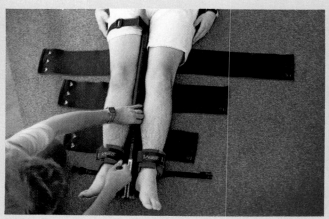

FIGURE 14-30 Sager in "set."

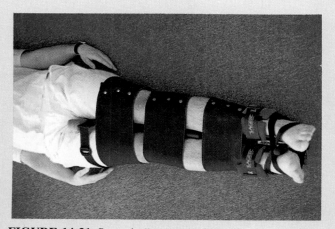

FIGURE 14-31 Sager in "secure position."

FIGURE 14-32 A pillow splint for a fractured patella or a dislocated knee.

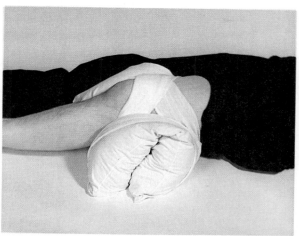

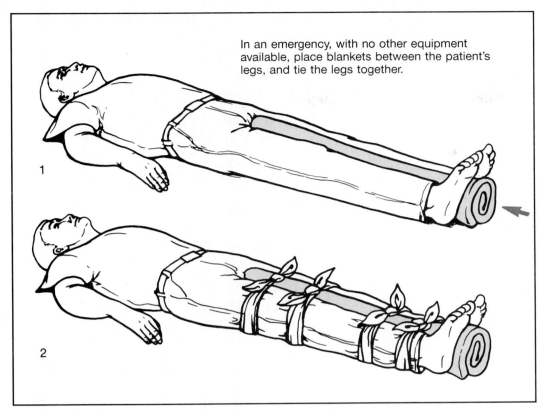

In an emergency, with no other equipment available, place blankets between the patient's legs, and tie the legs together.

FIGURE 14-33 Self-splint, using a blanket.

FIGURE 14-34 Fixation splints, using padded boards.

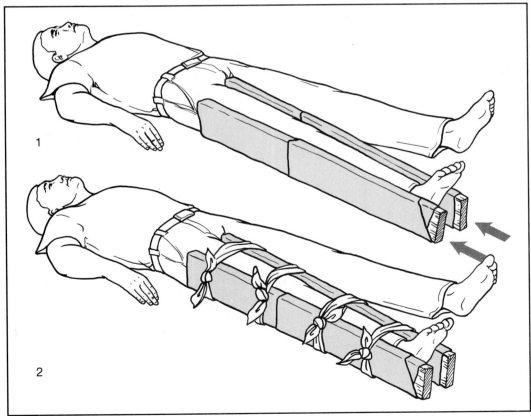

Emergency Care

Provide the following emergency care:

1. Have the patient lie down.
2. Carefully remove his or her shoes and socks, unless shoe removal will cause additional injury.
3. Do not try to reduce any deformity.
4. Elevate the limb.
5. Apply a dressing if the patient has an open wound.
6. Use an air splint (Figure 14-35), or wrap a pillow around the ankle and tie it to the ankle with cravat bandages (Figure 14-36).

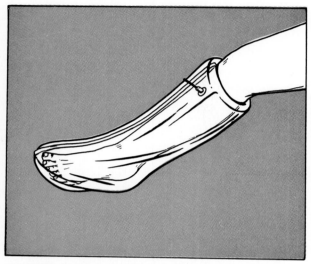

FIGURE 14-35 Immobilizing a fracture of the lower leg, ankle, or foot with a pneumatic splint.

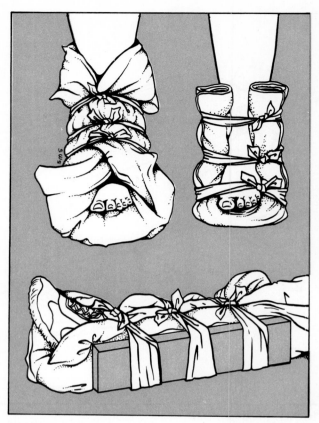

FIGURE 14-36 Immobilizing a fracture of the ankle and foot. Always untie laces if a shoe is left on the foot.

chapter 15

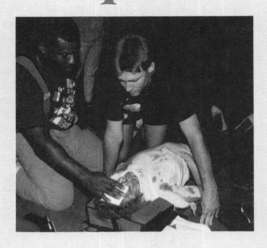

Head Injuries

✳ OBJECTIVES

- Identify the anatomical and functional components of the head and central nervous system that relate to head injuries.
- Recognize the signs and symptoms of head injury.
- Describe and demonstrate the necessary assessment procedures for a head-injured patient.
- Identify the common types of head and brain injuries.
- Describe and demonstrate the principles of treating head injury.

This chapter was written in conjunction with Thom Dick, EMS author, teacher, and full-time paramedic in La Mesa, California.

It is recommended that EMTs wear protective gloves whenever there is a possibility of coming in contact with a patient's blood, body fluids, mucous membranes, traumatic wounds, or sores. See Chapter 31.

☐ THE NERVOUS SYSTEM

Injuries of the head are some of the most serious and difficult that you will be required to handle. The patient is often confused or unconscious, making diagnosis difficult. And many injuries of the head are life-threatening; head injuries are one of the leading causes of death among this nation's young people. Someone in the United States suffers a head injury every fifteen seconds; a half-million of them require hospitalization, and one of them dies every five minutes. See Figure 15-1 for a summary of various causes of head injuries. Of those who survive, almost 100,000 are permanently disabled. If you handle a head-injured patient improperly, you can cause permanent damage or death. The outcome of a head injury depends not only on the severity of the injury, but accurate diagnosis and prompt and proper treatment. Most deaths from head injury occur at the time of the injury or within two hours of the time the patient reaches the hospital.

The brain, which takes up 80 to 90 percent of the space inside the skull, is surrounded by plates of large, flat bones that are fused together to form a helmetlike covering called the **cranial skull** (see Chapter 2). The remainder of the skull is made up of facial bones. Composed of fourteen irregularly shaped bones, it is made up of the cheek, nose, and jaw bones. The **basilar skull** (part of the cranium) is the weakest part of the skull because some of its bones are thin and some are perforated extensively by the spinal cord along with a number of nerves and blood vessels. A basilar fracture almost always involves intracranial bleeding because the fracture is likely to injure a blood vessel.

Within the skull, the brain is cushioned in a dense, serous substance called cerebrospinal fluid, which is produced by the brain and protects it against impact. The cerebrospinal fluid is clear and colorless, circulates

FIGURE 15-1

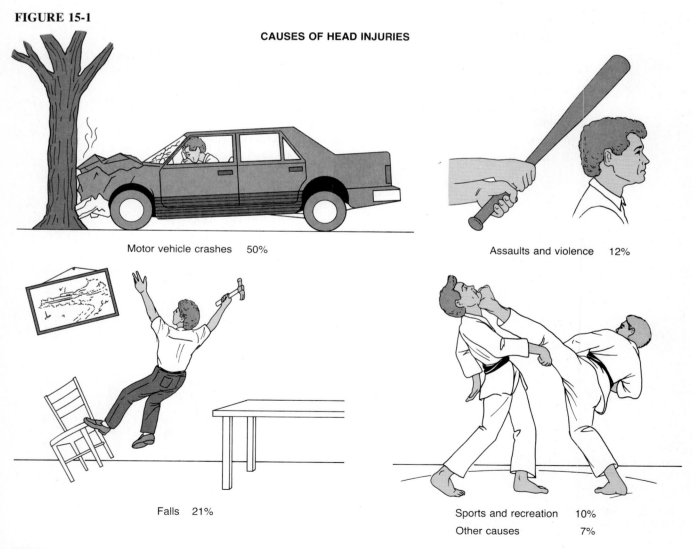

CAUSES OF HEAD INJURIES

Motor vehicle crashes   50%

Assaults and violence   12%

Falls   21%

Sports and recreation   10%

Other causes   7%

throughout the brain and spinal cord, and is reabsorbed by the circulatory system. The fluid provides a cushion between the brain and the skull, and between the spinal cord and the spinal column, protecting the brain and spinal cord from the adjacent bony structures. When both the skull and the membrane surrounding the brain are torn, cerebrospinal fluid leaks out through the nose and/or ears — cerebrospinal fluid leakage has become a classic sign of skull fracture and indicates a very serious injury; however, there can be serious head injury without cerebrospinal fluid leakage.

Inside the skull, the surface of the brain is protected from abrasion by the dura mater, the outermost of three meninges (or layers of tissue) that enclose the brain (Figure 15-2). Composed of a double layer of tough, fibrous tissue, the dura mater ("hard mother") is normally in contact with the skull; only a few millimeters of actual space lie between the dura and the surface of the brain. Any major bleeding, then, can compress the brain within just a few minutes.

Bleeding that occurs between the dura mater and the skull is called **epidural** (outside the dura) and usually involves the brain's outermost arteries. **Subdural** (beneath the dura) bleeding, on the other hand, is usually venous; recognized and treated early, it may not have permanent consequences.

FIGURE 15-2

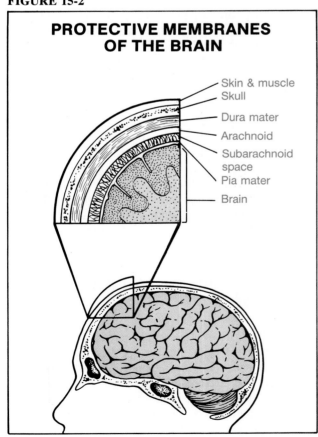

PROTECTIVE MEMBRANES OF THE BRAIN

Skin & muscle
Skull
Dura mater
Arachnoid
Subarachnoid space
Pia mater
Brain

Just beneath and in contact with the dura mater is a second membrane, the arachnoid; beneath that, and in contact with the brain, is the pia mater ("soft mother"). They are separated by a lattice of fibrous, spongy tissue with cerebrospinal fluid called the subarachnoid space, which provides most of the shock absorption for the brain. Bleeding that occurs between the arachnoid membrane and the surface of the brain is called subarachnoid hemorrhage; usually arterial, it can be rapidly fatal.

These three layers of tissue, or meninges, cover not only the surface of the brain, but also the **brain stem** and the spinal cord; these, too, are bathed constantly in cerebrospinal fluid. The cerebrospinal fluid not only cushions and protects, but performs a function similar to **lymph** in combatting infection and cleansing the brain and spinal cord.

The weakest part of the skull is the basal (or basilar) skull — the floor of the skull. Made up of many separate pieces of bone, it is perforated by numerous nerve trunks and blood vessels, including the spinal cord. A blow to the cranium often produces fractures not only in the area of the blow, but also in the basal skull.

While the interior surface of the cranium is smooth, the floor of the skull has an irregular surface. The major part of the brain (cerebrum) is not attached to the inside of the skull, but the brain stem is tethered in place by numerous nerves and vessels. As a result, a forceful blow on the head or a sudden change in its position (such as the deceleration that occurs in car accidents) can tear the brain stem or abrade the underside of the brain.

The brain is divided into three physical portions (Figure 15-3):

- The cerebrum, the largest part of the brain, comprises three-fourths of the brain's volume. Often called the "gray matter," it is made up of four distinct lobes. It is responsible for most conscious and sensory functions, the emotions, and the personality.
- The cerebellum, sometimes called the "little brain," controls equilibrium and coordinates muscular activity. Tucked underneath the cerebrum, it deals with muscular coordination, coordinates and integrates muscular movement, predicts when to stop movement, and coordinates the reflexes that maintain posture and equilibrium.
- The medulla, more commonly called the brain stem, is actually a *part* of the brain stem and is the most primitive but best protected part of the brain. It controls most automatic functions of the body, including cardiac, respiratory, and other functions vital to life.

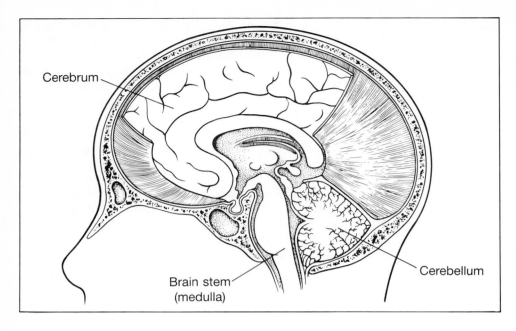

FIGURE 15-3 The three main divisions of the brain — cerebrum, cerebellum, and brain stem — with separating membranes.

☐ PHYSIOLOGY OF BRAIN INJURY

As already explained, the brain itself is enclosed in the skull — a rigid, unyielding case. If the brain tissue swells or if intracranial bleeding occurs, the brain at first tries to compensate for the lack of room in which to expand. Brain injury also increases the brain's metabolic needs — following brain injury, the brain needs more oxygen and glucose than usual.

Brain injury may be directly the result of trauma, or may be secondary — the brain becomes injured because of an injury to another body system (changes in blood pressure, for example, can affect perfusion of the brain). The injury may be either closed (the skull has not been fractured, even if the scalp is lacerated) or open (the skull is broken or cracked). One of the most common types of injury is "coup-contracoup," or acceleration-deceleration: the head comes to a sudden stop, but the brain continues to move back and forth inside the skull, resulting in massive injury.

When an area of the brain is injured, the blood vessels in the brain dilate so that more blood can flow to the injured area. If that fails, the blood vessels undergo further changes that cause serous fluid to leak into the affected area. As a result, the brain is diluted with water, thus lowering the level of carbon dioxide in the brain tissue.

When such leakage occurs, edema (swelling) results. The volume of the brain increases, leaving less space inside the skull for the blood and cerebrospinal fluid. At first, nothing happens: the brain stops producing cerebrospinal fluid, absorbs existing cerebrospinal fluid more rapidly, and employs several means of decreasing the amount of blood that it receives from the circulatory system.

However, the brain's compensation techniques can only go so far. Soon, intracranial pressure rises, and blood flow throughout the brain becomes inadequate. As a result, the brain cannot function normally, and swelling increases.

Typically, the respiratory center in the medulla reacts by causing the body to breathe more deeply and rapidly, lowering the levels of carbon dioxide in the bloodstream. Another area of the medulla — the **vasomotor center** — reacts to high levels of carbon dioxide by stimulating the heart and blood vessels to increase systemic blood pressure.

While one part of the vasomotor center is stimulating the heart to increase its output, another is reacting to messages that the blood pressure is too high. In response to those messages, the vasomotor center paradoxically slows the heart rate. As a result, a patient with excessive intracranial pressure will probably have a very high blood pressure and a very slow pulse — a grave sign in assessing the extent of head trauma.

☐ OBTAINING A PATIENT HISTORY

Critical to the patient's eventual recovery from a head or spinal injury is your ability to collect and relay an accurate sequence of what happened to the patient — both before you arrived on the scene and after you reached the patient. Remember that a brain-injured person who can answer your questions when you arrive might lose that ability by the time he reaches a hospital.

And even if bystanders can give you some information, most will not want to go to the hospital for further questioning. The primary sources of information will be your own observations, educated inferences, and accurate history-taking — *and the most important clue will be how the patient changes*.

Start by getting an immediate description of key signs and symptoms, and then watch constantly for changes (Figure 15-4). Note and record any changes, including the exact time the change occurred; the timing can impact later decisions regarding surgery. Key signs and symptoms include:

- Vital signs.
- Level of consciousness.
- Condition of the pupils.
- The patient's ability to move.
- The patient's pattern of speech.

When taking a history, try to get the following information:

- When did the incident occur?
- If the patient can communicate, what was his or her chief complaint when you arrived at the scene? Did the patient feel pain, tingling, numbness, or paralysis? Where? How has that complaint or those symptoms changed since the accident?
- What happened? How did the accident occur?

- What is the patient's pattern of mentation? Did he lose consciousness at any time? *This information is critically important in diagnosing brain injury.* How long was the period of unconsciousness? When did it occur in relation to the injury? Did the patient suddenly lose consciousness and then gradually reawaken, or did he or she pass out immediately, suddenly wake up, and then gradually lose consciousness again?
- Was the patient moved after the incident?

☐ PHYSICAL ASSESSMENT

Do a primary survey to detect any life-threatening problems and correct them. Immobilization of a spinal injury can wait, *but there must absolutely be no movement of the patient until you can immobilize him or her*. The primary assessment should be done in the following order:

Airway

Maintaining an adequate airway is the most vital element in the treatment of head injury, because the most serious complication is lack of oxygen to the brain. In correcting an airway, never hyperextend the neck (a high percentage of head injury is accompanied by cervical spine injury); use the modified jaw thrust or chin-lift maneuver to protect the cervical spine.

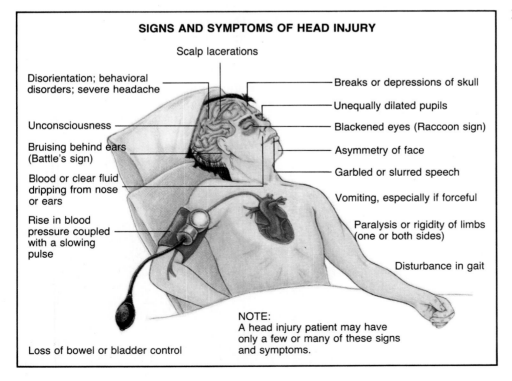

FIGURE 15-4

SIGNS AND SYMPTOMS OF HEAD INJURY

Scalp lacerations

Disorientation; behavioral disorders; severe headache

Unconsciousness

Bruising behind ears (Battle's sign)

Blood or clear fluid dripping from nose or ears

Rise in blood pressure coupled with a slowing pulse

Loss of bowel or bladder control

Breaks or depressions of skull

Unequally dilated pupils

Blackened eyes (Raccoon sign)

Asymmetry of face

Garbled or slurred speech

Vomiting, especially if forceful

Paralysis or rigidity of limbs (one or both sides)

Disturbance in gait

NOTE:
A head injury patient may have only a few or many of these signs and symptoms.

Vital Signs

Check and record vital signs every five minutes to stay aware of changes. The following vital signs should be recorded:

Blood Pressure

If blood pressure is high or rising, suspect pressure inside the skull; if it is low or dropping, suspect blood loss that has led to shock. Low blood pressure in a head-injured patient almost always is due to bleeding elsewhere, since head injury itself causes low blood pressure only in the final stages prior to death. As intracranial pressure increases, the patient's systolic blood pressure rises and the pulse pressure widens. Pulse pressure equals the difference between diastolic and systolic pressure.

Pulse

If the pulse is high or rising, suspect hemorrhage or neurogenic shock; if it is slow or dropping, suspect pressure inside the skull; if it is irregular, suspect rising blood pressure. A pulse of more than 160 will not provide adequate circulation to the brain.

Respiration

By simply noting a few specifics about the patient's breathing during primary assessment, you can alert yourself to the possibility of a serious neurologic disorder within the first twenty seconds of patient contact. At least six factors are critical: rate, depth, pattern, degree of effort, odor, and sound.

RATE   Slow breathing indicates that something is depressing the respiratory center in the brain stem. Common causes are direct trauma, bleeding, edema, drugs, or severe acidosis. Rapid, deep breathing can signal an imbalance of gases or the presence of a central nervous system stimulant in the bloodstream.

Monitor the patient's breathing and assess the respiratory rate frequently; changes and patterns provide important diagnostic information.

DEPTH   Like rate, the depth of a patient's breathing can signal whether the brain stem is depressed or stimulated.

PATTERN   Under normal conditions, there should be an even, constant pattern of inspiration and expiration. **Ataxic** respirations — irregularly spaced, occasional breaths with no particular rhythm — are serious and generally indicate damage to the medulla. Since they can also indicate airway obstruction, check to make sure that the airway is clear.

Deep, rapid breathing that does not return to normal may be a sign of high pressure within the cranium. Extremely shallow breathing can follow damage to the respiratory nerves, a depressed or dying respiratory center, or upper airway obstruction.

Evenly alternating cycles of deep and shallow or sometimes absent breathing (Cheyne-Stokes respirations) are often normal during sleep in children and the elderly. Under other circumstances, they can signal heart failure, uremia, drug-induced respiratory depression, and brain damage.

DEGREE OF EFFORT   Generally, the degree of effort required to breathe depends on the condition of the lungs, airway, and chest. However, there is an important exception: the **phrenic nerves,** which control most of the diaphragmatic breathing, emerge from the third, fourth, and fifth cervical nerve trunks (C3, C4, and C5). If a patient sustains spinal damage at or above the level of C3, he or she would have to depend on accessory muscles of respiration and exert greater effort to breathe.

Check the Head

Using extreme care, check the patient's head. Examining a head-injured patient requires extra effort to meticulously search the scalp under the patient's hair. Follow this procedure:

1. Look for depressions, fractures, lacerations, deformities, bruising around the eyes, bruising behind the ears, and other obvious problems. See Chapter 3.
2. Check the patient's pupils; are they equal? Are they constricted or dilated? Do they react to light? (Figure 15-5.)
3. The face should be the same on both sides; if it is not, the patient may have some paralysis.
4. Look to see whether blood and/or cerebrospinal fluid are dripping from the nose, ears, or mouth. If so, do not attempt to stop the flow; dress the dripping area lightly with sterile gauze to absorb the flow, but make sure that you do not create any

FIGURE 15-5 Assessing pupillary reaction.

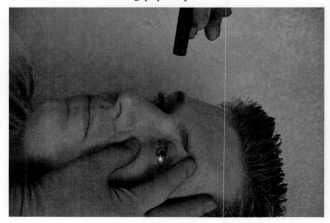

pressure (Figure 15-6). (Cerebrospinal fluid in blood can, but does not always, form a characteristic "targeting" pattern when the blood is dripped on a sheet, pillowcase, or sponge; it can rapidly form a double ring as the fluid migrates out of the blood.)

5. Look for signs of bruising that indicate skull fracture; they may occur immediately following injury, but sometimes don't appear for an hour or more. The most classic signs are Battle's sign (bruising behind the ears) and raccoon's sign (bruising of both eyes). Both indicate basilar skull fracture.

Check the Neck and Spine

To maintain light in-line stabilization, check the neck and spine for lacerations, bruises, swelling, protrusions, spaces, or other obvious deformities. (See Figure 15-7.)

Check the Extremities

Check the patient's arms and legs for paralysis or loss of sensation. Loss of function or sensation occurs below the point where the spine is injured, but you should

FIGURE 15-6 Blood and/or cerebrospinal fluid may come from the ears and/or nose of a victim of head injury. Turn patient's head to the side to allow drainage, and cover lightly with dressing. Do not block drainage.

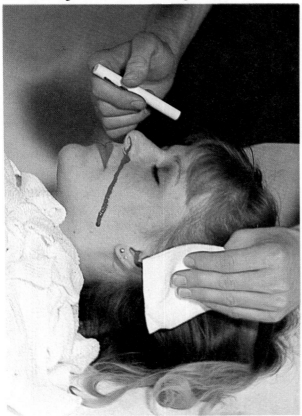

SPINAL INJURY PRECAUTIONS

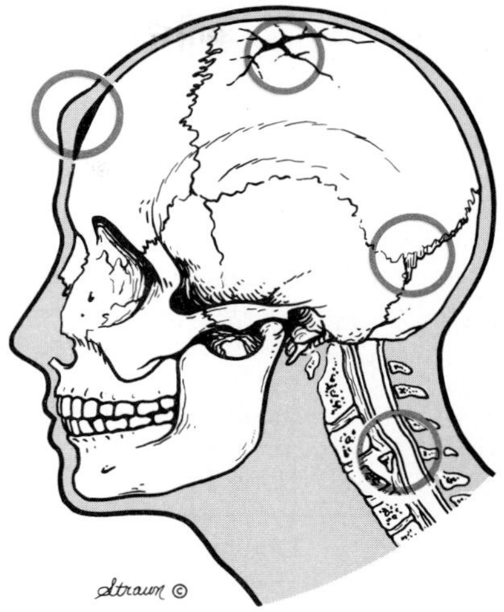

REMEMBER: Take spinal injury precautions in all cases of head trauma, as well as all cases of multiple trauma involving unconsciousness, particularly if resuscitative measures are required at the accident site.

FIGURE 15-7

check the arms even if the legs seem injured (the injury could be a fracture, not a spinal injury).

□ NEUROLOGIC ASSESSMENT

Every patient assessment should include a neurologic assessment — simply stated, an examination of the patient's neurologic functioning. You can use any format that is convenient, but it should include observations of the patient's level of responsiveness, sensory perception, and motor function, and a note of any special neurologic findings. Repeat your assessment several times to determine any changes, and remember that change, not the patient's status at any one time, is the most critical determinant in head and spinal injury. The Glasgow Coma Scale can be helpful for assessing brain injury in the field; it is explained in detail in Chapter 3. (See Figure 15-8).

Level of Responsiveness

You can usually assess a patient's mentation in terms of response to stimuli. A normally oriented, conscious patient should have a sense of humor; be capable of inde-

Glasgow Coma Scale

Eye opening	Spontaneous	4	
	To voice	3	
	To pain	2	
	None	1	
Verbal response	Oriented	5	
	Confused	4	
	Inappropriate words	3	
	Incomprehensible words	2	
	None	1	
Motor response	Obeys command	6	
	Localizes pain	5	
	Withdraw (pain)	4	
	Flexion (pain)	3	
	Extension (pain)	2	
	None	1	
Glasgow coma score total			

FIGURE 15-8 The Glasgow Coma Scale.

pendent thought and clear speech; and be able to identify the following about him or herself: identity, location and how he or she got there, and the date. The patient should be able to answer questions and obey commands appropriately. He or she should be able to localize pain and quickly withdraw any extremity from a painful stimulus. Movements should be purposeful, not random — he or she should push your hand away if pinched, for example.

A healthy, sleeping person should be easily aroused by hearing his or her name and should remain conscious and oriented without further stimuli. You should not have to shout or vigorously shake the patient awake; he or she should not drift back to sleep after being awakened. A healthy, sleeping person will flinch if you insert a nasal airway.

Sensorium

Find out what the patient can or cannot perceive about his surroundings by determining several factors about each of his senses, as follows.

Eyes

1. Check the patient's pupils with a bright light. Are they round and equal? Do they react equally? (See Figure 15-5.)

2. What about eye movements? Do the eyes track (follow movement normally)?

3. Do the eyes look normal? Is there any discoloration? A purplish discoloration of the soft tissues around one or both eyes — raccoon's sign — indicates intracranial bleeding with skull fracture. Raccoon's sign can often be seen within half an hour of injury but may not be apparent for up to a day.

Ears

1. Check both ears for leakage of blood or clear fluid; skull fracture or intracranial bleeding can cause both. (See Figure 15-6.)

2. Look behind the auricle of each ear for Battle's

sign, a purplish discoloration of the **mastoid** area that normally indicates basal skull fracture. Like raccoon's sign, Battle's sign can appear within half an hour to a day following trauma.

Nose

Check the **nares** for leakage of blood or clear fluid, which can indicate skull fracture or intracranial bleeding.

Mouth

Is the patient's airway clear? Does the patient taste anything abnormal, especially a bitter, sour, or metallic taste? A persistent salty taste can signal cerebrospinal fluid leakage. Do the teeth fit together normally?

Numbness

Does the patient have any numbness, especially of the face or the extremities?

Motor Function

1. Check the muscle tone of the patient's face by asking him or her to clench his teeth and grimace at you. Does the face seem symmetrical? If not, the patient may have suffered injury.
2. Ask the patient to grasp your index and third fingers of both hands simultaneously; assess the grip strength of the hands. Are they about the same (Figure 15-9.)?
3. Ask the patient to push against your palms with both feet, then pull upward with both feet against your palms (Figure 15-10). If you notice an inequality in muscle tone between the patient's left and right sides, ask if it is normal. Unequal muscle tone can signal brain damage or acute spinal cord injury. Motor function that is absent below some level of the patient's body (such as the nipple line) usually suggests spinal cord damage. (Checking foot strength should be done very cautiously; it can cause movement that can aggravate spinal injury, so if you suspect spinal injury, do not perform this test.)

Special Findings

Some special findings signal nervous system disorder or damage even if the assessment is otherwise good. Suspect nervous system problems if you find the following:

- Headache that is severe enough to be disabling or that is of sudden onset, even in the absence of trauma.

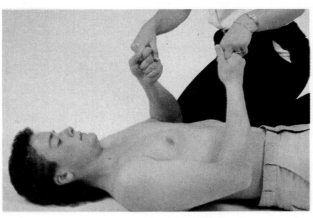

FIGURE 15-9 Assessing for grip strength.

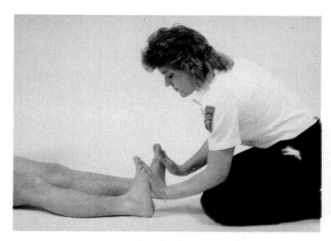

FIGURE 15-10 Assessing for foot strength.

- **Priapism** (persistent, emotionally unjustified erection of the penis), usually a sign of **lumbo-sacral** spinal injury.
- Forceful (projectile) vomiting, especially in adults, usually a sign of increased intracranial pressure.
- Widely dilated or inappropriately pinpoint-sized pupils, may indicate intracranial changes.
- **Incontinence** (of urine or feces), a loss of bowel or bladder control is usually a sign of spinal cord injury or nervous system disorder (such as seizure).
- Facial bruises, which suggest head and neck injury.
- Speech that is garbled and disordered in a conscious patient, or a conscious patient who cannot understand the speech of others or answer simple questions.
- Vital sign abnormalities that combine high blood pressure with slow pulse.
- Inappropriate flaccidity or rigidity in one or both extremities.

- Inappropriate nervousness, irritability, or anxiety, which can signal hypoxia, metabolic disturbances, high intracranial pressure, or cerebral irritability.

Scalp Injury

The scalp may be injured in the same way as any other soft tissue: it may be contused, lacerated, abrased, or avulsed. Because of the rich supply of blood vessels to the scalp, injuries of the scalp tend to bleed very heavily. In addition, the underlying fascia may be torn while the skin stays intact; bleeding then occurs under the skin and may confuse assessment attempts (the presence of blood under intact skin can mimic a depressed skull fracture).

☐ SKULL FRACTURE

Because of the skull's shape (spherical) and thickness (approximately $\frac{1}{4}$ inch), it is generally only fractured if the trauma is extreme. Skull fracture can be open or closed. The skull fracture itself does not cause disability and death; rather, it is the *underlying damage* that leads to serious consequences. Skull fracture itself presents no danger if it is not accompanied by brain injury, hematoma, cerebrospinal fluid leakage, or subsequent infection.

There are four basic types of skull fracture (Figure 15-11):

- **Depressed.** An object strikes the skull, leaving an obvious depression or deformity; bone fragments are often driven into the membranes or the brain itself by the force of the impact.
- **Linear.** The most common type of skull fracture (80 percent of all skull fractures are linear), it leaves a thin-line crack in the skull. Linear fractures are the least serious, and most difficult to detect, of all skull fractures.
- **Comminuted.** A comminuted fracture appears at the point of impact, with multiple cracks radiating from the center (it looks like a cracked eggshell).
- **Basal.** A basal skull fracture occurs when there is a break in the bed of the skull; it is often the result of a linear fracture that extends to the floor of the skull. Difficult to detect even by x-ray, a basal skull fracture often causes extensive damage.

Signs and Symptoms of Skull Fracture

The primary function of the skull is to protect the brain from injury. When the skull is fractured, part of the brain's protective armor is compromised, and serious brain injury can result.

You should suspect skull fracture with any significant trauma to the head. An open skull fracture is visible, but even a closed skull fracture will result in some signs and symptoms. Some are obvious, such as deformity or your ability to see the skull itself through lacerations. Skull fracture can exist without the usual signs, but you should look for the following (Figure 15-12):

- Obvious deformity of the skull.
- Visible damage to the skull, visible through lacerations in the scalp.
- Pain, tenderness, or swelling at the site of injury.
- Clear or pinkish fluid dripping from the nose, the ears, the mouth, or a wound in the head, or bleeding from any or all of these.
- Purplish discoloration or bruising over the mastoid process behind the ear (Battle's sign).
- Unequal pupil size.
- One eye misplaced in relation to the other eye.
- Purplish discoloration under or around the eyes in the absence of trauma to the eyes (raccoon's sign).

☐ INJURIES TO THE BRAIN

Injuries to the brain can be open or closed. In closed head injuries, the scalp may be lacerated, but the skull not exposed; there will be no opening to the brain. Brain damage, however, can nonetheless be extensive. The

FIGURE 15-11

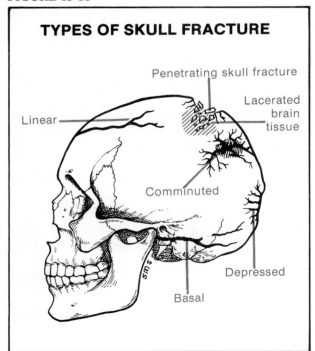

TYPES OF SKULL FRACTURE

Penetrating skull fracture

Lacerated brain tissue

Linear

Comminuted

Depressed

Basal

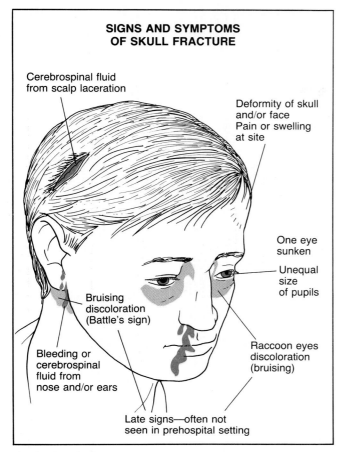

**SIGNS AND SYMPTOMS
OF SKULL FRACTURE**

Cerebrospinal fluid
from scalp laceration

Deformity of skull
and/or face
Pain or swelling
at site

One eye
sunken

Unequal
size
of pupils

Bruising
discoloration
(Battle's sign)

Bleeding or
cerebrospinal
fluid from
nose and/or ears

Raccoon eyes
discoloration
(bruising)

Late signs—often not
seen in prehospital setting

FIGURE 15-12

brain can be damaged whether or not the skull is fractured, since the amount of injury depends mainly on the mechanism of injury and the force involved. In general, however, brain tissue is susceptible to the same kinds of injury as any soft tissue — contusion, laceration, and puncture wounds (Figure 15-13).

Concussion

The most common and least serious brain injury is **concussion,** a temporary loss of the brain's ability to function that occurs when the brain sustains a blow, regardless of whether other injuries occurred. There is no detectable damage to the brain from a concussion — the patient remains "neurologically intact." Concussion is classified as mild, moderate, or severe, and the classification is based on the time between impact and the return of consciousness.

A concussion normally causes some disturbance or brain function ranging from momentary confusion to complete loss of consciousness, and it usually causes headache. If the patient loses consciousness, it is usually brief (lasting only a few minutes) and does not recur. Generally, any patient who is unconscious for more than five minutes is usually observed in the hospital for forty-eight hours to rule out serious injury.

Signs and Symptoms

Depending on where the force is absorbed in the brain, the signs of simple concussion might include the following:

- Momentary confusion.
- Confusion that lasts for several minutes.
- Inability to recall the incident and, sometimes, the period just before and after it (retrograde amnesia).
- Repeated questioning about what happened.
- Mild to moderate irritability or resistance to treatment.
- Combativeness.
- Verbal abuse.
- Inability to answer questions or obey commands appropriately.
- Persistent vomiting.
- Incontinence of urine or feces.
- Restlessness.
- Seizures.

The key distinguishing factor in concussion is that its effects appear immediately or soon after impact, and then they disappear, usually within forty-eight hours; recovery is complete. An injury that causes symptoms that develop several minutes after an incident or symptoms that do not subside over time is not a concussion, but a more serious injury.

Contusion

A contusion, or bruising and swelling of the brain tissue, can accompany concussion. If the level of consciousness remains altered for twenty-four hours after an injury, the patient has almost certainly suffered a contusion, not a concussion. A contusion causes bleeding into the surrounding tissues, which can be delayed (a stable patient may suddenly deteriorate), but may or may not cause increased intracranial pressure, even in cases of open head injury. Contusion is usually caused by **coup-contrecoup** or acceleration-deceleration injury (Figure 15-14). A patient with signs of concussion that do not clear up has probably suffered a contusion.

Signs and Symptoms

Signs and symptoms of contusion include the initial signs and symptoms of concussion plus one or more of the following:

- Loss of consciousness ranging from hours to months; upon return to consciousness, the patient will not be able to remember the incident or the events immediately preceding and following it.

HEAD INJURY AND BRAIN TRAUMA

Trauma

Primary injuries

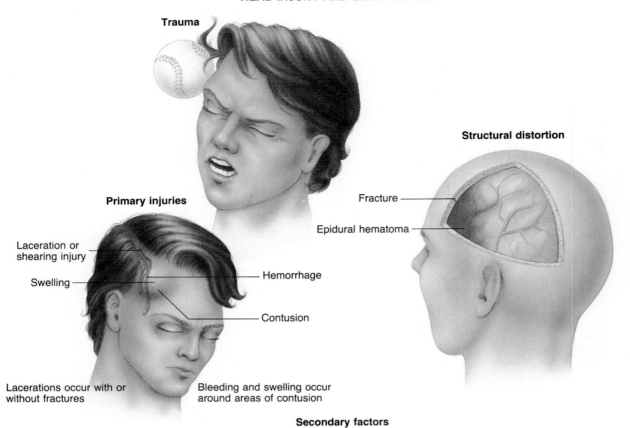

Structural distortion

Fracture

Epidural hematoma

Laceration or
shearing injury

Swelling

Hemorrhage

Contusion

Lacerations occur with or
without fractures

Bleeding and swelling occur
around areas of contusion

Secondary factors

Brain damage

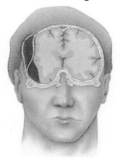

Contusions with pressure may
result in loss of consciousness

Respiratory and circulatory
changes may result from
primary brain injury

Subdural and/or epidural
hematomas and brain swelling
lead to increased pressure on
the brain

Signs & symptoms

- Deformity of the skull
- Drainage of spinal fluid or
  blood from nose and ears
- Black eyes
- Disorientation or confusion
- Unconsciousness or coma
- Unequal pupils or pupils that
  don't respond to light
- Partial or total paralysis

FIGURE 15-13

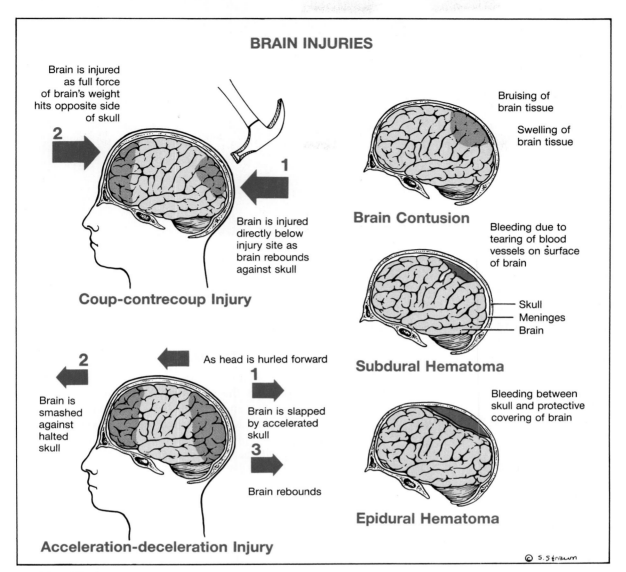

BRAIN INJURIES

Brain is injured as full force of brain's weight hits opposite side of skull

2

1

Brain is injured directly below injury site as brain rebounds against skull

Coup-contrecoup Injury

Bruising of brain tissue

Swelling of brain tissue

Brain Contusion

Bleeding due to tearing of blood vessels on surface of brain

Skull
Meninges
Brain

Subdural Hematoma

2

As head is hurled forward

1

Brain is slapped by accelerated skull

3

Brain rebounds

Brain is smashed against halted skull

Acceleration-deceleration Injury

Bleeding between skull and protective covering of brain

Epidural Hematoma

© S. Stnaum

FIGURE 15-14

- Paralysis, ranging from one-sided to total.
- Unequal pupils.
- Forceful or repeated vomiting.
- Alteration of vital signs.
- Profound personality changes.

Contusion can lead to swelling of the brain tissue, which can result in permanent disability or death. You can improve the patient's chances of recovery by vigorous airway management, hyperventilation of the patient, protection of the cervical spine, and positive-pressure ventilation (twenty-four to forty-eight breaths per minute).

Subdural Hematoma

A type of contusion, **subdural hematoma** (Figure 15-14) results when blood vessels on the surface of the brain are torn, causing bleeding between the brain and its protective covering. A layer of blood spreads over the brain; a subdural hematoma usually results from impact, which causes acceleration/deceleration injury. The bleeding associated with subdural hematoma is rarely arterial, and skull fracture is not usually present.

There are frequently no clinical signs of subdural hematoma; it may not be detected at the scene of the emergency. A very small hematoma may actually heal on its own. On the other hand, a severe hematoma may not cause signs at the scene, but later herniation of the brain may occur as the brain is displaced and it moves through openings in the bony skull. The survival of a hematoma patient is related to the size of the hematoma as well as the interval between injury and treatment.

Blood pooling causes pressure within the skull, and it displaces brain tissues as the bleeding spreads. The bleeding is always venous; the blood may clot quickly, and the displacement of brain tissue may be due to the clot. Subdural hematoma is the most common type of intracranial bleeding.

Signs and Symptoms

- Deterioration in level of consciousness.
- Vomiting.
- Dilation of one pupil.
- Abnormal respirations or apnea.
- Possible rising blood pressure.
- Slowing pulse.

While small subdural hematomas may resorb, a major subdural hematoma always requires surgical repair to close off bleeding vessels and relieve pressure within the skull.

Epidural Hematoma

Epidural hematoma (Figure 15-14) only accounts for about 2 percent of all head injuries that requires hospitalization. However, it is an extreme emergency that typically results from skull fracture. It most commonly occurs from low-velocity impact to the head or from deceleration injury. Approximately 20 percent of those with epidural hematoma die, even with rapid treatment.

In epidural hematoma, arterial bleeding pools between the skull and the protective covering of the brain. Bleeding is usually rapid, profuse, and severe. The bleeding expands rapidly in a small space, causing a dramatic rise in intracranial pressure.

Signs and Symptoms

Signs and symptoms include the following:

- Loss of consciousness followed by return of consciousness and then rapidly deteriorating consciousness.
- During periods of lucidity, the patient will have a severe headache.
- Pupil fixed and dilated on the side of impact.
- Seizures

Late signs can include fixed, dilated pupils, absent reflexes, and decreasing vital signs.

Immediate surgical repair is needed in cases of epidural hematoma. If it is treated early, the prognosis is generally good, since underlying brain damage is usually minimal.

Laceration

Like contusion, a laceration of brain tissue can occur in either an open or closed head injury; often it occurs when an object penetrates the skull and lacerates the

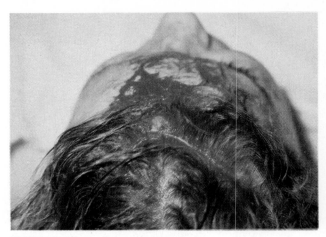

FIGURE 15-15 Open head injury.

brain. It is a permanent injury, almost always results in bleeding, and can cause massive disruption of the nervous system (Figure 15-15).

Puncture Wound

A puncture wound of the brain occurs when an object passes through the skull and enters the brain tissue, where it lodges in the brain. It is common in shootings and industrial accidents and often involves bullets, knives, or ice picks. An extreme emergency, it almost always results in long-term damage but is not necessarily fatal. *Never try to remove the object.* If an object is impaled in the head and is visible, immobilize it with soft bulky dressings and dress it with sterile dressings. If an object has penetrated the skull and you cannot see it, cover the wound lightly with sterile dressings. Permit drainage of blood in both cases, and position the patient for shock if bleeding is heavy. *Never apply firm pressure to the head following an injury that might have caused skull fracture.*

Open and Closed Head Injury

An open head injury is accompanied by a break in the skull, such as that caused by fracture or an impaled object (Figure 15-15). It involves direct local damage to the involved tissue, but it can also result in brain damage due to infection, laceration of the brain tissue, or punctures of the brain by objects that invade the cranium after penetrating the skull.

Closed head injury works a little differently. The skull is a nondistensible container with three contents whose individual volumes can vary, but whose total volume cannot: they include the brain tissue, the blood, and the cerebrospinal fluid. As mentioned earlier, the injured brain tries to compensate in a variety of ways by causing fluid levels to decrease. Basal skull fractures are likely to permit the leakage of cerebrospinal fluid through the nares or the external ear canals; under these circumstances, the cerebrospinal fluid is usually mixed with blood. If so, it can form a characteristic "target sign" when dripped on a sheet or pillowcase. But the rigid skull can hold only so much total volume, and if the brain tissue swells or bleeding occurs, pressure results, causing considerable damage.

□ EMERGENCY CARE FOR HEAD INJURY

Before beginning any emergency care for head injury, assess the patient's level of consciousness. Any patient who loses consciousness, no matter how briefly, must be evaluated at an emergency room. A patient who worsens needs *immediate* transport; he or she also needs continuous monitoring and assessment during transport. Urgent transport is vital: you should perform treatment on the way to the hospital.

Whenever you care for a victim of head injury, *always* assume that neck and/or spinal injury also exist. Handle the patient with extreme care, and immobilize the neck as early as possible; keep the neck stabilized and immobilized throughout the assessment and treatment. Keep the patient at rest throughout treatment.

General guidelines for emergency care include the following:

1. The top priority is establishing and maintaining an open airway with adequate oxygenation; oxygen deficiency in the brain is the most frequent cause of death following head injury (Figure 15-16). If the patient has sustained oral injuries, watch for blood and broken teeth, which can compromise the airway.

   • Use the modified jaw-thrust technique to open the airway without further injuring the spine.

   • Remove any foreign bodies from the mouth, and suction blood and mucus.

FIGURE 15-16 When treating a patient with a possible head injury, quickly assess the ABCs.

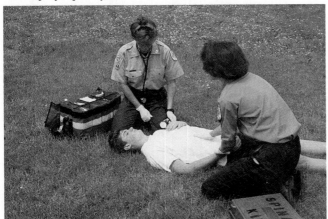

• Maintain neutral positioning of the head and neck by manual means until an **extrication collar** and head rolls can be applied and the patient can be fully fastened to a backboard or scoop stretcher.

• The patient may vomit, so protect against aspiration; have suction ready at all times and be prepared to roll the secured patient as necessary if vomiting occurs.

2. Closely monitor the patient's breathing; administer oxygen in as high a concentration as possible (if ventilation is necessary, use 100 percent oxygen at a rate of about forty times per minute) to minimize cerebral swelling. Provide resuscitation if necessary. Use hyperventilation on any head-injured patient: hyperventilation decreases the level of carbon dioxide in the blood, counteracting brain swelling and causing the brain tissues to constrict. Its effect is almost immediate, and it lasts for several hours. In some cases, hyperventilation alone may be enough to stabilize a head-injured victim for transport.

3. Face and scalp wounds may bleed heavily, but they are usually easy to control with pressure.

   • Guard against shock from blood loss.

   • Control bleeding from other wounds, but do not attempt to stop the flow of blood or cerebrospinal fluid from the ears or nose. If cerebrospinal fluid is leaking from the nose, ear, or head wound, cover loosely with a completely sterile gauze dressing to avoid introducing contaminants into the central nervous system; the dressing should absorb, but not stop, the flow.

   • For other wounds, use gentle, continuous direct pressure with sterile gauze only as needed to control bleeding.

4. If there is a protruding object:

   • Immobilize it with soft, bulky dressings and dress the wound with sterile dressings.

   • Never try to remove a penetrating object.

   • If the object is too long to allow for patient transport, cut it. Stabilize both sides of where the cut will be made, and use a tool that will not cause vibration or movement during cutting.

5. If the patient shows no sign of low blood pressure (systolic pressure below 80 to 90 mmHg), place him or her on a backboard and elevate the head of the backboard at least thirty degrees to reduce intracranial pressure. Never elevate only the patient's head and shoulders; tilt the entire upper body at a thirty- to forty-five-degree angle. If the patient shows signs of shock (high pulse rate, low blood pressure), elevate the foot of the backboard

or stretcher and inflate the antishock garment as needed — follow local protocol. *Note:* Shock is rarely caused by an isolated head injury — it always signals the possibility of additional injuries. However, it frequently results in brain damage or death. Avoid overheating; look for and treat other internal injuries.

6. At least 10 percent of those who are unconscious following a fall or car accident have also sustained cervical spine injury. In general, assume that all unconscious trauma patients have sustained spinal column injury.

   • Maintaining neutral positioning of the head and neck, apply a rigid extrication-type cervical collar to stabilize the cervical spine (Figures 15-17 and 15-18).

7. Monitor vital signs, watching for changes. Treat as appropriate.

8. Time is of the essence, but transport should be careful and smooth (Figures 15-19 and 15-20).

   • While en route, facial and scalp wounds can be dressed as necessary.

FIGURE 15-17 Maintain manual immobilization of the cervical spine while applying a rigid cervical collar.

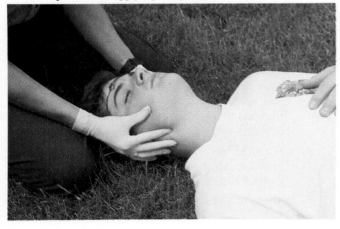

FIGURE 15-18 Apply a rigid cervical collar.

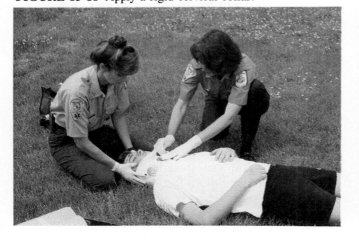

• Continue to monitor vital signs every five minutes and administer oxygen throughout rapid transport.

• Alert the receiving facility of the patient's exact condition and estimated time of arrival.

• Stay alert to the possibility of vomiting, and work quickly to prevent aspiration.

• The airway and neurological status should be continually monitored, and changes in the neurological status carefully documented.

FIGURE 15-19 Head-elevated position for conscious patient with minor closed-head injury and absolutely no signs of neck or spinal injury. Some EMS systems recommend placing the patient flat on his or her back. If this position is used, have suction equipment ready and monitor for vomiting.

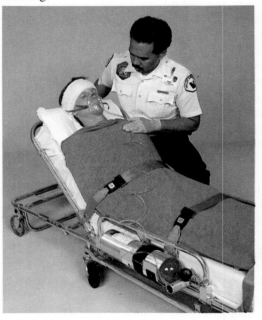

FIGURE 15-20 The patient with a head injury and possible neck or spinal injury should be immobilized on a spine board with the head end of the stretcher elevated six inches. Administer oxygen.

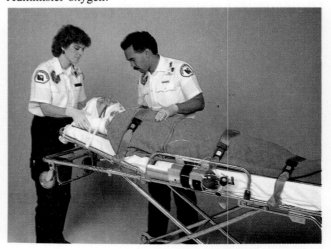

chapter 16

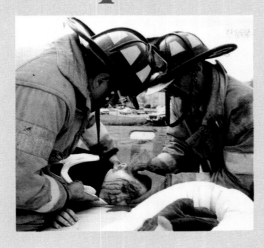

Injuries to the Spine

✳ **OBJECTIVES**

- Describe the general anatomy of the spine.
- Describe the common mechanisms of spinal injury.
- Demonstrate how to assess for spinal cord injury.
- Recognize the signs and symptoms of spinal injury.
- Demonstrate how to give emergency care for and immobilize a spine-injured patient.

This chapter was written in conjunction with Thom Dick, EMS author, teacher, and full-time paramedic, La Mesa, California.

It is recommended that EMTs wear protective gloves whenever there is a possiblity of coming in contact with a patient's blood, body fluids, mucous membranes, traumatic wounds, or sores. See Chapter 31.

265

Spinal cord injuries are some of the most formidable and traumatic injuries you will face: spinal cord injury affects most other organ systems, and improper handling may kill the patient.

Spinal injury can result from any force that pushes the spine beyond its normal weight-bearing ability or its normal limits of motion. Any trauma severe enough to cause injury to the brain (including a simple fall) can also cause injury to the spine. Especially prone to injury are the cervical and lumbar spine. You should always suspect spinal cord injury if head injury exists. If any vertebrae are crushed or displaced, the cord at that point may be severed, torn, compressed, or stretched, causing permanent damage.

The four top causes of spinal cord injury, in order, are car accidents, shallow-water swimming/diving accidents, motorcycle accidents, and other injuries and falls. Fifty percent of all spinal cord accidents result in paralysis from the neck down; the other half produce paralysis from the waist down.

Most victims of spinal injury are males (by a four-to-one ratio when compared to females) between the ages of fifteen and thirty. Approximately 43 percent are related to motor vehicle accidents, and another 21 percent are attributable to violent crimes. Many sports — including diving/swimming, skiing, sledding, and football — cause accidents that lead to spinal damage.

Some parts of the spine are far more susceptible to injury than others. Half of all spinal injuries occur in the neck, and half of those result in complete paralysis. Fewer injuries involve the thoracic vertebrae or the sacral and coccygeal vertebrae, which have little movement but are designed to bear weight.

Spinal injuries affect not only the spine, but often most other organ and bodily functions; improperly assessed and treated, they can result in catastrophic changes in a patient's quality of life. Obviously, proper emergency care is critical. Quick assessment and treatment are vital — there is little hope for recovery if the injury remains complete for seventy-two hours.

tebrae (neck area), but only 60 percent in the lumbar vertebrae (lower back area). (See Chapter 2).

The spinal cord is encased in a hollow, bony canal composed of thirty-three vertebrae which cushion the cord from injury. The thirty-three vertebrae are grouped in five categories (Figure 16-1).

- Seven cervical vertebrae are located in the neck and act to support the skull; because they are flexible and allow a wide range of motion, they are the most prone to injury.
- Twelve thoracic vertebrae are connected to the ribs; relatively rigid, they support the thorax.
- Five lumbar vertebrae are located in the lower back area; flexible but massive, they carry a large percentage of the body's weight.
- Five sacral vertebrae are fused together to form the sacrum; they form part of the pelvic girdle.
- Four coccygeal vertebrae are fused together at the tip of the spine to form the coccyx (some people have as few as two coccygeal vertebrae).

Between each vertebrae is a cartilage-like disc that helps to cushion and protect the vertebrae from injury.

FIGURE 16-1

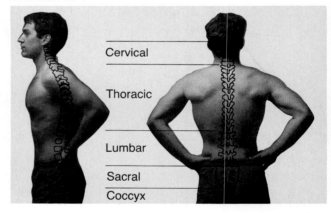

□ THE SPINAL CORD

While the spinal cord is composed of individual nerve cells, much of it is made up of nerves that extend from the brain. The cord is encased in a sheath of dura (protective membrane), which contains a cushioning layer of cerebrospinal fluid. The cord, which exits through a large opening at the base of the skull, carries messages from the brain to the various parts of the body through nerve bundles. The cord narrows as it goes: it fills 95 percent of the spinal column "canal" in the cervical ver-

(See Chapter 2). These discs are susceptible to injury themselves, however, usually from herniation, or slippage.

Most of the movement of the head is provided by the interface between the bottom of the skull and the top two cervical vertebrae (C1 and C2). Because their design also has to provide space for the routing of numerous nerve trunks from the spinal cord to other parts of the body, these two vertebrae are delicate. Any severe blow to the head should also be suspected of having fractured the basal skull, C1, and C2, or any combination of these, until a radiologist rules otherwise.

□ MECHANISMS OF SPINAL INJURY

The basic mechanisms that cause spinal injury include the following (Figure 16-2):

- Sudden compression (the weight of the body is driven against the head).

- Distraction (sudden "pulling apart" of the spine stretches and tears the cord).
- Excessive rotation.
- Excessive flexion or extension.
- Sudden, forceful lateral bending.

Bony spinal injuries occur when fragments of bone or pieces of disc injure the spine. They should always be suspected and managed in cases of motor vehicle accidents, head injury with loss of consciousness, blunt injury above the clavicles, falls (even from a standing position to the ground), motorcycle accidents or sports injury accidents that cause damage to helmets, hangings, unwitnessed drownings, diving accidents (especially in shallow water), violent injuries, violent assaults, and shootings (suspect spinal damage in all gunshot wounds to the head, neck, chest, and abdomen).

In addition, spinal cord injuries even in the absence of fractures are always a possibility in cases involving penetrating objects (especially stabbings and

FIGURE 16-2

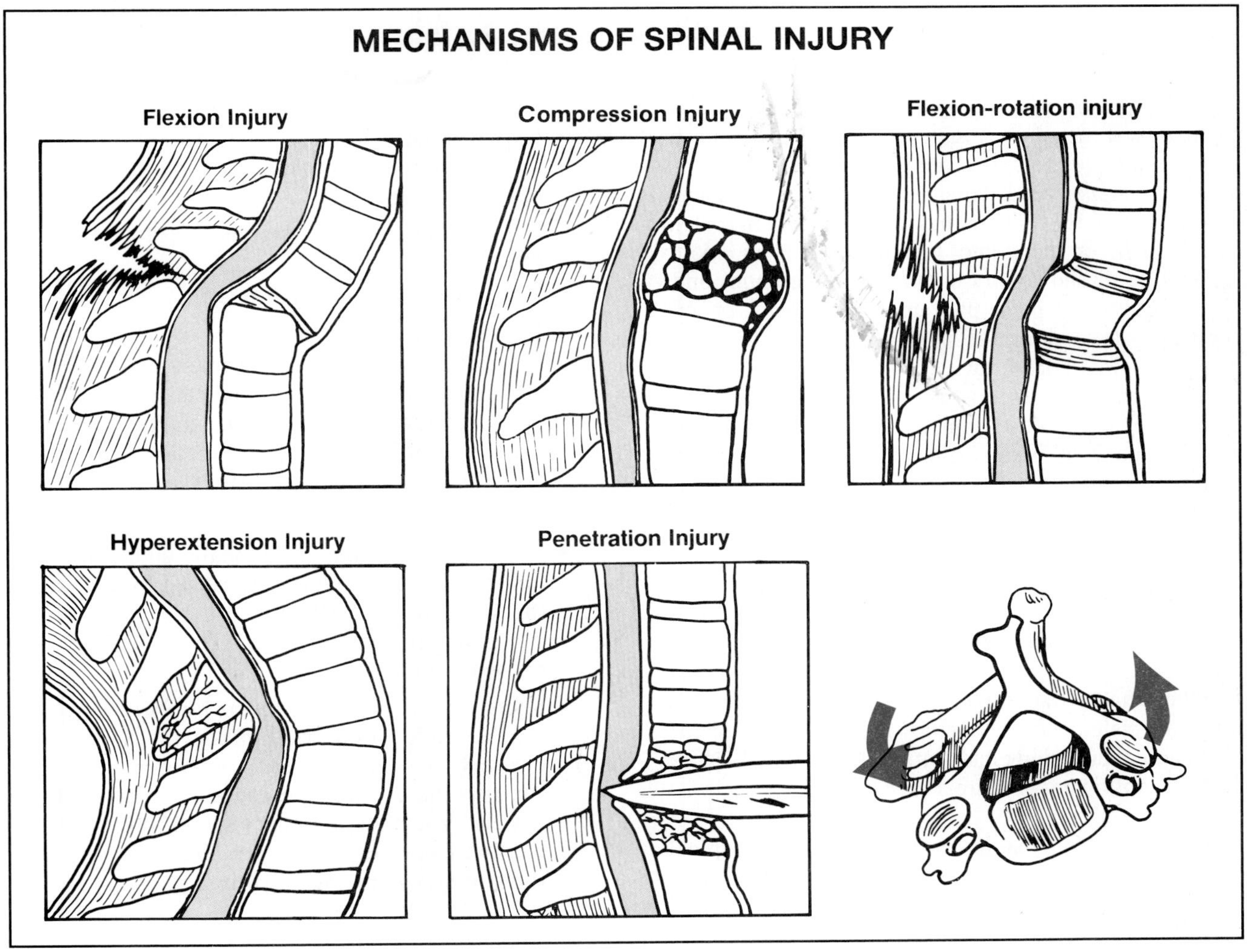

MECHANISMS OF SPINAL INJURY

Flexion Injury   Compression Injury   Flexion-rotation injury

Hyperextension Injury   Penetration Injury

shootings) and in any instance of sudden, unexplained loss of consciousness.

Spinal injuries occur in degrees: there may be an uninterrupted cord (the cord is still intact), incomplete cord injury (the blood supply to the cord is interrupted), or complete cord injury (there is severe interruption of cord function). Careless handling during assessment, treatment, and transport can make a once-intact spine sustain severe damage. Spinal injuries — which may or may not injure the spinal cord or nerves (only about 14 percent of all spinal fracture victims damage the cord) — can include disc injury (including compression), fracture, sprains (involving the ligaments), and dislocations. Suspect spinal injury with any serious injury, even injuries to the arms and legs; spinal injury often accompanies head, neck, and back injuries.

□ ASSESSMENT OF SPINAL CORD INJURY

The first step in assessment of spinal cord injury is to note the mechanism of injury — especially the type of movement and amount of force that was involved in the injury. The mechanism and its force can provide clues as to the extent of injury.

Remember that even if a patient can move or walk around, he or she may still be injured. Therefore, always treat as if spinal cord injury is present if the mechanism of injury suggests it, even if your assessment does not indicate spinal cord damage. *Always* suspect spinal cord damage if the patient has extreme discomfort in the neck, if he or she cannot turn his neck from side to side, or if he or she suffers numbness in the hands and/ or feet. Paralysis or pain, pain upon movement, or tenderness anywhere along the spine are reliable indicators of possible spinal cord injury.

If the patient is unconscious, assume that he or she has suffered spinal cord injury and treat accordingly. For a summary of assessment of both conscious and unconscious patients of spinal injuries, see Figures 16-3–16-13

□ SIGNS AND SYMPTOMS OF SPINAL INJURY

Remember that a fracture of one spot on the spine is usually associated with a fracture in other areas of the spine. The general signs and symptoms of spinal injury include the following (Figure 16-14):

- Pain that accompanies movement; suspect spinal injury if the patient complains of pain when moving an apparently uninjured neck, shoulders, or legs. Pain from spinal injury may be localized, and the patient should be able to indicate exactly where it hurts. *Never ask the patient to move, never allow him or her to move, and never move the patient yourself to test pain; base your assessment on any movement that occurred before you arrived on the scene.*

- Pain independent of movement. Such pain is generally intermittent instead of constant, and it may occur anywhere along the spine between the top of the head and the tops of the legs. If the lower spinal cord or column is injured, the patient may feel pain in his or her legs.

- Lacerations, cuts, punctures, or bruises over or around the spine (these indicate forceful injury). Injuries of the cervical spine may be accompanied by bruises or cuts on the head or face.

- Obvious deformity of the spine (not a usual sign). *Never have the patient remove his or her clothing in order to examine the back, since the movement may aggravate any existing injury. The clothing can be cut away.*

- Loss of response to pain or other stimuli.

- Numbness, tingling, or weakness in the arms and/ or legs.

- Weakness, loss of sensation, or paralysis below the level of injury. In a conscious patient, paralysis of the extremities is considered the most reliable sign of spinal injury.

- Loss of function in either the upper or lower extremities.

- Tenderness during gentle palpation.

- Impaired breathing, especially breathing that involves little or no chest movement and only slight abdominal movement (an indication that the patient is breathing with the diaphragm alone). The diaphragm may continue to function even though the chest wall muscles are paralyzed.

- Urinary or fecal incontinence.

- Priapism (a constant, emotionally unjustified erection of the penis, generally caused by damage to the spinal nerves that control the genitals). It occurs soon after injury and is a classic sign of cervical spine injury.

- Signs and symptoms of severe shock. Neurogenic shock, while often self-limiting, is severe when the nervous system has been injured and no longer controls the dilation and constriction of the blood vessels. You should suspect spinal injury in a patient with severe shock, even if there are no other signs or symptoms of spinal injury.

☐ Assessing Patients for Spinal Injuries

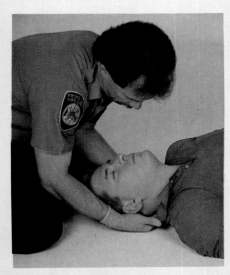

FIGURE 16-3 Point cervical tenderness and deformity.

SYMPTIONS AND SIGNS

Weakness, numbness.

Position or paralysis of arms.

Impaired breathing.

Shock.

Pain with movement or pain without movement.

Priapism.

Loss of bowel and bladder control.

CONSCIOUS — UPPER EXTREMITIES ASSESSMENT

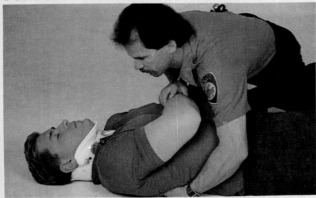

FIGURE 16-4 Point spinal column tenderness and deformity.

> **RESULTS:**
>
> Performance of all tests indicates little chance of damage in the cervical area but does not rule out all possibilities. Limited performance and pain — pressure on cord in cervical area. Failure to perform any test and negative lower extremity results — assume severe cord injury in neck.

CONSCIOUS — LOWER EXTREMITIES ASSESSMENT

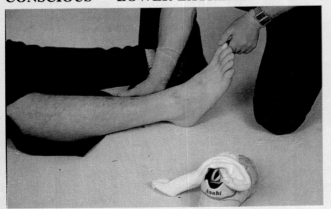

FIGURE 16-5 Touch toe.

> **RESULTS:**
>
> If the patient can perform these tasks, there is little chance of severe injury to the cord anywhere along its length; however, immobilizing the spine is called for since this test does not rule out all types of injuries, including vertebral fractures. If the tests can only be performed to a limited degree and with pain, there may be pressure somewhere along the cord. When a patient is not able to perform any of the test, you must assume that there is spinal iunjury damage.

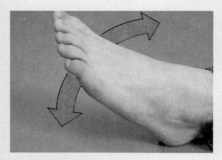

FIGURE 16-6 Foot wave.

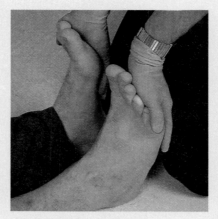

FIGURE 16-7 Foot push.

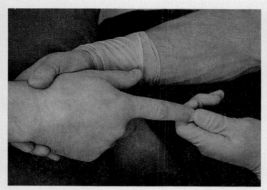

FIGURE 16-8 Touch finger.

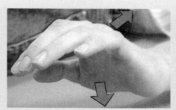

FIGURE 16-9 Hand wave.

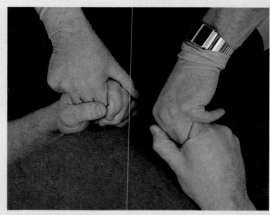

FIGURE 16-10 Hand squeeze.

UNCONSCIOUS PATIENTS:

Test the responses to painful stimuli (pinching) applied to the distal limb. If removal of shoes may aggravate existing injuries, apply the stimuli to the skin around the ankles.

FIGURE 16-11

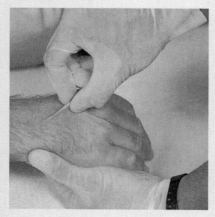

FIGURE 16-12

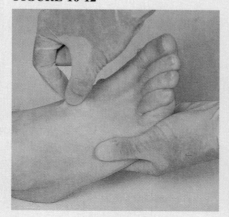

RESULTS:

Slight pulling back of foot—cord usually intact. No foot reaction—possible damage anywhere along the cord. Hand or finger reaction—usually no damage to cervical cord. No hand or finger reaction—possible damage to the cervical cord.

REMEMBER

It is difficult to survey the unconscious patient with accuracy. A deeply unconscious patient will not pull back from a painful stimulus. Should the mechanism of injury indicate possible spinal damage, or if the trauma patient is unconscious, assume that spinal injury is present.

FIGURE 16-13
SUMMARY OF OBSERVATIONS AND CONCLUSIONS

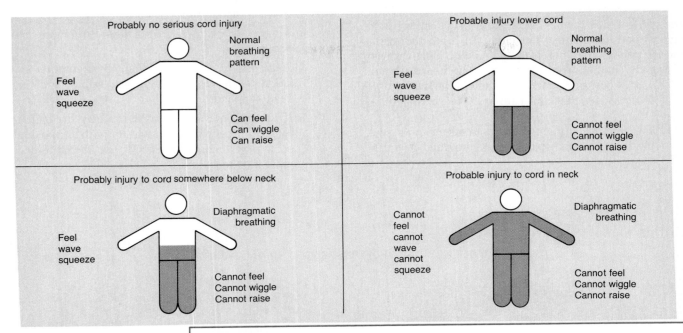

Probably no serious cord injury
- Normal breathing pattern
- Feel wave squeeze
- Can feel Can wiggle Can raise

Probable injury lower cord
- Normal breathing pattern
- Feel wave squeeze
- Cannot feel Cannot wiggle Cannot raise

Probably injury to cord somewhere below neck
- Diaphragmatic breathing
- Feel wave squeeze
- Cannot feel Cannot wiggle Cannot raise

Probable injury to cord in neck
- Cannot feel cannot wave cannot squeeze
- Diaphragmatic breathing
- Cannot feel Cannot wiggle Cannot raise

> **WARNING:**
>
> If the patient is unconscious or the mechanism of injury indicates possible spinal injury, assume that spinal injury is present.

FIGURE 16-14

SIGNS OF POSSIBLE SPINAL CORD INJURY

PAIN. The patient may be aware of unprovoked pain in the area of injury.

TENDERNESS. Gently touching the suspected area may result in increased pain.

DEFORMITY. Deformity is rare, although there may be an abnormal bend or bony prominence.

CUTS AND BRUISES. Patients with neck fractures may have cuts and bruises on the head or face. Patients with injuries in other areas of the spine will have bruises on the shoulders, back, or abdomen.

PARALYSIS. If the patient is unable to move or feels no sensation in some part of his body, he may have a spinal fracture, with cord injury.

PAINFUL MOVEMENT. If the patient tries to move, the pain may increase — never try to move the injured area for the patient.

STEPS FOR CHECKING SIGNS AND SYMPTOMS

CONSCIOUS PATIENTS	UNCONSCIOUS PATIENTS
■ Ask: What happened? where it hurt? can you move your hand and feet? can you feel me touching your hands (feet)? can you raise your legs and arms? ■ Look: For bruises, cuts, deformities. ■ Feel: For areas of tenderness, deformity, abnormal sensation. ■ The patient's strenght can be determined by having him squeeze the EMT's hand or by checking pressure against the foot.	■ Assess for breathing. ■ Look: For cuts, bruises, deformities. ■ Feel: For deformities, sensation. ■ Ask others: What happened? ■ Probe the soles of the feet, then the palms of the hands with a sharp object to check for response.

☐ EMERGENCY CARE FOR SPINAL INJURY

The general rule for management of spinal injury is to support and immobilize the spine, the head, the torso, and the pelvis. Your goal is to end up with a patient who is properly immobilized on a long spine board (Figure 16-15). It is best to overtreat than to risk further injury.

General guidelines for care are (Figure 16-16):

1. The first priority is to ensure an adequate air supply by maintaining an open airway and adequate ventilations.

- Unless the patient complains of pain when you do so, place the head in a neutral position and maintain that position manually until the patient can be fastened to a full-body immobilizer.
- Administer oxygen and assist ventilations as necessary.
- If the patient complains when you attempt to position the head, do not persist. Immobilize the head as found.
- If the patient's throat is blocked by his or her tongue, lift the chin straight up without moving or hyperextending the neck; use the modified jaw-thrust technique.

FIGURE 16-15

EMERGENCY CARE FOR SUSPECTED SPINAL INJURY

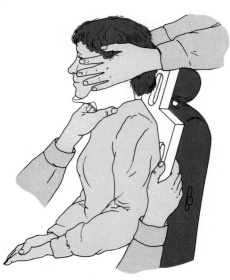

Take every precaution against converting a **spinal injury** into **cord damage.** In vehicular accidents, immobilize cervical spine before removing patient (spine board, cervical collar, rolled blanket, etc.). Advise the conscious patient **not to move the head.** A helmet should be removed unless there is difficulty in removing it. *Follow local protocol.* In such cases, immobilize on spine board with helmet in place.

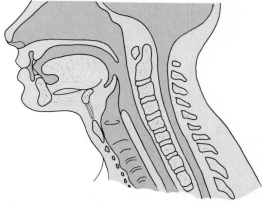

Is there respiratory difficulty? Remember that the airway has first priority. If resuscitative measures are indicated, support the head, immobilize the neck, and move the patient to a flat surface **with help.** Check the mouth for obstruction (dentures, tongue, etc.), and ventilate, giving all care to minimize motion of the neck. Control severe bleeding by direct pressure. If necessary, initiate CPR.

Keep in mind that respiratory paralysis may occur with cervical spine injury and that death may rapidly occur if respiratory assistance is delayed. Unless it is necessary to change a patient's position to maintain an open airway or there is some compelling reason, it is best to splint the neck or back in the original position of deformity.

Be alert for shock. If necessary, give oxygen and check with base physician about possible use of an antishock garment (PASG).

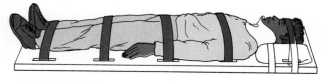

Immobilize patient before moving. As soon as possible, transfer to a firm stretcher or spine board and restrict head movement with tape, sandbags, collar, rolled towels, and/or blankets.

Provide emotional support, and transport to the hospital as carefully as possible.

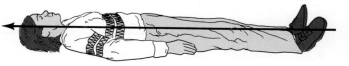

Always support the head in neutral alignment with body. Avoid flexion, extension, lateral movement, rotation, and traction.

NOTE:
Persons with neck injuries may have paralyzed chest muscles and damage to nerves affecting size of blood vessels. Breathing can then be accomplished only by the disphragm. Inadequate breathing and shock may occur.

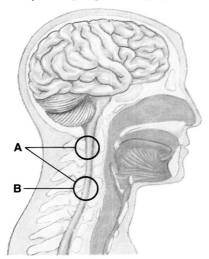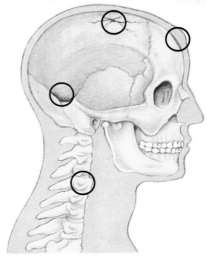

Spine injuries are most common at the cervical level. (A). The prime hazard is cord damage (B), which may result from trauma per se or from well-meaning but injudicious management **following** the accident. RULE: In all cases of neck injury, treat the patient as if there **is** a cervical fracture, until proven otherwise.

REMEMBER: Take spinal-injury precautions in **all** cases of head trauma, as well as all cases of multiple trauma involving unconsciousness, particularly if resuscitative measures are required at the accident site.

FIGURE 16-16

- If the patient is still not getting enough air, insert a nasopharyngeal airway and support ventilation.
- Ensure an adequate airway continuously throughout treatment and transport.

2. Administer high-concentration oxygen (50 to 100 percent), even if the patient appears to be breathing properly. Underventilation is the most serious problem in head and spinal injury.

3. Maintain a neutral position of the head and neck. If you encounter resistance, stablize the neck in the position in which you find it.

4. Check pulse and circulation; perform cardiopulmonary resuscitation if necessary; but do not move the patient.
   - Control any hemorrhage that is threatening life.
   - Never try to stop the flow of blood from the nose or ears — it could contain cerebrospinal fluid and cause a fatal buildup of pressure.
   - Never apply pressure to a bleeding head wound if you suspect skull fracture; you could push fragments of skull into brain tissue.

5. Stabilize the head and neck in normal anatomical position, and maintain manual immobilization until the patient's head is secured to a backboard. Holding the patient's hair out of the way and keeping the head and neck in normal anatomical position, apply a rigid cervical collar or extrication collar (Figures 16-17–16-24). *Do not use a soft collar* — it permits too much lateral movement, flexion, and extension. The collar will act as a temporary immobilizer and protect the patient's airway when you have inadequate manpower or multiple patients. *The collar is not enough by itself,* however — even after applying a collar, the patient must be secured to a backboard. (The collar also serves as a reminder and warning to medical personnel at the receiving facility that the patient has been exposed to a mechanism of injury that could have caused spinal injury). Remember that a collar is like most splints: it requires application by two rescuers — one to immobilize manually, and the other to apply the hardware. The goal of the collar is not to prevent the head from moving, but to prevent the head from moving in relationship to the spine.
   - Be sure to use a collar of the proper size for the patient. If you do, the patient's head will be in a

Injuries to the Spine **273**

EXTRICATION AND RIGID COLLARS

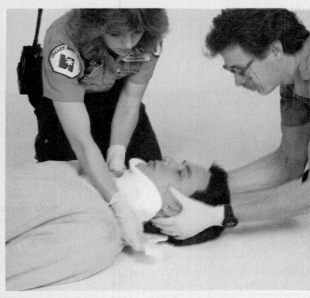

FIGURE 16-17 Stabilizing the head and neck while applying a rigid extrication collar.

NOTE:

Rigid cervical and extrication collars are applied to protect the cervical spine. *Do not* apply a soft collar.

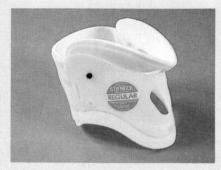

FIGURE 16-18 Stifneck™ — Rigid extrication.

FIGURE 16-19 Philadelphia Cervical Collar™. **FIGURE 16-20** Philadelphia Cervical Collar™ — Opened. **FIGURE 16-21** Nec-Loc™ — Rigid extrication. **FIGURE 16-22** Nec-Loc™ — Opened.

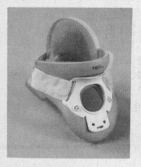
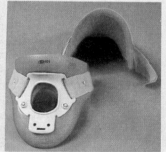
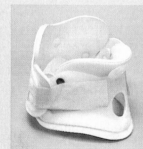
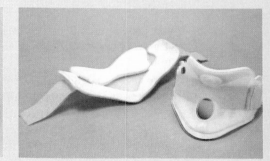

APPLYING MANUAL STABILIZATION

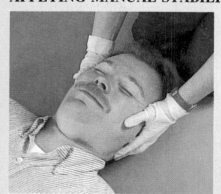

NOTE:

Do not apply traction to the head and neck, or pull and twist the head. You are trying to stabilize the head and neck.

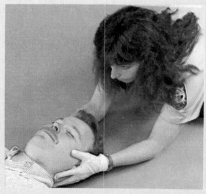

FIGURE 16-23 Properly position both hands.

FIGURE 16-24 Maintain stabilization — keep head in neutral alignment.

☐ Sizing and Application of a Rigid Extrication Collar (Stifneck®)

SIZING

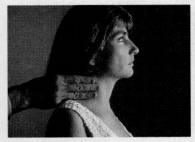

FIGURE 16-25

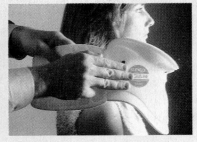

FIGURE 16-26

> **NOTE:**
>
> Using the chin piece as an anchoring point for the collar may cause hyperextension and be very detrimental to a patient with a cervical spine injury. Follow the steps as outlined in Figures 16-25–16-32. Rigid, extrication type collars should be used for spinal immobilization — not soft collars.

When immobilizing a patient with a rigid collar, it is critical for the rescuer to select the proper size. Too tall a collar can hypextend a patient's cervical spine, force the jaw closed, and limit access to the airway. Too short a collar can lead to inadequate immobilization, which may enable a patient's chin to slip off the chain piece and inside the collar into a hyperflexed position. If applied tightly, too short a collar may act as a constrictive band and impede venous blood flow.

SEATED APPLICATION

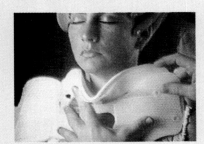

FIGURE 16-27

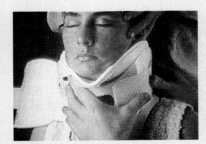

FIGURE 16-28

Once the proper size has been selected, it should be recognized that for optimal patient care, the patient's chin must be well-supported by the chin piece. To accomplish this, slide the collar up the chest wall of the patient. If the collar is pushed directly inward it may be difficult to properly position the chin piece and, therefore, to apply the collar tightly enough.

TIGHTENING

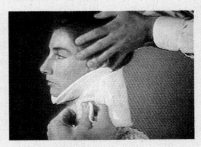

FIGURE 16-29

Tighten the collar and check that it fits according to the specific recommendations of the manufacturer. *Note:* Gripping the trach hole to anchor the collar can offset rotational forces that might occur during tightening.

SUPINE APPLICATION

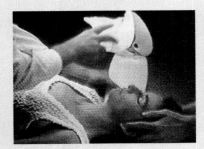

FIGURE 16-30

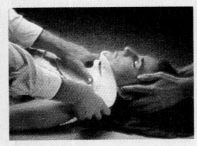

FIGURE 16-31

While it is relatively easy for the collars to be slid up the chest wall when a patient is in a sitting position, it can be a little trickier when a patient is in a supine position. Sliding the collar up the chest wall in a supine position is more of a pivoting action, which takes place after the back of the collar has been slipped underneath the patient's neck. The rescuer then rotates the collar up along the chest until the chin piece is properly positioned.

WARNING

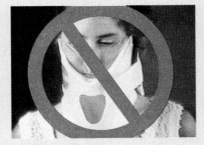

FIGURE 16-32

Improper sizing or application may allow a patient's chin to slip inside the collar. This must be prevented. Always check for neutral alignment and proper fit.

275

neutral position, but in order to talk to you he or she will have to speak with teeth clenched (Figures 16-25–32).

- If the collar is too small, it will not immobilize the patient's head unless you apply it too tightly — and if you do that, the patient's face will become flushed. Be aware of that sign and assess for it every few minutes; it indicates that the collar is restricting the outflow of blood from the head, thus raising the patient's intracranial pressure.

- If the collar is too large, it may cause extension of the patient's head, which can aggravate a spinal injury.

- If the patient is combative, one rescuer must manually hold the patient's neck in a neutral position and try to maintain alignment until the collar is applied.

6. Secure the patient to a long spine board as soon as all life-threatening conditions have been stabilized. (See Figures 16-33–16-54.)

- If you have to turn the patient over to get him or her on the backboard, log-roll the patient as a unit with the head aligned and without moving the neck. Maintain manual stabilization, keeping the body in alignment.

- To position the patient on the backboard, place the board parallel to the patient. Roll the patient on his or her side, maintaining neutral position of the head and neck; slide the board under the patient, and return him or her to a supine position on the board. Be sure to place a folded sheet or towel beneath the occiput of the patient's head — he or she may be lying on this immobilizer for several hours if the emergency department is busy!

- If the patient is standing, stabilize him or her manually and apply a rigid collar (Figures 16-55–16-57). Center a long spine board behind the patient's back. Adequate rescuers should grasp the board firmly and slowly lower the patient to a supine position. Once lowered, the patient should be fully immobilized and strapped to the backboard.

- If the patient is found in a sitting position, apply a cervical collar, then immobilize with **Ferno K.E.D. (Kendrick Extrication Device)** or other corset/vest-style extrication device) (Figures 16-58–16-64) or a short spine board; take care not to put the chin strap or chin cup on the patient (it prevents the patient from opening the mouth if he or she needs to vomit). (See pages 282–283.)

  To apply the KED, provide adequate immobilization while the device is being applied. Tape the head to the board; taping across the eye-

brows provides the greatest stabilization (to remove the tape, cut it down the center and remove it laterally). Secure the torso to the board with straps, Velcro, or tape, and cinch up the groin straps gently. Once extricated, move the patient directly onto the long board while he or she is still strapped to the KED or short board. Quickly loosen the groin straps and lower the legs. Strap the patient to the board at the shoulder, pelvis, and legs. Loosen straps immobilizing the patient to the KED so you can gain access to the chest and abdomen and to make the patient more comfortable.

- The KED and short spine board should be used *only* to immobilize a patient during extrication from a sitting position; the patient, should then be immediately placed on a long board. The KED cannot adequately immobilize the patient because it can't immobilize the surrounding joints of the head, spine, pelvis, and legs.

- While it is ideal to immobilize a patient to a KED prior to extrication, extrication should take no longer than two minutes. If immobilization is too cumbersome, lift the patient out, maintaining support of the head, torso, and legs.

- There are seven special warnings that must always be considered when applying a short board to a patient (Figures 16-65–16-73):

  1. *Warning:* Any assessment or reassessment of the back, scapulai, arms, or clavicles must be done before the board is placed against the patient. Assessment is not possible once the board is placed.

  2. *Warning:* The board should be angled to fit between the arms of the rescuer who is stabilizing the head. You *must* push the spine board as far down into the seat as possible. If you do not, the board may shift and the patient's cervical spine may compress during application of the board. To provide full cervical support, the top of the board should be level with the top of the patient's head. The uppermost holes must be level with the patient's shoulders. The base of the board should not extend past the coccyx.

  3. *Warning:* Never place a chin cup or chin strap on the patient. Such devices may prevent the patient from opening his or her mouth if he or she has to vomit.

  4. *Warning:* When applying the first strap to secure the torso, you *must not* apply the strap too tightly. This could cause abdomi-

□ Spinal Injuries — the Log Roll and the Long Spine Board

THE FOUR-RESCUER LOG ROLL

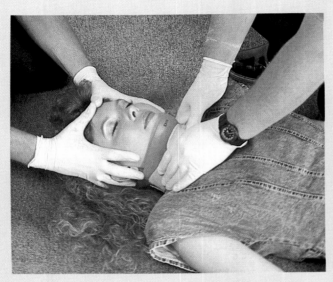

FIGURE 16-33 Activity around the patient is restricted. EMT 1 applies manual stabilization and the airway is opened by the jaw-thrust. EMT 2 places a rigid or extrication cervical collar around the patient's neck. EMT 1 maintains manual stabilization.

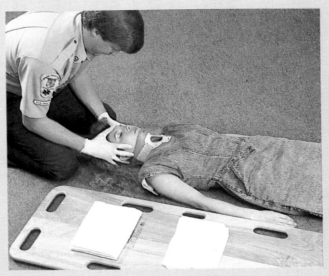

FIGURE 16-34 When possible, slide the board under the patient. If not, the board is placed parallel to the patient. When possible, padding is provided at the level of the neck, waist, knees, and ankles to help fill voids between the patient's body and the board.

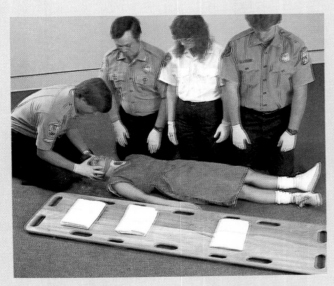

FIGURE 16-35 Three rescuers kneel at the patient's side opposite the board, leaving room to roll the patient toward them. Place one rescuer at the shoulder, one at the waist, and one at the knee. EMT 1 continues to stabilize the head.

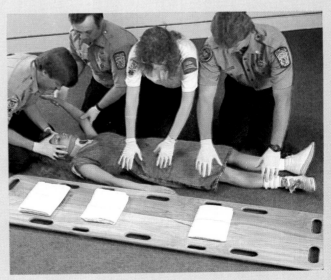

FIGURE 16-36 EMT 1 controls the move. The shoulder-level rescuer is directed to extend the patient's arm over the head on the side onto which the patient will be rolled.

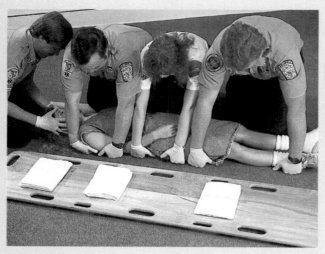

FIGURE 16-37 EMT 1 orders the rescuers to reach across the patient and take proper hand placements prior to the roll.

- The shoulder-level rescuer places one hand under the patient's shoulder and the other hand under the patient's upper arm.
- The waist-level rescuer places one hand on the patient's waist and the other hand under the patient's buttocks.
- The knee-level rescuer places one hand under the patient's lower thigh and the other hand under the midcalf.

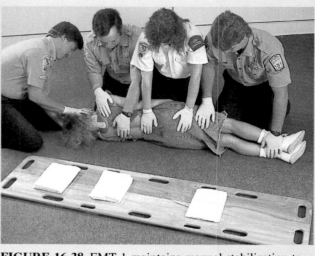

FIGURE 16-38 EMT 1 maintains manual stabilization to the head and neck. He or she directs the others to roll the patient, moving the patient as a unit.

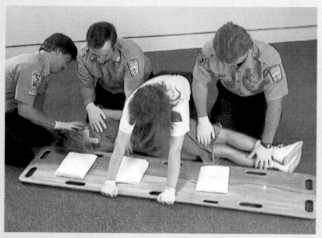

FIGURE 16-39 EMT 1 directs the waist-level rescuer to free hand to adjust the pads, grip the spine board, and pull it into position against the patient. (This can be done by a fifth rescuer.)

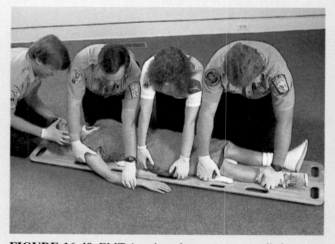

FIGURE 16-40 EMT 1 orders the rescuers to roll the patient onto the board.

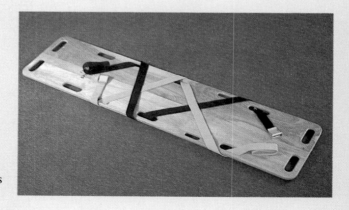

FIGURE 16-41 One strap is laced A-D-E. The other is laced B-C-F. Buckle A to B, E to F.

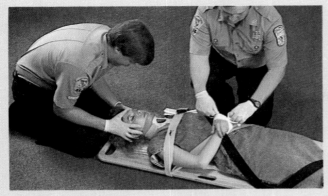

FIGURE 16-42 Patient's body is secured to board, wrists are loosely tied together.

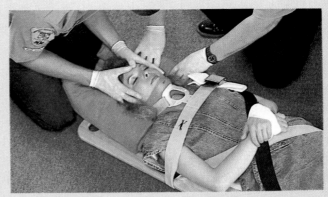

FIGURE 16-43 Center ten-inch-wide blanket roll over head. Roll ends toward patient's head. Commercial stabilizing devices may be used in place of the blanket.

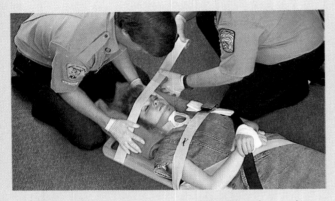

FIGURE 16-44 Use tape to secure forehead to long spine board.

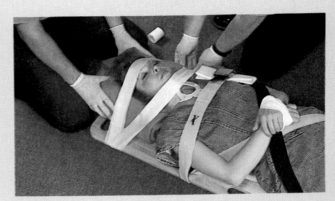

FIGURE 16-45 Complete process of securing the head and neck to the long spine board using tape.

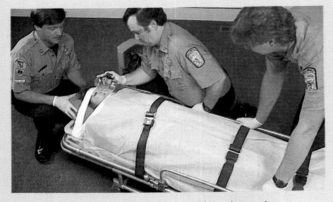

FIGURE 16-46 Transfer patient and board as unit.

☐ Three-Rescuer Log Roll for Spinal Injury

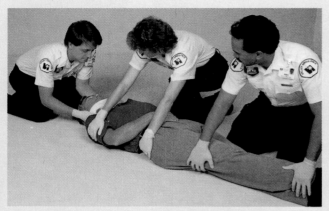

FIGURE 16-47 Maintain support for the head and neck while preparing for log roll.

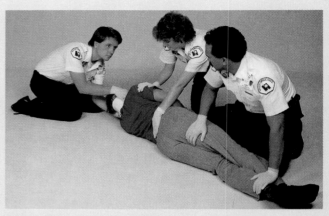

FIGURE 16-48 Roll patient onto side at command of EMT maintaining stabilization.

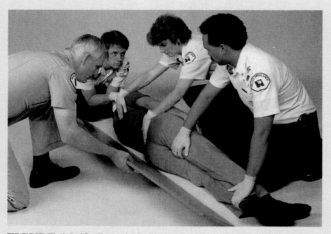

FIGURE 16-49 Examine the back, and move spine board into place.

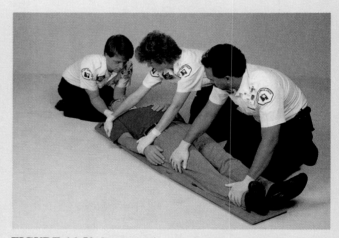

FIGURE 16-50 Lower patient onto spine board at command of EMT, maintaining in-line stabilization, and center patient on the board.

nal injury, aggravate existing abdominal injury, or limit respirations for the diaphragmatic breathing patient.

5. *Warning:* Some short spine boards have buckles with release mechanisms that can be accidentally activated during patient transfer operations. This is especially true of "quick-release" buckles. These buckles must be taped closed after the final adjustment of the straps.

6. *Warning: Do not* allow the buckles to be placed midsternum. Such a placement will interfere with proper hand placement should CPR become necessary.

7. *Warning: Do not* pad between the collar and the board. To do so will create a pivot point that may cause the hyperextension of the cervical spine when the head is secured. Instead, padding should be placed at the occipital region, but only enough to fill any void. This will help keep the head in a *neutral* position.

7. Strap the patient securely to the backboard; the torso should not be able to move or shift in any direction.

□ Two-Rescuer Immobilization of Spine-Injured Patient

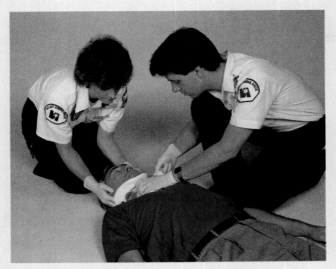

FIGURE 16-51 EMT 1 maintains an open airway and manual stabilization while EMT 2 applies an extrication.

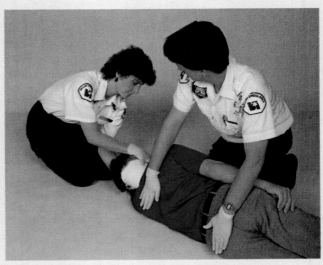

FIGURE 16-52 EMTs maintain in-line support while moving patient onto side.

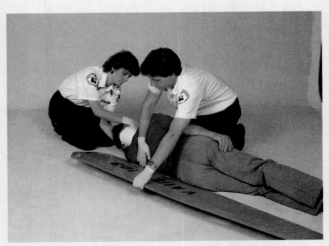

FIGURE 16-53 EMT 2 extends the patient's arm over the head and kneels at the patient's hips. EMT 1 orders the roll. Roll patient as a unit. After completing roll, EMT 2 pulls the board against the patient's back.

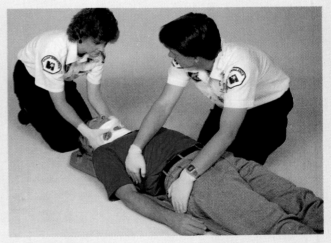

FIGURE 16-54 The patient is gently rolled onto the board. He is secured to the board in the usual manner. The hands are loosely tied together.

> **NOTE:**
>
> **Use extreme care. This method should be used only when dangers at the scene may threaten patients and rescuers.**

- The patient should be strapped at his or her shoulders, chest, hips, knees, and ankles with the wrists tied loosely together; make sure that straps do not cause pressure at the sites of other injury.
- Strap the patient's head down last so that any body movement during strapping will not cause movement in the neck.
- The strap across the chest should not be so tight that it inhibits movement of the chest muscles and impairs breathing.
- Use extreme caution during strapping so that you

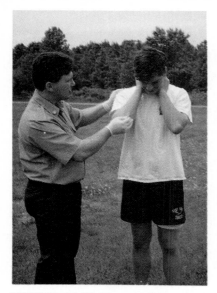

FIGURE 16-55 The standing patient complaining of neck pain following an injury should also receive spinal immobilization.

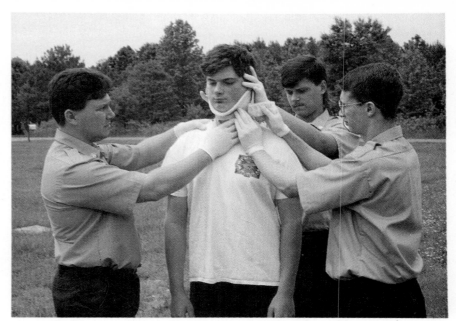

FIGURE 16-56 The cervical spine should be manually immobilized and a rigid cervical collar placed.

☐ The Ferno K.E.D. Extrication Device

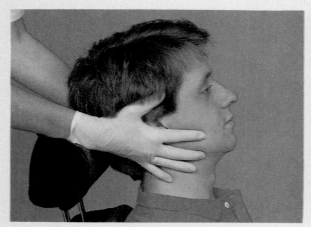

FIGURE 16-58 Stabilize head and neck.

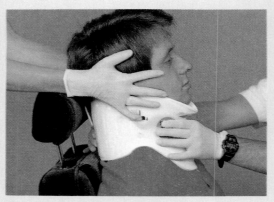

FIGURE 16-59 Apply a rigid collar.

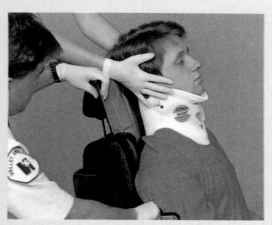

FIGURE 16-60 Slip KED behind patient. Center patient within device.

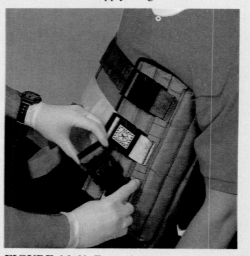

FIGURE 16-61 Fasten bottom and then middle chest straps.

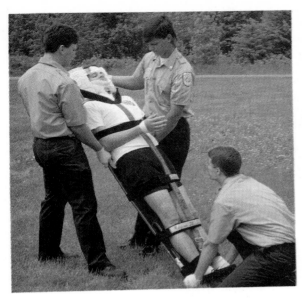

FIGURE 16-57 The long spine board can be applied while the patient remains standing.

do not rotate the patient when applying and tightening straps.

- The patient's head should be firmly strapped or taped to the board and surrounded with rolled towels, rolled blankets, or some other pliable objects. If you place light padding under the head, you can help prevent hyperextension of the neck; however, use caution not to flex the neck. Never place padding behind the neck itself. If the patient vomits, your strapping technique should be good enough to enable you to roll the patient onto his or her left side several times without any change in body position.

8. Treat for shock. Cover the patient to avoid heat loss, but do not allow overheating. Treat the patient by placing him or her in the Trendelenburg position by elevating the foot of the long board about twelve inches, unless head injury is suspected.

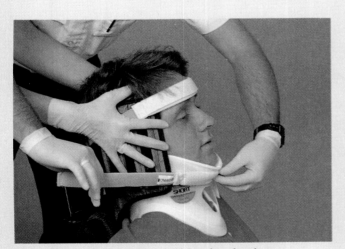

FIGURE 16-62 Secure head with velcro head straps.

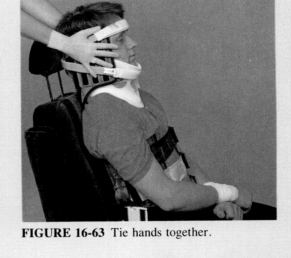

FIGURE 16-63 Tie hands together.

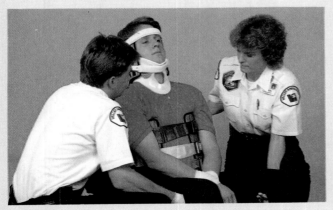

FIGURE 16-64 Lift the patient using the handles and locking hands under thighs.

NOTE:

Once the patient is extricated, the upper chest strap can be loosened if the patient is uncomfortable when breathing or displays signs of difficult or inadequate breathing.

☐ Applying a Short Spine Board

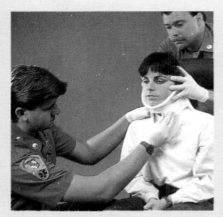

FIGURE 16-65 Stabilize the head and neck . . . apply manual stabilization. Secure extrication or rigid collar.

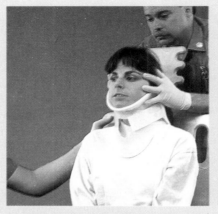

FIGURE 16-66 Position board behind patient, as far down into seat as possible. You may have to reposition patient.

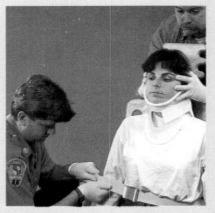

FIGURE 16-67 Secure the lower torso strap.

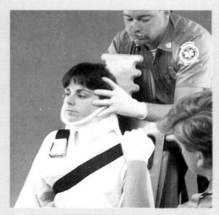

FIGURE 16-68 Cross the chest with the upper torso strap.

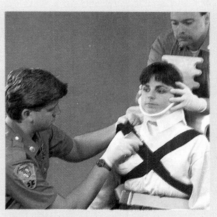

FIGURE 16-69 Recross the chest and buckle.

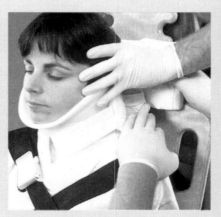

FIGURE 16-70 Fill voids between patient and board.

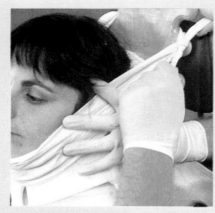

FIGURE 16-71 Secure the neck and lower head with 3-inch-wide cravat. Pass through upper notches and tie.

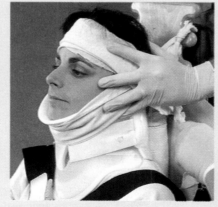

FIGURE 16-72 Secure the upper head with cravat. Pass through lower notches and tie.

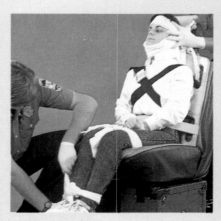

FIGURE 16-73 Loosely tie together the patient's wrists. Pad between the knees and tie together thighs and ankles.

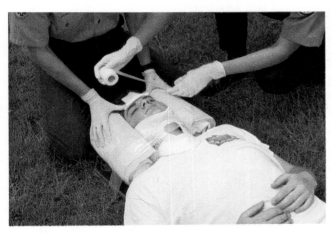

FIGURE 16-74 Stabilize the neck prior to transport.

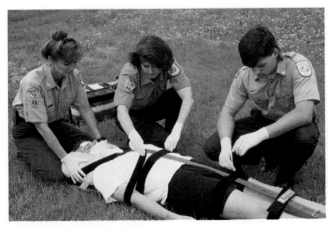

FIGURE 16-75 Secure the arms and legs.

9. Stabilize head and neck and secure arms and legs prior to transport (Figures 16-74 and 16-75).

10. If suctioning is required, turn the secured patient onto his or her side (Figure 16-76).

11. Move the patient onto the ambulance stretcher and secure him or her to it (Figure 16-77). A fully immobilized, spine-injured patient in preparation for transport is shown in Figure 16-78.

For all of the above procedures, various immobilization devices are available; some of them are shown in Figures 16-79 through 16-84.

☐ HELMET REMOVAL

The key to finding disorders of any kind is in looking for them in the first place. Thorough assessment is impossible as long as the patient is fully clothed, and that applies especially to protective headgear. The only time when a helmet should not be removed in the field is when the patient complains of pain during removal. *Follow local protocol regarding removing of helmets; it is controversial in some areas.*

Always involve at least two rescuers. Never attempt to remove a helmet yourself; wait for help. If the patient requires resuscitation in the meantime, remove the faceguard or shield and perform resuscitation without removing the helmet. As mentioned, if the patient complains of increased pain when you try to remove the helmet, leave the helmet on and immobilize the head.

The steps for removal of a full-face helmet are as follows (Figures 16-85–16-91):

1. If there is a chin strap, unfasten it.

FIGURE 16-76 If suctioning is required, turn immobilized and secured patient onto his or her side.

FIGURE 16-77 Move immobilized patient onto ambulance stretcher.

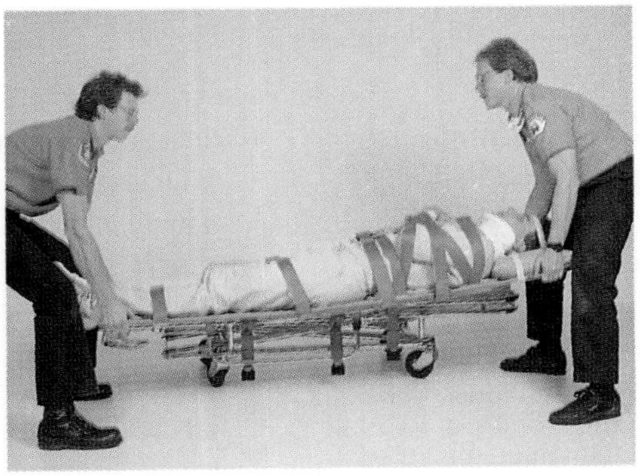

FIGURE 16-78 Fully immobilized, spine-injured patient on wheeled ambulance stretcher ready for transport. Head end of stretcher can be raised as shown for patient who is not in shock.

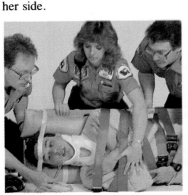

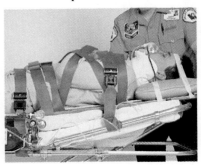

☐ Examples of Various Immobilization Devices

ALWAYS FOLLOW LOCAL PROTOCOL IN PURCHASING AND USING IMMOBILIZATION DEVICES.

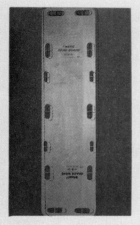

FIGURE 16-79 Long board.

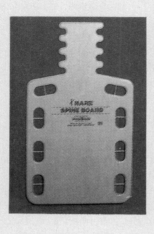

FIGURE 16-80 Short board.

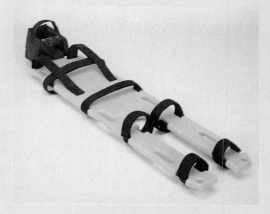

FIGURE 16-81 Full body splint.

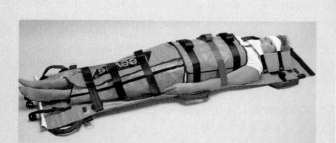

FIGURE 16-82 Fully body immobilizer.

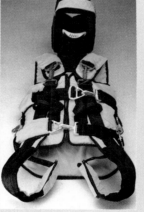

FIGURE 16-83 Corset-type half-back immobilizer.

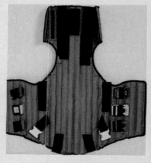

FIGURE 16-84 Corset-type Ferno KED immobilizer.

2. One rescuer applies manual neutral positioning for the head, while a second rescuer grasps the helmet and pulls both lower margins away from the patient's head. This provides added clearance for the patient's ears.

3. The second rescuer slips the helmet off of the patient's head, while the first rescuer continues to maintain neutral positioning.

4. The second rescuer sets the helmet aside (to be later transported with the patient), the helmet and assumes responsibility for neutral positioning of the head, while the first rescuer obtains and applies a firm cervical collar (extrication type) of the correct size. The patient's spine is then further immobilized by means of a backboard or scoop stretcher, straps, and a lateral immobilizer for the head (by standard means).

☐ Helmet Removal

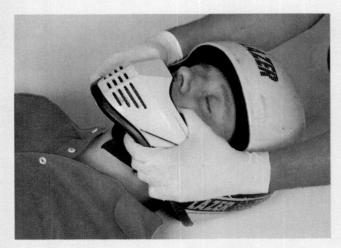

FIGURE 16-85 One rescuer applies stabilization by placing hands on each side of the helmet with the fingers on the patient's mandible. This position prevents slippage if the strap is loose.

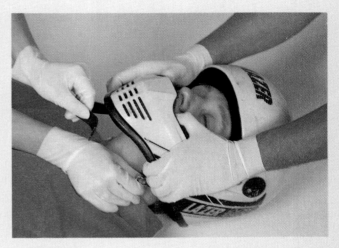

FIGURE 16-86 A second rescuer loosens the strap at the D-rings while maintaining stabilization.

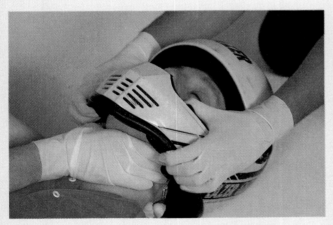

FIGURE 16-87 A second rescuer places one hand on the mandible at the angle, the thumb on one side, the long and index fingers on the other. With the other hand, the second rescuer holds the occipital region. This maneuver transfers the stabilization responsibility to the second rescuer.

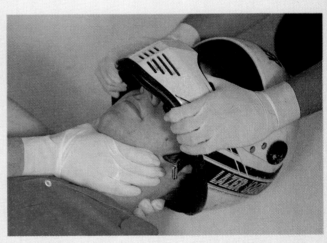

FIGURE 16-88 The rescuer at the top removes the helmet. Three factors should be kept in mind: (a) The helmet is egg-shaped and therefore must be expanded laterally to clear the ears; (b) If the helmet provides full facial coverage, glasses must be removed first; and (c) If the helmet provides full facial coverage, the nose will impede removal. To clear the nose, the helmet must be tilted backward and raised over it.

SUMMARY:

The helmet must be maneuvered over the nose and ears while the head and neck are held rigid: (a) Stabilization is applied from above; (b) Stabilization is transferred below with pressure on the jaw and occiput; (c) The helmet is removed; and (d) Stabilization is re-established from above.

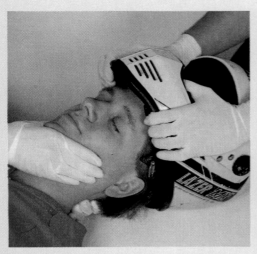

FIGURE 16-89 Throughout the removal process, the second rescuer maintains in-line stabilization from below in order to prevent head tilt.

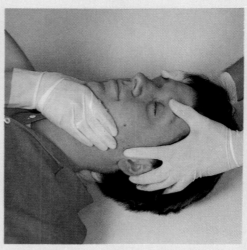

FIGURE 16-90 After the helmet has been removed, the rescuer at the top replaces his heads on either side of the patient's head with his palms over the ears, taking over stabilization.

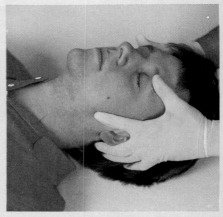

FIGURE 16-91 Stabilization is maintained from above until a cervical collar and a spine board are in place.

☐ Helmet Removal — Alternate Method

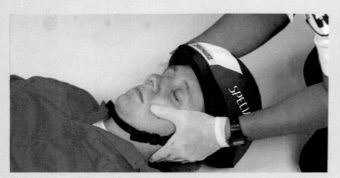

FIGURE 16-92 The first rescuer takes a position above or behind the patient and places hands on each side of the neck at the base of the skull; and applies steady stabilization with the neck in a neutral position. The rescuer may use the thumbs to perform a jaw-thrust while doing this.

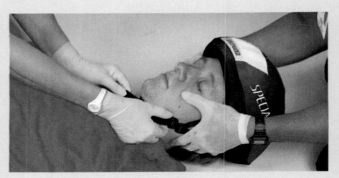

FIGURE 16-93 The second rescuer takes a position over or to the side of the patient and removes or cuts the chin strap.

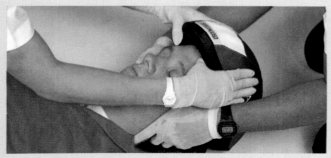

FIGURE 16-94 The second rescuer now removes the helmet by pulling out laterally on each side to clear the ears and then up to remove. Full face helmets will have to be tilted back to clear the nose (tilt the helmet, not the head). If the patient has glasses on, the second rescuer should remove them through the visual opening before removing the full face helmet. The first rescuer maintains steady stabilization during this procedure.

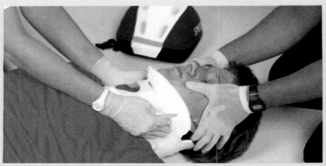

FIGURE 16-95 The second rescuer now applies a suitable cervical immobilization device, and the patient is secured to a long board.

chapter 17

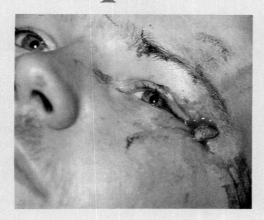

Injuries to
the Eye

✳ OBJECTIVES

- Outline the anatomy of the eye.
- Describe how to assess for eye injuries.
- Describe and demonstrate how to give appropriate emergency care for common eye injuries.
- Describe and demonstrate how to manage eye-injured patients wearing contact lenses.

It is recommended that EMTs wear protective gloves whenever there is a possibility of coming in contact with a patient's blood, body fluids, mucous membranes, traumatic wounds, or sores. See Chapter 31.

More than 1.5 million eye injuries occur each year in the United States, and they tend to be very urgent (Figure 17-1). Proper assessment and treatment can be instrumental in saving the patient's eyesight. It is important that you be well enough informed to suspect eye injuries in the appropriate settings. (See Chapter 2 for a review of eye anatomy and function.)

In general, you should always bandage *both* eyes to reduce movement of the injured eye; if one eye is left uncovered, it will continue to move, prompting sympathetic movement in the bandaged eye. Always close the patient's eyelids prior to bandaging to prevent drying of the eye tissues.

☐ ASSESSMENT OF THE EYES

Patients with injuries or medical problems involving the eye should be briefly but thoroughly questioned. When did the accident or pain occur? What did the patient first notice? Were both eyes affected? In what way?

Examine the eyes separately and together with a small penlight. Additional physical assessment of the eyes involves evaluation of:

- The **orbits** (eye sockets), for ecchymosis (bruising), swelling, laceration, and tenderness.

FIGURE 17-1

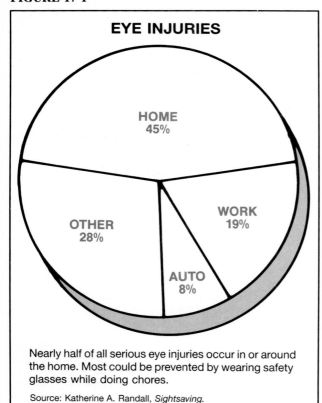

EYE INJURIES

HOME
45%

OTHER
28%

WORK
19%

AUTO
8%

Nearly half of all serious eye injuries occur in or around the home. Most could be prevented by wearing safety glasses while doing chores.

Source: Katherine A. Randall, *Sightsaving*.

- The lids, for ecchymosis, swelling, and laceration.
- The conjunctivae, for redness, pus, and foreign bodies.
- The **globe** (eyeball), for redness, abnormal coloring, and laceration.
- The **pupils,** for size, shape, equality, and reaction to light. They should be black, round, equal in size, and reactive to light.
- Eye movements in all directions, for abnormal gaze, paralysis of gaze, or pain on movement.

Suspect significant damage if the patient sustains visual loss that does not improve when he or she blinks; or if he or she loses part of the field of vision, has severe pain in the eye, has double vision, or is unusually sensitive to light.

☐ FOREIGN OBJECTS IN THE EYE

Foreign objects, such as particles of dirt, sand, cinders, coal dust, or fine pieces of metal, frequently are blown or driven into the eye and lodge there. They not only cause discomfort, but if not removed, may cause inflammation or possible infection, and/or may scratch the cornea. You can't always see corneal scratches, but signs and symptoms include pain, excessive tearing, and abnormal sensitivity to light. Fortunately, through an increased flow of tears, nature dislodges many of these substances before any harm is done. In no case should the eye be rubbed, since rubbing may cause scratching of the delicate eye tissues or force a foreign particle with sharp edges into the tissues, making removal difficult. It is always much safer for the EMT to transport the person to a physician than to attempt to remove foreign particles from the eye. An EMT should attempt removal of objects only in the **conjunctiva** (the transparent mucous membrane lining the eye and covering the outer surface of the eyeball), not those in the cornea.

However, if removal of a foreign particle is necessary, the procedure is as follows:

1. Flush the eye with clean water, if available, holding the eyelids apart (Figure 17-2). *Follow local protocol* — some EMS systems do not recommend flushing the eye except in cases of chemical burns.

2. Often, a foreign object lodged under the upper eyelid can be removed by drawing the upper lid down over the lower lid; as the upper lid returns to its normal position, the undersurfaces will be drawn over the lashes of the lower lid and the foreign body removed by the wiping action of the eyelashes.

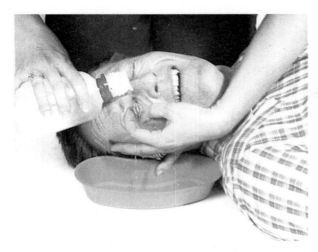

FIGURE 17-2 Flushing foreign particle out of the eye.

3. Particles lodged under the lower lid may be removed by pulling down the lower lid, exposing the inner surface (Figure 17-3). The corner of a piece of sterile gauze can be used to remove the foreign object.

4. A foreign object in the eye may also be removed by grasping the eyelashes of the upper lid and turning the lid over a cotton swab or similar object (Figures 17-4–17-7). The particle may then be carefully removed from the eyelid with the corner of a piece of sterile gauze.

Should a foreign object become lodged in the eyeball (Figure 17-8), do not attempt to disturb it, as it may be forced deeper into the eye and result in further damage. Place a bandage compress over *both eyes.*

Gentleness is essential in handling eye injuries. If difficulty is experienced in removing a foreign object from the eye, transport the patient to the hospital at once.

□ INJURY TO THE ORBITS

Trauma to the face may result in the fracture of one or several of the bones of the skull that form the orbits (eye sockets). A patient with an **orbital fracture** may complain of double vision and, due to nerve damage, may manifest loss of sensation above the eyebrow or over the cheek or upper lip. In some cases, massive nasal discharge may occur; in others, markedly decreased vision (Figure 17-9). Whenever the orbit has been fractured, assume that there is accompanying head injury.

Fractures of the lower socket are the most common and can cause paralysis of upward gaze (the patient's eyes will not be able to follow your finger upward). Hence, it is important to check all possible eye movements in the patient sustaining possible facial fractures.

Orbital fractures require hospitalization and possible surgery.

1. The patient should be transported in a sitting position.

2. If no associated injury to the globe (eyeball) is apparent, ice packs may be used over the injured area to reduce swelling.

3. However, if globe injury is suspected, or if you are in doubt, avoid using ice packs and transport the patient in a supine position if the globe has been punctured (this may prevent the loss of irreplaceable vitreous humor).

□ LID INJURIES

Lid injuries include **ecchymosis** (black eyes), burns, and lacerations (Figure 17-10 on page 293). They may also be characterized by a swollen or drooping eyelid or an

FIGURE 17-3 Gently attempt to remove objects in the white part of the eye. Using two fingers, gently pull down the lower eyelid while the patient looks up. Carefully pull up the upper eyelid as the patient looks down. An applicator swab can help you to grip the lid as shown.

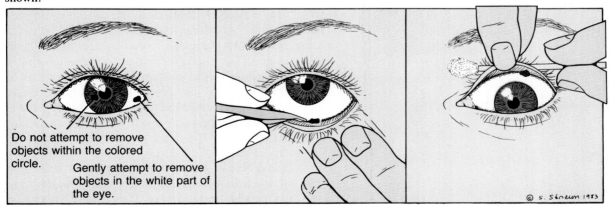

Do not attempt to remove objects within the colored circle. Gently attempt to remove objects in the white part of the eye.

© S. Stroem 1983

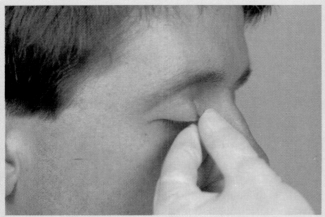

FIGURE 17-4 Grasp eyelash between thumb and forefinger while patient is told to look downward.

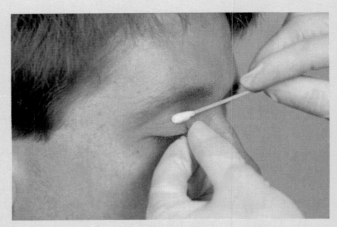

FIGURE 17-5 Place applicator swab along center of upper eyelid.

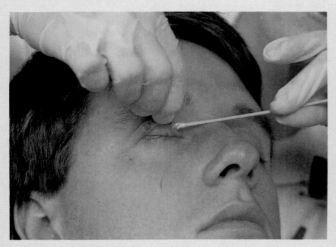

FIGURE 17-6 Pull eyelid forward and upward over applicator swab.

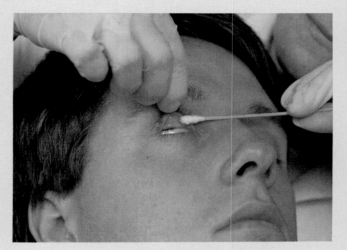

FIGURE 17-7 Undersurface of eyelid is exposed and foreign object can be gently removed with a sterile, moistened applicator swab.

FIGURE 17-8 Foreign object lodged in the eye.

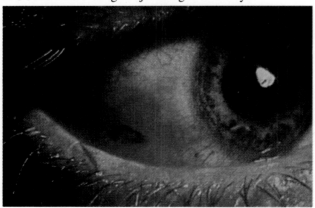

out of position eye. Because the eyelid is richly supplied with blood vessels, lacerations to the lid can cause profuse bleeding. Anything that lacerates the lid can also cause damage to the globe, so assess the injury carefully. In general, little can be done for these injuries in the field beyond gentle patching. Field care consists of controlling bleeding and protecting the injured tissue and underlying structures as you would any soft tissue injury. *Never* attempt to remove embedded material, such as gravel.

1. Eyelid bleeding can be profuse but can usually be controlled with light pressure. Only a light dressing should be used, and *no* pressure should be

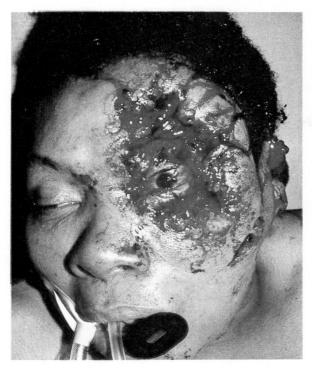

FIGURE 17-9 Eye orbit injury.

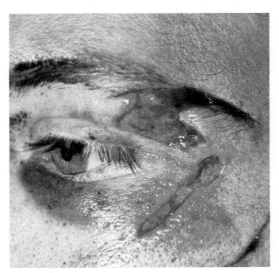

FIGURE 17-10 Eyelid injury.

used if the eyeball itself is injured. Use sterile gauze soaked in saline to keep the wound from drying out. If skin is avulsed, preserve and transport it with the patient for later grafting.

2. Cover the uninjured eye with a bandage to decrease movement of the injured eye.

3. Apply cold compresses to reduce swelling.

□ INJURIES TO THE GLOBE

Injuries to the globe include bruising, lacerations, foreign objects, and abrasions. Overnight use of contact lenses (even extended-wear lenses) can cause corneal abrasions, irritant conjunctivitis, and corneal ulcers; overnight use reduces oxygen to the cornea and increases risk of ulceration by fifteen times. Deep lacerations can cut the cornea, causing the contents of the eyeball to spill out. A ruptured eyeball can result from severe blunt trauma or projectile injury; signs include a pear- or irregular-shaped eyeball, laceration of the conjunctiva, or blood in the front chamber. (Do not use a patch or any kind of pressure if you suspect a ruptured eyeball, since pressure can force eye contents out.)

Injuries to the globe are best treated in the emergency room, where specialized equipment is available. Patches lightly applied to *both* eyes and keeping the patient in a supine position are all that is necessary in the field. Cold compresses may give some pain relief. The exceptions are chemical burns, especially **alkaline** burns, which rapidly lead to total blindness. In any patient suffering chemical burns to the eye, try to determine the cause of the burn and, if possible, bring the substance with you to the emergency room. Transport the patient flat on his or her back.

□ CHEMICAL BURNS OF THE EYE

Chemical burns of the eye (Figure 17-11) is one of the only eye injuries that is a dire emergency: permanent damage to the eye can ocur within seconds of the injury, and the first ten minutes following injury are crucial to the final outcome. Remember that burning and tissue damage will continue to occur as long as any substance is left in the eye, even if that substance is diluted.

FIGURE 17-11 Chemical burns of the eye.

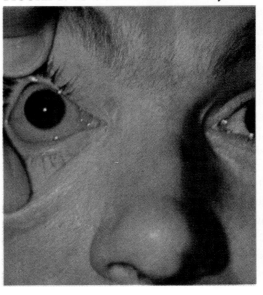

In general, alkali causes more serious damage than acid, because it burns more quickly and burns more deeply, affecting more layers. Generally, the higher the pH, the more severe the injury. If the injury involves alkali, you need to continue irrigation for at least an hour; irrigation should be done throughout transport and continued at the hospital.

The signs of chemical burns to the eye include irritated, swollen eyelids; redness of the eye or red streaks across the surface of the eye; blurred or diminished vision; excruciating pain in the eyes; and irritated, burned skin around the eyes.

In all chemical burns of the eye, begin immediate, continous irrigation with water or saline; it need not be sterile, but should be clean (See Figure 17-12.)

1. Holding the eyelids open so all chemicals can be washed out from behind the lids, continuously irrigate the eye with running water for at least thirty to sixty minutes, beginning as soon as you encounter the patient (Figure 17-13). Pour from the inside corner, across the eyeball to the outside edge. Take care not to contaminate the uninjured eye. If available at the site, have the patient irrigate the eye(s) with eye wash system (Figure 17-14).

2. Contact lenses must be removed or flushed out; if not, they will trap chemicals between the contact lens and the cornea. *Follow local protocol.* See the section on contact lens removal later in this chapter.

3. Remove any solid particles from the surface of the eye with a moistened cotton swab.

4. It may be easiest to place the patient on his side on the stretcher, with a basin or towels under his head, and to direct fluid continuously from IV bottles or clean water into the eye while gently holding the eyelid open.

5. You may have to force the lids open, since the patient may be unable to do so because of pain.

6. Irrigation should be continued throughout transport.

7. Do not use any irrigants other than saline or water.

8. Never irrigate the eye with any chemical antidote, including diluted vinegar, sodium bicarbonate, or alcohol.

9. If only one eye is affected, irrigate away from the unaffected eye.

10. Following irrigation, wash your hands thoroughly, using a nail brush to clean under your fingernails, to avoid contamination of your own eyes.

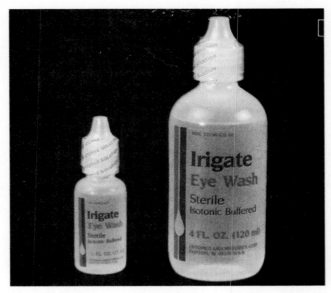

FIGURE 17-12 Commercial Irrigate eye wash.

FIGURE 17-13 Chemical burns of the eye should be continuously irrigated for thirty to sixty minutes.

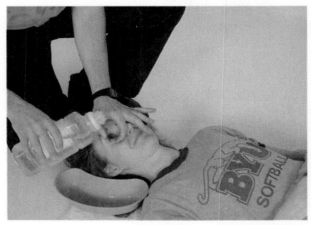

FIGURE 17-14 If possible, irrigate chemical burns of the eye in eye wash system. (*Courtesy of* Lab Safety Supply, Inc.. Jamesville. WI.)

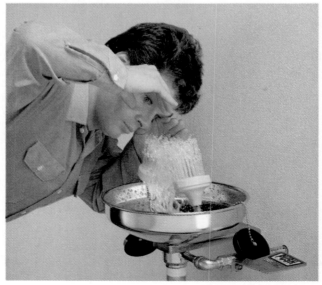

☐ IMPALED OBJECTS IN THE EYE

Objects impaled or embedded in the eye (Figure 17-15) should be removed only by a doctor. Penetrating objects must be protected from accidental movement or removal until the patient receives medical attention.

Impaled objects in the eye should be treated with great urgency.

To treat impaled objects in the eye:

1. Manipulate the eye as little as possible during treatment.

2. Tell the patient that both eyes must be bandaged to protect the injured eye.

3. Stabilize the head with sandbags or large pads, and always transport the patient on his back.

4. Encircle the eye with a gauze dressing or other suitable material, such as soft, sterile cloth; do not apply pressure. You can cut a hole in a single bulky dressing to accommodate the impaled object.

5. Position a metal shield, a crushed cup, or a cone over the embedded object. Do not use a styrofoam cup, since it can crumble. The object should not touch the top or sides of the cup (Figure 17-16).

6. Hold the cup and dressing in place with a self-adhering bandage compress or roller bandage that covers both eyes; do not wrap over the cup, since the pressure can push the cup down onto the impaled object. It is important to bandage both eyes to prevent movement of the injured eye (Figure 17-17).

7. Treat for shock. Give the patient nothing by mouth in case he or she needs general anesthesia when he or she reaches the hospital.

8. Never leave the patient alone, as he or she might panic with both eyes covered. Keep the patient in hand contact so that he or she will always know someone is there.

9. If the patient is unconscious, close the uninjured eye before bandaging to prevent drying of tissues, which can cause additional eye injury. Closing the eye allows normal tears to keep the eye moist.

☐ EXTRUDED EYEBALL

During a serious injury, the eyeball may be knocked out of the socket (extruded or avulsed) (Figure 17-18). Do not attempt to replace the eyeball into the socket.

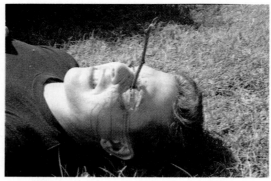

FIGURE 17-15 Impaled object in eye.

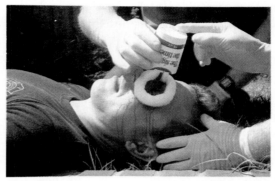

FIGURE 17-16 Dress and stabilize impaled object.

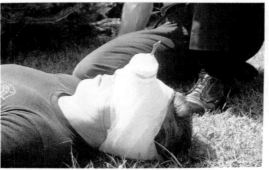

FIGURE 17-17 Bandage the cup in place.

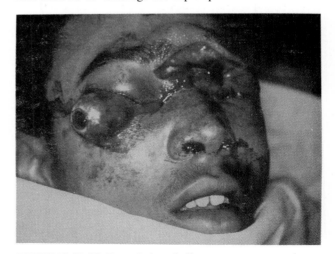

FIGURE 17-18 Extruded eyeball.

1. Cover the eye with a moist covering and a protective cup without applying pressure to the eye.

2. Apply a bandage compress or roller bandage that covers both eyes.

3. Transport the patient face up with the head immobilized.

☐ OTHER EYE INJURIES

In virtually all other medical emergencies involving the eye, you need only patch the affected eye and transport the patient to the hospital. While many of these represent critical emergencies, there is little that you can accomplish besides safeguarding the eye from further irritation. Such situations include:

- Eye infections — these are manifested by redness and discharge of pus.

- Acute **glaucoma** — the patient complains of eyeache, headache, nausea, and of seeing halos around lights. His eye is red, his pupil does not react to light, and his cornea is hazy. His eyeball is much harder — more swollen — than the "normal," soft-feeling eye. Glaucoma is an emergency that leads to blindness.

- **Retinal detachment** — the patient complains of a curtain blocking his field of vision, together with light flashes or dark spots in front of his eyes. In this situation, *gentle transport* is crucial. The patient should lie flat on his back on the stretcher, and every effort must be made to avoid bumps, bounces, or sudden stops.

- **Black eye** — any blow forceful enough to cause hemorrhage to the skin surrounding the eye may also damage the eye itself. There will be immediate swelling, tenderness, and discoloration. It is difficult to determine whether the eyeball has been injured. One way is to ask the patient details about his eyesight. Vision is blurred in the ordinary black eye. However, if the opposing eye is covered and the sight in the black eye is impaired, the eyeball has probably been damaged. Double vision with both eyes open also indicates eyeball damage. Transport the patient immediately.

- Cornea abrasion — depending on the severity of the scrape, the patient may require transport to an emergency room, usually to obtain medication for pain relief. Bandage both eyes; place a metal shield or cardboard over the injured eye to protect it. Any manipulation of the eye or the tissues surrounding it can cause permanent vision loss. Continue to calmly reassure the patient.

- **Light burns** — welding flash, **snow blindness. Ultraviolet light burns** of the cornea can be frighteningly painful, and they usually do not cause pain or signs and symptoms until three to six hours after exposure. The patient will complain of severe pain that feels like sand in the eyes. Symptoms will disappear in two to five days. These patients need treatment within six hours to fully restore eyesight. The patient should be kept in a dark room to avoid additional exposure. The pain may be decreased by closing the eyelids and covering both eyes with moist dressings and dark patches. Have the patient lie flat during transport to the hospital.

- **Heat burns** — the eyelids may be the only area burned in a heat burn. Do not attempt to open the eyelids if they are burned. The eye should be loosely covered with a sterile, moist dressing, and the patient should be transported immediately.

☐ BASIC RULES FOR EMERGENCY EYE CARE

Remember these basic rules when giving emergency eye care:

- Do not irrigate the injured eye. *The obvious exception is a chemical or detergent injury to the eye.* If the injury does not involve chemicals, you will only end up scratching the eye surface. If the eye has been perforated, damage incurred in washing it could be irreversible.

- Do not put salves or medicine into the injured eye. They will probably do more harm than good. The physician is better equipped to administer medication.

- Do not remove blood or blood clots from the eye. Blood contains antiseptics that will help the injured eye. Sponge blood from the face to help keep the patient comfortable. Leave the eye alone.

- Do not try to force the eyelid open unless you have to wash out chemicals.

- Have the patient lie down and keep quiet. Never let a patient with an eye injury walk without help, especially up or down stairs.

- Limit use of the *uninjured* eye; it is usually best to patch it along with the injured eye. Eyes move together, and if the patient is using one eye, chances are the other one is moving, too.

- Do not allow the patient to eat. In case general anesthesia is required at the hospital, food in the stomach will complicate the procedure.

- Never panic. It will upset the patient and cause you to lose valuable calmness needed in effective care.

- Any eye emergency should be seen by a physician.

☐ REMOVING CONTACT LENSES

An estimated 18 million Americans wear contact lenses of some type. Some patients wear a contact lens in only one eye, so be sure to examine *both* eyes carefully; do not dismiss the possibility of contact lenses after examining only one eye. Some patients, especially the elderly, wear both contact lenses and eyeglasses — so do not dismiss the possibility of contact lenses just because the patient is wearing eyeglasses. In most emergencies, the transport time will be short enough to allow emergency department personnel to remove the lenses.

To detect lenses, shine a penlight into the eye: a soft lens will show up as a shadow on the outer portion of the eye, while a hard lens will show up as a shadow over the iris.

Contact lenses should be removed if:

- There has been a chemical burn to the eye (the lens can trap chemicals and make irrigation difficult).
- The patient is unconscious and is wearing hard contact lenses, and if the transport time will be lengthy.

Contact lenses should *not* be removed if:

- There has been any injury to the eye. To do so may further aggravate the injury.
- The transport time is short enough to allow emergency department personnel to remove the lens.

Always follow local protocol in determining when and if contact lenses should be removed.

Different types of contact lenses are handled in different ways. Remember — do not use force, and be sure that your hands are clean.

Removing Hard Contact Lenses

Hard contact lenses are the most common. They are about the size of a shirt button and fit over the cornea. They can be removed by the following method (Figure 17-19):

1. Separate the eyelids.
2. Position the visible lens over the cornea by manipulating the eyelids.
3. Place your thumbs gently on the top and bottom eyelids, and open the eyelids wide.
4. Gently press the eyelids down and forward to the edges of the lens.
5. Press the lower eyelid slightly harder, and move it under the bottom edge of the lens.

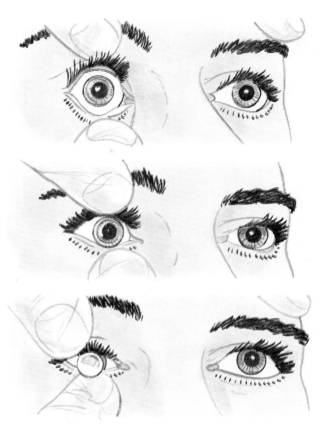

FIGURE 17-19 Removing hard corneal contact lenses.

6. Move the eyelids toward each other, with the lens sliding out between them.
7. Remove the lens, and put it in a safe place.
8. A suction cup moistened with saline can also be used to remove hard contact lenses (Figure 17-20).

Even though they are designed for extended wear, soft contact lenses can cause damage if left in for an extended time. Over time, they can gradually dehydrate and shrink, adhering to the cornea and making removal difficult.

Removing Flexible (Soft) Contact Lenses

These lenses are the second most common in use. They are just slightly larger than a dime and cover all of the cornea and some of the sclera. They are less dangerous than the hard lenses when left in the eye. They can be removed by placing several drops of saline on to the lens and then gently lifted off by pinching the lens between the thumb and index finger or in the following manner (Figure 17-21):

1. Place your middle fingertip on the lower lid, and pull down.

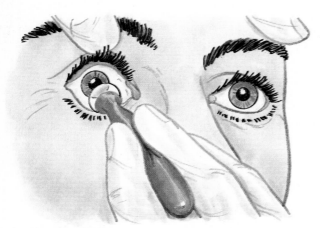

FIGURE 17-20 Using a moistened suction cup to remove hard contact lens.

2. Place your index fingertip on the lower edge of the lens, then slide the lens down to the sclera, or white of the eye.
3. Compress the lens gently between your thumb and index finger.
4. Gently pinch the lens, allowing air to enter underneath, and remove it from the eye.
5. Store in a water or saline solution.

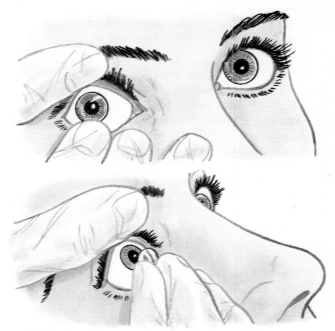

FIGURE 17-21 Removing flexible contact lenses.

6. If the lens has dehydrated, run sterile saline across the eye surface, slide the lens off the cornea, and pinch it up for removal.

chapter 18

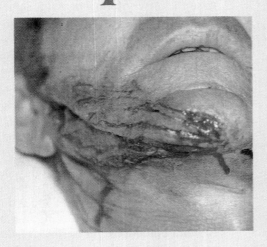

Injuries to the Face and Throat

✳ OBJECTIVES

- Describe how facial and throat injuries can lead to airway obstruction and spinal injury.
- Describe and demonstrate how to provide emergency care for various types of face and throat injuries, including care for avulsed teeth and facial fractures.
- Describe and demonstrate how to care for avulsed teeth.
- Describe and demonstrate how to care for facial fractures.

It is recommended that EMTs wear protective gloves whenever there is a possibility of coming in contact with a patient's blood, body fluids, mucous membranes, traumatic wounds, or sores. See Chapter 31.

☐ INJURIES TO THE FACE

The specialized structures of the face, prone to injury because of their location, can be permanently and irreversibly damaged. Injuries to the face are quite common: approximately 75 percent of all those involved in motor vehicle accidents sustain at least minor facial trauma. While some injuries to the face are minor, many face and throat injuries are life-threatening because they compromise the upper airway, impairing the patient's ability to breathe. In addition, many injuries of the face and throat stem from impacts strong enough to cause cervical spine damage or skull fracture (Figures 18-1 and 18-2).

In treating facial injury, it is helpful to determine the mechanism of injury, including the force and angle. While you should not waste precious time in the field conducting a thorough investigation, knowing the basic mechanism of injury can help you detect hidden injuries to facial bones.

Emergency Care

The greatest danger in facial wounds is compromise to airway and respiration. If the jaw is crushed or fractured, you may not have a clear path to the throat, which differentiates facial trauma from many other types of trauma. Care for injuries to the face the same way as for other soft-tissue injuries, with these distinctions:

1. Check the airway — foreign bodies, the tongue, fractures, swelling, and bleeding can all compromise the airway following facial injury. Suction as necessary to remove blood or foreign material.

2. Completely immobilize the neck to prevent aggravation of possible cervical spine injuries, which can accompany facial injuries.

3. Control bleeding with pressure; apply extremely gentle pressure if you suspect that bones beneath the wound may have been fractured or shattered (especially if the brain may be damaged by bone fragments).

4. Turn the patient prone or on one side, face down to facilitate drainage of blood; suction the patient as necessary. If you suspect spinal injury, immobilize the patient before turning him or her, or log roll and immobilize on his or her side.

5. Use dressings and pressure bandages for wounds of the face.

6. If nerves, tendons, or blood vessels have been exposed, cover them with a moist, sterile bandage.

7. Injuries to the mouth that involve bleeding are especially serious, because blood running down the throat can choke the patient or cause him or her to vomit.

☐ Injuries of the Face

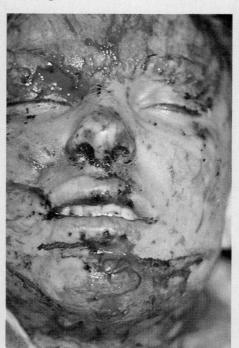

FIGURE 18-1

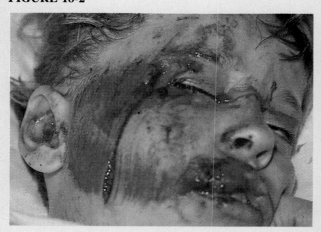

FIGURE 18-2

- Tilt the patient's head, and lift his or her chin to maintain the airway. Use modified jaw thrust to open airway if spinal injury is suspected.

8. Check for avulsed teeth, and salvage them if you can.

9. Monitor carefully for facial edema that could compromise breathing.
   - If the patient shows signs of respiratory distress (such as noisy breathing, cool skin, or cyanosis), position in a high **Fowler's position.**
   - Tilt the head forward to promote drainage.

   If the patient is unconscious:
   - Pull the tongue forward.
   - Insert a nasopharyngeal airway.
   - Administer humidified oxygen.

10. Remember that facial trauma can be very upsetting to the patient and brings with it fears of disfigurement. Treat the patient with understanding and reassurance.

Transportation of a Patient with Facial Injuries

Some facial injuries are relatively minor and require no special positioning of the patient. Since respiratory difficulty is often associated with this type of injury, the patient may be transported in the lateral recumbent position with the head low or tilted to aid drainage. If there are indications of spinal and/or neck injuries, fully immobilize the patient using a cervical collar and long spine board. Continuous suctioning may be required. When the facial soft tissues are injured, there may be underlying facial bone fractures. Take care to transport the patient so that no unnecessary pressure is placed on facial injury sites (Figure 18-3). Monitor the patient and be alert for airway problems.

☐ TRAUMA TO THE MOUTH AND JAW

In patients with trauma to the mouth and jaw, it is *essential* to immobilize the head and neck with a backboard, extrication collar, and **lateral immobilizer** (such as rolled towels) to protect against aggravation of cervical spine and spinal injuries, which commonly accompany this kind of trauma.

Patients who sustain significant trauma to the face may also have fractures of the jaw and damage to or loss of teeth. Therefore, you must examine the entire face and mouth carefully to determine the extent of injury (Figures 18-4–18-7). When the **mandible** (lower jaw) is fractured, it is generally broken in at least two places and will be unstable when you examine it. Bruising and swelling may be obvious.

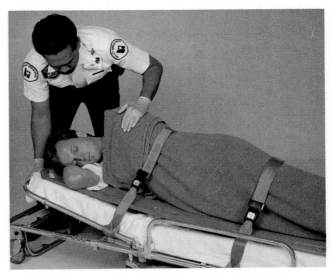

FIGURE 18-3 Transporting the conscious facial injury patient.

Fracture of the **maxilla** (upper jaw) is often accompanied by a "black eye." The face may appear elongated, and the patient's bite will no longer be even, but rather open. Again, swelling may be noticeable.

Emergency Care

In any case of severe facial trauma, suspect cervical spine trauma; immobilize the cervical spine early in treatment. An added benefit of cervical spine immobilization is the stabilization of facial bones. Emergency care in the field is aimed at insuring an airway.

1. Establish an airway. Artificial airways can force debris further down the throat and can aggravate existing injuries.
   - Inspect the mouth for small fragments of teeth or broken dentures, bits of bone, pieces of flesh, or fragments of foreign objects (such as pieces of broken glass) on which the patient might choke. Remove them as thoroughly as possible.
   - In facial injury, the tongue may lose its support structure and may flap back, covering the opening to the throat. If so, pull it forward to open the airway. If you have trouble grasping the tongue, you can accomplish the same goal by pulling the chin forward or by grasping the angle of the jaw and pressing it forward.
   - Suction any blood from the mouth and throat. The face, richly supplied with blood vessels, may bleed profusely and freely, even from a relatively minor wound. Suction the throat frequently throughout treatment and transport to keep it clear.

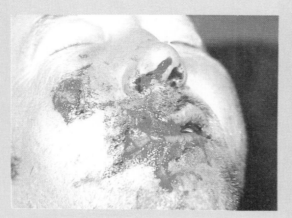

FIGURE 18-4

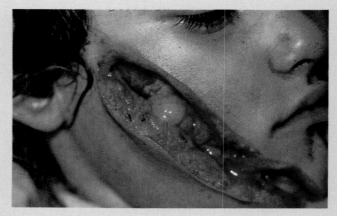

FIGURE 18-5

FIGURE 18-6

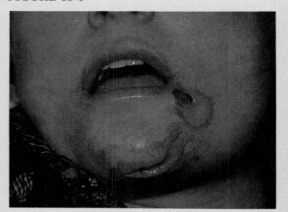

FIGURE 18-7

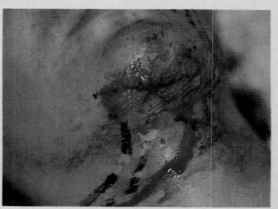

2. Control hemorrhage. Several major arteries run through the face, and they can bleed profusely and rapidly enough to cause death. Use compression and compression dressings to control bleeding from smaller wounds.

3. Examine the mouth for broken or missing teeth.

- If a tooth has been lost, try to find it. A surgeon can reimplant a tooth within two hours, and can use bone fragments to reconstruct the skull.

- If you find a missing tooth, save and transport it. If the patient is totally conscious, cooperative, and unhysterical, have the patient hold the tooth under the tongue until he or she reaches the hospital. Follow local protocol. In other situations, rinse the tooth with saline to gently remove any debris (**never** scrub the tooth). You can also transport the tooth wrapped in gauze that has been soaked in sterile saline. Never wrap the tooth in dry gauze, and guard against the tooth drying out.

- Never handle the tooth by the root; there may still be ligament fibers attached that could enable successful reimplantation.

- If you cannot find teeth that have been knocked out, assume that the patient has swallowed or aspirated them until proven otherwise.

- Control bleeding from the socket with a gauze pad.

- If dentures are in and unbroken, leave them in place — they can help support the structures of the mouth. If dentures are broken, remove them. Transport any dentures or pieces of dentures with the patient so the surgeon can use them to establish proper alignment when wiring the jaw.

☐ FRACTURES OF THE FACE AND LOWER JAW

Maxillofacial fractures may be simple — such as undisplaced nasal fractures — or extensive, involving severe lacerations, bony fractures, and nerve damage (Figure 18-8). Patients with maxillofacial injury will require assistance and transport to the hospital emergency room.

The first priority in caring for a patient with maxillofacial injury is establishing and maintaining the airway. Airway can be compromised in maxillofacial injury patients by blood, edema, or structural defects. Maxillofacial injuries are rarely life-threatening, but in major trauma, another part of the body may sustain a serious injury. Consider and examine the entire patient:

1. Before considering any care, examine the patient

FIGURE 18-8

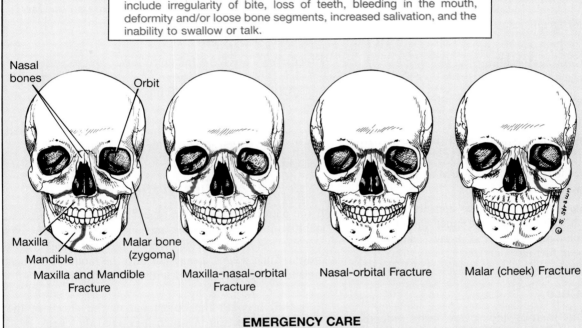

FACIAL FRACTURES

Facial fractures often result from impact injuries to the face. The main danger of facial fractures is airway problems. Bone fragments and blood may obstruct the airway. Common signs of a fractured jaw may include irregularity of bite, loss of teeth, bleeding in the mouth, deformity and/or loose bone segments, increased salivation, and the inability to swallow or talk.

Nasal bones
Orbit
Maxilla
Mandible
Malar bone (zygoma)

Maxilla and Mandible Fracture

Maxilla-nasal-orbital Fracture

Nasal-orbital Fracture

Malar (cheek) Fracture

EMERGENCY CARE

Emergency care is the same as for soft-tissue injuries with special attention to clearing the airway of any obstructing materials, teeth, blood, etc.

- Maintain open airway, allowing for drainage if necessary.
- If necessary, assist ventilation. Control bleeding with as little pressure as is necessary so as not to displace fractures. The use of the temporal and facial pressure points may be necessary.
- Always suspect and assess for spinal injuries, and take necessary immobilization precautions.
- Dress and bandage open wounds.
- Continually monitor airway.
- If necessary, immobilize mandible (lower jaw). However, if there is considerable bleeding in the mouth, it is best to not immobilize because it may compromise the airway.
- Keep patient quiet, and be very gentle so fracture areas will not displace or do further damage to other tissues.
- The patient who is not bleeding should be put in a semi-reclining position unless spinal injuries are suspected. Patients with bleeding facial injuries should be positioned on their sides with head turned down for draining.
- Assess for other possible injuries.
-

for possible cervical, thoracic, and lumbar spine fracture or injury.

2. Check for tearing or rupture of the eyeball — common in patients who wear contact lenses and who have suffered facial trauma.

3. Check for facial burns — they indicate pulmonary smoke and heat inhalation. Attempts at suctioning the throat can cause swelling, so be especially gentle.

The Face

Whenever there is significant laceration on the face, suspect underlying fracture. Signs and symptoms of maxilla fracture include movement of the maxilla, nosebleed, black eyes, numbness of the upper lip or cheek, and eyes that appear to be unlevel. The signs and symptoms of other facial fractures include:

- Distortion of facial features.
- Numbness or pain.
- Severe bruising and swelling.
- Bleeding from nose and mouth.
- Limited jaw motion.
- Teeth do not meet normally.
- Double vision when bone around the eye is fractured.
- Irregularities in the facial bones that can be felt before swelling occurs.
- The distance between the eyes appears too wide (the ligament that attaches the inner corner of the eyelid to the bone can break away, causing the eyes to appear further apart).

Emergency Care

Especially in blunt injuries and severe facial wounds, emergency care objectives are to control hemorrhage and clear the airway.

1. Clear the airway. With both conscious and unconscious patients if no neck injury exists, support the head with your hand, pull the jaw or jaw fragments upward, and hold the tongue down and forward. Remove dentures and foreign debris from the mouth.

2. Check for neck and spinal injuries.

3. After immobilizing for neck or spinal injuries, position the patient to allow for drainage.

4. Use suction to drain fluid from the back of the pharynx.

5. Place bandages carefully to allow for vomiting and blood drainage.

The Lower Jaw

Fracture to the lower jaw can result from a blunt instrument, a blow from the fist, an automobile accident, or a gunshot wound. Signs and symptoms of lower-jaw fractures are (Figure 18-9):

- The patient's mouth is usually open, but he may be unable to open the mouth.
- Saliva mixed with blood may flow from the corners of the mouth; the patient will find it difficult to stop drooling, since pain prevents him from swallowing.
- Talking is painful and difficult.
- Teeth are often missing, loosened, or uneven.
- Even if teeth are not missing, the patient will complain that teeth do not "fit together right."
- There may be pain in the areas around the ears.

Emergency Care

Emergency care for a fractured lower jaw requires:

1. Clearing and maintaining an open airway.
2. Caring for open wounds.
3. Carefully immobilize the lower jaw with cervical collar or cravats. Monitor for vomiting. *Follow local protocol.*

Objects Impaled in the Cheek

If the patient has a foreign object impaled in the cheek, stabilize it with bulky dressings and transport. *If the object has penetrated all the way through the cheek and is loose* (which means it may fall into the mouth, obstructing the airway), remove it with this method:

1. Pull or push the object out of the cheek in the same direction in which it entered the cheek.

FIGURE 18-9 Soft-tissue injuries and fracture of the lower jaw.

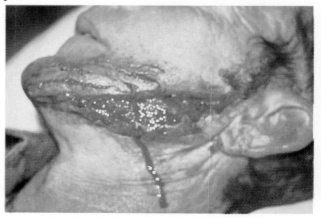

2. Pack dressing material between the patient's teeth and the wound; leave some of the dressing outside the mouth and tape it there to prevent the dressing from being swallowed. Monitor closely to make sure the dressing doesn't become loose and compromise the airway.

3. Dress and bandage the outside of the wound to control bleeding.

4. Suction frequently to remove blood.

□ INJURIES OF THE NOSE

Soft-tissue injuries of the nose should be cared for similar to other soft tissue injuries, with special care being taken to maintain an open airway and position the patient so that blood does not drain into the throat (Figures 18-10 and 18-11).

Nosebleeds

Nosebleeds are a relatively common reason for emergency calls. For complete information on managing nosebleed emergencies, see Chapter 7 on control of bleeding. Do not pack the nose; clear or bloody fluids can indicate skull fracture, and packing the nose can create dangerous pressure. In severe injury, be careful not to exert too much external pressure on the nose, which can push bone fragments deeper into the face.

Foreign Objects in the Nose

Foreign objects in the nose are usually a problem among small children. The best emergency care is to reassure and calm the child and parent, then transport the patient to the hospital.

Tissue damage and impaction can result from probing and inadequate attempts at removal. Special lighting and instruments available at the hospital minimize the risk of removal.

Nasal Fractures

The nose is the most commonly fractured bone in the face because of its delicate structure. A broken nose can usually be identified by swelling and deformity. To treat, apply ice compresses to reduce swelling, and transport.

□ INJURIES OF THE EAR

Cuts and lacerations of the ear occur frequently; occasionally, a section of the ear may be severed (Figures 18-12–18-13). Treat as for other soft tissue injuries. Save any avulsed parts and transport with the patient. Wrap avulsed parts in saline-soaked gauze. When dressing an injured ear, it is recommended that you place part of the dressing between the ear and the side of the head. As a general rule, don't probe into the ear.

Never pack the ear to stop bleeding from the ear canal. Clear or bloody fluid draining from the ear can indicate skull fracture. Place a loose, clean dressing across the opening of the ear to absorb blood, but do not exert pressure to stop the bleeding.

Foreign Objects in the Ear

Foreign objects in the **external ear** are a common problem among children. Some children have an irresistible

□ Injuries of the Nose

FIGURE 18-10

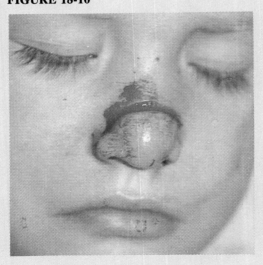

FIGURE 18-11

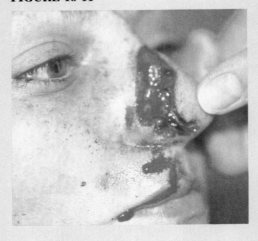

□ Injuries of the Ear

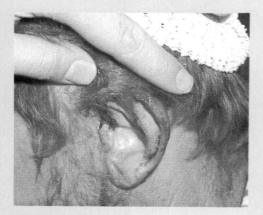

FIGURE 18-12

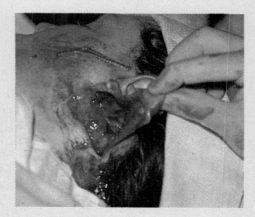

FIGURE 18-13

compulsion to stuff their ears with small objects, such as beans and peanuts. *Leave the ear alone,* and transport the patient to the hospital, where good lighting and appropriate equipment are available.

□ INJURIES OF THE THROAT

The throat can be injured by any crushing blow. Common causes include hanging (attempted suicide), impact with a steering wheel, or running or riding into a stretched wire or clothesline. The throat may also be lacerated, which may result in bleeding from a major artery or vein and air bubbles entering the blood vessels (Figures 18-14 and 18-15).

Besides obvious lacerations or other wounds, look for signs of an injured throat: displacement of the trachea to one side, obvious swelling or bruising, difficulty speaking (with crepitus sounds as air escapes from an injured larynx), loss of the voice, and airway obstruction that is not obvious from other sources (such obstruction is due to swelling of the throat).

Maintaining an airway is extremely important in

□ Injuries of the Throat

FIGURE 18-14

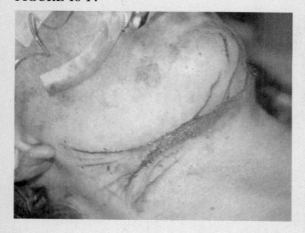

FIGURE 18-15

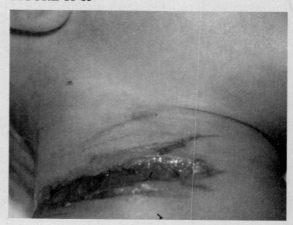

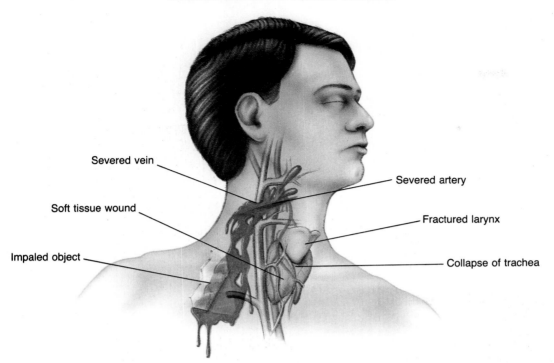

Severed vein

Soft tissue wound

Impaled object

Severed artery

Fractured larynx

Collapse of trachea

FIGURE 18-16

throat injuries, because blood clots when it is exposed to air and can threaten the airway (Figure 18-16).

Emergency Care

1. Suction out blood as needed, but keep suctioning time to an absolute minimum.
2. If breathing is impaired, give the patient 100 percent oxygen by face mask, and keep him or her calm. If necessary, assist the patient's breathing.
3. If tolerated by the patient and airway status, keep the patient lying down to lessen the chance of air entering the blood vessels. If you suspect venous bleeding, apply pressure above and below site to prevent air embolism.
4. Control bleeding with slight to moderate pressure and bulky dressings. If venous bleeding is profuse, some advocate use of an occlusive dressing with a figure-eight wrap of self-adherent roller bandage; *follow local protocol*. Be cautious of applying pressure — too much pressure will occlude carotid flow to the brain, slow heart rate due to vagal stimulation, or impede jugular outflow from the brain. Never apply pressure to both sides of the neck at the same time (Figures 18-17–18-25).
5. Position the patient on the left side with his head tilted downward at a fifteen-degree angle to trap any air bubbles that have entered the bloodstream.
6. Apply an occlusive dressing.
7. Treat for shock.
8. When treating bleeding wounds, never probe open wounds or use circumferential bandages which can interfere with blood flow on the uninjured side of the neck and can also impair respiration.
9. Transport the patient as soon as possible.

□ Emergency Care for Severed Neck Veins

NOTES:

1. For demonstration purposes, patient is upright.
2. Placing the patient on the left side in the Trendelenburg position will trap air emboli in the right atrium. Do not simply raise the legs. Tilt the entire body by 15°.
3. Bandaging should control bleeding without restricting breathing.
4. Dressing must be heavy plastic . . . sized to be no more than two inches larger in diameter than site.

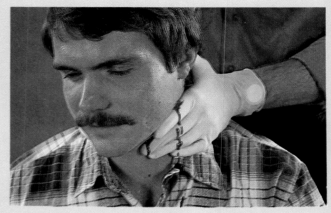

FIGURE 18-17 Do not delay! Place your gloved palm over the wound.

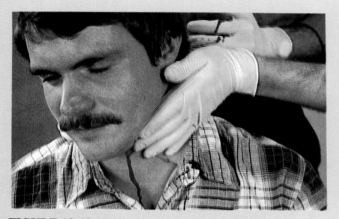

FIGURE 18-18 Apply pressure with a bulky dressing.

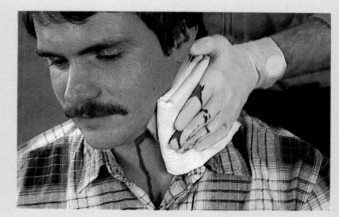

FIGURE 18-19 If venous bleeding is profuse, apply an occlusive dressing.

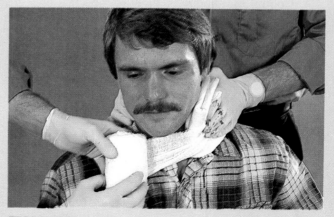

FIGURE 18-20 Start a figure-eight . . . bringing bandage over dressing.

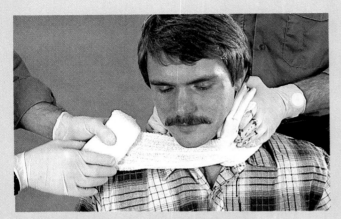

FIGURE 18-21 Cross over the shoulder . . .

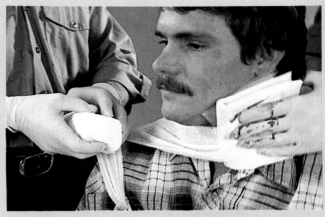

FIGURE 18-22 Bring bandage under the armpit.

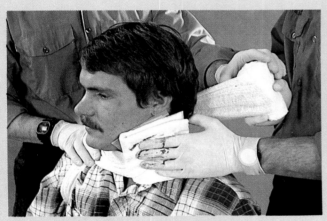

FIGURE 18-23 Cross back over shoulder and anchor several times to cover entire dressing.

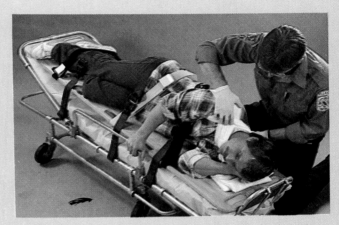

FIGURE 18-24 Place the patient on left side, tilting body to raise feet (Trendelenburg position).

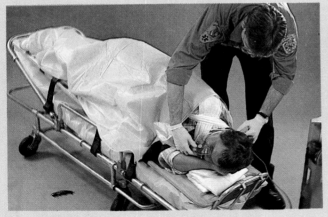

FIGURE 18-25 Care for shock and continue to administer a high concentration of oxygen.

chapter 19

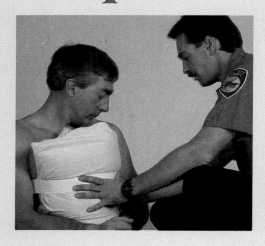

Injuries to the Chest

✳ OBJECTIVES

- ■ Review the anatomy of the chest cavity.
- ■ Identify signs and symptoms of chest injuries.
- ■ Describe the general emergency care principles for treatment of chest injuries.
- ■ Identify the specific types of chest injuries.
- ■ Describe appropriate emergency care for each type of chest injury.

□ ANATOMY OF THE CHEST

The chest is located in the upper part of the body, above the abdomen and below the neck, and is separated from the abdomen by the muscular wall of the diaphragm. The chest (thoracic) cavity contains the heart, lungs, and major blood vessels, which are protected by the bony cage of the ribs and the thoracic vertebrae. The ribs are connected to the vertebrae posteriorly, and all but two pairs are connected to the sternum anteriorly by cartilage. The esophagus and trachea pass through and into the chest from the throat, and the esophagus continues to the stomach (Figure 19-1).

Muscles between the ribs, called intercostal muscles, help change the size and shape of the rib cage and allow maximum expansion of the lungs during deep breathing. The rib cage encloses the lungs and heart. Damage to the ribs can result in injury to these organs, as can penetrating injuries that do not harm the ribs.

□ CHEST INJURIES

Chest injury is the second leading cause of death from trauma, second only to central nervous system injury. *All* chest injury should be considered life-threatening until proven otherwise, and you should always assume cardiac damage until it is ruled out. Victims of chest inury can look relatively fine, but can deteriorate suddenly and rapidly.

There are two general categories of chest injury: closed and open. In closed (blunt) chest injuries, the skin remains unbroken; it can be caused by a wide range of accidents, and commonly occurs from the blunt trauma of being struck by a falling object, being buried in a cave-in, or being thrown against a steering wheel in an automobile accident. Although the skin may not sustain any lacerations, serious underlying damage can occur, especially lacerations to the heart and lungs when deceleration forces them against the ribs. Any time the chest has fractures or wounds, suspect significant underlying injury.

Approximately 80 percent of all blunt trauma results from motor vehicle accidents. Blunt trauma, potentially deadly, distributes the force of trauma over a large area; it includes complications such as bruising of the heart and/or lung tissue, flail chest, pneumothorax, hemothorax, collapsed lungs, and injury to the aorta and other major vessels (Figure 19-2). If you suspect any of these, notify the receiving physician and transport immediately.

In an open (penetrating) chest injury, the skin is broken, usually by a bullet or knife or the end of a broken rib protruding through the skin. A bullet can cause substantial damage if it mushrooms, tumbles, or fragments in the body. A knife or other penetrating object damages the tissues and organs along the path of penetration; if it is dull, it tears or rips, and if sharp, it lacerates.

Remember: the most visually disturbing or alarming injuries are usually not the most life-threatening ones.

□ GENERAL SIGNS AND SYMPTOMS OF CHEST INJURY

Whether the injury is open or closed, certain signs and symptoms will occur in major chest trauma, many of them simultaneously. The major signs and symptoms of chest trauma include (Figure 19-3):

- Cyanosis (bluish coloring of the fingernails, fingertips, lips, or skin).
- Dyspnea (shortness of breath or difficulty in breathing).
- Rapid, weak pulse more than 120 beats per minute, indicating shock; people with pacemakers, cardiac injuries, cardiac medications, or central nervous system injury may not develop tachycardia, even though they are in severe shock.
- Tracheal deviation.

FIGURE 19-1 The rib cage encloses the lungs and heart, and damage to the ribs can result in damage to these organs, as can penetrating injuries that do not injure the ribs.

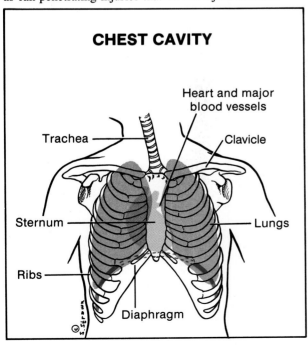

CHEST CAVITY

Heart and major blood vessels

Trachea

Clavicle

Sternum

Lungs

Ribs

Diaphragm

SIGNS, SYMPTOMS AND EMERGENCY CARE OF CHEST INJURIES

HEMOTHORAX

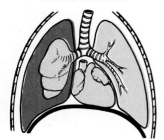

Blood leaks into the chest cavity from lacerated vessels or the lung itself and the lung compresses.

PNEUMOTHORAX

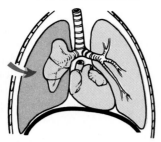

Air enters the chest cavity through a sucking wound or leaks from a lacerated lung. The lung cannot expand.

SPONTANEOUS PNEUMOTHORAX

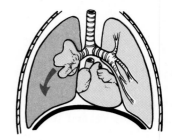

Air leaks into the chest from a weak area in the (nontrauma) lung surface and the lung collapses.

TENSION PNEUMOTHORAX

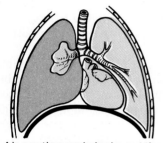

Air continuously leaks out the lung. It collapses, pressure rises, and the collapsed lung is forced against the heart and other lung.

MEDIASTINAL SHIFT

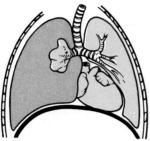

Usually caused by severe tension pneumothorax.

HEMOPNEUMOTHORAX

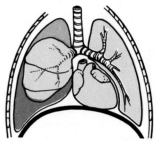

Air and blood leak into the chest cavity from an injured lung putting pressure on heart and uninjured lung.

GENERAL SIGNS AND SYMPTOMS

- Obvious trauma
- Chest or back pain at injury site
- Dyspnea: shortness of breath and difficulty in breathing
- Cough, with or without frothy blood
- Failure of chest to expand normally during respiration
- Marked cyanosis of fingernails and tips and/or tongue and lips
- Rapid weak pulse
- Low blood pressure
- Shock
- Sudden sharp pain which may be referred to shoulder, across chest and to abdomen
- Deviation of larynx and trachea from midline
- Distended neck veins
- Sucking sound when patient breaths
- Bloodshot and bulging eyes
- Purplish blue color of the head, neck and shoulders
- These signs may be indicative of serious emergency, however usually only few of the signs will be manifested at any one time.

FIGURE 19-2

LACERATED AORTA

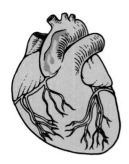

Lacerations of the great or major blood vessels.

TRAUMATIC ASPHYXIA

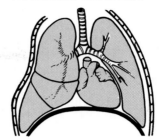

Severe chest compression puts pressure on heart and forces blood back into veins of the neck. It may cause severe lung damage.

PERICARDIAL TAMPONADE

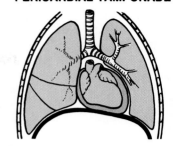

Blood or other fluid in the pericardial sac outside the heart exerts pressure on the heart.

TRAUMATIC EMPHYSEMA

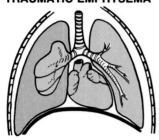

A sudden compression injury occurs when the glottis is closed. The air sacs (alveoli) in the lungs rupture and leak air.

LUNG CONTUSION

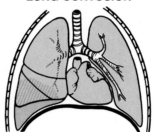

Usually caused by high velocity blunt trauma with bruising and bleeding from the lung.

RUPTURED DIAPHRAGM

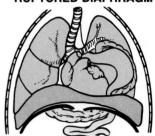

Usually caused by blunt trauma to one side or multiple trauma, often involving the pelvis.

EMERGENCY CARE

- Remove clothing to assess for open wounds; always check for an exit wound on back.
- Maintain an open airway and assist with ventilation.
- Administer high flow oxygen with a mask.
- Seal any open sucking wounds with an occlusive dressing (plastic wrap, aluminum foil, vaseline, gauze, etc.) leaving a corner untaped. *Follow local protocol*. If necessary, seal the wound with your gloved hands until proper dressing can be prepared.
- Be alert for tension pneumothorax. If it develops unseal the dressing for a few seconds to release pressure, then reseal.
- Do not remove impaled objects; stabilize with bulky dressings and bandage in place.
- Care for other bleeding and wounds with direct pressure and appropriate dressings, bandaged in place.
- Treat for shock.
- Continually monitor vital signs.
- Calm and reassure patient.
- Be alert for vomiting, coughing of blood and secretions from the mouth. Prevent aspiration and be ready for suctioning.
- Put the patient in semi-reclining position or lying on his injured side if breathing is easier and/or you suspect internal bleeding.
- Transport immediately.

S. Strawn © 1983

FIGURE 19-2 (Continued)

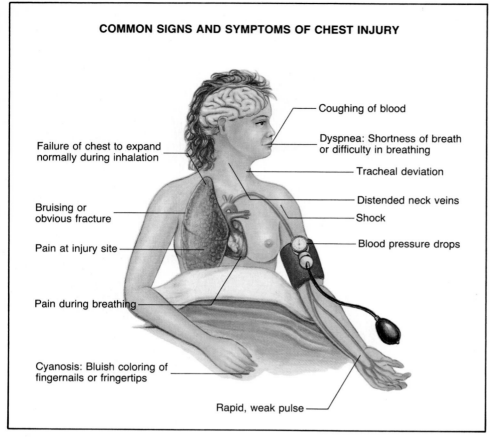

COMMON SIGNS AND SYMPTOMS OF CHEST INJURY

Failure of chest to expand normally during inhalation

Bruising or obvious fracture

Pain at injury site

Pain during breathing

Cyanosis: Bluish coloring of fingernails or fringertips

Coughing of blood

Dyspnea: Shortness of breath or difficulty in breathing

Tracheal deviation

Distended neck veins

Shock

Blood pressure drops

Rapid, weak pulse

FIGURE 19-3

- Pain during breathing.
- Distended neck veins.
- Pain at the injury site or pain near an injury that is made worse by breathing.
- Coughing up of blood **(hemoptysis),** usually bright red and frothy.
- Failure of chest (one or both sides) to expand normally during inhalation.
- Pale, cool skin, often moist (a sign of shock).
- Low blood pressure, indicating shock; blood pressure may remain high due to compensation until there is 20 percent blood loss.
- Bruising or obvious fracture.
- Changing mental status, including confusion, uncooperative behavior, irrational behavior, agitation, and restlessness.

Two of the most important signs are the respiratory rate and any change in the normal breathing pattern. Depending on the physical fitness of the patient, he or she breathes normally (in an uninjured state) from twelve to twenty times each minute without strain, pain, or difficulty. If a patient breathes more than twenty-four times per minute, experiences pain when breathing, or finds it difficult to take a deep breath, the patient has probably sustained a chest injury.

Broken ribs, bruising of the lungs, or severe lung disease can cause pain in the chest that is aggravated by breathing. Shortness of breath may be caused by failure of the chest to expand normally, fully, or properly; by obstruction of the airway; by compression of a lung (due to blood or air within the chest cavity); by loss of nervous control over breathing; or by lung disease (such as chronic obstructive pulmonary disease).

The failure of the chest wall to expand properly may result from direct injury to the chest wall, injury to the nerves that control the chest wall muscles, or injury to the part of the brain that controls respirations.

Laceration of lung tissue allows blood to seep into the lungs; the patient tries to clear it out by coughing. A patient coughing up blood may have lacerated tissue of the lungs or the bronchial tubes.

☐ GENERAL PRINCIPLES FOR TREATMENT OF CHEST INJURIES

Provide the following general emergency care for chest injuries:

1. Maintain an open airway; assess for obstruction from foreign objects (including broken teeth or

dentures), blood, mucus, or inflammation of the throat. Suction, and repeat the suction periodically, since the patient's status can change suddenly. Your first priority is to ensure adequate air circulation.

2. If necessary, administer mouth-to-mouth ventilation or supplemental oxygen and assist ventilations.

3. Control external bleeding; a patient who has sustained chest injury could be the victim of multiple injuries, so perform a quick assessment to detect *any* source of external bleeding.

4. Dress penetrating chest wounds as described later.

5. If there is an impaled object in the chest, stabilize and bandage in place.

   • Cut away clothing to expose the wound.

   • Dress the wound around the impaled object to control bleeding and prevent a sucking chest wound.

   • Stabilize the impaled object with rolls of self-adhering bandages or bulky dressings.

   • Tape bandages in place to stabilize the impaled object.

6. Transport the patient as soon as he or she is stabilized.

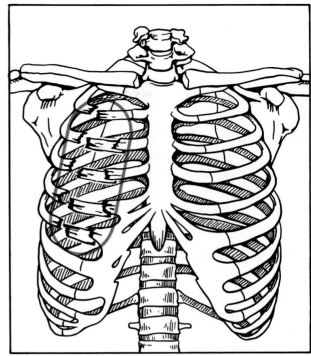

FIGURE 19-4 Flail chest occurs when blunt trauma causes fracture of two of more ribs, in more than one place.

□ FLAIL CHEST

Flail chest results when the chest wall becomes unstable due to fractures of the sternum (breastbone), the cartilage connecting the ribs to the sternum, and/or the ribs. It can affect the front, back, or sides of the rib cage. It most often occurs when two or more adjacent ribs are broken, each in two or more places; the segment of chest wall between them becomes free-floating. The free-floating segment is referred to as the "flail area," and the motion of that area is opposite the motion of the rest of the chest (Figure 19-4). When the patient inhales, the area collapses or does not expand; when he or she exhales, it protrudes while the rest of the chest wall contracts. This produces an unstable chest wall segment which markedly interferes with ventilation (**paradoxical breathing**) (Figure 19-5). The chest muscles may spasm and "splint" the chest, making it difficult to assess and notice paradoxical breathing.

Flail chest can be a life-threatening injury because it usually involves bruising of the lung tissues beneath the flail area and can lead to inadequate oxygenation of the heart. The fractured bone ends may also puncture a lung. Flail chest may involve serious intrathoracic bleeding from the costal arteries and veins, which can lead to shock. The patient must be stabilized and transported as rapidly as possible to a medical facility.

Signs and symptoms of flail chest include:

• Paradoxical breathing, almost always accompanied by severe pain.

• Swelling over the injured area.

• Signs of shock.

• Increasing airway resistance.

• Patient's attempt to splint the chest wall with his or her hands and arms.

• Pain and tenderness at the injury site.

• Possible crepitus from the bone ends rubbing together.

Signs that the heart has also been injured include cyanosis of the head, neck, shoulders, lips, and tongue; bulging neck veins; bulging, bloodshot eyes; and obvious deformity of the chest.

To check for flail chest, have the patient lie on his or her back. Place your hands gently on the patient's chest and neck for symmetry of the sides as he or she breathes. Bare his or her chest and stand at the patient's feet, watching for a seesaw motion of the chest while the patient breathes. It can be extremely difficult to detect flail chest in an obese or muscular person. Remember, flail chest can be excruciating — the patient may not want to relinquish guarding of his chest.

Injuries to the Chest   **315**

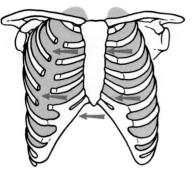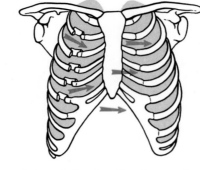

FLAIL CHEST: PARADOXICAL BREATHING

EXPIRATION	INSPIRATION
Injured chest wall moves out Uninjured chest wall moves in	Injured chest wall collapses in Uninjured chest wall moves out

EMERGENCY CARE

- Have patient lie on back.
- Remove clothing from chest area.
- Tape a small pillow or thick, heavy dressing over the injury site.
- Maintain open airway and assist ventilations as needed.
- Administer high concentration, positive-pressure oxygen.
- Treat for shock.
- Regularly monitor vital signs.
- Transport patient in semi-sitting position if you suspect internal bleeding; or if the patient has increased pain and discomfort in semi-sitting position, transport patient lying on the injured side.

FIGURE 19-5

Emergency Care

If you suspect that the heart has been injured, transport must be undelayed and rapid. To treat flail chest:

1. Maintain an open airway and administer high-concentration, positive-pressure, humidified oxygen. Vigorous oxygen therapy is often needed.

2. Use *gentle* palpation to locate the edges of the flail section.

3. Stabilize the flail site with a pad of dressings or a pillow; the stabilizing object must weigh less than five pounds (Figure 19-6). Secure it with wide cravats, straps, or tape to increase patient comfort. Keep the straps loose — restrictive dressings can impair breathing.

4. Position the patient with a flail segment against external support in a semi-sitting position or lying on injured side if sitting position causes discomfort (Figure 19-7).

5. Monitor vital signs closely; treat for shock.

6. Transport immediately. If you suspect internal bleeding, and the patient experiences severe pain lying on the injured side, transport in a semi-sitting position.

☐ PULMONARY (LUNG) CONTUSIONS

Pulmonary (lung) contusions are the most common potentially lethal chest injuries. They cause blood and edematous fluid to ooze into the lungs, resulting in a number of serious lung conditions, including collapse or compression of one or both lungs (see Figure 19-2). Oxygen and carbon dioxide exchange are compromised in the bruised area. Surgical repair is needed to relieve the condition.

Patients experiencing direct blows to the chest or severe blunt trauma to the chest probably have lung contusions; they can also result from crushing injuries, blast injuries, and rapid deceleration injuries. The amount of distress depends on the amount of damaged tissue. Look for signs of blunt trauma or other injuries, such as bruis-

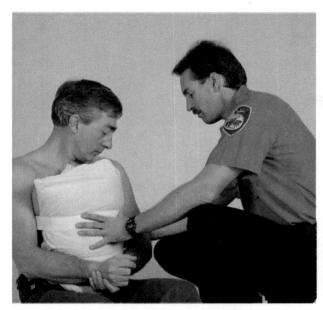

FIGURE 19-6 Stabilize flail chest by applying a pillow or bulky dressing and transport in a semi-sitting position.

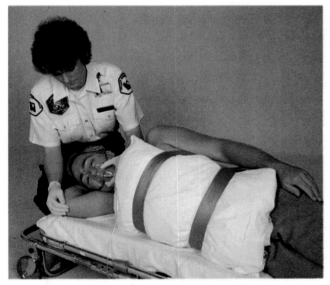

FIGURE 19-7 Position patient with flail chest in a lying position, on injured side, if sitting position causes discomfort.

ing, abrasions, and lacerations. Signs and symptoms include chest pain and the following:

- Severe shortness of breath.
- Rapid pulse.
- Cyanosis.
- Rapidly developing shock.

Emergency Care

The victim of pulmonary contusion invariably deteriorates — often rapidly. Because surgical repair is required, little can be done for the victim in the field.

Your main treatment goals should be as follows:

1. Maintain an open airway and administer positive-pressure oxygen as needed.
2. Stabilize the patient.
3. Transport immediately.
4. Report mechanism of injury if known.

☐ HEART (MYOCARDIAL) CONTUSION

The most common cardiac injury following blunt trauma to the chest is myocardial contusion, which involves actual bruising of the heart muscles. Such bruising disturbs the electrical conduction system of the heart, which controls the heart rate. You should always suspect myocardial contusion in a victim of blunt chest trauma who has pulse abnormalities (Figure 19-8).

Signs and symptoms of myocardial contusion are much like myocardial infarction, and include:

- Generalized chest pain.
- Obvious bruising on the chest wall.
- Angina.
- Rapid heartbeat.
- Irregular pulse.
- Dysrhythmias.

Emergency Care

To treat victims of myocardial contusion:

1. Stabilize the patient as rapidly as possible.
2. Transport immediately.
3. During transport, maintain an open airway, administer oxygen, and initiate CPR if necessary. Monitor pulse for abnormal rhythms.

☐ PERICARDIAL TAMPONADE

Any force great enough to bruise the heart muscle can also potentially lead to leakage of blood and other fluid from the heart into the pericardial sac surrounding the heart. The pericardial sac is relatively nondistensible; normally, it contains lubricating fluid, but if blood accumulates in it, the heart is squeezed until it cannot completely fill. If it reduces the heart's ability to pump blood, it is called a pericardial tamponade.

The most common cause of **pericardial tamponade** is a penetrating wound caused by a knife or bullet;

TRAUMATIC CARDIAC INJURIES

Trauma to the chest can induce three types of cardiac injury.
Determining the nature of the injury is difficult and emergency
care in the field is frequently limited to support of vital functions.

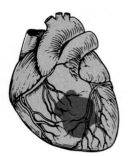

SIGNS AND SYMPTOMS

Cardiac Contusion

Injury to chest
Dislocation of chest wall
Weakness, rapid heart rate
Possible myocardial infarction
Possible sweating
Severe nagging pain not relieved with rest
    but may be relieved with oxygen

Penetrating Wound in Heart

In most cases, patient has a visible chest
    wound, caused by object like knife or
    bullet.
However, heart penetration can occur from
    bullet entering abdomen or back
Chest pain, bleeding
Drowsiness, loss of consciousness, possible
    agitation, combativeness, or confusion
    (Note: patient may appear intoxicated)
Distended neck veins, although these may
    not be present immediately
Pneumothorax or hemothorax (may not
    develop until several hours after the
    injury).
Hypovolemic shock

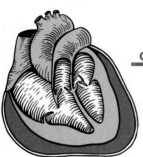

Cardiac Tamponade

Cardiac contusion, blunt trauma to anterior
    chest, penetrating chest wound, or recent
    cardiac surgery
Tamponade may also follow CPR
Dyspnea and possible cyanosis
Neck vein distention
Weak, thready pulse
Decreasing blood pressure
Shock (cardiogenic)
Narrowing pulse pressure

EMERGENCY CARE

- Transport patient to hospital immediately.
- Maintain open airway.
- Monitor and care for signs of shock.
- Stabilize any impaled object but do not remove.
- Control bleeding with direct pressure.
- Seal any sucking chest wound. Be alert for tension pneumothorax.
- Place patient in semi-reclining position unless vital signs worsen and
    improve with patient in lying position.
- Monitor the pulse rate throughout transportation.
- Provide 100% oxygen and ventilatory support, preferably with a demand
    valve.
- These are serious emergencies—do not delay in the field.

FIGURE 19-8

80 to 90 percent of all stab wounds to the chest cause pericardial tamponade. Suspect pericardial tamponade in any stab or bullet wound to the chest, upper abdomen, back, armpits, or neck. Blood loss at the scene may be minimal, which can mislead you and cause you to underestimate the seriousness of the condition.

Signs and symptoms of pericardial tamponade include:

- Variable stages of shock
- Weak pulse.
- Diastolic and systolic blood pressure measure-

ments becoming closer together during progressive blood pressure readings.

- Cyanosis of the face.
- Shortness of breath.
- Distended neck veins.
- Muffled heart sounds (almost imperceptible, even with the use of a stethoscope).

Emergency Care

Since surgical intervention is needed, you must act quickly. The highest priority is immediate and rapid transport. To treat victims of pericardial tamponade:

1. Establish an open airway. Vigorously administer 100 percent oxygen.
2. Transport *IMMEDIATELY,* notifying the receiving facility of pericardial tamponade. The patient needs immediate surgery to save his or her life.
3. Treat for shock, but do *NOT* use a PASG; it can elevate pressure on the chest and increase bleeding. Studies show that survival rates from pericardial tamponade are better without the PASG.

□ COMPRESSION INJURIES AND TRAUMATIC ASPHYXIA

A life-threatening emergency, severe and sudden compression of a patient's chest (such as when a person is thrown against a steering wheel) causes a rapid increase in intrathoracic pressure and results in a group of symptoms. Most serious, the sternum exerts sudden and severe pressure on the heart (see Figure 19-2).

Traumatic **asphyxia** occurs from a sudden compression of the chest wall; when it occurs, the blood is forced the wrong way out of the heart (from the right side of the heart rather than the left side) and back into the veins, particularly those of the head and shoulders. Signs and symptoms of traumatic asphyxia include:

- Severe shock.
- Distended neck veins.
- Bloodshot, protruding eyes.
- Cyanotic tongue and lips.
- **Hemoptysis** (coughing up blood) or vomiting blood.
- Swollen, cyanotic appearance of the head, neck, and shoulders.

Rib fractures and flail chest may also be caused by the sudden impact.

Emergency Care

To treat compression injuries and traumatic asphyxia:

1. Maintain an open airway.
2. Administer 100 percent, positive-pressure oxygen before and during transport.
3. Control any bleeding that results from the trauma.
4. Monitor the patient closely and watch for complications. Put the patient in a semi-reclining position or on his injured side if breathing is easier and/or you suspect internal bleeding.
5. Transport immediately.

□ BROKEN RIBS

While broken ribs themselves are not life-threatening, they can cause injuries that *are.* While rib fracture is uncommon in children, because children's ribs have more resilient cartilage, direct blows or blunt trauma to the chest often result in fractured ribs in adults. The ribs most often fractured are the fifth through the tenth (those in the middle of the rib cage). The upper ribs are difficult to fracture because they are protected by the bony shoulder girdle. Fracture of the upper ribs is usually a dire emergency, because it generally indicates injury to the head, neck, spinal cord, lungs, or great vessels. Mortality is usually about 50 percent. Pneumothorax, hemothorax (see Figure 19-2), subcutaneous emphysema, and lacerated intercostal vessels are common potential complications of rib fracture.

The most common symptom of rib fracture is pain at the fracture site (Figure 19-9). It usually hurts the patient to move, cough, or breathe deeply. The patient may assume a characteristic stance, leaning toward the injured side and holding it gently. The patient will probably take shallow breaths and will likely want to hold his hand over the area, since immobilization often offers some pain relief (Figure 19-10). Other signs and symptoms, which may or may not be present, include:

- Grating sound upon palpation.
- Chest deformity.
- Shallow, uncoordinated breathing.
- Crackling sensation near the fracture site.
- Bruising or lacerations at the suspected fracture site.
- Frothy blood at the nose or mouth, indicating that the broken rib has lacerated or punctured a lung.

Emergency Care

If only one rib has been fractured and no danger exists of heart or lung laceration, you should usually not bind

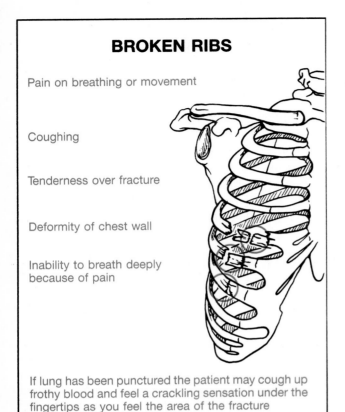

BROKEN RIBS

Pain on breathing or movement

Coughing

Tenderness over fracture

Deformity of chest wall

Inability to breath deeply because of pain

If lung has been punctured the patient may cough up frothy blood and feel a crackling sensation under the fingertips as you feel the area of the fracture (Subcutaneous emphysema)

FIGURE 19-9

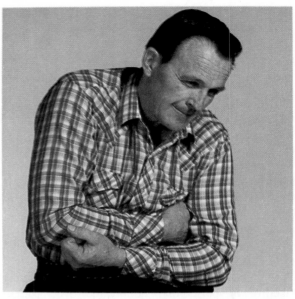

FIGURE 19-10 Typical "guarded" position of patient with rib fractures.

the chest. However, since x-ray examination is necessary for diagnosis, you should always assume that multiple ribs have been broken and immobilize liberally.

The greatest priority in treatment is to make sure that the patient can breathe adequately by providing oxygen and splinting the chest as needed. Give the pa-

tient a pillow or blanket to hold against the fractured ribs for support (Figure 19-11).

□ TRANSECTION OF THE GREAT VESSELS

In some cases of profound, deceleration-type chest injury, one of the several large blood vessels — including the major artery leading from the heart to the trunk, abdomen, and lower extremities — may be lacerated, resulting in massive life-threatening hemorrhage. The acceleration/deceleration injury of an automobile accident

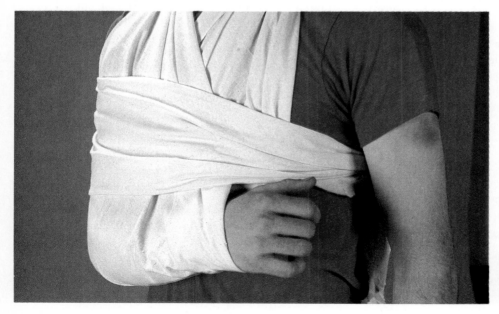

FIGURE 19-11 Care for simple rib fractures. Apply a sling and swathe to hold the arm against the injured side of the chest.

causes the ascending aorta to move forward while the descending aorta remains fixed; the result is tearing. Fatal 90 percent of the time, such an injury requires immediate surgical intervention. Once rare, it is now much more common due to the advent of high-speed automobile travel.

Signs and symptoms of **transection** include:

- Burning or tearing pain in the chest or back, with pain in the chest that radiates to the back.
- Rapidly falling blood pressure; blood pressure may be high in the upper extremities and low in the lower extremities.
- Rapid loss of consciousness.
- Shock.

Emergency Care

Remember that surgical intervention is required, and time is critical. To treat a victim of transection:

1. *Transport without delay,* treating shock and monitoring vital signs closely during transport.
2. Administer positive-pressure oxygen during transport.
3. Transport as quickly as possible without risking an accident; radio the receiving facility with your assessment so that a team will be ready to receive the patient.

☐ HEMOTHORAX

Like pneumothorax, hemothorax fills up the chest cavity with blood (rather than air) and creates pressure on the heart and lungs. The lungs cannot expand, and the same process occurs as with pneumothorax. In addition, severe bleeding can cause shock (see Figure 19-2).

Hemothorax occurs as a result of blunt or penetrating trauma to the chest caused by either open or closed chest wounds. It often accompanies pneumothorax. The blood usually originates from lacerated blood vessels in the chest wall or chest cavity; in rare cases, it results from a lacerated lung. The severity of the hemothorax depends on the amount of blood lost into the chest cavity.

If the hemothorax is small, it may be asymptomatic. Otherwise, the signs and symptoms of hemothorax are similar to those of pneumothorax, except there are no bulging neck veins due to blood loss; the following may or may not be present:

- Shock (due to blood loss).
- Rapid heartbeat.
- Rapid, shallow breathing.

- Absent breath sounds on the injured side.
- Tightness of the chest.
- Weak, thready pulse.
- Bruising over the injured area.
- Confusion and anxiety.
- Hemoptysis (coughing up blood) or blood flecks on the patient's lips.
- Frothy or bloody sputum.

Emergency Care

Priorities are to ventilate and control bleeding. To treat a victim of hemothorax:

1. *Do not waste time with prolonged assessment in the field;* transport the patient immediately in a semi-reclining position unless shock is suspected.
2. During transport, give the patient oxygen and assist breathing if necessary.
3. Control bleeding from any external wounds with a pressure dressing during transport.
4. Treat for shock.

☐ TENSION PNEUMOTHORAX

Next to pericardial tamponade, tension pneumothorax is the most life-threatening chest injury. In tension pneumothorax, air continuously leaks out of the lung and becomes trapped in the pleural space. Once the process of compression within the chest cavity due to the presence of air begins, it worsens progressively with each breath until the lung on the affected side is reduced to the size of a small ball (sometimes only a few inches in diameter). Even after the lung can be compressed no more, air continues to leak into the pleural space and the pressure continues to rise, pressing the collapsed lung against the heart and the lung on the opposite side (see Figure 19-2). The remaining lung then starts to collapse. The extreme pressure in the chest cavity prevents blood from returning to the heart through the veins, and the blood is no longer pumped out. Death can occur rapidly, sometimes within minutes.

Signs and symptoms of tension pneumothorax include:

- Obvious and increasing difficulty in breathing.
- Bulging of neck veins with tracheal deviation.
- Bulging of the chest wall above the collarbone and between the ribs.
- Reduced breathing sounds on one side of the chest and eventually on both sides.

- Tracheal deviation to the uninjured side.
- Falling blood pressure and narrowing pulse pressure.
- Rapid, weak pulse.
- Uneven chest movements during breathing; decreased or absent chest expansion on the affected side.
- Cyanosis.
- Extreme anxiety.

Emergency Care

Tension pneumothorax is one of the few emergencies in which seconds strictly count. Treatment is aimed at transporting the patient rapidly to a facility where he can receive surgical help and at relieving the increasing pressure in the pleural cavity. To treat, do the following:

1. Transport immediately, monitoring the patient continuously during transport and radioing the receiving facility with your assessment.
2. If you have bandaged a sucking chest wound, try releasing the dressing for a few seconds; if there is a tension pneumothorax, air will rush out of the wound. Release the dressing during expiration of air, and reapply it during inspiration; leave one corner untaped to allow for release of pressure.
3. During transport, administer 100 percent oxygen; assist ventilation as necessary.
4. Treat for shock.

□ PNEUMOTHORAX

Pneumothorax occurs when air from a wound site enters the chest cavity but not the lung; pneumothorax is usually due to blunt or penetrating trauma. The pressure of the air in the chest cavity presses against the lung, separating it from the chest wall and causing it to collapse (see Figure 19-2). The volume of the lung is reduced, resulting in respiratory arrest.

Air can enter the chest cavity in one of two ways: either from a sucking wound that allows air to enter from the outside (open pneumothorax), or from air that leaks out of a lung due to laceration. Once the lung is ruptured, it does not expand properly with breathing, and within minutes the patient suffers from a lack of oxygen.

In some cases, called **spontaneous pneumothorax,** the lung does not collapse because of injury, but because a congenitally weak area on the surface of the lung ruptures (see Figure 19-2). The weakened lung loses its ability to expand, and the patient experiences sharp chest pain and mild to severe respiratory distress.

Spontaneous pneumothorax is common among smokers or emphysema patients, especially if they are emaciated.

Suspect pneumothorax if a patient suffers a sudden shortness of breath without an obvious cause. Other signs and symptoms include:

- Sudden, sharp chest pain.
- Failure of the lung to expand with inhalation, causing decreased or absent breath sounds on the affected side.
- Severe respiratory distress with dyspnea.

Emergency Care

Treatment for pneumothorax includes the following:

1. Clear and maintain an open airway.
2. Administer high-concentration oxygen with a bag-valve mask (other positive-pressure devices may create tension pneumothorax).
3. Cover any open chest wounds. If necessary, use your hand; preferably, apply an occlusive dressing to cover the wound (the dressing should be at least two inches wider than the wound on all sides). Tape the dressing to the chest on three sides, leaving one corner untaped to allow release of pressure (otherwise, it can become a tension pneumothorax).
4. Monitor the patient closely; a pneumothorax can become a tension pneumothorax (described above) if pressure builds. If tension pneumothorax develops, briefly remove the occlusive dressing (see page 323).
5. Transport the patient as soon as possible.

□ SUBCUTANEOUS EMPHYSEMA

When the lung or part of the bronchial tree is lacerated (usually from broken ribs or from a penetrating chest injury), air from the lungs escapes into the soft tissues of the chest wall. Small bubbles or air invade the subcutaneous tissues, and the entire chest, neck, and face can be affected (see Figure 19-2).

Signs and symptoms of subcutaneous emphysema include:

- Impaired breathing.
- Slight cyanosis.
- Crackling sound when pressure is exerted on the skin.

Emergency Care

Immediate surgical intervention is needed to repair the laceration and restore normal respiration. To treat subcutaneous emphysema:

1. Transport the patient as soon as possible in a semi-reclining position or lying on his or her injured side if breathing is easier and/or you suspect internal bleeding.
2. During transport, maintain an open airway.
3. During transport, administer 100 percent oxygen and assist ventilation if necessary.
4. Radio the receiving facility with your assessment so that a team can be ready to administer care to the patient upon arrival.

☐ SUCKING CHEST WOUNDS (OPEN PNEUMOTHORAX)

In open chest wounds, air from the environment sometimes enters the chest cavity when the chest is expanded during the patient's normal breathing. It moves through the wound as the patient inhales; when the patient exhales, air is forced back out of the wound. Each time the patient breathes, a moist sucking or bubbling is produced as the air passes in and out of the wound. In addition, there will be decreased breath sounds (Figure 19-12).

☐ Sucking Chest Wound

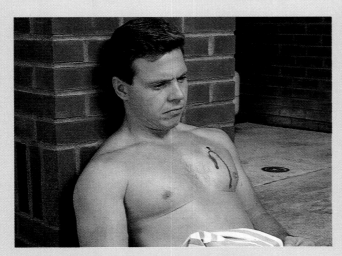

FIGURE 19-12 Sucking chest wound and possible pneumothorax.

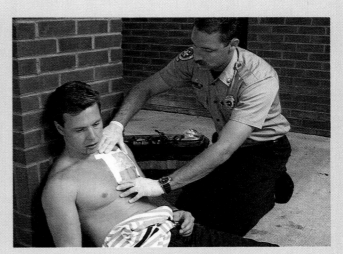

FIGURE 19-13 Position occlusive covering, which should contact the chest wall directly.

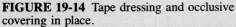
FIGURE 19-14 Tape dressing and occlusive covering in place.

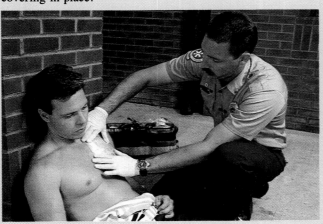

FIGURE 19-15 Position patient to ease breathing.

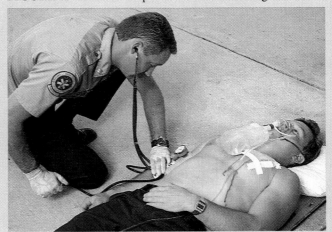

323

Pneumothorax results when air enters the chest cavity but does not enter the lung from the wound site. The pressure of the air in the chest cavity presses against the lung, causing it to collapse.

Emergency Care

To treat open pneumothorax:

1. Apply an occlusive dressing over the sucking wound *immediately* to prevent serious respiratory problems (Figure 19-13). Household plastic wrap is not strong enough and can be sucked into the wound — use gauze, aluminum foil, an IV bag, or Vaseline gauze held in place with a pressure dressing. Your goal should be to create an airtight seal over the wound and prevent air from passing through the wound. The dressing must be large enough so that it is not sucked into the wound; there should be at least two inches of overlap on all sides. If the tape won't stick to the skin, cover it with bulky dressings and a cravat. If there is both an entrance and an exit wound, both must be dressed.

2. Tape the dressing to the chest, leaving one corner or side untaped to prevent a buildup of pressure (Figures 19-14—19-17). *Follow local protocol.*

3. Administer oxygen.

4. Transport as soon as possible, with the patient either sitting up or in some other position of comfort that is least painful and allows for the least labored breathing.

On inspiration, dressing seals wound, preventing air entry

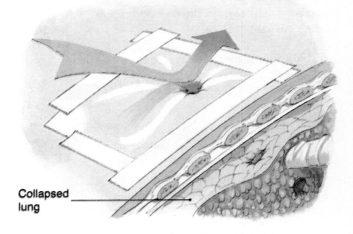

Collapsed lung

Expiration allows trapped air to escape through untaped section of dressing

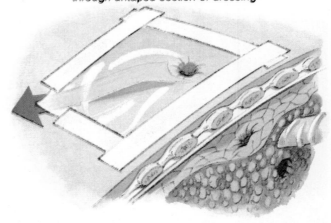

FIGURE 19-16 Creating a flutter valve to relieve tension pneumothorax.

chapter 20

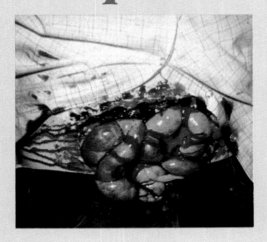

Injuries to the Abdomen and Genitalia

✳ OBJECTIVES

- ■ Review the anatomy of the abdominal cavity, the genitourinary system, and the male and female genitalia.
- ■ Recognize the common signs and symptoms of abdominal and genitalia injuries.
- ■ Describe and demonstrate the appropriate emergency care for specific injuries of the abdomen.
- ■ Describe the appropriate emergency care for specific injuries of the genitalia.

It is recommended that EMTs wear protective gloves whenever there is a possibility of coming in contact with a patient's blood, body fluids, mucous membranes, traumatic wounds, or sores. See Chapter 31.

A wide range of accidents, from motor vehicle accidents to shootings or blunt trauma, affect the organs of the abdomen. And because the abdominal cavity contains not only vital organs but a rich supply of blood vessels, major abdominal injuries are life-threatening and demand prompt and proper prehospital treatment.

Injuries to the **genitalia,** while embarrassing and frightening, are seldom life-threatening. However, you have an important duty to protect the patient from public embarrassment and to provide emotional support.

□ THE ABDOMINAL CAVITY

The abdominal cavity contains the major organs of the gastrointestinal tract, and in a woman it also contains the internal sex organs — the ovaries, fallopian tubes, and uterus. The abdominal cavity is separated from the thoracic cavity by the diaphragm.

The abdominal cavity is well protected above by the thorax, below by the heavy ring of pelvic bones, and at the sides and in the back by thick tough muscles, the lower ribs, and the spinal column. It is protected in front by flat muscular layers, which for greater strength run in different directions in the abdominal wall.

The **peritoneum** is a sheathlike membrane in the abdominal cavity that consists of two layers. The outer layer **(parietal)** lines the walls of the abdominal cavity, and the inner layer **(visceral)** surrounds and helps support the abdominal organs. Where the surfaces of these two layers contact each other, they secrete peritoneal fluid, a lubricant that prevents the layers from sticking together to form **adhesions.**

The abdomen contains both hollow and solid organs. The hollow organs include the stomach, gallbladder, **duodenum,** large intestine, small intestine, and urinary bladder. If the hollow organs rupture or are lacerated, partially digested food, enzymes, feces, gastric juices, or other matter can spill out into the abdominal cavity, causing immediate peritonitis. (Signs and symptoms of peritonitis can include fever, abdominal pain, chills, pain radiating to the shoulder, and absent bowel sounds.)

The solid abdominal organs include the spleen, liver, pancreas, ovaries, and kidneys; most are covered by a strong membrane or muscle capsule, and if they are ruptured, they will hemorrhage into the capsule for some time before blood spills into the abdominal cavity. If solid organs rupture or are lacerated, severe life-threatening hemorrhage can result.

□ ABDOMINAL INJURIES

Patients involved in fights, falls, or automobile accidents should always be suspected of having sustained injury to the abdominal area. Injuries might range from severe hemorrhage, resulting in shock, to a rupture of the diaphragm, which forces abdominal organs into the chest cavity. Almost all injuries to the abdominal area require surgical repair. Monitor the patient closely during transport.

Blunt trauma is serious, because it can involve any of the vascular organs surrounding and adjacent to the abdomen. Injuries to the liver, kidneys, pancreas, spleen, and gallbladder may cause severe hemorrhaging that can result in death. Certain medications — including aspirin, **ibuprofen,** blood thinners, and many **steroids** — will increase the bleeding. If a patient has suffered abdominal trauma, assume that he or she has also suffered chest trauma until proven otherwise (Figure 20-1).

The pneumatic antishock garment (PASG) offers definitive improvement in emergency care for patients suffering abdominal injuries. The PASG also can help prevent shock and may increase survival rates. Such care should be used only under direction of the receiving physician. If you are not specially trained, equipped, and allowed by local protocol for administering such care, provide basic emergency care and transport the patient immediately.

Open Wounds

A wound in which the skin is broken and the abdominal cavity is penetrated is extremely dangerous because of possible damage to internal organs. The stomach or intestine may be perforated, internal bleeding may occur, and infection may develop. Bacteria may be introduced into the **peritoneal cavity** from the outside or from a perforated intestine.

It is sometimes difficult to determine whether internal organs have been injured; in the presence of open abdominal wounds, assume that organ damage has occurred. Generally, signs and symptoms include:

- Severe abdominal tenderness.
- Abdominal muscle rigidity.
- Abdominal distention.
- Intense pain.
- Severe shock.
- Paralysis of bowels (absence of bowel sounds).
- Nausea and/or vomiting.
- Abdominal muscle spasm due to the presence of irritating substances, including blood.

Closed Wounds (Internal Injuries)

In closed abdominal wounds, the abdomen has been damaged by a severe blow or crushing injury, but the skin remains unbroken. Such wounds may be extremely dangerous, because serious injury to the internal organs,

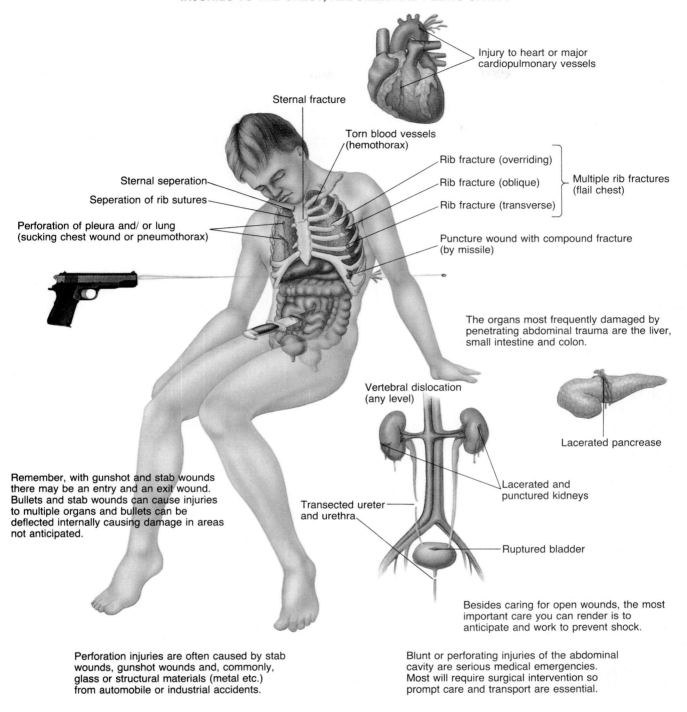

Injury to heart or major cardiopulmonary vessels

Sternal fracture

Torn blood vessels (hemothorax)

Rib fracture (overriding)

Rib fracture (oblique)

Rib fracture (transverse)

Multiple rib fractures (flail chest)

Sternal seperation

Seperation of rib sutures

Puncture wound with compound fracture (by missile)

Perforation of pleura and/ or lung (sucking chest wound or pneumothorax)

The organs most frequently damaged by penetrating abdominal trauma are the liver, small intestine and colon.

Vertebral dislocation (any level)

Lacerated pancrease

Lacerated and punctured kidneys

Remember, with gunshot and stab wounds there may be an entry and an exit wound. Bullets and stab wounds can cause injuries to multiple organs and bullets can be deflected internally causing damage in areas not anticipated.

Transected ureter and urethra

Ruptured bladder

Besides caring for open wounds, the most important care you can render is to anticipate and work to prevent shock.

Perforation injuries are often caused by stab wounds, gunshot wounds and, commonly, glass or structural materials (metal etc.) from automobile or industrial accidents.

Blunt or perforating injuries of the abdominal cavity are serious medical emergencies. Most will require surgical intervention so prompt care and transport are essential.

FIGURE 20-1

internal hemorrhage, and shock may occur. Obviously, a number of medical conditions can also cause abdominal pain; however, in the field, it is generally not useful or feasible to try to distinguish among all the so-called acute abdomen conditions (see Chapter 29).

To assess a patient for the presence of a closed abdominal injury, have the patient lie supine with knees flexed and supported. Remove or loosen clothing over the abdominal area. Assess by looking, listening, and feeling as follows:

Injuries to the Abdomen and Genitalia   **327**

1. Inspect for lacerations, open wounds, bruising, impaled objects, or protruding abdominal organs.
2. Watch abdominal movement as the patient breathes.
3. Gently palpate all four quadrants; watch for guarding, rigidity, pain, and tenderness (Figure 20-2).
4. If transport is delayed or while in transport, check bowel sounds by listening carefully with a stethoscope for at least one minute in each of the four abdominal quadrants. In a healthy patient, bowel sounds should occur every five to fifteen seconds (they will sound gurgling).

General Signs and Symptoms of Abdominal Injuries

As with chest wounds, the amount of blood is not necessarily indicative of the severity of injury. Deep underlying damage may not result in much external hemorrhage. Patients with abdominal injuries may exhibit any of the following (Figure 20-3):

- The abdomen may be distended or irregularly shaped.
- There may be bruising of the abdomen or back due to blood leaking into the retroperitoneal cavity.
- The abdomen may be rigid and tender wih pain felt in an area other than the site of injury.
- The patient may have pain that begins as mild discomfort and then progresses to an intolerable pain.
- The patient may protect his or her abdomen.
- The patient prefers to lie still with legs drawn up in the **fetal position** (Figure 20-4).
- Pain may radiate to either shoulder.
- There may be abdominal cramping.

FIGURE 20-2 In closed abdominal wounds, gently palpate the abdominal quadrants, watch for guarding, rigidity, pain, and tenderness.

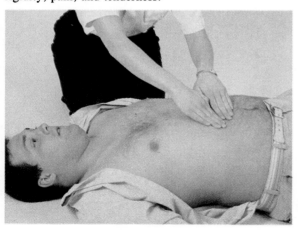

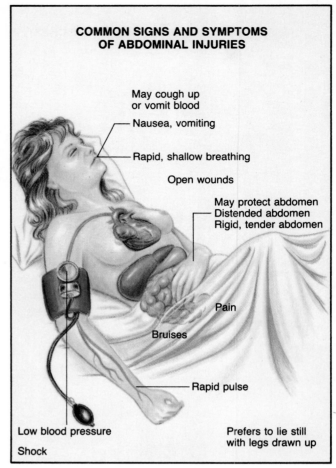

COMMON SIGNS AND SYMPTOMS OF ABDOMINAL INJURIES

May cough up or vomit blood
Nausea, vomiting
Rapid, shallow breathing
Open wounds
May protect abdomen
Distended abdomen
Rigid, tender abdomen
Pain
Bruises
Rapid pulse
Low blood pressure
Shock
Prefers to lie still with legs drawn up

FIGURE 20-3

- There may be rapid, shallow breathing.
- The pulse may be rapid and the blood pressure low.
- Open wounds and penetrations may be evident.
- The patient may be nauseated and may vomit.

FIGURE 20-4 Patients with abdominal injuries often lie with their legs drawn up in the fetal position.

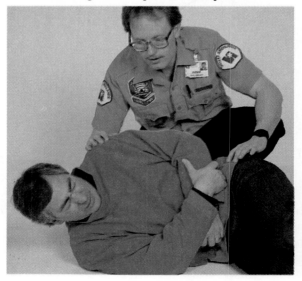

- Organs may protrude through open wounds (**evisceration**) (Figure 20-5).
- Fractures may be evident.
- There may be obvious lacerations and puncture wounds in the abdomen.
- There may be blood in the urine.
- The patient may be in shock.
- The patient may be vomiting blood.
- Back pain may be present if the kidneys have been injured.
- The patient may be very weak or very thirsty.

General Emergency Care for Abdominal Injuries

As with all injured patients, top priorities are airway, breathing, and circulation. Additionally, provide the following emergency care for abdominal injuries:

1. Remove or cut away clothing from the abdominal area to allow for adequate assessment.
2. Suspect shock with any abdominal injury, and work diligently to prevent it. Keep the patient warm, but do not overheat. Check with the base physician about the possible use of a pneumatic antishock garment (PASG).
3. Control bleeding and dress all open wounds with a dry, sterile dressing.
4. If organs are protruding, do not touch them and do *not* attempt to replace them within the abdominal cavity. Cover them with a sterile dressing and keep the dressing moistened with sterile saline solution; apply an occlusive dressing to retain moisture and protect from contaminants.
5. A patient with abdominal injury is usually most comfortable lying on his or her back with knees flexed; elevate the feet if possible.
6. Be alert for vomiting. Maintain an open airway by suctioning or positioning the patient for adequate drainage.
7. Constantly monitor vital signs and abdominal condition.
8. Do not remove penetrating or impaled objects. Cut away clothing that surrounds the impaled object. Dress the wounds around the impaled object to control bleeding; stabilize the impaled object with bulky dressings, and bandage in place to prevent movement.
9. Immobilize the patient if you suspect pelvic fracture.
10. Do not give the patient anything by mouth.

11. Administer high-flow oxygen through a nonrebreather mask, especially if the patient is shocky.
12. Transport as quickly as possible, monitoring constantly during transport.

Abdominal Eviscerations

An evisceration bandage is used when an abdominal laceration wound has resulted in a protrusion of the abdominal contents. In such cases (Figures 20-5–20-9):

1. Administer oxygen.
2. Suspect shock and work to prevent it.
3. Constantly monitor vital signs.
4. Do *not* try to replace organs within the abdomen.
5. Cover the organs with a clean, moist, sterile dressing. Use sterile gauze compresses if available, and moisten them with clear water or saline. *Never* use absorbent cotton or any material that clings when wet, such as paper towels or toilet tissue.
6. Cover the moist dressing with an occlusive material such as clean aluminum foil or plastic wrap (follow local protocol) to retain moisture and warmth.
7. Gently wrap the dressing in place with a bandage or clean sheet.
8. Transport the patient as soon as possible in a supine position with knees flexed and supported.
9. Provide supportive treatment as appropriate during transport.

Rupture or Hernias

The most common form of rupture or hernia is a protrusion of a portion of an internal organ through the wall of the abdomen. Most ruptures occur in or just above the groin, but they may occur at other places over the abdomen. Ruptures result from a combination of weakness of the tissues and muscular strain.

The signs and symptoms of a rupture are as follows:

- Sharp, stinging pain.
- Feeling of something giving way at the site of the rupture.
- Swelling.
- Possible nausea and vomiting.

To treat (Figure 20-10):

1. Lie the patient on his or her back with the knees well drawn up.
2. Place a blanket or similar padding under the knees.

☐ Abdominal Evisceration

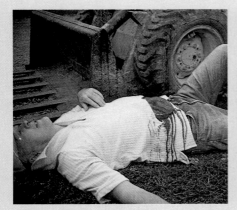

FIGURE 20-5 Abdominal evisceration — an open wound resulting in protrusion of intestines. Administer oxygen.

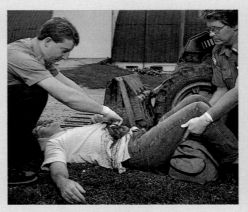

FIGURE 20-6 Cut away clothing from wound and support knees in a flexed position.

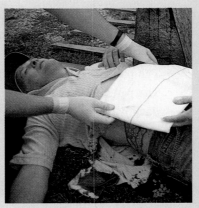

FIGURE 20-7 Place dressing over wound. *Do not attempt to replace intestines within abdomen.*

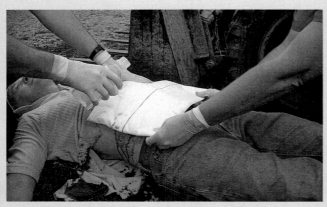

FIGURE 20-8 Moisten dressing with saline. It is best to premoisten before application. Note: In some EMS areas, dry dressings are recommended. Follow local protocol.

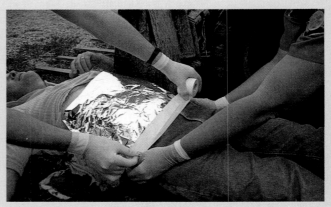

FIGURE 20-9 Gently and loosely tape the dressing in place, then apply an occlusive material such as aluminum foil (follow local protocol) or plastic wrap. Tape loosely over dressing to keep dressing moist.

FIGURE 20-10 Emergency care for a rupture or hernia.

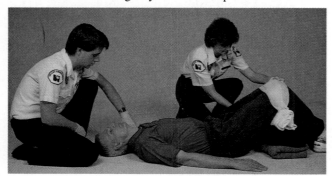

3. Never attempt to force the protrusion back into the cavity.
4. Cover the patient with a blanket.
5. Transport the patient in this position.
6. Treat the patient for shock if it is present.

☐ GENITOURINARY SYSTEM INJURIES

Review the anatomy and physiology of the urinary and reproductive systems in Chapter 2.

Kidney Injuries

Injuries to the kidneys themselves are not common, because the kidneys lie in a well-protected area of the upper abdomen. Intense, forceful, blunt trauma to the lower rib cage or flank is required to injure the kidneys. Occasionally, a fractured rib may lacerate a kidney, causing severe hemorrhage; however, even that is not common, since the lower ribs are not particularly vulnerable to fracture.

Signs and symptoms of kidney injury include:

- Blood in the urine.
- Mild to severe pain, which may radiate to the groin or the thigh on the affected side.
- Tenderness to the touch over the kidney area.
- Deep bruising over the kidney area.
- Signs of shock.

To treat suspected kidney injury:

1. Treat the victim for shock. Keep the patient warm, but do not overheat.
2. Transport as soon as possible; kidney injury requires surgical intervention. Monitor vital signs during transport, and be alert for complications.

Bladder Injuries

While kidney injuries are relatively uncommon, bladder injuries occur in approximately half of all crushing injuries to the pelvis. In addition, bladder injuries are common with pelvic fracture, blunt trauma to the lower abdomen, penetrating injuries to the lower abdomen, and sudden deceleration injuries.

The bladder, a hollow organ, is rarely injured when it is empty. When a full bladder is injured, urine spills into the surrounding tissues and can cause peritonitis if not surgically treated promptly.

Signs and symptoms of bladder injury include:

- Blood in the urine.
- Blood visible at the urethral opening.
- Pain during urination, an urge to void, or an inability to void.
- Distended abdomen.
- Nausea and/or vomiting.
- Pallor.
- Fever and/or chills.
- Obvious trauma to the lower abdomen.

To treat bladder injuries:

1. Treat the patient for shock. Keep the patient quiet and warm, but do not overheat.

2. Administer oxygen as needed.
3. Transport as soon as possible; bladder injuries require surgical intervention. Monitor vital signs closely during transport.

Male Genitalia

While injuries to the external male genitalia — lacerations, avulsions, abrasions, penetrations, and contusions — are excruciatingly painful, they are not necessarily life-threatening. However, the amount of pain involved and the nature of the injury can cause great concern to the patient.

Injuries to the external male genitalia can be extremely embarrassing to the patient. Act in a calm, professional way. Protect the patient from onlookers; help protect his privacy by using sheets, towels, or other material as a drape over the genital area.

Penis

The skin of the penis can be torn or avulsed, particularly in an uncircumcised patient, and most commonly in an industrial accident. To treat:

1. Wrap the penis in a soft, sterile dressing moistened with sterile saline solution.
2. Apply an ice bag to the penis to relieve pain and reduce swelling.
3. If you can find the torn skin, wrap it in sterile gauze that has been moistened with sterile saline solution; transport it in a cooled container when you transport the patient.
4. Never remove penetrating objects; stabilize them with bulky dressings prior to transport.
5. Always preserve avulsed parts, but do not delay treatment or transport in search for avulsed parts.
6. In some cases, the penis itself may be partially or completely amputated, and blood loss may be significant. Apply direct pressure with a sterile pressure dressing to the remaining stump of the penis to control blood loss. If necessary, apply tourniquet until direct pressure can bring bleeding under control. Transport as quickly as possible.
7. If you can find the amputated penis, wrap it in a sterile dressing moistened with sterile saline solution, place it in a plastic bag, and transport it in a cooled container when you transport the patient.
8. If you suspect that the patient cut off his own penis, be prepared to deal with his hostile emotions.
9. Maintain close monitoring and control of bleeding during transport.

During particularly active sexual intercourse or

blunt trauma, the structures that support the penis may be "fractured" (lacerated), resulting in swelling, bruising, and intense pain. The patient may have heard a loud "snap" at the time of injury. Upon examination, you may see evidence of bleeding into the surrounding tissues, usually on only one side of the penis.

To treat:

1. Transport the patient as quickly as possible to the hospital; surgical repair is needed.
2. During transport, apply ice to reduce swelling, control bruising, and relieve the pain.
3. If there is bleeding into the tissues, apply local pressure with a sterile dressing to control bleeding.
4. Splint the penis.

Tears of the **foreskin** or laceration of the skin just underneath the ridge can result in heavy bleeding. To treat:

1. Use pressure to control the bleeding.
2. Apply ice to reduce swelling and relieve pain.
3. Transport.

Sometimes the penis gets caught in the zipper of pants, an injury that usually occurs among children. To treat:

1. If only one or two teeth of the zipper are involved, try to gently unzip the pants and free the penis. It may be easiest to cut off the zipper fastener and gently separate the teeth.
2. If the patient is unusually upset or if a long section of skin is caught, cut the zipper out of the pants to make the patient more comfortable.
3. Apply ice to reduce swelling and relieve pain.
4. Transport.

Scrotum and Testicles

A direct blow to the **scrotum** can cause the testes to rupture, or can result in a pooling of blood around them, causing tremendous pain and a feeling of pressure.

To treat:

1. Apply ice to the entire crotch area to reduce swelling, bleeding, and pain.
2. Transport the patient.
3. If scrotal skin becomes avulsed, try to find it. Wrap it in moist, sterile gauze, and transport it with the patient to the hospital.
4. Dress the scrotum itself in a sterile dressing moistened with sterile saline solution, and control bleeding with pressure.
5. Make the patient as comfortable as possible during transport.

Occasionally testicles will become ruptured due to severe trauma to the groin. However, because of their tendency to withdraw easily and quickly into the abdominal wall, injury to the testicles is uncommon. When a testicle does rupture, the most serious manifestation is severe bleeding, often causing accumulation of blood in the scrotal sac around the testicle in the peritoneal cavity (due to leakage of blood).

To treat:

1. Apply ice packs to the area.
2. Transport the patient immediately to a hospital, where surgical intervention is necessary for repair.

Female Genitalia

Injuries to the external female genitalia are rare but can follow **straddle injuries,** sexual assault, blows to the perineum area, abortion attempts, lacerations following childbirth, or foreign bodies inserted into the vagina. Because the area is richly supplied with blood vessels and nerves, the injury can cause blinding pain and considerable bleeding; however, it is usually not life-threatening. To treat:

1. Control bleeding with local pressure, using moist compresses. Apply pressure over an external laceration. If bleeding is severe and uncontrolled, use a PASG if local protocol allows and with approval of medical control.
2. Dress the wounds, and keep the dressing in place with a diaper-type bandage. Stabilize any impaled objects or foreign bodies.
3. Use ice packs over the dressing to relieve pain and reduce swelling.
4. *Never* place dressings or packs inside the vagina.
5. Treat for shock.
6. Monitor vital signs.
7. Transport as soon as possible; major bleeding will have to be controlled surgically.

If the patient is the victim of a sexual assault, respect her modesty. Provide a cover, and do not question her about the incident. Do not touch or examine the genitalia unless there is life-threatening bleeding. To help preserve evidence:

- Do not allow the victim to bathe or douche.
- Do not allow the victim to wash her hair or clean under her fingernails.
- If possible, do not clean wounds.
- Handle the victim's clothing as little as possible.
- Bag all items of clothing and other items separately; if there is blood on any item, do *not* use plastic bags.

chapter 21

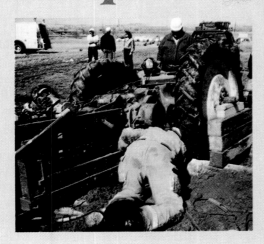

Farm, Rural, and Industrial Accidents

✳ **OBJECTIVES**

■ Understand the factors responsible for the high rate of injury and fatality in farm, rural, and industrial accidents.

■ Identify the types of farm machinery and related objects that are responsible for the majority of farm injuries.

■ Describe the precautions and appropriate emergency care for specific farm-related injuries.

■ Describe the principles of disentanglement from farm equipment.

■ Describe principles and priorities for responding to an industrial accident.

It is recommended that EMTs wear protective gloves whenever there is a possibility of coming in contact with a patient's blood, body fluids, mucous membranes, traumatic wounds, or sores. See Chapter 31.

While 73 percent of the nation's population lives in urban areas, the death rate from unintentional trauma is the highest in rural areas. And those who are injured in rural settings are notoriously undertreated.

Rural trauma includes farm accidents, nonurban motor vehicle accidents, off-road motor vehicle accidents, recreational accidents, drownings, and firearm accidents (usually associated with hunting). Rural motor vehicle accidents have a higher fatality rate than those occurring in urban areas: they involve irregular terrain, high rates of speed, lack of the helmets, and remote distances from hospitals and trauma centers.

The most common farm accidents involve farm machinery, poisoning (from hazardous chemicals), electrocution, suffocation (in grain bins and silos), falls, and animals (both falls from animals and animal assaults).

According to the National Safety Council, farming is now considered the nation's most hazardous occupation; in recent years, 61 out of every 100,000 farmers died in on-the-job accidents, and 58 of every 1,000 farmers were disabled, either permanently or temporarily. Many accident victims were children, since they comprise a significant percentage of the farm work force. The highest farm injury rate is in children between the ages of five and fourteen. According to a study conducted at the Mayo Clinic, there are 300 children killed on farms each year, and an additional 23,500 seriously injured.

The number of accidents per man-hour worked is five times higher in agriculture than the national average for major industry. Unfortunately, there is little EMS training regarding the specifics of common farm injury, even though some form of agricultural activity exists in *every* state. Agricultural-type injuries can even occur in urban areas, as heavy farm machinery is used for snow removal. Augers, too, are used in many nonfarm applications, such as grinding meat in restaurants or grocery stores.

□ WHY FARM AND RURAL ACCIDENTS ARE SO SERIOUS

Farm accidents can be among the most difficult to manage, even for experienced EMTs. Why are farm accidents so serious? Consider the following:

- Family farms often fail to follow general safety standards — and few are regulated by government

safety agencies, since they do not meet the required minimum number of employees.

- Many farmers lack formal training in how to operate farm machinery; they lack familiarization and experience.

- Farm equipment is designed to cut, tear, shred, and mash — and it does, often human flesh.

- There is often delay in notification — there is often no phone at the scene, and someone may have to walk some distance in order to find a telephone. Many rural areas do not have 911 service and do not have a central dispatch; others are staffed only by volunteer teams. Victims are often not discovered for hours — rural roads are often two-lane asphalt roads in residential areas. Many are unlit, lack proper shoulders, have poorly controlled intersections, have frequent unmarked railroad crossings, and have animals on the road.

- The fatigue factor is tremendous: the machinery, noise, and workload all contribute. Farmers rarely are able to take breaks or vacations, and often work into the night to complete a job. Overnight entanglement is very common in rural areas.

□ CAUSES OF FARM ACCIDENTS

The object or agent that causes the farm accident generally falls into one of four broad categories:

1. Agricultural tractors.
2. Farm machinery. Deaths from farm machinery have increased 44 percent in the last 50 years, while nonfarm machinery deaths decreased 79 percent in the same period.
3. Product storage and handling equipment.
4. Chemicals and toxins.

Some injuries and mechanisms of injury are related to specific kinds of farm machinery (Figures 21-1–21-6).

Tractors

Tractors (Figure 21-7) are the most common cause of farm-related fatalities, with 83 percent of all tractor fatalities caused by crushing injuries (a tractor can weigh up to fifteen tons). Many fatal accidents involve tractors overturning — these cause more deaths than any other factor on the farm. Most often they involve adolescents and adults, but sometimes children are involved, too — children are killed in one-third of all tractor rollovers. Some farmers are run over by their tractors, and others

The farm section in this chapter was written by Mike Smith, Director of the Paramedic Training Program, Tacoma Community College, and Ray Andrews, Emergency Rescue Technician Instructor and Chief, Pleasant Valley Fire Department.

□ Injuries Sustained from Farm Machinery

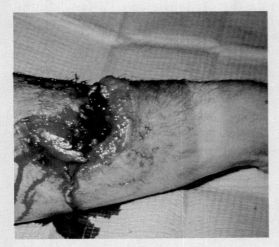

FIGURE 21-1 Arm in power takeoff.

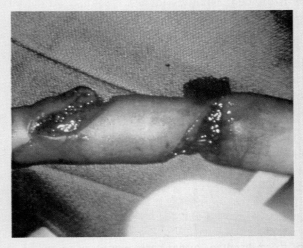

FIGURE 21-2 Arm in auger.

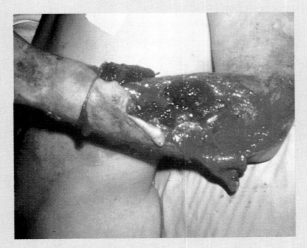

FIGURE 21-3 Arm in auger.

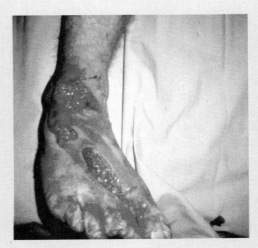

FIGURE 21-4 Foot in auger.

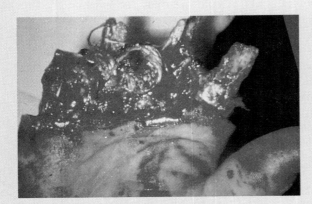

FIGURE 21-5 Hand in snapping rolls.

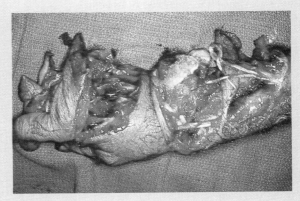

FIGURE 21-6 Hand and arm in hay baler.

are injured in power takeoff accidents, falls from tractors, and other causes. Most tractor accidents occur in the spring and summer months. Recent estimates from the National Safety Council indicate that 33 percent of all farm accident fatalities involve tractors, with most involving turnovers.

The rubber-tired tractors used today fall into two major categories: two-wheel drive and four-wheel drive. Engines may be fueled by gasoline, diesel, or liquid propane; fuel leaks and potential fire/explosion hazards result from tractor accidents, so fire protection is critical during rescue.

The tractor engine *must* be shut down before rescue can occur. Shut down the engine even if it is not running — it can suddenly start up again during rescue. After the engine has been shut down and the fuel situation modified, you will need to stabilize the tractor before you can begin rescue. If you are unfamiliar with the equipment always call for assistance.

Tractor Stabilization

To stabilize:

1. Lock up the tractor's rear wheels with two one- or two-ton cable hoists and three chains.
2. Wrap one chain around the rear tire and through the rim "high," and the second chain around the same wheel and through the rim "low"; the third chain should be attached to the front of the tractor and stretched to a hoist.
3. Attach the other hoist to the two rear chains.
4. If the tractor does not have slots in the rims, the hoist and chains must be stretched across the rear tire to a strong point on the rear of the tractor.
5. Care must be taken not to lift the secure tire off the ground during rescue.
6. It is important to take time to lock up the rear wheels even if the machine is upright.

Emergency Care

Call for at least two rescue teams in any tractor accident; one should be capable of handling fire, since there will almost certainly be spilled fuel and hot hydraulic fluid. Once you have stabilized the tractor, treat the patient as follows:

1. Assess the patient, and determine potential injuries. Since approximately 85 percent of all tractor overturns are to the side, expect crushing injuries to the head, chest, and abdomen, as well as multiple lacerations.
2. Quickly determine whether any immediate life-threatening injuries exist; give aggressive management to airway, breathing, and circulation problems.
3. Common tractor rollover injuries include burns from spilled engine coolants, transmission fluid, hydraulic fluid, or battery acid. Pay special attention to the eyes, and assess for chemical burns. If present, irrigate as described in Chapter 17, "Injuries to the Eye."
4. Pay immediate attention to possible chest injuries, including pneumothorax, sucking chest wounds, and so on.
5. Treat for shock; use a pneumatic antishock garment (PASG) if indicated and if local protocol suggests it.
6. Stabilize all injuries; splint and immobilize all fractures.
7. When possible, lift or remove the tractor from the patient once the patient is stabilized.

Lifting Operations

During any lifting operation, a cross-crib capable of supporting the machine must be built in case lifting devices fail or if the machine has to be set down and repositioned for another lift. The **crib** should be as wide as possible and is normally limited by the storage space available in the rescue vehicle. Also, the cribbing and lifting devices need a solid surface from which to work and function properly. This is sometimes difficult in a soft field or ditch. The rescue squad should carry several one-quarter-inch tread plates about eighteen by twenty-four inches with two-by-six's attached to the smooth side. The plates will serve as a firm lifting surface on soft ground or on blacktop.

High-pressure **airbags** (approximately 90 to 120 psi) are the best tools available at this time to lift a heavy, irregularly shaped machine. The bags must be placed carefully, keeping in mind the machine's center of gravity. Even though the bags appear to be indestructible, they are not, and you must take time to build a cross-crib as the bags are inflated. Bags may be stacked to get a higher lift, but they become increasingly unstable as they are inflated. An airbag is most efficient during its first three to five inches of lift. Whenever possible, a crib should be built to get the bag within one to two inches of the object to be lifted. A steel plate should be placed between the bag and the crib to keep the crib from being knocked apart during inflation.

Cranes, wreckers, and boom trucks can also be utilized (if readily available), especially if you are dealing with a very large tractor. (Some of today's largest tractors weigh over 30,000 pounds!) Regardless, cribs should still be built to protect the patient and rescuers from equipment failure or operator error.

In lifting or removing an overturned tractor from an operator, follow these basic rules:

1. Always build a crib to guard against equipment failures or operator errors.

2. Always try to determine the center of gravity of the tractor and watch during the lift to ensure that the part to be lifted is moving properly and that another part is not putting more pressure on the patient.

3. Anytime more than one lifting device has to be used, use extra care in coordinating the lift to keep loads from shifting.

Lifting a tractor is *not* like lifting an automobile; a tractor is usually heavier and, due to its varied shape, is difficult to stabilize, since many of the accidents occur in remote locations on soft ground. To be sure, a tractor rollover presents a difficult challenge. However, if safe rescue principles are employed and patient care is provided aggressively in conjunction with the extrication activities, this complex situation can be handled with confidence.

Power Takeoff Shafts

The **power takeoff (PTO)** shaft is a drive shaft that connects a tractor to farm implements such as balers, mowers, corn pickers, forage harvesters, and so on (Figure 21-8). The PTO shaft is the second most common cause of accidents, and the accidents most often occur in fall in fall or winter when a farmer's heavy clothing gets caught in the shaft and pulls the farmer in. The farmer can get wrapped around the shaft, resulting in fatal injuries. Power takeoff shaft injuries are not common — comprising only about 8 percent of all farm injuries — but they are characteristically fatal.

To shut down a PTO, turn off the tractor that is providing the power. (Shutdown procedures are discussed in detail later in this chapter). Some PTOs will free-wheel in either direction when the power is shut off, while some lock up immediately.

To disentangle the patient, do the following:

1. If the patient is wrapped on the shaft clear of the coupling device, you might uncouple the shaft, slide it apart, and take the section with the patient to the hospital.

2. If you cannot uncouple the shaft, cut it with a power saw, porta-band saw, gasoline-powered circular saw, or hack saw.

   • When cutting is shaft, take extreme care to prevent if from spinning by locking it in place with a bar through the universal joint on both ends.

   • Avoid the last six inches, since it is more solid and extremely difficult to cut.

3. As you remove the patient, make sure that all rescuers and onlookers stand clear to avoid further injury.

4. Locate any amputated parts and transport them with the victim.

5. Always assume that the victim has sustained neck or back injuries; immobilize prior to transport.

Silo Injuries

When crops are stored in silos, gas is formed by the natural chemical fermentation; fermenting crops can release high levels of carbon monoxide, methane, and nitrogen dioxide. These can cause serious injury or death at relatively low concentrations.

Silo gas has a strong bleach odor and usually causes yellow, red, or dark brown fumes. The greatest danger of silo gas is just after harvest, but fumes can persist and occur when a silo is opened months later to unload.

Most silo injuries occur when a victim falls into the silo and either becomes trapped in the unloading device or is overcome by silo gas. Some suffer cardiac arrest in the silo. Unfortunately, silo gas causes little immediate pain, and a victim may not realize he has been injured — only to die hours later during sleep because his injured lungs fill with fluid.

Two teams are usually required to rescue victims from a silo. Rescuers should be lowered in, and the victim raised out through the top on a litter. Always use a self-contained breathing apparatus when doing rescue work at a silo.

Manure Storage Ponds

Injuries at manure storage ponds are generally either from drowning or from toxic fumes. Manure storage areas generally put off ammonia, carbon monoxide, methane, and hydrogen sulfide — and underground storage ponds put these off in very high concentrations.

The primary goal of rescue is to provide ventilation. Always use back-up rescuers, and always wear a self-contained breathing apparatus.

Other Equipment

Other types of farm equipment and the injuries they may cause include the following:

Combines

The **combine** (Figure 21-9), as we know it today, is a machine used to harvest and thresh all kinds of grain. Combines commonly cause partial or complete amputation.

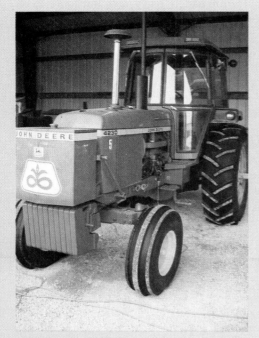

FIGURE 21-7 Diesel tractor.

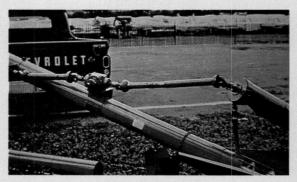

FIGURE 21-8 Power takeoff shaft.

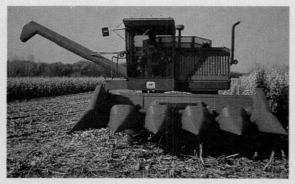

FIGURE 21-10 Auger and hopper with protective cage.

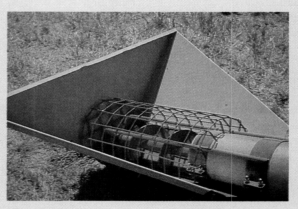

FIGURE 21-9 Combine with corn head.

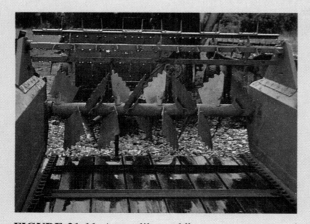

FIGURE 21-11 Auger-like paddles on manure spreader.

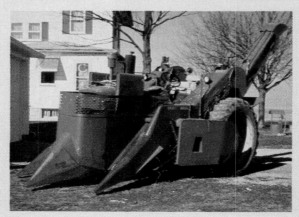

FIGURE 21-12 Corn picker.

Grain Tanks and Augers

Grain tanks and **augers** (Figures 21-10 and 21-11) are used to move the threshed, separated, and cleaned grain from the cleaning shoe to the grain tank, and then from the grain tank to the wagon or truck for transport. Augers are generally four to six inches in diameter with flights three to five inches apart. The elevator has a series of rubber or steel paddles attached to a drive chain that moves at about 350 feet per minute. Augers can pull in victims with extreme force.

Augers often cause complete amputation, usually of the hands and arms, but sometimes of the feet and legs. Auger accidents often involve children, who are not experienced enough to avoid accident. Entanglement in augers is so severe that it often cannot be handled in the field; you may need to cut the auger free and transport it with the patient. If amputation is complete, you may be able to slowly rotate the auger in its natural direction until the amputated part emerges at the end. If you need to cut the auger in cases of incomplete amputation, cut it five feet from the patient's body, taking care to avoid excessive vibration or movement.

Never reverse an auger — it can cause increased tissue damage.

Victims who fall into grain tanks risk death from suffocation. *Always assume that a victim in a grain tank is alive,* even if he has been trapped for hours. *Do not use the gravity gate or auger to release the grain* — instead, cut uniform holes around the base of the tank, four to six feet above the ground.

If the victim is only partially submerged and you can see the victim from the top of the tank, lower a rescuer on a harness. Establish an airway and clear the area around the victim's head so it is possible to breathe; use plywood, sheets of metal, or a 55-gallon drum with both ends removed to keep grain away from the victim's face.

Corn Pickers

Corn pickers (Figure 21-12) use a system of rollers, belts, and blades to remove corn from the stalk and then to shear the corn away from the cob. Power for corn pickers, whether tractor-mounted or pull-behind, is taken from the tractor PTO and hydraulic systems.

Accidents involving corn pickers usually involve a hand that is crushed when a farmer tries to free trapped material in the picker. Traumatic amputation is rare, but the hand is often lost as a result of damage or infection. Extrication is extremely difficult, since the machinery is in heavy metal housings and cannot be reversed.

Snapping Rolls

Snapping rolls, which move at twelve feet per second when operating at normal speed, generally cause severe crushing injuries to the hand. Most often, a weed or stalk can catch between the rolls and stop. A farmer who tries to remove the trapped weed or stalk can cause the snapping rolls to start up again with the slightest movement of the trapped material — and the snapping rolls move more quickly than the farmer can let go.

Hay Baler

The **hay baler** compacts straw and hay into bundles; some are small rectangular bundles, and others are massive rounded ones. The hay baler exerts force of up to 1,300 pounds between spring-loaded rollers; amputations often result. Hay balers also commonly cause compression, avulsion, and wringer injuries. Because the springs can be released and the belts cut, it is not as difficult to free a patient from a hay baler as from other farm equipment.

☐ OPERATIONAL CONTROLS

Becoming familiar with operational controls on farm machinery can save you time and frustraton during rescue attempts. Levers, knobs, or switches may be used to control the various components of farm machinery. Some manufacturers use different colors or shapes to help the operator quickly identify the controls.

Common color codes include:

- Red — combine movement controls (throttle, gearshift, ground speed control).
- Yellow — auxiliary power controls (separator control, cylinder speed control, header drive control).
- Black — miscellaneous function controls.

☐ EQUIPMENT SHUTDOWN

The first step in shutting down farm machinery is to stabilize it. You can use one of several methods:

- Block or chock the wheels.
- Set the parking or operational brakes.
- Tie the machine to another vehicle.
- Solicit help from neighbors or family members — they can probably tell you how to shut down the machinery.

Once the machine is stabilized, shut it down with the following procedure:

1. Enter the cab, if possible, and look at the controls.
2. Locate the ignition switch or key and throttle

lever. If you have any doubt that you have located the right controls, do *not* touch them.

3. Slow the engine down with the throttle; switch off the key.

4. If the machine is fueled with diesel, the key may not shut off the engine. Locate a fuel or air shutoff lever; again, if you are in doubt, do *not* touch the lever.

5. Pull the knob or lever to shut down the engine.

6. If you cannot shut down the engine in the cab, try at the fuel tank area.

7. If all other attempts at shutting down the machine fail, locate the air intake and discharge a 20-pound CO_2 or Halon fire extinguisher into the air intake; make sure that you hold the trigger of the extinguisher until the engine comes to a complete stop.

☐ PATIENT ASSESSMENT AND EMERGENCY CARE

Most emergency care for farm accidents is the same as for any other injury; some specifics you should look for, however, include the following:

1. If fingers have been injured, stabilize the wrist joint; it, too, is probably injured but may be overlooked in an attempt to save the fingers.

2. If you cannot exert direct pressure right on a wound to control bleeding, use direct pressure over the nearest pressure point. (Farm equipment and entanglement may prevent you from having clear access to the wound.)

3. Remember priorities of airway, breathing, and circulation. Disentanglement can take up to an hour; do not neglect breathing and maintenance of a clear airway while you are waiting for the victim to be freed. Administer high-flow oxygen throughout.

4. Constantly monitor vital signs so that you will not lose a patient to an undetected injury.

5. In some injuries, the equipment itself will help control bleeding because of the pressure exerted on the injury. In these cases, it might be wise to transport the patient in the equipment instead of disentangling; most equipment can be cut to a manageable size.

6. Preserve amputated parts, despite their appearance. Rinse amputated parts with sterile saline or clean water, wrap in a moist towel, put the wrapped part in a water-tight plastic bag, mark the bag with the contents, and place the bag on top of a cold pack or sealed bag of ice. Transport the part

with the victim. *Never submerge the part in water or place it directly on ice.*

Disentanglement

Begin disentanglement once the machine has been stabilized, the engine has been shut down, other hazards (such as leaking fuel) have been controlled, the patient has been stabilized, and a medical team is standing by to provide necessary medical support during extrication. Disentanglement requires appropriate training and assistance at the scene.

☐ INDUSTRIAL RESCUE

Like rural emergencies, industrial emergencies are anything but routine: there are often hazardous materials at the scene, multiple injuries, heavy machinery, or victims who are in unusual positions (crushed beneath fallen debris, or trapped at high angles, for example).

Your first priority in responding to the scene of an industrial accident is to protect your own safety. If there are hazardous materials or chemical spills at the scene, you will need to assure that all rescue units are protected. You may also need to stabilize part of a structure to prevent further injury to both victims and rescuers. If victims are trapped in confined spaces, make sure all rescuers use a self-contained breathing apparatus to prevent being overcome by toxic fumes.

Call multiple response teams, including teams who can fight fire and who are experienced in handling hazardous materials. If the site is large, designate an area where responding units should report; assign a rescuer to stand at the gate or site to meet incoming units and to direct them to injured victims.

If victims are buried by heavy debris, call specialty teams who can hoist the heavy objects — such as concreate, steel reinforcements, heavy machinery, or roofing materials — from the victims so you will have access. *A member of an EMT team should supervise removal of heavy objects,* since those working to remove the objects probably do not have medical training. Removal should be closely monitored to prevent further injury to the victims.

If the victim has been contaminated by hazardous materials, direct a HazMat team to begin immediate decontamination; other rescuers should not assess or treat a contaminated victim, or they may become contaminated themselves. Generally, the victim should be flushed with plenty of running water; clothing (including underwear) should be removed and bagged for disposal; and the victim should be dressed in clean clothes before being assessed and treated. In cases of gross contamination, specially equipped rescuers may need to scrape or dissolve chemicals from the victim before assessment and treatment can take place.

If the victim is trapped at a high angle, mobilize sufficient rescuers *who are properly equipped for the rescue*. Secondary safety belts, full-body harnesses, and rappelling harnesses can be used in high-angle rescues. Victims who are not severely injured can be lowered with full-body harnesses and rappelling harnesses; those who are more severely injured or who require immobilization prior to lowering can be lowered in a Stokes basket. Regardless of which method is used, a rescuer must be lowered alongside the victim to monitor the victim's condition and provide reassurance during descent.

If the industrial accident involves multiple injuries, standard triage procedure should be immediately employed to categorize and prioritize victims for care and transport.

chapter 22

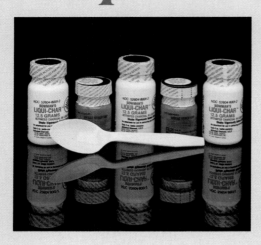

Poisoning Emergencies

✱ OBJECTIVES

- Describe the incidence and seriousness of poisoning and various ways in which poisons can enter the body.
- Identify the common signs and symptoms of ingested, inhaled, and absorbed poisons.
- Describe the appropriate emergency care for specific types of poisoning.

Each year in the United States, thousands of people die from suicidal or accidental poisonings. Poisoning is now the fifth most common cause of accidental death in the United States and ranks first among children (Figure 22-1). Each year, it is estimated that 3 percent of all children in the United States require treatment for poisoning.

In addition to the fatalities, approximately eight million cases of nonfatal poisoning occur each year because of exposure to substances such as industrial chemicals, cleaning agents, plant and insect spray, and medications — in fact, two-thirds of all poisonings in all age groups involve drugs. More than 90 percent of all poisonings occur at home; the most common involve cleaning substances, painkillers, and cosmetics. Two-thirds of all calls to Poison Control Centers involve children. As a result, EMTs are very likely to encounter poisoning emergencies, especially those involving children.

A poison is any substance — liquid, solid, or gas — that impairs health or causes death by its chemical action when it is introduced into the body or onto the skin surface. Some substances that are otherwise harmless become deadly if used incorrectly. Some can be fatal in very low doses, such as pesticides, caustics, preparations containing alcohol, theophylline, clonidine, tricyclic antidepressants, and prenatal vitamins (or other nutritional supplements that contain iron). It is critical that you learn to recognize signs and symptoms of poisoning and that you become able to administer effective emergency care.

Poisons may enter the body in the following ways:

- **Ingestion,** or through the mouth (medication, household cleaners, agricultural products, and chemicals).
- Inhalation in the form of noxious dusts, gases, fumes, or mists (**carbon monoxide, chlorine, ammonia,** insect sprays, chemical gases).

FIGURE 22-1 Poisoning is the number-one cause of accidental death among children.

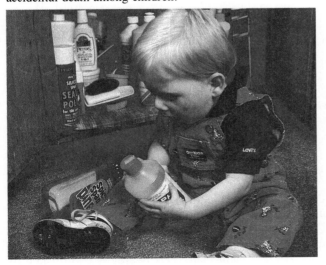

- Injection into the body tissues or bloodstream by hypodermic needles or as bites of rabid animals, poisonous snakes, or poisonous insects (snakebite, spider bite, insect sting).
- Absorption through the skin (as with mercury or certain other poisonous liquids) or contact with the skin (as with poisonous plants and certain fungi).

☐ INGESTED POISONS

In the United States alone, eight to ten million poisonings each year occur in the form of ingestion; thousands of those victims die. The most common agents involved are **salicylates** (aspirin), **acetaminophen,** alcohol, detergents/soaps, and petroleum distillates. Children are frequently poisoned by eating houseplants or outdoor plants, such as oleander, dieffenbachia, lily of the valley, foxglove, rhododendron, or bleeding heart. Half of all plant poisonings are caused by mushrooms.

Ingested poisons usually remain in the stomach only a short time; the stomach absorbs substances only minimally. Rather, absorption takes place after the poison has passed into the small intestine. Thus, much of the management of poisoning is aimed at trying to rid the body of the poison before it gains access to the intestinal tract.

The chief causes of poisoning by ingestion are:

- Overdose of medicine (intentional or accidental).
- Medicines, household cleaners, and chemicals within the reach of children.
- Combining drugs and alcohol.
- Storing poisons in food or drink containers.
- Carelessness.

Importance of Taking a History

Getting a history from a victim of poisoning can be difficult, and the history that you do obtain might not necessarily be accurate: the victim himself may be misinformed, he or she may be deliberately trying to deceive you, or may be subject to a drug-induced confusion. However, to manage the poisoned patient correctly, you need a relevant history. If the patient is a child, other children in the household may have also eaten the poison, so assess all children carefully. Interview family members and witnesses. To begin, look for clues at the scene — overturned or empty medicine bottles, scattered pills or capsules, recently emptied containers, spilled chemicals, spilled cleaning solvents, an overturned plant or pieces of plant, the remains of food or drink, or vomitus.

To get as much history as you can, ask the patient or bystanders the following questions:

- What was ingested? Bring the container and all of its remaining contents, the plant portions or parts that might have been ingested, or other specimens to the hospital or emergency room. Remember to bring all possible containers — the most obvious open container may not be the one that was used. If a plant was ingested, find out what part was involved (roots, leaves, stem, flower, or fruit). If vomiting has occurred, save a sample of the vomitus in a clean, closed container, and transport it with the patient.

- When was the substance taken? Decisions regarding **emesis** (inducing vomiting) will depend significantly upon how much time has elapsed since ingestion. Is there a possibility that other substances were taken along with it?

- How much was taken?

- Has the patient or any bystanders made an attempt to induce vomiting? Has anything been given as an **antidote?**

- Does the patient have a psychiatric history that might suggest a suicide attempt?

- Does the patient have an underlying medical illness, allergy, chronic drug use/abuse, or addiction?

Signs and Symptoms

The signs and symptoms of poisoning by ingestion are variable, depending on the substances involved. *A seriously poisoned person may show few or no symptoms,* so don't gauge the severity of the emergency on symptoms alone. The most common signs and symptoms are:

- Dilated or constricted pupils.
- Nausea, retching, vomiting, and diarrhea.
- Severe abdominal pain, tenderness, distension, and cramps.
- Slowed or abnormal respiration and circulation.
- Excessive salivation or foaming at the mouth.
- Excessive sweating.
- Excessive tear formation.
- Burns or stains around the mouth, pain in the mouth or throat, pain upon swallowing (corrosive poisons may corrode, burn, or destroy the tissues of the mouth, throat, and stomach) (Figure 22-2).
- Unusual breath or body odors.
- Signs of shock.
- Characteristic chemical odors on the breath (such as that left by turpentine).

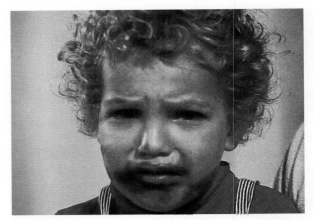

FIGURE 22-2 Skin discoloration — possible poisoning.

- Unconsciousness or varying levels of consciousness.
- Convulsions or seizures.

Physical Examination

The physical examination is especially important in poisoning cases, because the history you obtain is likely to be inaccurate. In addition to the standard procedures for primary and secondary surveys, be especially alert for certain signs (Figure 22-3):

- Observe the patient's skin for cyanosis, pallor, needle marks, abscesses, excessive perspiration, or unusual hues (such as blue-gray, yellow, gray, brown, or black).

- Smell the patient's breath for the characteristic odors of petroleum products, alcohol, or other suggestive odors. Inspect the patient's mouth for signs of caustic burns, excessive salivation, or absence of the gag reflex.

- Assess the level of consciousness; do a complete neurological examination. Check for seizures, muscle spasticity, impairment of central nervous system function, **delirium,** mental disturbances, or signs of coma.

- Assess pupillary reaction; look for impairment of vision or blurring of vision.

- Assess blood pressure.

- Assess pulse and respirations.

- Assess the appearance and odor of any vomitus or diarrhea.

Poison Centers

Poison control centers have been set up across the U.S. and Canada to assist in the treatment of poison victims. Officials at the center can help you decide which first aid measures are a priority and can help you formulate an effective treatment plan. This is usually coordinated by

POSSIBLE INDICATORS OF CHILDHOOD POISONING

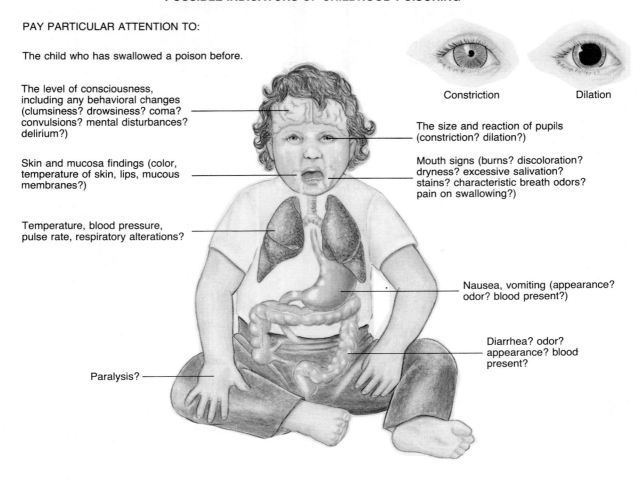

PAY PARTICULAR ATTENTION TO:

The child who has swallowed a poison before.

The level of consciousness, including any behavioral changes (clumsiness? drowsiness? coma? convulsions? mental disturbances? delirium?)

Skin and mucosa findings (color, temperature of skin, lips, mucous membranes?)

Temperature, blood pressure, pulse rate, respiratory alterations?

Paralysis?

Constriction   Dilation

The size and reaction of pupils (constriction? dilation?)

Mouth signs (burns? discoloration? dryness? excessive salivation? stains? characteristic breath odors? pain on swallowing?)

Nausea, vomiting (appearance? odor? blood present?)

Diarrhea? odor? appearance? blood present?

FIGURE 22-3

your medical control. The poison center can also provide information on any available antidote that may be appropriate for your patient.

Tell officials at the center the patient's approximate age and body weight. Summarize the patient's condition, including level of consciousness, level of activity, skin color, vomiting, and so on. Give as many specifics about the poison as you can — estimate how much was ingested, and give the brand name of a household product if you can.

Call to poison centers are toll-free, and most are staffed twenty-four hours per day to assist prehospital personnel as well as the public. Staffed by experienced professionals, each center is also connected to a network of consultants nationwide who can answer questions about almost any toxin. In addition, information on the poison center's computer is updated every ninety days to provide the latest information on treatment options and antidotes. Finally, centers provide followup telephone calls, monitoring the patient's progress and making treatment suggestions until the patient is either hospitalized or asymptomatic.

Contacting the poison center in case of ingested poisoning is safer and more reliable than following manufacturer's label cautions, especially since label information may be incomplete, too generic, or too outdated to be effective. However, initial patient assessment, treatment, and/or transport should not be delayed to accommodate a call to the poison center. Follow local protocol.

Emergency Care for Ingested Poisons

The priorities in managing ingested poisons are airway, breathing, and circulation. Follow these guidelines:

1. **Maintain the airway.** This cannot be overemphasized! Be prepared for an emergency — the patient's status can change suddenly. The sleepy or comatose patient is in constant danger of aspira-

Poisoning Emergencies **345**

tion — maintaining the airway is one of your primary responsibilities. The first choice for managing the airway in ingested poisoning is the nasopharyngeal airway. Avoid unprotected mouth-to-mouth resuscitation, since you can inadvertently be poisoned yourself by residue on the patient's lips and mouth.

2. **Keep the airway clear with suctioning.** Secretions may be profuse following the ingestion of certain poisons, so be prepared. If the patient is in a coma, has no gag reflex, and is suffering seizures, insert an airway (nasal or oral).

3. **Induce vomiting.** If the patient has ingested poison within less than thirty minutes, is fully awake and alert, and if he has a gag reflex, the general rule is to induce vomiting to empty the stomach. *Follow local protocol.* There are some important exceptions for which you should *never* induce vomiting; they are itemized under number 4 in this list. The method of choice of inducing vomiting is to use **syrup of ipecac** (Figure 22-4). Syrup of ipecac works to induce vomiting by irritating the lining of the stomach and triggering the vomiting center in the brain. However, there is some controversy about using ipecac in the field. Follow local protocol, and use it only if instructed to do so by the Poison Control Center and confirmed by your dispatch. To induce vomiting:

   • Have the patient drink water, juice, or a carbonated beverage; an adult needs eight to sixteen ounces, a child four to eight ounces. The liquid must be clear to allow for examination of the vomitus.

   • Administer syrup of ipecac. *Make sure that you are using syrup of ipecac, NOT ipecac fluid extract, which is fourteen times more potent — and it can be fatal at the listed doses* (Figure 22-5). Syrup of ipecac doses are: adult, two tablespoons (thirty cubic centimeters); children one year and older, one tablespoon (15 cubic centimeters); infants under twelve months, one to two teaspoons (five to 10 cubic centimeters). Follow an infant's dose with one bottle of water, a child's with one to two glasses of water, and

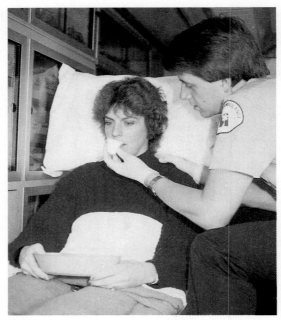

FIGURE 22-5 If directed, induce vomiting with syrup of ipecac and water.

an adult's with two to three glasses of water (Figure 22-6). When possible, it is recommended that children under twelve months be "ipecaced" in a health-care facility, since they can't control their head and neck muscles and are at increased risk of aspiration. Follow local protocol.

• If the patient begins to get stuporous after ipecac has been given, take all necessary measures to protect the airway and prevent aspiration.

• Have the patient sit and lean forward to prevent vomitus from being aspirated into the lungs. Place an infant or small child on his or her stomach with the head lower than the rest of the body, face pointed downward (Figure 22-7).

• Do not delay transport while waiting for the patient to vomit. Syrup of ipecac may take up to twenty minutes to work; vomiting almost always occurs after one dose if you allow enough time for it to work. While a second dose is seldom necessary, you can repeat your initial dosage *once* if the patient does not vomit after fifteen to twenty minutes and if the patient is still awake and alert. Stimulate the gag reflex with a tongue blade before giving the second dose; that alone may cause vomiting.

• If the patient does not vomit after the second dose, you must transport rapidly so that a physician can perform gastric **lavage.** Syrup of ipecac is toxic to the heart if it is not eliminated.

• When the patient stops vomiting from the ipecac, give him or her **activated charcoal** if di-

FIGURE 22-4 Emergency care kit for poisoning includes syrup of ipecac and activated charcoal.

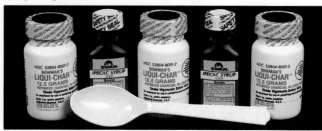

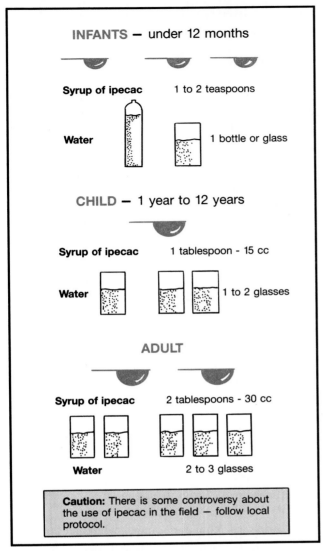

INFANTS — under 12 months

Syrup of ipecac   1 to 2 teaspoons

Water   1 bottle or glass

CHILD — 1 year to 12 years

Syrup of ipecac   1 tablespoon - 15 cc

Water   1 to 2 glasses

ADULT

Syrup of ipecac   2 tablespoons - 30 cc

Water   2 to 3 glasses

Caution: There is some controversy about the use of ipecac in the field — follow local protocol.

FIGURE 22-6 How to induce vomiting.

FIGURE 22-7 Position patient for vomiting and save all vomitus.

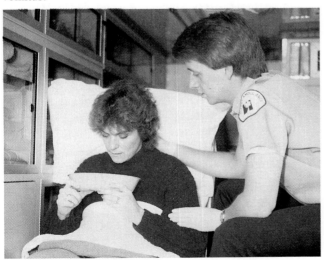

rected to do so by medical control — a special distilled charcoal that because its surface is covered with pores can absorb many times its weight in contaminants. Activated charcoal binds to the poisons in the stomach (it will not bind to alcohol, kerosene, gasoline, caustics, or metals, such as irons) and enhances elimination of these poisons. It is best when used promptly, but can still be effective after several hours (and up to four hours for some poisons). Mix at least two tablespoons of dry charcoal in a glass of tap water to make a slurry. (Many poison antidote kits contain a premixed charcoal slurry that should *not* be mixed with water.) Give the mixture to children in an opaque container, since they may be reluctant to drink it. *Never give activated charcoal before or together with syrup of ipecac, because the charcoal will inactivate the ipecac and render it ineffective. Many feel that activated charcoal should not be used in a pre-hospital setting — follow local protocol.*

- Save part of the vomitus so it can be evaluated by a toxicologist if necessary.
- Give the patient nothing by mouth for one hour following emesis.
- Never allow the patient to fall asleep in a supine position after vomiting; vomiting could recur, and the patient could aspirate.

4. As mentioned, *there are times when you should NOT induce vomiting* — follow local protocol. As a general rule, you should never induce vomiting in the following cases (Figure 22-8):

- Significant vomiting has already occurred.
- The patient has swallowed a substance that may reduce his or her level of consciousness.
- The patient has swallowed a sharp object (such as a nail, pin, razor blade, broken glass).
- The patient is younger than six months of age.
- The patient is stuporous or comatose; the vomitus may be aspirated into the lungs, causing pneumonia.
- The patient has no gag reflex.
- The patient is having or has had seizures.
- The patient shows signs or symptoms of acute myocardial infarction.
- The patient has ingested corrosives (strong acids or alkalis). These include many household cleaners that can damage the esophagus and lining of the mouth as they are ejected.
- The patient has ingested petroleum distillates or products (such as kerosene, gasoline, lighter fluid, or furniture polish). You may be instructed to induce vomiting anyway if the patient has in-

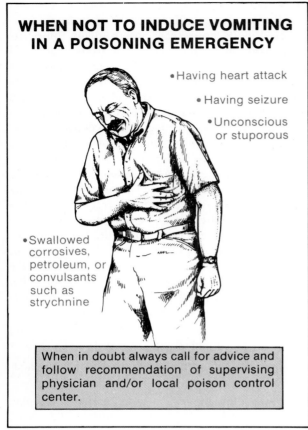

WHEN NOT TO INDUCE VOMITING IN A POISONING EMERGENCY

- Having heart attack
- Having seizure
- Unconscious or stuporous
- Swallowed corrosives, petroleum, or convulsants such as strychnine

When in doubt always call for advice and follow recommendation of supervising physician and/or local poison control center.

FIGURE 22-8

gested excessive amounts or if he or she has swallowed an extremely toxic product, such as a pesticide or one containing heavy metals. Check with your local poison center.

- The patient has ingested a convulsant, such as **strychnine** (often found in mouse poisons); vomiting may induce convulsions.

- The patient is pregnant or lactating.

- When in doubt, call for advice, follow local protocol, and follow the recommendations of the poison center.

5. If a child has handled or been poisoned by a corrosive substance, always wash his or her hands and fingers thoroughly to prevent any damage to the eyes if the child rubs them. Rinse the child's lips and mouth with clean water to remove traces of poison. If in doubt, flush his or her eyes with water.

6. Be prepared to manage shock, coma, seizures, and cardiac arrest as detailed in other chapters of this book. Mouth-to-mouth resuscitation may be dangerous if the patient still has poison on his or her lips, tongue, or the skin surrounding the mouth. Use a bag-valve-mask unit, positive pressure ventilations, or a pocket face mask.

7. Do not give mustard or salt to induce vomiting.

8. If syrup of ipecac is not available, *as a last resort* you can induce vomiting by using the end of a napkin- or handkerchief-padded spoon to tickle the back of the throat and stimulate the gag reflex. Vomiting may be more effectively induced if you first give the patient several glasses of warm water. If the patient is a child, administer a cup of water and place him face down across your knees before tickling the throat.

9. Transport the patient in a lateral recumbent position to allow for drainage.

All poisoned patients need to see a physician, even if it appears that all signs and symptoms have been controlled and the emergency is over.

□ INHALED POISONS

Almost 8,000 people die each year in the United States as a result of inhaling poisonous vapors and fumes, some of which are present without any sign. Most toxic inhalation occurs as a result of fire. It is critical that care be immediate, because the body absorbs inhaled poisons rapidly. The longer the exposure without treatment, the poorer the prognosis.

Common sources of inhaled poison include:

- Carbon monoxide.
- Carbon dioxide from industrial sites, sewers, and wells.
- Chlorine gas (common around swimming pools).
- Fumes from liquid chemicals and sprays.
- Ammonia.
- **Sulphur dioxide** (used in the home and commercially to make ice).
- Anesthetic gases (ether, nitrous oxide, chloroform).
- Solvents used in dry cleaning, degreasing agents, or fire extinguishers.
- Industrial gases.
- Incomplete combustion of natural gas.
- **Hydrogen sulfide** (sewer gas).

Signs and Symptoms of Inhaled Poisoning

The general signs and symptoms of inhaled poisoning include the following:

- Severe headache.
- Nausea and/or vomiting.

348   *Chapter 22*

- Cough, stridor, wheezing, or rales.
- Shortness of breath.
- Chest pain or tightness.
- Facial burns.
- Signs of respiratory tract burns, including singed nasal hairs, soot in sputum, or soot in throat.
- Burning or tearing eyes.
- Burning sensation in the throat or chest.
- Cyanosis.
- Confusion.
- Dizziness.
- Varying levels of consciousness.

Carbon Monoxide

The most common gas that causes poisoning is carbon monoxide — present in paint remover, aerosols, coal, charcoal briquettes, tobacco, gasoline, insulating materials, building materials, exhaust fumes of internal combustion engines (such as cars), lanterns, sewer gas, charcoal grills, and gas that is manufactured for cooking and heating. Carbon monoxide poisoning causes half of all poisoning deaths in the United States; more than 3,800 people die each year from carbon monoxide poisoning, and at least 10,000 others are injured badly enough to cause illness.

Carbon monoxide is completely nonirritating, tasteless, colorless, and odorless. It is formed by the incomplete combustion of gasoline, coal, kerosene, plastic, wood, and natural gas. The primary sources of carbon monoxide are home-heating devices (including furnaces and wood-burning fireplaces) and exhaust fumes from automobiles. Other common sources are tobacco smoke (which contains enough carbon monoxide to cause symptoms), barbecue grills, kitchen stoves, gas lamps, recreational fires, propane-powered industrial equipment, and faulty water heaters, kerosene heaters, and space heaters.

The signs and symptoms of carbon monoxide poisoning are very similar to those of the flu, but there are no accompanying fever, general body aches, or swollen or tender lymph glands.

The initial symptoms of poisoning include headache, weakness, agitation, confusion, and slight dizziness. As the poisoning progresses, the patient suffers dim vision, spots before the eyes, sensitivity of the eyes to light, temporary blindness or hearing loss, and, eventually, convulsions, coma, and death. If the patient is not removed from the source quickly, he will become unconscious and will have trouble breathing. It takes only a few minutes to die from carbon monoxide poisoning. Death is so certain, in fact, that more than half of all suicides in the United States each year are committed with automobile exhaust, which is 7 percent carbon monoxide.

Carbon monoxide causes asphyxia because it binds with the hemoglobin of the blood 200 times more readily than oxygen does. The blood, therefore, carries less and less oxygen from the lungs to the body tissues. In addition, the hemoglobin doesn't release the oxygen as easily, and carbon monoxide also interferes with the transfer and processing of oxygen in the cells. The greatest and most rapid effect of carbon monoxide is on the organs with the greatest concentration of oxygen: the brain and the heart.

You should consider carbon monoxide poisoning as a possibility whenever you encounter unexplained flu symptoms, such as headache, nausea and vomiting, and confusion — especially if other family members or coworkers are suffering from the same symptoms. The signs and symptoms of acute carbon monoxide poisoning are the same in adults and children and depend on the percentage of carbon monoxide in the blood. They may range from subtle central nervous system effects to coma and death. The signs and symptoms often come and go and vary throughout the day (as the patient unwittingly moves away from the source and into fresh air). The signs and symptoms are usually shared by others in the same environment, including pets. The range of signs and symptoms includes the following (Figure 22-9):

FIGURE 22-9

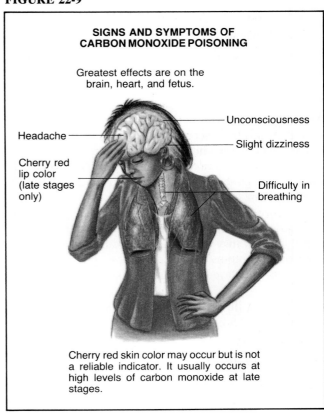

SIGNS AND SYMPTOMS OF
CARBON MONOXIDE POISONING

Greatest effects are on the brain, heart, and fetus.

Headache

Cherry red lip color (late stages only)

Unconsciousness

Slight dizziness

Difficulty in breathing

Cherry red skin color may occur but is not a reliable indicator. It usually occurs at high levels of carbon monoxide at late stages.

Low Levels of Carbon Monoxide

- Reduced exercise tolerance in patients with chronic obstructive pulmonary disease.
- Angina in patients with pre-existing heart conditions.
- Throbbing headache.
- Shortness of breath with little exertion.
- Nausea.
- Irritability, confusion, loss of judgment, and difficulty concentrating.

Moderate Levels of Carbon Monoxide

- Severe headache.
- Severe nausea and vomiting.
- Dizziness.
- Yawning.
- Visual disturbances.
- Confusion and difficulty thinking.

High Levels of Carbon Monoxide

- Lethargy and stupor.
- Syncope on exertion.
- Heart arrhythmias and chest pain.
- Temporary loss of vision.
- Convulsions.
- Pulmonary edema.
- Coma.

Note: Skin color is normal at first, but becomes pale and then cyanotic as poisoning progresses. In late stages at very high levels, mucous membranes and skin become bright cherry-red in color, sometimes blistering. Cherry-red lips are not commonly seen, and occur only when very high levels of carbon monoxide are in the patient's system.

Approximately 10 to 30 percent of all carbon monoxide poisoning victims have a delay in the onset of symptoms that may be several weeks. If such a delay occurs, the symptoms are usually irreversible. Signs and symptoms of delayed poisoning include:

- Flu-like illness (look for a persistent flu-like illness without fever or upper respiratory infection).
- Irritability.
- Memory loss.
- Inability to concentrate.
- Inability to think abstractly.

- Personality changes.
- Uncontrolled crying.

Emergency Care for Inhaled Poisons

1. *Protect yourself first!* Safeguarding your own health, get the patient into fresh air immediately, removing him or her from the source of the poison. If the patient is in a closed garage or room or some other small or closed space, call a rescue squad or the fire department. Remember — the presence of carbon monoxide is difficult to detect. Do not delay unnecessarily in an area that may be contaminated. If there are no contraindicating injuries, have the patient lie down with the head elevated.

2. Loosen all tight-fitting clothing, especially around the neck and over the chest.

3. If the patient is not breathing, start artifical ventilation immediately, and continue while transporting or until the patient is breathing on his or her own. Do not interrupt the artificial ventilation for any reason. If necessary, administer CPR.

4. If the patient's breathing is noisy, he or she may have laryngeal edema; use a nasopharyngeal airway to protect the airway.

5. As soon as possible, administer 100 percent humidified oxygen by non-rebreathing mask (Figure 22-10). Use a device that delivers the highest possible concentration of oxygen. Assist respirations if necessary (i.e., bag-valve-mask).

6. If the patient is vomiting, fainting, suffering respiratory problems, undergoing cardiac irritability, or comatose, or if the patient's blood pressure

FIGURE 22-10 Administer 100 percent oxygen by mask for a victim of inhaled poison.

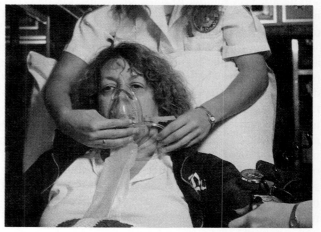

drops below 50 mmHg, use the PASG if allowed by local protocol.

7. Treat the patient for shock and keep him or her completely inactive and quiet throughout transport.

8. All victims of carbon monoxide poisoning *must* have medical care; 45 percent of all carbon monoxide victims develop delayed neurological complications after initial recovery. Transport the patient immediately, even if he seems to have recovered (awakening or seeming alertness can be false signs of recovery).

9. Contact the poison control center for further instructions.

□ ABSORBED POISONS

Absorbed poisons — usually chemicals or poisonous plants that enter through the skin — generally cause burns, lesions, and inflammation. Rarely, absorbed poisons will not cause irritation of the skin; in those cases, you will need to rely on bystanders and the patient to determine the source and presence of poisoning. Corrosives or other chemicals that are splashed into the eyes cause extreme burning pain, excessive tearing, and the inability to open the eye.

Skin reactions range from mild irritation to severe chemical burns; there may be redness, heat, itching, rash, inflammation, and burning. Systemic signs and symptoms of absorbed poisons include headache, abnormal breathing, irregular or abnormal pulse, and possible anaphylactic shock.

Emergency Care for Absorbed Poisons

Whenever a patient has corrosives or chemicals on the skin or in the eyes, contact the regional poison center immediately. Depending on the poison, there may be a true medical emergency; you need to act quickly and transport immediately. Guidelines for treating chemical burns of the eyes are found in Chapter 35, "Burn Emergencies." General guidelines for treating other absorbed poisons are as follows:

1. Move the patient from the source of poisons, protecting your own hands with gloves. Blot dry any liquid toxins on the patient's skin.

2. Brush any dry chemicals or solid toxins from the patient's skin, taking extreme care not to abrade the skin and not to spread the contamination.

3. Before you remove the patient's clothes, irrigate all parts of the body copiously with running water when possible (a shower or garden hose is ideal).

Make sure that you protect bystanders and the patient from further contamination.

4. After the first washing, remove all of the patient's clothing, including shoes and jewelry. Wash the patient a second time with plenty of running water. Some experts advocate the use of soap during the second washing; follow local protocol.

5. Carefully check "hidden" areas, such as the nailbeds, skin creases, areas between the fingers and toes, and any hair.

6. Transport, keeping the patient warm during transport.

□ POISONOUS PLANTS

Ingestion of a Poisonous Plant

A number of common backyard and household plants are poisonous if they are eaten. The United States Public Health Service estimates that 12,000 children eat potentially poisonous plants every year; the ingestion of poisonous plants is an extremely common poisoning emergency, especially in children under the age of five years. And the plants involved are not exotic — they include morning glory, rhubarb leaves, buttercup, daisy, daffodil, lily of the valley, narcissus, tulip, azalea, English ivy, mistletoe berries, iris, hyacinth, laurel, philodendron, rhododendron, wisteria, delphinium, and certain parts of the tomato, potato, and petunia plants.

Signs and symptoms of plant ingestion depend, of course, on the plant that was ingested; each one has individual toxins. The most common signs and symptoms of poisonous plant ingestion include:

- Intense burning of the tongue and mouth.
- Nausea and vomiting.
- Diarrhea.
- Watering of the mouth, nose, and eyes.
- Seizures.
- Excessive sweating.
- Weakness.
- Paralysis.
- Stomach pain.
- Dilated pupils.
- Fever.
- Hallucinations.
- Abdominal cramps.
- Respiratory depression.
- Central nervous system depression.
- Cardiac arrhythmias.

Emergency Care for Ingestion of Poisonous Plants

Treatment for ingestion of poisonous plants consists of the following:

1. Induce vomiting with syrup of ipecac. Follow the guidelines listed under ingested poisons.
2. Administer activated charcoal after all vomiting has stopped.
3. Provide basic supportive care; apply cold compresses to the mouth to ease pain and itching.
4. Transport as quickly as possible.

Skin Contact with a Poisonous Plant

Poison ivy (Figure 22-11) thrives in sun and in light shade. It usually grows in the form of a trailing vine that sends out numerous kinky brown footlets that are slightly thickened at the tips. It can also grow in the form of a bush and can attain heights of ten feet or more. You don't need direct contact with the plant in order to have a reaction from poison ivy: the poisonous element, urushiol, can be carried on animal fur, tools, and clothing. If poison ivy is burned, particles of urushiol are contained in the smoke and can be breathed in or can contaminate the skin. **Poison sumac** (Figure 22-12) is a tall shrub or slender tree, usually growing along swamps and ponds in wooded areas. **Poison oak** (Figure 22-13) resembles poison ivy, with one important difference: the poison oak leaves have rounded, lobed leaflets instead of leaflets that are jagged or entire. Poison oak is found mostly in the Southeast and West. Other plants that can cause mild to severe **dermatitis** include stinging nettle, crown of thorns, buttercup, mayapple, marsh marigold, candelabra cactus, brown-eyed Susan, shasta daisy, and chrysanthemum.

Patients with allergic reactions to urushiol (approximately 75 percent of all Americans) will have much more severe reactions to contact with poison ivy. Signs and symptoms of contact with a poisonous plant generally include the following:

- Fluid-filled, oozing blisters at the site of contact (it generally takes two to seven days for the rash to form, but severe contact can cause a rash within twelve hours) (Figure 22-14).
- Itching and burning.
- Swelling.
- Pain if the reaction is severe.
- Other areas of contact can cause conjunctivitis, asthma, and other allergic reactions.

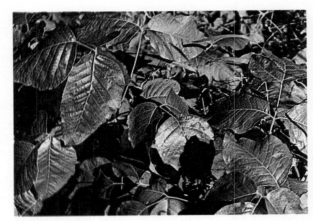

FIGURE 22-11 Poison ivy.

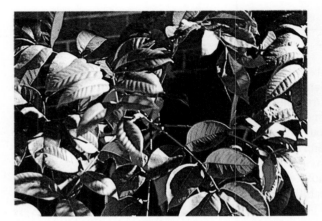

FIGURE 22-12 Poison sumac.

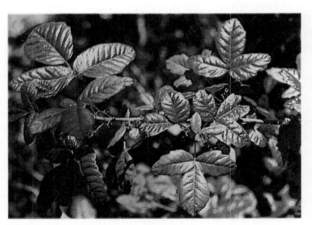

FIGURE 22-13 Poison oak.

If the rash is scratched, secondary infections can occur. The rash usually disappears in one to two weeks in cases of mild exposure, and up to three weeks when exposure is more severe.

Toxin on the hands may spread the rash to other parts of the body, but the clear fluid that weeps from the rash will not spread the rash or infect new sites.

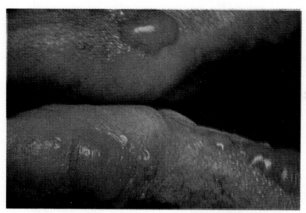

FIGURE 22-14 Blisters from poisonous plant contact.

Emergency Care for Skin Contact with a Poisonous Plant

The following emergency care is recommended:

1. Remove any clothing that may have plant oils on it. Be careful not to spread contamination as you remove the patient's clothing, and protect your own skin from exposure.

2. Wash the exposed skin thoroughly as soon as possible after contact to limit the spread of plant oils. Speed counts! Wash within five minutes, if possible. Do not use soap — it causes plant oils to spread. Ideally, you should pour rubbing alcohol over the area and rinse it with cool water. Then flood the exposed skin with cool water and pat — do not rub — dry. Make sure to scrub under the fingernails to remove any plant oils there.

3. Apply cold compresses to help reduce swelling and irritation.

4. Apply soothing lotions to help reduce swelling and irritation; use **calamine** or calamine/antihistamine, but steer away from others, since they can worsen the allergic reaction.

5. Keep the area clean and dry, and instruct the patient not to scratch the rash.

6. If a severe exposure does not respond to the above-outlined treatment, transport the patient.

☐ FOOD POISONING

The incidence of food poisoning is increasing rapidly. Each year some 33 million Americans are affected (Figure 22-15).

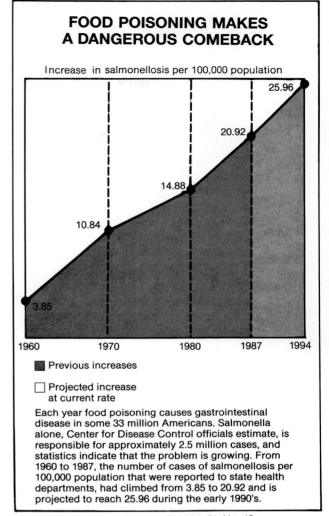

FOOD POISONING MAKES A DANGEROUS COMEBACK

Increase in salmonellosis per 100,000 population

25.96
20.92
14.88
10.84
3.85

1960   1970   1980   1987   1994

☐ Previous increases

☐ Projected increase at current rate

Each year food poisoning causes gastrointestinal disease in some 33 million Americans. Salmonella alone, Center for Disease Control officials estimate, is responsible for approximately 2.5 million cases, and statistics indicate that the problem is growing. From 1960 to 1987, the number of cases of salmonellosis per 100,000 population that were reported to state health departments, had climbed from 3.85 to 20.92 and is projected to reach 25.96 during the early 1990's.

Adapted from: Paul L. Cerrato, *RN*, Vol. 51, No. 10.
FIGURE 22-15

Food poisoning occurs when food that contains bacteria or the toxins that bacteria produce is eaten. Illness can be caused either by the bacteria itself or by the toxins produced by the bacteria.

Food poisoning is difficult to detect since symptoms and signs vary greatly. Usually, you will note abdominal pain, nausea and vomiting, gas and loud, frequent bowel sounds, and diarrhea.

Emergency care consists of transporting and following general guidelines for ingested poisons and giving care for shock. Do not give the patient anything to eat or drink. Extremely young or old patients may need to be hospitalized to control dehydration.

chapter 23

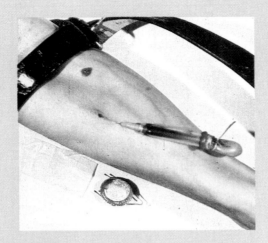

Drug and Alcohol Emergencies

✱ OBJECTIVES

- Know the general terminology relating to drug/alcohol dependency.
- Explain how to determine if an emergency is drug/alcohol related and the factors that may make it life-threatening.
- Review the various drug groups, including alcohol, and identify the signs and symptoms associated with their use.
- Describe the general guidelines for managing a drug/alcohol emergency, including the talk-down technique.
- Describe emergency care and special precautions for dealing with the PCP user.
- Describe the major medical problems associated with cocaine use and know the emergency response to cocaine intoxication.

Drugs and alcohol are misused and abused by a variety of individuals. **Alcoholism** — which is treatable, but not curable, and is fatal if not treated — strikes all classes and almost every age group. In the United States alone, there are ten million alcoholics. Alcohol is the most abused drug in the United States: two-thirds of all adults are "social drinkers," and there are more than 100 million drinkers, 20 percent of whom are alcoholics.

Alcohol is directly involved in approximately 30,000 deaths and 500,000 injuries each year as a result of automobile accidents. It is a factor in half of all motor vehicle accidents, and in 78 percent of all fatally injured drivers over the age of twenty-five. It is a factor in half of all arrests for criminal activity. Because of its deleterious effects on the liver, pancreas, central nervous system, and other body organs, alcohol reduces the average life span of an alcoholic by ten to twelve years (Figures 23-1–23-9).

As an emergency medical technician, it is important that you become familiar with the various categories of commonly abused drugs, learn their effects on the body, recognize signs and symptoms of **overdose** and **withdrawal,** and know the principles of emergency care.

Background information concerning each drug group is provided in Table 23-1 format to help you understand the seriousness and complexity of drug and alcohol emergencies. It is not expected that you will remember everything about each of the drug groups. The

□ Alcohol and Drug Abuse Disorders

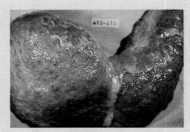

FIGURE 23-1 Fungal damaged heart from drug injection.

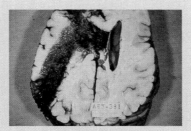

FIGURE 23-2 Bullet wound to brain, alcohol-related.

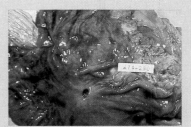

FIGURE 23-3 Chronic gastric ulcer from alcohol use.

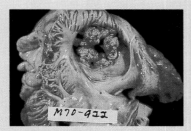

FIGURE 23-4 Alcoholic cirrhosis of the liver.

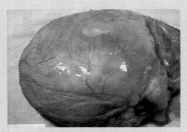

FIGURE 23-5 Enlarged, weak heart, alcohol-induced.

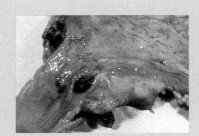

FIGURE 23-6 Ruptured vein in esophagus, causing severe internal bleeding. Alcohol-induced.

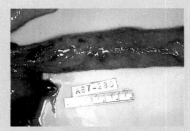

FIGURE 23-7 Dilated esophageal veins from chronic alcohol use.

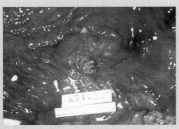

FIGURE 23-8 Internal bleeding from an ulcer caused by chronic alcohol use.

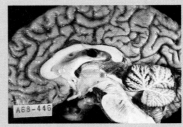

FIGURE 23-9 Brain damage (cerebellum) from chronic alcohol use.

TABLE 23-1
Emergency Consequences of Commonly Abused Drugs

DRUG CLUSTER	MOST COMMON DRUG OF ABUSE	CONSEQUENCE OF ABUSE
STIMULANTS AND APPETITE SUPPRESSANTS	AMPHETAMINES Caffeine Cocaine Ephedrine Methylphenidate Nicotine Over-the-Counter Preparations	Moderate dosages cause increased alertness, mood elevation, excitation, euphoria, increased pulse rate and blood pressure, insomnia, loss of appetite. "Recreational" use of cocaine, even in small doses, can cause severe cardiac toxicity, including angina pectoris, arrhythmias, and myocardial infarcts. Overdoses can cause agitation, violence, paranoia, increase in body temperature, hallucinations, convulsions, possible death. Cocaine overdose cause excitement, euphoria, rapid respiration, elevated blood pressure, cyanosis, paralysis, loss of reflexes, and can lead to circulatory failure and death. Although the degree of physical addition is not known, sudden withdrawal can cause apathy, long periods of sleep, irritability, depression, disorientation.
CANNABIS PRODUCTS	Hashish Marijuana THC (Tetrahydrocannabinol)	Moderate dosages cause euphoria, relaxed inhibitions, increased appetite, dry mouth, disoriented behavior. Overdoses can cause fatigue, tremors, paranoia, possible psychosis. Although the degree of physical addition is not known, sudden withdrawal can cause insomnia, hyperactivity, and decreased appetite is occasionally reported.
DEPRESSANTS — NARCOTICS AND OPIATES	Codeine Heroin Methadone Morphine Opium (90% of opiate-dependent abusers will have a mixed overdose)	Moderate dosages cause euphoria, drowsiness, lethargy, respiratory depression, constricted pupils, constipation, nausea. Overdoses can cause slow and shallow breathing, clammy skin, convulsions, coma, possible death. Sudden withdrawal results in watery eyes, runny nose, yawning, restlessness, rapid pulse, elevated blood pressure, diarrhea, loss of appetite, irritability, tremors, panic, chills and sweating, cramps, nausea, needle tracks.
DEPRESSANTS — SEDATIVES AND TRANQUILIZERS	Alcohol Antihistamines Barbiturates Chloralhydrate Other Non-Barbiturate, Nonbenzodiazepine, Sedatives Over-the-Counter Preparations Diazepam and Other Benzodiazepines Other Major Tranquilizers Other Minor Tranquilizers	Moderate dosages can result in slurred speech, drowsiness, impaired thinking, incoordination, disorientation, drunken behavior without odor of alcohol. Overdose can result in CNS depression, shallow respiration, cold and clammy skin, dilated pupils, weak and rapid pulse, coma, respiratory/circulatory failure, possible death. Aggressive and suicidal behavior may also occur. Sudden withdrawal results in anxiety, insomnia, tremors, delirium, convulsions, possible death.
PSYCHEDELIC DRUGS (Hallucinogens)	DET (N, N-Diethyltryptamine) DMT (N, N-Dimethytryptamine) LSD (Lysergic Acid Diethylamide) Mescaline MDA (3, 4 Methylenedioxyamphetamine) PCP (PHENCYCLIDINE) STP (DOM-2, 5-Dimethoxy, 4-Methylamphetamine)	Moderate dosages can result in motor disturbances, anxiety, paranoia, delusions of persecution, illusions and hallucinations, poor perception of time and distance. Overdose can result in longer, more intense "trip" episodes, psychosis or exacerbation of a pre-existing psychiatric problem, and possible death. Flashbacks can occur months or years after the original dose. PCP may also cause paralysis, violence, rage, status epilepticus.
INHALANTS	Aerosol Propellants Gasoline and Kerosene Glues and Organic Cements Lacquer and Varnish Thinners Lighter Fluid Medical Anesthetics	Moderate dosages cause excitement, euphoria, feelings of drunkenness, giddiness, loss of inhibitions, aggressiveness, delusions, depression, drowsiness, headache, nausea. Overdoses can cause loss of memory, delirium, glazed eyes, slurred speech, drowsiness, hallucinations, confusion, unsteady gait, and erratic heart beat and pulse are possible. Sudden withdrawal results in insomnia, decreased appetite, depression, irritability, headache. Death can result from suffocation or from a phenomenon called SSD ("sudden sniffing death"), which is still poorly understood but which might follow myocardial infarction.

information that is most important for you to remember concerns emergency care for drug and alcohol abuse and overdose.

☐ GENERAL TERMINOLOGY

Drug abuse is defined as the self-administration of drugs (or of a single drug) in a manner that is not in accord with approved medical or social patterns. **Compulsive drug use** refers to the situation in which an individual becomes preoccupied with the use and procurement of the drug. Compulsive drug use usually leads to **addiction** characterized by physical and/or psychological dependence.

Physical dependence is defined by the appearance of an observable **abstinence syndrome** or withdrawal following the abrupt discontinuation of a drug that has been used regularly. Physical dependence signs and symptoms are different for different drug classes (such as **narcotics, depressants,** or **stimulants),** but physical dependence can always be identified by the presence of abstinence syndromes.

A physically dependent person will usually have one set of signs and symptoms due to drug use and an opposite set when the drug is withheld. **Opiates,** for example, reduce gastrointestinal activity. When a person who is physically dependent on opiates is denied the drug, he or she suffers the opposite effect of increased gastrointestinal activity.

Physical dependence is not a "normal" physiological condition. It represents adaptation by the bodily systems to the presence of the drug. When a person becomes physically dependent, then, the absence of the drug has a significant physiological impact.

Psychological dependence refers to a condition in which the patient experiences a strong *need* to use the drug repeatedly, even in the absence of physical dependence. The state of psychological dependence is sometimes called **habituation.**

While most drug therapy has traditionally centered on treating physical dependence, psychological dependence is often more compelling and critical. Some drugs produce no physical dependence at all but produce intense psychological dependence.

One of the difficulties with psychological dependence is that the patient is "rewarded" for taking the drug. He or she becomes motivated, feels good, and thinks that he or she is capable of doing marvelous things. In many cases, the drug is used to escape feelings of depression.

Tolerance refers to a situation in which, after repeated exposures to a given drug, achieving the desired effect requires larger doses. The magnitude of tolerance can be measured by comparing the results obtained from the initial dose of the drug with those obtained from subsequent doses.

In many instances, tolerance works within a drug class, i.e., tolerance to one **barbiturate** produces a tolerance to all barbiturates. In addition, tolerance may develop in response to only some actions of a particular drug. Tolerance to the different effects of a drug does not necessarily develop at the same rate or with the same degree.

The extent of tolerance and the rate of its development depend on the individual, the drug, the dose, the frequency of dose, and the method of administration. Most tolerance results from frequent and continuous exposure to the drug. An increase in dosage will again produce the desired results. With some drugs, however, the patient reaches a plateau, and the desired effect cannot be obtained with *any* dosage. Remember — with **street drugs,** there is no quality assurance. A "dime bag" that produces moderate euphoria today could be a lethal dose tomorrow!

Addiction involves physical and psychological dependence, tolerance, and compulsive drug use. It is characterized by overwhelming involvement in the use of a drug.

☐ HOW TO DETERMINE IF AN EMERGENCY IS DRUG/ALCOHOL RELATED

Because abuse of drugs and alcohol produces signs that mimic a number of system disorders or diseases, it is often difficult to properly assess a condition as a drug or alcohol emergency. This is especially true if a patient is unconscious.

If you suspect that an unconscious patient might be experiencing a drug or alcohol emergency, do the following:

- Inspect the area immediately around the patient for evidence of drug or alcohol use — empty or partially filled pill bottles, syringes, empty liquor bottles, and so on. Be sure to check the patient's pockets.
- Check the patient's mouth for signs of partially dissolved pills or tablets that may still be in his or her mouth. (If present, remove.)
- Smell the patient's breath for traces of alcohol. (Be sure that you do not confuse a musky, fruity, or acetone odor for alcohol — all three can be indicative of diabetic coma.)
- Ask the patient's friends or family members, if they are nearby, what they know about the incident.
- Ask any witnesses who might have seen the pa-

tient lose consciousness if they can offer any suggestions about what might have happened.

- Remember — many serious diseases (such as diabetes and epilepsy) resemble drug overdose or abuse. Do not make the mistake of assuming that ingested drugs are the only reason a person may be struporous or have slurred speech. *Never jump to conclusions*.

Many emergencies that will be seen in the field will involve drug overdose — an emergency that involves poisoning by a drug (whether the drug is legally sold or illegally obtained). Most drug overdoses in the field involve habitual drug users, but drug overdose can also be accidental, the result of miscalculation, the result of confusion, the result of using more than one drug, or intentional (usually as the result of a suicide attempt).

☐ HOW TO DETERMINE IF AN ALCOHOL/DRUG EMERGENCY IS LIFE-THREATENING

If you suspect drug or alcohol ingestion at a dangerous level, observe the patient briefly for these six signs and symptoms that indicate a life-threatening emergency (Figure 23-10):

- **Unconsciousness.** The patient cannot be awakened, or, if can be awakened, lapses back into unconsciousness almost immediately. The patient appears to be in a deep sleep or coma.

- **Breathing difficulties.** The patient's breathing may have stopped, may be weak and shallow, or may be weak and strong in cycles. The patient's exhalations may be raspy, rattling, or noisy. The patient's skin may be cyanotic, indicating that he or she is not receiving enough oxygenated blood.

- **Fever.** Any temperature above 100°F. (38°C.) may indicate a dangerous situation when drugs and/or alcohol are involved.

- **Abnormal pulse rate or irregular pulse.** Normal range for pulse rate is between 60 and 100 beats per minute for an adult; any pulse that is below or above that acceptable range may indicate danger, as does a pulse that is irregular (not rhythmical).

- **Vomiting while not fully conscious.** A person who is stuporous, semiconscious, and who vomits runs a high risk of aspirating the vomitus, creating serious breathing difficulties.

- **Convulsions.** An impending convulsion may be indicated by twitching of the face, trunk, arms, or legs; muscle rigidity; or muscle spasm. A patient who is experiencing a series of violent jerking movements and spasms is having a convulsion.

☐ SIGNS AND SYMPTOMS OF DRUG ABUSE

Each of the drug classes has unique effects, signs and symptoms of withdrawal and overdose, and patterns of tolerance. See Table 23-1.

Drug abusers are more prone to certain injuries, illnesses, and infectious diseases. Most prominent among these are AIDS, hepatitis, endocarditis, phlebitis, paranoia, depression, suicide, homicide, and injuries from falls.

Confronted with a patient who may have a drug-related condition, how can you determine which drug is involved? Sometimes it is just not possible in the field to make that determination; in many cases, you will simply have to treat general signs and symptoms and provide transport. You might be able to make a determination based on some classical signs of specific drug use: **cocaine** users often pick at their skin or clothing to get rid of imaginary "bugs," and **phencyclidine (PCP)** users are usually very easily agitated by even the slightest noise.

Another factor that makes it very difficult to determine *which* drug was used is that many users take a combination of drugs (sometimes without knowing it), and many drugs purchased on the street are adulterated with white, powdery substances such as starch, talc, sugar, or sawdust. Some estimate that cocaine sold on the street is often diluted up to 75 percent with sucrose, talc, or starch. Even if the patient can tell you what he or she took, it might not be accurate — the patient may have been misled by the person who sold the drug. For example, only about 3 to 4 percent of all the drugs that contain PCP are actually sold on the street as PCP.

☐ OBSERVATION AND ASSESSMENT

The most important information to be gathered from the emergency drug/alcohol patient concerns the level of consciousness and vital signs. The severity of the intoxication can be determined by observing the following:

- Whether the patient is awake and will answer questions.
- Whether the patient withdraws from painful stimuli.
- Whether respirations are adequate.

DRUG AND ALCOHOL EMERGENCY INDICATORS

If any of the following six danger signs are present, no matter what caused the crisis, the patient's life may be threatened and there is an immediate need for emergency care and medical assistance.

1

Unconsciousness:
The patient cannot be awakened from what appears to be a deep sleep or coma. If awakened for a short period of time, he almost immediately relapses into unconsciousness.

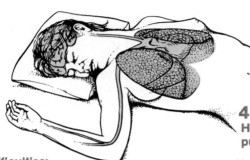

3

Raised temperature:
As a guide it may be stated that any temperature above 100° F. or 38° C. falls into this category.

4

High or low pulse rate, or an irregular pulse:

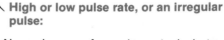

Normal range for pulse rate is between 60 and 100 beats per minute for an adult; any pulse that is below or above that acceptable range indicates danger, as does a pulse that is irregular (not rhythmical).

2

Respiratory difficulties:
The patient's breathing may be very weak, strong and weak in cycles, or may stop altogether. Inhalation or expiration may be noisy. If the patient's skin is bluish (cyanotic), he is almost certainly not receiving enough oxygen, but the absence of cyanosis does not necessarily mean that respiratory difficulties are not severe.

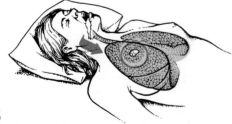

5

Vomiting while semi-conscious or unconscious:
If the patient vomits while semi-conscious or unconscious the prime danger consists of the possibility that he may breathe vomitus back into his lungs, causing further respiratory difficulties.

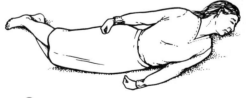

6

Convulsions or seizures:
Muscle rigidity, spasm, or twitching of face, trunk muscles, or extremities may indicate an impending convulsion with a series of violent muscle spasms and jerking movements.

FIGURE 23-10

- Whether the circulatory system is functioning properly (blood pressure, pulse, skin color).

Typically, most patients will fall into one of three categories:

1. Awake, claiming to have ingested a medicine — the patient answers questions and is alert and aware.
2. Semicomatose — the patient will respond appropriately to verbal or noxious stimuli but fall asleep when the stimulus is removed.
3. Comatose — the patient cannot be aroused to consciousness by verbal or noxious stimuli.

Adulteration of a drug with starch, talc, sugar, sawdust, or other white, powdery substance can further complicate the emergency by introducing bacteria. During the primary survey, look for medical complications of drug use such as sepsis or pulmonary emboli.

After your primary survey, supportive care should be initiated as soon as possible. It is obvious that many of the procedures can and should be carried out simultaneously by various members of the emergency team. In any case, the immediate objective is to assess cardiopulmonary functioning and to stabilize basic life support functions. If the EMT is confronted with a comatose patient who is not breathing and whose pulse is absent, CPR must be started immediately.

Once the patient's vital signs have been obtained and stabilized, a secondary survey should be completed.

☐ ALCOHOL EMERGENCIES

At low doses, alcohol causes general excitement, stimulation, and a reduction of natural inhibitions. But don't let that initial response obscure the fact: alcohol is a central nervous system depressant that in moderate doses causes stupor — and that in large doses can cause coma or death.

Alcohol is a major cause of automobile accidents. Alcohol ingestion, even in smaller doses, is also a major factor in drug overdoses, homicides, burns, drowning, and general trauma.

Alcohol is completely absorbed from the stomach and intestinal tract within two hours from the time it is ingested — and sometimes as quickly as within thirty minutes. Once absorbed from the stomach, it is relatively quickly distributed to all body tissues. It is concentrated, however, in the blood and brain, with brain concentrations rapidly approaching those found in the blood.

The alcoholic syndrome usually consists of problem drinking, during which alcohol is used frequently to relieve tensions or other emotional difficulties, and the stage of true addiction, in which abstinence from drinking causes major withdrawal symptoms. The form in which alcohol is ingested is irrelevant; the heavy beer drinker is as much as **alcoholic** as the patient who indulges in too much hard liquor. Alcoholics use alcohol in all its forms: Sterno®, moonshine, grain alcohol, antifreeze, and rubbing alcohol, to name a few. Frequently, alcoholics are dependent on other drugs as well, especially those in the sedative, barbiturate, and tranquilizer categories.

Alcoholism occurs in all social strata. Many alcoholics have underlying psychiatric disorders (especially **schizophrenia**). The alcoholic differs from the true social drinker in that he or she usually begins drinking early in the day, is more prone to drink alone or secretly, and may periodically go on prolonged binges characterized by loss of memory ("blackout periods"). Abstinence from alcohol is likely to produce withdrawal symptoms, such as tremulousness, anxiety, or **delirium tremens (DTs).** As the alcoholic becomes more dependent upon drinking, his performance at work and relationships with friends and family are likely to deteriorate. Absences from work, emotional disturbances, and automobile accidents become more frequent (Figure 23-11).

One of the most serious disorders associated with alcoholism is **Wernicke-Korsakoff syndrome,** a chronic brain syndrome resulting from the toxic effect of alcohol on the central nervous system combined with the malnutrition common among alcoholics. Common signs and symptoms of the syndrome include paralysis of the eyes, dementia, hypothermia, the inability to sort fiction from reality, and eventual coma.

The alcoholic is also more prone to the following illnesses:

- Hypertension.
- Brain damage due to liver malfunction.
- Cirrhosis of the liver.
- Liver failure (the liver degenerates to fatty material).
- **Pancreatitis** (including inflammation, abscesses, and necrosis).
- Cardiomyophathy.
- **Peritonitis.**
- Suppression of the bone marrow's ability to produce red and white blood cells.
- Upper gastrointestinal hemorrhage due to varicose veins in the esophagus (a common cause of death among alcoholics).
- Seizures.
- Subdural hematoma, due to the fact that alcohol damages the liver and interferes with its ability to synthesize clotting factors (alcohol suppresses

ALCOHOL EMERGENCIES

CAUTION These signs can mean illnesses or injuries other than alcohol abuse (e.g. epilepsy, diabetes, head injury).

It is therefore especially important that the person with apparent alcohol on his breath (which can smell like the acetone breath of a diabetic) not be immediately dismissed as a drunk.

He should be carefully checked for other illnesses/injuries.

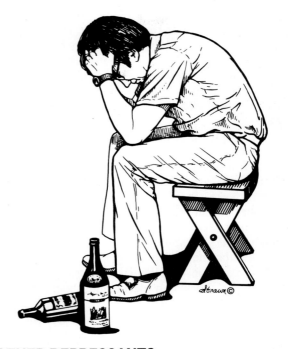

SIGNS

The signs of alcohol intoxication are familiar to all:
- Odor of alcohol on breath
- Swaying/unsteadiness
- Slurred speech
- Nausea/vomiting
- Flushed face

EFFECTS

Alcohol affects a person's judgement, vision, reaction time and coordination. In very large quantities, it can cause death by paralyzing the respiratory center of the brain.

DEPRESSANT

Alcohol is a depressant, not a stimulant. Many people think it is a stimulant since its first effect is to reduce tension and give a mild feeling of euphoria or exhilaration.

ALCOHOL COMBINES WITH OTHER DEPRESSANTS

When alcohol is taken in combination with analgesics, tranquilizers, antihistamines, barbiturates, etc., the depressant effects will be added together and, in some instances, the resultant effect will be greater than the expected combined effects of the two drugs.

MANAGEMENT

The intoxicated patient should be given the same attention given to patients with other illnesses/injuries.

The intoxicated patient needs constant watching to be sure that he doesn't aspirate vomitus and that he maintains respirations.

WITHDRAWAL PROBLEMS

An alcoholic who suddenly stops drinking can suffer from severe withdrawal problems. Sudden withdrawal will often result in DT's (delerium tremens).

Signs include:
1. Shaking hands
2. Restlessness
3. Confusion
4. Hallucinations
5. Sometimes maniacal behavior

The patient must be protected from hurting himself.

FIGURE 23-11

eleven of the twelve clotting factors produced in the liver).

- Fractures of the ribs and extremities due to repeated falls.
- **Hypoglycemia.**
- **Pruritis.**

Acute Intoxication

Acute **intoxication** depends on the amount of alcohol consumed. The signs are similar to those of overdosage with any other CNS depressant: drowsiness, disordered speech and gait, and behavior that is violent, destructive, or erratic. But beware — *this picture may be precisely mimicked by the diabetic patient in* **insulin shock.** Therefore, be suspicious and when in doubt give sugar. If the patient is not diabetic, no harm will be done; many nondiabetic alcoholics have significant **hypoglycemia** anyway.

Also be alert to the possibility that the patient may have taken a combination of alcohol and sedative drugs. Check the patient's pockets and surroundings for evidence of medications, which may significantly complicate the picture.

The primary concern in acute intoxication is maintaining an airway. Give the alcoholic in a coma the same emergency care you would give any other comatose patient. Monitor the patient carefully. In severe cases of acute intoxication, respiratory depression, cardiac arrhythmias, or shock may occur and should be managed as in any other patient.

It is possible to drink a lethal dose of alcohol, but it is not common, since vomiting generally occurs first.

Withdrawal Syndrome

Withdrawal syndrome occurs after a cutback in the amount of alcohol a person is used to; there may not necessarily be total abstinence. Withdrawal syndrome can also occur when blood alcohol levels begin to fall after severe intoxication. Withdrawal syndrome is dose-dependent: the more the alcoholic was drinking, the more severe the syndrome will be.

There are four general stages of alcohol withdrawal: Stage 1 occurs within about eight hours and is characterized by nausea, insomnia, sweating, and tremors. Stage 2, which occurs within eight to seventy-two hours, is characterized by a worsening of Stage 1 symptoms plus vomiting and illusions or hallucinations. Stage 3, which usually occurs within forty-eight hours, is characterized by major seizures, and Stage 4 is characterized by delirium tremens. See Figure 23-12.

Withdrawal syndrome mimics a number of psychiatric disorders, but, as mentioned above, comprises a wide spectrum of signs and symptoms ranging from acute anxiety and tremulousness to DTs. The most common signs and symptoms include:

- Insomnia.
- Muscular weakness.
- Fever.
- Seizures.
- Disorientation, confusion, and thought-process disorders.
- Hallucinations.
- Anorexia.
- Nausea and vomiting.
- Sweating.
- Rapid heartbeat.

Early withdrawal almost always begins within one or two days after the last drink; it is very frightening to the patient but is rarely life-threatening. DTs — a severe, life-threatening condition with a mortality rate of approximately 15 percent — can occur between one and fourteen days after the patient's last drink, most commonly within two to five days. A single episode of DTs lasts between one and three days; multiple episodes can last as long as one month.

DTs are characterized by severe confusion, loss of memory, tremors, restlessness, extremely high fever, dilated pupils, profuse sweating, insomnia, nausea, diarrhea, and almost always hallucinations, mostly of a frightening nature (snakes, spiders, or rats, for example). DTs should be suspected in any patient with delirium of unknown cause; reassurance is all that is necessary in the field.

Seizures are very common in alcoholic withdrawal, but not in DTs. The seizures tend to occur early in the withdrawal period, usually during the first forty-eight hours of abstinence; 90 percent of all alcohol-induced seizures occur within seven to forty-eight hours after the patient's last drink. Nearly half have only one seizure. One-third of all who have seizures in early withdrawal will progress to DTs if left untreated or if treated inadequately.

End-stage alcoholism is characterized by hypothermia, cirrhosis, liver failure, **dementia,** permanent CNS damage (**Wernicke-Korsakoff syndrome**), esophageal **varices,** gastrointestinal bleeding, and coma.

Signs That Medical Attention Is Needed Immediately

When you encounter an alcohol abuse patient, certain signs indicate that medical attention is needed *immediately:*

- Nervous system depression — sleepiness, coma, **lethargy,** and decreased response to pain.

ALCOHOL WITHDRAWAL SYNDROME

Delirium tremens constitutes the most extreme form of alcohol withdrawal syndrome. Less severe forms include alcoholic tremulousness, alcoholic hallucinosis, and withdrawal seizures, which generally (but not always) precede delirium tremens.

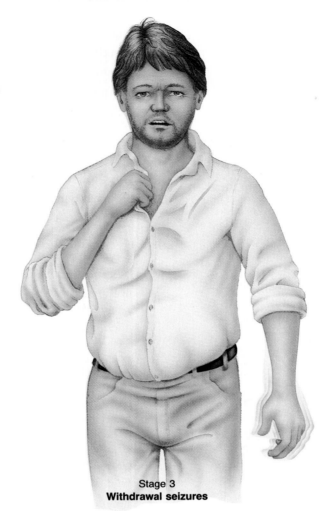

Stage 1
Alcoholic tremulousness

Difficulty concentrating

Restlessness

Irritability

Insomnia

Sweating

Nausea, vomiting

Tremors

Stage 2
Alcoholic hallucinosis

Visual, auditory, and/or tactile hallucinations

Stage 4
Delirium tremens

Confusion

Inattentiveness

Disorientation

Fever

Nausea, vomiting

Incoherence

Hyperirritability

Relentless insomnia

Stage 3
Withdrawal seizures

These are characterized by muscle rigidity and relaxation that usually alternate rhytmically in rapid succession and in groups of 2–6.

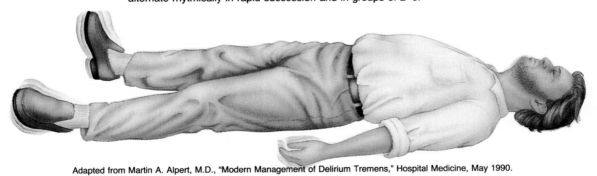

Adapted from Martin A. Alpert, M.D., "Modern Management of Delirium Tremens," Hospital Medicine, May 1990.

FIGURE 23-12 Stages of withdrawal.

- Tremors (especially if the patient is suffering withdrawal).
- Extremely low blood pressure.
- Withdrawal that has become painful.
- Digestive upsets, including **gastritis,** vomiting, bleeding and dehydration.
- Excessively slow or absent breathing.
- Grand mal seizures.
- Delirium tremens (terrifying mental confusion, constant tremors, fever, dehydration, rapid heartbeat, and fumbling movements of the hands). DTs generally require more than seventy-two hours of aggressive treatment.
- Disturbances of vision, mental confusion, and muscular incoordination.
- Disinterested behavior and loss of memory.
- Injury to bones and joints that is unexplained and that is in various stages of healing.

The three major causes of death with alcohol withdrawal are infections, trauma, and other intoxication.

□ GENERAL GUIDELINES FOR MANAGING A DRUG/ALCOHOL CRISIS

Crisis intervention is by definition short term; it involves alleviating the pain and confusion of a specific event or circumstance. The conscious patient with drug- or alcohol-related emergency problems is often experiencing severe emotional stress. In such instances, the most important crisis intervention tools are the verbal and nonverbal communication skills of the attending EMT.

The goal of crisis intervention is to establish and maintain rapport, create trust, and build a short-term working relationship that will lower anxiety, produce a clearer understanding of the problem at hand, and identify the resources necessary to cope with it.

The following guidelines may be helpful in reducing emotional overreaction by helping the patient make sense out of what is happening to him or her:

1. Provide a reality base.
   - Identify yourself and your position.
   - Use the patient's name.
   - Anticipate the concerns of the patient, family, and friends.
   - Based on the patient's response, introduce as much familiarity as possible, e.g., persons, objects, newspapers, TV programs.

- Be calm and self-assured.
2. Provide appropriate nonverbal support.
   - Maintain eye contact.
   - Maintain a relaxed body posture. Be quiet, calm, and gentle.
   - Touch the patient if it seems appropriate.
3. Encourage communication.
   - Communicate directly with the patient, not through others.
   - Ask clear, simple questions.
   - Ask questions slowly, one at a time.
   - Try not to ask questions that require a simple "yes" or "no."
   - Tolerate repetition; do not become impatient.
4. Foster confidence.
   - Be nonjudgmental. Do not accuse the patient.
   - Help the patient gain confidence in you.
   - Listen carefully.
   - Respond to feelings; let the patient know that you understand his or her feelings.
   - Identify and reinforce progress.

Obtaining a history may also be helpful. You should ask the following questions:

- What was taken? The drug container and all its contents should be brought to the emergency department. Its label may help identify the drug, and the number of pills remaining may give a clue as to how much was ingested.
- When was it taken?
- How much was taken?
- Was anything else taken (other drugs or alcohol)? Particularly among today's drug culture, overdoses are rarely "pure" and usually represent a combination of agents.
- What has the patient or bystanders done to try to correct the situation? Has vomiting been induced? Street resuscitation procedures are frequently as dangerous as the overdose itself, and exactly what has been done for the patient is very important. The most common form of street resuscitation is "stimulation" — cold showers, vigorous slapping, and so forth. Check for broken teeth, blood in the mouth, or other signs of injury. If the patient has overdosed on barbiturates, his or her friends may have tried to reverse this by giving the patient **speed (methedrine** or **dexedrine).** There is also a myth prevalent on the streets that salt or milk given intravenously will reverse an overdose. In fact, salt may cause pulmonary edema, and milk can induce **lipid** pneumonia. All of these street

remedies will complicate the picture, so you should learn as much as possible about what has been done.

☐ MANAGING THE VIOLENT DRUG PATIENT

In managing the violent patient (also see Chapter 40, "Crisis Intervention"):

1. Do not approach a potentially violent patient alone. Do so only with a law enforcement official or a sufficient number of people to control an outbreak of violence. EMTs should not create a situation in which they may be injured.

2. Avoid aggressive actions unless there is the immediate possibility of serious injury. In all other circumstances, only defensive techniques, e.g., holding the arms or legs, or rolling in a blanket, should be permitted.

3. If you are assaulted, it is possible that you ignored the many signals of impending loss of control presented by the patient. These include high degrees of agitation, sweating, and excessive talking while struggling with violent impulses, etc. Control your own anxiety, be alert to such signals, and take evasive action (leaving the room or calling in other people) before the patient's impulses are translated into action. There is nothing wrong with running from a room occupied by a physically threatening patient, armed or unarmed.

4. If you can, transport the patient to the hospital immediately. If possible, keep something familiar with the person — a family member, a friend, a coat, or some other possession.

5. Let the person sit near the door of the room; do not place any obstacle (person or furniture) between the person and the door. In other words, do not block the route of escape. A person who feels trapped will likely become more anxious, which will exaggerate his or her hostility and violence. Make absolutely certain to protect your own route of escape.

6. If the patient is armed, the police must be called. If there are not enough personnel to ensure control of an unarmed but violent patient, the police should also be called. Once they have neutralized the threat, assessment and emergency care can be resumed.

7. The patient must be protected while in the emergency setting. Needles, sharp instruments, drugs, etc. should not be in the immediate proximity of the patient. Also, the patient should be observed at all times while in transport.

☐ DEALING WITH HYPERVENTILATION PATIENTS

Hyperventilation is common in drug-abusing patients. It can be a manifestation of acute anxiety, but it also may indicate metabolic acidosis, severe pain, drug withdrawal, or aspirin poisoning.

Hyperventilation in a drug emergency should be cared for as a medical disorder and *not* as anxiety hyperventilation. *Do not* have the patient breathe into a paper bag.

Often it is difficult to provide a quiet, reassuring environment in an emergency setting. The hyperventilating patient should be removed from the crisis situation as soon as possible. Hyperventilating patients should not be left alone. You should listen (in a nonjudgmental way) to the problems of the patient and respond to the patient's questions regarding his or her condition in a calm, professional manner.

☐ GENERAL PROCEDURES FOR OVERDOSE

Several major medical problems can result from drug overdose; among the most common are respiratory problems, central nervous system depression, internal injuries, cardiac arrest, and hyperthemia or hypothermia.

You may face a problem as well: a victim of drug overdose may become violent. Your first goal is protect yourself from danger; know and follow your local protocols regarding leaving a patient and waiting for more help to arrive.

An increasing "overdose" problem has grown out of the practice of using "mules" or "body packers." These are people who swallow latex containers filled with pure cocaine in an attempt to smuggle the cocaine across international borders. They commonly use surgical gloves, latex balloons, or condoms; the package of cocaine may be as large as a golf ball.

In most cases, the package passes through the intestinal system and out of the body without causing damage, but sometimes it breaks. If it ruptures, the system is flooded with a massive dose of pure cocaine. The ensuing toxic emergency requires aggressive life support measures and rapid transport.

The general goals in handling a patient with overdose are to protect the patient and yourself, to calm the patient without harming him or her, and to prevent physical injury, aspiration, and **hyperthermia.** An overdose of almost any drug will cause poisoning and should be cared for at once. Emergency care is limited for a person suffering from drug poisoning, but the following procedures can be done. Your two primary goals should be to monitor the patient's vital signs and to provide basic life support. The following guidelines apply to treatment in all drug and alcohol emergencies:

- Call the Poison Control Center for advice on overdose.
- Be prepared for cardiac arrest. Constantly monitor vital signs; *your primary priority is to maintain an open airway.*
- Do not panic. Treat the patient calmly. Squelch your impulses to throw cold water on the patient or to move him around. Of course, you should move a patient if he or she is inhaling a harmful substance or if he or she is in immediate danger (for instance, if a patient has lost consciousness near a burning building).
- If conscious, try to get the patient to sit or lie on a stretcher. Do not use restraints unless the patient poses a risk to safety.
- Quickly assess the situation. Because symptoms of drug abuse resemble those of other diseases, it is important that you obtain as much information as possible. If the patient is conscious, ask what he has taken. If the patient is unconscious, ask friends or family members who may know what has happened. Whatever you do, do not spend a lot of time finding out what has happened at this stage; there may be life-threatening symptoms that need to be handled directly. You can always come back for further assessment once the patient is under control.
- Establish and maintain a clear airway. Remove anything from the mouth or throat that might pose a breathing hazard, including false teeth, blood, mucus, or vomitus.
- Administer high-flow oxygen and artificial ventilation if needed.
- Turn the patient's head to the side and downward toward the ground in case of vomiting.
- Should vomiting occur, suctioning may be necessary. Use great care to prevent aspiration of vomitus.
- Report any blood in the vomitus; bright red blood in the vomitus can be a sign of ruptured blood vessels in the stomach or esophagus.
- Monitor the patient's vital signs frequently. Various drugs can cause changes in respiration, heart rate, blood pressure, and central nervous system functions. In case of respiratory or cardiac complications, treat the life-threatening situations immediately.
- Watch overdose patients carefully; they can be

conscious one minute and lapse into unconsciousness the next.

- Try to maintain proper body temperature.
- Monitor the body temperature; if it goes over 104°F., sponge the patient with tepid water.
- Take measures to correct or prevent shock. **Hypovolemic shock** can result from vomiting, profuse sweating, or inadequate fluid intake. Be alert for allergic reactions.
- If the patient is conscious, induce vomiting *only under the direction of medical control.* Vomiting should be induced particularly if the drug was ingested within the last thirty minutes. This course of action depends, however, on where the crisis occurred and the drug was taken. If the patient can be taken to a hospital within minutes, induced vomiting is unnecessary. On the other hand, in an isolated setting where medical care is not promptly available, induced vomiting is useful. Of course, if the drug has been taken intravenously or by inhalation (sniffing), induced vomiting will not help. Nor should vomiting be induced in stuporous patients who may become comatose within minutes because the danger of aspiration of vomitus is too great. Do not induce vomiting if the victim does not have a good gag reflex, has taken phenothiazine (a tranquilizer), is having seizures, or is pregnant. For directions on induced vomiting, see Chapter 22, "Poisoning Emergencies."
- If the patient is conscious, reassure him of his well-being, and explain thoroughly who you are and that you are trying to help. (Figure 23-13).
- Speak firmly to the patient. Be understanding and assuring. Have an accepting, nonjudgmental attitude toward the patient; *never* ridicule or criticize a patient. (Figure 23-14).
- Obtain a brief history so that you know what kind of drug or alcohol was consumed. Perform a brief physical assessment to eliminate possibilities of complications or other injuries.
- Transport the patient as soon as his or her condition is stabilized.
- If there is time prior to transport, search the area around the patient for tablets, capsules, pill bottles or boxes (especially empty ones), syringes, other drug paraphernalia, ampules, prescriptions, hospital attendance cards, or physician's notes that might help you identify what drug the patient has taken. Have any such evidence transported to the hospital along with the patient.
- Reduce stimuli as much as possible; lower the lights if you can, and let the patient rest in a calm, quiet atmosphere.

☐ The Overdose Patient

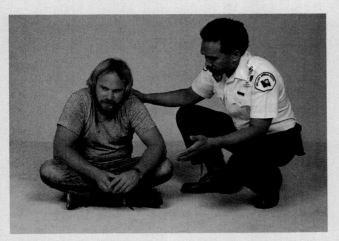

FIGURE 23-13 Explain thoroughly who you are and that you are trying to help.

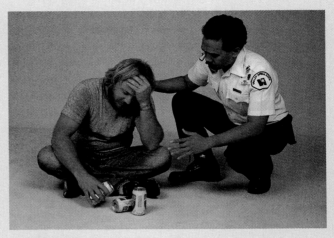

FIGURE 23-14 Maintain a nonjudgmental attitude and do not leave intoxicated patients alone.

- If the patient is agitated, move him or her to a quiet place where he or she can be observed and where there will be little interaction with others. It is critical that you calm the patient who seems to be agitated or paranoid. Carefully explain each step of care so that you can help reduce **paranoia.**

- Encourage deep breathing exercises to help the patient stay calm.

- If the patient becomes increasingly excited and approaches or reaches a delirious phase, be firm but friendly. Some patients will be in an excited phase when the emergency team arrives. This is a common problem with overdoses of amphetamines, antidepressants, and some over-the-counter medications. If necessary, make proper efforts to restrain such patients to protect them from themselves, and try to obtain help, especially en route to the hospital. Always try human restraint first and mechanical restraint as a last resort.

- *Do not* jump to conclusions — do not make decisions based solely on the patient's personal appearance, the fact that you detect an alcoholic odor, or the patient's companions.

- *Do not* accuse or criticize the patient.

- *Do not* leave intoxicated patients alone; make sure that they are attended and observed at all times. They should not be left alone even in a jail cell.

The Talk-Down Technique

The dangers associated with the **hallucinogens** and **marijuana** are primarily psychological in nature. These may be evident as intense anxiety or panic states (**bad trips**), depressive or paranoid reactions, mood changes, disorientation, and an inability to distinguish between reality and fantasy. Some prolonged psychotic reactions to psychedelic drugs have been reported, particularly with persons already psychologically disturbed.

The **talk-down technique** has been established as the preferred method for handling bad trips. This technique involves nonmoralizing, comforting, personal support from an experienced individual. It is aided by limiting external stimulation, such as intense light or loud sounds, and having the person lie down and relax.

Never use the talk-down technique for patients who have used PCP, because it may further aggravate them.

The goal of talking-down is to reduce the patient's anxiety, panic, depression, or confusion. Follow these steps:

1. Make the patient feel welcome. Remain relaxed and sympathetic. Because a patient can become suddenly hostile, have a companion with you. Be calm, but be authoritative.

2. Reassure the patient that his or her strange mental condition is a result of ingestion of the drug and that he or she *will* return to normal. Help the patient realize that he or she is not mentally ill.

3. Identify yourself clearly. Tell the patient who you are and what you are doing to help. Be careful not to invade the patient's "personal space" until you have established rapport; try to stay approximately eight to ten feet away until you sense that the patient has some trust in you. Never touch the patient until he or she gives you permission *unless*

Drug and Alcohol Emergencies **367**

he or she suddenly poses a threat to your safety or to his or her own safety.

4. Help the patient verbalize what is happening to him or her. Review for the patient what is going on in his or her trip; ask questions. Outline the probable time schedule of events.

5. Reiterate simple and concrete statements. Repeat and confirm what the patient says so that he or she knows you are listening. Orient the patient to time and place: be absolutely clear in letting the patient know where he or she is, what is happening, and who is present. Help the patient identify surrounding objects that will probably be familiar, a process that helps with self-identification. Listen for clues that will let you know whether the patient is anxious; if so, discuss those anxieties with him. Help the patient work through them and to conquer guilt feelings.

6. Forewarn the patient about what will happen as the drug begins to wear off. He will probably be confused one minute and experience mental clarity the next. Again, help the patient understand that this is due to the drug, not to mental illness.

7. Once the patient has been calmed, transport him to the hospital.

☐ PHENCYCLIDINE (PCP)

One of the most dangerous hallucinogens — and one that deserves separate treatment — is phencyclidine (PCP, known by at least forty-six names, is also called angel dust, killer weed, supergrass, crystal cyclone, hog, elephant tranquilizer, PeaCe Pill, embalming fluid, horse tranquilizer, mintweed, mist, monkey dust, rocket fuel, goon, surfer, KW, or scuffle). Nothing has so bewildered and amazed researchers as phencyclidine — a drug that is cheap, easy to make, and easy to take and that is related to horrible psychological effects (some of which can last for years).

PCP is stored in body fat; if a user suddenly loses weight, the drug can be released into the bloodstream and can cause a reaction even if the drug has not been recently taken.

Physical signs and symptoms of moderate PCP intoxication include extreme agitation, involuntary horizontal and vertical movement of the eyes, unresponsiveness to pain, severe muscular rigidity, production of excessive bronchial and oral secretions (leading to choking in some cases), and hypertension. Signs and symptoms during moderate intoxication tend to come in spurts — a patient may seem to have no reaction and may suddenly flare into frantic activity (physical and mental).

All the physical and psychological signs and symptoms present with a moderate dose will be present with a high dose but in a much exaggerated state. A high dose of phencyclidine — 10 to 20 milligrams — can lead to death. Physical signs and symptoms include disruptions in heart rhythm, marked increases in blood pressure, marked decreases in blood pressure, decreased urinary output, convulsions, respiratory arrest or decrease in respiration, coma, and vivid visual hallucinations. A user may be intermittently in and out of a coma for weeks and months following severe intoxication. Acute muscle rigidity occurs, and eyes are often fixated open with a blank stare. In some cases, **laryngospasm** (spasm of the throat muscles) may occur. Excessive sweating, drooling, and vomiting are characteristics of severe intoxication.

Three of the most severe reactions stemming from high doses of PCP are psychological ones: schizophrenia, paranoia, and memory loss (**amnesia**) — in some cases, permanent. Behavioral manifestations of PCP use include violence, agitation, and bizarre behavior.

Emergency Response for PCP Overdose

The PCP patient may be combative and require restraint. Your first priority is to protect yourself; if you are injured, you will not be able to help the patient! It is critical that you provide reassurance that will not frighten or further upset the patient. Most patients will be confused and upset; adverse emergency care efforts can increase psychological harm. Keep the patient in a quiet, nonstimulating environment. *Talking-down — a method recommended for other victims of hallucinogenic drugs — should not be used with PCP patients, since it will probably further aggravate them.*

Since PCP acts as an anesthetic, the patient will probably be unaware of any injuries sustained. Check quickly to determine whether there are any injuries that need attention. If there are, administer emergency care before continuing with psychological care. Restrain a patient who attempts to harm others. Keep the lights in the room as dim as you can (they will need to be bright enough, however, for medical personnel to monitor signs and otherwise care for the patient). Do whatever you can to minimize the confusion. Most PCP patients will require minimal medical care, but vital signs will still need to be monitored regularly. Therefore, you should transport the patient as quickly as possible while you work to establish calm.

☐ COCAINE

Another drug that deserves special mention is cocaine — partly because of its widespread use, and partly because of the devastating medical complications of its use. Cocaine is now the drug most often involved in emergency room visits.

Cocaine use in the United States has reached epidemic proportions: it is estimated that 5 million Americans are regular users, and that an additional 30 million have experimented with it. It has become known as the "equal opportunity drug" because of its widespread use and acceptance in all age, racial, ethnic, and socioeconomic groups. Cocaine is inhaled through the nose, injected into the veins, and injected into the muscles; in its "freebase" form, it is also smoked. Unfortunately, that widespread use may be due in part to the common misconception that cocaine is not addictive and that it is relatively safe.

Neither is the case. Cocaine is highly addictive. And in addition to the host of medical problems associated with its use, cocaine overdose can be fatal.

The major medical problems associated with cocaine use that may be seen by an EMT include the following:

- Cardiac disease, angina pectoris, myocardial infarction, arrhythmias, fibrillation, and sudden death (these can occur after even small doses, and in people who do not have pre-existing heart disease).

- Aortic dissection (probably resulting from the fact that cocaine increases blood pressure dangerously).

- Stroke — cocaine causes cerebral infarction, cerebral hemorrhage, and rupture of cerebral aneurysms (you should suspect cocaine use in any young adult who suffers a stroke, until proven otherwise).

- Seizures (these can also affect people who inhale the smoke of crack without using it themselves).

- Severe headache, unrelated to head injury, that cannot be relieved with analgesics.

- Respiratory problems, including hyperventilation, shortness of breath, rapid respiration, **Cheyne-Stokes respiration,** and respiratory arrest.

- Neurological problems, including loss of vision, headache, convulsions, tremors, dizziness, and depressed reflexes.

- Psychiatric problems, including anxiety, agitation, euphoria, psychosis, paranoia, hallucinations, suicides, and depression.

Emergency Response to Cocaine Intoxication

Before treating any suspected victim of cocaine intoxication, make certain you take measures to prevent the spread of hepatitis, AIDS, and other infectious diseases. These are becoming prominent among cocaine users as intravenous use gains popularity.

Immediately monitor vital signs; cocaine intoxication can cause rapidly progressing cardiac and respiratory complications that can lead to cardiac or respiratory arrest. Maintain heartbeat and respirations, using life support as necessary.

If the patient begins to experience seizures, treat as you would for any other convulsing patient. Move any obstacles that might cause injury, and monitor vital signs after the seizure has stopped.

Cocaine intoxication causes disturbances in body temperature, and patients tend to become hyperthermic. Monitor core body temperature and initiate cooling measures if temperature increases.

Remember that patients with cocaine intoxication may become psychotic, agitated, or suicidal; exercise caution in protecting yourself and others at the scene from injury. Call for additional help, if needed, to keep the patient from hurting anyone. Limiting the amount of stimulation to which the patient is exposed can help prevent the onset of psychiatric complications. Keep the patient in a quiet place with lights dimmed, and talk to him or her in a quiet, reassuring way.

Because medical complications of cocaine intoxication can progress rapidly, transport the patient as quickly as possible to a medical facility.

chapter 24

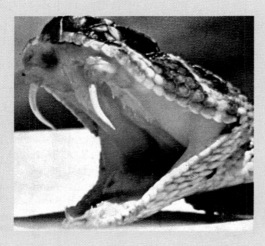

Bites
and Stings

✳ OBJECTIVES

■ Distinguish between poisonous and nonpoisonous snakes and indicate those that are most dangerous.

■ Describe the signs and symptoms of and emergency care for a pit viper bite and a coral snake bite.

■ Identify the signs and symptoms of and emergency care for insect bites, black widow bites, brown recluse bites, tick bites, and scorpion stings.

■ Explain the signs and symptoms of and emergency care for insect stings, including care for an allergic reaction.

■ Describe the signs and symptoms of and emergency care for poisoning by common marine life.

It is recommended that EMTs wear protective gloves whenever there is a possibility of coming in contact with a patient's blood, body fluids, mucous membranes, traumatic wounds, or sores. See Chapter 31.

Insect bites and stings are common, and most are considered minor. It is only when the insect is poisonous or when the patient has an allergic reaction and runs the risk of developing anaphylactic shock that the situation becomes an emergency. Even under those conditions, accurate diagnosis and prompt treatment can save lives and prevent permanent tissue damage.

□ SNAKEBITE

About 45,000 people every year are bitten by snakes in the United States; of those, 7,000 involve poisonous snakes, and of those treated, only about fifteen die.

More than half of the poisonous snakebites involve children, and most occur between April and October during daylight hours.

About 20 of the 120 species of snakes in the United States are poisonous; they include rattlesnakes, coral snakes, water moccasins, and copper heads (Figures 24-1–24-8). There are poisonous snakes in every state except Alaska, Hawaii, and Maine. Of the poisonous bites in the United States, 55 percent are from rattlesnakes, 34 percent from copperheads, 10 percent from water moccasins, and 1 percent from coral snakes. Almost all of the fatalities are from rattlesnake bites, and between 95 and 98 percent of the bites occur on extremities (Figures 24-9 and 24-10).

□ Common Poisonous Snakes

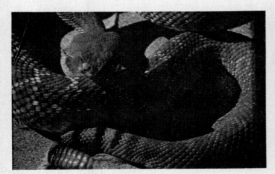

FIGURE 24-1 Rattlesnake.

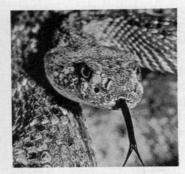

FIGURE 24-2 Rattlesnake.

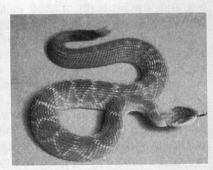

FIGURE 24-3 Rattlesnake.

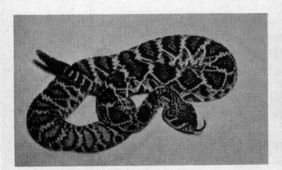

FIGURE 24-4 Rattlesnake.

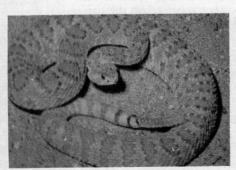

FIGURE 24-5 Rattlesnake.

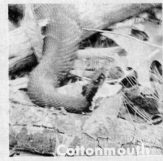

FIGURE 24-6 Cottonmouth.

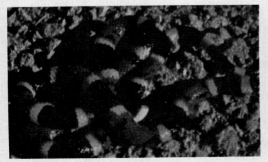

FIGURE 24-7 Coral snake.

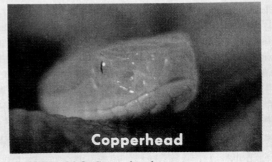

FIGURE 24-8 Copperhead.

371

□ Common Snakebite Sites

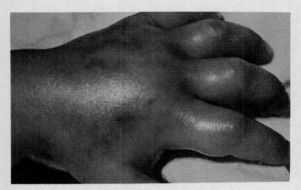

FIGURE 24-9 Snakebite to the hand.

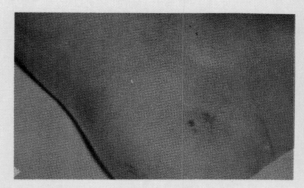

FIGURE 24-10 Snakebite to the heel.

Nonpoisonous snakebites are not considered serious and are generally treated as minor wounds; only poisonous snakebites are considered medical emergencies. Symptoms generally occur immediately, but only about one-third of all bites manifest symptoms. When no symptoms occur, probably no venom was injected into the victim. In 50 percent of coral snake bites, no venom is injected because the coral snake has to "chew" the skin for envenomation to occur. In as many as 25 percent of all venomous pit viper bites, no venom is injected, possibly because the fangs are injured, the venom sacs may be empty at the time of the bite, or the snake may not use the fangs when it strikes.

Poisonous snakebite venom contains some of the most complex toxins known; venoms can affect the central nervous system, brain, heart, kidneys, and blood. Simply stated, a snake's venom is its digestive enzyme, and the venom tends to "digest" any tissue into which it is injected. Signs that indicate a poisonous snakebite include:

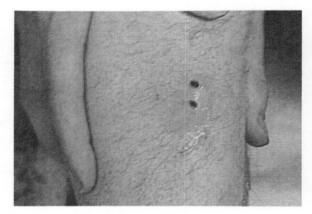

FIGURE 24-11 Rattlesnake bite.

almost immediately, but always within four hours of the incident.

The wound begins to swell and discolor usually immediately, but always within four hours. Most poisonous snakes have the following characteristics:

- Large fangs; nonpoisonous snakes have small teeth. The two fangs of a poisonous snake are hollow and work like a hypodermic needle. (The exception is the coral snake, a poisonous snake that does not have fangs.)
- Elliptical pupils (vertical slits, much like those of a cat); nonvenomous snakes have round pupils.
- Presence of a pit. Venomous snakes (often called pit vipers) have a telltale pit between the eye and the mouth. The pit, a heat-sensing organ, makes it possible for the snake to accurately strike a warm-blooded victim, even if the snake cannot see the victim.

- The bite consists of one or two distinct puncture wounds (Figure 24-11). Nonpoisonous snakes usually leave a series of small, shallow puncture wounds because they have teeth instead of fangs. (The exception is the coral snake, which leaves a semicircular marking from its teeth.) The presence of teeth marks does not rule out a poisonous bite, but the presence of fang marks *always* confirms poison (Figure 24-12). While the bite pattern is a good general guide, it is not without error and can sometimes be misleading: teeth marks can accompany fang marks, for example. In addition, there may be an inaccurate strike or varied marks due to shedding and replacement of fangs.
- The patient experiences severe pain and burning

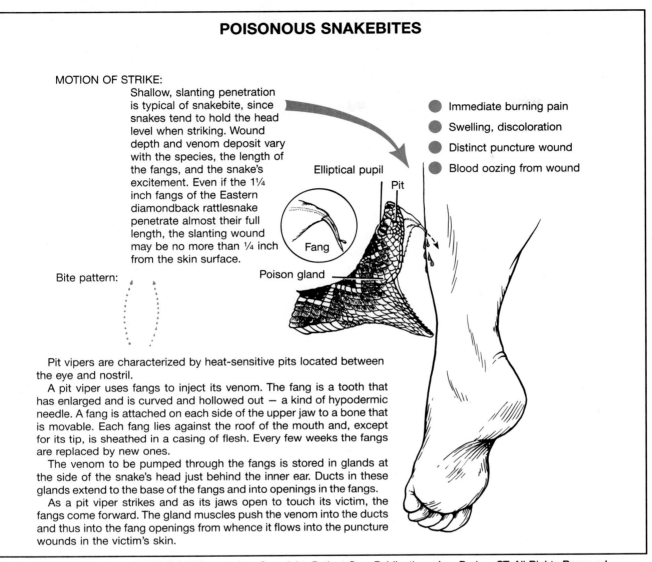

POISONOUS SNAKEBITES

MOTION OF STRIKE:

Shallow, slanting penetration is typical of snakebite, since snakes tend to hold the head level when striking. Wound depth and venom deposit vary with the species, the length of the fangs, and the snake's excitement. Even if the 1¼ inch fangs of the Eastern diamondback rattlesnake penetrate almost their full length, the slanting wound may be no more than ¼ inch from the skin surface.

Bite pattern:

Elliptical pupil

Pit

Fang

Poison gland

Immediate burning pain

Swelling, discoloration

Distinct puncture wound

Blood oozing from wound

Pit vipers are characterized by heat-sensitive pits located between the eye and nostril.

A pit viper uses fangs to inject its venom. The fang is a tooth that has enlarged and is curved and hollowed out — a kind of hypodermic needle. A fang is attached on each side of the upper jaw to a bone that is movable. Each fang lies against the roof of the mouth and, except for its tip, is sheathed in a casing of flesh. Every few weeks the fangs are replaced by new ones.

The venom to be pumped through the fangs is stored in glands at the side of the snake's head just behind the inner ear. Ducts in these glands extend to the base of the fangs and into openings in the fangs.

As a pit viper strikes and as its jaws open to touch its victim, the fangs come forward. The gland muscles push the venom into the ducts and thus into the fang openings from whence it flows into the puncture wounds in the victim's skin.

FIGURE 24-12

- A variety of differently shaped blotches on backgrounds of pink, yellow, olive, tan, gray, or brown skin.
- A triangular head that is larger than the neck, such as in the diamondback rattlesnake.

There is one exception to all of this: the coral snake, a highly poisonous snake that resembles a number of nonpoisonous snakes, does not have fangs and has round pupils. Because its mouth is so small and its teeth are short, most coral snakes inflict bites on the toes and fingers. Coral snakes are small and are ringed with red, yellow, and black; the red and yellow touch each other.

Chances for recovery are great if the patient receives care within two hours of the bite. Antivenin is available for a number of poisonous snake bites, but it is effective only against venom that is still circulating in the bloodstream. Antivenin cannot reverse damage that has already occurred.

Snakebite is rarely fatal, but it can be made much worse by improper treatment. Close adherence to accepted treatment guidelines can greatly improve the patient's prognosis following snakebite.

Emergency Care

The care for a snakebite depends on whether the patient was bitten by a pit viper (rattlesnake, copperhead, or cottonmouth) or coral snake. Remember to protect yourself against snakebite. If the snake has already been killed, handle it with great care: the fangs of a dead or even decapitated snake can still inject venom. Snakes can often be found within a twenty-foot radius of the area in which the bite occurred.

Pit Viper

The severity of a pit viper bite is gauged by how rapidly symptoms develop, which depends on how much poison was injected. As a general rule, you can safely assume that the patient has not been poisoned if the burning pain characteristic of pit viper bite does not develop within one hour of the time the patient was bitten.

Signs and symptoms of pit viper bite include the following:

- Immediate and severe burning pain and swelling around the fang marks, usually within five minutes. The entire extremity generally swells within eight to thirty-six hours.
- Purplish discoloration around the bite, usually developing within two to three hours.
- Numbness and possible blistering around the bite, generally within several hours.
- Nausea and vomiting.
- Rapid heartbeat, low blood pressure, weakness, and fainting.
- A minty, metallic, or rubbery taste in the mouth.
- Numbness and tingling of the tongue and mouth.
- Excessive sweating.
- Fever and chills.
- Muscular twitching.
- Convulsions.
- Dimmed vision.
- Headache.

Consider the bite to be severe if the patient develops signs or symptoms of shock, paralysis, blurred vision, or convulsions, or if he or she becomes unconscious.

Priorities are to maintain basic life support — airway, breathing, and circulation. Follow these guidelines:

1. Move the patient away from the snake to prevent repeated bites.
2. Have the patient lie down, and keep him or her calm and quiet. Keeping the patient at rest reduces the circulation and absorption of venom in the body tissues. Maintain direct eye contact, and speak in a soothing, reassuring voice. Remember that many snakebite victims will be hysterical — snakebite can cause tremendous psychological trauma. Continually reassure the patient as you give emergency care. Never allow a snakebite victim to drink alcohol. Activity increases circulation, and circulation increases the absorption of venom.
3. Keep the bitten extremity lower than the heart, and immobilize it in a functional position. Remove any rings, bracelets, or other jewelry that could impede circulation if swelling occurs.
4. Wipe the wound area with alcohol, soap and water, hydrogen peroxide, or other mild antiseptic. *Follow local protocol.* Take special care not to scrub or tear the tissues; cleanse the area very carefully, since envenomation makes the tissues extremely fragile. Irrigate the entire wound area with clean water.
5. Find the fang marks. Wrap a flat band that is at least three-fourths of a inch wide around the extremity two to four inches above the fang marks, between the bite site and the heart. *Follow local protocol.* The band should be tight enough to stop the flow of blood through the veins but not through the arteries. You should be able to slip two fingers between the patient's skin and the constricting band (Figure 24-13). *Make sure that you adjust the constricting band as swelling occurs so that it does not become too tight.* Never place constricting bands on either side of a joint, around a joint, or around the head, neck, or trunk.
6. Apply suction to the wound directly over the fang marks. *Follow local protocol.* An extractor from a snakebite kit is ideal (Figure 24-14). The suction must be strong and be applied within the first five minutes to be effective. After thirty minutes, the venom is diffused and cannot be removed by suction.
7. The most effective recommendation for snakebite treatment is to transport the patient to a medical facility for antivenin therapy.

FIGURE 24-13

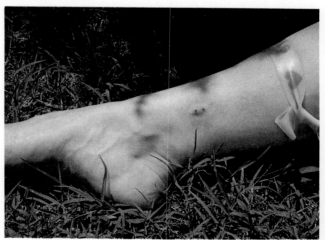

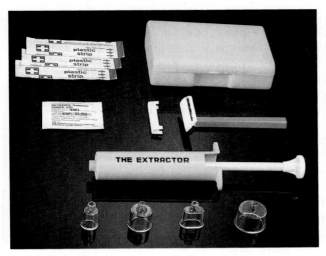

FIGURE 24-14 An extractor kit for suctioning venom.

8. Use basic life support procedures as appropriate, and treat the patient for shock. Monitor vital signs, keep the patient warm and lying down, and administer oxygen. Give the patient nothing by mouth.

9. Transport the patient to the hospital as soon as possible, even if there are no signs of envenomation. Symptoms worsen with time, and the greatest damage and poorest prognosis occur when treatment is delayed by a few hours. Be prepared to perform CPR during transport.

10. It's best if the bitten area can be kept cool, but many experts now recommend against the use of ice or cold under any conditions. Follow local protocol.

Coral Snake

Coral snakes — and other **neurotoxic** snakes like the cobra, mamba, sea snake, and krait — are the most poisonous of all snakes. Fortunately, they account for only 1 to 2 percent of all snakebites in the United States. Instead of having fangs like the pit vipers, the coral snake has several pairs of short, grooved, fanglike teeth in its upper jaw. Thus, it chews its victims instead of striking with a clean blow. The venom from a coral snake is absorbed rapidly into the bloodstream and is disseminated quickly throughout the body.

Signs and symptoms of a coral snake bite are completely different from those of a pit viper. Rather than leaving two distinct fang marks, the coral snake leaves one or more tiny scratch marks in the area of the bite. While a pit viper bite causes immediate burning pain, little pain or swelling occurs with a coral snake bite; if pain does occur, it is generally confined to the local bite area. The patient's tissue usually does not turn black and blue. Usually, in fact there is *no* pain or swelling at the bite site; in some cases numbness or weakness can develop at the bite site within an hour or so.

Coral snake venom has its effects on the central nervous system. One to eight hours after the bite, the patient will experience blurred vision, drooping eyelids, slurred speech, increased salivation and sweating, and drowsiness. As time passes, the patient may develop nausea and vomiting, shock, difficulty in breathing, paralysis, convulsions, and coma. Depending on the size and age of the patient, total central nervous system shutdown can occur in as few as ten minutes.

Emergency care for a coral snake bite:

1. Remove the patient's rings, bracelets, or any other jewelry that could impede circulation if swelling occurs.

2. Flush the bite area with warm, soapy water to wash away any remaining poison; use at least several quarts of water.

3. Apply a coolant bag to the bite. Never pack the bite area in ice, since you may cause frostbite.

4. Immobilize the extremity, treat the patient for shock, and give nothing by mouth.

5. *Never incise or suction a coral snake bite.*

6. *Transport the patient as quickly as possible; monitor vital signs during transport.*

☐ INSECT BITES

General Emergency Care

In most cases of insect bite, emergency care consists of:

1. Washing the wound thoroughly with soap and water.

2. Covering the wound with a loose dressing to discourage the patient from scratching it.

3. Applying cold compresses to the wound to reduce swelling and ease itching. *Never* pack ice directly on the skin.

Itching should subside within a few hours. If itching persists beyond two days, or if signs of infection develop, seek medical help.

Any patient who develops signs and symptoms of an allergic reaction following an insect bite should be seen by a physician. The signs and symptoms of allergic reaction include:

- Burning pain and itching at the bite site.
- Itching on the palms of the hands and soles of the feet.
- Itching on the neck and the groin.

- General body swelling.
- A nettlelike rash over the entire body.
- Breathing difficulties.

Anaphylactic shock, a life-threatening medical emergency, may follow insect bite. If any of the following signs or symptoms develop, transport the patient immediately and perform basic life support measures (see the anaphylactic shock section of Chapter 8):

- Faintness, weakness.
- Nausea.
- Shock.
- Unconsciousness.

Special Care for Specific Bites

Bites of certain insects — including the black widow spider, brown recluse spider, scorpion, and tick — require special care.

Black Widow Spider

The black widow spider is characterized by a shiny black body, thin legs, and a crimson red marking on its abdomen, usually in the shape of an hourglass or two triangles (Figure 24-15). Do not be confused by appearances, however — of the five species in the United States, only three are black, and not all have the characteristic red marking.

The female black widow spider, larger than the male, is one of the largest spiders in the United States. Males generally do not bite; females bite only when hungry, agitated, or protecting the egg sac. Contrary to folklore, the black widow spider is not aggressive; many bites, in fact, occur when a finger or hand enters the web and is mistaken as prey. Black widow spiders are usually found in dry, secluded, dimly lit areas. The spider is known for its extremely strong, funnel-shaped web. More than 80 percent of all bite victims are adult men.

FIGURE 24-15 Black widow spider.

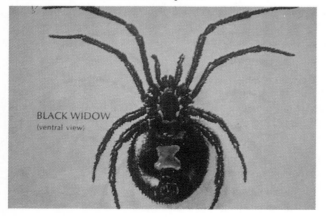

BLACK WIDOW
(ventral view)

Black widow spider bites are the leading cause of death from spider bites in the United States. The venom — fourteen times more toxic than rattlesnake venom — is a neurotoxin that causes little local reaction but that results in pain and spasm in the large muscle groups within thirty minutes to three hours. Severe bites cause respiratory failure, coma, and death.

Those at highest risk for developing severe bites are children under the age of sixteen, the elderly over the age of sixty, people with chronic illness, and anyone with hypertension.

The most common signs of black widow spider bite is high blood pressure, flushing, sweating, and grimacing of the face within ten minutes to two hours. Other signs and symptoms include:

- A pinprick sensation at the bite site, becoming a dull ache within thirty to forty minutes.
- Pain and spasms in the shoulders, back, chest, and abdominal muscles within thirty minutes to three hours.
- Rigid, boardlike abdomen.
- Restlessness and anxiety.
- Fever.
- Rash.
- Headache.
- Vomiting or nausea.

The symptoms of black widow spider bite generally last from twenty-four to forty-eight hours; the weakness and headache, however, may linger for months.

Prehospital care is generally not effective in the long-term treatment of black widow spider bite. The general goal of prehospital care is general wound care and transport. Follow these treatment guidelines:

1. Reassure the victim.
2. Administer care for shock.
3. Apply a cold compress to the bite area; do *not* apply ice.
4. Transport the patient to the hospital as quickly as possible.

Brown Recluse Spider

The brown recluse spider is generally brown but can range in color from yellow to dark chocolate brown (Figure 24-16). The characteristic marking is a brown, violin-shaped marking on the upper back. The bite of the brown recluse spider is a serious medical condition: the bite is nonhealing and **necrotic** and requires surgical skin grafting to repair (Figure 24-17).

Unfortunately, most brown recluse spider bite vic-

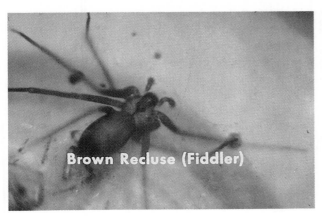

FIGURE 24-16 Brown recluse spider.

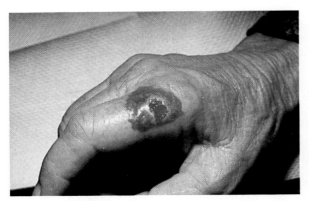

FIGURE 24-17 Brown recluse spider bite.

tims are unaware that they have been bitten, since the bite is often painless at first. Several hours after the bite occurs, the following signs and symptoms result:

- Within a few hours, the bite is a bluish area with a white periphery, gradually becoming surrounded with a red halo (a "bulls-eye" pattern).
- Within twenty-four hours, the patient develops:
  — Fever (usually of 103°F.)
  — Joint pain.
  — Nausea and vomiting.
  — Chills.
- Within seven to ten days, the bite becomes a large ulcer.

Emergency care consists of the following:

1. Administer care for shock.
2. Administer mouth-to-mouth ventilation or oxygen if needed.
3. Transport the patient as soon as possible.
4. If practical it is important to positively identify the spider so that surgical incision can be done as soon

as possible. If you can, bring the spider to the hospital with the patient.

Scorpion

Of the three species of scorpion in the United States that sting and inject poisonous venom, only one is generally fatal (Figure 24-18). The severity of the sting depends on the amount of venom injected. Ninety percent of all scorpion stings occur on the hands.

Signs and symptoms of scorpion stings include:

- Sharp pain at the sting site.
- Swelling at the sting site, which spreads gradually.
- Discoloration at the sting site.
- Nausea and vomiting.
- Restlessness.
- Drooling.
- Poor coordination.
- Incontinence.
- Seizures.

Emergency treatment of scorpion stings consists of the following:

1. Apply a flat, constricting band two inches above the sting if it is on an extremity. The band should be tight enough to stop venous, but not arterial, flow; you should be able to slip two fingers between the band and the patient's skin.
2. Apply a cold compress to the sting site to slow the spread of the venom and to reduce swelling. Never use ice.
3. Transport the patient immediately.

FIGURE 24-18 Scorpion.

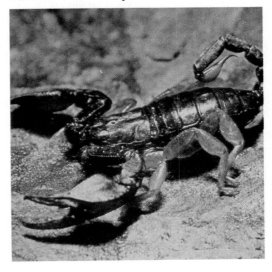

Fire Ants

Most common in the southeastern United States, fire ants get their name not from their color (which may range from red to black), but from the intense, fiery, burning pain their bite causes.

Fire ants bite down into the skin, then sting downwardly as they pivot; the result is a characteristic circular pattern of bites. Fire ant bites produce extremely painful vesicles that are filled with fluid (Figure 24-19). At first the fluid is clear; later it becomes cloudy. The bite causes a sharp. stinging pain followed by swelling.

Fire ant bites can also cause a large local reaction, characterized by swelling, pain, and redness affecting the entire extremity. There is also the threat of anaphylactic shock and secondary infection.

There is no specific prehospital care for fire ant bites. Provide care for systemic and allergic reactions, if any, and transport. Cold compressess can help reduce pain and swelling.

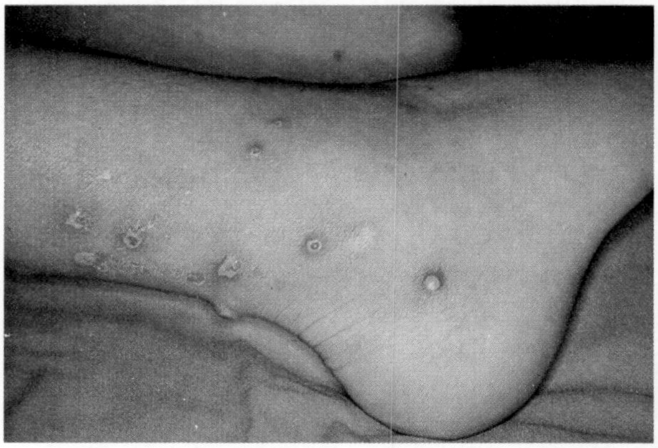

Ticks

Ticks (Figure 24-20) can cause a serious problem because they can carry tick fever, **Rocky Mountain spotted fever,** and other bacterial diseases. In addition, a prolonged attachment of an infected female tick can cause progressive paralysis that mimics polio; 10 percent of all victims die as a result.

Ticks are visible after they have attached themselves to the skin. However, since they often choose warm, moist areas, you should carefully inspect the patient's scalp, other hairy areas, the armpits, the groin, and skin creases. *Never* pluck an embedded tick head out of the skin — you may force infected blood into the patient.

To remove a tick, follow these guidelines:[1]

1. Remove a tick as soon as you discover it. The longer the tick remains attached to the skin, the more likely it is that an infection will result.

2. Use tweezers when removing a tick, or cover your fingers with a tissue; if you touch the tick, you may contaminate yourself. However, if you do not have tweezers and cannot cover your fingertips, pull the tick off right away rather than waiting and looking around for an appropriate implement.

3. To remove a tick, grasp it as close as possible to the point where it is attached to the skin. Pull firmly and steadily until the tick is dislodged, then flush it down the toilet. Do not twist or jerk the tick, since this may result in incomplete removal.

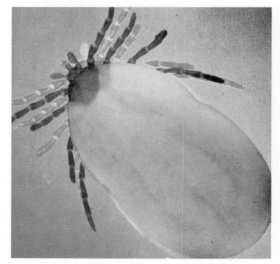

FIGURE 24-19 Fire ant bites.

FIGURE 24-20 Engorged tick.

Avoid squashing an engorged tick during removal: infected blood may spurt into your eyes, mouth, or a cut on the surface of your skin.

4. Once the tick is removed, wash your hands and the bite area thoroughly with soap and water, and apply an antiseptic to the area to prevent a bacterial infection.

5. Remember to have the patient mark the date on his or her calendar. It documents the exact time of exposure and will serve as a reminder if the patient needs to seek medical care.

6. If the patient develops fever with chills, headache, or muscle aches after being exposed to a tick, immediate treatment from a physician should be sought.

One of the most serious complications of tick infestation is Rocky Mountain spotted fever, which can occur in patients who are unaware that they have a tick. Signs and symptoms generally develop within seven to

[1] Reproduced with permission from *Patient Care*, June 15, 1988. Copyright © 1988, *Patient Care*, Oradell, NJ.

ten days of tick infestation and include nausea and vomiting, abdominal pain, headache, generalized weakness, flaccid paralysis, and respiratory failure.

Transport as rapidly as possible, providing basic life support during transport.

Lyme Disease

A growing health threat related to tick bites is Lyme disease, or Lyme borreliosis. First recognized in 1975, it is named after Lyme, Connecticut, where the disease was first identified. It is caused by the bite of an infected deer tick, which can be no larger than a poppy seed — many victims don't remember being bitten by a tick. The geographic range of infected ticks is fairly limited: more than 90 percent of all cases have occurred in only eight states (Massachusetts, Rhode Island, Connecticut, New York, New Jersey, Pennsylvania, Wisconsin, and Minnesota). A few cases have been reported in the Pacific states and north central states. (See Figure 24-21.)

The most common sites of deer tick bite are the upper arms and legs, trunk, armpits, groin, and buttocks.

Pregnant women who contract Lyme disease can transmit it to the fetus in utero.

Signs and Symptoms

The signs and symptoms of Lyme disease differ dramatically between the early stage (within four weeks after the bite) and the late stage (up to years after the bite).

FIGURE 24-21

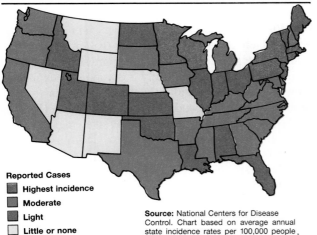

Reported Cases
 Highest incidence
Moderate
Light
Little or none

Source: National Centers for Disease Control. Chart based on average annual state incidence rates per 100,000 people.

Lyme disease, named for Old Lyme, Connecticut, where the first case was observed in 1975, has now been reported in 43 states, according to the National Center for Disease Control. States with the largest number of cases reported: New York, New Jersey, Pennsylvania, Connecticut, Massachusetts, Rhode Island, Wisconsin and Minnesota.

Reprinted from: *Mayo Clinic Health Letter,* October, 1989, with permission of Mayo Foundation for Medical Education and Research, Rochester, Minnesota.

Early signs and symptoms are characterized by a spreading, ring-like rash with a bright-red border at the bite site (in dark-skinned victims, the border will appear bluish). The rash can be painful or itchy, and will probably feel warm.

A second characteristic sign of early Lyme disease is flu-like symptoms, including nausea and vomiting, fever, chills, fatigue, muscle aches, sore throat, headache, and swollen glands.

Within four to six weeks, victims of Lyme disease may develop nervous system disorders, including Bell's palsy and meningitis.

Antibiotic therapy is generally needed, and some patients may require hospitalization. The only appropriate treatment in the field is *prompt removal of any tick;* prompt removal can prevent infection.

☐ INSECT STINGS

The-normal reaction to an insect sting is a sharp, stinging pain followed immediately by an itchy, swollen, painful **wheal.** Swelling may persist for several days but usually subsides within twenty-four hours. Redness, tenderness, and swelling at or around the sting site — even if severe — in the absence of other symptoms are considered to be a local reaction. Local reactions are rarely serious or life-threatening and can be treated successfully with cold compresses.

But allergic reactions are another story: approximately fifty people die each year in the United States as a result of insect stings — more than all other bites combined, including snakebite. Thousands of people are allergic to the sting of bees, wasps, and hornets, and for those people, stings may cause death — on the average, within ten minutes of the sting, but almost always within the first hour. According to some estimates, 0.5 percent of the U.S. population is at risk because of severe allergic reactions.

The stinging insects that most commonly cause allergic reactions in patients are a group of the **Hymenoptera** — the insects with membranous wings. These consist of the honeybee, the wasp, the hornet, and the yellow jacket.

In determining care for a patient, it is important to identify what kind of insect inflicted the sting. Clues in habitat and stinging habit can help in identification. Honeybees leave the stinger and venom sac behind, embedded in the skin; hornets and wasps do not. Hornets prefer trees and shrubs, and yellow jackets stay close to the ground — both hornets and yellow jackets build their nests near the ground. Wasps love attics and build their nests high off the ground in sheltered places, usually under eaves. Honeybees cluster around flowers and flowering shrubs, including the flowering clover in lawns.

Signs and Symptoms of Anaphylaxis

Signs and symptoms of anaphylaxis include the following (also see the anaphylactic shock section of Chapter 8):

- Faintness.
- Dizziness.
- Generalized itching.
- Hives.
- Flushing.
- Generalized swelling, including the eyelids, lips, and tongue.
- Upper airway obstruction.
- Difficulty swallowing.
- Shortness of breath, wheezing, or stridor.
- Labored breathing.
- Abdominal cramps.
- Confusion.
- Loss of consciousness.
- Convulsions.
- Low blood pressure (60/40).

In some patients, anaphylactic symptoms may be delayed for as long as two weeks. In those cases, signs and symptoms include:

- Rash.
- Fever.
- Joint pain.
- Neurological problems.
- Secondary infections.

Emergency Care for Insect Stings

If the victim of an insect sting carries a "sting kit," help him or her use it, following the manufacturer's instructions and local protocol.

Emergency care for individuals who experience allergic reactions to stings consists of the following (Figure 24-22):

1. Lower the affected part below the heart.
2. If the sting was inflicted by a honeybee and the stinger is still in the skin, remove the stinger by gently scraping against it with your fingernail, with the edge of a knife, or with a credit card (Figure 24-23). Be careful not to *squeeze* the stinger. The venom sac will still be attached, and you will eject additional venom into the area. Make sure that you remove the venom sac — it can continue to secrete venom even though the stinger is detached from the insect.
3. Apply a commercial cold pack or ice bags to the site to relieve pain and swelling.
4. If the patient develops breathing difficulty, oxygen may help. If respirations are not adequate with oxygen, give mouth-to-mouth ventilation.
5. Keep the patient warm. Have him or her lie down, and elevate the legs and lower the head if the patient shows signs and symptoms of (or danger of lapsing into) shock.
6. Transport the patient immediately.
7. Make sure that the patient will be under strict observation for the first twenty-four hours to eliminate the possibility of later breathing problems or hemorrhage. Tell family members to take the patient to the hospital immediately if any suspicious signs and symptoms develop.
8. If you know that the patient is allergic to stings, do not wait for the signs and symptoms to occur — delay can be fatal. If the patient has a history of severe allergic reactions and has an insect sting kit, assist him or her in administering the contents of the kit (Figure 24-24). *Follow local protocol.* Transport the patient to the hospital immediately.

□ MARINE LIFE POISONING

Four-fifths of all organisms on the earth live in the ocean, which covers 71 percent of the earth's surface. Venomous organisms are naturally part of that vast life form. There are approximately 2,000 poisonous marine animals; while they usually live in temperate or tropical waters, they can be found in virtually all waters (Figures 24-25–24-36). Most are not aggressive; in fact, most marine life poisoning occurs when a victim swims into or steps on an animal.

There are differences between the stings and bites of aquatic organisms and those of land organisms. First, the venom of aquatic organisms may produce more extensive tissue damage. (See Figures 24-37 and 24-38.) Common signs and symptoms include a burning pain, swelling, and hives. Systemic signs and symptoms can include general weakness, dizziness, sweating, headache, pallor, rapid heartbeat, respiratory distress, abdominal pain and cramping, and nausea or vomiting. Such injuries should be treated as soft-tissue injuries. Second, venoms of aquatic organisms are destroyed by heat; therefore, heat, rather than ice, should be applied to such stings and bites.

ALLERGIC REACTION TO INSECT VENOM

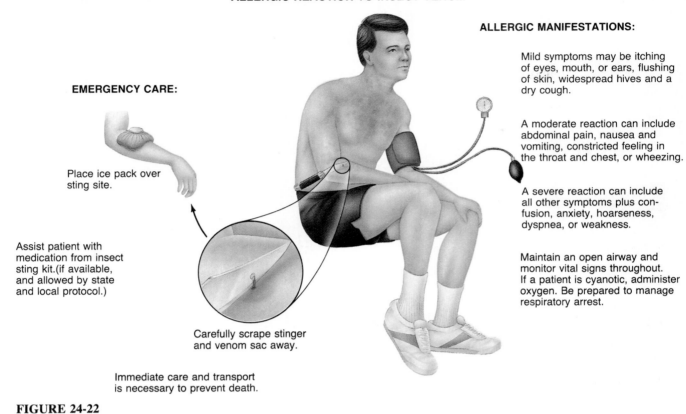

ALLERGIC MANIFESTATIONS:

Mild symptoms may be itching of eyes, mouth, or ears, flushing of skin, widespread hives and a dry cough.

A moderate reaction can include abdominal pain, nausea and vomiting, constricted feeling in the throat and chest, or wheezing.

A severe reaction can include all other symptoms plus confusion, anxiety, hoarseness, dyspnea, or weakness.

Maintain an open airway and monitor vital signs throughout. If a patient is cyanotic, administer oxygen. Be prepared to manage respiratory arrest.

EMERGENCY CARE:

Place ice pack over sting site.

Assist patient with medication from insect sting kit.(if available, and allowed by state and local protocol.)

Carefully scrape stinger and venom sac away.

Immediate care and transport is necessary to prevent death.

FIGURE 24-22

FIGURE 24-23 Scraping a honeybee sting away with the edge of a credit card.

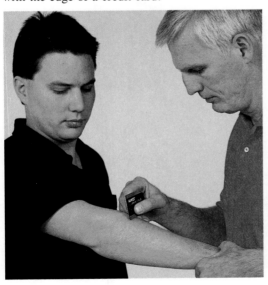

FIGURE 24-24

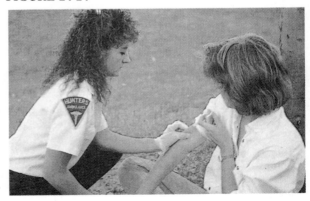

☐ Common Sources of Marine Life Stings and Wounds

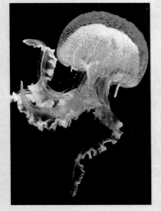

FIGURE 24-25 Jellyfish.

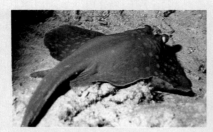

FIGURE 24-26 Stingray.

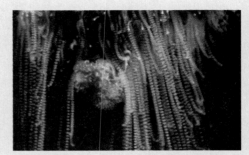

FIGURE 24-27 Tentacles of Portuguese Man-of-War.

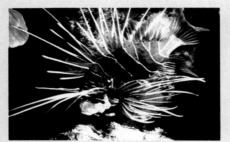

FIGURE 24-28 Lionfish.

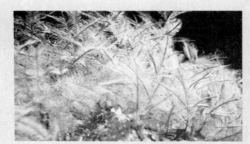

FIGURE 24-29 Feather hydroid.

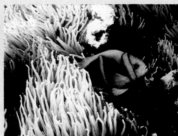

FIGURE 24-30 Sea anemone and clownfish.

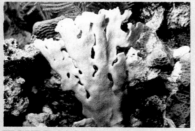

FIGURE 24-31 Fire coral.

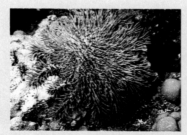

FIGURE 24-32 Crown-of-Thorns starfish.

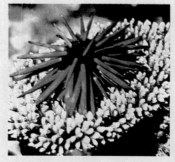

FIGURE 24-33 Sea urchin.

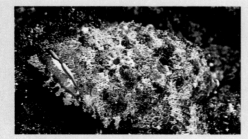

FIGURE 24-34 Scorpion fish.

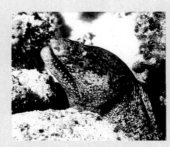

FIGURE 24-35 Moray eel.

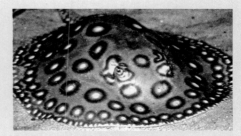

FIGURE 24-36 Stingray.

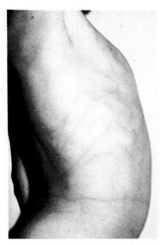
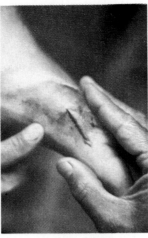

FIGURE 24-37 Jellyfish sting.

FIGURE 24-38 Stingray sting.

Emergency Care

Treat large bites (such as those from a shark) like any other major trauma:

1. Control bleeding.
2. Treat for shock.
3. Give basic life support.
4. Transport.

Try to identify the marine animal; some very effective antivenins are available. In cases of poisonous injuries, patients may have a wide variety of symptoms, ranging from a minor injury to death. If anaphylactic shock develops, follow general guidelines for treating anaphylaxis. General care for injuries inflicted by most sea animals consists of the following:

1. Apply a constricting band above the sting or bite. Check for a pulse in the limb to ensure that the constricting band is not too tight. It should be tight enough to restrict the flow of blood through the veins but not through the arteries.
2. Remove with **forceps** any material that sticks to the sting site on the surface of the flesh.
3. Irrigate the wound thoroughly with water.
4. If the skin is unbroken, wash the wound with a mild agent such as Alcoholic Zephiran, strong soap solution, or ammonia. *Never scrub the area.*

Make sure that washings from the irrigation and the oxidizing agent flow away from the body.

5. Remove stingers and barbs the same way in which you remove bee stingers. Wear latex or surgical gloves to prevent injury to yourself. Be careful not to squeeze more venom into the wound. If the stinger is barbed perpendicular to the wound and you are unable to remove it without excessive force, support the stinger or barb, bandage it in place, and wait for surgical removal. Immobilize the area to help prevent venom from spreading.
6. Apply heat and maintain the injured area at a temperature of 110° to 114°F. for thirty minutes or while in transport. Apply heat for another thirty minutes if symptoms recur. Follow local protocol.
7. Transport the patient immediately to a hospital. Position the patient so that gravity does not force return of the venom.

To treat tentacle stings, such as those inflicted by jellyfish, corals, hydras, and anemones, follow these guidelines:

1. Remove the patient from the water.
2. Carefully remove dried tentacles if possible.
3. If available, pour vinegar on the affected area to denature the toxin.
4. If available, sprinkle the affected area with meat tenderizer to destroy the toxin.
5. If available, sprinkle the affected area with talcum powder.
6. Transport.

To treat puncture wounds, such as those inflicted by stingray spines and spiny fish, follow these guidelines:

1. Remove the patient from the water.
2. Remove any spines you can see unless they are embedded in joints or neurovascular structures or are deeply embedded (these require surgical removal). Immobilize the injured part.
3. Soak the affected area in hot water for at least thirty minutes, changing the water frequently to maintain its temperature.
4. Transport the patient while soaking the injured part.

Bites and Stings   **383**

chapter 25

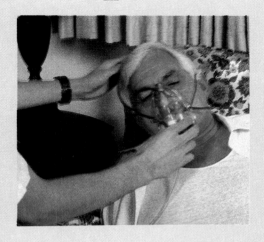

Respiratory Emergencies

✻ OBJECTIVES

- Explain the anatomy and physiology of the respiratory system.
- Identify the common causes of dyspnea, including chronic obstructive pulmonary disease (emphysema, bronchitis, and asthma), pneumonia, pulmonary embolism, pulmonary edema, and hyperventilation.
- Recognize the signs and symptoms that may accompany the various types of emergencies that cause dyspnea.
- Describe and demonstrate how to administer emergency care for each of the causes of dyspnea.

It is recommended that EMTs wear protective gloves whenever there is a possibility of coming in contact with a patient's blood, body fluids, mucous membranes, traumatic wounds, or sores. See Chapter 31.

Vital to survival is the body's ability to deliver sufficient amounts of freshly oxygenated blood to all cells. Without enough oxygen, some cells — such as those in the heart and brain — can die within minutes. Review the respiratory system in Chapter 2, and Chapter 4 and refer to Figure 2-13.

A variety of disease and injury conditions can impact the body's ability to get enough oxygen. The need for rapid treatment in these cases is essential to saving life and preventing cell death from oxygen starvation.

☐ DYSPNEA (SHORTNESS OF BREATH)

Dyspnea, one of the most common medical complaints, is defined as a sensation of shortness of breath — a feeling of air hunger accompanied by labored breathing. Two major sets of circumstances generally accompany dyspnea: in one, air cannot pass easily into the lungs; in the other, air cannot pass easily out of the lungs. Most commonly, there is resistance in either the airway (from obstruction or an inflamed, swollen epiglottis) or in expansion of the lungs. Most is due to anxiety or pain.

Dyspnea is not a disease in itself but is a symptom of a number of diseases. Breathing will generally be rapid and shallow, but patients may feel short of breath whether they are breathing rapidly or slowly. Remember that shortness of breath is normal following exercise, fatigue, coughing, or the production of excess sputum. In these cases, the condition is not considered true dyspnea.

Dyspnea can be a gradual process, or it may occur suddenly. Common causes include pulmonary embolism, chronic heart disease, myocardial infarction with cardiac failure, congestive heart failure, **pleurisy,** pneumonia, inhalation injury, aspiration of a foreign body, asthma, pneumothorax, hemothorax, thoracic spine abnormalities, infection, burns, anaphylaxis, flail chest, mouth/neck tumors, **goiter,** rib fracture, chronic bronchitis, and emphysema. As a general rule, dyspnea due to chronic heart disease is usually associated with fluid buildup (edema) in the lungs or the legs; breathlessness in such patients is usually relieved by sitting or by elevation of the head of the bed.

Emergency treatment of dyspnea is aimed at treating the *cause* of the shortness of breath, not the dyspnea itself. If you cannot readily determine the cause, take the following steps:

1. Maintain an open airway. Administer oxygen as soon as possible. Dysnea may be caused by aspiration of a foreign body; immediately check for aspiration, and clear the airway if necessary.

2. Treat for shock.

3. Transport as rapidly as possible. Enroute, administer oxygen at a rate of at least six liters per minute (ten to twelve liters per minute if using a nonrebreather mask).

☐ CHRONIC OBSTRUCTIVE PULMONARY DISEASE (COPD)

Obstructive airway diseases are characterized by diffuse obstruction to air flow within the lungs. The most common are emphysema, chronic bronchitis, and asthma. The most reversible is asthma, while the most irreversible is emphysema; chronic bronchitis falls somewhere in between. The incidence of chronic obstructive pulmonary disease is high; up to 20 percent of the adult population in the United States suffers from some form of it (Figure 25-1).

Emphysema

Emphysema is characterized by distension of the air spaces (groups of alveoli) beyond the bronchioles, with destructive changes in their walls. Basically, the alveoli lose their elasticity, become distended with trapped air, and stop functioning. Air is trapped in the alveoli, causing the small walls to eventually break down. As a result, the total number of alveoli decreases, making it more difficult for the patient to breathe.

The patient with emphysema is often thin, with the chest often barrel-shaped, and with evidence of weight loss; a significant number of calories are used for breathing. He or she generally gives a history of increasing dyspnea on exertion, with progressive limitation of his activity. Coughing may not be a prominent problem; if he or she does cough, usually only small amounts of mucus are produced. Exhalation is prolonged and difficult, and the patient's lungs remain expanded even after exhalation. Patients with emphysema are not usually cyanotic, and for this reason they are sometimes referred to as **"pink puffers."**

The same procedure that destroys the alveoli also destroys the pulmonary airways, eventually increasing air resistance and making breathing more difficult. Most deaths from emphysema result directly from cardiac arrhythmias, right heart failure, or massive infections.

Chronic Bronchitis

Chronic bronchitis is characterized by inflammation, edema, and excessive mucus production in the bronchial tree. The patient uses his neck and chest muscles to assist his breathing. By definition, chronic bronchitis features a productive cough that has persisted for at least three months out of the year over the past two consecutive years.

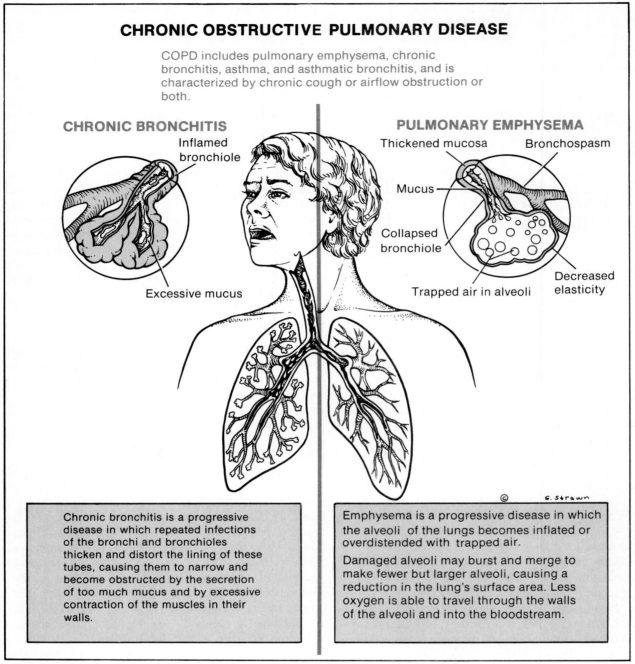

CHRONIC OBSTRUCTIVE PULMONARY DISEASE

COPD includes pulmonary emphysema, chronic bronchitis, asthma, and asthmatic bronchitis, and is characterized by chronic cough or airflow obstruction or both.

CHRONIC BRONCHITIS

Inflamed bronchiole

Excessive mucus

PULMONARY EMPHYSEMA

Thickened mucosa

Bronchospasm

Mucus

Collapsed bronchiole

Trapped air in alveoli

Decreased elasticity

© S. Strawn

Chronic bronchitis is a progressive disease in which repeated infections of the bronchi and bronchioles thicken and distort the lining of these tubes, causing them to narrow and become obstructed by the secretion of too much mucus and by excessive contraction of the muscles in their walls.

Emphysema is a progressive disease in which the alveoli of the lungs becomes inflated or overdistended with trapped air.

Damaged alveoli may burst and merge to make fewer but larger alveoli, causing a reduction in the lung's surface area. Less oxygen is able to travel through the walls of the alveoli and into the bloodstream.

FIGURE 25-1

Because chronic bronchitis occurs in the bronchi, the alveolar gas exchange is normal; however, the alveoli do not expand fully because the air cannot get past the diseased bronchi. To make matters worse, recurrent infections leave scar tissue, which further narrows the bronchi.

The typical patient with chronic bronchitis has almost invariably been a heavy cigarette smoker with many respiratory infections. The bronchitis gets worse with exercise. The patient is usually somewhat short and overweight, with a plethoric, usually bluish complexion — features that have given rise to the term **"blue bloater"** to describe the patient.

The patient with chronic bronchitis often has a tendency toward associated heart disease and right heart failure, which causes the cyanosis. The disease also causes peripheral edema and distended neck veins, and most patients experience associated congestive heart failure.

On examination, the chronic bronchitic is often coughing, and rhonchi and wheezes can be heard in the chest. High-pitched wheezing occurs during both inhalation and exhalation as the patient struggles to get air in and out of the lungs; low-pitched snoring sounds occur during both inhalation and exhalation as air flows through the narrowed and secretion-choked passageways of the bronchial tree.

Signs and Symptoms of Emphysema and Chronic Bronchitis

Victims of COPD have a tendency to frequent infections from colds and flu. They also become easily winded under conditions that do not tax most healthy people (such as walking on a level surface). The other signs and symptoms of emphysema and chronic bronchitis may include:

- Gasping for air and shortness of breath
- Sitting, leaning forward in an attempt to breathe (Figure 25-2).
- Distended neck veins.
- Audible rales, rhonchi, or wheezes.
- Cyanosis.
- Prolonged exhalation with pursed lips.
- Barrel-shaped chest.
- Cough.

Emergency Care

Management of COPD patients in acute decompensation is aimed primarily at relieving hypoxemia. Most of us breathe because the carbon dioxide level in our system has become too high, not because the oxygen level has dropped too low. Only a very small minority of COPD patients have hypoxic drive. For those COPD patients with hypoxic drive, however, levels of carbon dioxide are chronically high, which means that they lose the normal drive to breathe in response to a high carbon dioxide level. Instead, they breathe because oxygen levels have become too low.

This is *not* a justification to withhold oxygen from a COPD victim, because he may die without it. But you must remain alert to the fact that oxygen administration may depress the patient's own respiratory drive; therefore, you must at all times be ready to assist ventilations. Monitor respirations constantly.

Despite the mix-up with the hypoxic drive, the number-one goal of COPD treatment is to enhance oxygenation; without it, the patient may die. The major threat to life in COPD is a lack of oxygen. To treat the COPD patient in the field, do the following:

1. Establish an airway.
2. The patient will probably be most comfortable in a sitting tripod or semi-sitting position to assist the accessory breathing muscles. Keep him or her in a sitting position with his legs dangling over the side of the stretcher.
3. Administer oxygen. Monitor respirations. If the patient is unconscious, use any possible method of ventilation, following local protocol (Figure 25-3).
4. Monitor the patient's respiratory rate and depth, and assist ventilations if respiration becomes depressed. *Watch the patient closely for changes in rate and depth*.
5. Maintain the patient's body temperature.
6. Encourage the patient to cough up his secretions.
7. Loosen any restrictive clothing as you comfort and reassure the patient.
8. Transport as soon as possible.

FIGURE 25-2 Victims of emphysema and chronic bronchitis often lean forward in an attempt to breathe.

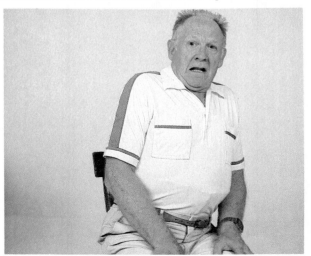

FIGURE 25-3 Administering oxygen to a patient with chronic obstructive pulmonary disease (COPD). In some areas, a venturi mask is recommended. Follow local protocol.

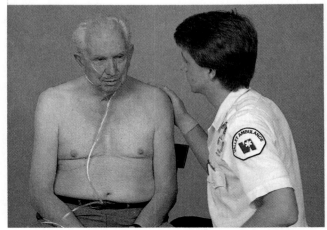

Asthma

Bronchial asthma is characterized by an increased sensitivity of the trachea, bronchi, and bronchioles to various stimuli, with widespread reversible narrowing of the airways (**bronchospasm**). The airway is obstructed by the bronchospasm; in addition, the mucous membranes lining the bronchioles swell, and the bronchi become obstructed with thick mucus. There are generally two different degrees of asthma: acute or chronic asthma, with periodic attacks and symptomatic periods between attacks; and status asthmaticus, with a prolonged and life-threatening attack.

There are also generally two different kinds of asthma. Extrinsic asthma, or "allergic" asthma, is usually a reaction to dust, pollen, or other irritants in the atmosphere; it is often seasonal, occurs most often in children, and often clears up after adolescence. Intrinsic, or "nonallergic," asthma is most common in adults and is not due to allergic reaction, but often to infection. It is not seasonal, and is often chronic. Most often, it is caused by emotion, inhaled fumes, viral infections, aspirin, cold air, or some other irritant.

The acute asthmatic attack varies in duration, intensity, and frequency. It reflects airway obstruction due to:

- Bronchospasm (generalized spasm of the bronchi).
- Swelling of the mucous membranes in the bronchial walls.
- Plugging of the bronchi by thick mucus secretions.

The typical acute attack, usually accompanied by a recent respiratory infection, may feature the following signs and symptoms:

- Patient sits upright, often leaning forward, fighting to breathe.
- Spasmodic, unproductive cough (the cough may actually be productive, but because of bronchospasm, the sputum or mucus stays trapped in the bronchial tree, making the cough appear to be unproductive).
- Whistling, high-pitched wheezing, usually audible during exhalation; may also be present on inhalation.
- Very little movement of air during breathing; may produce quiet breath sounds.
- Hyperinflated chest with air trapped in the lungs because of increased obstruction during exhalation.
- Rapid, shallow respirations.
- Rapid pulse (usually exceeding 120 beats per minute).
- Fatigue.

Emergency Care for Acute Asthma Attack

The three goals of asthma treatment are to improve oxygenation, relieve bronchospasm, and improve the patient's ventilation. Follow these guidelines:

1. Establish an airway.
2. Administer high-flow humidified oxygen until cyanosis abates (Figure 25-4). Dry oxygen tends to worsen the problem of thick secretions.
3. Stay calm, and keep the patient as calm as possible; stress and emotional intensity both worsen the asthma (Figure 25-5). Keep the patient in a position of comfort.
4. Transport as quickly as possible.

Status Asthmaticus

Status asthmaticus is a severe, prolonged asthmatic attack that does not respond to aggressive treatment and that represents a *dire medical emergency*. Wheezing is not a reliable sign of status asthmaticus: there may be no wheezing at all — and, in fact, the breath sounds may be almost absent. Signs and symptoms of status asthmaticus may include the following (Figure 25-6 on page 390):

- Severe inflation of the chest due to continued trapping of air.

FIGURE 25-4 Administering oxygen to an asthma patient.

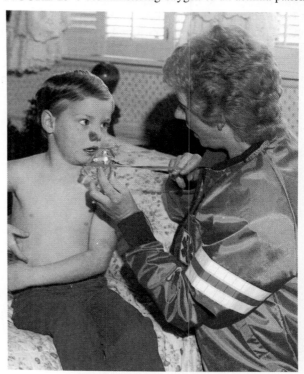

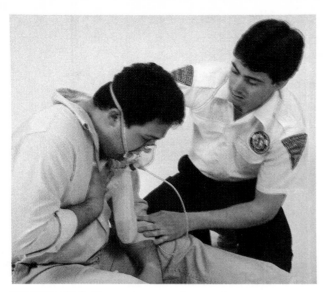

FIGURE 25-5 Reassuring an asthma patient.

- Cyanosis.
- Walking and talking only with the greatest effort.
- Extremely labored breathing, with the patient fighting to move air and using accessory muscles of respiration.
- Inaudible breath sounds and wheezes due to negligible movement of air.
- Exhaustion.
- Dehydration.

Do not be fooled by a patient who seems to be suffering from status asthmaticus but who then seems to begin to recover. *He or she could still be in grave danger.*

To treat status asthmaticus, follow the same general guidelines as with acute asthma, but increase your urgency in establishing care and transporting the patient to the hospital. If the attack has lasted for longer than twelve hours, administer high-flow, humidified oxygen throughout transport. Be sure to maintain a calm, reassuring attitude.

A note of caution: all that wheezes is not asthma. Many other diseases cause diffuse wheezing, such as acute left heart failure **(cardiac asthma),** smoke inhalation, chronic bronchitis, anaphylaxis, and acute pulmonary embolism.

☐ PNEUMONIA

Pneumonia is the medical term used to describe a group of illnesses that are characterized by lung inflammation and fluid- or pus-filled alveoli, leading to inadequately oxygenated blood. Pneumonia is most frequently caused by a bacterial or viral infection, but it can also be caused by inhaled irritants (such as chemicals or smoke) or aspirated materials (such as vomitus).

Signs and Symptoms

Victims of pneumonia generally appear very ill; most complain of fever and chills "that shake the bed." Signs and symptoms may be influenced by the area of the lung that is affected — pneumonia in the lower lobes may not produce cough but usually causes abdominal pain. Look for the following signs and symptoms:

- Lung inflammation and obstruction:
  — Chest pain, usually made worse when breathing.
  — Dyspnea.
  — Noisy breathing.
  — Rapid respiration.
  — Respiratory distress.
  — Productive cough with purulent yellow sputum or mucus, sometimes streaked with blood.
- Systemic response to infection:
  — Fever (usually exceeding 101°F.)
  — Chills.
  — Hot, dry skin.

Emergency Care

1. Position the patient so that he or she is comfortable and can breathe with the least amount of distress; most pneumonia patients will prefer to sit upright or in a semi-sitting position.
2. Administer oxygen.
3. Transport as soon as possible.

☐ PULMONARY EMBOLISM

Pulmonary embolism is the sudden blocking of a pulmonary artery or one of its branches by a clot or other small particle carried by the blood. Pulmonary emboli arise from a number of different sources:

- Air may enter the circulation through an open wound.
- Blood clots form in a vein, break loose, and are moved through venous circulation through the right side of the heart, becoming impacted in the progressively narrowing network of pulmonary arteries.
- Fat particles may enter the bloodstream from the ends of broken bones.

Each year, there are more than one-half a million cases of pulmonary embolism in the United States. Unfortunately, 70 percent of all cases of pulmonary em-

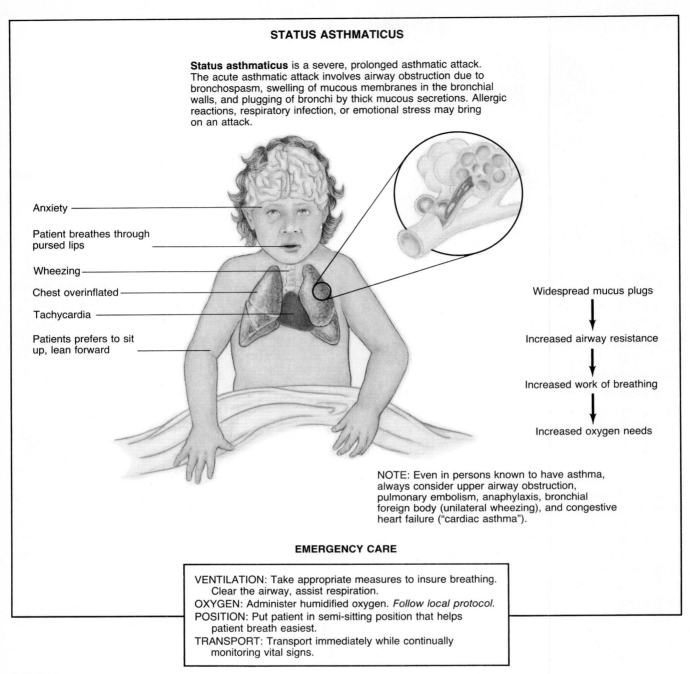

STATUS ASTHMATICUS

Status asthmaticus is a severe, prolonged asthmatic attack. The acute asthmatic attack involves airway obstruction due to bronchospasm, swelling of mucous membranes in the bronchial walls, and plugging of bronchi by thick mucous secretions. Allergic reactions, respiratory infection, or emotional stress may bring on an attack.

Anxiety

Patient breathes through pursed lips

Wheezing

Chest overinflated

Tachycardia

Patients prefers to sit up, lean forward

Widespread mucus plugs

↓

Increased airway resistance

↓

Increased work of breathing

↓

Increased oxygen needs

NOTE: Even in persons known to have asthma, always consider upper airway obstruction, pulmonary embolism, anaphylaxis, bronchial foreign body (unilateral wheezing), and congestive heart failure ("cardiac asthma").

EMERGENCY CARE

VENTILATION: Take appropriate measures to insure breathing. Clear the airway, assist respiration.
OXYGEN: Administer humidified oxygen. *Follow local protocol.*
POSITION: Put patient in semi-sitting position that helps patient breath easiest.
TRANSPORT: Transport immediately while continually monitoring vital signs.

FIGURE 25-6

bolism are misdiagnosed and, as a result, are not treated rapidly enough; an estimated one-third of the misdiagnosed victims die. In any patient presenting with the symptoms of pulmonary embolism (listed below), first rule out myocardial infarction and then *immediately* suspect and treat for pulmonary embolism.

Factors which may lead to pulmonary embolism include:

• Surgery.

• Prolonged immobilization and long periods of physical inactivity, which cause the blood to become stagnant in the lower extremities. Immobilization of a lower extremity in a cast can have the same effect.

- Smoking.
- Traumatic or difficult childbirth.
- **Thrombophlebitis,** or inflammation of the veins, especially in the legs and pelvis, usually characterized by calf pain and tenderness.
- Pregnancy.
- COPD.
- Congestive heart failure.
- Tumors, especially those of the gastrointestinal tract.
- Use of certain drugs, most notably oral contraceptives (at particularly high risk are women over the age of thirty who take oral contraceptives).
- Chronic atrial fibrillation.
- Multiple fractures.
- Open wounds involving the arteries or veins, especially those of the neck.

Signs and Symptoms

The signs and symptoms of pulmonary embolism depend on the size of the obstruction: if a large clot lodges in a pulmonary vessel, gas exchange will be severely impaired, and the patient will show signs of respiratory distress. The signs and symptoms of pulmonary embolism are much like those of congestive heart failure, and may or may not include chest pain. *Suspect pulmonary embolism in any person at high risk who suddenly develops explained dyspnea or chest pain.*

In general, the signs and symptoms of pulmonary embolism may include the following (Figure 25-7):

- Sudden, severe, unexplained dyspnea (occurs in 80 percent of the victims).
- Respiratory distress.
- Sharp chest pain, possibly made worse by coughing and deep breathing. It is usually focal and is described as stabbing. (While chest pain is present in 85 to 90 percent of all cases of pulmonary embolism, you should be aware that it does not *always* exist.)
- Cough (present in about 50 percent of all cases); the patient may cough up blood.
- Rapid heartbeat.
- Falling blood pressure; because patients have difficulty maintaining blood pressure, they may faint when they stand up.
- Distended jugular veins.
- Less commonly, the patient may experience fever, tenderness in the calf or elsewhere, edema, or cyanosis.

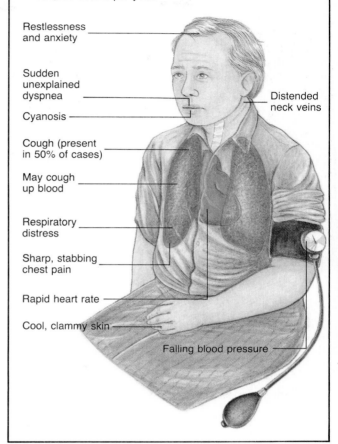

SIGNS AND SYMPTOMS OF PULMONARY EMBOLISM

Pulmonary embolism is a clot or embolus that blocks a pulmonary artery. It is a serious problem accounting for 200,000 deaths per year.

Restlessness and anxiety

Sudden unexplained dyspnea

Cyanosis

Distended neck veins

Cough (present in 50% of cases)

May cough up blood

Respiratory distress

Sharp, stabbing chest pain

Rapid heart rate

Cool, clammy skin

Falling blood pressure

FIGURE 25-7

Emergency Care

Emergency care in the field is largely supportive, since definitive therapy requires hospitalization. To treat pulmonary embolism in the field:

1. Establish an airway.
2. Assist ventilations as needed.
3. Administer oxygen in the highest possible concentration.
4. Monitor vital signs.
5. Transport without delay.

☐ ACUTE PULMONARY EDEMA

Acute pulmonary edema occurs when an excess of fluid builds up in the extravascular tissues in the spaces of the lungs. There are two general kinds of pulmonary

Respiratory Emergencies **391**

edema. Cardiogenic edema ocurs gradually, usually —
but not always — when the blood vessels in the lungs
are damaged. This damage most often results from disease, heavy cigarette smoking, myocardial infarction,
congestive heart failure, hypertension, or pulmonary
embolus. Non-cardiogenic edema is generally caused by
near-drowning, aspiration pneumonia, smoke inhalation, or inhalation of toxins.

Generally, acute pulmonary edema is caused by
myocardial infarction, sudden increases in the blood
pressure, failure to take cardiac medications, arrhythmias, too much salt, too much exercise, pregnancy,
anemia, and too-rapid infusion of intravenous fluids.

Signs and Symptoms

Look for the following signs and symptoms (Figure 25-8):

- Dyspnea.
- Rapid, labored breathing (in severe cases).
- Crackling or wheezing sounds.
- Cyanosis.
- Frothy pink, blood-tinged sputum (a late sign).
- Distended jugular veins.
- Rapid pulse.
- Cool, clammy skin.
- Restlessness.
- Anxiety.
- Patient appears completely exhausted.

Emergency Care

1. *Vigorous oxygen therapy is essential.* Administer
   high-flow, humidified, positive-pressure oxygen;
   monitor breathing and other vital signs carefully
   and throughout transport. Carefully suction airway
   as needed.
2. Keep the patient's head and shoulders elevated; if
   he is comfortable, allow him to sit upright and
   support his back and shoulders with pillows. Drop
   the legs to encourage venous pooling (Figure 25-9).
3. Keep the patient calm, and allow little or no
   movement; do whatever is necessary to preserve
   the patient's strength.
4. Transport as soon as possible.

☐ HYPERVENTILATION

Hyperventilation is a condition characterized by "overbreathing" or breathing too rapidly. It is normal for
most people occasionally (such as a situation of great

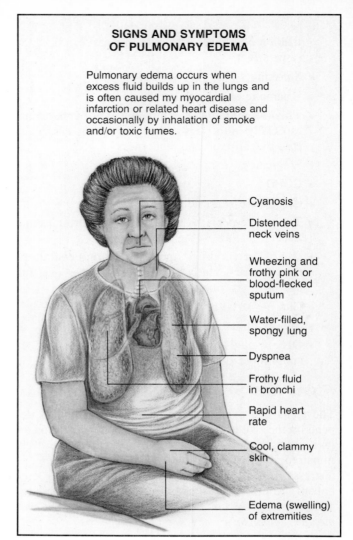

**SIGNS AND SYMPTOMS
OF PULMONARY EDEMA**

Pulmonary edema occurs when
excess fluid builds up in the lungs and
is often caused my myocardial
infarction or related heart disease and
occasionally by inhalation of smoke
and/or toxic fumes.

Cyanosis

Distended
neck veins

Wheezing and
frothy pink or
blood-flecked
sputum

Water-filled,
spongy lung

Dyspnea

Frothy fluid
in bronchi

Rapid heart
rate

Cool, clammy
skin

Edema (swelling)
of extremities

FIGURE 25-8

surprise), and remains normal as long as breathing
quickly returns to a normal rate. Hyperventilation syndrome, on the other hand, is an abnormal state in which
rapid breathing persists. It is a common disorder, and is
usually associated with anxiety; as the victim becomes
more anxious, he or she breathes more rapidly, which in
turn heightens the anxiety, and so on — creating a vicious cycle. Hyperventilation syndrome is characterized
by rapid, deep, or abnormal breathing. The lungs are
overinflated, and the victim blows off too much carbon
dioxide, resulting in **alkalosis.** The causes of hyperventilation syndrome are varied, but usually involve psychological stress. When caused by anxiety, hyperventilation is usually benign; if caused by an underlying
medical condition, the outcome can be catastrophic —
so it is important to try to establish a cause. It typically
is associated with aspirin overdose, diabetic coma,
pneumonia, asthma, pulmonary edema, pulmonary embolism, and increasing intracranial pressure. Most victims are young, anxious patients, most of whom are unaware that they are breathing abnormally. Not everyone
who is breathing rapidly or deeply is hyperventilating.

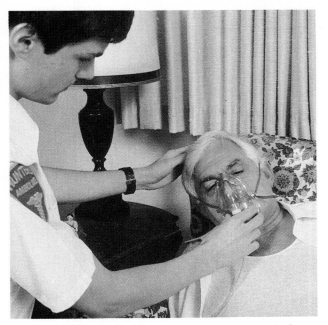

FIGURE 25-9 Allow the acute pulmonary edema patient to sit upright, and administer high-flow, warm, humidified, positive-pressure oxygen.

Signs and Symptoms

Whatever the cause of the hyperventilation syndrome, overbreathing can lower the arterial carbon dioxide to an abnormal level. The resulting **alkalosis** causes the signs and symptoms of the syndrome, which can include the following:

- Air hunger.
- Giddiness or unusual behavior.
- Fatigue.
- Abdominal discomfort or bloating.
- Marked anxiety, escalating to panic.
- Dyspnea.
- Dizziness or lightheadedness.
- Blurring of vision.
- Dryness or bitterness of the mouth.
- Numbness and/or tingling of the hands and feet or the area around the mouth.
- Tightness or a "lump" in the throat.
- Pounding of the heart with stabbing pains in the chest.
- A feeling of great tiredness or weakness.
- A feeling of being in a dream.
- A feeling of impending doom.
- Drawing-up of the hands at the wrist and knuckles, with flexed fingers (**carpopedal** spasm — can be common but may occur in severe attacks only).
- Fainting.
- Deep, sighing, rapid respirations with rapid pulse.

Emergency Care

Prior to beginning treatment, rule out any organic causes for rapid breathing, such as diabetic coma, pulmonary embolism, trauma, or asthma. If you are certain that none of these life-threatening conditions exists, follow these guidelines to help control hyperventilation syndrome:

1. Remain calm and reassuring; listen carefully, show understanding consideration, and try to help the patient calm down.
2. Try to talk the patient into slowing the respiratory rate.
3. In uncomplicated anxiety hyperventilation, help the patient build the blood carbon dioxide level back up by having him or her breathe into an oxygen mask that is not connected to oxygen, causing him to rebreathe his or her own exhaled air (Figure 25-10). Do *not* use this method if you suspect that there is a medical cause for the rapid respiration.
4. Explain to the patient what happened.
5. Transport the patient to an emergency room, where he can be further examined by a physician.
6. If in doubt about the cause of the symptoms, administer low-flow oxygen; it will *not* make the hyperventilation worse.

FIGURE 25-10 For anxiety hyperventilation, have the patient breathe into an oxygen mask that is not connected to oxygen. *Do not use* this method if there is a medical cause for the hyperventilation.

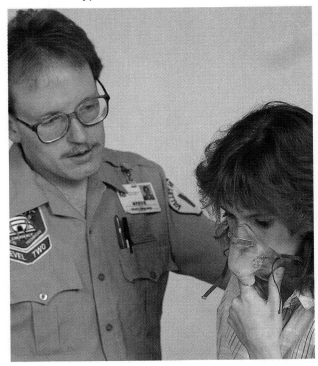

chapter 26

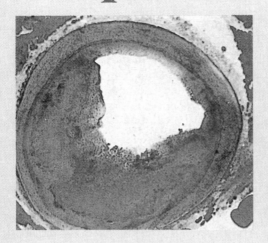

Heart Attack and Other Cardiac Emergencies

✻ OBJECTIVES

- Outline the anatomy and function of the heart.
- Describe coronary artery disease and related risk factors.
- Describe the cause, signs and symptoms, and emergency care for angina, congestive heart failure, and myocardial infarction.
- Explain the basic components of patient assessment for cardiac emergencies.

It is recommended that EMTs wear protective gloves whenever there is a possibility of coming in contact with a patient's blood, body fluids, mucous membranes, traumatic wounds, or sores. See Chapter 31.

Heart attacks and associated heart disease are the number-one killer in the United States today. Almost half a million Americans die each year of cardiovascular disease before they can reach a hospital, and almost 29 million more Americans suffer from some form of cardiovascular disease. The most common problem is coronary artery disease, which usually leads to angina pectoris and may eventually lead to acute myocardial infarction (heart attack) if left untreated.

Because of the critical nature of heart disease emergencies, you should treat every adult with chest pain as a heart attack victim until proven otherwise.

☐ CARDIAC ANATOMY AND PHYSIOLOGY

The heart is in the center of the chest, and about two-thirds of it lies on the left side. The base of the heart points toward the right shoulder, while the apex points toward the left hip.

A four-chambered, muscular organ about the size of a fist, the heart receives unoxygenated blood from the veins and pumps oxygenated blood through the vascular system. An electrical conduction system causes the myocardium to contract. The electrical impulse originates in the right atrium and spreads through both atria, causing them to contract. The impulse continues down to a special spot in the heart called the **atrioventricular node** (located between the atria and the ventricles), and then through special fibers to the ventricles, causing them to contract.

The heart muscle is made up of three layers: the **endocardium,** or innermost layer; the middle layer, or myocardium; which does the greatest amount of work; and the outermost layer, or **epicardium.** See Chapter 2.

The right side of the heart receives unoxygenated blood into the right atrium, and the right ventricle pumps the blood to the lungs, where it is oxygenated. The freshly oxygenated blood enters the left atrium, moves to the left ventricle, and is pumped systematically throughout the rest of the body.

The heart's chambers propel blood by contraction, and the four valves ensure that the blood moves in only one direction (forward).

- The **tricuspid valve,** located between the right atrium and the right ventricle, prevents the return of blood from the ventricle to the atrium.
- The **pulmonary valve,** located at the base of the pulmonary artery, prevents blood from returning to the right ventricle from the pulmonary artery.
- The **bicuspid valve** (also known as the mitral valve) is located between the left atrium and the left ventricle and prevents the return of blood to the left atrium from the left ventricle.

- The **aortic valve,** at the base of the aortic artery, prevents blood from returning to the left ventricle from the aorta.

Like the rest of the body, the heart is nourished by blood that is carried through the arteries of the circulatory system. The three main **coronary arteries** that are the first to branch off the aorta and that provide nourishment to the heart are the right coronary artery, the left coronary artery, and the anterior descending branch (which comes off of the left coronary artery).

☐ CORONARY ARTERY DISEASE

As the name implies, coronary artery disease affects the arteries that supply the heart with blood by injuring the inner lining of the arterial walls. The two types of coronary artery disease are **arteriosclerosis** and **atherosclerosis,** which is a form of arteriosclerosis, and patients commonly have both kinds.

Atherosclerosis results when fatty substances and other debris (called **plaque**) are deposited on the inner lining of the arterial wall (Figure 26-1). As a result, the

FIGURE 26-1 Fatty deposit buildup in arteries. The deterioration of a normal artery is seen as atherosclerosis develops and begins depositing fatty substances and roughening the channel lining until a clot forms and plugs the artery to deprive the heart muscle of vital blood, which results in heart attack.

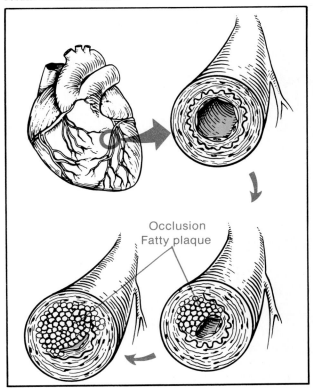

Occlusion
Fatty plaque

lumen (opening) of the artery is narrowed, reducing the flow of blood through the affected artery. Another form of arteriosclerosis occurs when **calcium** is deposited in the walls of the arteries, resulting in loss of arterial elasticity and an increase in blood pressure. Arteriosclerosis generally affects other arteries in addition to the coronary arteries, and may lead to hypertension, kidney disease, or stroke.

In coronary artery disease, the lumen of the coronary artery is narrowed, restricting the amount of blood that can reach and nourish the heart muscle. Roughened surfaces on the artery cause buildup of additional plaque, further narrowing the artery. At some point, the patient may experience angina pectoris (chest pain) or a myocardial infarction (death of part of the myocardium) because the coronary artery eventually becomes blocked (occluded) (Figures 26-2–26-5).

□ CARDIAC RISK FACTORS

Researchers have identified a number of cardiac risk factors that predispose an individual to coronary artery disease and eventual heart attack. The major risk factors include (Figure 26-6):

- Heredity (a family history of coronary artery disease or heart disease).
- Diabetes mellitus that is not controlled.
- Sex (males are affected more than females).
- Age (signs and symptoms generally develop after the age of forty).
- Race.
- High serum cholesterol and triglycerides (may be

□ Cardiovascular Disease

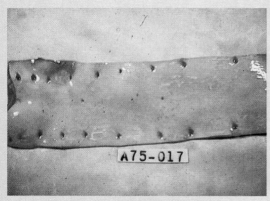

FIGURE 26-2 Inside surface, normal artery.

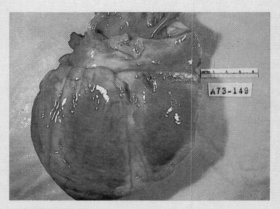

FIGURE 26-3 Myocardial infarction.

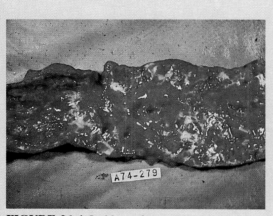

FIGURE 26-4 Inside surface, severe atherosclerosis.

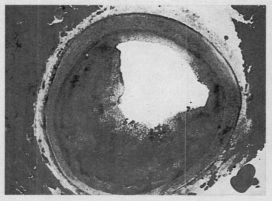

FIGURE 26-5 Artery cross-section, atherosclerosis.

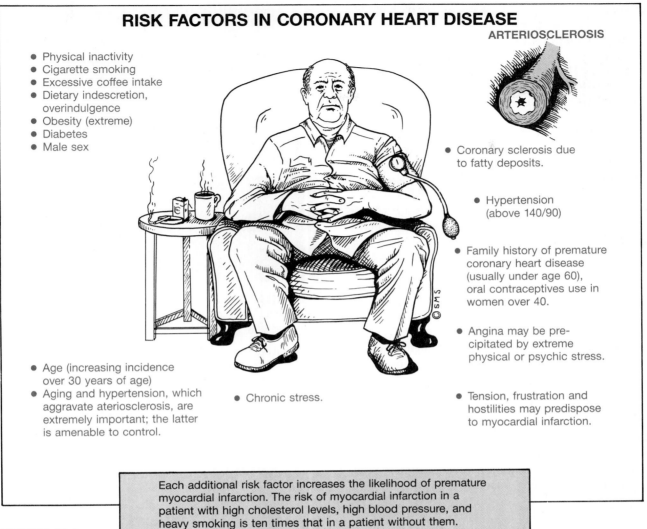

RISK FACTORS IN CORONARY HEART DISEASE

ARTERIOSCLEROSIS

- Physical inactivity
- Cigarette smoking
- Excessive coffee intake
- Dietary indescretion, overindulgence
- Obesity (extreme)
- Diabetes
- Male sex

- Coronary sclerosis due to fatty deposits.

- Hypertension (above 140/90)

- Family history of premature coronary heart disease (usually under age 60), oral contraceptives use in women over 40.

- Age (increasing incidence over 30 years of age)
- Aging and hypertension, which aggravate ateriosclerosis, are extremely important; the latter is amenable to control.

- Chronic stress.

- Angina may be precipitated by extreme physical or psychic stress.

- Tension, frustration and hostilities may predispose to myocardial infarction.

Each additional risk factor increases the likelihood of premature myocardial infarction. The risk of myocardial infarction in a patient with high cholesterol levels, high blood pressure, and heavy smoking is ten times that in a patient without them.

FIGURE 26-6

related to eating foods that are high in saturated fats).

- Hypertension.
- Smoking.
- Sedentary lifestyle.
- Poorly handled stress.

Obviously, the first five factors cannot be controlled; however, with awareness and determination, an individual can change the last four factors and decrease the risk of developing coronary artery disease.

☐ ANGINA PECTORIS

Angina pectoris literally means a "pain in the chest," but is actually a set of signs and symptoms that can occur in a patient with serious coronary artery disease. In essence, angina occurs when the heart's demand for oxygen is temporarily greater than what it is receiving.

There are several possible causes of angina pectoris. Because of coronary artery disease, the coronary arteries may be narrowed, and only a limited supply of oxygen-rich blood can be delivered to the heart. Angina pectoris can also occur if the coronary arteries have an abnormal spasm (called "Prinzmetal's angina"). It can also occur if the blood supply to the heart is slowed by the presence of a thrombus or clot, or if the blood loses its ability to carry adequate amounts of oxygen (such as happens in anemia).

Like any muscle, the heart relies on a constant supply of oxygen to function. When the demand for oxygenated blood is greater than the diseased or constricted arteries can provide, the patient experiences angina pectoris, a brief feeling of pain or discomfort that signals the heart's need for oxygen.

Angina pectoris does not always manifest itself as

pain — it may be a feeling of tightness, gripping, heaviness, squeezing, burning, or a dull constriction. The pain is usually on the left side of the chest but may radiate to the jaw, neck, shoulder, arm, or hand (usually on the left side). The pain is sometimes accompanied by nausea, vomiting, and shortness of breath. Angina pectoris is often mistaken for indigestion, and misdiagnosis is frequent.

Most often angina pectoris occurs because the patient has increased the heart's demand for oxygen by an increased workload, usually by physical activity or emotional excitement, and most often in cold weather. The heart rate may increase as a result of physical activity beyond the patient's limit, emotional stress, or being outdoors in extreme weather (hot, cold, or windy). When the heart's workload is increased, it needs greater amounts of blood — which the diseased arteries are unable to deliver. When there is not enough blood to meet the metabolic needs of the cardiac cells, angina pectoris results. Less commonly, angina may occur without exertion, as in unstable angina or angina that is the result of spasms in the coronary arteries.

Approximately 80 percent of all angina victims are men in their fifties or sixties; angina is reversible and produces no permanent damage to the heart. Pain is generally relieved by rest, usually within a few minutes after the patient stops the activity, calms down, moves indoors, or takes nitroglycerin as prescribed by a physician. In some cases, angina results from valvular or congenital heart disease, both of which increase the heart's need for oxygen; even healthy coronary arteries occasionally cannot meet the demand.

Signs and Symptoms

The most common complaint of angina is chest pain that may range from a mild ache to a severe crushing pain. (See Figure 26-7.) It appears suddenly but is usually associated with physical exertion. The pain is located substernally but may also radiate to the jaw, neck, left shoulder, left arm, and left hand. Other common signs and symptoms include (Figure 26-8):

- Dyspnea.
- **Diaphoresis.**
- Lightheadedness.
- Palpitations.
- Nausea and/or vomiting.
- Pale and cool skin.

Remember — it is impossible in the field to differentiate between the pain of angina pectoris and the pain of myocardial infarction. While angina is a transient episode that leaves the heart undamaged, it *is* an indication of coronary artery disease and needs to be treated

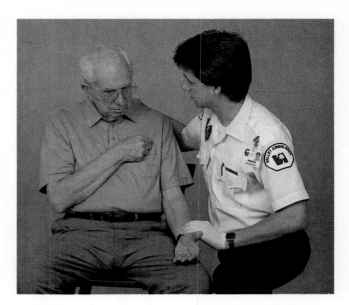
FIGURE 26-7 The most common complaint of angina is chest pain.

by a physician. Left untreated, it may eventually cause myocardial infarction.

If the patient has nitroglycerin tablets or spray, help him or her use it; nitroglycerin reduces the heart's work and need for oxygen and helps to dilate the coronary arteries so that more oxygenated blood flows to the heart. For more detailed instructions on helping patients with nitroglycerin, see the guidelines for general emergency care of cardiac patients at the end of this chapter.

☐ ACUTE MYOCARDIAL INFARCTION (AMI)

Called a "heart attack" by the lay person, acute myocardial infarction means death of the myocardium (heart muscle). When blood supply to part of the heart is significantly reduced or stopped completely, the affected part dies (Figure 26-9). Myocardial infarction is most often associated with coronary artery disease — most frequently with a thrombus or clot in coronary arteries already diseased by atherosclerosis. It can also result from a spasm in the coronary arteries or when the heart's need for oxygen exceeds its supply for an extended period of time.

Because of the configuration of the coronary arteries and the pressure involved in the heart, it is often the left ventricle that sustains the myocardial infarction.

- **Sudden death.** Nearly one-half a million people die each year in this country from myocardial infarction before they ever reach a hospital. Most of them die within two hours of first experiencing signs and symptoms of myocardial infarction.

DISTINGUISHING ANGINA PECTORIS FROM MYOCARDIAL INFARCTION

	ANGINA PECTORIS	MYOCARDIAL INFARCTION
Location of Pain	Substernal or across chest	Same
Radiation of Pain	Neck, jaw or arms	Same
Nature of Pain	Dull or heavy discomfort with a pressure or squeezing sensation	Same, but maybe more intense
Duration	Usually lasts 2 to 10 minutes rarely longer	Usually lasts longer than 30 minutes
Other Symptoms	Usually none	Perspiration, weakness, nausea, pale gray color
Precipitating Factors	Extremes in weather, exertion, stress, meals	Often none
Factors Giving Relief	Stopping physical activity, reducing stress, nitroglycerin	Nitroglycerin may give incomplete, or no relief

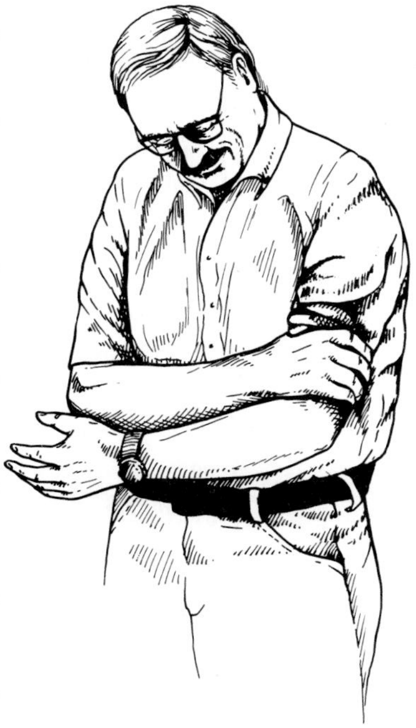

If in doubt as to which condition the patient has, always treat as if it is an acute myocardial infarction.

FIGURE 26-8

Sudden death occurs because myocardial infarction often causes dysrhythmias.

- **Cardiogenic shock.** If 40 percent or more of the left ventricle is damaged after a myocardial infarction, severe impairment of the heart's pumping action results, leading to inadequate circulation of blood. The mortality rate from cardiogenic shock is 80 percent. In cardiogenic shock, the heart is both inefficient and inadequate.

- **Congestive heart failure.** Congestive heart failure may develop between three and seven days after a myocardial infarction because the heart's pumping ability is impaired, but the heart can still meet the demands of the body.

- **Cardiac dysrhythmias.** Cardiac dysrhythmias are abnormal heart rhythms that occur following a myocardial infarction, generally caused by an **irritable heart** or by injury to the electrical conduction system of the heart.

Signs and Symptoms

The signs and symptoms of myocardial infarction vary depending on the amount of pump damage and how the autonomic nervous system responds to the damage.

The major symptom of a myocardial infarction is chest pain that may range from mild discomfort to a severe crushing pain — *but it should be noted that 25 percent of all myocardial infarction patients have no chest pain at all* (usually the elderly or diabetics). Myocardial infarctions without pain are called "silent myocardial infarctions." The pain of myocardial infarction lasts for longer than thirty minutes, and the classical location is substernal radiating to the neck, jaw, left shoulder, and left arm.

Pain may or may not be present, however — and the pain may not necessarily be aggravated by exertion. Remember, too, that pain associated with myocardial infarction can be experienced in a great number of ways, and it often feels exactly the same as the pain of angina

MYOCARDIAL INFARCTION
(Heart Attack)

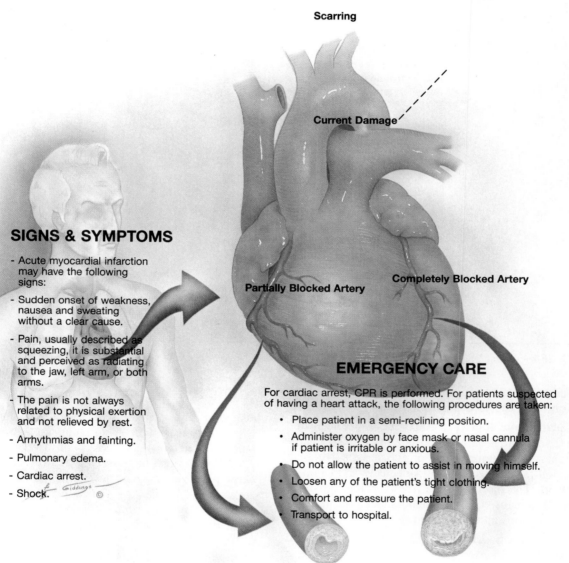

PHYSICAL FINDINGS

- Pulse usually increases, but occasionally will slow.
- Blood pressure falls.
- Respiration is normal unless pulmonary edema develops; then respiration is rapid and shallow.
- Patient appears frightened and may be sweaty and pale gray in color.

Scarring

Current Damage

SIGNS & SYMPTOMS

- Acute myocardial infarction may have the following signs:
- Sudden onset of weakness, nausea and sweating without a clear cause.
- Pain, usually described as squeezing, it is substantial and perceived as radiating to the jaw, left arm, or both arms.
- The pain is not always related to physical exertion and not relieved by rest.
- Arrhythmias and fainting.
- Pulmonary edema.
- Cardiac arrest.
- Shock.

Partially Blocked Artery

Completely Blocked Artery

EMERGENCY CARE

For cardiac arrest, CPR is performed. For patients suspected of having a heart attack, the following procedures are taken:

- Place patient in a semi-reclining position.
- Administer oxygen by face mask or nasal cannula if patient is irritable or anxious.
- Do not allow the patient to assist in moving himself.
- Loosen any of the patient's tight clothing.
- Comfort and reassure the patient.
- Transport to hospital.

FIGURE 26-9

pectoris. *Any adult with chest pain should be suspected of myocardial infarction until proven otherwise.*

Other common signs and symptoms of myocardial infarction include the following (Figures 26-10 and 26-11):

- Dyspnea.
- Diaphoresis.
- Cool and pale skin.
- Possible cyanosis.

EARLY SIGNALS OF A HEART ATTACK

PAIN, in one form or another, usually accompanies a heart attack and ranges from a mild ache to unbearable severity. When severe, pain is often felt as constricting, like a vise on the chest. Pain also often includes the burning and bloating sensations that usually accompany indigestion. Pain may be continuous and then might subside, but don't ignore it if it does. Pain could occur in any one or combination of locations shown below.

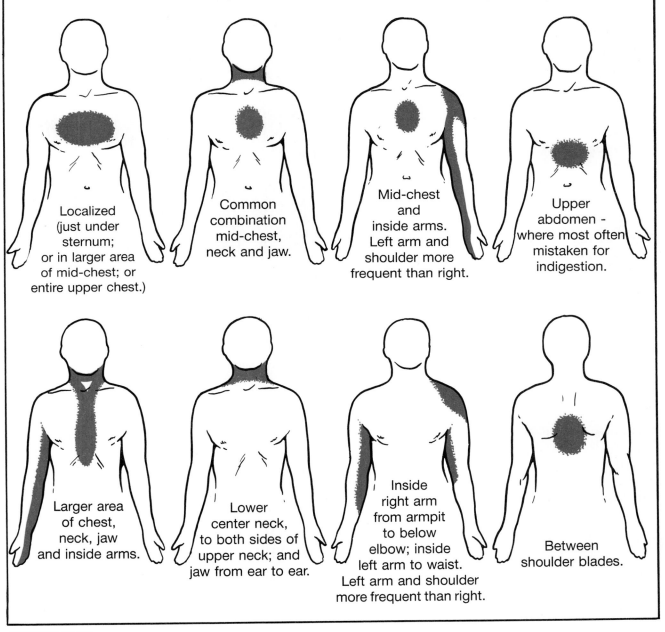

Localized (just under sternum; or in larger area of mid-chest; or entire upper chest.)

Common combination mid-chest, neck and jaw.

Mid-chest and inside arms. Left arm and shoulder more frequent than right.

Upper abdomen - where most often mistaken for indigestion.

Larger area of chest, neck, jaw and inside arms.

Lower center neck, to both sides of upper neck; and jaw from ear to ear.

Inside right arm from armpit to below elbow; inside left arm to waist. Left arm and shoulder more frequent than right.

Between shoulder blades.

FIGURE 26-10

- Nausea and/or vomiting.
- Weakness.
- Lightheadedness.
- Anxiety.

- Feeling of impending doom.
- Variable blood pressure (low with cardiogenic shock).
- **Syncope** (fainting).

Heart Attack and Other Cardiac Emergencies   **401**

☐ Acute Myocaridal Infarction (AMI)

SYMPTOMS AND SIGNS MAY INCLUDE:

Respiratory:

- Dyspnea—shallow or deep respirations.
- Cough that produces sputum.

Behavioral:

- Anxiety, irritability, inability to concentrate.
- Depression.
- Feeling of impending doom.
- Mild delirium, personality changes.
- Fainting.
- Occasional thrashing about and clutching of the chest.

Circulatory:

- Signs of shock.
- Increased pulse rate, sometimes irregular.
- Some patients may have a slowed pulse rate.
- Reduced blood pressure in 50% of the patients. Normal blood pression in 25% of patients. Increased blood pressure in 25% of patients.

Pain:

- 15% to 20% are painless ("silent") attacks.
- Marked discomfort that continues when at rest rather than a sharp or throbbing pain.
- Usually not alleviated by nitroglycerin.
- May last 30 minutes to several hours.
- Originates under sternum and may radiate to arms, neck, or jaw.

An AMI Can Lead to:

- Mechanical heart failure with pulmonary edema.
- Shock (usually within 24 hours).
- Congestive heart failure (immediately, or up to a week or more later).
- Cardiac arrest (40% die before they reach the hospital).

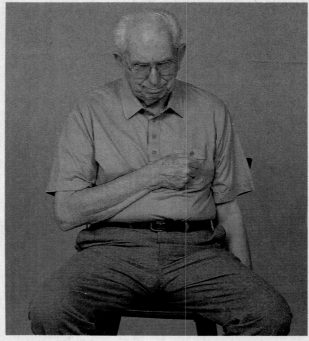

FIGURE 26-11

AMI — EMERGENCY CARE

FOR THE UNCONSCIOUS PATIENT

- Establish and maintain an airway.
- Provide pulmonary resuscitation or CPR if needed. If respiratory or cardiac arrest develops, deliver oxygen with a bag-valve-mask unit or a demand value resuscitator.
- Administer high concentration of oxygen.
- Loosen restrictive clothing.
- Conserve body heat, but do not allow overheating.
- Transport immediately—quiet transport.
- Monitor vital signs.

FOR THE CONSCIOUS PATIENT

- Keep the patient calm and still—*do not* allow patient to move himself to the ambulence stretcher.
- Take history and determine vital signs.

WARNING!
TREAT ALL SUSPECTED ANGINA AND AMI PATIENTS AS IF THEY ARE HAVING AMIs.

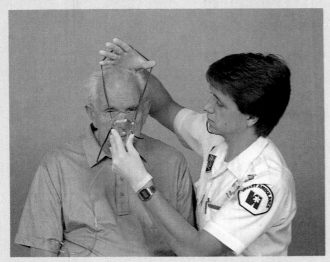

FIGURE 26-12

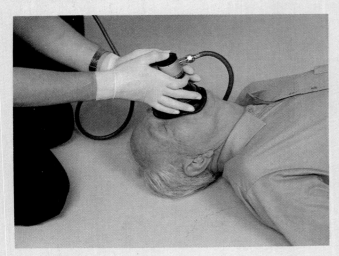

FIGURE 26-13

- Help patient with medication.
- Administer high concentration of oxygen.
- Conserve body heat.
- Transport as soon as possible in a semi-reclined or sitting position. Provide quiet transport.
- Monitor vital signs during transport.

Emergency care may be complicated by many factors. If the patient is conscious, his or her irritability, restlessness, and feeling of impending doom may make the patient uncooperative and unwilling to settle down, even though it is vital that the patient do so. Many AMI patients will resist the placement of a face mask for oxygen delivery. If the patient resists after an explanation of the importance of oxygen, use a nasal cannula at 6 liters/minute. Provide needed oxygen, but do not upset the patient.

- The pulse may be weak or bounding, fast or slow, regular or irregular, depending on the type and extent of damage. A pulse of less than 60 per minute is alarming.

Emergency Care

Time is critical in the treatment of myocardial infarction: the first few minutes after the myocardial infarction begins are critical to survival. If CPR is started within four minutes, there is a dramatic difference in the survival of the patient.

For all possible cases of myocardial infarction, provide the following care (Figures 26-12–26-18):

1. Assess for airway, breathing, and circulation. Assist as necessary; begin CPR if needed.

2. Administer oxygen at six liters per minute by nasal cannula or at ten liters per minute by face mask. Adjust the rate based on patient color (degree of cyanosis) and comfort (Figure 26-12—13).

3. Do not let the patient move on his own; restrict all unnecessary movement, and provide comfort and reassurance to calm the patient.

4. Place the patient in the position of greatest comfort and ease of breathing. A sitting or semi-reclined position with the head elevated thirty degrees is preferred by most patients.

5. Monitor vital signs continuously, and notify the receiving facility of the patient's status. Continue to monitor vital signs throughout transport.

6. Transport immediately to the closest appropriate facility.

☐ CONGESTIVE HEART FAILURE

Congestive heart failure currently affects more than two million Americans; one-half million are diagnosed each year in this country, and more than a third die each year. Congestive heart failure symptoms can be treated, but the underlying condition is almost never curable.

Congestive heart failure results when the heart's pumping output does not meet the needs of bodily tissues; i.e., perfusion is inadequate. While there are a number of causes, the most common include myocardial infarction, hypertension, chronic obstructive pulmonary disease, coronary artery disease, and heart valve damage. Congestive heart failure represents a true medical emergency; a stable patient can suddenly and rapidly deteriorate without warning.

Congestive heart failure is usually the result of myocardial infarction that has damaged the heart muscle. It can also be caused by thombosis, disease, or infection that damages the heart or its valves.

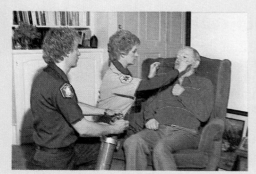

FIGURE 26-14 Reassure patient with chest pain and administer oxygen.

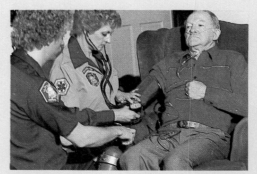

FIGURE 26-15 Check vital signs. Obtain patient history.

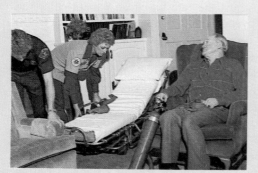

FIGURE 26-16 Prepare for transport.

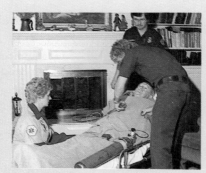

FIGURE 26-17 Secure patient and oxygen.

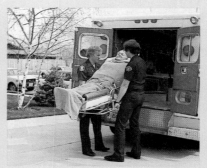

FIGURE 26-18 Load patient into ambulance.

As congestive heart failure progresses, fluid builds up behind the failing left heart, in the pulmonary network. This increases pressure in the pulmonary capillaries, causing plasma to seep out of the capillaries into the surrounding lung tissue — a condition called pulmonary edema. As a result, pink, frothy sputum may be coughed up (a sign of severe pulmonary edema). If not corrected, severe respiratory distress follows. Congestive heart failure gradually reduces the lung's oxygen capacity, and death occurs.

Signs and Symptoms

Pain may or may not occur with congestive heart failure, usually depending on whether myocardial infarction has also occurred. The most dramatic sign of congestive heart failure is pulmonary edema, resulting in severe dyspnea (and often resulting in spasmodic coughing that produces pink frothy sputum). In addition to shortness of breath, the patient may experience the following (Figure 26-19):

- Wheezing (due to airway spasm that results from fluid in the lungs).
- Noisy lung sounds.
- Diaphoresis.
- Rapid heart rate (tachycardia).
- Increased respiratory rate with fast, labored breathing.
- Engorged liver and spleen.
- Apprehension or agitation, often accompanied by the feeling of being smothered.
- Paleness or cyanosis.
- Difficulty breathing while lying flat.
- Normal to high blood pressure.
- **Pedal** and lower extremity edema.
- Anxiety.
- Mild to severe confusion.
- A desire to sit upright.
- Abdominal distention.
- Distended neck veins.

Remember — while these signs and symptoms are the most common, the patient may have any combina-

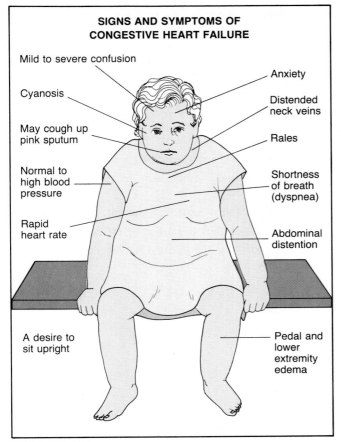

SIGNS AND SYMPTOMS OF CONGESTIVE HEART FAILURE

Mild to severe confusion

Cyanosis

May cough up pink sputum

Normal to high blood pressure

Rapid heart rate

A desire to sit upright

Anxiety

Distended neck veins

Rales

Shortness of breath (dyspnea)

Abdominal distention

Pedal and lower extremity edema

FIGURE 26-19

tion of them, and some patients may have only one or two. Congestive heart failure with respiratory difficulty is life-threatening and requires immediate care.

Emergency Care

In any patient experiencing severe dyspnea, with or without severe pulmonary edema, care for it as follows:

1. Sit the patient upright on the stretcher, legs dangling over the side; this position encourages the flow of fluid out of the lungs and into the extremities. *Never lay the patient flat.*
2. Administer 100 percent high-flow oxygen (by mask if the patient tolerates it); assist respirations if necessary with demand-valve.
3. Transport rapidly.

☐ PATIENT ASSESSMENT FOR CARDIAC EMERGENCIES

Note: Information-gathering is recommended and can be helpful in treatment of cardiac patients, but you should *never* delay treatment or transport in order to gather in-

formation about the patient. If you are able to gather information while positioning the patient, administering oxygen, and taking vital signs, you might determine the following:

- The location and radiation of the pain, its mode of onset, duration, severity, character, and any associated symptoms (such as nausea).
- Whether and how the patient has attempted to alleviate the pain, and whether these efforts were successful.
- Whether the patient has ever experienced similar pain. Was it of the same duration and intensity? Under what circumstances did the pain occur? Are the current circumstances different than circumstances that caused the pain in the past? If there was a past occurrence, what was wrong then? What was the diagnosis?
- Whether there is dyspnea, and under what conditions it exists. Does it awaken the patient? Does any body position (sitting, lying down) make it better or worse? Has it ever happened before, and, if so, under what circumstances? Are there any other associated symptoms?
- Whether the patient is cyanotic.
- Whether the patient's mental state is impaired. Is the patient confused, disoriented, restless, anxious, or agitated?
- Whether the patient has fainted or lost consciousness.
- Whether the patient noticed any palpitations (abnormalities in heartbeat, often reported as feeling the heart "skip a beat"). What were the onset, frequency, and duration? Has it ever happened before? What were the circumstances then? Did they differ from the present circumstances?
- Whether and why the patient is taking any medication. Be especially alert for nitroglycerin, digitalis, **diuretics,** any other medications prescribed for chest pain, or medications prescribed to suppress chronic arrhythmias.
- Whether the patient is under treatment for any serious illnesses.
- Whether the patient has ever had hypertension, diabetes, **rheumatic fever,** lung disease, or a previous episode of heart attack or heart failure.

Be as brief as possible in gathering information and again, *do not delay treatment or transport in order to perform extended assessment.* Relay any information that you are able to gather to the receiving facility staff to help the physician determine the appropriate treatment for the patient.

☐ GENERAL EMERGENCY CARE FOR CARDIAC PATIENTS

A patient with a heart disease emergency can be given the following general care (see Figures 26-14–26-18):

1. Have the patient cease all movement.

2. Place the patient in a semi-reclining or sitting position, or position of comfort. Keep the patient at rest to reduce anxiety.

3. If the problem is a suspected angina attack, ask the patient if he has nitroglycerin. If the patient has tablets and has not already taken them, place one tablet underneath the tongue. The nitroglycerin may also be in spray form, which is also used under the tongue. This is not allowed in some areas — *follow local protocol.*

4. Make sure that the airway is open, and administer high-flow oxygen with a face mask. If this is not possible because the patient is anxious and irritable, use a nasal cannula at no more than six to eight liters per minute. If the patient is in respiratory or cardiac arrest, use a demand value or bag-valve-mask resuscitator.

5. Loosen constricting clothing.

6. Maintain body temperature as close to normal as possible.

7. Comfort and reassure the patient.

8. Administer CPR if cardiac arrest occurs.

9. Transport to the closest advanced life support facility.

chapter 27

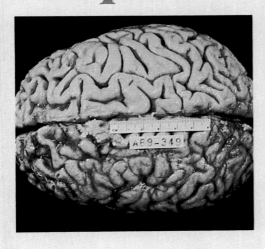

Stroke

✳ OBJECTIVES

- Understand the types of circulation disturbance in the brain that can cause a stroke.
- List the common signs and symptoms of stroke.
- Describe and demonstrate the appropriate emergency care for stroke patients.

It is recommended that EMTs wear protective gloves whenever there is a possibility of coming in contact with a patient's blood, body fluids, mucous membranes, traumatic wounds, or sores. See Chapter 31.

Stroke is defined as any disease process that impairs circulation to the brain. The third most common cause of death in this country, stroke affects approximately half a million Americans each year. More than half of those die, and many others suffer permanent neurological damage as a result of the stroke. The prognosis among those who survive for the first few minutes is improved with rapid transport, proper treatment en route, advances in patient care, and new techniques for rehabilitation.

Stroke, also known as cerebrovascular accident (CVA), occurs when the blood flow to the brain is interrupted long enough to cause damage, resulting in the sudden onset of brain dysfunction. The characteristics of stroke, which range from the unnoticed to those causing coma, depend on the extent of the stroke, the site of the stroke, and the amount of brain damage that results.

The outcome of stroke — regardless of its cause — depends on the age of the patient, the location and function of the brain cells that were damaged, the extent of the damage, and how rapidly other areas of brain tissue are able to take over the work of the damaged cells (brain cells do not regenerate). Without treatment, recurrence among survivors of stroke is common; with appropriate treatment, recurrence is not common.

According to the American Heart Association Council on Stroke, the most likely candidate for stroke has high blood pressure and a history of brief, intermittent stroke episodes called **transient ischemic attacks (TIAs).** Other predisposing factors in general include diabetes and hardening of the arteries in the heart, neck, and legs. The stroke patient often smokes heavily and has high levels of cholesterol or other fats in the blood. Some have a high red blood cell count or **gout.**

□ GENERAL CAUSES OF STROKE

The four general causes of interference of the blood supply to the brain are:

- **Thrombus.**
- **Embolus.**
- **Hemorrhage.**
- **Compression (Figure 27-1).**

Thrombus

The most common cause of stroke occurs when a cerebral artery is blocked by a clot (thrombus) that forms inside the artery; 75 to 85 percent of all strokes are caused by a thrombus. This condition is called by several names, including **cerebral thrombosis, cerebral infarction,** and **ischemic stroke.** Cerebral thrombosis usually occurs in those over the age of fifty, and the in-

cidence generally increases with age. The major cause is atherosclerosis. Approximately 60 percent of cerebral thrombosis victims have hypertension, 25 percent have diabetes, and up to half also have some type of vascular disease.

Clots do not generally form in healthy arteries, but rather around the hardened, thickened arterial walls damaged by atherosclerosis. As the deposits build up along the arterial walls and narrow the passageway, blood flow slows substantially; the deposits eventually form clots. If they become large enough, they can completely stop the flow of blood through that artery, thereby reducing the blood supply to areas of brain tissue and nerves. The brain tissue then rapidly dies from a lack of glucose and oxygen. Less commonly, the clot may also cause the artery to constrict due to spasm, which also cuts off the blood supply to the brain.

Up to 75 percent of all thrombus strokes are preceded by one or more transient ischemic attacks, brief "spells" similar to strokes that result when the blockage is incomplete or lasts only a few minutes. In the case of a TIA, the brain cells are injured but they do not die. (If the brain cells are deprived for a longer period, resulting in death, a full-blown stroke has occurred.)

TIAs often occur in a series over a period of many days, usually getting worse with time. While most TIAs are warning of a possible future stroke, they *can* occasionally occur without being followed by a stroke. As mentioned, they result in no permanent brain damage.

The symptoms of a TIA last for less than twenty-four hours and usually for less than one hour. All are temporary, leaving no permanent effects; often, only one symptom may be present. The most common symptoms of TIAs include:

- Blindness in one eye.
- Headache.
- Dizziness.
- Lightheadedness.
- Fainting.
- Difficulty in performing familiar acts.
- Temporary paralysis of the face.
- Temporary paralysis of one side of the body.
- Difficulty pronouncing and/or understanding words.
- Inability to recognize familiar objects.

TIAs do *not* cause nausea or vomiting, and often headache is not present.

Whether or not it is preceded by a TIA, a thrombotic stroke usually occurs gradually, occurring in steps and getting worse over time as the blockage slowly increases. When TIAs are present, they tend to progressively worsen as more and more brain tissue becomes involved.

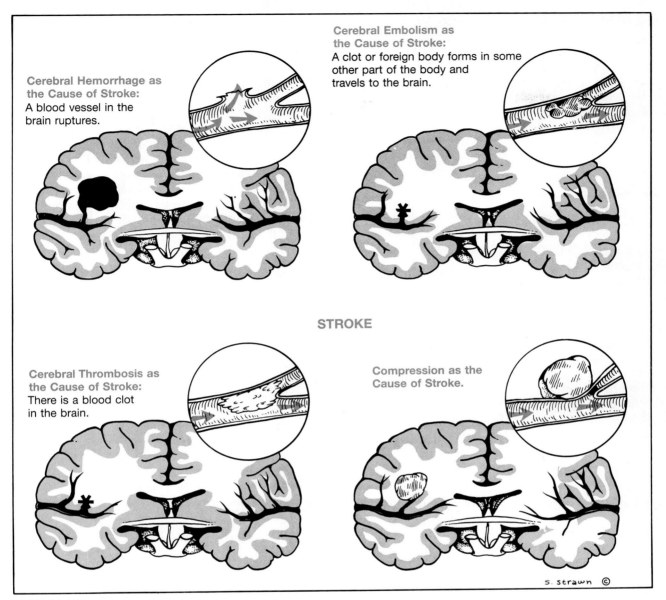

Cerebral Hemorrhage as the Cause of Stroke: A blood vessel in the brain ruptures.

Cerebral Embolism as the Cause of Stroke: A clot or foreign body forms in some other part of the body and travels to the brain.

STROKE

Cerebral Thrombosis as the Cause of Stroke: There is a blood clot in the brain.

Compression as the Cause of Stroke.

S. strawn ©

FIGURE 27-1

Embolus

A stroke may also result when a clot develops elsewhere in the body, travels through the bloodstream, and becomes lodged in one of the cerebral arteries — a condition called cerebral embolism. While embolism strokes are probably much less common than thrombus strokes, they occur much more rapidly; of all strokes, in fact, they have the most rapid onset. They often occur in young or middle-aged adults.

Emboli are most often found in people who have existing heart disease that results in uncontrolled and ineffective beating of the heart.

When a clot — either a thrombus (formed at the site in the brain) or an embolus (formed elsewhere and carried to the brain) — plugs up a cerebral artery, the condition is called cerebrovascular occlusion. Remember that occlusion may also be caused by a foreign body.

Hemorrhage

In 15 to 25 percent of all strokes, the stroke occurs when a diseased blood vessel in the brain bursts, flooding the surrounding brain tissue with blood (Figures 27-2 and 27-3). Bleeding can either be into the brain tissue itself (generally resulting from hypertension) or into the spinal fluid that surrounds the brain (generally resulting from rupture of an **aneurysm,** or weak spot in the vessel). Hemorrhage is the most dramatic form of stroke, and 80 percent of its victims die.

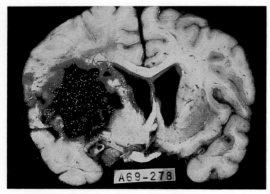

FIGURE 27-2 Cerebrovascular accident (stroke) from cerebral hemorrhage.

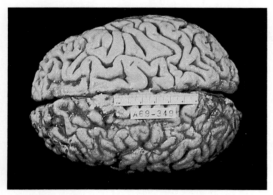

FIGURE 27-3 Stroke-damaged brain — one side.

Onset is abrupt, and it rapidly and progressively worsens as more brain tissue becomes involved; however, it does *not* occur in steplike stages, as does thrombotic stroke.

The artery involved in the hemorrhage can no longer carry blood to the starving tissues and nerves in the brain, and the accumulation of blood can cause great pressure within the brain. The blood then displaces and compresses brain tissue, causing it to die. While headache is not as common with thrombotic or embolism strokes, up to half of all hemorrhage stroke victims experience severe headache; vomiting is common.

Either the resulting clot or the accumulation of blood itself causes dangerous pressure to the brain, damaging and eventually killing adjacent brain tissue. The major causes of hemorrhage stroke are trauma (head injury), hypertension, and aneurysms that rupture. While aneurysms may be congenital (present from birth), they account for only 8 percent of all strokes; most aneurysms are caused by the damage that results from arteriosclerotic disease. The aneurysms — weak spots in the arterial walls — become filled with blood, balloon out, and eventually burst, surrounding the adjacent tissue with blood. With atherosclerosis, the damaged blood vessel is prone to breakage and leakage. Hypertension is also found in more than half of all stroke victims.

One of the newest risk factors for stroke is cocaine use. While all the physiological reasons are not known, it is known that cocaine increases blood pressure and can also cause cerebral infarction.

Cerebral hemorrhage is most likely to occur when the patient suffers from a combination of hypertension and atherosclerosis. While other forms of stroke usually occur in patients over forty years of age, cerebral hemorrhage can affect patients of any age (in younger people, it is usually caused by bursting of a congenital aneurysm). However, while it can occur at any age, the incidence does increase progressively over the age of fifty. In fact, the risk of stroke doubles for every decade of life past the age of forty-five.

Compression

A very small percentage of strokes occur when extreme pressure is applied to a cerebral artery, cutting off blood supply to the adjacent brain tissue and nerves. This pressure — or compression — can be caused by a brain tumor by displaced cerebral tissue following hemorrhage elsewhere in the brain or following head trauma, or by a clot that forms outside the artery as a result of blood leakage elsewhere in the brain. Compression can also result if a cerebral artery goes into spasm; however, spasms are usually so brief that resulting damage is rarely permanent.

☐ SIGNS AND SYMPTOMS OF STROKE

The signs and symptoms of stroke depend on the location, size, and severity of the stroke. Most signs of stroke come on suddenly and are focal in nature. The worst strokes are signalled by rapid and progressive signs and symptoms that are accompanied by the development of new signs and symptoms. Remember that other medical problems — such as epilepsy — can mimic stroke.

The precise signs and symptoms that accompany a stroke depend on the cause. A stroke caused by clotting (thrombus) results in lessening of bodily functions without accompanying pain or seizures; onset is gradual and progresses in a steplike way. A stroke caused by hemorrhage produces a sudden, excruciating headache followed by a rapid loss of consciousness. A stroke caused by an embolus is marked by possible sudden convulsions, paralysis, and abrupt loss of consciousness. A severe headache may occur explosively, although it is possible that no headache at all may occur.

The general signs and symptoms of stroke occur suddenly and may include the following (Figure 27-4):

- An alteration of the level of consciousness:

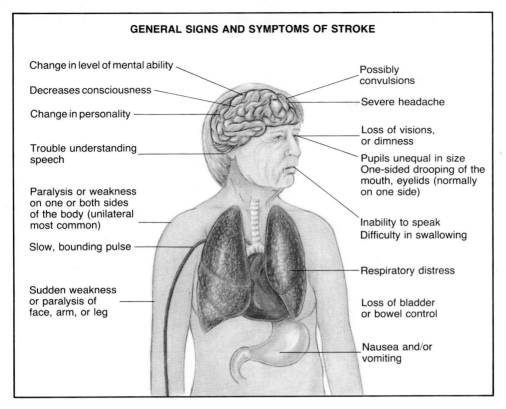

GENERAL SIGNS AND SYMPTOMS OF STROKE

Change in level of mental ability

Decreases consciousness

Change in personality

Trouble understanding speech

Paralysis or weakness on one or both sides of the body (unilateral most common)

Slow, bounding pulse

Sudden weakness or paralysis of face, arm, or leg

Possibly convulsions

Severe headache

Loss of visions, or dimness

Pupils unequal in size One-sided drooping of the mouth, eyelids (normally on one side)

Inability to speak Difficulty in swallowing

Respiratory distress

Loss of bladder or bowel control

Nausea and/or vomiting

FIGURE 27-4 Note: Even though a variety of signs/ symptoms may appear in a stroke victim, one may be sufficient reason to begin emergency care.

— Unexplained dizziness, confusion, or unsteadiness.
— A change in personality.
— A change in the level of mental ability, including concentration ability.
— Decreased consciousness, ranging from dizziness to coma.
— Convulsions.
- Effects on motor function:
— Weakness of the arms, legs, or face.
— Numbness or paralysis of the face, arms, or legs, often on only one side.
— One-sided weakness or numbness that gradually evolves to general weakness or numbness.
— Paralysis or weakness on one or both sides of the body; unilateral weakness or paralysis is most common.
— Mouth drawn to one side of the face or drooping on one side; paralysis of facial muscles, resulting in loss of facial expression and drooping eyelid.
- Effects on sensory function and changes in vision:
— Loss of vision or temporary dimness of vision, particularly in one eye.
— Double vision.
- Altered communication abilities:

— Inability to speak or trouble in speaking or understanding speech.
- Other symptoms:
— Headache accompanied by a stiff neck (caused by hemorrhage).
— A sudden severe headache or a change in the pattern of headaches normally experienced by the patient.
— Flushed or pale face.
— Respiratory distress.
— Pupils unequal in size or reaction or constricted.
— Loss of bowel or bladder control.
— Nausea and or vomiting.

If the stroke occurs on the left side of the brain, the damage is noticeable on the right side of the body; if the stroke occurs on the right side of the brain, the damage is evident on the left side of the body.

If a family member or friend is with the patient, it is helpful to obtain a brief history of the patient's medical problems. A young patient with a history of rheumatic heart disease or an older patient with a history of heart disease probably has an embolus that has lodged in a cerebral artery.

It is important to note the patients state of consciousness. Only massive strokes or those involving the brain stem render the patient completely unconscious. These, of course, are the most serious and require the most extensive medical care. Coma and neck rigidity are usually caused by cerebral hemorrhage (generally not massive in nature); a patient suffering from thrombosis or embolism generally will not have a stiff neck. The most critical stroke patient is the one who loses consciousness completely and becomes flaccid (limp) on the involved side; these signs indicate major brain injury. Remember — it is not important to spend time at the scene attempting to determine what type of stroke occurred; emergency care is the same regardless.

□ EMERGENCY CARE

The following steps should be initiated (See Figures 27-5 and 27-6):

1. Handle the patient calmly and carefully; be particularly gentle with paralyzed parts. Maintain a considerate, optimistic and hopeful attitude. Remember that the patient can hear you, even if he is not able to communicate back, so be careful about what you say in the patient's presence.

2. Position the patient on his or her back with his or her head and shoulders slightly raised (about twenty to thirty degrees) to relieve intracranial pressure. Keep the head in a neutral, forward-facing position to maintain arterial and venous flow to and from the head. Use a simple head tilt to keep the tongue from falling back and blocking the throat. If the patient is unconscious, use a nasal or oral airway. Administer high flow oxygen.

3. Assess the patient's airway and respiration.

□ Emergency Care of Stroke Patients

CONSCIOUS PATIENT:

- Ensure an open airway.
- Keep patient calm.
- Administer high concentration of oxygen.
- Monitor vital signs.
- Transport in semi-reclined position.
- Give nothing by mouth.
- Keep warm.
- Sit in front of the patient. Keep eye contact, and speak slowly and clearly.

UNCONSCIOUS PATIENT:

- Maintain open airway.
- Provide high concentration of oxygen.
- Monitor vital signs.
- Transport in lateral recumbent position. Keep paralyzed side down and well-protected with padding.

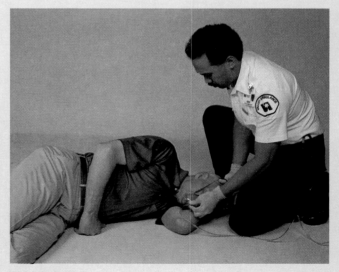

FIGURE 27-6

FIGURE 27-5

- Clear the airway of any foreign matter, food, or vomitus with a gauze-wrapped finger.
- Administer oxygen with a nasal cannula; if using a mask, watch carefully for aspiration.
- If the patient manifests breathing difficulty; use a soft nasopharyngeal airway to avoid respiratory obstruction (especially if the patient has lost consciousness); remember that a flaccid tongue can fall back and block the throat.
- Remove all dentures and dental bridges.
- Assist breathing if necessary.
- If you believe that the patient may choke on vomitus or mucus, turn his head to the side to facilitate drainage.

4. Take vital signs. Take both carotid and radial pulses; lack of regularity may signal heart disease. Note whether pulses are equal bilaterally. High blood pressure accompanied by a slow pulse is an indication of marked or ongoing swelling of brain tissue; immediate transport to a hospital is critical.

5. If the patient develops further difficulty in breathing or becomes unconscious, turn the patient on his or her side, preferably with the paralyzed side down and well cushioned. If the unconscious patient begins to vomit, turn the patient on his or her side, clear the airway by suctioning, and administer high-flow oxygen. Transport the patient on his or her side.

6. If the patient's eyelid is affected, gently close the lid and loosely tape it closed to prevent eye membranes from drying out.

7. Keep the patient warm, but do not overheat; excessive heat speeds brain damage.

8. Keep the patient absolutely quiet; shield him or her from curious onlookers.

9. Never give the patient anything to eat or drink; paralysis of the pharynx is common. Never use any kind of stimulant, such as smelling salts.

10. Transport the patient as gently and quickly as possible, avoiding unnecessary movement (it can aggravate the stroke). As you prepare for transport, carefully support the paralyzed limbs as you lift and move the patient. If paralysis is present, transport with the paralyzed side down, with limbs well protected with ample padding (such as rolled or folded towels).

Remember — even though patients may be unresponsive, they may be able to hear and understand what you are saying and what goes on around them. It is critical that you avoid saying anything that will increase a patient's anxiety, because anxiety can aggravate and worsen a stroke considerably. Remain hopeful and optimistic, and provide moral support to the patient, even if he or she seems unresponsive.

chapter 28

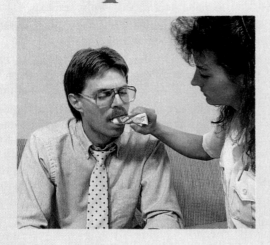

Diabetic Emergencies

✳ OBJECTIVES

- Describe the types of diabetes.
- Explain the causes of diabetes, including the role of blood sugar (glucose) and insulin.
- Distinguish between diabetic coma and insulin shock.
- Identify the signs and symptoms of diabetic coma.
- Identify the signs and symptoms of insulin shock.
- Describe how to assess and give emergency care for diabetic emergencies.

It is recommended that EMTs wear ptotective gloves whenever there is a possibility of coming in contact with a patient's blood, body fluids, mucous membranes, traumatic wounds, or sores. See Chapter 31.

Conservatively estimated, there are more than six million diabetics in the United States. Probably another five million have diabetes but without obvious signs and symptoms; therefore, these victims are completely unaware of their disease. Unfortunately, the first indication of the disease may be a life-threatening medical emergency (such as diabetic coma), and you may not know from any previous diagnosis that diabetes is the cause.

There are two basic types of diabetes: Type I (insulin-dependent, but historically called juvenile diabetes) tends to begin in childhood when a patient has little or no ability to produce insulin. Such an individual requires regular insulin injections to maintain body function. Type II (noninsulin-dependent but historically referred to as maturity-onset diabetes) tends to develop in adulthood when a patient may produce enough insulin but may not be able to utilize it. This type of diabetes is usually controlled by diet and/or oral medication.

Diabetes has long been recognized as a serious metabolic disorder, but in recent years it has come to be understood as a far more complex disease than originally conceived. Not only does diabetes impair the ability of the body to utilize carbohydrates — once thought to be its only mode of attack, and still its most immediate and apparent one — but it also involves fat and protein metabolism and causes varied manifestations in all bodily systems.

Diabetes seems to be transmitted genetically and, until a few years ago, was presumed to be inherited as a recessive characteristic. Now most specialists regard the exact mode of transmission as unclear; many believe that other complex causes may be involved.

□ CAUSES OF DIABETES

Diabetes seems to be caused by a problem (resulting from injury, infection, or genetic defects) in the tiny islets of Langerhans, the area of the pancreas where insulin is formed. Insulin is a hormone needed by the body to facilitate the movement of glucose (sugar) out of the bloodstream, across the cell membrane, and into the cell. Without glucose, the cells are not able to meet their energy needs. Therefore, when insulin is insufficient or absent, as in the case of the diabetic, the blood glucose level increases because it accumulates in the bloodstream (insulin does not move it into the body cells). This causes a paradoxical situation: the diabetic has an extremely elevated blood glucose level but a severely depleted supply of glucose in the cells due to the absence of insulin. All organ systems are affected.

Insulin also prevents amino acids from being used as fuel. Therefore, when insulin levels are too low, proteins are used as fuel, eventually robbing the muscles and vital organs of their mass.

When glucose cannot be used, it builds up in the blood, causing **hyperglycemia,** a significant sign of diabetes. The kidneys, whose function is to filter out excesses from the bloodstream and discard them, start spilling sugar into the urine. A large amount of sugar in the urine causes the kidneys to eliminate considerable water simply to wash the sugar away — a condition that leads to **polyuria** (frequent passing of large amounts of urine). This combination leads both to the tremendous thirst that affects hyperglycemic diabetics and to the danger of dehydration (Figure 28-1).

Diabetics may lose from 500 to 2,000 calories a day through glucose eliminated in the urine, which is why the advanced diabetic is extremely hungry, tends to eat all the time to satisfy his hunger, and still loses weight. The caloric loss also contributes to serious fatigue.

Diabetics face a grave physical situation when their blood glucose level is too high or too low: either condition (hyperglycemia or hypoglycemia) can cause coma, and both can be life-threatening if not treated promptly.

If you encounter a person who is unconscious, look for signs of diabetes: a medical alert tag, bracelet, or card; signs of insulin injection (needle marks in the thigh or abdomen); signs of oral diabetic medication (bottles in the house); signs of poor circulation or amputation of the toes, feet, or lower leg; or other telltale signs of diabetes.

□ DIABETIC COMA (KETOACIDOSIS AND HYPERGLYCEMIA)

Diabetics who go untreated, who fail to take their prescribed insulin, or who undergo some kind of stress (such as infection) may become comatose with a condition referred to as diabetic coma (**ketoacidosis or diabetic acidosis**). Diabetic coma, the most frequent cause of hospitalization in diabetics under the age of thirty, is basically a condition of too little insulin and too much blood sugar — in other words, there is not enough insulin to cover the food intake.

Direct causes of imbalance that result in diabetic coma include:

- Infection — the most common cause of diabetic coma is several days of infection, such as viral respiratory infection.
- Failure of the patient to take prescribed insulin, or taking an insufficient amount of insulin.
- Eating too much food that contains or produces sugar.
- Stresses (such as heart attack).

It is critical that you search for and determine any

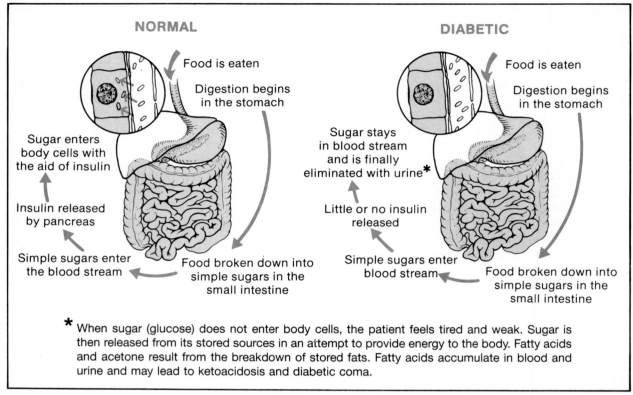

* When sugar (glucose) does not enter body cells, the patient feels tired and weak. Sugar is then released from its stored sources in an attempt to provide energy to the body. Fatty acids and acetone result from the breakdown of stored fats. Fatty acids accumulate in blood and urine and may lead to ketoacidosis and diabetic coma.

FIGURE 28-1 Normal versus diabetic use of sugars.

underlying causes for the diabetic coma. For example, it is possible to miss a heart attack if you are merely concerned with the coma itself. Similar coma can result from endocrine disorders not related to diabetes; treatment of the coma is the same.

Signs and Symptoms of Diabetic Coma

Many victims of diabetic coma appear intoxicated. *Never* automatically assume that someone is drunk until you have ruled out diabetic coma. Signs and symptoms of diabetic coma include the following (Figure 28-2):

- Acidosis:
  — Labored respirations and exaggerated air hunger (**Kussmaul's respirations,** the body's attempt to compensate for the acidosis).
  — Sweet or fruity (acetonic) odor on the breath caused by excess ketones as they are eliminated through the lungs.
  — Frequent severe and intense abdominal pain.
  — Varying degrees of responsiveness, from restlessness to complete coma; decreasing levels of consciousness correspond to the degree of dehydration; confusion and disorientation are common.

- Dehydration:
  — Flushed, dry, warm skin.
  — Sunken eyes.
  — Rapid, weak pulse.
  — Intense thirst.
  — Lack of normal skin tone (pinched skin does not return to normal).
  — Anorexia.
  — Frequent urination at first; scanty or no urine as dehydration progresses.
  — Dizziness.
  — Irritability.

- Hyperglycemia:
  — Weakness.
  — Weight loss.
  — Fatigue.

- Other symptoms:
  — Abdominal pain, loss of appetite, nausea, and vomiting (common).
  — Fever (may occur simultaneously with coma).

In the early stages, diabetic coma is characterized by excessive hunger, thirst, and urination. The onset of

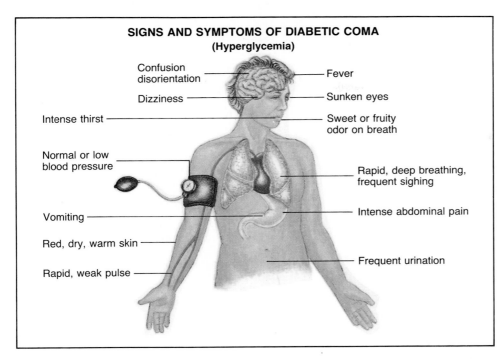

SIGNS AND SYMPTOMS OF DIABETIC COMA
(Hyperglycemia)

Confusion disorientation

Dizziness

Intense thirst

Normal or low blood pressure

Vomiting

Red, dry, warm skin

Rapid, weak pulse

Fever

Sunken eyes

Sweet or fruity odor on breath

Rapid, deep breathing, frequent sighing

Intense abdominal pain

Frequent urination

FIGURE 28-2

diabetic coma is gradual, developing in most cases over a period of twelve to forty-eight hours. The patient appears extremely ill and becomes sicker and weaker as the condition progresses. If untreated, the patient dies; with treatment, improvement is gradual, occurring six to twelve hours after insulin is administered and metabolic acidosis is treated.

Emergency Care

To treat diabetic coma, do the following (Figure 28-3):

1. Monitor vital signs carefully every few minutes; rule out heart attack, stroke, or other cardiac emergencies as the cause of the coma.

2. Check for signs of head or neck injury. If they are present, treat as indicated.

3. Follow the procedure for any comatose patient with regard to airway maintenance and oxygen. Hyperventilate the patient; it helps combat acidosis. Insert an airway if needed. Give CPR support if needed. Be alert for vomiting, and have suction ready at all times during treatment and transport.

4. Treat the patient for shock. Keep the patient lying down flat or with his or her head and shoulders elevated slightly unless he or she is in shock. Make sure that the patient stays warm.

5. Continue careful monitoring of vital signs.

6. If you can find them quickly, take any pre-measured insulin vials or bottles with the patient to the hospital; they will help the emergency room per-

sonnel determine what kind of treatment is needed.

7. Transport the patient as soon as possible.

□ INSULIN SHOCK (HYPOGLYCEMIA)

Insulin shock occurs when a diabetic has had too much insulin or too little sugar. Insulin shock results from treatment for diabetes, not from the diabetes itself. The glucose moves out of the bloodstream and into the cells more rapidly than it is produced, resulting in an insufficient blood sugar level to maintain normal brain function. Nerve cells are deprived of glucose, and they die. Because the brain is as dependent on glucose as it is on oxygen, and because the brain is the first organ to react to low blood sugar, permanent brain damage or death can result from insulin shock if emergency care is not given immediately (see Figure 28-3).

Insulin shock has a rapid onset, and it happens more often in children because of their broadly varied activity and diet levels. Insulin shock can be caused by several different factors:

• The diabetic skips a meal but takes the usual amount of insulin.

• The diabetic vomits a meal after taking insulin.

• The patient takes more than the prescribed dosage of insulin, or the normal dosage is accidentally administered in a vein.

Diabetes is a condition in which the body is unable to use sugar
  normally.
Body cells need sugar to survive.
Insulin in the body permits sugar to pass from the blood stream to
  body cells.
If there is not enough insulin, sugar will be unable to get to body cells
  and they will starve.
If there is too much insulin, there will be insufficient sugar in the blood
  stream and brain cells will be damaged since they need a constant
  supply of sugar.

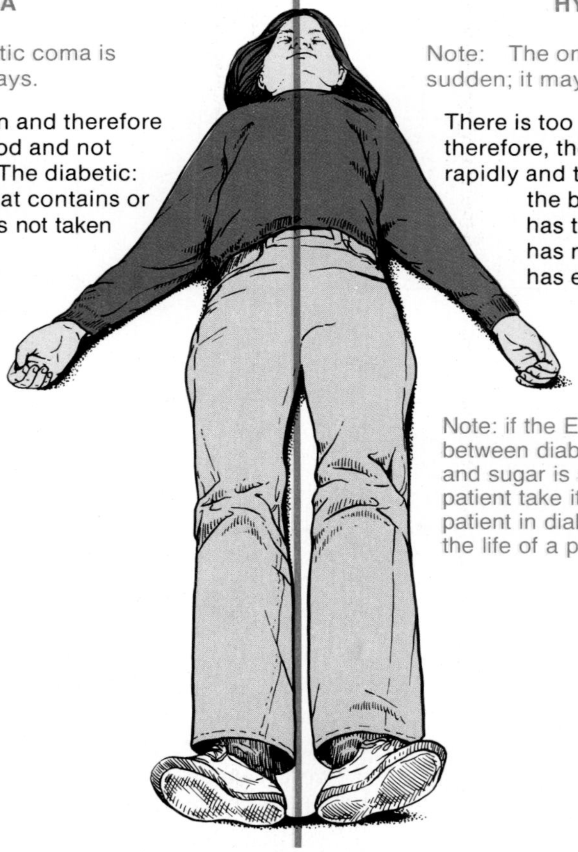

DIABETIC COMA
HYPERGLYCEMIA

Note: The onset of diabetic coma is
gradual over a period of days.

There is insufficient insulin and therefore
too much sugar in the blood and not
enough in the body cells. The diabetic:
  has eaten too much that contains or
  produces sugar, or has not taken
  his or her insulin.

INSULIN SHOCK
HYPOGLYCEMIA

Note: The onset of insulin shock is
sudden; it may occur within minutes.

There is too much insulin in the body;
therefore, the sugar leaves the blood
rapidly and there is insufficient sugar for
the brain cells. The diabetic:
  has taken too much insulin, or
  has not eaten enough food, or
  has exercised excessively.

Note: if the EMT cannot distinguish
between diabetic coma and insulin shock
and sugar is available, have the conscious
patient take it. It can't appreciably hurt the
patient in diabetic coma and may save
the life of a patient in insulin shock.

© 1983 S. Strawn

EMERGENCY CARE

This patient needs immediate
  transportation to a medical facility.
Monitor vital signs.
Follow procedures for any comatose
  patient regarding airway
  maintenance and oxygen.
Keep patient lying flat with head and
  shoulders slightly elevated.
If vomiting occurs put in coma position
  with head turned to aid draining and
  prevent aspiration.

This patient desperately needs sugar
before brain damage and death occur.
Sugar in any form can be given
to a conscious patient. He or she
needs immediate transportation to a
medical facility.

FIGURE 28-3

- The patient exercises strenuously or excessively.
- The patient is subject to severe emotional excitement or exertion.
- The patient is exposed to severe cold.
- The patient's insulin dosage or diet has been changed, and the patient does not adapt well to the changes.

Reactions begin five to twenty minutes after the injection of too much insulin, or several hours after other forms of oral medication are taken. The patient appears extremely weak. Insulin shock develops suddenly and progresses rapidly, usually over a period of just a few minutes. *It is a dire medical emergency* that can cause death within a few minutes.

Signs and Symptoms of Insulin Shock

The signs and symptoms of insulin shock often mimic those of cerebrovascular accident (stroke) or alcohol or drug intoxication. The most common include (Figure 28-4):

- Headache.
- Extreme muscle weakness and incoordination.
- Dilated pupils.
- No unusual odor on the breath.
- Nausea and/or vomiting.

- Pale, moist skin.
- Hunger.
- Normal or shallow breathing.
- Weakness or paralysis of one side of the body.
- Shakiness (sometimes involving the entire body).
- Normal blood pressure or low blood pressure.
- Normal or rapid pulse; may be full and bounding.
- Double vision and other visual disturbances.
- Apathy, anxiety, combativeness, or irritability.
- Confusion leading to disorientation, eventual unconsciousness, and coma.
- Absence of thirst.
- Profuse drooling from the mouth.
- Tremors.
- Convulsions in late stages.
- Tingling and numbness in the extremities, mostly the fingers and feet.
- Dizziness or lightheadedness.
- Diminished levels of consciousness, including syncope (fainting).
- Profuse sweating (diaphoresis).
- Speech difficulties.
- Disturbances in behavior (the patient may appear to be drunk, hostile, or belligerent).

FIGURE 28-4

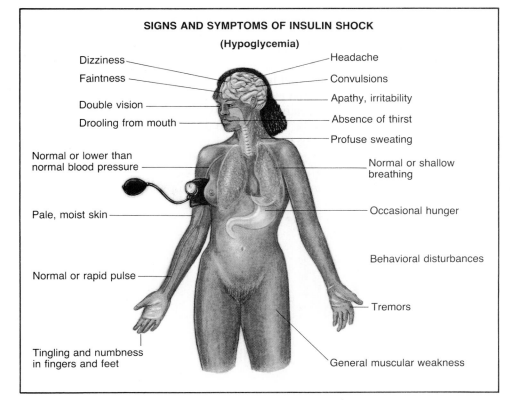

SIGNS AND SYMPTOMS OF INSULIN SHOCK
(Hypoglycemia)

Dizziness
Faintness
Double vision
Drooling from mouth
Normal or lower than normal blood pressure
Pale, moist skin
Normal or rapid pulse
Tingling and numbness in fingers and feet

Headache
Convulsions
Apathy, irritability
Absence of thirst
Profuse sweating
Normal or shallow breathing
Occasional hunger
Behavioral disturbances
Tremors
General muscular weakness

If you suspect that the patient might be entering a state of insulin shock, ask him two critical questions:

1. Have you eaten today?
2. Have you taken your insulin today?

If the person has taken insulin but has not eaten, he or she may be going into insulin shock. If he or she has eaten but has not taken insulin, he or she may be going into diabetic coma. Beware, however, that these guidelines do not always apply.

Emergency Care

Emergency care for a patient in suspected insulin shock should be as follows (see Figure 28-3 and 28-6):

1. If the patient is conscious, give a commercially available glucose paste or orange juice with one to two teaspoons of sugar, soft drinks that contain sugar, corn syrup, honey, jelly, life-savers, gumdrops, sugar cubes, or candy to help increase the carbohydrate level (Figure 28-5). If nothing else is available, give simple table sugar.
2. If the patient is unconscious, establish an airway and administer oxygen.
3. Never give an unconscious person anything to eat or drink.
4. Watch for complications, such as shock or convulsions, and treat appropriately.
5. Transport immediately, even if the patient seems to be completely recovered.

Improvement is usually fairly rapid following the administration of sugar, but it is still important to transport. Do not worry about the amount of sugar given to the patient, as the doctor will balance the need for sugar against insulin production when the patient arrives at the hospital.

It is important to note that diabetics are not the only patients who are prone to hypoglycemia. Alcoholics, patients who have ingested certain poisons, and others may develop the same syndrome. Therefore, do

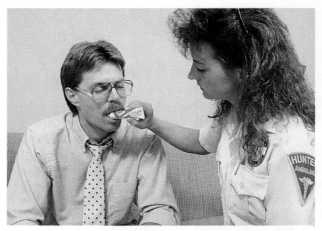

FIGURE 28-5 Administering a concentrated sugar source to a conscious insulin shock (hypoglycemic) patient.

not discount the possibility of hypoglycemia in a comatose patient, just because he is not known to be a diabetic.

The general rule to remember about emergency care for a conscious diabetic patient is: *When in doubt, give sugar.* You will not harm a hyperglycemic patient by giving sugar (the amount administered is trivial compared to what he already has in his blood), but you may save the life of a hypoglycemic patient by this emergency care.

Most diabetics are counseled to carry cards in their wallets describing their condition and listing the name and telephone number of a doctor who is familiar with the patient's medical history. One card in common use reads: "If unconscious or behaving abnormally, I may be having an insulin reaction or my blood sugar may be too low. If I can swallow, give me sugar, candy, fruit juice, or a sweetened drink. If I am unable to swallow or if recovery does not take place quickly, call a physician or send me to a hospital at once."

DIABETIC COMA (Hyperglycemia)

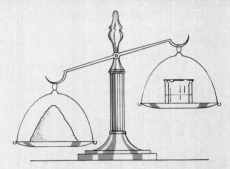

CAUSES:

- The diabetic's condition has not been diagnosed and/or treated.
- The diabetic has not taken his insulin.
- The diabetic has overeaten, flooding the body with a sudden excess of carbohydrates.
- The diabetic suffers an infection that disrupts his glucose/insulin balance.

EMERGENCY CARE:

- Administer a high concentration of oxygen.
- Immediately transport to a medical facility.

SYMPTOMS AND SIGNS:

- Gradual onset of symptoms and signs, over a period of days.
- Patient complains of dry mouth and intense thirst.
- Abdominal pain and vomiting common.
- Gradually increasing restlessness, confusion, followed by stupor.
- Coma, with these signs:
  - Signs of air hunger—deep, sighing respirations
  - Weak, rapid pulse.
  - Dry, red, warm skin.
  - Eyes that appear sunken.
  - Normal or slightly low blood pressure.
  - Breath smells of acetone—sickly sweet, like nail polish remover.

INSULIN SHOCK (Hypoglycemia)

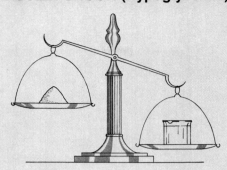

CAUSES:

- The diabetic has taken too much insulin.
- The diabetic has not eaten enough to provide his normal sugar intake.
- The diabetic has overexercised or overexerted himself, thus reducing his blood glucose level.
- The diabetic has vomited a meal.

EMERGENCY CARE:

- Conscious patient—Administer sugar. Granular sugar, honey, lifesaver or other candy placed under the tongue, orange juice, or glu-tose.
- Avoid giving liquids to the unconscious patient; provide "sprinkle" of granulated sugar under tongue.
- Turn head to side or place in lateral recumbent position.
- Provide oxygen.
- Transport to the medical facility

SYMPTOMS AND SIGNS:

- Rapid onset or symptoms and signs, over a period of minutes.
- Dizziness and headache.
- Abnormal hostile or aggressive behavior, which may be diagnosed as acute alcoholic intoxication.
- Fainting, convulsions, and occasionally coma.
- Normal blood pressure.
- Full rapid pulse.
- Patient intensely hungry.
- Skin pale, cold, and clammy; perspiration may be profuse.
- Copious saliva, drooling.

SPECIAL NOTES: DIABETIC COMA AND INSULIN SHOCK

When faced with a patient who may be suffering from one of these conditions:

- Determine if the patient is diabetic. Look for medical alert medallions or information cards; interview patient and family members.
- If the patient is a known or suspected diabetic, and insulin shock cannot be ruled out, assume that it is insulin shock and administer sugar.

Often a patient suffering from either of these conditions may simply appear drunk. Always check for other underlying conditions—such as diabetic complications—when treating someone who appears intoxicated.

FIGURE 28-6

chapter 29

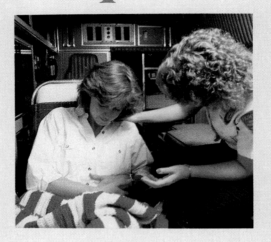

Acute Abdominal Distress and Related Emergencies

✳ OBJECTIVES

■ Describe the common causes of acute abdominal distress and other related gastrointestinal emergencies.

■ Identify the signs and symptoms of acute abdominal distress and ruptured esophageal varices.

■ Explain special examination procedures necessary when assessing a patient with acute abdominal distress.

■ Describe and demonstrate appropriate emergency care for:

— acute abdominal distress

— ruptured esophageal varices

— prolonged vomiting.

It is recommended that EMTs wear protective gloves whenever there is a possibility of coming in contact with a patient's blood, body fluids, mucous membranes, traumatic wounds, or sores. See Chapter 31

422

Acute abdominal distress features pain that may stem from the cardiac, gastrointestinal, genitourinary, reproductive, or other systems — or pain that may be referred from elsewhere. The pain due to trauma is usually very localized, and the patient should be able to point to it accurately with one or two fingers unless bleeding is heavy, which usually causes diffuse pain. Pain in the abdomen that is due to organ dysfunction, however, is often vague and may be referred; the patient may point to it with an entire fist or even an open hand, vaguely indicating a larger area of the body.

□ CAUSES OF ABDOMINAL PAIN

According to medical reference guides, there are approximately one hundred different causes of abdominal pain. Pain localized to the abdomen usually means an abdominal problem. Sudden onset of acute pain in a previously healthy person that lasts more than six hours usually indicates a condition that requires surgery.

For ease in assessment, the abdomen is divided into four "quadrants," or sections (see Chapter 2). Pain above the umbilicus is considered in the upper right or left quadrant; pain below the umbilicus is considered in the lower right or left quadrant. The location, direction, and characteristics of abdominal pain are important indicators.

Upper abdominal pain usually is due to conditions of the stomach, upper small intestine (duodenum), pancreas, or **bile ducts.** Specific causes include food poisoning, gastritis, **gastroenteritis,** gastric and duodenal ulcer, stone in the bile duct, and inflammation of the pancreas. The upper right quadrant contains most of the liver, the gall bladder, half of the pancreas, the right kidney, the duodenal section of the small intestines, the upper ascending colon, and half of the transverse colon. Upper abdominal pain in the right quadrant usually signifies a spasm in the colon, duodenal ulcer, a gall bladder attack, or a problem of the muscular wall of the abdomen. Other causes would include hepatitis and pneumonia.

The upper left quadrant contains the stomach, spleen, most of the pancreas, a small section of the liver, the left kidney, the small intestine, half of the transverse colon, and the upper descending colon. Upper abdominal pain in the left quadrant is usually due to pneumonia, gastritis, ruptured spleen, perforated colon, aortic aneurysm, or pancreatitis.

The lower right quadrant contains the small intestine, half of the bladder, the appendix, large intestine, part of the ascending colon, right ovary and fallopian tube, half of the uterus, and the cecum. A common cause of lower abdominal pain on the right side is appendicitis, which often begins as a vague pain across the abdomen and gradually shifts to the right side. Other causes would include muscular strain, kidney stone, **diverticulitis,** perforated bowel, intestinal obstruction, or hernia (including a strangulated hernia). Such pain in women may be caused by a twisted ovary, inflamed fallopian tubes, ovarian **cyst,** or an **ectopic pregnancy.**

The lower left quadrant contains the small intestine, half of the bladder, part of the descending colon, the cecum, the sigmoid colon, the rectum, the left ovary and fallopian tube, and half of the uterus. Pain in the left lower abdomen can occur from the causes stated in the previous paragraph, as well as acute diverticulitis (a type of colitis). Although appendicitis rarely causes pain on the left side, it cannot be ruled out.

Pain across the entire lower abdomen or especially at the midline may be caused by colitis or bowel obstruction. When the pain is mild and not associated with diarrhea, it usually is due to intestinal spasms or excessive intestinal gas. Other causes would include a urinary bladder inflammation **(cystitis),** pelvic inflammatory disease, ectopic pregnancy, and menstrual cramps in women.

Causes of abdominal pain with no specific localization can include diabetic coma, intoxication, food poisoning, uremia, mononucleosis, sickle cell anemia, and influenza.

When the peritoneum becomes inflamed (a condition called peritonitis), excruciating pain results. In most cases, peritonitis is due to pus, urine, blood, gastric contents, **stool,** or dead tissue coming into contact with the peritoneum. A steady, severe pain that is aggravated by even slight movement accompanies peritonitis, which is also characterized by fever. Possible causes of peritonitis include an ulcer that erodes through the stomach or duodenum, spilling digestive juices into the peritoneum; pancreatitis, which causes enzymes to leak; rupture of an organ (such as the spleen or the bladder); and infection.

Every patient with abdominal distress should be considered life-threatening until proven otherwise. *Abdominal pain should be considered very serious if the pain is associated with lowered blood pressure, syncope, or toxic appearance.*

□ SIGNS AND SYMPTOMS OF ABDOMINAL DISTRESS

Any severe abdominal pain should be considered an emergency; any abdominal pain that lasts longer than six hours, regardless of its intensity, should be considered an emergency. A patient with an **acute abdomen** appears very ill; general signs and symptoms of acute abdominal distress include:

- Abdominal pain (local or diffuse).
- Colicky pain (cramplike pain that occurs in waves).
- Local or diffuse abdominal tenderness.
- Anxiety and reluctance to move.
- Rapid, shallow breathing.
- Rapid pulse.
- Nausea and/or vomiting.
- Low blood pressure.
- Tense, often distended abdomen.
- Signs of shock, especially if peritonitis is present.
- Signs of internal bleeding: vomiting blood (bright red or coffee-grounds) or blood in the stool (bright red or tarry black).

A patient with acute abdominal distress often adopts a position on his or her side with knees drawn up toward the abdomen (Figure 29-1).

□ SPECIAL EXAMINATION PROCEDURES

In assessing a patient with acute abdominal distress, your number-one priority should be to look for signs of shock — rapid, thready pulse; restlessness; cold, clammy skin, and falling blood pressure. Shock is common with internal bleeding, peritonitis, or diarrhea, all of which cause substantial fluid loss. Because the abdomen may be very tender and the patient will be guarded — and because even slight palpation can aggravate existing pain — follow these general guidelines when examining the acute abdomen:

1. Determine whether the patient is restless or quiet, and whether movement causes pain.
2. Look to see whether the abdomen is distended. Confirm the abnormal contour with the patient (Figure 29-2).
3. Feel the abdomen *very* gently to determine whether it is tense or soft and whether any masses are present. If you know that a specific quadrant is causing the pain or the majority of the pain, examine that quadrant last (Figures 29-3 and 29-4).
4. Determine whether the abdomen is tender when touched and whether the patient can relax his or her abdominal wall upon request. Note any abdominal guarding.
5. Determine the location and quadrant of the pain.

Note: If the patient is a child, suspect the need for surgery if there is tenderness or guarding on palpation.

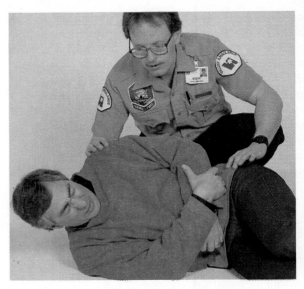

FIGURE 29-1 Typical "guarded" position for patient with acute abdominal distress.

In a patient with abdominal pain, do not waste time with extensive palpation of the abdomen prior to transport. Extensive palpation can worsen the pain and aggravate the medical condition that causes it.

□ EMERGENCY CARE FOR ACUTE ABDOMINAL DISTRESS

The goals of field management for acute abdominal distress are to prevent any possible life-threatening complications (such as hemorrhage or shock), to make the patient comfortable, and to transport as quickly as possible for diagnostic care by a physician. A patient with acute abdominal distress must *always* be transported, because many need surgery; the sooner the patient is transported and evaluated by a physician, the better the outcome. Follow these treatment guidelines:

1. Keep the airway clear; be alert for vomiting and possible aspiration. If the patient is nauseated, position him or her on the left side if it does not cause too much pain; keep a suction and an emesis basin ready. If the patient vomits, save and transport some of the vomitus for testing at the hospital.
2. Position the patient as comfortably as possible. If there are signs of volume depletion (lowered blood pressure, increased pulse) place the patient supine with the lower extremities elevated. If there are no signs of volume depletion, allow the patient to determine the most comfortable position unless it interferes with emergency care. Most patients prefer

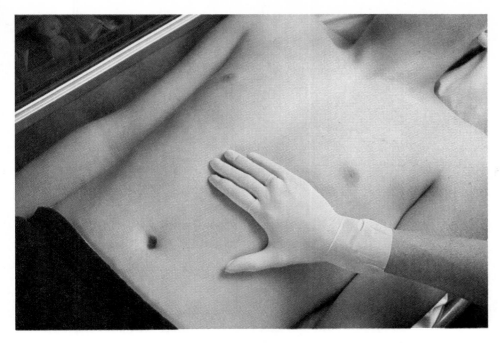

FIGURE 29-2 Inspection of the abdomen.

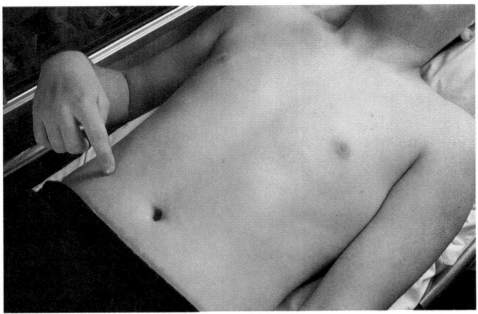

FIGURE 29-3 Have the patient point to the site of pain. Leave examination of this quadrant until last.

FIGURE 29-4 In the abdominal distress patient, gently determine if the abdomen is tense or soft and whether any masses are present.

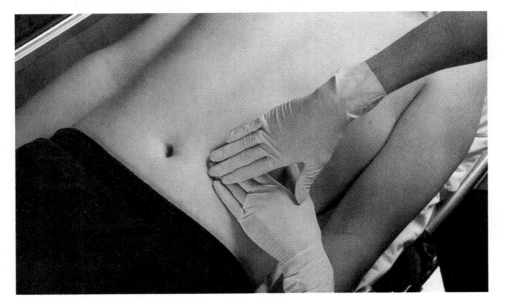

to lie on their sides or backs with their knees drawn up toward the abdomen.

3. Administer high flow oxygen through a nasal cannula at four to six liters per minute.

4. Comfort and reassure the patient (Figure 29-5).

5. *Never give anything by mouth.*

6. Do not give the patient any medications by any route or allow him or her to take medications; medications may mask symptoms and complicate the physician's diagnosis and treatment.

7. Prevent shock; if shock already exists, treat it.

8. Record the signs and symptoms and the patient's description of his condition — time of onset, direction, characteristics of the pain (steady, dull, sharp, stabbing), body temperature, and any unusual body changes. Make your record brief, and do not delay transport to make it.

9. Transport as efficiently as possible. Protect the patient from any rough handling, and try to make the ride as smooth as possible.

□ RUPTURED ESOPHAGEAL VARICES

Esophageal varices — bulging, engorged, and weakened blood vessels lining the wall of the lower one-third of the esophagus — can potentially develop in any patient due to increased pressure in portal circulation (the circulation that drains from the intestine to the liver), but are most common among heavy alcohol drinkers, patients with liver disease (such as cirrhosis or hepatitis), patients with chronic liver dysfunction, patients with an enlarged liver, or victims of jaundice. They are usually characterized by painless gastrointestinal bleed-

FIGURE 29-5 Reassure and monitor the abdominal distress patient while in transport.

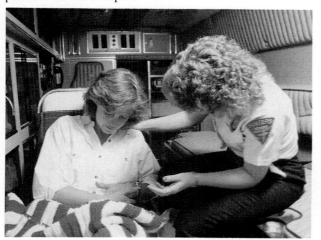

ing. When one or more of these varices rupture, bleeding is profuse and severe and can be fatal within minutes unless the patient has prompt treatment.

Look for the following signs and symptoms of esophageal varices:

- Vomiting of profuse amounts of bright red blood.
- Blood welling up in the back of the throat, with or without vomiting.
- Absence of pain or tenderness in the stomach.
- Rapid pulse (usually exceeding 120 beats per minute).
- Respiratory distress.
- Pallor.

Since esophageal varices are most common among patients with liver disease, additional signs and symptoms may include jaundice, an enlarged liver, or dilated veins just below the skin's surface.

Emergency Care

The victim of ruptured esophageal varices needs rapid blood replacement and surgical procedures aimed at stopping the bleeding. Your priorities in the field are to secure and maintain the airway, prevent aspiration, treat or prevent shock, and transport without delay. Follow these guidelines:

1. Immediately secure an open airway; use a mechanical airway if needed. Give oxygen.

2. Suction the patient's mouth, throat, and nose frequently to remove blood and excess saliva. Maintaining a clear airway is critical to the patient's survival.

3. Treat the patient for shock. Position him or her on the left side, face pointed downward to facilitate drainage and help prevent aspiration.

4. Transport without delay to the nearest facility, continuing suction and monitoring vital signs throughout transport. Radio the receiving facility to prepare personnel for the arrival of a critical patient.

□ ABDOMINAL AORTIC ANEURYSM

An **abdominal aortic aneurysm** occurs when the wall of the aorta in the abdomen weakens, dilates, and eventually ruptures. One of the most lethal conditions that causes abdominal pain, it is most common in those with atherosclerosis. It is estimated that approximately 20 percent of all men over the age of fifty have abdominal aortic aneurysms.

The pain from abdominal aortic aneurysm is very sudden in onset. Signs and symptoms include sudden, severe, constant pain in the abdomen or back; the pain tends to radiate to the lower back, flank, or pelvis. There may be nausea and vomiting. Characteristic signs include mottled abdominal skin, pale legs, and decreased or absent femoral and pedal pulses. If the abdomen is soft, you will be able to detect a pulsating abdominal mass that is palpable; if the aneurysm has burst, the abdomen will likely be hard and rigid.

Emergency Care

If you suspect abdominal aortic aneurysm, do the following:

1. Palpate the abdomen *very* gently; pressure or firm palpation can aggravate the emergency and cause further dissection of the artery.
2. Treat the patient for shock.
3. *Transport the patient without delay;* radio ahead to the receiving facility so that a surgical team can be prepared.

☐ VOMITING

Vomiting — the stomach's response to an infection, irritation, obstruction, or other disease process — is one of the most common gastrointestinal complaints or emergencies. Most vomiting is caused by self-limiting infection and clears up within a day or two. Vomiting becomes a medical emergency when it is prolonged enough to cause dehydration, when it is aspirated, or when it signals serious medical conditions.

Medical emergencies can result, however, when vomiting is prolonged enough to cause substantial fluid loss and **electrolyte** imbalance (a condition that can develop as rapidly as within twenty-four hours in infants and young children or the elderly). Infants or children who continue to vomit over a period of one day and adults who continue to vomit for several days may lose significant fluid volume and develop electrolyte imbalances serious enough to cause shock.

Another problem occurs when a sleepy, stuporous, semiconscious, unconscious, or comatose patient vomits: the normal gag reflex protection is depressed or absent, and the patient may aspirate vomitus into the lungs. Because the cough reflex is usually also absent or depressed, the patient does not cough to clear the lungs of the aspirated material. The gastric juices contained in vomitus literally eat away the delicate lung tissue, resulting in rapid tissue destruction, massive infection, and life-threatening pulmonary abscesses.

Emergency Care

If a patient has vomited enough to cause shock or is in such a condition as to be at high risk of aspiration, follow these guidelines:

1. Take immediate measures to secure a patent airway and to maintain it. Place the patient on the left side, head lower than the feet, and point the head downward to facilitate drainage should vomiting occur.
2. Use large-bore suction catheters to rapidly clear the pharynx, nose, and mouth of any vomitus or saliva that accumulates.
3. Use the manual jaw thrust technique to help keep the airway clear.
4. If the patient has aspirated vomitus, he or she will probably be breathing rapidly, secreting excessive saliva, and be cyanotic. Assist breathing if necessary, and administer 100 percent, positive-pressure oxygen. Transport the patient without delay, administering oxygen and monitoring vital signs during transport. Surgical removal of the aspirated material within thirty to sixty minutes can usually save the patient's life.
5. If the patient has vomited enough to cause shock (signalled by low blood pressure, dehydration, and a rapid, thready pulse), administer oxygen, treat for shock, and transport immediately.
6. If possible, determine how much has been vomited, how often the patient has vomited, what the vomited material contains, and whether the vomiting was forceful or projectile. If you can, collect some of the vomitus to transport with the patient for diagnosis at the receiving facility.

☐ ESOPHAGEAL REFLUX (HEARTBURN)

Esophageal reflux — commonly referred to as heartburn — can be frightening and excruciating for the patient but does not constitute a medical emergency unless it is symptomatic of a serious medical problem, such as myocardial infarction.

Esophageal reflux results when gastric juices spill from the stomach into the esophagus, irritating the esophageal lining. Because the lining does not produce mucus, it cannot protect itself against the corrosive effects of the gastric juices. In most cases, esophageal reflux results in only mild irritation; in extreme cases, deep ulcers or perforations can occur. The resulting pain is called heartburn because of the burning sensation it causes.

While heartburn may cause problems if perforation results or if it signals other, more serious, medical problems, most cases can be controlled by antacids and changes in the diet. Unless the patient is in danger of developing shock, appears to have a more serious medical problem, or begins to vomit blood, refer him to a physician and limit field management to reassuring the patient. Make sure that you do not confuse heartburn with cardiac pain; to be certain, assess for cardiac problems.

☐ DIARRHEA AND CONSTIPATION

Diarrhea is defined as an abnormally large number of loose, watery stools; **constipation** is defined as stools that are dried, hardened, or extremely difficult to pass. Not medical problems in themselves, diarrhea and constipation are symptomatic of other medical problems that range in seriousness from **influenza** to cancer.

Among the most common causes of diarrhea are the following:

- Bacterial or viral infections.
- Severe infections (such as dysentery).
- Gastroenteritis and other conditions that irritate the lining of the intestine.
- **Parasitic** infestations.
- **Fecal impaction** (obstruction of the intestines caused by dried, impacted stool matter that lodges in the intestinal tract, allowing only liquids to pass).
- Ulcerative colitis and other inflammatory bowel diseases.
- Severe anxiety or stress.
- Extreme emotional reactions.

In itself, diarrhea is rarely a medical emergency. The only cause for concern is when diarrhea has persisted for several days and the patient has become dehydrated or has lapsed into hypovolemic shock as a result of fluid, and electrolyte loss.

A patient who is weak, lethargic, dehydrated, and shocky should be treated for shock and transported to a hospital for further treatment.

Chronic constipation occurs most commonly in the elderly, usually as a result of changes in diet and activity level. Those who may have difficulty chewing and swallowing food often rely on a diet of bland, soft foods — which, in turn, tend to produce a small, hard stool that is difficult to pass. Those who are not in good health sometimes stop trying to pass difficult stools, and the fecal matter accumulates in the bowel, causing significant abdominal distention.

As with diarrhea, constipation itself rarely presents a medical emergency. But because chronic constipation can be a symptom of a serious medical disorder — such as cancer of the colon — those complaining of chronic constipation should be transported so that they can be evaluated by a physician.

chapter 30

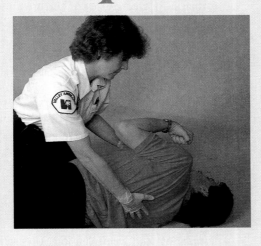

Epilepsy, Dizziness, and Fainting

✴ OBJECTIVES

- Explain the common causes of epilepsy-related seizures.
- Explain the common causes of dizziness.
- Explain the common causes of fainting.
- Identify the various types of epileptic seizures.
- Recognize the common signs and symptoms of a grand mal seizure.
- Describe and demonstrate how to assess and give appropriate emergency care for seizures and fainting.

It is recommended that EMTs wear protective gloves whenever there is a possibility of coming in contact with a patient's blood, body fluids, mucous membranes, traumatic wounds, or sores. See Chapter 31.

Neurological emergencies, basically involving a disturbance in the chemical or electrical activity of the brain, are generally more frightening than they are life-threatening. With quick recognition of the condition and vigorous airway management to prevent oxygen deprivation, you can generally prevent a major medical emergency. A patient who passes from one **seizure** to another without regaining consciousness first, however, *does* represent a life-threatening medical emergency.

□ SEIZURES AND EPILEPSY

A seizure is an involuntary, sudden change in sensation, behavior, muscle activity, or level of consciousness and results from irritated, overactive brain cells. In general, seizures are caused by an abnormal discharge of electrical energy in the brain; they are sudden in onset, usually occurring after only very brief, if any, warning. Any condition that affects the structural cells of the brain or alters its chemical metabolic balance may trigger seizures.

Evidence suggests that the tendency toward seizures runs in families. More than 12 million Americans suffer seizures each year — and they are one of the most common emergencies seen by EMTs.

Causes of Seizures

A significant cause of seizures is epilepsy, one of the most common and puzzling of central nervous system disorders (see Figure 30-1). Epilepsy is a chronic brain disorder characterized by recurrent seizures with or without a loss of consciousness. It includes approximately twenty different seizure disorders. More than 2 million Americans suffer from epilepsy.

Other suspected causes of seizures include the following:

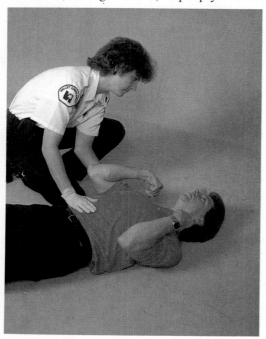

FIGURE 30-1 Epilepsy is one of the most common causes of seizures

- Spurts in growth.
- High fever (febrile seizures); the highest percentage of seizures due to high fever occur among children, and most children who seize in response to fever stop by the time they reach adolescence.
- Open or penetrating head injury, usually accompanied by unconsciousness, or head injury that causes deep tissue damage or concussion.
- Cerebrovascular accident (stroke).
- Childhood illnesses, including measles, mumps, and chicken pox.
- Pregnancy and complications of pregnancy, such as **eclampsia** and **toxemia.** Eclampsia begins with seizures; almost half of all women with epilepsy experience increased seizures during pregnancy.
- Illnesses such as constipation, diarrhea, diabetes, arrhythmias, minor urinary infections, upper respiratory infections, kidney failure, liver failure, brain tumor, **anemia,** fluid disturbances, and electrolyte imbalances.
- In general, infections of any kind can, under the right circumstances, cause seizures.
- Scar tissue, lesions, or tumors that take up space in the brain and/or exert pressure on brain tissue.
- Central nervous system infections, such as **meningitis** or **encephalitis.**
- Endocrine disturbances, such as **hypothyroidism, ovulation, menstruation,** or **menopause.**
- Genetic malformations of the brain.
- Alcohol or drug withdrawal.
- Extreme variations in sleep habits or patterns, including sleep deprivation.
- Birth injury.
- Apnea.
- Hypoglycemia.
- Swelling of the brain tissue, regardless of cause.
- Hyperventilation caused by athletic activity, sexual intercourse, or acute anxiety.
- Extreme emotional reactions.
- Ingestion of certain drugs or poisons, including heavy metals (such as lead).
- **Alzheimer's disease** and other degenerative diseases.

Types of Seizures

For a complete listing of seizures, see Table 30-1. The most common types of seizures encountered in the field include the following:

Grand Mal Seizures

Grand mal seizures (also known as major motor seizures), characterized by convulsions, always produce a loss of consciousness. Caused by uncontrolled electrical activity that spreads across the entire brain, they often precipitate a change in mood, confusion, blurred vision, or gastrointestinal distress just prior to the seizure.

The origin of the seizure is usually in the frontal or temporal lobes, but it spreads rapidly. Patients experiencing grand mal seizures manifest an arched back, alternating contraction and relaxation of the extremities, frothing of the mouth, and clenching of the jaws. Breathing stops because the diaphragm is seizing during the phase of prolonged muscle contraction, and cyanosis may result. The patient may become incontinent (lose bowel and bladder control).

Petit Mal Seizures

Often called **absence attacks, petit mal seizures** do not involve convulsions, may be inherited, and almost always occur among children (most often between the ages of four and eight and most often among girls, although they may occur as late as age twenty).

Petit mal seizures feature brief periods — usually only five to thirty seconds — during which the patient appears to be daydreaming or staring; the eyelids may flutter rapidly. The victim of a petit mal seizure does not lose consciousness, but he *does* lose contact with his environment, however briefly. The patient usually returns to normal quickly and is often not aware of the attack. Many patients experience more than one attack in a single day, some as many as one hundred in a single day.

Several other types of seizures common in children include atonic and infantile spasms (Table 30-1).

Psychomotor Seizures

Psychomotor seizures usually originate in the temporal lobe. They typically occur in adults and are characterized by the repetition of inappropriate acts (such as climbing up and down stairs or pulling off clothing) that may be mistaken as neurotic behavior.

Febrile Seizures

Caused by high fever (either by the high temperature itself or by the speed of its onset), **febrile seizures** are most common in infants and children from six months to four years of age. The average age for febrile seizures is twenty-three months, and they occur more frequently in boys than in girls. They tend to occur more often in a child whose family has a history of febrile seizures, and are commonly associated with otitis media, tonsillitis, pharyngitis, gastrointestinal infections, pneumonia, and recent immunizations. Approximately 3 to 5 percent of all children under the age of five suffer from febrile seizures. Febrile seizure is the most common neurological disorder of childhood.

Withdrawal Seizures

Withdrawal seizures occur when a patient who has been dependent on a drug for a long period suddenly quits using the drug, including alcohol. Prolonged seizures often occur in rapid succession.

Status Epilepticus

While most seizures stop within five minutes (even though the patient may remain unconscious for several minutes longer), **status epilepticus** is a series of seizures that occur in rapid succession and that do not allow for a period of lucidity between seizures. *Status epilepticus is a dire medical emergency;* approximately 1,500 Americans have status epilepticus seizures a year, and half of them die as a result.

Status epilepticus may result from any worsening of whatever caused the seizures in the first place, or it may occur as a result of a new condition in any patient. It is often the result of improper drug therapy for an epileptic patient. In approximately half of all cases of status epilepticus, the cause is unknown; in children, it may be the result of febrile seizures that develop into status epilepticus. Because of the length of the prolonged or recurrent seizures, the brain is deprived of oxygen; irreversible brain damage can result, as well as complications of the cardiac, respiratory, and renal systems. In prolonged status epilepticus, cells accumulate calcium and eventually die. Common complications of status epilepticus include cardiac arrhythmias, hypoxia, hyperthermia, compromised airway, and aspiration pneumonia.

Signs and Symptoms

Most seizures are self-limiting (except for status epilepticus), and most last only about five minutes — although the patient may experience residual drowsiness for several hours. The signs and symptoms of a grand mal seizure (including epileptic seizure) occur in stages, and include the following (Figure 30-2).

Progression of a Grand Mal Seizure

Grand mal seizures have a specific progression of events. It is descriptively convenient to refer to this

TABLE 30-1
Epilepsy: Recognition and Emergency Care

SEIZURE	WHAT IT LOOKS LIKE	OFTEN MISTAKEN FOR	WHAT TO DO	WHAT NOT DO DO
GRAND MAL (Convulsive) (Generalized tonic-clonic)	Sudden cry or moan, rigidity, followed by muscle jerks, frothy saliva on lips, shallow breathing or temporarily suspended breathing, bluish skin, possible loss of bladder or bowel control, usually lasts 2-5 minutes. Normal breathing then starts again. There may be some confusion and/or fatigue, followed by return to full consciousness.	Heart attack Stroke. Unknown but life-threatening emergency	Look for medical identification; protect from nearby hazards; loosen ties or shirt collars; place folded jacket under head. Turn on side to keep airway clear. Reassure when consciousness returns. If single seizure lasted less than 10 minutes, ask if hospital evaluation wanted. If multiple seizures, or if one seizure lasts longer than 10 minutes, take to emergency room.	Don't put any hard implement in the mouth. Don't try to hold tongue; it can't be swallowed. Don't try to give liquids during or just after seizure. Don't use artificial ventilation unless breathing is absent after muscle jerks subside or unless water has been inhaled. Don't restrain.
PETIT MAL (Non-convulsive)	A blank stare, lasting only a few seconds, most common in children. May be accompanied by rapid blinking, show chewing movements of the mouth. Child having the seizure is unaware of what's going on during the seizure, but quickly returns to full awareness once it has stopped. May result in learning difficulties if not recognized and treated.	Day dreaming. Lack of attention. Deliberate ignoring of adult instructions.	No emergency care necessary, but medical evaluation should be recommended.	
JACKSONIAN	Jerking begins in fingers or toes, can't be stopped by patient, but patient stays awake and aware. Jerking may proceed to involve hand, then arm, and sometimes spreads to whole body and becomes a convulsive seizure.	Acting out bizarre behavior.	No emergency care necessary unless seizure becomes conclusive, then first aid as above.	
SIMPLE PARTIAL (also called sensory)	May not be obvious to onlooker, other than patient's preoccupied or blank expression. Patient experiences a distorted environment. May see or hear things that aren't there, may feel unexplained fear, sadness, anger or joy. May have nausea, experience odd smells, and have a generally "funny" feeling in the stomach.	Hysteria. Mental illness. Psychosomatic illness. Parapsychological or mystical experience.	No action needed other than reassurance and emotional support.	

TABLE 30-1
Epilepsy: Recognition and Emergency Care

PSYCHOMOTOR (Complex Partial)	Usually starts with blank stare, followed by chewing, followed by random activity. Person appears unaware of surroundings, may seem dazed and mumble. Unresponsive. Actions clumsy, not directed. May pick at clothing, pick up objects, try to take clothes off. May run, appear afraid. May struggle or flail at restraint. Once pattern established, same set of actions usually occur with each seizure. Lasts a few minutes, but post-seizure confusion can last substantially longer. No memory of what happened during seizure period.	Drunkedness. Intoxication on drugs. Mental illness. Indecent exposure. Disorderly conduct. Shoplifting.	Speak calmly and reassuringly to patient and others. Guide gently away from obvious hazards. Stay with person until completely aware of environment. Offer help getting home. Don't grab hold unless sudden danger (such as a cliff edge or an approaching car) threatens. Don't try to sustain. Don't shout. Don't expect verbal instructions to be obeyed.
MYOCLONIC SEIZURES	Sudden, brief, massive muscle jerks that may involve the whole body or parts of the body. May cause person to spill what they were holding or fall off a chair.	Clumsiness. Poor coordination.	No emergency care needed, but should be given a thorough medical evaluation.
ATONIC SEIZURES (also called drop attacks)	The legs of a child between 2-5 years of age suddenly collapse under him and he falls. After 10 seconds to a minute, he recovers, regains consciousness, and can stand and walk again.	Clumsiness. Lack of good walking skills. Normal childhood "stage."	No emergency care needed (unless he hurt himself a he fell), but the child should be given a thorough medical evaluation.
INFANTILE SPASMS	Starts between 3 months and 2 years. If a child is sitting up, the head will fall forward, and the arms will flex forward. If lying down, the knees will be drawn up, with arms and head flexed forward as if the baby is reaching for support.	Normal movements of the baby, especially if they happen when the baby is lying down.	No emergency care, but prompt medical evaluation is needed.

Source: Epilepsy Foundation of America

433

GRAND MAL SEIZURES

A Grand Mal Seizure is a sign of an abnormal release of impulses in the brain. It is a physical, not a psychological, disorder.

1
The patient may have an "aura" or premonition which is part of the seizure. An aura is often described as an odd or unpleasant sensation that rises from the stomach toward the chest and throat.

For some patients the aura is always the same, such as numbness or motor activity (like turning of head and eyes, spasm of a limb) or it may consist of a peculiar sound or taste.

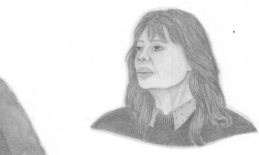

2
Loss of consciousness follows the aura. The forced expulsion of air caused by contraction of the skeletal muscles may cause a high pitched cry sound. The patient may be pale at this point with possible spasms of various muscle groups causing the tongue to be bitten.

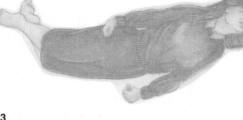

3
The patient will usually fall with convulsions and lose consciousness. Cyanosis may accompany the seizure because breathing stops during the phase of prolonged muscle contraction. Within seconds the patient will manifest an arched back and alternating contraction and relaxation of movements in all extremities (clonic convulsive movements). The attack usually lasts from about 30 seconds to five minutes. The patient may lose bladder and bowel control.

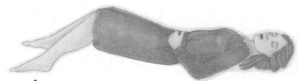

4
Gradually the clonic phase (convulsions) subsides. It is followed by a **postictal state**, characterized by a deep sleep with gradual recovery to a state of transient confusion, fatigue, muscular soreness, and headache. The patient should be encouraged to rest since activity could precipitate another attack.

EMERGENCY CARE

- If the patient seems to stop breathing, monitor airway and assist ventilation if necessary. The situation becomes life-threatening if the patient passes from seizure to seizure without regaining consciousness (status epilepticus). This situation requires transport and medical attention.
- The major requirements of the EMT are the ABC's and to protect the patient from hurting himself during a seizure.
- The patient should not be physically restrained in any way unless he is endangering his own welfare.
- Move objects, not the patient.
- Position the patient to allow for drainage and suctioning.
- Loosen tight clothing.
- If status epilepticus occur or breathing ceases assist breathing with bag-valve-mask and oxygen, record vital signs, and transport immediately.
- Keep patient from being a spectacle.
- Reassure and reorient patient following the seizure.
- Allow him to rest.
- An ambulance is often called for a grand mal seizure, but if the patient responds normally he may not need transport. If in doubt always transport to a medical facility. Follow local protocol and check with base physician.

FIGURE 30-2

progression as ranging from warning phase to period of recovery.

1. *Aura.* An aura is a subjective sensation preceding seizure activity. The aura may precede the attack by several hours or only by a few seconds. An aura may be of a psychic or a sensory nature, with olfactory, visual, auditory, or taste hallucinations. Some common types include hearing noise or music, seeing floating lights, smelling unpleasant odors, feeling an unpleasant sensation in the stomach, or experiencing tingling or twitching in a given body area. Not all seizures are preceded by an aura.

2. *Loss of consciousness.* The patient will become unconscious after the aura sensations.

3. *Tonic phase.* This is a phase of continuous motor tension, characterized by tension and contraction of the patient's muscles.

4. **Hypertonic phase.** The patient experiences extreme muscular rigidity including hyperextension of the back.

5. *Clonic phase.* The patient experiences muscle spasms marked by muscular rigidity and then relaxation.

6. *Post-seizure.* The patient progresses into a coma.

7. *Postictal.* The patient will awaken confused, fatigued, may complain of a headache, and experience some neurological deficit.

Assessment

Because a patient himself will rarely remember the seizure, you will need to obtain a history of the seizure from bystanders unless you witnessed the seizure yourself. If possible, determine the following:

- What was the seizure like? Does the patient have a history of seizures? How frequently do they occur? Does he take medication for seizures? If so, did he take his regular medication yesterday/today? Do certain things seem to cause the patient to have seizures? Did any of those things happen today?

- Get a careful description of the onset of the seizure if you did not witness it. Was it preceded by an aura? Did it begin in one area of the body and progress? In which direction did the eyes deviate — left or right? Did the patient bite his tongue or lose control of bladder/bowel functions? Note the time of onset and the duration of the seizure. Observe the behavior after the seizure.

- Does the patient have a recent or remote history of head injury?

- Does the patient have a history of alcohol or drug abuse? If so, when and how much was ingested?

(Seizures often occur during withdrawal from alcohol and certain drugs.)

- Does the patient have a history of diabetes (that might predispose him to hypoglycemia), heart disease (irregular heartbeat can cause oxygen deficiency to the brain), or stroke (scars from old strokes sometimes irritate brain tissue)?

- Has the patient had a recent fever, headache, or stiff neck, which might be indicative of meningitis?

In performing the physical assessment, pay particular attention to:

- Signs of injury to the head, tongue, or elsewhere on the body.

- Completion of a thorough neurological examination.

- Signs of alcohol or drug abuse (alcohol on the breath, needle tracks, and so on).

- Irregular heartbeat; if present, monitor vital signs.

- **Medalert tag** or other identifying medal or bracelet.

- Fever.

Emergency Care

Although seizures are generally not life-threatening, all who experience a first-time seizure should be evaluated by a physician. Regardless of whether the seizure is the patient's first, observe him or her carefully throughout; document the patient's appearance, the duration of the seizure, any aura that occurred, any injuries that occurred, any incontinence, and the time and place the seizure occurred. The following specific management techniques can help the patient:

1. Stay calm. If conscious, reassure the patient. Reassure others who are with the patient, explain what is happening, and try to keep them calm.

2. Stay with the patient until the seizure has passed. If you need help, send someone else to get it. If you leave to get equipment or additional help, the patient may become injured aspirate, or asphyxiate while you are gone.

3. Help the patient lie down on the floor so that the patient will not fall and become injured. Do not move the patient unless near a dangerous object that cannot be moved (such as a hot radiator); instead, move objects that are near the patient so that injury will not occur during the course of the seizure (Figure 30-3).

4. *Never try to force anything between a patient's clenched teeth.* Doing so may break the patient's

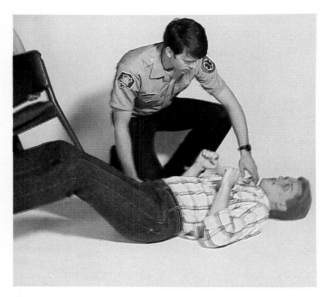

FIGURE 30-3 Assessing a patient experiencing a grand mal seizure. Move objects away from the patient rather than trying to move him or her.

teeth, force his or her tongue back so that it occludes the airway, cause other injury to the patient, or cause injury to you. *Some EMS directors do not recommend the use of bite sticks — follow local protocol.*

5. Remove or loosen any tight clothing and remove eyeglasses.

6. Turn the patient on his or her side (preferably the left side) with the head extended and the face turned slightly downward so that secretions and vomitus can drain quickly out of the mouth (Figure 30-4). This position also prevents the tongue from falling back and tends to prevent choking.

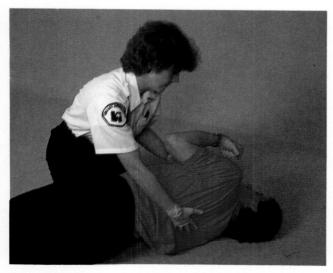

FIGURE 30-4 Turn the patient on his or her side to allow drainage of secretions.

7. Maintain an airway and if necessary administer oxygen through a nasal cannula at a moderate flow of four to six liters per minute. Some protocols call for non-rebreathing mask at ten to fifteen liters per minute. *Follow local protocol.* Suction out the patient's mouth periodically if the teeth are not clenched.

8. If the patient stops breathing, open the airway; use a mechanical airway if necessary. Remove anything that might impair breathing.

9. Watch what you say during the seizure; even though the patient appears asleep or stuporous, he or she will probably retain the sense of hearing.

10. Do not attempt to restrain the patient unless in immediate danger from objects that cannot be moved.

11. If possible, keep the patient from becoming a spectacle. If a screen or other barrier is available, place it around the patient. Ask onlookers and bystanders to leave.

12. Cover the patient with a blanket for warmth and to spare him embarrassment once the seizing is over.

13. Following the seizure, reassure and reorient the patient. Speak slowly and calmly in a normal tone of voice. Allow the patient to rest, and make him or her as comfortable as possible. Administer oxygen if needed; determine flow by skin color and condition.

14. Check for and stabilize any injuries that may have occurred during the seizure.

15. If the patient lapses into a second seizure without regaining consciousness from the first one (status epilepticus), transport immediately and consider his or her condition a grave medical emergency. Follow additional guidelines listed below.

16. If the patient is a feverish infant or child, cool the fever with room-temperature (not cold) wet towels or a sponge bath in tepid water. *Follow local protocol.*

17. Never give the patient anything to eat or drink; food or drink may mask symptoms, cause vomiting, and interfere with the physician's followup examination.

18. Transport the patient in a supine position.

If the patient experiences status epilepticus, *you are dealing with a dire medical emergency.* Your number-one goal is oxygenation. Follow these steps:

1. Place the patient on the floor or bed, away from other furniture. Do not try to restrain.

2. Clear and maintain the patient's airway; use a me-

chanical airway if possible. Turn head sideways to prevent aspiration.

3. Administer oxygen with a nasal cannula or nonrebreather mask. *Follow local protocol.* Assist breathing if necessary. Even though it can be extremely difficult to administer oxygen to a seizing patient, you must do it — lack of oxygen due to impaired breathing during seizure activity is the most serious threat to life. Monitor for vomiting to prevent aspiration.

4. Record and carefully monitor vital signs.

5. Transport the patient without delay to the hospital. If you have only one assistant, you may wish to ask a bystander to accompany you in the back of the ambulance to assist in preventing the patient from become injured while you maintain the airway. **Note:** *Oral airways are frequently involved in breakage of teeth among seizure patients; a nasopharyngeal airway is recommended. Follow local protocol.*

☐ DIZZINESS, FAINTING, AND UNCONSCIOUSNESS

Two of the most common medical complaints are dizziness (a term used by patients to describe a broad variety of very different symptoms) and syncope, or fainting. Actually, dizziness and fainting are not medical conditions at all, but are symptoms that can result from a large number of diseases.

Dizziness

Most patients are not experiencing true dizziness, or **vertigo** — instead, they may feel woozy, light-headed (especially when they stand up), or as though they are in a dream. They also may have blurred vision. True vertigo involves a hallucination of motion: the patient feels as though he is spinning around or, more commonly, that the room is whirling in circles. Some feel as though they are being pulled to the ground; there is a tilting, rocking, veering sensation. Others feel that the room has tilted enough so that they can no longer stand up in it. True vertigo is an actual disturbance of the patient's sense of balance.

Vertigo usually occurs in episodes that are almost always quite brief. Vertigo is usually accompanied by nausea, vomiting, sweating, paleness, and uncontrollable back-and-forth darting of the eyes. It is often accompanied by tinnitus (ringing of the ears) and hearing loss.

There are two different types of vertigo, and both stem from a disturbance of the vestibular system (the system that maintains our sense of balance). The vestibular system registers the direction that gravity is coming from and registers the speed and direction the head is turning in. Each type of vertigo causes very different signs and symptoms. **Central vertigo,** the less common of the two, is also the most serious, because it usually signifies a dramatic medical problem involving the central nervous system (such as **multiple sclerosis,** cerebrovascular accident, seizure disorders, or brain tumor). The signs and symptoms of central vertigo include dysfunction of the eye muscles, unequal pupil size, and facial droop. In some cases, central vertigo may mimic a TIA or cerebrovascular accident (stroke). Patients with central vertigo do not experience nausea, vomiting, hearing loss, or a whirling sensation.

Labyrinthine vertigo, much more common, occurs as a result of disturbance of the **labyrinthine system,** the major system of balance in the inner ear. Patients with labyrinthine vertigo experience nausea, vomiting, **nystagmus** (rapid, involuntary twitching of the eyeball), and a whirling sensation. Most — if not all — of the symptoms are made worse by even the slightest movement. In an attempt to avoid any movement at all, the patient may appear to be in a coma, with head and neck held rigid, eyes tightly shut, skin pale and sweaty, the heartbeat rapid. Upon examination, though, you will find that the patient is awake and alert but terrified to move. Some forms of labyrinthine vertigo (such as **Meniere's disease**) are hereditary and involve hearing loss; episodes can last for hours and recur over a period of many years. It can also be caused by infection of the ear or the nerve in the inner ear, allergy, a blow to the head, migraine headaches, a middle ear cyst, and high doses of antibiotics (especially streptomycin).

A patient may also suffer from what has been called "positional vertigo," or a sensation of dizziness that occurs in only one position. Positional vertigo does not involve hearing loss, and usually goes away on its own within a few months.

Management of dizziness in the field is limited to administering oxygen, if needed, reassuring the patient, and transporting him with as little movement as possible. Conduct a thorough assessment to rule out any immediately life-threatening conditions, and avoid the temptation to diagnose in the field. Most cases of true vertigo require extensive laboratory testing for proper diagnosis.

Fainting

Fainting, or **syncope,** is a sudden and temporary loss of consciousness that results when, for some reason, the brain is temporarily deprived of oxygen. It is often due to irregular heart rhythm or a sudden drop in blood pressure. Some patients feel as though everything is going dark, and then they suddenly lose consciousness. Syncope almost always occurs when the patient is standing up or when the patient suddenly stands up from a sitting position. A deathlike collapse follows that puts the body in a horizontal position, allowing blood circulation to the brain to improve. As a result, the patient rapidly regains consciousness. For a few moments after regaining consciousness, the patient may feel confused and anxious; many will not remember the fainting episode at first.

Again, fainting itself is not a disease, but it can be symptomatic of a wide range of conditions and diseases; most commonly, severe emotion, emotional stress, seizures, heat exhaustion, strenuous activity, a severe coughing attack, fright, certain drugs, profound pain, hypoglycemia, or cardiac arrhythmias (usually when the heartbeat is below 30 or over 180 beats per minute). It's important to evaluate a patient with syncope, because it can be due to a serious heart problem that needs to be treated.

Some patients experience warning signs that they are about to experience syncope. Especially if the syncope is due to extreme emotion or fright, the patient may feel nauseated, lightheaded, weak, cold, and shaky. Some experience deep abdominal pain or a pounding pain in the head. One method of preventing a patient who is experiencing these warning signs from actually fainting is to have the patient, seated, lower the head to knee-level (Figure 30-5).

Fainting in children is often caused by breath-holding. Other common causes include hypoglycemia (low blood sugar), dehydration, myocardial infarction, epilepsy, cardiac arrhythmias, congenital heart disease, valvular heart disease, and congenital heart failure.

To give emergency care for syncope, follow these guidelines:

1. If the patient has not fainted but tells you that he or she feels faint, place him or her in a seated position, lowering the head to a level between the knees. Do not do this with patients with fractures, possible neck or spine injuries, or head injuries. If a patient is having trouble breathing have him or her lie down; elevate the legs.

2. If the patient has already fainted, keep him or her in a supine position and elevate the legs ten to twelve inches. If the patient falls against furniture, a wall, or some other obstacle and does not get into a flat position, the patient will not regain consciousness because the blood flow to his brain will not improve. *Do not allow a person who has fainted to sit up right away.*

3. Until proven otherwise, assume that the brain has been deprived of oxygen. Establish an airway and administer oxygen by nasal cannula or face mask if the patient is conscious; monitor for possible vomiting.

4. Loosen any tight clothing that may restrict free breathing.

5. Make a rapid assessment for any life-threatening condition that may have caused the fainting; if you determine that the patient has a serious medical codition, initiate appropriate emergency care.

6. Check for any injuries that may have been sustained during the fall, and treat appropriately.

7. Transport the patient to the hospital in a supine position (Figure 30-6); do not allow a patient who has fainted to get up and walk around after regaining consciousness.

FIGURE 30-6 Conscious fainting patient prepared for transport. Monitor for vomiting.

FIGURE 30-5 Fainting may be prevented by having a seated patient lower his or her head to a level between the knees.

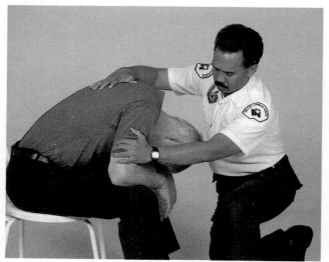

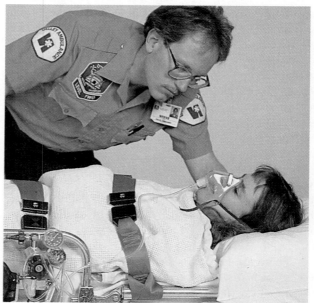

chapter 31

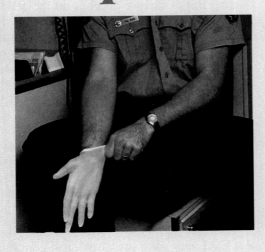

Infectious Disease Control

✱ OBJECTIVES

- Explain the infectious disease process with special emphasis on modes of transmission.
- Identify the infectious diseases of concern in an emergency setting.
- Describe the nature of AIDS and learn the universal precautions to prevent the spread of AIDS.
- Describe the general guidelines for preventing the spread of other infectious diseases, including protective procedures, recommended protective clothing, and the cleansing/disinfecting of patient care equipment and of the emergency response vehicle.

It is recommended that EMTs wear protective gloves whenever there is a possibility of coming in contact with a patient's blood, body fluids, mucous membrances, traumatic wounds, or sores.

□ BACTERIA, VIRUSES, AND THE IMMUNE SYSTEM

An infectious, or communicable, disease is one that can be transmitted from person to person, or from an infected animal or the environment to a person. Illness results when the **bacteria, viruses,** or other agents invade and multiply in the host (the person's body) and as a result cause specific diseases.

Illness and the development of resulting disease depend primarily on the causative agent and on the reaction of the body's immune system. Basically, bacteria or viruses can invade the body without causing the signs and symptoms of disease if the body's immune system responds adequately. Only when the bacteria or viruses overpower the immune system do the signs and symptoms of disease develop.

When bacteria enter the body, they attack normal cells by secreting toxins that damage or kill the cells and by competing with the cells for nutrients. Bacteria are self-contained, living cells that reproduce rapidly if not checked by the immune system or appropriate medication. While bacteria are self-contained, living organisms, viruses are inert particles that are not capable of reproducing until they have entered a **host** cell. The virus has a protective outer coating that enables it to bind securely to host cells; once the virus has penetrated the cell's lining, the coating dissolves, allowing the virus to alter cellular function as it attacks from inside the cell. When the cell regenerates itself, it reproduces a cell that has been genetically altered by the virus.

Obviously, the immune system has to fight bacteria and viruses in two different ways. With a bacterial infection, the body's **B-lymphocytes** recognize the bacteria and produce **antibodies** — proteins that search out and kill the bacteria. (Some less-sophisticated B-lymphocytes produce antibodies that search out and kill anything foreign, not just specific bacteria.)

B-lymphocytes can fulfill the same immune response to viruses *only while the viruses are still free-floating in the bloodsteam.* Once a virus invades a cell, the B-lymphocytes become compromised: in order to kill the virus, they also have to kill the body's own cell that is serving as host. Because the B-lymphocytes are incapable of this type of action, the immune system calls up its second line of defense — the **T-lymphocytes,** which can identify and destroy cells occupied by viruses.

The function of the immune system and its production of antibodies is what enables researchers to identify disease. If study of a patient's blood shows that antibodies to a certain illness are present, the physician can be certain that the patient has either been exposed to the illness or developed it.

□ TRANSMISSION OF INFECTIOUS DISEASE

The spread of disease depends on the ability of the infecting organism to survive outside its **reservoir** (source). A reservoir may be an infected person (whether or not he has symptoms of illness), an animal, an insect, or even an inert object. Transmission also depends on the ability of the infecting organism to move from one place to another. Some, such as the common cold, are very easily transmitted; others, such as tuberculosis, are relatively difficult to transmit. Factors that increase susceptibility to infection include inadequate nutrition, poor hygiene, living in crowded unsanitary conditions, and stress.

How Transmission Affects the EMT

An EMT may have actual physical contact with an infected patient, or he or she may pick up or spread the infection through contaminated equipment and instruments. Airborne transmission, while not as great a concern, may also affect EMTs who are treating patients.

As of February 1990, the Occupational Safety and Health Administration (OSHA) has mandated guidelines for infection control for emergency medical personnel. These requirements include gloves; gowns and protective eyewear if splashes are likely; and ventilation equipment such as a pocket mask should be used when possible when performing mouth-to-mouth resuscitation.

□ IDENTIFYING PATIENTS WITH INFECTIOUS DISEASES

Organisms that produce disease in man range in size from the submicroscopic viruses to the fish tapeworm, which can grow to over thirty feet in length. Microorganisms can be single-celled or multi-celled and are found in both plants and animals. The **pathogen,** or disease-causing agent, lives and multiplies at the expense of the body and its tissues, often destroying tissue cells completely.

Identification of infectious diseases in the field can be very difficult. Since the EMT will not have the diagnostic tools necessary, a potentially infectious patient will need to be identified by certain signs and symptoms. A patient should be considered infectious if he displays any of the following:

• Fever.

- A rash, open sores, or skin lesions anywhere on the body.
- Diarrhea.
- Vomiting.
- Coughing or sneezing, especially with chest pain.
- Draining wounds (pus, blood, or other matter oozing from open wounds anywhere on the body).
- Profuse sweating.
- Abdominal pain.
- Headache accompanied by a stiff neck.
- Signs of jaundice (yellowish discoloration of the skin or sclera of the eyes).

Obviously, these signs and symptoms may indicate a wide range of diseases, many of which are not infectious, but they should alert you of the need to exercise protective measures.

□ DISEASES OF CONCERN IN THE EMERGENCY SETTING

See Table 31-1 for a complete listing of diseases and recommended protective measures.

□ ACQUIRED IMMUNODEFICIENCY SYNDROME (AIDS)

One of the most terrifying and difficult infectious diseases currently posing a health hazard is acquired immunodeficiency syndrome, or AIDS. Within a few years of the first identified, isolated cases of AIDS, the disease has spread globally. At this time there is treatment, but no known cure.

Unfortunately, it is extremely difficult to get an accurate picture of the AIDS situation. The incubation period is unknown but may be as long as ten years, so researchers estimate that as many as two million Americans may be infected without knowing it and, therefore, may be spreading the disease in alarming proportions. In fact, researchers estimate that for every diagnosed case of AIDS, there are at least fifty undiagnosed Americans with the disease. The numbers with **ARC, or AIDS-related complex** (an AIDS-like illness that does not fit the rigid standards the CDC has established for diagnosing AIDS), is estimated to be two to five times greater than the number with AIDS itself.

In what is considered an alarming trend, the demographics of AIDS is changing considerably. It was once considered almost exclusively a disease of homosexual men; however, according to former Surgeon General C. Everett Koop, the total number of cases of AIDS is expected to increase ninefold over the next five years, *while the cases among heterosexuals will skyrocket*. A disproportionately high percentage of blacks and Hispanics are infected. And while the initial pockets of AIDS cases were pretty much isolated to San Francisco, Los Angeles, and New York City, researchers estimate that soon more than 80 percent of all AIDS cases in America will be in other areas of the country.

Because the disease was primarily one affecting homosexual men and IV drug users, experts and researchers tended to ignore its impact on women other than prostitutes. But women may account for a startling amount of growth in new AIDS cases, according to an open letter circulated at the Third International Conference on AIDS in Washington, D.C. According to the letter, women are proportionately the fastest growing group of AIDS patients in the United States. Half of those with the disease are intravenous drug users, half are black, and almost another one-fourth are Hispanic. Nearly one-third contracted the disease through heterosexual contact, a category in which women clearly outnumber men. And, according to the figures cited in the letter, AIDS is now the leading cause of death for women aged twenty-five to twenty-nine in New York City.

What is AIDS?

Simply stated, AIDS is a disease that renders the immune system ineffective. The AIDS virus (which has been named HTLV-III, LAV, ARV, and HIV by various groups of researchers) enters the body and affects the immune system's T-lymphocytes. As discussed earlier, the T-lymphocytes identify and destroy cells that are occupied by viruses. There are actually two types of T-lymphocytes:

- "Helper" T-lymphocytes stimulate the immune system to combat disease.
- "Suppressor" T-lymphocytes tell the immune system to shut down when its work is no longer needed.

In the normal body, there are about twice as many helper T-lymphocytes as suppressor T-lymphocytes. The AIDS virus kills the helper T-lymphocytes and renders the remaining ones ineffective. The body can no longer recognize and respond to foreign cells, like viruses and cancer cells, and as a result can no longer fight disease.

At that point, AIDS victims become infected with what researchers have called **opportunistic infections** — serious illnesses that either do not occur among people with healthy immune systems or that produce

TABLE 31-1
Diseases and Recommended Protective Measures

DISEASE	MODES OF TRANSMISSION	RECOMMENDED PROTECTIVE CLOTHING	RECOMMENDED PROTECTIVE PROCEDURES	RECOMMENDED VEHICLE/ EQUIPMENT CLEANING/ DISINFECTING
Aids	Blood and body fluids Sexual contact Infected needles Blood/blood products Maternal/child	Disposable mask Double utility gloves Eyeglasses/protective eyewear Waterproof apron, gown, or shoe covering if massive trauma All cuts, lesions, scratches, hangnails, or other open wounds on hands bandaged	Wash hands thoroughly Use extreme care in suctioning Never perform unprotected CPR Use only disposable needles; do not cut, bend, or recap; seal in a clearly labeled, rigid, puncture-proof bag	Wash vehicle surfaces with hospital-approved germicidal, rinse with diluted bleach solution Soak and disinfect all non-disposable equipment Immediately clean up any spills of blood or body fluids; disinfect Double-bag all soiled refuse; dispose of properly Soak linens/clothing in hydorgen peroxide; launder for 25 minutes in hot soapy water; bleach
Hepatitis B	Blood and body fluids	Disposable gloves All cuts, lesions, scratches, hangnails, or other open wounds on hands bandaged	Get Hepatitis B vaccination Have injection of HBIG within two weeks of exposure, and second injection one month later Use disposable needles; do not cut, bend, or recap; seal in a clearly labeled, rigid, puncture-proof bag Avoid mouth-to-mouth ventilation if possible	Clean vehicle and non-disposable equipment with a diluted bleach solution Double-bag and seal all soiled refuse; dispose of properly Double-bag all soiled clothing and linens; launder in hot soapy water and bleach
Meningitis	Contaminated food/water Direct contact with oral or nasal secretions Droplet spread	Disposable mask	Wash hands thoroughly Use extreme care in suctioning	Scrub all vehicle parts or surfaces contacted by the patient Launder clothing/linens in hot soapy water and diluted bleach
Herpetic Whitlow	Oral secretions	Disposable gloves Bandage open wounds on hands	Wash hands with germicidal soap	Scrub vehicle surfaces and launder clothing contaminated by oral secretions
Tuberculosis	Droplet spread (usually continual) Direct contact with oral or nasal secretions	Disposable mask	Wash hands thoroughly Avoid mouth-to-mouth ventilation (use mechanical devices) Use respiratory protection (Figure 31-1)	Scrub vehicle surfaces/equipment contaminated by secretions Launder clothing/linens contaminated by secretions in hot soapy water and bleach Incinerate all disposable equipment used on patient
Influenza	Droplet spread	Disposable mask	Wash hands thoroughly Use care in suctioning mouth/nose	Scrub surfaces of vehicle contacted by patient Disinfect all non-disposable equipment used for patient Launder contaminated clothing/linens in hot soapy water
Infectious Mononucleosis	Direct contact with oral/nasal secretions	Disposable mask if suctioning	Wash hands thoroughly Use care in suctioning mouth/nose	Scrub vehicle surfaces contaminated by oral secretions Disinfect all non-disposable equipment used for patient Launder contaminated clothing/linens in hot soapy water
Common Childhood Diseases	Droplet spread Oral/nasal secretions Indirect contact (Rubella) Direct contact with skin lesions (chickenpox)	Disposable mask Disposable gloves (chickenpox)	Get vaccination if not already immune (Measles/Mumps/Rubella) Use caution in suctioning mouth/nose Avoid touching skin lesions (chickenpox)	Scrub vehicle surfaces and non-disposable equipment contaminated with secretions or lesions Boil non-disposable equipment Launder contaminated clothing/linens in hot soapy water. Boil clothing/linens contaminated by patients with chickenpox or scarlet fever

only very mild illness when the immune system is functioning as it should. The serious infections caused by viruses, bacteria, parasites, and fungi enable researchers to identify a person with AIDS.

The Centers for Disease Control in Atlanta has indicated that in order to be officially diagnosed with AIDS, an individual must test positive with the AIDS virus and must have either two types of **malignancy** or one of the twelve specific infections now associated with AIDS (such as **pneumocystis carinii pneumonia, Kaposi's sarcoma, cytomegalovirus, cryptosporidium enterocolitis, candida albicans esophagitis,** and so on).

Another category of patients are those with AIDS-related complex (ARC). These patients have the AIDS virus but do not have any of the opportunistic infections required for classification as AIDS patients. Instead, they must have three or more clinical symptoms that have lasted longer than three months (symptoms such as fever of more than 100°F., weight loss of greater than 10 percent or fifteen pounds, persistent diarrhea, night sweats, debilitating fatigue, and persistent **lymphadenopathy**). They must also have laboratory confirmaiton of a number of abnormalities, including a reduced number of helper T-lymphocytes and an abnormal helper/suppressor T-lymphocyte ratio. Even though many ARC cases develop into full-blown AIDS cases, the ARC cases are not included in the statistics as AIDS victims. Still others are infected with the HIV but do not develop symptoms. *Remember: even those without symptoms are contagious.* Former Surgeon General Koop estimates this number to be between 1.5 and 3 million in the United States alone.

Modes of Transmission

The AIDS virus can be transmitted by a person who is ill with AIDS, by a person who has AIDS-related complex, or by a person who carries the AIDS virus but does not have symptoms. HIV is extremely fragile and unable to survive very long outside the human body, so it cannot be transmitted casually. Researchers have confirmed that the only way AIDS can be transmitted is by intimate contact with the body fluids (such as blood, semen, and vaginal secretions) of an infected individual (even though the infected individual may not realize that he or she is sick). The virus is found in the highest concentrations in blood and semen.

While the AIDS virus has been found in saliva, there have been no documented cases of the disease being passed solely through deep or open-mouthed kissing. *AIDS cannot be transmitted by shaking hands, coughing, sneezing, sharing meals, sharing eating utensils, or any other casual contact.* You cannot get AIDS from toilet seats, towels, office equipment, eating utensils, or other objects casually handled by infected persons. *AIDS transmission requires intimate contact with the bodily fluids (mostly semen, blood, and cervical secretions) of infected persons.* Although not common, it is theoretically possible that AIDS could be transmitted through urine, saliva, tears, cerebrospinal fluid, peritoneal fluid, pericardial fluid, pleural fluid, synovial fluid, amniotic fluid, and breast milk.

The identified modes of transmission include the following:

Sexual Contact

More than two-thirds of AIDS victims in the United States are believed to have acquired the virus through sexual contact; some researchers believe that the figure is closer to three-fourths. Any sexual contact — homosexual or heterosexual — that involves the exchange of semen, saliva, blood, urine, or feces can result in AIDS. Vaginal intercourse can transmit AIDS, but anal intercourse (common among homosexuals) seems particularly effective in transmitting the virus, possibly because it causes small tears in the rectal lining that allow the infected semen to enter the bloodstream readily.

Studies show that both men and women can transmit AIDS to their sexual partners, although female-to-male transmission is much less common in this country. The chances of becoming infected with AIDS become greater the more sexual partners a person has; it is also greater if there are sores, abrasions, lesions, or other open wounds in the rectum or genital tract, although these are not necessary for transmission of the virus.

Infected Needles

Use of an infected needle is also a major source of infection; in some cities (such as New York City), persons sharing needles have outnumbered homosexual or bisexual men as the fastest-growing new AIDS cases. Those who most often share needles — such as intravenous drug users and athletes who inject steroids — are at highest risk. Tattooing may also be responsible, and some cases may have occurred in poverty-stricken areas where needles are reused for medical or immunization purposes.

Infected Blood or Blood Products

Prior to 1985, blood donated by infected persons was passed to noninfected persons, facilitating transmission of the AIDS virus. Particularly at risk were hemophiliacs, who, because of their increased needs, must receive donated plasma that is pooled from as many as several thousand donors at a time. Others receiving blood transfusions following surgery or trauma also became infected. Since 1985, donated blood has been carefully screened to prevent infected blood from being given in hospitals or other settings. In addition, blood used for hemophiliacs is heat-treated to destroy the AIDS virus.

Maternal-Child Transmission

The AIDS virus can be transmitted from a mother to her child as early as the twelfth week of gestation, during the birth process, or following birth (usually through breast milk). Only about half the babies born to AIDS mothers will become infected themselves. Babies infected in utero are usually born with characteristic malformations, such as **microcephaly** (abnormally small heads) and facial malformations (such as abnormally full lips and flat noses).

High-Risk Groups

More than 90 percent of all identified AIDS cases have occurred among people in high-risk groups, as identified by the Centers for Disease Control. These groups include the following:

- Homosexual or bisexual men (65 percent of all adult cases).
- Intravenous drug users (17 percent of all adult cases).
- Blood transfusion recipients (2 percent of all adult cases and 12 percent of all pediatric cases).
- Heterosexual partners of high-risk individuals (2 percent of all adult cases).
- Children of parents at high-risk for AIDS (80 percent of all pediatric cases).
- Hemophiliacs (1 percent of all adult cases and 6 percent of all pediatric cases).
- Female prostitutes.
- Haitians.

Some researchers are now concentrating on high-risk behaviors instead of high-risk groups because *any* member of *any* group is at risk of contracting AIDS if he or she practices certain behaviors. Those behaviors include:

- Having multiple sexual partners.
- Needle-sharing or use of contaminated needles.
- Using hypodermic needles or syringes not sealed in the orginal package.
- Having anal intercourse.
- Emergency medical personnel who do not follow recommended protective guidelines are considered to be at risk for becoming infected with AIDS. Direct contact — defined as contaminated needle-stick injury, mucous membrane exposure, instrument-stick injury, or contact with a patient's open lesions — can result in transmission of the disease *if* precautions are not taken. *If you follow recommended guidelines for personal protection,* *you can significantly reduce your risk of becoming infected with the AIDS virus as a result of rendering patient treatment.*

Signs and Symptoms of AIDS

AIDS is a systemic infection that can involve many body organs and systems, resulting in what is probably a countless array of symptoms and signs. Death usually results from overwhelming and numerous infections or from loss of the ability to breathe. Some commit suicide. In general, the most common signs and symptoms include the following:

- Persistent, low-grade fever.
- Night sweats.
- Swollen lymph glands.
- Loss of appetite.
- Nausea.
- Persistent diarrhea.
- Headache.
- Sore throat.
- Fatigue.
- Weight loss.
- Muscle and joint aches.
- Rash.
- Various opportunistic infections, obviously, cause their own signs and symptoms.

Not everyone infected by the AIDS virus will develop AIDS or ARC, but they are still capable of transmitting the virus to others regardless of whether they themselves have signs or symptoms. As many as half of those infected will not develop signs or symptoms. About one-fifth will have only minor signs and symptoms that may be mistaken for a cold, influenza, or mononucleosis.

Universal Precautions for AIDS

Universal precautions are called "universal" because they mean exactly that: you must assume that *all* patients you treat are infected with AIDS.

Since medical history and examination cannot reliably identify all patients infected with the AIDS virus or with blood-borne diseases, the following blood and body fluid precautions should be consistently used for *all* patients. This approach, previously recommended by the Centers for Disease Control and referred to as "universal blood and body-fluid precautions" or "universal precautions," should be used in the care of *all* patients, especially those in emergency-care settings in which the risk of blood exposure is increased and the infection status of the patient is usually unknown.

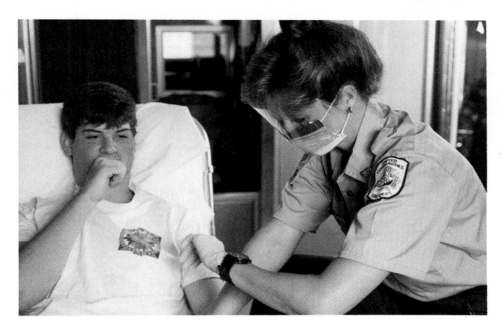

FIGURE 31-1 Use respiratory protection if a respiratory infectious disease, such as tuberculosis, is suspected.

• All health-care workers should routinely use appropriate barrier precautions to prevent skin and mucous membrane exposure when contact with blood or other bodily fluids of any patient is anticipated. You can pick up the virus if you touch blood or body fluids and your hands are chapped, abraded, or affected with a dermatologic condition (such as eczema). Gloves should be worn for touching blood and body fluids, mucous membranes, tissues, or non-intact skin of all patients, and for handling items or surfaces soiled with blood or body fluids. Gloves should be latex, not vinyl — vinyl allows more than two times the penetration of bacteria and viruses. Gloves should be changed after contact with each patient. Masks and protective eyewear (goggles or safety glasses) or face shields should be worn during procedures that are likely to generate droplets of blood or other body fluids to prevent exposure of mucous membranes of the mouth, nose, and eyes. Gowns or aprons should be worn during procedures that are likely to generate splashes of blood or other body fluids (Figure 31-2).

• Hands and other skin surfaces should be washed immediately and thoroughly with soap and water if contaminated with blood or other body fluids. Hands should be washed immediately after gloves are removed. If possible, wash with an antimicrobial agent.

• All health-care workers should take precautions to prevent injuries caused by needles, scalpels, and other sharp instruments or devices during procedures; when cleaning used instruments; during disposal of used needles; and when handling sharp

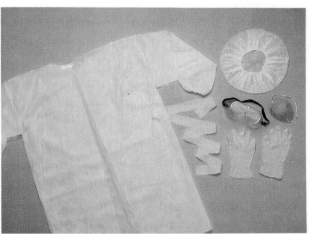

FIGURE 31-2 An infection control kit can be used for infectious disease cases and/or for situations where risk of body fluid contamination is present.

instruments after procedures. To prevent needle-stick injuries, needles should not be recapped, purposely bent or broken by hand, removed from disposable syringes, or otherwise manipulated by hand. After they are used, disposable syringes and needles, scalpel blades, and other sharp items should be placed in rigid-wall, puncture-resistant containers for disposal. The rigid-wall, puncture-resistant containers should be located as close as practical to the use area. Large-bore reusable needles should be placed in a rigid-wall, puncture-resistant container for transport. If there is no available container, you should use the one-handed needle recap technique — with one hand, slide the needle into the cap and then push it down (Figure 31-3).

Infectious Disease Control **445**

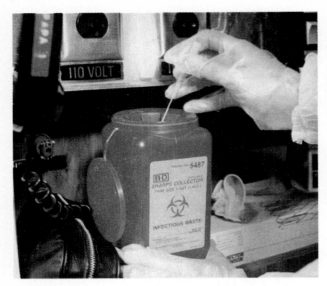

FIGURE 31-3 After using syringes or other sharp instruments used for invasive procedures, place in a rigid-wall puncture-resistant container.

- Although saliva has not been implicated in HIV transmission, minimize the need for emergency mouth-to-mouth resuscitation by carrying pocket masks, mouthpieces, resuscitation bags, or other ventilation devices in areas in which the need for resuscitation is predictable.
- Health-care workers who have lesions or weeping dermatitis should refrain from all direct patient contact and from handling patient-care equipment until the condition is gone.
- Pregnant health-care workers are not known to be at greater risk of contracting HIV infection than health-care workers who are not pregnant; however, if a health-care worker develops HIV infection during pregnancy, the infant is at risk of infection resulting from prenatal transmission. Because of this risk, pregnant health-care workers should be especially familiar with and should strictly adhere to precautions to minimize the risk of HIV transmission.

The most recent guidelines call for "universal body-substance isolation," an expanded form of universal precautions that protects against exposure to all body fluids, not just blood. Universal body-substance isolation calls for creativity on the part of the EMT, and applies to *all* patients. Some suggestions include double-gloving and wearing structural gloves over latex gloves if there is any broken glass at the scene of an accident.

□ PREVENTING INFECTION SPREAD DURING CPR

As an EMT, you undoubtedly will be faced with performing mouth-to-mouth ventilation on cardiac arrest victims about whom you have little or no medical infor-

mation. On the other hand, a lay person who performs mouth-to-mouth ventilation is most likely to do so in the home (where approximately 80 percent of all cardiac arrests occur), is most likely to know the cardiac arrest victim, and often knows the victim's health status. For that reason, the greatest concern over the theoretical risk of disease transmission from mouth-to-mouth ventilation is directed at people who perform CPR frequently, such as health-care and public safety personnel and prehospital emergency health-care providers.

According to an article first published in the *Journal of the American Medical Association* and reprinted by the U.S. Public Health Service, providers of prehospital emergency health care include the following: paramedics, emergency medical technicians, law enforcement personnel, firefighters, life-guards, and others whose jobs might require them to provide first-response medical care. The risk of transmission of infection from infected persons to providers of prehospital emergency health care should be no higher than that for other health-care workers, the article says, providing that appropriate precautions are taken to prevent exposure to blood or other body fluids.

According to the article, no transmission of hepatitis B virus infection during mouth-to-mouth resuscitation has been documented. However, because of the theoretical risk of salivary transmission of the AIDS virus during mouth-to-mouth resuscitation, special attention should be given to the use of disposable airway equipment or resuscitation bags and the wearing of gloves when in contact with blood or body fluids. The AIDS virus can be transmitted if the patient or rescuer have breaks in the skin around the lips or in the soft tissues of the mouth. (The risk is even greater for airborne diseases.) Resuscitation equipment and devices known or suspected to be contaminated with blood or other bodily fluids should be used once and disposed of or be thoroughly cleaned and disinfected after each use. *The general guideline is to avoid performing mouth-to-mouth resuscitation if there is any other immediate method of ventilation available.*

Clear plastic face masks with one-way valves are available for use during mouth-to-mouth ventilation (Figure 31-4). These masks provide diversion of the victim's exhaled gas away from the rescuer and may be used by health-care providers and public safety personnel properly trained in their use during two-person rescue, in place of mouth-to-mouth ventilation, the article continues. The need for and effectiveness of this adjunct in preventing transmission of an infectious disease during mouth-to-mouth ventilation are unknown. If this type of device is used as reassurance to the rescuer that a potential risk might be minimized, the rescuer must be adequately trained in its use, especially with respect to making an adequate seal on the face and maintaining a

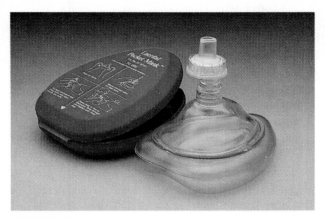

FIGURE 31-4 Pocket masks with one-way valves can be used to reduce the risk of cross-contamination. Many disposable types are also available.

patent airway. As an additional precaution, the rescuer may elect to wear latex gloves, since saliva or blood on the victim's mouth or face may be transferred to the rescuer's hands.

□ GUIDLINES FOR HANDWASHING

Handwashing — defined as a vigorous, brief rubbing together of all surfaces of lathered hands, followed by rinsing under a stream of water — is the *single most important procedure* in preventing the spread of infection. According to the U.S. Public Health Sevice, most contaminants can be removed from the skin with ten to fifteen seconds of vigorous lathering and scrubbing. Make sure to remove all jewelry before washing your hands — rings hinder thorough hand-washing and harbor bacteria. Pay attention to all creases and crevices, the areas between the fingers, and use a brush to scrub under and around the fingernails. Keep the nails short and unpolished. If your hands are visibly soiled, more time may be required for handwashing. Hands should then be thorough rinsed under a stream of running water and dried with a clean cloth or disposable towel. *Make sure you wash your hands even if you were wearing gloves.*

Unless otherwise indicated, plain soap can be used for handwashing. Handwashing with plain soap or detergent (as opposed to antimicrobial-containing products) suspends microorganisms and allows them to be rinsed off. If you are in the field, you can temporarily use a foam or liquid handwashing agent that requires no water. If you were exposed to high-risk fluids, use an antimicrobial agent.

□ GUIDELINES FOR PROTECTIVE CLOTHING

Recent figures show that those who wear protective gear run a 62 percent less chance of becoming infected with AIDS or hepatitis B by patients. Current guidelines suggest that the following protective clothing be used to help prevent the spread of AIDS:

- Gloves should be worn whenever there is the possibility of coming in contact with the patient's blood, body fluids, mucous membranes, traumatic wounds, or sores. The purpose of the glove is to prevent blood from reaching the skin of the health-care worker; therefore, the health-care worker does not need a high-quality surgeon's latex glove. If a glove is accidentally torn while in use, remove it as soon as patient safety permits, wash your hands, and replace the glove with a new one.

- During any invasive procedure, a face mask or face shield should be worn to protect against blood splashing into the nose and mouth.

- If the patient has sustained heavy bleeding or there is the possibility of heavy bleeding, additional protective clothing — such as gowns, aprons, or shoe coverings — should be worn as appropriate to prevent widespread contamination by infected blood or body fluids.

□ EQUIPMENT CLEANING, DISINFECTING, AND STERILIZATION

The AIDS virus is relatively fragile, and can be detroyed within a few minutes by heat, disinfectants, alcohol, household bleach, and drying.

Officials at the CDC emphasize that no case of AIDS transmission has been documented that involved contaminated patient-care equipment. Nevertheless, the following precautions should be used routinely in the care of *all* patients.

Standard sterilization and disinfection procedures of patient-care equipment currently recommended for use in a variety of health-care settings are adequate to sterilize or disinfect instruments, devices, or other items contaminated with blood or other body fluids from persons infected with AIDS. Use the following guidelines:

- Whenever possible, use disposable equipment. Disconnect any disposable equipment from nondisposable equipment while wearing gloves; sterilize the nondisposable equipment according to guidelines, and properly dispose of the rest.

- Noncritical items that do not ordinarily touch the patient or that touch only intact skin (such as blood pressure cuffs) rarely, if ever, transmit disease. Simple sponging, wiping, or washing with regular detergent is usually all that is required. Rinse with clear water and allow to air dry thoroughly. Wash backboards, cervical collars. PASGs, and other similar equipment with hot soapy water.

- All pieces of equipment that are to be disinfected or sterilized should first be thoroughly cleaned to remove all organic matter (blood and tissue) and other residue.

- Patient-care equipment that enters normally sterile tissue or that touches mucous membranes must be sterilized before each use and subjected to high-level disinfection. Chemical germicides that are registered with the U.S. Environmental Protection Agency (EPA) as "sterilants" may be used either for sterilization or for high-level disinfection. You also can use a solution of household bleach diluted in water (concentrations ranging from 1:10 to 1:100) to disinfect equipment and surfaces. Clean all organic matter and other debris off of the equipment before disinfecting, and follow manufacturer's instructions for disinfecting any equipment. Be sure to clean any visible blood and secretions out of all cracks and crevices.

To further reduce the risk of spreading AIDS, use disposable equipment whenever possible, and dispose of it promptly and properly.

□ DISPOSING OF INFECTIOUS WASTES

There is no evidence to suggest that most hospital waste is any more infectious than residential waste. However, wastes (including disposable equipment) contaminated with the blood and body fluids of any patient should be considered to carry some risk of spreading the AIDS virus. The following guidelines should be used when dealing with wastes contaminated with blood or body fluids:

- Dispose of all needles and other sharp instruments (such as lancets and scalpels) in rigid, puncture-proof containers *immediately* after you use them. *Never recap needles.* Keep a rigid, puncture-proof container next to the patient throughout treatment.

- Following treatment and transport of a patient, gather all disposable equipment (such as gloves, paper towels, and so on) that has been soiled by blood or body fluids and place it in a separate container (such as a large plastic garbage bag). Seal the container and label it as infectious waste (Figure 31-5).

- Sheets and pillowcases should be folded from the edges to the middle; place, but do not throw, them into the laundry bag.

- All infectious waste should be either incinerated or **AUTOCLAVED** before disposal in a sanitary landfill.

- Bulk blood, suctioned fluids, excretions, and secretions can be carefully poured down a drain connected to a sanitary sewer. Sanitary sewers may also be used to dispose of other infectious wastes capable of being ground and flushed into the sewer.

□ GUIDELINES FOR CLEANING THE VEHICLE

Although microorganisms are a normal contaminant of walls, floors, and other surfaces, these environmental surfaces rarely are associated with transmission of infec-

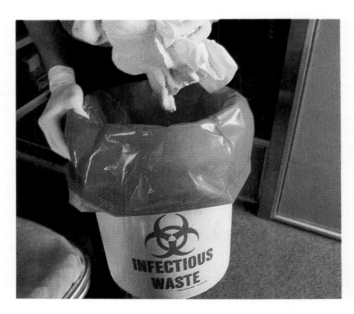

FIGURE 31-5 Bag all linen and label if infectious.

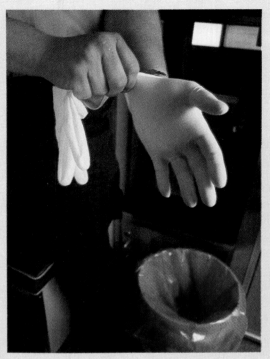

FIGURE 31-6 Always wear protective gloves.

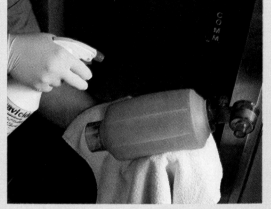

FIGURE 31-7 Using an approved antiseptic solution, clean any equipment that potentially contacted the patient.

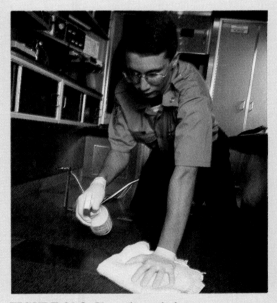

FIGURE 31-8 Clean the ambulance compartment.

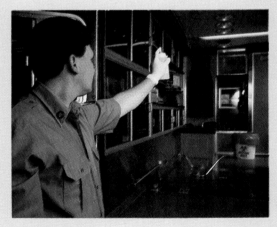

FIGURE 31-9 Use antiseptic sprays and ventilate the ambulance.

tions to patients or personnel. Therefore, extraordinary attempts to disinfect or sterilize the surfaces of your vehicle are not necessary.

Routine cleaning of the vehicle is recommended, and removal of blood and body fluids should be done as soon as possible. "Routine cleaning" should consist of completely wiping down the ambulance interior and stretchers every twenty-four hours with a hospital-grade disinfectant or a 1:10 solution of household bleach and water. Keep the vehicle well ventilated during cleaning. The following guidelines are recommended (Figures 31-6–31-9):

- Wear disposable gloves and eye protection during all cleaning and decontamination procedures.
- Remove any blood, body fluids, or other matter with paper towels or disposable linens; dispose of these properly and immediately. Wherever blood was found, clean with a disinfectant or bleach solution.
- Scrub the soiled area with any hospital-grade disinfectant-detergent registered by the DPA; follow manufacturer's directions carefully.
- Rinse and let dry.
- Walls, window coverings, and other nonhorizontal surfaces do not need routine cleaning but should be cleaned if visibly soiled.

□ RECOMMENDED IMMUNIZATIONS FOR EMTS

Before you begin active duty, make sure that you are adequately protected against common communicable diseases. You should have a tuberculin skin test (tine test) annually while on duty; have the test more often if you are in an area of concentrated tuberculosis cases. Your physician can advise you.

In addition to the tuberculin skin test, you should have the following:

- Hepatitis B vaccination.
- Influenza vaccination (annually).
- DPT (diphtheria/pertussis/tetanus), with a tetanus booster every ten years.
- Polio immunization.
- Rubella (German measles) vaccination.
- Measles vaccination.
- Mumps vaccination

□ GENERAL GUIDELINES FOR PREVENTING THE SPREAD OF INFECTION

In addition to the specific guidelines listed in Table 31-1 and in the section on AIDS, follow these general guidelines to prevent the spread of infection when working with infectious disease patients:

- *Wash your hands thoroughly after every call.* If running water is not available, use a commercial germicidal hand rinse to clean your hands. If you need to clean or disinfect any equipment or the ve-

hicle, thoroughly wash your hands again afterward.
- Whenever possible, use disposable equipment and supplies on patients with infectious diseases. When you have finished, bag all used equipment in a clearly labeled bag that has been sealed to prevent leakage; follow local protocol for appropriate disposal.
- Have disposable gloves, masks, gowns, and shoe coverings on hand at all times. If you suspect that you may be splattered with blood or body secretions, wear appropriate disposable gear (Figure 31-10). Follow the procedure outlined above to dispose of any soiled gloves, masks, gowns, or shoe coverings. (Soiled refuse from AIDS or hepatitis B patients should be double-bagged and sealed.)
- Always wear disposable gloves when working with or cleaning up blood.
- If you need to transport an infectious patient on a stretcher, first cover the stretcher with disposable sheets. After treating the patient, dispose of the linens appropriately.
- *Never* reuse disposable equipment — it should be discarded after use on one patient. If you suspect that a patient may have a communicable disease, place soiled (used) disposable equipment in a clearly labeled plastic bag and seal it. (Used equipment from AIDS or hepatitis B patients should be double-bagged).
- Disassemble and disinfect all nondisposable equipment after every use. Thoroughly clean equipment first to remove blood, vomitus, or other soil; then wash in a strong disinfectant and let the disin-

FIGURE 31-10 EMT wearing appropriate infection-control gear while treating a patient with an infectious disease.

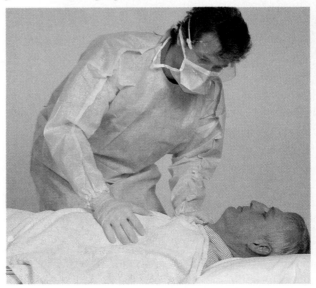

fected equipment soak. Rinse in a disinfectant solution, then in clean water, and allow to dry thoroughly.

- Bag all tissues, dressings, and other disposable paper items that were contaminated with infectious material in a clearly labeled plastic bag sealed to prevent leakage. (Refuse from AIDS or hepatitis B patients should be double-bagged.) Follow local protocol for disposal.

- Dump any secretions, blood, or vomitus from suction devices down the drain or hopper at the hospital; wash thoroughly into the sewer system.

- If your uniform becomes soiled with infectious material (such as pus, blood, oral secretions, or mucus), remove it as soon as possible, bag it and label it, take a hot shower, and wash with germicidal soap. Rinse thoroughly. Your uniform should be washed for at least twenty-five minutes in hot, soapy water and diluted bleach solution if bleach will not harm your uniform.

- Remove all equipment and linens from the ambulance and wash all ambulance surfaces contacted by the patient with strong soap and water; follow by scrubbing with disinfectant (make sure that you use a disinfectant approved for use in hospitals). Remember to disinfect resuscitation bags, humidifiers, and other equipment used during the call. There is no need to routinely clean the vehicle walls, windows, or floors unless they have been visibly soiled. Rinse with plenty of clear water (a hose works well). Let the ambulance air-dry thoroughly, and restock it with clean supplies.

- After you have finished all cleaning of equipment and the ambulance, wash your hands again *thoroughly*.

- Document in your logbook or on your flowsheet the cleaning you have done.

- For infection control, consider a commercially packaged infection-control kit. These contain protective equipment, germicidal rinses, and other products that can help prevent the spread of infection. They are available under a variety of names from several different manufacturers. Carefully follow written manufacturers' directions; a weaker solution or briefer immersion time may not disinfect or sterilize.

- Promptly report any suspected exposure, including the date and time of the exposure, the type of fluid involved, the amount of fluid, and details of the exposure.

chapter 32

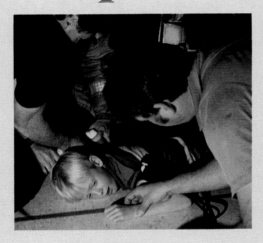

Pediatric Emergencies

✱ OBJECTIVES

- List the physiological differences between adult and child organs, blood volume, and systems.
- Describe how to deal with parents in an emergency.
- Explain how to assess children and interpret their reactions.
- Demonstrate how to obtain a pediatric medical history and take the vital signs of children.
- Discuss how to manage a pediatric trauma patient.
- Describe the impact of children's physiology on the types of emergencies that are likely.
- Identify and discuss how to respond to common emergencies in children.
- Demonstrate how to transport infants and children properly.

It is recommended that EMTs wear protective gloves whenever there is a possibility of coming in contact with a patient's blood, body fluids, mucous membranes, traumatic wounds, or sores. See Chapter 31.

Every day in the United States, approximately forty-one children die from trauma, and 4,000 more are admitted to hospital emergency rooms with injuries. The leading causes of fatal injuries in children under fourteen are trauma (particularly motor vehicle accidents), drownings, burns, poisonings, and falls. As an EMT, you can plan on approximately 10 percent of your patients being children.

Children can be categorized in the following groups, although these categories are not hard-and-fast pigeonholes.

- "Infant" refers to a child up to the age of twelve months.
- "Child" usually refers to an individual between one and twelve years of age.
- "Adolescent" refers to someone between twelve and eighteen years of age.

Each age group has different emotional and physical characteristics that can complicate your care. Children are *not* just little adults. There are important psychological and physical differences. (Figure 32-1). This chapter focuses on those differences to supplement the emergency care information in other chapters. Remember, however — a breathing problem is a breathing problem; a bleeding wound is a bleeding wound. How you approach it in a baby is a little different from how you approach it in the adult, but the basic treatment and goals are the same.

□ DEALING WITH PARENTS

When a child is ill or injured, you usually have more than one patient: the child and either or both parents. Some parents are calm, cooperative, and supportive, especially if they are experienced. If their child's condition is perceived as threatening, they are naturally more agitated. It is normal for parents to be upset, to cry, to blame themselves, or to get mad at someone else —

FIGURE 32-1

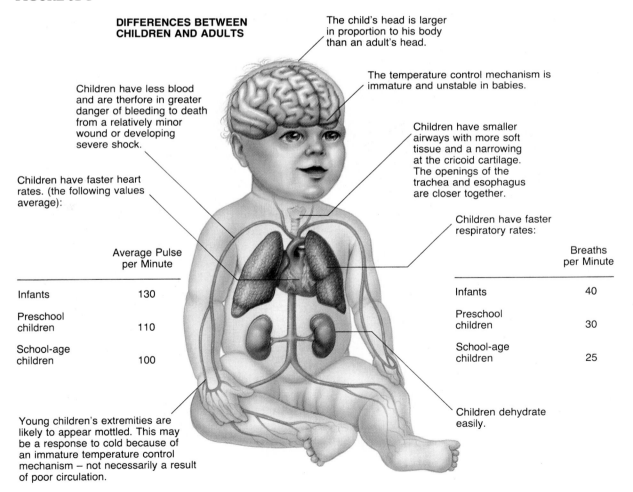

DIFFERENCES BETWEEN CHILDREN AND ADULTS

The child's head is larger in proportion to his body than an adult's head.

The temperature control mechanism is immature and unstable in babies.

Children have less blood and are therfore in greater danger of bleeding to death from a relatively minor wound or developing severe shock.

Children have smaller airways with more soft tissue and a narrowing at the cricoid cartilage. The openings of the trachea and esophagus are closer together.

Children have faster heart rates. (the following values average):

	Average Pulse per Minute
Infants	130
Preschool children	110
School-age children	100

Children have faster respiratory rates:

	Breaths per Minute
Infants	40
Preschool children	30
School-age children	25

Young children's extremities are likely to appear mottled. This may be a response to cold because of an immature temperature control mechanism – not necessarily a result of poor circulation.

Children dehydrate easily.

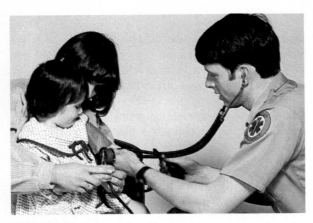

FIGURE 32-2 A good pediatric assessment involves the parent and must take the needed amount of time.

even you. You need to listen carefully to these feelings and remain nonjudgmental. While taking the history and inquiring about the circumstances of the event, allow the parent(s) to verbalize their emotions (Figure 32-2). Conclude with something brief and supportive like, "Thanks for telling me this. We'll do the very best we can for your little boy."

If the parents are hysterical or have been badly injured themselves, they will not be much help. In fact, they will need emergency care themselves. Make the parents your allies if at all possible. If the parent can hold the child or be present and within view, the child will probably be calmer. Generally, the more intact the family unit remains, the more effective the care will be.

In addition to the guilt, anger, concern, and apprehension natural to all parents of an ill or injured child, be aware that most parents will not understand emergency medical procedures. You do not want them to grab your arm and yell, "What are you doing to my baby?" when you are listening to breath sounds. Forestall such problems by explaining in brief, simple terms what you are doing. Usually it is best to keep your language simple and jargon-free but use your judgment. Some parents, especially if they are professional or are highly educated, may feel more reassured if you use technical terminology.

You will probably need to question the parents and other witnesses or care-givers to get a history of the incident. Remember to ask them how their child normally acts and whether a particular item that you discover during the examination is normal for this child. If the child sees his or her parents calm and cooperative, it will do wonders toward reassuring the child. This approach also allows the parents to feel that they are participants in their child's care and are not just bystanders.

□ DEALING WITH THE CHILD

It is difficult to assess pain in children because they lack both the body awareness to describe the exact location of the pain and the vocabulary to describe the nature of

the pain. Usually pain, and especially bleeding, is so frightening that they cannot separate the emotional component from the physical. Ask the parents, if possible, how the child usually responds to pain to get some idea of how typical the reactions are.

During your first look at the child, ask yourself these questions:

- How is he or she breathing?
- Does he or she look sick?
- Is he or she in shock?
- Is he or she in extreme pain?

Serious conditions mean that you will concentrate on immediate management and transport. The more experienced you are, the more you will be able to tell about the child's condition by that first visual assessment.

Reactions by Age

What you can expect from a pediatric patient depends to some degree on age:

Infants

Up to six months, a baby will usually let you undress him or her and put him or her on a flat surface as long as he or she is warm and you touch the baby with warm hands. Between six and eight months, a baby will almost always cry if separated from his parents. If possible, let the baby's mother or father (or older brother or sister) hold him or her while you examine the baby.

You will be able to remove clothing without much trouble. Start your examination somewhere besides the head for children up to school age, since little children do not like having their faces touched by strangers. One suggestion is to conduct a toe-to-head survey, which will still produce a complete survey. (This is assuming that the ABCs are intact.) Typical sources of trauma in infants are the improper use of equipment such as cribs or car seats, burns, and scalds.

Toddlers

Up to about age five, and particularly around ages two and three, children to not like having their clothing removed, do not like being touched, are frightened easily, and overreact to pain. You are not necessarily doing something wrong if a toddler is screaming and thrashing around during your assessment (Figure 32-3).

Remain calm, speak soothingly, and try to distract the child or engage his or her interest. Decide which parts of the physical assessment are essential and get through them as best as you can. Explain medical procedures in terms they can understand: "Now I'm going to press on your tummy to see if everything's okay. Tell me if it hurts." (But pay equal attention to flinching).

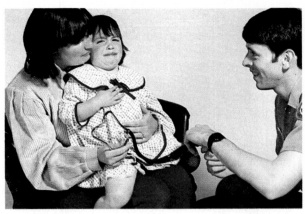

FIGURE 32-3 Two- to three-years-olds are often difficult to assess. Decide which parts of the physical assessment are essential.

"Now I'm going to shine my light in your right ear." Allow the child to see your equipment in full view before you use it, if possible, and let the child touch the stethoscope or other equipment. Put it first on the child's leg or the parent's hand so that the patient can see it is not threatening. If you use a rubber ring on the diaphragm, it will not be cold.

Have a parent present if possible. Have the parent hold the child in his lap; otherwise, the child will almost certainly squirm, thrash, and even try to run away. Set a few ground rules: "It's okay to cry. I know this hurts. But biting and kicking are not okay."

Children this age are aware of death and are afraid of many things. They may also feel that their illness or injury is a punishment for something they have done. Explain gently, "Accidents can happen to everyone, even when they're careful. It's too bad you forgot to look, but I'm not angry with you. I just want to help you as much as I can." Be sensitive to a child who is toilet trained and becomes overwhelmed with a bowel or bladder accident brought on by the illness or injury.

Be tactful and direct in dealing with physical fears (Figure 32-4). Cover bleeding injuries as soon as possible. Explain the obvious: "Your arm is broken, but it can be fixed. We'll take you to the hospital where they can help fix you." Let the child take a favorite "reassurance" toy like a teddy bear or a blanket. In an accident where separation from parents is necessary, a small personal item of one of the parents (e.g., dad's handkerchief) may help. Typical sources of trauma in this age group are drowning, or near-drowning, injuries from toys, and falls.

Children from Age Six

Usually children from this age on are cooperative and curious. It is easy to engage their interest in the procedures or your equipment. Remember, though, that illness or injury may cause children to regress. A ten-year-old may behave like a six-year-old after an accident. On the other hand, the child may act exceptionally mature.

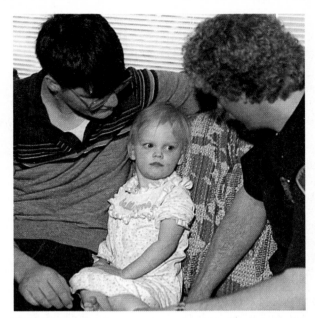

FIGURE 32-4 Three- to five-years-olds live in a world of fears. Extreme patience and tact are required.

Honesty is very important with children this age. Treat them with respect. Make them partners in their care. Information is reassuring to them, so explain each procedure in detail.

Children this age and even younger know that they need to take care of their clothes and sometimes get very anxious if you cut their clothes. Explain gently but firmly, "I need to cut this sleeve off so that I can look at your arm. Your mom won't get mad about your shirt because this is an emergency. Can you see the special scissors I'm using?" (Be sure that you do not let the undressed child get cold).

Typical sources of trauma in this age group are pedestrian accidents, bicycle accidents, sports injuries, and gunshot wounds.

Adolescents

Adolescents also regress. They need the respect accorded to adults and the support given to sick children. A good procedure is to reassure as though to a child but answer questions factually as for an adult.

Some experts suggest a relaxed rather than a professional approach, especially if the situation involves conflict with an authority figure like a schoolteacher, a police officer, or a parent. Smile, speak softly, and speak slowly. Record everything that the adolescent says and express no skepticism, even if it is obviously untrue. If the adolescent trusts you, he or she will be more likely to give you straight information during transport to the hospital.

Most adolescents, either patients or their peers, will be reluctant to disclose information about their sexual history, drug use, personal habits, and illegal activities; ask for only the information that you need and explain why you need it.

Do not be surprised if peers tease the patient. It may be normal and even reassuring. If it disturbs your patient, however, intervene. Acknowledge the patient's friends, let them help by notifying parents, holding equipment, and so on, and be honest but tactful in telling them about the patient's condition if they ask.

Adolescents are preoccupied by their bodies. An injury intensifies this preoccupation. If possible, use the exam to reassure them about what is normal. "I'm checking the pulse in your ankle to see if the heart is getting enough blood down here. Yes, it's about 73, normal range for pulse," or "Your lungs are certainly in good shape." They may not ask about their greatest fears; for example, whether a facial cut will leave a scar or whether a broken shoulder means that they can never ski again.

Because adolescents are often extremely concerned about modesty, they need calm, professional treatment. Always explain what you are doing and why. Have a responder of the same sex conduct the physical assessment, if possible. Sometimes the presence of a peer, parent, or close friend is both physically and emotionally reassuring. Use your judgment, however. If the adolescent feels that he or she has to "play" to a peer, either by being extra brave or flippant, then privacy is more important. You may need to explain that it is all right to react to pain, since you need to know what hurts.

Save examination of the genital area for last. Explain what you are doing in a calm, professional way.

Typical sources of trauma among adolescents are motor vehicle accidents, bicycle accidents, sports injuries, and gunshot wounds.

☐ GENERAL PROCEDURES

With all age groups, follow these procedures:

1. If possible, have only one EMT deal with the child. Introduce yourself. "Hi, My name is Jerry. What's yours? Well, Lucy, I'm trained to help hurt children." Perhaps nothing is emotionally harder than a sick or injured child, but prepare yourself psychologically so that you can radiate confidence, competence, and friendliness. Avoid "baby talk." Remember that you are a stranger. Children between one and six seldom like strangers, especially if their parents are not there.

2. Get as close as possible to the child's eye level. Sit down next to the child if possible.

3. With children under school age, keep instruments inconspicuous at first, do not use instruments when you begin the examination, and keep the most painful parts of the examination for the end.

4. Explain what you are doing in terms they can un-

derstand. Follow up on questions. Speak in a calm, quiet voice and maintain eye contact as much as possible. Even infants will respond to a calm voice, and an apparently unconscious child may actually absorb much of what you say. Never become impatient or lose your temper. Switch off with a partner or take a brief time out if you need to.

5. Involve the parents (or a familiar person) as much as possible during care and transport. If the case involves an automobile accident and injury to parents, it is still less frightening to a child to be with an injured parent than to be separated. Of course, you must make your decision based on the seriousness of the injury and the necessary treatment. If the parent is uninjured, have him handle the instruments to minimize the child's fear.

6. Be honest. "It will hurt when I touch you here, but it will only last a minute. If you feel like crying, it's okay." Children can tolerate pain if they are prepared for it and are given adequate support. Ask children for their help and assure them that they are doing a good job. Some services keep toys, stickers, or other "rewards" to console and encourage a child.

7. Be gentle. Use all appropriate measures to reduce the amount of pain that a child must endure. If you must restrain a child, be sure that it is absolutely necessary, and use only a minimum degree of restraint to be safe and allow you to provide good care.

☐ OBTAINING A MEDICAL HISTORY

In obtaining a history, use the following procedures:

1. If a child has a life-threatening illness or injury, conduct the preliminary survey rapidly and manage serious conditions promptly. If the condition is not life-threatening, take more time to talk with the child, engage interest in your instruments and procedures, and involve the parent in the procedure.

2. Having anxious, upset parents and a screaming child can be unnerving, but do not get rattled, and do not take shortcuts.

3. Interview witnesses if time allows. (See "Taking a History" in Chapter 3, Patient Assessment.) If the case is an illness, ask:

   • When did the symptoms develop?

   • How have they progressed?

   • Have the care/medications already given been effective?

   • When was the last meal?

4. If the case involves injury, also determine:
   - The details of the accident.
   - The mechanism of injury.
   - The time of the accident.
   - Emergency care already given.

☐ VITAL SIGNS FOR CHILDREN

Table 32-1 lists normal pulse, blood pressure, and respiratory rates for children from birth through age ten. Younger children will generally have lower blood pressures, higher pulses, and higher respiratory rates. Each degree centigrade of fever in a child is normally accompanied by a 10 percent increase in pulse and respirations.

Check and record a child's vital signs more frequently than you would an adult's. Pay attention, however, to your subjective impression of the child. Your overall impression of how the child looks and acts can be more important and tell you more about the status of the child than any one vital sign (e.g., the child may be cyanotic, yet still be distracted by toys and cooing).

Children have marvelous compensatory mechanisms that conceal physiological insult for some time. It is only after exhaustion of this mechanism that you may see indicative changes in the vital signs. The changes may then occur very quickly, and the child's condition may deteriorate rapidly.

Always scan the child's skin for signs of injury. If the child seems dehydrated, feel the extremities with the back of your hand. Hands and feet will be cold in case of shock, but warmer closer to the trunk. Also note skin color. Cyanosis is abnormal, except for the mottled color of hands and feet in the newborn.

If capillary refill in a child takes as long as five or six seconds, it is a sign that the blood volume is acutely low.

Respirations

Check respirations by placing your hand on the infant/child's stomach. Children breathe faster than adults, with the range of an infant (sixty-four per minute) to an eight-year-old (twenty-three per minute). The key is to take respiratory rates frequently. An increase over the previous rate may be significant. Also, the quality of breathing (adequate, inadequate, noisy, etc.) is as important as the rate.

Blood Pressure

Be sure that you check the blood pressure with a correct-size cuff; it should cover about two-thirds of the upper arm. A too-wide cuff will give you an erroneously low reading, while a too-narrow cuff will produce an erroneously high reading. If you do not have a pediatric cuff, use an adult-size cuff and take the reading on the thigh. (Take blood pressure only if appropriate equipment is available.)

Because children's vessels constrict so efficiently, the earliest warning signals of shock may be prolonged capillary refill (when you press a nail, then release it) and tachycardia (rapid heartbeat). Losing 10 percent of blood volume will cause an increase in the heart rate by twenty beats per minute. Twenty percent blood loss will increase the heart rate thirty beats per minute.

Pulse

It is very difficult to feel a carotid pulse in infants and toddlers because their necks are short. The most reliable pulse to check is the apical pulse. A child's heart is somewhat higher and more central in the chest than an adult's. Place your stethoscope below the scapula on the left side of the back and count each "lub-dub" as one beat.

To check circulation or to take a pulse more rapidly after the initial reading, use the radial pulse in a child, but the brachial pulse in an infant. If the radial pulse is not clear, check the brachial pulse above the el-

TABLE 32-1
Normal Pulse, Respiration, and Blood Pressure Rates for Children

AGE	WEIGHT Lbs.	WEIGHT Kg.	PULSE ( ) INDICATES AVERAGE	RESPIRATION	BLOOD PRESSURE AVERAGE SYSTOLIC	BLOOD PRESSURE AVERAGE DIASTOLIC
Newborn (1–28 days)	7.4	3.4	94–145 (125)	30–60	80	46
3 Months	12.5	5.7	110–140 (120)	24–35	89	60
6 Months	16.5	7.4	100–140 (120)	24–35	89	60
1 Year	22.0	10.0	98–160 (120)	20–30	89	60
2 Years	27.0	12.4	90–140 (110)	20–30	96	64
3 Years	31.0	14.5	80–120 (100)	20–30	96	70
4 Years	33.6	16.5	65–132 (100)	12–26	96	70
5 Years	41.0	19.0	80–110 (100)	12–26	96–98	70
6 Years	47.0	21.5	75–100 (100)	12–25	96–98	56
10 Years	71.0	32.3	70–110 (90)	12–21	110	60

bow. Feel for the point on the medial side of the humerus, mid-shaft in the groove between the biceps and triceps.

Rapid pulse may be caused by shock, fever, or oxygen deficiency. It may also be normal in scared or overly excited children. Tachycardia (rapid pulse) may be normal considering the circumstances; however, bradycardia (slow pulse) in a child is a worrisome sign.

Slow pulse may be caused by pressure in the skull, depressant drugs, or some comparatively rare medical conditions. Ask the parent what is normal for the child. As you assess the pulse, take note that the farther away from the heart the peripheral pulse can be detected, the better the cardiac output.

Temperature

Children's temperatures are much more important than adult temperatures as warning signals because they can change so quickly. Feeling the toe temperature during the secondary survey will give you a good idea of the infant's cardiac output.

If it is necessary to get an accurate temperature in the field, take it rectally for children under six or for any child who is too disoriented or upset to hold the thermometer safely and consistently under the tongue or in the axillary region. Rectal thermometers are like oral thermometers in degrees marked but usually have a distinguishing knob on the end without the mercury. To take a rectal temperature:

1. Shake down the mercury.
2. Coat the thermometer with a water-based lubricant like K-Y jelly.
3. Turn the child on his side or on the stomach, and insert the thermometer approximately one inch into the recturm.
4. Hold it in place for two to five minutes.

Young children can develop fevers of up to 105°F. (40.6°C.) quickly. Causes of high temperature are infection and heatstroke (from being left in a hot car, for instance). Some pediatric physicians are allowing temperatures to remain elevated at a moderate level for a time. (Follow local protocol).

To lower the body temperature:

1. Give the child fluids by mouth. Follow local protocol.
2. Sponge-bathe the face, hands, feet, etc. or, if necessary, remove the child's clothes and sponge-bathe him or her in tepid (98°F) water. Do not use alcohol — the body will absorb it, and it may cause hypothermia.
3. You may also wrap the child in a wet sheet and use fans.

4. If the child begins shivering, stop the bathing. The body's shivering mechanism will generate more heat than you can dissipate with tepid bathing.

These measures are not particularly helpful for children if the cause of the fever is something besides heatstroke. Rather, treat the cause of the fever.

The two most common results of high fever are dehydration and convulsions. Dehydration is an abnormal loss of fluids and electrolytes. Symptoms include nausea, loss of appetite, vomiting, and possible fainting. A dehydrated child's pulse will be weak and rapid, the skin pale, the eyes sunken, and the tongue shrunken. When you pinch the skin, it will stay "tented." Dehydration in the infant also results in a sunken fontanelle.

To treat dehydration, place the child flat and treat for shock. An IV of normal saline needs to be started as soon as possible by IV-certified (consider calling backup if possible) personnel. Transport the child immediately to a medical facility. However, do not delay transport to have an IV started.

A child under five years may have convulsions if the temperature rises rapidly. See the discussion on convulsions later in this chapter.

Abnormally low temperatures are signs of shock or some other low metabolic state, near-drowning, or exposure. Treat such cases by doing the following:

1. Passively warm the child by removing wet clothes. Wrap in blankets during transport. Skin contact with a warm individual in an emergency situation may be helpful. (Core warming performed in a medical facility is the treatment of choice.)
2. Wrap the child in blankets after the initial warming.

Abdomen

In conducting your physical assessment of the critically ill child, look for signs of trauma, asymmetries, herniae, or marked distention in the abdominal area. Gently palpate. If this causes pain, or if a cooperative child has a rigid abdomen accompanied by tenderness, transport quickly to a hospital.

Also listen to the abdomen with a stethoscope; perforations and obstructions will greatly reduce bowel sounds.

☐ NEUROLOGICAL ASSESSMENT OF CHILDREN

Almost 80 percent of all children with significant trauma suffer neurological injury; it is the cause of death at least two-thirds of the time.

Assessing possible neurological damage in children is similar to the process for adults, but the stimuli must be more simplified (Table 32-2). Check for:

- Level of consciousness — if the child's consciousness seems lowered, check with the parents to see how typical or unusual this response is. You will be able to reconstruct a Glascow Coma Scale later if you check the following:
- Pupils — of equal size? Do they respond to light?
- Check the head, neck, and chest to observe for signs of trauma.
- Response to verbal and/or painful stimuli? Pinch the skin between the child's thumb and forefinger.
- Ability to recognize familiar objects and people?
- Ability to move extremeties purposefully?
- Clear or bloody fluid draining from ears?

Try to classify the child as alert, oriented, or disoriented, and as responsive or unresponsive (the AVPU method). This technique works in the following way:

1. Your patient is alert and oriented if he or she can focus on you and answer these questions. If not, he or she is disoriented:
   - What is your name?
   - What happened to you?
   - Where are you?
2. Your patient is responsive if he or she seems to be unconscious but:
   - Will open his or her eyes if you speak to him or her or will try to answer the question.

TABLE 32-2
Pediatric Coma Score*

Eye Opening:

4 = Spontaneous
3 = To speech
2 = To pain
1 = None

Best Motor Response:

6 = Spontaneous
5 = Localizes pain
4 = Withdraws to pain
3 = Flexion to pain (decorticate)
2 = Extension to pain (decerebrate)
1 = No response

Best Verbal Response:

5 = Oriented/Smiles
4 = Confused/Cries (consolable)
3 = Inappropriate, persistent cry
2 = Incomprehensible/Restless
1 = No response

*The score indicates level of consciousness. A score of 3, describing coma, to a score of 15, describing a fully conscious state.

- Tries to avoid pain. Pinch the skin between the thumb and index finger. If he or she tries to pull the hand away or push you away, the patient is responsive to painful stimuli.
- Displays pupillary response and eye movement.
- Displays muscular strength. Ask the child to "squeeze the ball as hard as you can" or "pretend you're pedaling your bike."
- Has normal reflexes.

If the child is young and/or badly frightened, ask the mother or father to perform the tests under your direction, if possible. Engage a young child in games of "pattycake" or "peekaboo" during the test.

□ TRAUMA

The number-one killer of American children is the automobile. Each year, between 20,000 and 25,000 children die from injuries sustained from automobile accidents. Four times this number are permanently disabled, and a hundred times more are incapacitated for two weeks or longer. Furthermore, these statistics have remained unchanged for three decades. Fifty percent of deaths from trauma occur within the first hour after an accident.

Children may experience trauma while riding bikes, all-terrain vehicles, and motorcycles, even as pedestrians on busy roads and during recreational activities. Basic trauma management in children is the same as for adult basic life support!

1. Establish an airway, and stabilize the cervical spine. Follow all of the basic rules for managing the patient with a head, neck, or spine injury.
2. Make sure that the child is breathing and has a heartbeat. If not, perform artificial ventilation or CPR.
3. Control bleeding.
4. Treat for shock.
5. Immobilize any neurological and musculoskeletal injuries.

Pediatric Field Scoring

A useful tool for rapidly determining the severity of injury in a child is the Pediatric Trauma Score (PTS), devised by J. J. Tepas, M. D., and validated by Diane Threadgill Alred, R.N.[1] Familiarity with and use of this tool will provide a schedule of priorities in evaluating major body systems. It works by assigning a numeric score to each system.

[1] Diane Threadgill Alred, "Pediatric Field Scoring," *Emergency*, October 1987, pp. 18–23. This summary is adapted from her article by permission.

Weight

Other field scoring systems do not take into consideration the differences caused by a child's weight. A toddler struck by a car fender will be injured more severely than a ten-year-old. "Multisystem injury is the rule, rather than the exception."

Size/weight assessed:

- ☐ +2 Heavier than twenty kilograms (forty-four pounds).
- ☐ +1 Between ten and twenty kilograms (twenty-two to forty-four pounds).
- ☐ −1 Less than ten kilograms (twenty-two pounds).

Airway

- ☐ +2 No assistance needed besides being sure that an unconscious child's head does not flex forward on the chest.
- ☐ +1 Constant observation required to maintain the patient's position or open airway. Also if supplemental oxygen is needed.
- ☐ −1 Invasive techniques required, such as endotracheal intubation.

Systolic Blood Pressure

Pressures greater than 90 mmHg are adequate, and pressures of 50 mmHg or less are immediately life-threatening. Children with pressures between these two points may be in hypovolemic shock, but their blood vessels can constrict so efficiently that their blood pressure will not drop until they lose approximately one-fourth of the circulating blood volume. Monitor these in-between children closely.

Circulatory assessment:

- ☐ +2 Systolic blood pressure greater than 90 mmHg.
- ☐ +1 90 to 50 mmHg.
- ☐ −1 Less than 50 mmHg.

If the proper-sized cuff is not available, use this circulatory assessment instead:

- ☐ +2 Pulse palpable at the wrist.
- ☐ +1 Pulse palpable at groin.
- ☐ −1 No pulses palpable.

Central Nervous System

Any child who loses consciousness in any degree as a result of injury may have sustained damage to the central nervous system either from a direct blow or from secondary injuries. Two out of three trauma fatalities in children involve head injury, many of them after the accident as a result of undiagnosed and untreated cerebral damage.

- ☐ +2 Fully alert, no loss of consciousness.
- ☐ +1 Loss of consciousness in any degree for any length of time.
- ☐ −1 Comatose and unresponsive.

Wounds

These include abrasions, burns, lacerations, penetrating injuries, or missile injuries.

- ☐ +2 No wounds.
- ☐ +1 Minor wounds, including abrasions and lacerations.
- ☐ −1 Major open wounds, penetrating wounds, burns, tissue loss, or avulsions.

Fractures

- ☐ +2 No fracture.
- ☐ +1 Simple closed fracture, tibia-fibula.
- ☐ −1 Open fracture(s), multiple fractures.

What the PTS Score Means

With a PTS of 0, the child will certainly die, even though the scores can go as low as −6. A PTS of +6 means that the child has a 30 percent chance of dying, and a PTS of +8 means a 1 percent chance. If the PTS is +8 or lower, rapidly transport the child to a trauma center if one is available. All traumatized children should be transported to a hospital.

☐ SPECIAL SITUATIONS FOR CHILDREN

Most emergencies involving children are managed in the same way as those involving adults. However, the different size and physiological development of children mean that you must treat some emergencies differently.

For instance, blunt trauma is the most common injury in children. Quite frequently, a child will be severely injured but display no early, obvious signs. On accident scenes, try to reconstruct the accident and understand the mechanism of injury. Remember that in a trauma situation, "load-and-go" is better than "stay-and-play" once you have quickly assessed for injuries that could be life-threatening within the next twenty minutes.

When you are treating a child, be aware of the following special conditions and situations:

- Infants have proportionally large tongues. If a tongue relaxes, it can block the airway, which is about one-third the diameter of a dime in a newborn.
- The PASG is not usually recommended for use on a child. It may cause chest compression and reduce the child's ability to breathe. Abdominal compression may cause vomiting and aspiration. Follow local protocol.
- Small children and infants have heads that are large in proportion to their bodies, making head injuries more likely. Pediatric head injuries account for 250,000 hospitalizations and 4,000 deaths annually. Assume cervical damage if a child has an injury above the clavicles, is unconscious, has a mechanism of injury that suggests cervical injury, or has an undefined area of injury. Falls are the most common type of nonfatal injury in young children, and 75 percent of them involve some kind of head injury.
- Because the liver, spleen, and kidneys of children are not as well protected as those of adults, and because they occupy a larger ratio of the abdominal cavity, they are more susceptible to blunt trauma. Children are not as likely as adults to suffer broken ribs but are more likely to have internal chest injuries.
- A child's skin surface is large compared to his or her body mass, making children more susceptible to hypothermia and dehydration.
- Infants younger than nine months cannot yet fully support their own heads. Always support a baby's head when you pick it up.
- Because the fontanelles are not closed on the baby's skull, check them during your assessment. You can see visible pulses at the anterior fontanelle. It will bulge when the baby cries or if there is pressure inside the skull. If the baby is dehydrated, the fontanelle will be depressed.
- Most children involved in trauma will have gastric dilation. Their stomachs will enlarge, pressing up on the left side of the diaphragm until the pressure significantly reduces the amount of air they can breathe. There is a risk of vomiting and potential aspiration.
- Figure a child's blood volume at eighty milliliters per kilogram. A one-year-old child who weighs about ten kilograms (twenty-two pounds) will have an approximate blood volume of 800 milliliters. This means that you must stop bleeding as quickly as possible, since comparatively small blood loss in an adult would constitute a major hemorrhage for a child. Open fractures in children tend to bleed considerably.

- Children's necks are sometimes too short for you to determine accurately if the trachea is deviating from midline.
- In children's lungs, the breathing sound from the "good" lung can easily be confused as sound coming from the collapsed lung.
- Sixty-four percent of bicycle-related deaths in the United States involve children; nearly 90 percent involve motor vehicles, and 50 percent of them occur between Friday afternoon and Sunday evening. Head and neck injuries are involved in three-fifths of all pediatric hospital admissions for bicycle-related injuries.
- In very rare cases, prolonged days of high concentrations of oxygen administered to premature babies soon after birth may permanently damage the **retinal vessels** inside the eyeball, damaging the eyesight. However, this condition occurs from oxygen in the bloodstream, not from oxygen contacting the cornea. Furthermore, older infants and children are not susceptible to this danger in the same way. You need not be afraid to administer oxygen, even to a baby, when it is needed. A "blue" child is not being oxygenated. Give enough oxygen to keep the lips and mucous membranes pink.
- Children often get arms, legs, hands, feet, or heads trapped under or in rigid structures. The child is sometimes in pain and is almost certainly panicky. Calm him or her first and see if he or she can extricate himself by moving slowly. Lubricate skin surfaces if helpful, and slowly saw or cut away obstructions if necessary. Check for abraded skin and lacerations.
- In car accidents involving children, suspect blunt trauma to the abdomen if the child was wearing a lap-belt only.

☐ COMMON PEDIATRIC EMERGENCIES

Respiratory Emergencies

The National Pediatric Trauma Registry has reported that 30 percent of all pediatric trauma deaths are related to inappropriate airway management. According to the American Heart Association, more than 90 percent of deaths from foreign-body aspiration among children occur in children under five; 65 percent occur in infants. Yet an estimated 96 percent of cases of asphyxia associated with trauma could be saved by earlier identification. Furthermore, respiratory disease is the primary cause of all pediatric deaths from cardiopulmonary arrest not associated with trauma.

When attempting to clear the airway in infants and small children, place the airway in a neutral position. *Caution:* hyperextention may reduce the effective size of the airway in an infant.

Take respiration rates frequently; an increase may be significant. Respiration rates in children alter easily from emotional and physiological reasons, so one respiration count is not sufficient. Respiratory distress, even if the airway is intact, will exhaust the child rapidly, and you will need to work fast to save him or her. The following are some dangerous conditions.

Rapid Breathing

In cases of rapid breathing (tachypnea), look for breathing through the mouth, flaring of the nostrils, and/or using the chest muscles excessively. Also check for bluish lips and emotional distress like apprehensiveness and irritability.

Possible causes of rapid breathing are:

- Fever, which raises the metabolic rate, increasing the need for oxygen. Each degree of fever increases the respiratory rate by about four breaths per minute.
- Diabetes.
- Oxygen deficiency.
- Aspirin overdose and other forms of poisoning.
- Head injury.
- Stress or fear.

Noisy Breathing

Children normally breathe more loudly than adults because of anatomical differences. Children under five frequently have "rattling" breath sounds. Check with a parent if you hear an unusual sound to determine whether it is normal.

The following is a checklist of sounds characteristically produced by problems (Figure 32-5):

- Coughing, gagging, or gasping will be violent when the child breathes in a foreign body or bodily secretions.
- Rales — fine, crackling sounds that resemble the noise of rolling a few strands of hair near the ear — are commonly heard in **bronchiolitis** and pneumonia.
- Wheezes, caused by air moving at a high rate through restricted passages, are more "musical" than rales and may sometimes be a whistle. If you hear wheezes on inhalation, the child probably has a partial obstruction high in the airway. If you hear them on exhalation, they may signify a partial obstruction in the lower airway, asthma, or bronchiolitis. Wheezing sounds are caused by

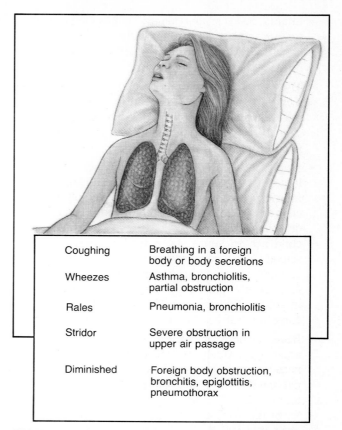

Coughing	Breathing in a foreign body or body secretions
Wheezes	Asthma, bronchiolitis, partial obstruction
Rales	Pneumonia, bronchiolitis
Stridor	Severe obstruction in upper air passage
Diminished	Foreign body obstruction, bronchitis, epiglottitis, pneumothorax

FIGURE 32-5 Sounds indicating breathing difficulties in a child.

asthmatic bronchospasm or inhalation of blood, vomitus, stroke, or foreign objects.

- Stridor — a harsh, high-pitched sound that occurs typically during inspiration — results from severe obstruction in the upper air passage, as in the case of laryngeal edema. Because stridor occurs only with upper airway problems, if it is absent, the cause of the emergency is more likely bronchiolitis, asthma, pneumonia, or a foreign body.

Diminished Breathing

The causes of diminished breathing can include obstruction, pneumonia, bronchiolitis, epiglottitis, and pneumothorax. If the upper airway is obstructed, the breathing will sound croupy.

Obstructed Airway

Children are more susceptible to respiratory problems than adults because they have smaller air passages and less reserve air capacity. An infant or young child's trachea is held open by soft cartilage, which means that hyperextension of the neck can make the trachea collapse, closing the windpipe. Also, because the tongue is proportionately large, it can shift backward and block the airway.

Correct either of these problems in an older child

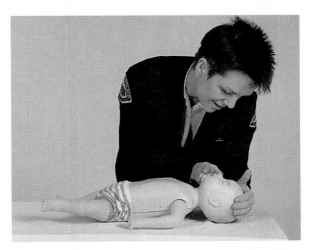

FIGURE 32-6 Airway obstruction may be relieved in an infant or small child by keeping the head in neutral position, not hyperextended.

by rolling the child on his or her side, lifting the shoulders, and placing a rolled towel under them so that the nose is elevated in the "sniffing" position. In a toddler or infant, airway obstruction may be relieved by keeping the neck straight, placing your hand on the forehead, and putting the finger of your other hand just under the infant's chin (Figure 32-6).

In caring for an obstructed airway, follow the procedure discussed in Chapter 4. (Figure 32-7)

Croup

Infectious croup is a common infection of the upper airway, usually caused by a virus, but sometimes by bacteria. It is most common in children between one and five years of age.

The infection causes swelling beneath the glottis and progressively narrows the airway (Figure 32-9). Inhalation produces a peculiar whooping sound, or stridor; high-pitched squeaking sounds may also be present. The child is typically hoarse and frequently coughs with a harsh "seal bark." As the condition worsens, further obstructing the airway, you will see the classic signs of respiratory distress: nasal flaring, tugging at the throat, retraction of muscles around the rib cage, restlessness, a rising pulse rate, and bluish coloring. About 10 percent of children with infectious croup require hospitalization.

Infectious croup may be confused with spasmodic croup. In spasmodic croup, the child is typically recuperating from a cold or other infection, and he or she appears fairly well during the day except for hoarseness. After going to bed, however, he develops a harsh, metallic cough. After a few hours, it becomes an alarming, barking sound. The child insists on sitting up, struggling for breath. In any event, consult medical command and transport.

Severe attacks can be dangerous and should be treated by:

1. Giving humidified oxygen by a mask held slightly

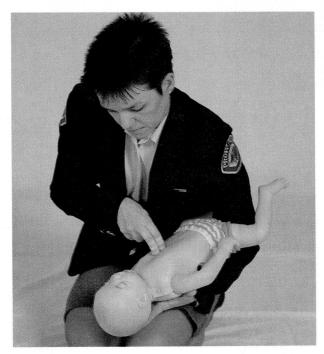

FIGURE 32-7 Expel a foreign body in an infant with complete airway obstruciton by positioning the infant as shown and applying four chest thrusts.

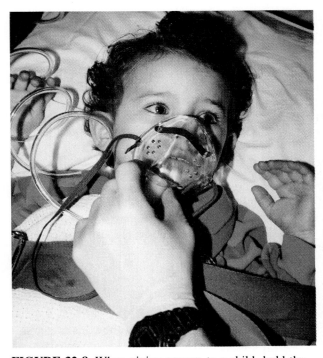

FIGURE 32-8 When giving oxygen to a child, hold the mask slightly away from the child's face instead of placing it right on the face. The mask giving high flow oxygen will enrich the air the child breathes in.

away from the child's face, *not* placed over the mouth. (Figure 32-8)

2. Keeping the patient in a comfortable position, either propped up or in a parent's arms.

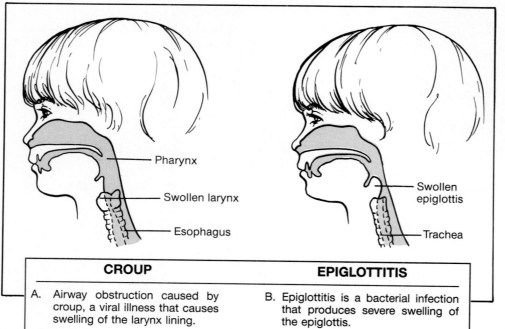

CROUP	EPIGLOTTITIS
A. Airway obstruction caused by croup, a viral illness that causes swelling of the larynx lining.	B. Epiglottitis is a bacterial infection that produces severe swelling of the epiglottis.

FIGURE 32-9

3. Transporting him or her to the hospital with as little disturbance as possible.

Be aware that cool night air will nearly always shrink the swollen membranes, bringing relief. You may need to explain original signs to emergency department personnel if the child appears much better after transport.

Epiglottitis

Epiglottitis is caused by a bacterial infection that inflames the epiglottis and causes it to swell. The condition looks much like croup (see Figure 32-9). Epiglottitis is life-threatening; if left untreated, it has a 50 percent mortality rate.

Signs of epiglottitis are:

- Pain on swallowing.
- High fever (102 to 104°F., 38.9 to 40°C.)
- Drooling (the patient cannot swallow his or her saliva).
- Mouth breathing.
- Changes in voice quality.
- The patient insists on sitting up and leaning forward.
- The patient's chin is thrust outward.
- The child is usually not hoarse and does not struggle to breathe, although there may be a short "croak" during inhalation.

- Speaking is painful.
- As the attack worsens, the patient may appear strikingly still.

The major signs of epiglottitis can be remembered by the three Ds:

1. Drooling.
2. Dysphasia (difficulty in speaking).
3. Difficulty in swallowing.

If you suspect epiglottitis, be calm and gentle. Do *not* attempt to place an oropharyngeal ariway, as it can cause laryngospasm. Try to keep the child relaxed while you prepare him or her for transport, but take him or her directly and with all possible speed to an emergency room. Keep him upright during transport.

Do not try to examine the child's throat, make him or her lie down, suction the throat, or put an oxygen mask on him or her that uses cold, moist air at a high rate. If the child chokes or coughs from any of these irritations or from anxiety, the larynx may spasm, completely blocking the airway. At this point, only a direct airway into the trachea will prevent death.

Provide oxygen if possible. Let the child hold the mask, or turn it on full and hold it a few inches away from the child's face. Be careful that it does not cause irritation or coughing.

For more information in comparing croup and epiglottitis, see Table 32-3.

TABLE 32-3
Comparison Chart for Epiglottitis and Croup

VARIABLE	CROUP	EPIGLOTTITIS*
Age	Any age (peak, 2 to 5 yr)	6 mo to 3 yr
Season	None	Fall/winter
Time of day	Throughout the day	Night/early am
Cause	*Haemophilus influenzae*	Virus
Clinical		
Onset	Rapid	Insidious
Fever	High	<103°F.
Toxic	Yes	No
Sore throat	Yes	Variable
Drooling	Yes	Yes
Stridor	Inspiratory	Inspiratory/expiratory
Position	Sitting	Variable
Epiglottis	Cherry red epiglottis	Normal epiglottis

*In adults, epiglottitis commonly presents as the "worst sore throat of the patient's life" and less commonly accompanies stridor.

Asthma

Asthma is common in children, particularly those with allergies. Every asthmatic attack should be regarded as a serious medical emergency.

Acute asthmatic attack occurs when the bronchioles spasm and constrict, causing the bronchial membranes to swell and congest. Thick mucus blocks the airways, interfering especially with exhalation. As a result, air is trapped in the lungs at the end of each exhalation, the chest becomes overly inflated, breathing becomes increasingly impaired, oxygen deficiency causes more distress to the child, and dehydration makes the mucous plugs thicker. This vicious cycle must be broken to reverse the process.

Get the patient's history from the parents:

- How long has the child been wheezing?
- How much fluid has he taken during this period?
- Has he had a recent cold or other infection, particularly one involving the respiratory tract?
- Has he had any medication for this attack? What is it? When? How much? It is especially important to ask about inhalant medications.
- Does he have any known allergies to drugs, foods, pollens, or other inhalants?
- Has he ever been hospitalized for an acute asthmatic attack? How recently? How often?

During the physical assessment, pay particular attention to:

- General appearance. How distressed does the patient appear to be? What is his physical position? Children with mild attacks often appear agitated and prefer to sit but will lie. Children with severe attacks seem exhausted and unable to move. Frequently they prefer to lean forward, bracing themselves on their elbows. Children under the age of two often show no agitation and will lie on their backs, even when this increases their difficulty in breathing. They may be blue from lack of oxygen but will still smile and be distracted by toys and cooing. They may also breathe quickly and shallowly — between sixty and eighty respirations per minute.
- Level of consciousness. Sleepiness, and changes in level of consciousness are progressively more serious signs of oxygen deficiency and acidosis (retention of carbon dioxide).
- Vital signs. As an attack worsens, the pulse grows faster and weaker. Blood pressure may fall. Cardiac arrhythmias are an ominous sign.
- Skin and mucous membranes. Pinch the skin to look for evidence of dehydration ("tenting"). Check the lips and nailbeds for bluishness, indicating insufficient oxygen.
- Respiration. Even deep chest movements do not indicate that the child is getting enough oxygen. Listen for rales and wheezes. A mild to moderate attack is characterized by loud breathing sounds, loud wheezes and occasional rales. As the attack worsens, the breath sounds become less audible and are completely absent in a severe attack. Listen to the entire chest. Localized wheezes suggest a foreign obstruction; asthma causes generalized wheezes.

Treat asthma attacks by giving the child fluids and humidified oxygen by mask. Allow the child to assume a position of most comfort. Usually, you will need to transport the patient for further care. Because of the emotional component of asthma, try to be as calm and reassuring as possible. A severe attack that cannot be broken with medication is called status asthmaticus and is extremely serious. Consider paramedic back-up, if possible.

Bronchiolitis

Bronchiolitis is easily confused with asthma but is caused when the bronchioles (small bronchi) in the lungs become inflamed after viral infections. During exhalations, the child will wheeze loudly and have other signs similar to those of asthma. Usually, however, age can be a clue. Children under one almost never have asthma; children over two almost never have bronchiolitis.

Collect the same history and perform the same assessment that you would for asthma. For treatment:

1. Give humidified oxygen by mask, and assist breathing as necessary.

2. Let the child semi-sit with his or her neck slightly extended if this position is more comfortable.

3. Monitor the pulse rate while you transport the child to the hospital.

Cardiac Arrest

If your patient is a child with no heartbeat, he or she may be experiencing **ventricular standstill** or **ventricular fibrillation.** The most frequent causes of ventricular standstill are severe croup, aspiration of a foreign body, or drowning. The most common causes of ventricular fibrillation are electrical shock or drowning. Other causes of cardiac arrest in children are severe blood loss, allergic reactions that produce anaphylactic shock, or congenital heart or lung disease.

Ninety-five percent of cardiac arrests in children come from airway obstruction and respiratory arrest; the other 5 percent are caused by shock. It is extremely important to prevent both conditions before they become established and to provide breathing assistance.

As with all cases of cardiac arrest, call for help if you are alone and follow protocols for speed, orderly direction, cooperative efforts, and continuous monitoring. Your goal must be to keep the brain alive. Unless too much time has elapsed between the arrest and artificial ventilation, the child can be neurologically normal, even following comparatively long periods of arrest.

Signs of cardiac arrest in a child are (Figure 32-10):

- Unresponsiveness.
- Convulsions.
- Gasping or no respiratory sounds.
- No audible heart sounds.
- Chest is not moving.
- Pale or blue skin.

- Absent brachial pulse.
- Muscle contractions.

For CPR techniques and emergency care, see Chapter 6.

Convulsions

Convulsions may be caused by any condition that would also produce seizures in adults: head injury, meningitis, oxygen deficiency, drug overdose, and hypoglycemia. Adults seldom have convulsions caused by fever, but children may. The risk of convulsions is high among children up to age two but decreases in children up to age six. Approximately 5 percent of children have febrile convulsions. Although these childhood convulsions are frightening, they generally leave no adverse permanent effects.

During the seizure, the child's arms and legs become rigid, the back arches, the muscles may twitch or jerk in spasm, the eyes roll up and become fixed, the pupils dilate, and the breathing is often irregular or ineffective; the patient may lose bladder and bowel control, and he or she is completely unresponsive. If the seizure lasts long enough, the skin will turn blue. The spasms will prevent the child from swallowing, and he or she will push the saliva out of the mouth. Saliva is more copious during the seizure as well. The patient will appear to be frothing at the mouth. If saliva is trapped in the throat, the child will make bubbling or gurgling sounds.

In obtaining the history, ask:

- Has the child had seizures before? How often? Have they always been associated with fever, or do they occur when he or she is well? Did others in the family have convulsions as children. (Febrile convulsions seem to occur frequently in families.)
- How many seizures has the child had within the

FIGURE 32-10

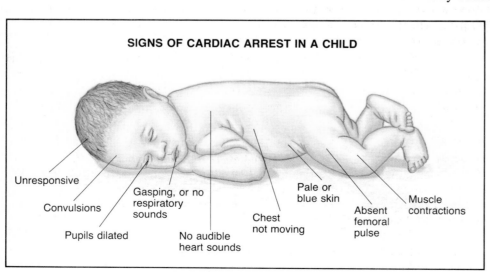

SIGNS OF CARDIAC ARREST IN A CHILD

Unresponsive

Convulsions

Pupils dilated

Gasping, or no respiratory sounds

No audible heart sounds

Chest not moving

Pale or blue skin

Absent femoral pulse

Muscle contractions

last twenty-four hours, and what was done for them?

- Has the child had a head injury, a stiff neck, or a recent headache? Does he or she have diabetes?
- Is the child taking any medications?
- What did the seizure look like? Did it start in one part of the body and progress? Did the eyes go in different directions? If yes, which directions?

A simple convulsion is self-limiting, ends within fifteen minutes, and most often within two or three minutes, is grand mal (all muscles involved) in nature, and does not recur. If the child has a single convulsion, all you need to do is maintain an airway and be sure that he or she does not injure himself. Transport as soon as possible after the single seizure.

Emergency care for childhood convulsions is:

1. Examine the child for state of consciousness, evidence of fever or dehydration, and signs of injury. Pay particular attention to the neurologic examination or those portions that you can conduct.

2. During a seizure, the tongue may relax and shift backward, decreasing the size of the air passage. To prevent this, turn the child onto his or her side. This will also help prevent aspiration of fluids if he or she has mucus or is frothing.

3. During the jerky spasm, do not hold the child down, but place the child where he or she will not fall or strike something. A crib with padded sides is excellent; so is a rug on the floor. If a bed does not have sides, watch to make sure that he or she does not fall off.

4. Loosen any clothing that is tight and restricting.

5. If periods of slow or absent breathing occur during a single convulsion, suction the airway, administer oxygen, and assist ventilations with a bag-valve-mask. Most deaths from seizures are due to oxygen starvation.

6. If the child is feverish, sponge him or her with lukewarm water (98°F).

In complex febrile convulsions, usually one part of the body is more strongly affected than others. These convulsions last longer than fifteen minutes and may recur without a recovery period (status eilepticus). *This condition is a true medical emergency.* Give a child oxygen during a prolonged seizure; he or she is at risk for severe combined metabolic and respiratory acidosis. Transport him to the hospital, paying particular attention to maintaining the airway and protecting the patient from injury. Consider paramedic backup en route.

Shock

Severe shock in children is unusual because their blood vessels constrict so efficiently. However, when blood pressure drops, it will drop so far and so fast that the child may go into cardiac arrest. Monitor blood pressure often, visually checking also for collapsed neck veins.

The major causes of shock in children are blood loss, acute infection **(sepsis),** and heart failure. These conditions are most commonly caused by major trauma — being hit by a car, or extensive burns.

Newborns will go into shock due to loss of body heat. They cannot shiver or warm themselves through activity (apparent shivering is really due to hypoglycemia), and their surface area is large in relation to their body weight. Be sure to keep infants warm during transport. Preheat an **incubator** or your ambulance to at least 80°F. (27°C.) for full-term babies. Preheat it to 85°F. (30°C.) for premature babies. If you have no incubator, wrap the baby in warm blankets (prewarmed, if possible), then aluminum foil to preserve body heat. Be sure that the baby's head (but not face) is covered.

Remember that all children are more susceptible to hypothermia from shock or blood loss than adults because of their smaller body size. Be sure that they are in a heated environment, that you use thermal or space blankets, that the oxygen in the mask is warmed with a heated nebulizer, that all IV fluids are warmed if used, and that you use hot packs on the trunk, head, and extremities (use caution to prevent burns).

Signs and symptoms of shock in children are pallor, coldness, sweatiness, low blood pressure, a rapid, thready pulse, lack of vitality, extreme anxiety, or unconsciousness (Figure 32-11).

To provide emergency care for shock:

1. Have the child lie flat.
2. Keep him or her warm and as calm as possible.
3. Monitor his or her vital signs often, especially breathing and heart function.
4. Provide additional oxygen when indicated.
5. Transport to a medical facility.

Infectious Diseases

Meningitis

In meningitis, the lining of the brain and spinal cord are infected from either bacteria or viruses. These infections can be fatal rapidly, so they must be assessed promptly and treated appropriately. Some protocols suggest that each case of documented fever in a child younger than three months should be considered meningitis until proven otherwise.

Signs of meningitis in children include recent ear or respiratory tract infection, high fever, lethargy, irritability, a severe headache, or a stiff neck. Infants generally do not have stiff necks but are lethargic and will not eat. The fontanelle may be bulging unless the child is dehydrated. Movement is painful.

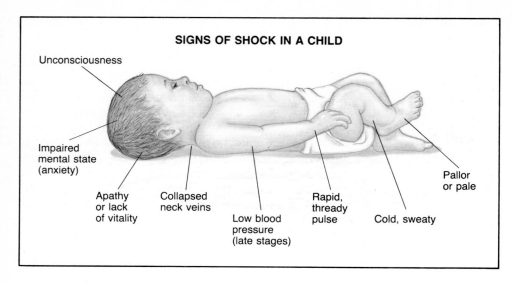

SIGNS OF SHOCK IN A CHILD

Unconsciousness

Impaired
mental state
(anxiety)

Apathy
or lack
of vitality

Collapsed
neck veins

Low blood
pressure
(late stages)

Rapid,
thready
pulse

Cold, sweaty

Pallor
or pale

FIGURE 32-11

If you suspect meningitis, you should complete the assessment rapidly and transport to the hospital. If the child is in shock, treat with oxygen and intravenous fluids.

Septicemia

Septicemia is a systemic infection (usually bacterial) in the bloodstream. It is usually serious, since it can rapidly develop into septic shock. Signs include a focus of infection (pneumonia, ear infections, or an infected wound), illness, fever, lethargy, irritability, or shock. Infants' fontanelles are usually flat.

You should administer supplemental oxygen, and anticipate shock.

Reye's Syndrome

The cause of Reye's syndrome is not clear, but it occurs among children between the ages of five and fifteen, with younger children being at higher risk, more frequently in the fall and winter, and less frequently in urban children after the age of one. Often cases will be associated with influenza B, chicken pox, the use of aspirin, and gastroenteritis in infants.

It cannot be diagnosed in the field but should be considered a serious disease and can result in death. Complications include respiratory failure, cardiac arrhythmias, and acute pancreatitis.

Pay particular attention to the respiratory system during assessment, and transport rapidly while administering supplemental oxygen if necessary. Use support ventilation if necessary.

Sudden Infant Death Syndrome

Sudden infant death syndrome (SIDS) is defined as the sudden and unexpected death of an infant or young child in which an **autopsy** fails to identify the cause of death. SIDS is a post-mortem diagnosis, *not* one that can be made in the field. While the facts behind SIDS will be outlined here, do not make a firm diagnosis to family members; you can only guess about the cause of death based on the evidence you see.

What is SIDS?

SIDS, commonly known as crib death or cot death, is the number-one cause of death among infants between one month and one year of age. About 6,500 babies die of SIDS every year in the United States (two per 1,000 live births). It occurs in both poor and wealthy neighborhoods and in both urban and rural communities.

SIDS cannot be predicted or prevented. It almost always occurs while the baby is sleeping. The typical SIDS case involves an apparently healthy infant, frequently born premature, and usually between the ages of four weeks and seven months, who suddenly dies overnight in his or her crib. No illness has been present, though the baby may have had recent cold symptoms. There is usually no indication of struggle. Sometimes, though, the child has obviously changed position at the time of death.

There is much confusion about SIDS among both the general public and the medical profession. Not until recently has serious medical research on SIDS been conducted. However, its exact cause is still unknown. One of the hypotheses generally accepted by physicians is that death in SIDS victims occurs as the result of a complete upper airway obstruction. The death, which takes place suddenly, is not believed to cause pain or suffering. Another theory is that, due to incomplete development of the respiratory center in the medulla, a SIDS child may simply "forget" to breathe (Figure 32-12).

The *only* way in which SIDS can be conclusively diagnosed is by autopsy. Diagnosis is made by exclusion; that is, the autopsy reveals no evidence of a rapidly fatal infectious disease, such as pneumonia or meningi-

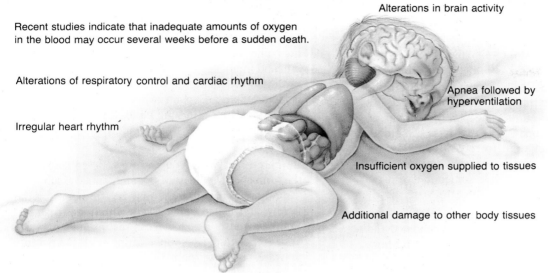

CAUSES OF SUDDEN INFANT DEATH

Recent studies indicate that inadequate amounts of oxygen in the blood may occur several weeks before a sudden death.

Alterations in brain activity

Alterations of respiratory control and cardiac rhythm

Apnea followed by hyperventilation

Irregular heart rhythm

Insufficient oxygen supplied to tissues

Additional damage to other body tissues

FIGURE 32-12

tis, or a previously unsuspected abnormality. Knowledge about the cause of death obtained from a thorough autopsy can ease the family's concern and intense guilt feelings.

What SIDS Is Not

- SIDS is not caused by external suffocation. It is not uncommon for victims to be found wedged into the corner of their cribs or with their heads covered by blankets. Under such circumstances, it is natural to assume that the baby smothered. However, SIDS also occurs under conditions when there is no possibility of suffocation.

- SIDS is not caused by vomiting and choking. Sometimes milk or blood-tinged froth is found around the mouth or in the bedding. This usually occurs after death.

- SIDS is not contagious. One twin may succumb to SIDS, while the other remains healthy. SIDS is less common after the first year of life, so older children and adults are not at risk. The common viruses that seem to be associated with SIDS do not survive outside of living bodies.

- SIDS does not cause pain or suffering to the infant. SIDS can occur within five minutes and is probably instantaneous. Its victims do not cry out and often do not show any trace of having been disturbed in their sleep.

- SIDS cannot be predicted, even if the baby saw a doctor the day of the event.

Managing the SIDS Situation

Do the following in a SIDS emergency:

1. If the child is obviously dead, immediately initiate resuscitative efforts. Begin infant CPR, and continue it during transport; determine whether parents made any first-aid efforts. (Follow local protocol.)

2. A child may display the obvious characteristics of death (such as rigor mortis); under normal circumstances, you would be required to leave the body undisturbed and contact proper authorities. A SIDS case, however, is not "normal." The extreme emotional condition of the parents makes them your patients as much as the infant, and the best way to "treat" them is to make them feel that something was done. Many parents cling to the hope that their infant is not dead and that he can be resuscitated, even when death is apparent. By starting CPR on the obviously dead baby, you at least allow the family to have the memory that professional intervention was attempted. Leave no room for "if"s and "maybe"s. *Follow local protocol.*

3. Obtain a brief medical history of the infant, including:

- Physical appearance of the baby.
- Position of the baby in the crib.
- Physical appearance of the crib.
- Presence of objects in the crib.
- Unusual or dangerous items in the room (such as plastic bags).
- Appearance of the room/house.
- Presence of medication, even if it is for adults.
- Behavior of persons present.
- Circumstances concerning discovery of the unresponsive child.
- Time the baby was put to bed or fell asleep.

- Problems at birth.
- General health.
- Any recent illnesses.
- Date and results of last physical exam.

4. Encourage the parents to talk and tell their story.

5. When the time comes to transport the infant to the hospital, make sure that you tell the parents where you are taking the child. The parents should be encouraged to accompany their baby in the ambulance; if they do not want to, give them clear directions regarding where you are taking their baby. Encourage them to have someone else drive them, and remind them to arrange for care of any siblings.

6. Once you deliver the baby into the hands of the emergency department staff, there is nothing more you can do for him or her. Your attention is now turned to your other "patients" — the family of the SIDS victim.

Aiding Family Members in SIDS Emergencies

The reactions of family members to the SIDS incident will be varied. Many factors can affect these reactions: the situation of the child's death, the meaning that the child had to the individual, the marriage relationship, or the cultural background. You must not misinterpret or read into these reactions.

One of the most common immediate reactions of parents to SIDS is shock and disbelief. This may cause family members to become immobilized — incapable of making decisions. Or this may cause them to act as if they are cold and unfeeling. It is not that they do not care, just that they are having a hard time facing reality.

It will be difficult for you to deal with extreme reactions. Some parents may physically act out their emotions, resulting in hysteria, crying, or wailing. Parents may be confused and overwhelmed with guilt feelings, unfairly venting their anger and frustration on you. When anger is aimed at you, or perhaps your professional capabilities are questioned, your natural tendency is to retaliate with your own angry remarks, which only compounds the problems.

All too often, EMTs are quick to dismiss the parents because they are not their patients in the traditional sense of the word. You tend to ignore the mother's barrage of questions concerning her child and politely tell her to go away. You are there to deliver medical care in an emergency situation, not to get "involved." Do not become personally involved, but understand that these parents and family members need your care also. Their need may not be as obvious to you as an open wound, but the hurt is there and is very real. If left untreated, it may scar or never heal at all.

How can you help the SIDS survivors in this difficult situation?

1. First, you must be in command of your own feelings and behavior at all times. Act in a calm, efficient manner, exhibiting kind concern. While in the home, make the parents feel that something is being done. Explain what you are doing and where you are taking the child. Take command of the situation and try to keep the parents informed of the child's status (Figure 32-13).

2. Be careful of what you say to your colleagues at the hospital. Casual comments such as "smothered" or "injured" may be overheard by the family and cause unnecessary emotional distress. Small, often nonverbal, gestures on your part are very important. By simply sitting with the parents you are showing them that someone cares. Offer to be of assistance to them — to make phone calls or to get them coffee. A sympathetic ear may be all these parents need.

3. Be careful not to "diagnose" the child's problem or to speculate on the outcome. Let all medical information come from the emergency room physician. If you have any questions or comments, or wish confirmation that the child is a SIDS victim, discuss these matters privately with emergency room personnel. If SIDS is indicated by the emergency physician as the cause of death, you could explain to the parents about the syndrome. Help to reassure them that they are in no way responsible for the death. Your time with the family may be

FIGURE 32-13 While in the home of a SIDS victim, make the parents feel that something is being done. Explain what you are doing and where you are taking the child.

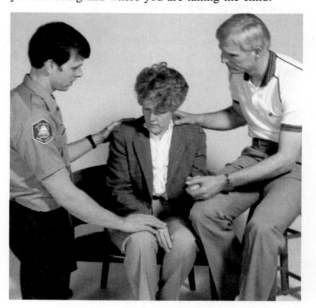

brief, but it can greatly influence their recovery. Communication with the parents concerning their SIDS baby is often done by ER personnel or the hospital chaplain.

It is very common for rescuers to experience emotional turmoil after a SIDS call. Ignoring emotions like anxiety, guilt, or anger will not cause them to go away and may have a serious negative impact on your own mental health.

A debriefing session after a SIDS case by a professional is very helpful. You should talk out your feelings with colleagues, spouses, etc., and *not* hold them inside.

Child Abuse and Neglect

Estimates of the children who are abused and/or neglected annually in the United States range between 500,000 and 4 million; between 2,000 and 4,000 die each year as the result of physical abuse. In fact, homicide by child abuse has been the only major cause of pediatric death to increase in the last thirty years. An estimated 10 percent of the children under age five treated in emergency departments for injuries are victims of physical abuse. The proportion of severe and fatal injuries has been going up in recent years, increasingly at the hands of unrelated male companions of the child's mother.

The adult (usually a parent) who abuses a child often behaves in an evasive manner, volunteering little information or giving contradictory information about what happened to the child. The parent may show outright hostility toward the child or toward the other parent and rarely shows any guilt.

Regardless of the behavior of the parent, certain circumstances should evoke suspicion that a child has been abused.

Identifying Abuse

Abuse may be physical, emotional, sexual, or may fall under the category of neglect. Each type of abuse has distinct characteristics — physical and behavioral indicators — that may allow you to identify the child as an abuse victim.

Be aware of the risk patterns: The classic at-risk groups are boys, blacks, and urban children, although the higher percentages may result from tracking these three groups more closely. Premature infants or twins are at higher risk. Children under five are at higher risk than older children; children between birth and age five sustain a disproportionately high percentage — 74 percent — of fatal injuries. Handicapped, developmentally delayed, uncommunicative (that is, autistic), or "disappointing" (wrong gender, wrong looks) children are also at higher risk.

When sexual abuse is involved, stepdaughters are six times more likely to be abused by stepfathers than by biological fathers and are also at risk from other male companions of their mothers. Men are responsible for 95 percent of the sexual abuse of girls and 80 percent of the sexual abuse of boys.

See Table 32-4, "Physical and Behavioral Indicators of Child Abuse and Neglect," for specific information.

In many cases, a child will be victim of a combination of physical, emotional, and sexual abuse and neglect. While Table 32-4 spells out specifics, you should generally look for abrasions, lacerations, incisions, bruises, broken bones, multiple injuries in various stages of healing, injuries on both the front and back or on both sides of the child, unusual wounds (such as circular burns), a fearful child, or a child who has injuries to the head, back, and abdomen, including the genitals (Figures 32-14–32-19). Especially look for situations where the injuries do not match the mechanism of injury described by the parents or the patient.

Bruises that are true accidents are often found on the lower arms, knees, shins, iliac crests, forehead, and under the chin. "Suspicious" bruises are found on the buttocks, genitalia, thighs, ears, side of face, trunk, and upper arms. The presence of multiple bruises in various stages of healing suggests abuse.

Emergency Care for Child Abuse

While emergency care is a complicated psychological process, you should be familiar with some immediate steps that can be taken promptly upon being called to a possible abuse situation.[2] The following guidelines assume that a parent is the abuser — remember that a child may also be abused by a stepparent, grandparent, babysitter, sibling, or neighbor.

1. Gain entry to the home and access to the child. If the parents placed the emergency call you can probably accomplish this without difficulty. If the call came from outside the family, the parents may resist, and entry should be handled by the police. If you are asked to help the child, calm the parents and suggest by your actions that you are there to help and render emergency care to the child. Tell them that if the child does happen to be injured, from whatever cause, you are prepared to help with the injuries. Speak in a low, firm voice.

2. Focus attention on the child while you administer emergency care. Speak softly to the child. Call the child by his or her first name. *Do not* ask the child

---

[2] H. L. P. Resnick et al., *Emergency Psychiatric Care — The Management of Mental Health Crises* (Bowie, Md: The Charles Press Publishers, 1975), pp. 135–37.

TYPE OF ABUSE/NEGLECT	PHYSICAL INDICATORS	BEHAVIORAL INDICATORS
PHYSICAL ABUSE	Unexplained Bruises and Welts: • on face, lips, mouth • on torso, back, buttocks, thighs • in various stages of healing • clustered, forming regular patterns • reflecting shape of article used to inflict (electric cord, belt buckle) • on several different surface areas • regularly appear after absence, weekend, or vacation • especially about the trunk & buttocks • be particularly suspicious if there are old bruises in addition to fresh ones Unexplained Burns: • cigar, cigarette burns, especially on soles, palms, back or buttocks • immersion burns (sock-like, glove-like doughnut shaped on buttocks or genitalia) • patterned like electric burner, iron, etc. • rope burns on arms, legs, neck or torso Unexplained Fractures (particularly if multiple): • to skull, nose, facial structure • in various stages of healing • multiple or **spiral fractures** Unexplained Lacerations or Abrasions: • to mouth, lips, gums, eyes • to external genitalia	Wary of adult contacts Apprehensive when other children cry Behavioral extremes: • aggressiveness, or • withdrawal Frightened of parents Afraid to go home Reports injury by parents The child who is apathetic who *may not* cry despite his or her injuries The child who has been seen by emergency personnel recently for related complaints The child whose injury occurred several days before you were called
PHYSICAL NEGLECT	Consistent hunger, poor hygiene, inappropriate dress Consistent lack of supervision, especially in dangerous activites or for long periods Unattached physical problems or medical needs Abandonment	Begging, stealing food Extended stays at school (early arrival and late departure) Constant fatigue, listlessness, or falling asleep in class Alcohol or drug abuse Delinquency (e.g., thefts) States there is no caretaker
SEXUAL ABUSE	Difficulty in walking or sitting Torn, stained, or bloody underclothing Pain or itching in genital area Bruises or bleeding in external genitalia, vaginal, or anal areas Venereal disease, especially in pre-teens Pregnancy	Unwilling to change for gym or participate in Physical Education class Withdrawal, fantasy, or infantile behavior Bizarre, sophisticated, or unusual sexual behavior or knowledge Poor peer relationships Delinquent or run-away Reports sexual assault by caretaker
EMOTIONAL MALTREATMENT	Speech disorders Lags in physical development Failure-to-thrive	Habit disorders (sucking, biting, rocking, etc.) Conduct disorders (antisocial, destructive, etc.) Neurotic traits (sleep disorders, inhibition of play) Psychoneurotic reactions (hysteria, obsession, compulsion, phobias, hypochondria) Behavior extremes: • complaiant, passive • aggressive, demanding Overly adaptive behavior: • inappropriately adult • inappropriately infant Developmental lags (mental, emotional) Attempted suicide

> **NOTE: Much of the above will not be obvious in the field—but the information can help you understand what may have precipitated the emergency.**

☐ Child Abuse and Neglect

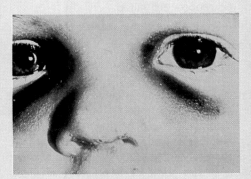

FIGURE 32-14 Child physical abuse.

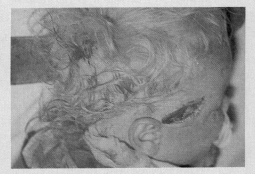

FIGURE 32-15 Child physical abuse.

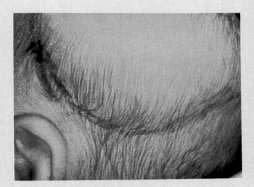

FIGURE 32-16 Child neglect from lack of appropriate medical care.

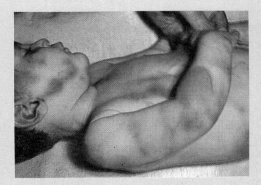

FIGURE 32-17 Child abuse death from multiple injuries.

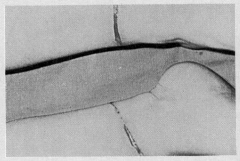

FIGURE 32-18 Physical abuse — restraining by tying.

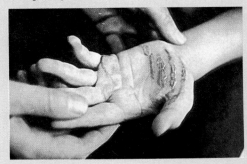

FIGURE 32-19 Physical abuse — burns from hand held onto an electric stove.

to re-create the situation while he or she is still in the crisis environment, with the abuser still present. If the scene is dangerous, request law enforcement to be dispatched.

3. Emergency care begins with recognizing that the child may have been abused. Once you have reason to suspect this — based on the history and the primary survey — examine the child from head to toe, searching for abrasions, bruises, lacerations, and evidence of internal injury. Look also for signs of head trauma, closely examining the ears and nose for blood or cerebrospinal fluid and the eyes for pupillary changes. Conduct the examination in a matter-of-fact fashion, and keep your suspicions to yourself. Make careful note, in addition, of all that you have observed at the scene (condition of the home, any objects that might have been used to hurt the child, such as a belt or straps).

4. Do not question the adults in front of the child or the child in front of the adults.

5. After administering emergency care, tell the parents that the child should be taken to the hospital for X-rays and further care. Ask the parents to notify the hospital that the child will be arriving shortly. In a room adjoining the room where the child is resting, ask the parents to describe how the injury occurred. Do not glare at the parents. Do not respond with disbelief to their explanation. Simply gather information concerning the injuries like you would for any other problem. Do not question the parents about abuse or make any insinuation — that is not your role.

6. It is also *not* your responsibility to confront the parents with the charge of child abuse. You must be tactful and discreet. Being supportive and non-judgmental with the parents will help them be more receptive to the other members of the health care team.

7. Transport the child to an emergency room. Depending on the child's injuries, and if the child is frightened or the parents are threatening, place the child on the seat next to you, and ask the parents to follow in their own car. When this is not possible (if the parents do not have access to a car, for instance, or if they do not want to drive), the child should be seated next to you in the front seat (if possible), and the parents should be asked to sit in the back seat, out of the child's sight. Try to prevent the child from turning around and looking at his parents. In the ambulance, make sure that the child can see only the EMT, not his parents. (Insurance policy may not allow this form of transportation. Know your insurance coverage.)

8. Talk to the child. Tell him that you know that he or she is in pain but that you are doing what you can to stop it. Touch the child's arm lightly, or maintain some other kind of physical contact. Speak in a low, deliberate, kind, and reassuring manner.

9. When you reach the hospital, *privately* convey your suspicions and findings to the physician. It will be of particular value to him or her to learn what you have observed in the home, since this information is otherwise unavailable to the physician.

10. *Always* report your suspicions of child abuse.

11. Maintain total confidentiality regarding the incident; do not share it with your family or friends.

It is critical that you be aware of the reporting laws in your own state and the reporting protocols for your EMS system. Aspects of the law to learn are:

- Who must report the abuse.
- What types of abuse and neglect should be reported.
- To whom the reports are made.
- What information a reporter must give.
- What immunity he is granted.
- Criminal penalties for failing to report.

Child-abuse cases are particularly painful for EMTs. Be sure you talk out your feelings to someone you can trust. Feelings of anger, revulsion, frustration, and helplessness are normal and must be dealt with. In most instances, there is no "perfect" solution, whether the child remains in the home or is placed elsewhere. But good interviewing and reporting skills can make a positive difference, even in bad situations.

Other Emergencies

See Chapter 22 on how to deal with poisoning emergencies, Chapters 35 and 38 on burns and drowning, respectively; Chapter 24 on bites, and Chapter 7 on bleeding.

☐ TRANSPORTING THE CHILD

You should transport the traumatized child when he or she:

- Has serious injury to one or more body systems.
- Is in shock.
- Has fractures.
- Has suspected or actual spinal injury.
- Has a head injury.
- Has respiratory difficulties or unequal chest expansion.
- Has lost consciousness for more than one minute or experiences disorientation.
- Has seizures following a head injury.
- Has a penetrating injury above the elbow or above midthigh.
- Has been hit by a car traveling more than ten miles per hour, strongly enough to damage the car, and/or hard enough to throw him more than five feet.
- Has been run over by, dragged by, or thrown from a car.
- Has been in a car accident involving a rollover, one in which the passenger space was invaded, or one in which another passenger was killed or seriously injured.

☐ A Pediatric Immobilization System

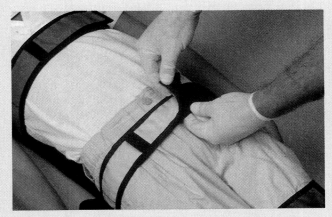

FIGURE 32-20 Adjust the color-coded straps to fit the child.

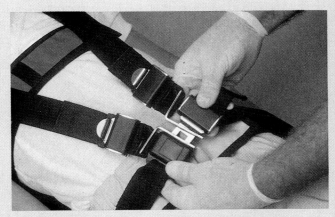

FIGURE 32-21 Attach the four-point safety harness.

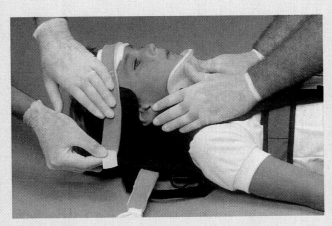

FIGURE 32-22 Fasten the adjustable head support system.

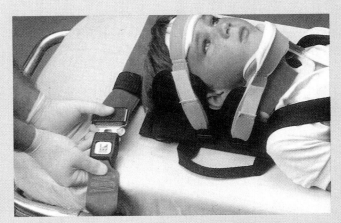

FIGURE 32-23 Fastern the loops at both ends to connect to cot straps.

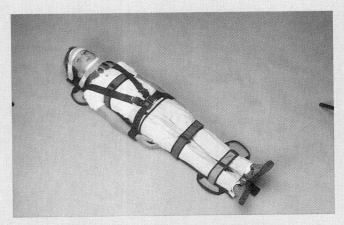

FIGURE 32-24 The child patient completely immobilized.

Because of child-restraint laws in many states, you will encounter an increasing number of children involved in motor vehicle accidents who are in child safety seats. These seats, if properly installed, are designed to hold a child in place during impact, particularly from head-on or rear-end collisions. Their effectiveness in broadside or rotating accidents is not yet clear.

You may transport small children in their own car seats under some circumstances. Often the child is reassured by being in his or her familiar seat. If your ambulance is not equipped with a pediatric spine board, consider using the child's seat as long as the plastic shell is not cracked and the metal tubes do not have jagged metal edges exposed.

You can immobilize a child in the seat by bracing his or her head between two rolled towels and passing a band of tape across his or her forehead and around the seat. A folded blanket placed on the abdomen and taped in place around the seat can immobilize the trunk. Be sure that you can still adequately evaluate respiration. Do not use the small sandbags usually kept with ambulance equipment, since they press downward on the shoulders, may impede breathing, and may destabilize clavicle injuries. Position the seat so that the child can see his or her parent without turning his or her head.

Remember that almost any child under age five will violently protest being restrained. Do not be disturbed by crying if restraint is necessary, but try to minimize the emotional stress on the child by having a parent close enough to maintain eye contact with the child, talk to the child, and touch the child.

If you suspect cervical or spinal injury, be sure that the head is immobilized. If you do not have a cervical collar the correct size, improvise one by rolling up a towel, taping it, lying it in a horseshoe shape over the neck, and taping down the ends. Young patients, even though immobilized, will sometimes struggle against the restraint. Sometimes laying a hand gently on the forehead will keep the patient from fighting against the straps. Very often, however, you must count on keeping the cervical spine in line manually until the emergency department personnel take over.

Child-size restraining boards (such as the **mummy board**) are commercially available. A pediatric immobilization system is shown in Figures 32-20–32-24.

☐ TAKE CARE OF YOURSELF

Almost half of the 15,000 children in the United States who die from accidents are pronounced dead either at the scene or at the hospital. The sudden and violent death of a child, either just before you arrive or while he is in your care, is emotionally wrenching. As a professional EMT, you need to control your emotions so that you can render the best possible assistance and be supportive of other victims, but after the case is over, you need to deal with those feelings. If your unit has a counselor or standard "talk-it-over" groups, use them. If not, find a trusted friend who will listen without cutting you off either to reassure you or give you advice about what to do next time.

If you cannot find some way to talk through your feelings and instead try to suppress them, a typical pattern of worry about your own children, nightmares, or burnout may develop.

chapter 33

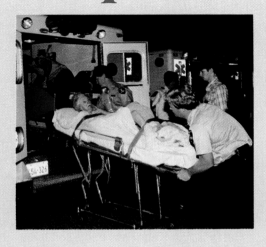

Geriatric Emergencies

✳ OBJECTIVES

- Outline how the various body systems change as a person ages.
- Recognize how some common signs and symptoms may differ in the elderly.
- Describe special communication concerns that need to be considered when caring for geriatric patients.
- Describe special assessment and examination considerations for geriatric patients.
- Describe the common medical problems of the elderly.

It is recommended that EMTs wear protective gloves whenever there is a possibility of coming in contact with a patient's blood, body fluids, mucous membranes, traumatic wounds, or sores. See Chapter 31.

More than one-third of your calls as an EMT will involve patients over the age of sixty-five. In the United States, there are currently more people over the age of sixty-five than there are under the age of fourteen — and the fastest growing segment of the population are those aged eighty-five and older.

People over the age of sixty-five present some special challenges to the EMT. While the elderly represent only 10 percent of the population, they take 30 percent of all prescription drugs, and they account for 25 percent of all fatal injuries. They have an average of three coexisting chronic diseases. They take three times as many medications as the general population. And the physiology of aging itself changes the signs and symptoms of the elderly, and you may need to modify some of your field treatment techniques accordingly.

The leading causes of death and medical problems in the geriatric population are heart disease, cancer, stroke, cirrhosis, fractures, chronic obstructive pulmonary disease, pneumonia, diabetes, confusion, and misuse of drugs. The functioning of the elderly patient's organs may be markedly altered as a result of normal aging (with or without illness), chronic illness, and symptoms masked by various psychiatric/neurologic disorders. As a result of these changes, the geriatric patient's response to illness is changed. In general, the geriatric patient needs to be assessed and treated carefully. Especially at risk are those who are seventy-five or older, living alone, incontinent, immobile, recently hospitalized, recently bereaved, and/or demented. Any delay in recognizing health-care needs and providing care may have devastating, irreversible consequences.

☐ HOW BODY SYSTEMS CHANGE WITH AGE

Body systems change with age, affecting the signs and symptoms manifested in common medical emergencies. To complicate matters, many elderly people suffer from malnutrition: they are on a fixed income, can't go shopping, get little fresh produce, have failing vision, and have a failing sense of taste and smell. Most elderly patients will have not one, but a combination of different disease processes in varying stages of development. Because the aging body has fewer reserves with which to combat disease, it is essential that you recognize these changes so that you can provide prompt, appropriate care for elderly patients in the field (Figure 33-1).

FIGURE 33-1 Differing signs and symptoms in the elderly.

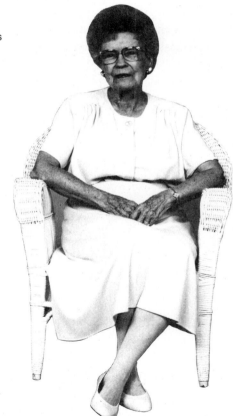

Immune System
Fever often absent in conditions that would cause fever in younger patients

Neurological System
Approximately one-fifth of people over 65 suffer some form of dementia

Cardiovascular System
Blood vessels lose elasticity
Heart pump less volume
Hypertension common
Heart rhythm changes

Musculoskeletal System
Osteoporosis
Osteoarthritis

Respiratory System
Less air enters lungs
Lungs lose elasticity
Muscles used in breathing lose strength and coordination
Dehydration increases tendency for respiratory infection

Renal System
Drug toxity problems common because of changes in the kidneys

Gastrointestinal System
Chronic heart burn is common
Periodontal disease cause tooth loss
Less salivary flow
Possible bowel incontinence
Fecal impaction, constipation common

Skin
Becomes thinner, tears more easily
Less perspiration
Sense of touch dulled

Cardiovascular System

With age, calcium is progressively deposited in areas of wear-and-tear, especially around the valves of the heart. A yellowish pigment called **lipofuscin** is deposited on the myocardium, and the fibrous tissue throughout the cardiovascular system becomes generally thickened. Arteries lose their elasticity, creating greater resistance against which the heart must pump. The aorta loses its elasticity, increasing the patient's blood pressure. In turn, however, the heart pumps out less volume, even during exercise. Heart rhythm increases, but there are fewer electrical conducting cells ("pacemaker cells") as the heart grows older. There is a general decline in the maximum heart rate, which means that the heart may not increase even when there is infection, shock, or stress.

The Musculoskeletal System

The most significant change due to aging is **osteoporosis,** resulting in susceptibility to fractures and delayed healing. The osteoporosis itself is not especially a problem, but resulting immobility can lead to illness and death. **Osteoarthritis** also accompanies aging and may be due to infection, trauma, and metabolic changes as well as the changes of aging. Again, immobility is the most serious problem associated with osteoarthritis.

The Immune System

There are actual changes in the components of the immune system with aging. There are also associated conditions that make the immune system weaker. The skin breaks down and there is a tendency for sores, which allow microorganisms to enter the body. The elderly are more prone to diabetes, which compromises the immune system. And the normal flora of the body changes, making the elderly susceptible to entirely different infections.

Overall, the body's response to infection is not the same as it was when younger. A young person experiences a fever as the white blood cell count skyrockets to handle infection; among the elderly, white blood-cell increases is much lower, and many do not experience fever at all. (Even when it does exist, fever may not be detected because of the elderly person's lower basal body temperature.)

As the body's immune system slows down, the elderly person may suffer a recurrence of a disease that he or she had when he or she was much younger.

The Neurological System

While the aging process itself does not cause dementia, many of the conditions that accompany aging — such as malnutrition, the use of a variety of drugs, and common medical problems such as hypertension — may aggravate dementia. Approximately one-fifth of the people over the age of sixty-five suffer from some form of dementia, and many more suffer clinical depression.

Gastrointestinal System

Changes in the gastrointestinal system contribute to various medical conditions as well as to malnutrition. The structures in the mouth deteriorate, **periodontal disease** causes tooth loss, and degeneration of the salivary glands causes less salivary flow. The smooth muscle contractions of the esophagus decrease, and the opening between the esophagus and the stomach loses tone, resulting in almost chronic heartburn as gastric acid enters the esophagus from the stomach. The liver decreases in size and weight, and loses its ability to aid in digestion and the metabolizing of some drugs. Smooth muscle contractions throughout the rest of the gastrointestinal tract are slowed; therefore, it takes much longer for food to move through the system. Because the lining of the small intestine degenerates, nutrients are not as readily absorbed, further aggravating any malnutrition problems. Fecal impaction and constipation are common because smooth muscle contractions of the large intestine diminish. In some, degeneration of the rectal **sphincter muscle** causes bowel incontinence.

The Renal System

As a result of the normal aging process, the kidneys become smaller and the arteries that supply them become hard and brittle. In general, the kidneys lose a certain percentage of their ability to filter the blood. Since many drugs (including antibiotics) are filtered out by the kidneys, it is common for the elderly to have drug toxicity problems if they take too much medication or take it too frequently.

The Skin

During the aging process, the skin undergoes tremendous changes. It becomes thin, and tears easily, and there is less attachment tissue between the dermis and epidermis. Cells are produced less rapidly, so wounds heal more slowly and skin is slow to replace itself. Less perspiration is produced, and the sense of touch is dulled. Because the skin is more prone to tear or become injured, it becomes less of a protective barrier as part of the immune system in keeping contaminants out of the body.

The Respiratory System

With age, calcium deposits and other changes in the rib cage make it more difficult for the lungs to expand. Less air enters the lungs, and less gas exchange occurs; part of the alveolar surface degenerates, and the bronchial tree enlarges to compensate. The lungs lose elasticity, and many of the muscles used in breathing lose their strength and coordination. Certain parts of the immune system change, and the cilia are no longer as mobile, allowing the lungs to be much more prone to infection. Dehydration, common in the elderly, exaggerates the tendency for respiratory infection.

☐ DIFFERING SIGNS AND SYMPTOMS IN THE ELDERLY

While many medical problems present a basic or standard set of signs and symptoms in the general population, the changes involved in the aging process lead to different or altered signs and symptoms among the elderly. Be alert for the following differences as you assess patients over the age of sixty:

- In myocardial infarction, pain is less common as age increases; the most common symptoms of myocardial infarction in the elderly are shortness of breath, fainting, severe confusion, and stroke. While one-third of the elderly victims never experience pain, aching shoulders and indigestion are common.

- In congestive heart failure, little or no dyspnea is present; dyspnea in the elderly is much more common as a sign of obesity, pulmonary edema, or chronic obstructive pulmonary disease.

- In pneumonia, the classic symptom of fever is usually absent. Chest pain is much less common among the elderly, as is cough. Most cases of pneumonia among those over sixty are due to aspiration, not infection.

☐ SPECIAL ASSESSMENT CONSIDERATIONS

Assessment of the elderly patient may be difficult due to factors that complicate clinical evaluation (Figure 33-2). These factors include the following:

- The elderly become debilitated much more rapidly than do young people. A minor problem may become a major one in a period of a few hours.

- It can be very difficult to take a history: the patient may have diminished hearing, sight, and cognitive abilities. You will probably need to rely more heavily on family members to give you important information.

- The patient may be taking a number of medications, some of which may be very potent. These

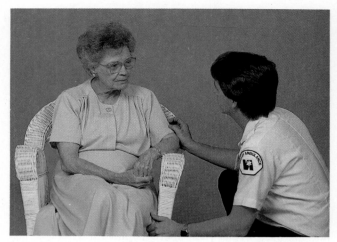

FIGURE 33-2 Special assessment considerations are often necessary when caring for an elderly patient.

may change or mask signs and symptoms; drugs may also mask the onset of shock.

- As many as one in four elderly have psychiatric disorders, which may be the cause of some symptoms, such as clouding of consciousness. However, you need to *assume that mental status is normal until proven otherwise,* usually as a result of information from family members.

- It may be difficult to separate the effects of aging from the consequences of disease.

- The chief complaint may seem trivial (e.g., constipation).

- The patient may fail to report important symptoms.

- The EMT may fail to note important signs or symptoms.

- The geriatric patient is likely to suffer from more than one disease (or problem) at a time. Chronic illness may make assessment for acute problems difficult, and signs and symptoms of chronic illness may be confused with signs and symptoms of acute problems.

- Aging may change the individual's response to illness and injury. Pain may be diminished or absent (e.g., silent myocardial infarction), and consequently the patient or EMT may underestimate the severity of the patient's condition.

- The temperature-regulating mechanism may be depressed, leading to minimal or absent fever with severe infection and making the geriatric patient prone to environmental thermal syndromes.

- Social and emotional factors may have greater impact on the health of the geriatric patient than on any other age group.

- Communication problems are common in the

older patient (see the next section in this chapter). The senses diminish; the patient may have glaucoma, cataracts, blindness, or poor vision. Hearing diminishes, as well as general mental skills. The geriatric patient is much more likely to experience depression than younger patients.

- Common complaints of the geriatric patient that may not be specific to any one disorder include fatigue and weakness, dizziness/vertigo/syncope, falls, headache, insomnia, **dysphagia,** loss of appetite, inability to void, and constipation/diarrhea.

□ SPECIAL COMMUNICATION CONSIDERATIONS

Diminished Sight or Blindness

You can expect increased patient anxiety because of an inability to see surroundings, coupled with an inability to exert control over the situation. You must talk calmly and be positioned so that the patient can best see you if he or she has any sight at all. Explain your procedures carefully; if the patient has them, make sure he or she is wearing his eyeglasses.

Diminished Hearing or Deafness

Many elderly people cannot hear high-frequency speech, especially consonants. Obtaining a history can be difficult if the patient cannot hear questions. Do not assume that the patient is deaf without first inquiring with the family or bystanders. If the patient is wearing a hearing aid, make sure that it is turned on. Do not shout, as it distorts sounds if the patient has some hearing, and it does not help if the patient is deaf. However, an increase in voice volume may help with the hearing-impaired. You may also try placing your stethoscope in the patient's ears and speaking into the diaphragm.

Note writing may help, too. If the patient can lip read, speak slowly and directly toward the patient. Whenever possible, verify the history with a reliable friend or relative, or seek assistance from these individuals in communicating with the patient.

Diminished Mental Status

Many elderly patients have normal mentation; some may be unable to remember details, while others may be routinely confused. Other elderly patients may have experienced an acute onset of diminished mentation.

Attempt to determine if the patient's mental status is normal for him or her, or if it represents a significant change. Do not assume that the confused, disoriented patient is "just senile." It is your responsibility to provide a complete assessment of the patient, checking for possible underlying physiological abnormalities.

Noise of radios, an ECG, or strange voices may add to the patient's confusion. Attempt to explain or reduce the noise.

Depression

Depression is common and may mimic **senility** or **organic brain syndrome.** Depression may be the reason why the patient is acting in an uncooperative manner. In addition, the patient may be malnourished, dehydrated, overdosed, contemplating suicide, or simply imagining physical ailments for attention.

□ SPECIAL EXAMINATION CONSIDERATIONS

Be alert to the following difficulties when examining an elderly patient:

- The patient may be fatigued easily.
- The patient commonly wears layers of clothing—this may hamper the physical assessment.
- You need to explain actions clearly before examining the elderly patient.
- The patient may minimize or deny symptoms due to fear of being bedridden, institutionalized, or losing his sense of self-sufficiency.
- Peripheral pulses may be difficult to evaluate.
- You must distinguish between signs and symptoms of a chronic disease(s) and the acute problems:
  — The geriatric patient may have **nonpathological** rales (rales not caused by disease or infection).
  — Loss of skin elasticity and mouth breathing may give the false appearance of dehydration.
  — Edema may be caused by varicose veins, inactivity, and position rather than congestive heart failure.

□ SPECIAL TRAUMA CONSIDERATIONS

Situations that would be basic in other age groups call for aggressive care in the elderly. And the elderly are at greater risk for experiencing a traumatic injury (primarily due to falls) because of the following factors:

- They may have slower reflexes, failing eyesight and hearing, arthritis, blood vessels that are less elastic and more subject to injury, and fragile tissues and bones.

- They are at high risk for trauma from criminal assault.
- They are prone to head injury, even from relatively minor trauma. Signs and symptoms of brain compression may develop more slowly, sometimes over days or weeks; the patient may have forgotten that he or she was even injured.
- They often have a significant degree of **cervical spondylosis** (a degenerative disease of the cervical vertebrae). Changes of the vertebrae gradually compress the nerve roots to the arms, or possibly to the spinal cord itself. If injury occurs to the cervical spine, the cord is more likely to be injured. Sudden neck movement, with or without fracture, may cause spinal cord injury.

☐ COMMON MEDICAL PROBLEMS IN THE ELDERLY

Myocardial Infarction

The elderly are at increasing risk for myocardial infarction and its complications, including cerebrovascular accident (stroke), cardiovascular disease, and lowered blood pressure.

The elderly tend to experience a lot of chest pain, *but most chest pain in the elderly is not associated with myocardial infarction.* As mentioned, myocardial infarction in the elderly is most often accompanied by shortness of breath, and only one-third of the time accompanied by chest pain.

Pulmonary Embolus

The elderly are at increasing risk of pulmonary embolus, due to coronary heart failure, trauma to the lower extremities, decreasing heart output, and prolonged bed rest that results from injuries or illness.

The most classic signs and symptoms of pulmonary embolus may not be seen in the elderly. The most common signs in the elderly are shortness of breath and a worsening of pre-existing heart disease.

Pneumonia

Aspiration pneumonia is much more common in the elderly, and it often results from accidental aspiration of vomitus.

The elderly pneumonia victim may be insensitive to pain, and may not manifest the classic signs and symptoms of pneumonia. In the elderly, watch for increased respiration rate, lowered blood pressure, lowered body temperature, and clouded consciousness as the most common signs and symptoms of pneumonia.

Shock

Because the heart and the arteries of an elderly person don't respond well, shock progresses much more rapidly in the elderly than in any other age group. Loss of even a small amount of blood can drive an elderly person into shock.

Hypothermia

The elderly aged seventy-five and older are at greater risk of hypothermia than any other age group; elderly men run three to four times the risk of hypothermia as do elderly women. These people can become hypothermic even if they never go outside.

A number of situational factors make the elderly more prone to hypothermia: living on a fixed income, many cannot afford to keep their homes adequately heated. Because of physical impairments, they may not be able to move around much, so they get colder much more easily. And, because of impaired cognition, they simply may not realize how cold it is.

The physiological changes associated with aging also make the elderly more prone to hypothermia. These factors include a smaller insulating layer of fat, reduced muscle mass, a lower basal metabolism, impaired reflexes, decreasing blood flow (especially to the extremities), and a reduced shivering response.

Syncope

Syncope—a "transient loss of consciousness reversed when the patient lies down," sometimes called *fainting* — is *extremely* common in the elderly. Caused by a reduced blood flow to the brain, it can be a sign of a number of underlying diseases as well as a side effect of medications.

Syncope is often caused by changes in heart rhythm or by problems with the heart. It can also be caused by hypoglycemia, hyperventilation, seizures, low blood pressure, or transient ischemic attacks. Interestingly, its cause remains undiagnosed in more than half of all elderly patients.

Falls

Falls are responsible for half of all accidental deaths in the elderly. Among the elderly, deaths from falling are more common than deaths from all other accidents combined. Three-fourths of the elderly who fall are women.

There are sometimes environmental reasons why the elderly fall — these may include stairways without handrails, slippery bathtubs, slippery rugs, steep steps, or improperly fitting footwear. There are also a number of medical reasons why the elderly fall: the most common are dizziness, side effects from medications, heart rhythm problems, spinal weakness, syncope, transient ischemic attacks, low blood pressure, internal bleeding, and poor vision. An estimated 40 percent of all falls among the elderly are caused by medical problems.

Many elderly people who fall do not develop life-threatening injuries and do not die as a result of the fall. But certain injuries are common among those who fall; make sure you check for hip fracture, head injuries, chest and abdominal injuries, spinal fractures, and fractures of the hand, wrist, and forearm (caused by falling on an outstretched hand).

Drug Toxicity

The elderly are more at risk for drug toxicity for a simple reason: as mentioned, they comprise only 10 percent of the nation's population, but they take approximately one-third of the prescription drugs. They also buy the greatest number of over-the-counter medications. That's not all: they tend to have a number of coexisting diseases, so they are at greater risk for drug interaction.

Some drug toxicity is caused by error in doses: the elderly person may take a wrong dose because of poor eyesight (can't read the label on the bottle), confusion (can't remember what the doctor said to do), forgetfulness (forgets the medicine was just taken a few minutes ago), or a tendency to take the medication after it's no longer needed.

Elder Abuse

Abuse of the elderly is most frequent in care centers and other institutions, but it can — and does — happen at home; any elderly person is at risk if he is cared for by a provider who is under stress from other sources. Abuse of the elderly can be physical, financial, or mental (usually involving threats or insults). At highest risk are those elderly who are bedridden, demented, incontinent, frail or those who have disturbed sleep patterns.

Signs of abuse can include bruises, bite marks, bleeding beneath the scalp (indicative of hair-pulling), lacerations on the face, trauma to the ears, broken bones, deformities of the chest, cigarette burns, and rope marks.

Dementia and Alzheimer's Disease

Dementia in the elderly can be acute or chronic; often, it is irreversible. It is normal for the mental processes to undergo changes as a person ages, but approximately 15 percent of those over the age of sixty-five develop full-blown dementia.

Dementia is often caused by medications, especially analgesics, sedatives, tranquilizers, and medications to reduce blood pressure or ease the symptoms of Parkinson's disease. Other common causes in the elderly include brain lesions, heart disease, constipation, urinary retention, infection, depression, alcohol use, chronic pain, and other underlying diseases.

The characteristic results of dementia are chronic changes, including loss of short-term memory, decline in intellectual abilities, and decline in judgment, math ability, and abstract thought.

Believed to affect more than two million Americans, **Alzheimer's disease** causes more than 100,000 deaths each year in this country. It is the fifth-largest killer in the United States; while it doesn't directly cause death, its patients stop eating, become immobile, and eventually become racked with infections. It is the most common cause of dementia in the elderly, and accounts for two-thirds of all dementia in people over the age of sixty-five.

Its cause is unknown; we do know that it is a disease of the nerve cells, not the circulation. While it is often a disease of the elderly, it can affect people as young as forty. Scientists believe that Alzheimer's disease may have a hereditary link that causes degeneration of the brain tissue. The brain cells literally atrophy and die. Alzheimer's disease is both progressive and global.

The signs and symptoms of Alzheimer's disease mimic many other conditions, sometimes eluding proper diagnosis until the disease is in its later stages. The disease causes confusion, emotional depression, irritability, and violence between lucid intervals. There is a progressive loss of appetite and a decreasing ability of the patient to care for his or her own needs. Eventually, the patient does not recognize loved ones; in late stages, the patient becomes childlike. Many Alzheimer's disease victims attempt or commit suicide.

Symptoms of Alzheimer's disease can also result from diabetes, so administer sugar. Provide oxygen and transport, using soft restraints if necessary.

chapter 34

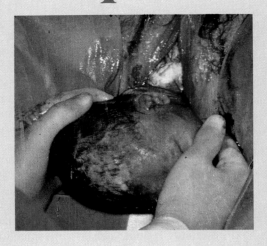

Childbirth and Related Emergencies

✳ OBJECTIVES

- Discuss the basic anatomy of the female reproductive system and the development of a fetus.
- Describe the process of childbirth and the specific stages of labor, including onset.
- Describe how to assess the need for emergency delivery vs. transport.
- Describe the proper equipment and preparation for a normal delivery.
- Demonstrate how to assist the mother in delivering the baby and placenta. Discuss how to care for the baby and mother properly during and after delivery.
- Demonstrate how to assist in childbirth outside a home (i.e., automobile).
- Discuss complications of pregnancy and delivery and how to give care.
- Discuss complications in newborns and demonstrate how to give care.
- Discuss common causes of trauma to the pregnant woman that may have implications for the child, and demonstrate how to treat.

> It is recommended that EMTs wear protective gloves whenever there is a possibility of coming in contact with a patient's blood, body fluids, mucous membranes, traumatic wounds, or sores. See Chapter 31.

EMTs are frequently called upon to assist pregnant women. Too often a pregnant woman is transported to a medical facility in great haste, the primary reason being the EMT's fear of the mother giving birth en route to the hospital. Although some babies are born at homes or in ambulances, in most circumstances there is no need for haste. Childbirth is a normal, natural process. In only a few situations involving complications do you need to transport rapidly. All EMTs should be familar with the nature, signs, symptoms, and emergency care of normal childbirth and obstetric complications.

□ NORMAL PREGNANCY AND STAGES OF LABOR

Physiology of Pregnancy

The Uterus

The uterus is a smooth muscle; during pregnancy its wall becomes thin, and its muscle fibers stretch and thicken to accommodate the developing fetus, the **placenta,** the **fetal membranes,** and the **umbilical cord** (Figure 34-1). The special arrangement of smooth muscle and blood vessels in the uterus allows for great expansion during pregnancy, for forcible contractions during labor and delivery, and for rapid contraction after delivery that will constrict blood vessels in the uterus and prevent hemorrhage. During pregnancy, the **cervix** (neck of the uterus) contains a mucous plug that is discharged during labor. The expulsion of this mucous plug is known as the **bloody show,** and appears as pink-tinged mucus in the vaginal discharge.

The Placenta

After fertilization in the fallopian tube occurs, the zygote (fertilized ovum) attaches itself to the uterine wall, and the placenta (a disk-shaped inner lining attached at one surface to the uterus and at the other to the umbilical cord) begins to develop. Rich in blood vessels, the placenta provides nourishment and oxygen from the mother's blood and absorbs waste products from the baby into the mother's bloodstream. The exchange of nutrients and wastes occurs through a special sieve-like mechanism in the placenta; the baby's and mother's blood do not mix.

The placenta also produces hormones such as **estrogen** and **progesterone** to sustain the pregnancy. At full term, the placenta is about eight inches wide, one inch thick, and weighs about one pound, varying in size and weight with the baby (it is about one-sixth of the baby's weight). After the birth, the placenta separates from the uterine wall and is delivered as the **afterbirth.**

Fetal Membranes

The **fetal membranes** consist of an **amniotic sac,** or **bag of waters,** filled with amniotic fluid, in which the baby floats. The amount of fluid varies, usually from 500 to 1,000 milliliters. The plastic-like sac of fluid insulates and protects the baby during pregnancy. During labor, part of the sac is usually forced ahead of the baby, serving as a resilient wedge to help dilate the cervix.

Umbilical Cord

The umbilical cord is the unborn baby's lifeline that attaches the baby to the placenta. The cord contains one vein and two arteries in a spiral arrangement and a pro-

FIGURE 34-1 Anatomy of the placenta.

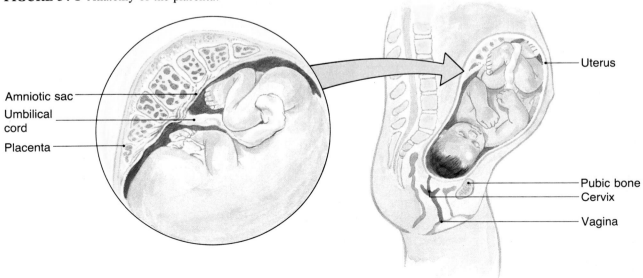

Amniotic sac

Umbilical cord

Placenta

Uterus

Pubic bone

Cervix

Vagina

tective, gelatin-like substance called **wharton's jelly.** The vein carries oxygenated blood to the fetus, while the arteries carry deoxygenated blood back to the placenta. The structure of the cord and the blood traveling through it at about four miles per hour keep the cord from kinking, which would obstruct the vital blood flow to and from the placenta. When the baby is born, the nerveless cord resembles a sturdy rope; it is about twenty-two inches long and about one inch in diameter.

The Birth Canal

Toward the end of a full-term pregnancy, the baby has usually positioned itself head down, with its buttocks toward the upper end of the uterus. The head-down position, with the baby's head already descended through the broad, upper inlet of the mother's pelvis, brings the uterus downward and forward. Mothers can feel the difference and say that the baby has "dropped." This position is most favorable for the baby's passage through the cervix to the vagina.

Stages of Labor

Labor is the term used to describe the process of childbirth. It consists of contractions of the uterine wall that force the baby and, later, the **afterbirth** (placenta) into the outside world. Normal labor is divided into three stages; the length of each stage varies greatly in different women and under different circumstances (Figure 34-2).

First Stage (Dilation)

During this first and longest stage, the cervix becomes fully dilated to allow the baby's head to progress from the body of the uterus to the **birth canal.** Through uterine contractions, the cervix gradually stretches and thins until the opening is large enough to allow the baby to pass through.

The contractions usually begin as an aching sensation in the small of the back; within a short time, they become cramp-like pains in the lower abdomen that recur at regular intervals. Each contraction lasts thirty to sixty seconds; the pain disappears when the uterus relaxes. At first, the contractions occur ten to twenty minutes apart and are not very severe; they may even stop completely for awhile, then start again. Appearance of the mucous plug, discussed earlier, may occur before or during this stage of labor.

Stage one may continue for eighteen hours or more for a woman having her first baby. Women who have had a previous baby may only experience two or three hours of early labor.

Second Stage (Expulsion)

During this period, the baby moves through the birth canal and is born. Contractions are closer together and last longer — forty-five to ninety seconds. As the baby moves down the birth canal, the mother experiences considerable pressure in her rectum, much like the feeling of a bowel movement. This means that the baby is moving downward.

When the mother has this sensation, she should lie down and get ready for the birth of her child. The tightening and bearing-down sensations will become stronger and more frequent, and the mother will have an uncontrollable urge to push down, which she may do. There will probably be more bloody discharge from the vagina at this point. Soon after the baby's head appears at the opening of the birth canal (**crowning**), the shoulders and the rest of the body will follow (Figures 34-3–34-13).

Third Stage (Placental)

During this stage, the placenta separates from the uterine wall, and the placenta and its attached fetal membranes are expelled from the uterus.

FIGURE 34-2

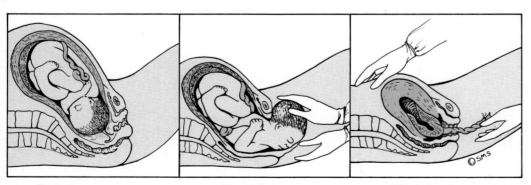

First stage:

First uterine contraction to dilation of cervix

Second stage:

Baby enters birth canal and is born

Third stage:

Delivery of placenta

☐ MANAGING AN OBSTETRICS CALL

Remember that pregnancy and childbirth are neither illnesses nor diseases. They are, however, physically traumatic events, and complications can be life-threatening.

It is important that someone concentrate on supporting the mother — your partner, the husband, or another woman. This person should be able to remain calm and focused on the woman. If not, she is better off alone with you. This support person should hold the woman's hand, speak encouragingly and calmly to her, help her concentrate on breathing regularly with the contractions, wipe her face, give her ice chips, or help her drink clear fluids if she is thirsty. The mother should not eat anything once labor starts.

Determining When to Transport

Your first task is to decide whether you have time to transport the mother safely to the hospital. As a general guideline, there are three cases in which you should *not* try to transport the mother to a hospital or doctor:

1. When you have no suitable transportation.
2. When the delivery of the baby can be expected within five minutes.
3. When the hospital or doctor cannot be reached (due to a natural disaster, bad weather, or some kind of catastrophe).

It is important that you time the contractions in order to determine whether or not you should transport the patient. Place your hand on the mother's abdomen, just above her navel, so that you can feel the involuntary tightening and relaxation of the uterine muscles. Time the contraction (in seconds) from the moment that the uterus first tightens until it is completely relaxed. Time the interval (in minutes) from the start of one contraction to the start of the next. You can tell how intense the contraction is by how hard the uterus feels during the contraction. With an intense (strong) contraction, your fingers cannot indent the surface of the abdomen.

If the contractions are more than five minutes apart, you will usually have time to transport the mother to a close hospital safely, providing traffic is not a problem. If they are two minutes apart, you probably do not. If they are between two and five minutes, you should make your decision based on these factors:

- How soon can you reach the hospital?
- Is this the patient's first delivery? If it is, even hard contractions will not usually result in birth as quickly as if she has had other children.

- Has the mother's amniotic sac ruptured, and if so, when? If rupture has occurred, birth of the baby is usually very soon.
- Has the mother felt the baby move? When was the last time she felt any fetal movement? (Fetal movement in the last trimester can be a very important indication of fetal health.)
- Does the mother feel as though she has to move her bowels? This sensation is caused by the baby's head in the vagina pressing against the rectum and indicates that delivery is imminent. Do not let her go to the bathroom. The sensation is a false signal, and the baby could be delivered while she is trying to move her bowels.
- Visually examine the mother's vagina to see whether the crown of the baby's head is visible. If so, the baby is about to be born, and you will not have time to transport before delivery. Be professional and reassuring during this examination. Be sensitive to the mother's modesty. Explain exactly what you are doing and why. Do not touch the genital area to reduce the risk of contamination.

Transporting a Woman in Labor

If you think that time will permit, transport the mother in the following manner:

1. Bring the stretcher to your patient and transport her to the ambulance on it.
2. Keep her lying down during transport, and remove any underclothing that might obstruct delivery.
3. Place a folded blanket, sheet, or other clean object underneath her buttocks and lower back.
4. Have the mother bend her knees and spread her thighs apart so that you can watch for the crown of the baby's head in the birth canal. Safeguard her modesty, and be sure that she is not unduly exposed.
5. Never ask the mother to cross her legs or ankles, and never tie or hold her legs together in an attempt to delay delivery. Never try to delay or restrain delivery in any way, since the pressure may result in death or permanent injury to the infant.
6. In case of vomiting, turn the mother's head to one side and clean out her mouth, either manually or by suction.

Assisting with Delivery

If there is not time to transport the woman before birth, prepare to assist with the delivery. Be alert to the possibility of **supine hypotensive syndrome.** The pregnant woman near term has a large, heavy mass in her abdo-

The cord should definitely *not* be cut in the field unless it is causing a breathing problem for the baby. The placenta contains healthy, oxygenated blood, and the uterine contractions continue to pump it into the baby. If necessary, wait until the placenta is delivered to cut the cord.

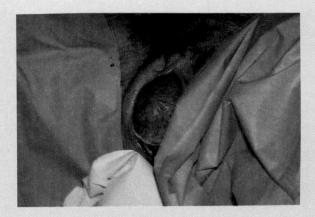

FIGURE 34-3 Late crowning.

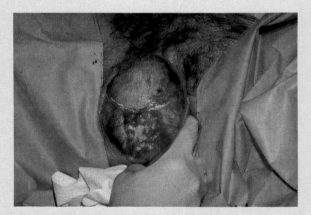

FIGURE 34-4 Head delivering.

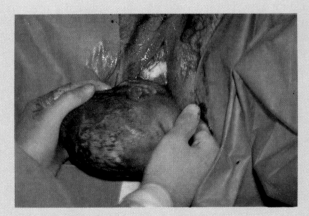

FIGURE 34-5 Head delivers and turns.

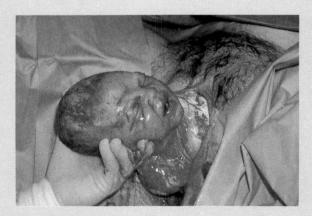

FIGURE 34-6 Shoulders deliver.

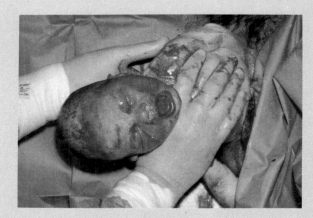

FIGURE 34-7 Chest delivers.

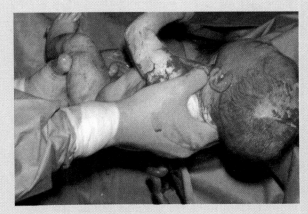

FIGURE 34-8 Infant delivered.

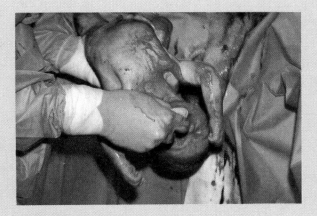

FIGURE 34-9 Suctioning airway.

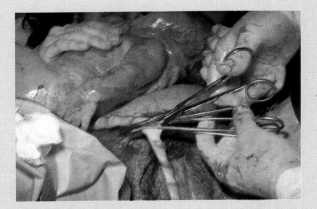

FIGURE 34-10 Cutting of cord.

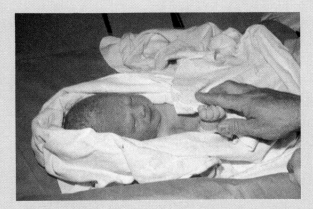

FIGURE 34-11 Wrap the baby after wiping dry with a towel.

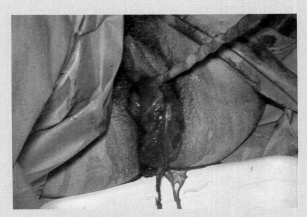

FIGURE 34-12 Placenta begins delivery.

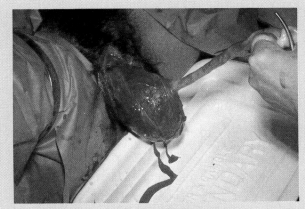

FIGURE 34-13 Placenta delivers.

men. When she lies flat on her back (supine), the uterus, fetus, and placenta compress the inferior vena cava, the major vein of the body. Return of deoxygenated blood to the heart is thereby impaired, and the amount of circulating blood is decreased. These changes are especially pronounced when the mother's blood supply is already marginal (e.g., when she experiences bleeding before delivery). Place the mother on her left side, and treat her for shock.

☐ EMERGENCY HOME DELIVERY

Basic Guidelines

The following procedures assume a home delivery. See the section "Other Emergency Deliveries" in this chapter for instructions about deliveries in the ambulance or at another setting.

1. Be calm. Reassure the mother that you are there to help her with the delivery.

2. Use sterile techniques to the greatest extent possible under the circumstances.

3. Be prepared to administer emergency care to both the mother and the baby, which may include respiratory and cardiac resuscitation for the baby, and shock prevention and control of bleeding for the mother.

4. Ensure the mother's comfort, modesty, and peace of mind as much as possible. Provide a quiet environment, undistracted by children, noise, TV, etc.

5. Properly protect yourself from disease transmission, because the amount of blood and body fluid exposure during delivery can be significant. Several diseases (e.g., AIDS) can be transmitted in these fluids if the mother has the disease. Scrub your hands and nails, even if you have sterile gloves, since you may tear the latex during delivery. If possible, wear latex or vinyl gloves, a cover gown, and a face mask. Handle blood and body fluid-soaked dressings, pads, and linens carefully. Place them in separate bags that prevent leakage. Seal and label the bags. See Chapter 31 for a more complete discussion.

6. Probably the first stage of labor will be over by the time you are involved. If for some reason it is not, and transportation is not possible, concentrate on helping the mother stay in control. Fear will make her tense against the contractions, causing pain. During the early stages of labor, if she can be relaxed, she will sense the contractions as pressure, but not as pain.

7. Most birthing techniques are based on training the woman to respond by controlled breathing. If she does not know how to do this, help her by holding her hand, maintaining eye contact, and saying, "Now, let me know when a contraction starts by nodding your head. Okay, breathe out, two, three, in, two, three." When the mother breathes in, her muscles tighten. Have her blow out with each contraction. Keep the rate of breathing slow but comfortable for her. Tell her that she is doing a good job and that her symptoms are normal.

8. The mother should not strain or push at all during the early stages of labor. The pressure may cause a swollen cervix that cannot dilate, and a Caesarean section may become necessary. During the second stage, the contractions will change, and even for an inexperienced mother, the urge to "bear down" will be unmistakable. At this point, pushing is normal.

9. At any point before or during labor, the bag of waters (amniotic fluid) that surrounds the baby may rupture, causing about a pint of fluid to gush out. (If this occurs before labor has begun, the woman should call her doctor and lie down, since the cord may slip through the cervix unless the baby's head is snug against it. Determining this condition requires vaginal examination under sterile conditions, which you should *not* attempt.)

10. If the patient feels more comfortable walking, sitting, reclining, or assuming some other position during first-stage labor, let her do so.

11. When contractions recur at regular three- to four-minute intervals, last from fifty to sixty seconds each (or longer), and feel very hard, the mother is in the latter part of the first stage of labor, and the cervix is probably dilating rapidly. She should lie down, preferably on her left side with her right arm slightly elevated so that the baby's weight is not lying against the mother's aorta and vena cava. The second stage will probably follow quickly. Do not leave the patient.

12. If the membranes have not already ruptured to release the amniotic fluid, they may do so now. Some blood-tinged mucus may also appear. As labor progresses, the watery fluid and bloody mucus will probably increase. Do not wipe the vaginal area unless you have a sterile towel. If a clean towel is available, place it under the mother's buttocks to absorb moisture.

13. When the contractions are about two minutes apart, they are usually very hard. The patient will not be able to breathe through them; instead, she will want to bear down and push. The mother should not bear down until the top of the baby's head is visible. A sensation of pressure on the rectum is also normal at this point. The cervix is

probably fully dilated, the baby's head is in the birth canal, and delivery will occur within a few minutes.

14. When she is bearing down, remind her not to arch her back, but rather to curve it and bring her chin to her chest to avoid excessive straining. While bearing down, she should hold her breath for seven to ten seconds, while slowly releasing air through slightly parted lips. She should not hold her breath longer: it can cause hypotension and excess straining. Excess straining can cause hemorrhoids, broken blood vessels at the surface of the skin, and possibly a too-fast delivery that will lacerate the perineum.

Desirable Equipment

A basic sterile **obstetric pack** should be available in every ambulance dispatched to an emergency maternity call or in every dispensary subject to such an emergency call (Figures 34-14 and 34-15).

The recommended equipment includes the following items, contained in a sterile pack:

- ☐ 3 sheets.
- ☐ 5 towels.
- ☐ 1 dozen 4-by-4-inch gauze pads or sponges.
- ☐ 2 to 3 sanitary napkins, individually wrapped.
- ☐ 1 rubber suction syringe — ear syringe, rubber bulb type.
- ☐ 1 baby receiving blanket.
- ☐ 4 pairs sterile rubber gloves.
- ☐ Foil-wrapped germicidal wipes.
- ☐ Surgical scissors (for cutting the cord).
- ☐ Wide umbilical tape or sterilized cord.
- ☐ 2 cord clamps or ties.
- ☐ 2 large plastic bags.
- ☐ 1 set of **hemostats.**

FIGURE 34-14 Disposable obstetrical kit.

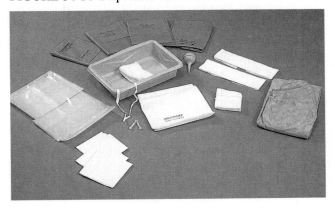

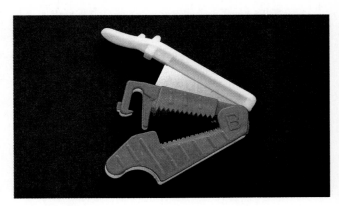

FIGURE 34-15 Umbilical cord cutter/clamp.

Preparation for a Normal Delivery

Follow these procedures in preparing for a normal delivery:

1. Assist the patient to recline. Her knees will naturally be separated by the bulge of the abdomen. Do not pull on them to separate them further. Her feet should be flat on the surface beneath her so she can brace herself.

   - Try to provide a firm surface padded with folded sheets, towels, or blankets so that she can push against it. Waterbeds are much too flexible, so the patient may need to be moved onto the floor.

   - It is easier for you if the surface can be elevated. Most of the time the mother will be in a bed. Try placing chairs underneath the bed legs to elevate the bed, and make it firmer by putting a solid object (such as a piece of plywood, an ironing board, or table leaves) between the mattress and the box springs.

   - Try to protect the mattress from the blood and amniotic fluid. Use a waterproof sheet, if one is available or keep a thick layer of newspapers next to the mattress.

   - Place a draw sheet underneath the mother on the bed.

   - Lift the mother's buttocks about two inches off the surface with a pad of folded sheets, blankets, or towels.

   - Support her head, neck, and shoulders with pillows so that she does not feel like she is lying "downhill."

   - Position the mother so that at least two feet of surface extend beyond her vagina. This surface will support the slippery baby.

2. Remove any constricting clothing, or push it above the mother's waist.

3. Wash your hands very thoroughly with soap and water.

4. Place the obstetric pack where it will be convenient for you, and open it. Remove one sheet, touching only the corners. Between contractions, when the mother can concentrate on what you are telling her to do, ask her to raise her hips. Place one fold of the sheet well underneath her hips, and unfold it toward her feet. If time permits, use a second sheet to cover the mother's abdomen and legs, leaving the birth canal area uncovered. If you do not have sheets, use a sterile towel.

5. Have the best possible light directed toward the mother's genital area. Watch for gaping of the vagina and bulging of the skin in the **perineum** (the area between the vagina and the anus). With each contraction, the baby's head may be visible as the **labia** (lips of the vagina) open wider.

6. If equipment is available, place it on the table next to the mother; keep it away from the birth canal so that it will not be contaminated by the gush of amniotic fluid. Cleanse your hands with germicidal wipes. Put on sterile gloves if you have them.

7. Do not touch the vagina at any time.

8. Watch for the baby's head to emerge at the vagina. Be prepared to support the baby's head as it emerges.

9. If the amniotic sac has not broken earlier, pinch it with your fingernails to rupture it. This will prevent the baby from inhaling amniotic fluid. Clear fluid can be absorbed harmlessly through the baby's lungs; but if the water is greenish or brownish, it means that the baby has suffered distress and had a bowel movement in the uterus. The color comes from meconium in the baby's bowel and can cause pneumonia if aspirated.

10. As delivery becomes imminent (when the baby's head crowns), get the mother to pant with contractions, rather than pushing down. Permit the head to deliver between contractions, if at all possible, to avoid tearing of the mother's skin between the vagina and the anus and to prevent injury to the infant's head from sudden release of pressure. The EMT's applying gentle pressure to the perineum will also help to prevent tearing.

11. When the baby's head appears, place one hand below his or her head, then spread the fingers of the other hand evenly and gently around the head. Stay away from the fontanelles, or soft spots. Allow the head to emerge, but not "pop" out.

Delivery of the Baby

Follow these procedures to deliver the baby (Figure 34-16):

1. In a normal presentation, the baby's head faces down; the baby then usually turns so that his nose is toward the mother's thigh.

2. As soon as the baby's head is visible, support the head with one hand and pick up the rubber bulb syringe. Compress the syringe *before* you bring it to the baby's face. When it is compressed, insert the tip about 1 to 1.5 inches into the baby's mouth. Then slowly release the bulb to allow mucus and other fluid to be drawn into the syringe. Remove the syringe and discharge the contents onto a towel. If possible, suction each nostril at this time as well. Babies breathe through their noses so the nostrils must be clear.

3. When the head is born, check to see if the umbilical cord is around the baby's neck. If it is, use two fingers to slip the cord over the shoulder; clamp and cut the cord only if you cannot dislodge it.

4. The upper shoulder will be born first. To help the lower shoulder out, support the head in an upward position. As the shoulders emerge, be prepared for the rapid appearance of the rest of the baby's body — the head and shoulders are the widest parts and take the longest to emerge.

5. As the abdomen and hips emerge, place your other hand under these areas. You should now have two hands supporting the baby.

6. No attempt should be made to pull the baby from the vagina. Avoid touching the mother's anus during the delivery. When born, the baby will be bluish and covered with a whitish, cheesy, slippery substance known as the **vernix caseosa.** Handle the slippery body carefully; do *not* put your finger in the baby's armpits, because pressure on the nerve centers there can cause paralysis.

7. Use a sterile towel (or the cleanest cloth available) to receive the baby. If possible, note and record the time of birth.

8. As soon as the baby is completely delivered, place the baby on his or her back on a towel. Keep the baby's head slightly lower than the rest of the body, and turn the head slightly to one side to allow mucus and fluid to drain from the nose and mouth. Keep the baby at the same level as the mother's vagina.

9. Wipe away any blood and mucus from the nose and mouth with sterile gauze or a gloved finger, maintaining a firm hold to prevent the baby from slipping. Use the rubber syringe again to suction the nostrils first, then the mouth. Be sure to squeeze the bulb *before* inserting the tip, then place the tip in the baby's nostrils and mouth, and release the bulb slowly. Expel the contents into a waste container, and repeat suctioning as needed

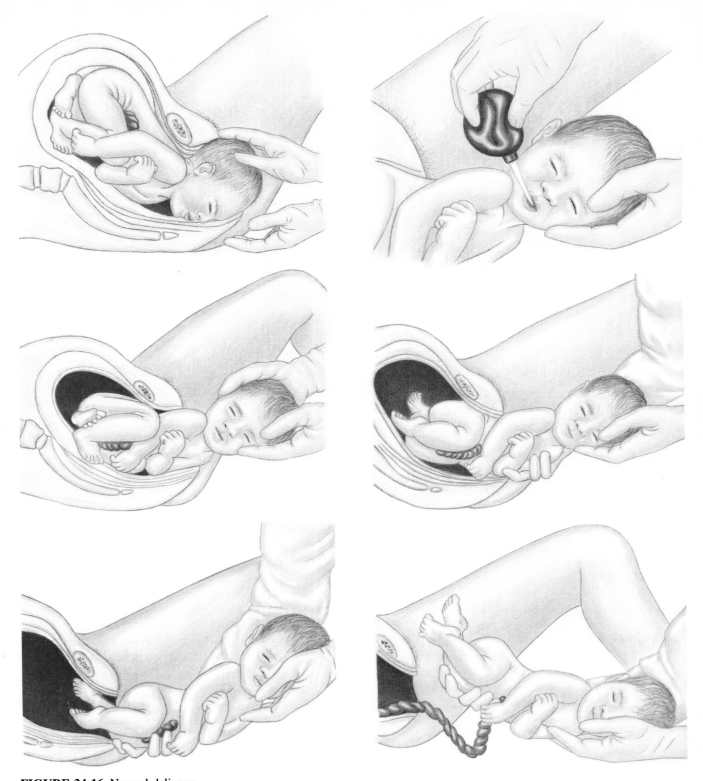

FIGURE 34-16 Normal delivery.

(Figure 34-17). Keep the baby's head lowered and to the side when clearing mucus by finger or syringe. Do not suction longer than ten seconds; monitor the heart rate continually.

10. Do *not* pull on the cord when picking up the baby. Raise the baby's hips *slightly* higher than the head

for drainage, and lay the baby on his or her side at the level of the birth canal or lower (not on the mother's abdomen at this time). Extend the head slightly backward while lifting the chin slightly upward to keep the airway clear. The baby will probably breathe and cry almost immediately.

Childbirth and Related Emergencies **493**

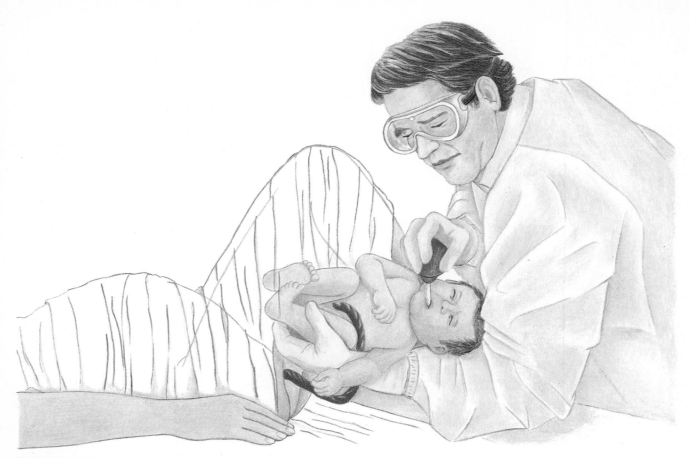

FIGURE 34-17 Suctioning the mouth of the newborn is accomplished by squeezing the bulb, then inserting the tip into the infant's mouth. The bulb is released to suction, then the tip is removed from the mouth and the bulb is squeezed to remove its contents.

Soon after this cry, the cord will become limp and will no longer pulsate — the blood flow ceases, since changes occur in the baby's circulatory system flow after he is born.

11. If the baby does not breathe on his or her own at this point, stimulate the baby by rubbing the back gently or by slapping the soles of his feet (Figure 34-18). If you still get no response, start mouth-to-mouth ventilation (see Chapter 4), bearing in mind that a baby's lungs are very small and require very small puffs. Never use mechanical ventilation devices on a newborn infant. If the baby finally begins breathing on his or her own, administer oxygen by mask (four liters or less) until the baby's skin color is pink. If breathing is still absent, however, and no pulse is present, begin cardiac compressions (see Chapter 6) and continue until you arrive at the hospital. Keep the baby wrapped in a blanket as much as possible.

12. As soon as the baby is breathing and crying, dry him or her vigorously with a towel (do not wipe off the vernix) and wrap the baby in a blanket or infant swaddle. If possible, the blanket should be heated to about 90°F. Wrap the baby so that only his or her face is exposed (Figure 34-19). Do not pull on the cord, and do not tie the cord. The cord will usually be long enough for you to place the baby on the mother's abdomen; help her to hold the baby there in a side-lying position.

13. To cut the cord (check local protocol), check the cord for pulsation. If the umbilical cord has a pulse, wait a few minutes until the pulsation stops. Then place two clamps or tapes on the cord about three inches apart, positioned about six to nine inches from the baby's navel. Cut the cord between the two clamps, using sterile surgical scissors (Figure 34-20). Periodically check the ends of the cord for bleeding, and control any bleeding that may occur. A premature infant is likely to develop severe shock from just a "little" loss of blood.

14. If there are complications, you may transport the mother before the placenta is delivered.

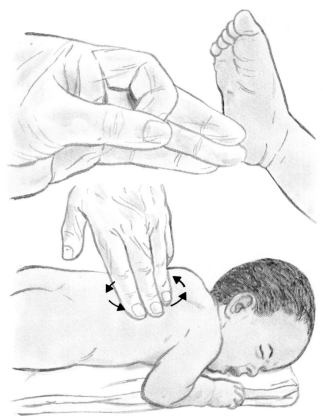

FIGURE 34-18 It may be necessary to encourage the newborn to breathe.

FIGURE 34-19 An infant swaddle to warm the baby.

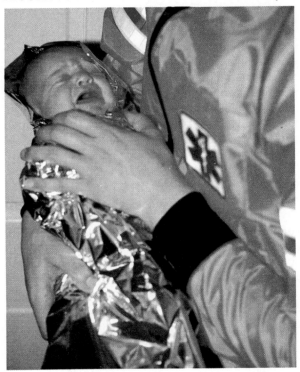

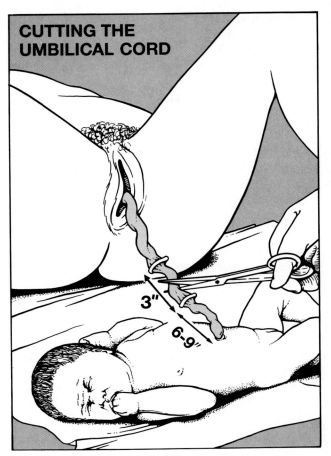

3"

6-9"

FIGURE 34-20

Delivery of the Placenta

Follow these procedures for delivery of the placenta:

1. If there are no complications and cutting the cord is accepted local protocol, observe the appearance of the cord and its location at the vagina. As the placenta separates from the uterus, the cord will appear longer.

2. Place one hand on the mother's abdomen, and feel for a definite contraction. The contracting uterus should feel like a hard, grapefruit-sized ball.

3. Wait for the delivery of the placenta. The placenta is usually delivered in less than ten minutes, but most will deliver within twenty minutes. Never pull on the cord to check for separation of the placenta. As the uterus contracts, encourage the mother to bear down to expel the placenta and membranes. Some bleeding may be expected as the placenta separates.

4. When the placenta appears at the vagina, grasp it gently, and rotate it. Do not pull, but slowly and gently guide the placenta and the attached membranes (fetal sac) from the mother's vagina.

5. If you have not cut the cord, wrap the placenta in a sterile towel, and place it next to the baby. Wrap the baby and the placenta together in the third sterile sheet from the pack, and place both in the mother's arms.

6. If you have cut the cord, place the placenta in a plastic bag to be taken to the hospital, where it may be examined for completeness; retained pieces of placenta will cause persistent bleeding and may require surgical intervention.

7. Check the amount of vaginal bleeding. One or two cups, or less than 500 milliliters, are normal.

8. Examine the skin between the anus and the vagina for lacerations, and apply pressure to any bleeding tears. If there is a tear, let the mother know that this is normal and that it will be taken care of at the hospital.

9. Remove the soiled sheet. Save all evidence of blood loss (stained sheets or towels) for the physician to examine.

10. Place two sanitary napkins over the vaginal and perineal area, touching only the outer surface and placing the napkins from the vagina toward the anus. Help the mother place her thighs together to hold the napkins in place.

11. Elevate the feet if needed.

12. Locate the uterus again, and massage the lower abdomen to help contract the uterus, thereby controlling bleeding. Rub with a circular motion, using the flat of your four fingers cupped around the uterus, until you feel it firm up. Encourage the mother to nurse the baby during this process, because this will help to control bleeding by stimulating contraction of the uterus. It also benefits the baby: it keeps the baby warm, triggers the baby's rooting and suckling reflexes, and bonds him or her to the mother. If a baby does not suckle within the first few hours, it may be difficult for the baby to learn it. The mother's breasts will not produce milk for two or three days, but the colostrum already present is a thin, yellow fluid with easily digestible protein and important antibodies.

13. Continue to give the mother comfort and emotional support.

14. Cover the mother and baby for warmth. The mother will chill easily after giving birth. She will also need to urinate frequently. Remember — complications are more likely to develop in a cold, stressed infant. Prepare both for transportation to the hospital.

15. Transport carefully. Lights and siren and undue speed are not necessary.

□ NEWBORN CARE

The body surface area of infants is proportionately greater than that of older children or adults; therefore, infants are likely to lose more heat. Protecting newborn infants against heat loss preserves their energy and avoids the complex problem that hospital personnel must face in dealing with the warming of a cold infant.

The most practical steps to take in preventing heat loss are:

1. Immediately dry a wet infant, paying particular attention to the head, which has a large surface area.

2. Quickly wrap the infant in warmed blankets or in a plastic **bubble bag swaddle.** The bubble bag allows observation and effectively prevents heat loss by all mechanisms. (Do not put an already cold infant in a plastic swaddle.)

3. Skin-to-skin contact with the mother will also warm the baby. Cover both of them.

4. Transport the adequately wrapped baby in the mother's arms.

5. Do not administer oxygen unless respiratory difficulties occur. Oxygen in a cylinder is much colder than room air.

□ EVALUATING THE NEWBORN

The **Apgar scoring system** for evaluating infants at birth can be used to an advantage in emergencies. This procedure assigns a numerical score of zero to ten; the more vigorous the infant, the higher the score. A number of zero to two is scored to each sign; the total of the five individual assessments is the Apgar score. This method of evaluation provides a good overall indication of an infant's condition. Table 34-1 uses A-P-G-A-R as a memory device.

A total score of zero to three represents severe distress; four to six indicates moderate distress; and seven to ten indicates mild or no distress. Infants are ordinarily evaluated at one and five minutes after delivery, but you should score the infant as soon as you see him or her, even if hours have elapsed since delivery. Most newborns score seven to eight at one minute and eight to ten at five minutes. If the infant scores seven or less at five minutes, repeat the test at ten minutes. The signs are evaluated as follows:

1. The least important sign is color (appearance)
   - Very few infants are completely pink or typical newborn color and receive a score of two.

TABLE 34-1
The Apgar Scoring Chart

	Sign	0	1	2	Rating 1 Min.	Rating 5 Min.
A	1. Appearance (Color)	Blue, pale	Body pink, hands and feet blue	Completely pink		
P	2. Pulse (Heart rate)	Absent	Slow (below 100)	Over 100		
G	3. Grimace (Irritability)	No response	Some motion, cry	Vigorous cry		
A	4. Activity (muscle tone)	Flaccid, limp	Some flexing of extremities	Active motion		
R	5. Respiratory Effort	Absent	Slow, irregular	Good, crying		

- Most babies score one because their hands and feet are blue for a while following birth.
- Paleness and blue color over the entire body are rated zero.

2. The heart rate (pulse) is the most important sign and the best way to determine whether oxygen is reaching the tissues after birth. A rate below 100 beats per minute is extremely serious. Count the heart rate for at least thirty seconds. If a stethoscope is not available, feel the pulse of the umbilical cord where it joins the skin of the abdomen.
   - Score two if the rate exceeds 100.
   - Score one if the rate is below 100.
   - Score zero if there is no detectable heartbeat.

3. "Grimace" refers to reflex irritability. Flick the sole of the baby's foot.
   - If the infant cries, score two.
   - Score one for a weak cry or slight motion of the head.
   - Score zero for no response.

4. Activity refers to reflexes or degree of flexion of the arms and legs and the resistance to straightening them. The normal infant's elbows, knees, and hips are flexed, and you will encounter some degree of resistance in trying to extend them.
   - Score two for normal muscle tone.
   - Score one for muscle tone that is intermediate between normal and limp.
   - An oxygen-starved infant is limp, and there is no resistance to straightening the extremities. Score this condition zero.

5. The second most important sign is the respiratory effort.

- Score two for regular respirations and a vigorous cry.
- Score one when respirations are irregular, shallow, or gasping.
- Score zero if breathing is absent.

Once you memorize the scoring system, you can evaluate an infant in thirty seconds. The Apgar score determines how intense your resuscitative efforts need to be, and it is an important item to report on an emergency childbirth record (Figure 34-21) upon arrival at the hospital.

☐ OTHER EMERGENCY DELIVERIES

Sometimes a baby will be born in your ambulance, or you will be called to assist at a birth at a roadside, at an accident scene, or under other emergency conditions. Basically, try to follow the procedures as outlined previously, adapting as needed to the emergency situation.

- Shield the mother from onlookers. Try to keep her as warm and comfortable as possible.
- If no sterile equipment is available, use the cleanest items that you have — towels or part of the mother's clothing. If newspapers are available, place some underneath the mother. When possible, place a raincoat or blanket underneath her if she must lie on the ground.
- If the mother is in an automobile and lying on the seat, have her place one foot on the floorboard.
- In an emergency situation, do not try to wipe away secretions from the vagina, since you may contaminate the birth canal.
- Be sure to record time of birth.

The following is a form that is very helpful in carrying information to the receiving physician. It can be quickly and easily filled out and given to the attending physician or nurse when the EMT delivers the mother and baby to the hospital.

1. TIME OF BIRTH _____

2. TYPE OF PRESENTATION (such as head or feet) _____

3. DATE _____

4. CORD AROUND THE NECK? _____ Yes _____ No   NUMBER OF TIMES _____

5. AMNIOTIC MEMBRANES RUPTURED AT _____

6. APGAR SCORE _____   ONE MINUTE   FIVE MINUTES

   HEART RATE   _____   _____

   RESPIRATORY EFFORT   _____   _____

   MUSCLE TONE   _____   _____

   REFLEX IRRITABILITY   _____   _____

   COLOR   _____   _____

7. TIME PLACENTA DELIVERED _____

   APPEARANCE _____

   NUMBER OF VESSELS IN CORD (if cut) _____

8. INFANT RESUSCITATION (if necessary) _____

   TIME _____ REMARKS _____

   _____

   _____

FIGURE 34-21

☐ COMPLICATIONS OF PREGNANCY

Although women are at risk for the same causes of lower abdominal pain as men (for example, appendicitis and diverticulitis), assume that any woman between ages twelve and fifty who is complaining of severe lower abdominal pain, with or without vaginal bleeding, is having a complication of pregnancy. Other complaints with similar signs are seldom life-threatening; complications of pregnancy almost always are.

Toxemia of Pregnancy

A common condition affecting about one out of every twenty mothers is **toxemia of pregnancy.** It occurs most frequently in the last trimester and is most likely to affect women in their twenties who are pregnant for the first time.

Women at risk are those with a history of diabetes, heart disease, kidney problems, or hypertension. You should also ask the patient if her mother or sisters had high blood pressure during pregnancy.

Toxemia is characterized by high blood pressure and swelling in the extremities. Any of the following signs and symptoms may occur:

• Sudden weight gain (two pounds a week or more).
• Blurred vision or spots before the eyes.
• Pronounced swelling of the face, fingers, legs, or feet. Some swelling in the feet and legs is normal.
• Decrease in urinary output.
• Severe, persistent headache.

- Persistent vomiting.
- Elevated blood pressure (140/90 or higher mmHg); an increase of 15 mmHg or more in the diastolic pressure is very serious.
- Mental confusion or disorientation.
- Protein in the urine.
- Abdominal pain in the right upper quadrant.
- Hypertension.

She may also suffer kidney damage, liver damage, and/or cerebral edema, although these signs must be diagnosed in the hospital. The only known cure for these conditions is delivery of the fetus, although drug therapy to reduce blood pressure gradually (sudden drops are very dangerous to the baby) is sometimes effective.

The two stages of toxemia are:

- **Preeclampsia:** A previously normal pregnant patient develops hypertension, edema, headaches, and visual disturbances.
- **Eclampsia:** In addition to any or all of the other signs and symptoms of pre-clampsia, the patient has convulsions, a sudden fever, and irritated reflexes. Eclampsia is one of the most severe complictions of pregnancy. The death rate for mothers is from 5 to 15 percent; for babies, it is about 25 percent. Death can occur from cerebral hemorrhage, respiratory arrest, renal failure, or circulatory collapse. During a seizure, the placenta can separate from the uterine wall.

Eclampsia can usually be prevented if you keep the mother quiet, which will aid in keeping her blood pressure down. If you encounter a toxemic woman:

1. Contact your base physician immediately.
2. Position the patient on her left side; this will prevent vena caval obstruction and allow her to breathe more easily, thus supplying the baby with more oxygen.
3. Keep the patient calm and quiet.
4. Administer oxygen, and keep suction close at hand. During a seizure, the mother's body, and hence the baby's, will become oxygen-deprived.
5. Transport the patient as gently as possible to the hospital.
6. Do not use sirens or flashing lights, which can bring on seizures. Anticipate seizures at any moment.
7. Check for respirations; they should start within one minute after the seizure. When the seizure subsides and the patient regains consciousness, elevate her head and shoulders. This will allow her to breathe more easily and will make her more comfortable. Administer high flow oxygen.

Spontaneous Abortion

Abortion is defined as loss of pregnancy before the twentieth week of gestation; it is often referred to as a **miscarriage.** There are three major classifications of abortion.

- **Spontaneous abortion** is an abortion that occurs naturally.
- **Criminal abortion** is an illegal attempt to produce an abortion, often under highly unsterile conditions. This type of abortion is usually hazardous to the mother's life.
- **Therapeutic abortion** is a legal abortion that is performed in an authorized medical setting.

Abortions are further classified according to the stage.

Signs and Symptoms of Spontaneous Abortion

In general, signs and symptoms of spontaneous abortion include (Figure 34-22):

- The patient's knowledge or suspicion that she is pregnant.
- Vaginal bleeding (often heavy).
- Cramp-like pains in the lower abdomen (similar to menstrual cramps or labor contractions).
- Passage of tissue.
- Inability to feel the uterus.
- Uterus located below the woman's navel.

Emergency Care

In cases of spontaneous abortion:

1. Provide life support for the woman.
2. Treat her for shock.
3. Transport her as soon as possible to the hospital.
4. Take any passed tissue or evidence of blood loss (bloody sheets, towels, underwear) to the hospital for the examining physician.
5. Provide emotional support. Intense grief is normal and to be expected for both the parents.

Ectopic Pregnancy

In a normal pregnancy, the **egg** is implanted in the uterus; in an ectopic pregnancy, the egg is implanted outside the uterus — in the abdominal cavity, in the fallopian tube (95 percent of the time), on the outside

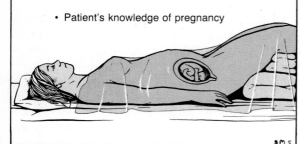

SIGNS AND SYMPTOMS OF SPONTANEOUS ABORTION

- Passage of tissue
- Heavy vaginal bleeding
- Inability to feel the uterus
- Cramplike pains in lower abdomen
- Uterus located below woman's navel
- Patient's knowledge of pregnancy

FIGURE 34-22 Diagram depicts a patient who is cramping and bleeding, threatening abortion.

wall of the uterus, on the ovary, or on the outside of the cervix. Ectopic pregnancy is a severe medical emergency, because the placenta eventually invades the surrounding tissue, causes rupture of a blood vessel, and results in severe abdominal bleeding and internal hemorrhage. It is the leading cause of first trimester maternal deaths and occurs in one of 200 pregnancies, terminating the pregnancy usually between the sixth and twelfth weeks.

The signs are very similar to those of ruptured ovarian cysts, but the treatment is also similar in the prehospital setting. The major difference is that the cyst rupture usually occurs one week before the period is due to begin while an ectopic pregnancy will rupture the fallopian tube about six weeks after the last period.

Signs and Symptoms of Ectopic Pregnancy

Signs and symptoms of ectopic pregnancy include:

- Sudden, sharp abdominal pain, localized on one side. If the bleeding is extensive, the pain will become more diffuse.

- Vaginal spotting.
- Missed menstrual period.
- Pain under the diaphragm.
- Pain radiating to one or both shoulders.
- Tender, bloated abdomen.
- A palpable mass in the abdomen; it may either be the developing embryo or a blood clot resulting from the internal bleeding.
- Weakness when the mother is sitting.
- Decreased blood pressure.
- Increased pulse.
- Shock.
- (Rarely) bluish discoloration around the navel.

Because the internal bleeding is not readily apparent and because external bleeding through the vagina is usually slight, you will not be able to detect immediately why the mother is in shock. Suspect ectopic pregnancy in any woman of childbearing age, especially if any of the above listed signs and symptoms are present.

Emergency Care

1. Place the patient on her back with knees elevated to treat for shock.
2. Keep her warm.
3. Administer oxygen.
4. In severe cases, you may need to use the PASG on only the legs to reverse the drop in blood pressure (under a physician's direction).
5. Transport the patient to the hospital immediately for surgery.

Placenta Previa

Placenta previa refers to abnormal positioning of the placenta within the uterus. Usually, **implantation** of the developing embryo occurs in the upper one-third of the uterus; in placenta previa, implantation is abnormally low (Figure 34-23). During labor, the placenta separates from the uterus, severely impairing the baby's circulation and endangering the lives of the mother and baby.

When the cervix dilates or as the fetus moves from the uterus, the placenta tears. This is painless but results in serious hemorrhage of the mother. Signs include severe bleeding from the vagina and shock.

Emergency Care

1. Elevate the legs and maintain body temperature.
2. Apply the PASG, but inflate *only* the leg sections (under a physician's direction).
3. Deliver 100 percent oxygen with a mask.
4. Transport gently but quickly to an appropriate medical facility. Diagnosis must be made by **ultrasound.**

Abruptio Placenta

Abruptio placenta (see Figure 34-23) is another major cause of predelivery hemorrhage, and it occurs more frequently than placenta previa. It is life-threatening for the mother and fetus; therefore, it needs to be recognized and cared for rapidly. Abruptio placenta occurs in only 1 percent of pregnancies but accounts for 15 to 20 percent of fetal deaths. Abruptio placenta is the leading cause of fetal death after blunt trauma.

There are several causes of abruptio placenta, including toxemia and trauma. For whatever reason, during the last three months of the pregnancy the normally implanted placenta separates from the uterine wall. Spontaneous bleeding begins, although in 20 percent of the cases, the bleeding occurs behind the placenta with no external signs. Shock to the mother and inadequate oxygenation to the fetus may result.

The signs and symptoms include external vaginal bleeding, though not necessarily in great quantities, and severe, localized abdominal pain. Abdominal rigidity and shock signs will also occur.

Emergency Care

1. Monitor vital signs carefully.
2. Assess the mother for thirst, pallor, diaphoresis, and an altered mental state.
3. Administer 100 percent oxygen by mask.
4. Treat for shock.
5. Transport gently but quickly.

FIGURE 34-23

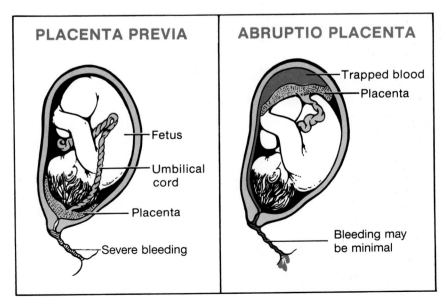

PLACENTA PREVIA

ABRUPTIO PLACENTA

Fetus

Umbilical cord

Placenta

Severe bleeding

Trapped blood

Placenta

Bleeding may be minimal

Ruptured Uterus

As the uterus enlarges during pregnancy, the uterine wall becomes extremely thin, especially around the bottom. **Ruptured uterus** (Figure 34-24) may be caused by any of the following (Figure 34-25):

- The patient has a weak uterine scar from a previous **Cesarean section** or surgical operation.
- The patient has had many previous pregnancies, a situation that considerably weakens the uterine wall.
- The baby is too large for the pelvis.
- Labor is extended and forceful. (In instances in which the baby is too large to be born through the vaginal opening, an extended, forceful labor may force the baby out through the uterine wall.)

Signs and Symptoms of Ruptured Uterus

Signs and symptoms of a ruptured uterus include (See Figure 34-25):

- A tearing sensation in the abdomen, which may show an hourglass appearance.
- Constant and severe pain.
- Nausea.
- Shock.
- Usual minimal vaginal bleeding.
- Cessation of noticeable uterine contractions (the uterus relaxes *during* the contraction).
- Ability to feel the baby in the abdominal cavity through palpation and examination.
- Contraction of the uterus until it is located below the navel.

FIGURE 34-24

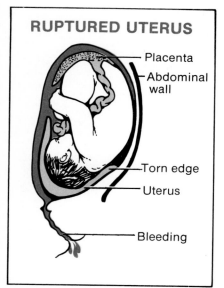

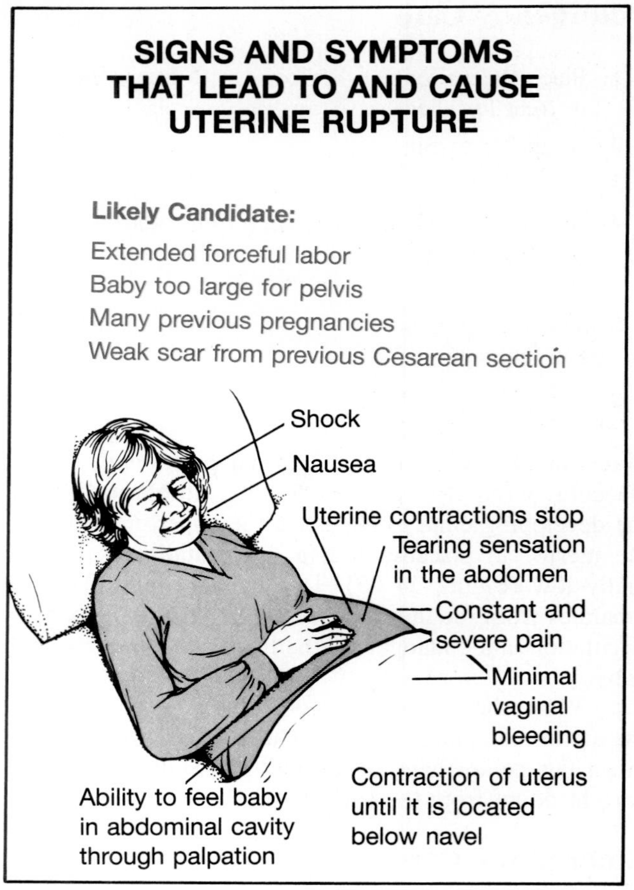

RUPTURED UTERUS

- Placenta
- Abdominal wall
- Torn edge
- Uterus
- Bleeding

SIGNS AND SYMPTOMS THAT LEAD TO AND CAUSE UTERINE RUPTURE

Likely Candidate:

Extended forceful labor
Baby too large for pelvis
Many previous pregnancies
Weak scar from previous Cesarean section

- Shock
- Nausea
- Uterine contractions stop
- Tearing sensation in the abdomen
- Constant and severe pain
- Minimal vaginal bleeding
- Ability to feel baby in abdominal cavity through palpation
- Contraction of uterus until it is located below navel

FIGURE 34-25

Emergency Care

1. Immediately treat for shock.
2. Keep the patient warm.
3. Do not administer anything by mouth since the mother must have emergency surgery.
4. Transport the patient immediately. Patient mortality rate from a ruptured uterus is usually 5 to 20 percent; the infant mortality is over 50 percent.

Prepartum Hemorrhage

Prepartum hemorrhage means bleeding before the birth of the baby. It is generally caused by placenta previa, abruptio placenta, or a ruptured uterus.

Emergency Care

Emergency care of third-trimester prepartum hemorrhage complications includes:

1. Place the mother in a shock position.
2. Provide high concentrations of supplemental oxygen.

3. Apply a PASG, inflating the *legs only* (follow local protocol).

4. Transport her rapidly to the nearest medical facility.

5. Continue to monitor vital signs.

6. Estimate the amount of visible blood loss.

Prolapsed Umbilical Cord

Prolapsed umbilical cord (Figures 34-26 and 34-27) refers to the situation in which the cord comes out of the vagina before the baby. It is most common in **breech births.** The baby is in great danger of suffocation, since the cord is compressed against the birth canal by the baby's head, cutting off the baby's supply of oxygenated blood from the placenta.

Emergency Care

Emergency care is urgent (see Figures 34-26 and 34-27):

1. Place the mother either in a knee-chest position, or have her lie down with her hips and legs elevated on a pillow. Keep her warm, and have her lie on her left side if possible.

2. Administer high-flow oxygen.

3. With a gloved hand, gently push the baby up the vagina far enough so that the head is off the umbilical cord. (Certainly it is potentially dangerous to the baby during the final stages of labor when the baby's head is crowning and the contractions are extremely forceful. Clear this with medical command.)

FIGURE 34-26 Prolapsed cord.

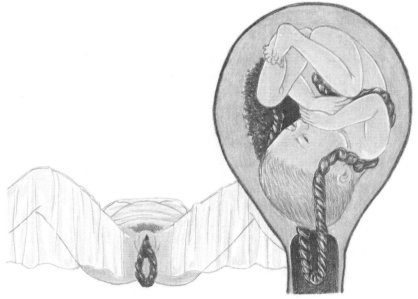

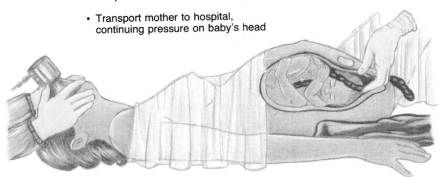

- Elevate hips, administer oxygen and keep warm

- Keep baby's head away from cord

- Do not attempt to push cord back

- Wrap cord in sterile moist towel

- Transport mother to hospital, continuing pressure on baby's head

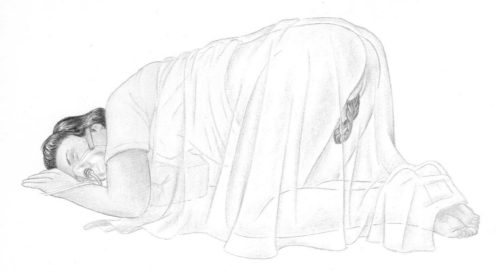

FIGURE 34-27 Patient positioning for prolapsed cord.

4. Do not attempt to push the cord back into the vagina. Cover the cord with a sterile towel moistened with a saline solution.

5. Transport the mother and the baby to the hospital at once, maintaining pressure on the baby's head.

Uterine Inversion

Inversion, or turning inside-out, of the uterus may occur from extensive pressure on the uterus or from pulling on the umbilical cord to deliver the placenta. Shock commonly accompanies this condition. Should **uterine inversion** occur, care for it as follows:

1. Keep the patient flat.
2. Administer oxygen.
3. If the placenta is still attached to the uterus, do not remove it.
4. Pack all protruding tissues lightly with moist, sterile towels, and transport the patient rapidly to the hospital.

Excessive Bleeding after Delivery

Internal bleeding can result when placental tissue is left in the uterus, when uterine contractions are inadequate, or when the mother develops clotting disorders. If bleeding is profuse, continue uterine massage, and put the baby to the mother's breast. If bleeding persists, transport the mother rapidly to the hospital while giving her care in the usual way for shock. Administer high-flow oxygen. Avoid vaginal examination or packing of the vagina. Continue gentle uterine massage during transport.

External bleeding from tears in the skin between the vagina and the anus can be managed with firm pressure. It may be necessary to open the labia to place packs at the bleeding site. Consider the use of PASG and IV administration if trained personnel are available.

Pulmonary Embolism

Sudden shortness of breath, rapid heartbeat, and/or low blood pressure in the mother after delivery may be signs of pulmonary embolism, either from a blood clot or from amniotic fluid. Emergency care is the same as for any patient with pulmonary embolism: administer high-flow oxygen and transport the patient to the hospital immediately.

Medical Emergencies

Two medical emergencies that may be associated with pregnancy are:

1. Convulsions: A pregnant woman may have a seizure as a result of eclampsia or for any usual reason: epilepsy, high fever, or a blow to the head. For treatment, see the discussion under "Eclampsia."

2. Heart-lung complications: A pregnant woman may experience breathing difficulties due to asthma, allergies, or cardiac arrest. Treat the emergency condition and administer oxygen while transporting as quickly as is safely possible.

☐ COMPLICATIONS OF DELIVERY

Breech Birth

Breech birth refers to a delivery in which the baby's feet or buttocks appear first instead of the head. All efforts should be made to get the mother to the hospital, but when transport is not possible, follow these rules for a buttocks presentation. (Figure 34-28):

1. Position the mother as usual, and prepare her for delivery.

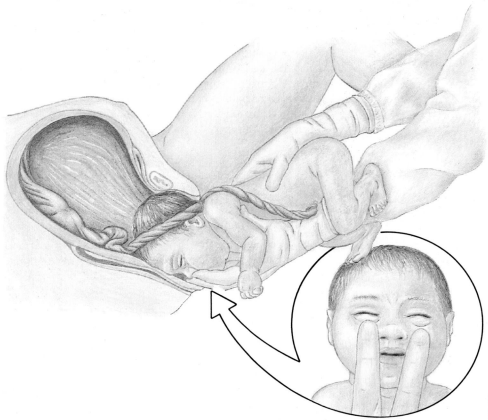

FIGURE 34-28 Provide and maintain an airway during a breech birth.

2. Let the buttocks and trunk of the baby deliver on their own.

3. Place your arm between the baby's legs, and support the baby's back with the palm of your hand. Let the baby's legs dangle astride your arms. The head should follow on its own.

4. If the head takes longer than three minutes to delivery after the waist and trunk have delivered, you must take steps to prevent the baby from suffocating, since the head will compress the umbilical cord inside the vagina and cut off circulation.

   - Place your middle and index fingers, gloved if possible, along the infant's face with your palm toward the face.
   - Reach into the vagina to the baby's nose.
   - Form an airway as you push the vagina away from the baby's face until its head is delivered slowly. Hold the baby's mouth open a little with your finger so that it can breathe.

5. Never attempt to pull the baby from the vagina by the legs or trunk.

6. When the head has delivered, give the mother and infant normal postdelivery care.

7. If the head does not deliver within three minutes, transport the mother to a medical facility either with her buttocks elevated or in a knee-chest posi-

tion. Deliver high-flow oxygen to the mother. Maintain the baby's airway throughout transport.

Umbilical Cord around the Neck

If the umbilical cord is wrapped around the baby's neck in the birth canal:

1. Try to slip it gently over the baby's shoulders or head.

2. If you cannot slip it over the baby's head, and if it is tight around the neck, place clamps or ties on the cord three inches apart, and cut between them quickly; unwrap the cord from around the neck.

3. Deliver the shoulders and body, supporting the head at all times.

Brow Presentation

In the face or brow presentation, the baby's face is next to the cervix and the neck is extended. Labor may be delayed, and a cesarean section may be necessary. Transport immediately.

Limb Presentation

If an arm or leg is first to emerge from the vagina, transport the mother *immediately* to the hospital. A limb presentation means that the baby has shifted so much in

Childbirth and Related Emergencies **505**

the uterus that a normal delivery is impossible; the baby will have to be delivered by surgical technique. Delay can be fatal. *Do not* pull on the baby by an arm or leg.

Wedged Shoulders

If the baby's shoulders become wedged in place after the head has been delivered:

1. Do *not* pull on the baby.
2. Suction the baby's mouth and nose.
3. Make sure that the baby is breathing.
4. Transport mother and baby to the hospital.
5. Constantly monitor the mother and baby during transport.

Multiple Births

One pregnancy in about eighty-six results in twins. Non-identical, or fraternal, twins each have their own placentas. Identical twins share one placenta. **Multiple births** generally present no problems, and twins are delivered in the same manner as single babies, one after another.

Even if the mother is unaware of the fact, you may suspect a multiple birth if the abdomen is still very large after one baby is delivered. There will be more strong uterine contractions, and the baby's size will be out of proportion to the mother's abdomen. Labor contractions start again about ten minutes after the first baby is born.

To manage a multiple-birth situation:

1. When the first baby is born, clamp and cut the cord (as described earlier) to prevent hemorrhage to the second baby. Contractions will continue, and the second and subsequent babies should be born within minutes. About one third of the second twins will be breech. Handle the baby as you would for a single birth.
2. If the second baby has not delivered within ten minutes of the first, transport the mother and the first baby to the hospital for delivery of the second twin. After the babies are delivered, the placenta or placentas will be delivered normally.
3. Expect hemorrhage after the second birth.
4. Keep the babies warm. Twins are often born early and may be small enough to be considered **premature.** Special precautions should be taken to prevent a fall in temperature.

Premature Births

A premature baby may weigh less than five and one-half pounds and is born before thirty-six weeks of **gestation.** You can judge by the baby's appearance or from the his-

tory given by the mother whether the baby is premature.

Premature babies are more susceptible to respiratory diseases and infection and must be given special care. Thinner, smaller, and redder than a full-term baby, a premature baby also has a larger head in proportion to his or her body. Take these steps to care for a premature baby:

1. Keep the baby warm with a blanket or infant swaddle. Use aluminum foil as an outer wrapping for extra insulation if you lack other supplies.
2. Keep the baby's nose and mouth clear of fluid by gentle suction with a bulb syringe.
3. Prevent bleeding from the umbilical cord; a premature infant cannot tolerate losing even minute amounts of blood without being at high risk for shock.
4. Administer supplemental oxygen by blowing oxygen across the infant's face; do not blast the oxygen directly into the baby's face. Never deprive a premature infant of oxygen for fear of toxicity.
5. Premature infants are highly susceptible to infection. Prevent contamination and do not let anyone breathe into the baby's face.
6. If you have the facilities in your vehicle, warm the baby during transport by placing covered hot water bottles in the bottom and along the sides of a crib. Make sure that you wrap the baby securely and that the bottles are covered completely, since the skin of a premature infant burns easily.

□ COMPLICATIONS IN NEWBORNS

Resuscitation

Some infants require resuscitation after birth, and this is the most frequent reason why EMTs are summoned in the event of planned home delivery. At all times, give attention to the **ACT** of newborn resuscitation: **airway/breathing** (supplying the blood with oxygen), **circulation,** and **temperature.** To avoid injuring the infant, use the least amount of care necessary to maintain the infant. Heart rate can determine how hard you will have to work to resuscitate the newborn.

If the heart rate is above 100:

1. Airway/breathing:
   - Gently suction the infant's mouth with a bulb.
   - Place the neck in a neutral position; do not hyperextend.
   - Stimulate respirations as necessary by gently flicking the soles of the feet with a finger or by

rubbing the back. Avoid traumatic stimulation, such as beating on the back.

2. Circulation: No specific measures are required. Monitor the heart rate continuously.

3. Temperature: Maintain body heat as described using previously detailed measures.

If the heart rate is less than 100:

1. Airway/breathing:
   - Follow the above outlined steps.
   - Administer oxygen by mask.
   - If breathing is absent or very irregular, assist breathing.

2. Circulation: Monitor pulse carefully and prepare to begin external cardiac compressions if the heart rate does not respond to oxygen and quickly drops below eighty beats per minute.

3. Temperature: Lack of heat prolongs or prevents recovery. In addition to ensuring immediate survival, the goal of resuscitation must be to prevent central nervous system impairment.

If there is no heart rate:

1. Airway/breathing:
   - Clear the airway. Use mechanical suction only as a last resort. Use only gentle pressure.
   - Immediately assist breathing, usually with mouth-to-mouth and mouth-to-nose resuscitation.

2. Circulation: Absence of a heart rate is a grim sign. Begin external cardiac compressions immediately.

3. Temperature: Continue to warm the infant and guard against hypothermia.

Breathing Assistance and Cardiac Compression

In the infant, bag and mask or mouth-to-mouth and mouth-to-nose ventilation are usually adequate to assist breathing. The baby should be on a flat, firm surface. Fold a small towel and place it underneath the baby's shoulders to keep the head in a neutral position. The normal rate of respiration in the newborn is forty breaths per minute. Short, quick puffs of air should be given at the rate of forty per minute; too large a volume can over-expand or burst the baby's lungs. Remember — the baby breathes through his nose.

Cardiac compressions should be performed for an absent heartbeat or for a heart rate less than eighty that does not respond to oxygen or assisted breathing. Compress the baby's midsternum with two fingers while supporting the back. The rate of cardiac compressions is

four or five for each breath, or two per second. Continue resuscitation until you arrive at an emergency medical center or until the baby has been pronounced dead by a physician. Do not give up. Many babies survive even long periods of nonspontaneous breathing without brain damage if they have good CPR.

Dead or Dying Infants

Occasionally, a baby will be born dead; you should not attempt resuscitative efforts if the baby has obviously been dead for at least several hours prior to birth. Such a baby may have large blisters covering its body, may have an extremely soft head, and may smell rotten. Your main consideration should be the parents' grief and disappointment. Regardless of your religion, you can baptize the baby of Christian parents at their request, or they may perform the rite themselves. One approach is to sprinkle a few drops of water on the baby's bare skin and repeat these words, "I baptize you in the name of the Father, and of the Son, and of the Holy Spirit." Ask the parents the procedure they wish to follow.

You or they may also want to baptize a baby who is obviously dying. Continue resuscitative efforts during the baptism and during transport until you reach the hospital or until a physician officially declares the baby dead.

Do not lie to the mother. Many death and dying experts believe that she should see the dead baby if she wishes; it will help her accept and deal with the trauma more easily. If she has poor vital signs, is in shock, has experienced excessive blood loss, or in emotionally unstable, gently tell her that she can see the baby later but that it died before birth.

Meconium Passage

Meconium passage means that the child has experienced distress and has had a bowel movement inside the amniotic sac. The amniotic fluid will be a greenish color. Breathing in some of the fluid may cause possible infection and pneumonia. Meconium passage is common during breech births.

The important emergency care is to clear the oral and nasal passages before the baby takes a first breath. Suction the nose and mouth with a small suction catheter as soon as the head is born if at all possible.

☐ PREGNANCY AND TRAUMA

A baby in the uterus is remarkably well protected. Direct fetal injuries are, therefore, comparatively rare, and the baby's greatest risk of danger is from the mother's injury or illness.

Typically a pregnant patient will be very concerned that your procedures might injure her unborn child. Reassure her that you know she's pregnant, that your procedures will not harm the child, and that keeping her safe and stable is the best way to ensure her baby's safety.

Some conditions in pregnancy place the woman at a higher risk for accidents:

- She is off-balanced and more likely to fall.
- Because she weighs more, she is more likely to suffer sprained wrists from trying to break a fall.
- During the later stages of pregnancy, joints and ligaments have relaxed, making for general, though minor, weakness and unsteadiness.
- She is more subject to fatigue, fainting, and hyperventilation.
- Late pregnancy can push the diaphragm up as much as an inch, causing difficulty in breathing for the mother.
- Her blood volume increases by 30 to 50 percent; as a result, she may not show clinical signs of hemorrhage until she has lost 30 to 50 percent of her blood volume. During shock, blood flow to the uterus can decrease by 10 to 20 percent with no change in the mother's vital signs.
- Her pulse rate and blood pressure usually go up, and she is at greater risk for shock and hemorrhage.
- The uterus lies in front of the other abdominal organs, but the liver and spleen may become distended, compressed, or displaced, making them more vulnerable to injury or rupture. The bladder also rises so that it is not protected by the pelvis, as in nonpregnant women.
- Pelvic fracture is the most common fracture in pregnant women and is particularly dangerous because the increased chance of hemorrhage leads to increased risk of shock. Even minor abdominal trauma can cause major hemorrhage. Pelvic fractures are also most potentially lethal to the infant in the form of skull fracture. During the end of the last trimester, the head is lodged in the pelvis and the amniotic fluid cushions it less effectively.
- During car accidents, impact or even lap belts can cause bruises quite easily (common and not serious) and internal damage to the uterus, fetus, or placenta (rare but very serious). In a nonpregnant woman, you would check for absent bowel sounds or rebound tenderness as danger signals, but the stretching of the abdominal wall during pregnancy alters its response and may make guarding altogether absent. The safest way for a pregnant woman to ride in a vehicle is with a combination seat and chest restraint so that the force of impact is not concentrated over the uterus.

- Unlike the uterus, the placenta lacks elastic fibers and is particularly vulnerable to shearing forces. You should consider abruptio placenta a possibility in every case of blunt abdominal injury to a pregnant woman.
- Babies seem particularly susceptible to electric shock. Even comparatively mild shocks from household equipment that do not leave burns can result in stillbirths, possibly because the amniotic fluid channels much of the current through the baby.

Twenty-two percent of all deaths during pregnancy are trauma-related, with the leading cause being motor vehicle accidents. When a pregnant woman is involved in an accident, you should delay treating pregnancy–related problems until you have run through the priorities for any trauma patient: airway, breathing and circulation, and bleeding.

If a significant mechanism of injury is present, assume the potential of serious injury, whether or not outward signs are present. The most common life-threatening conditions related to abdominal trauma in pregnant women are splenic rupture, liver lacerations, abruptio placenta, and pelvic fracture.

Emergency Care

Use the following guidelines in caring for a pregnant patient in trauma:

1. Routinely give supplemental oxygen to counteract the inevitable oxygen reduction to the uterus if there is any stress.
2. Place the patient on her left side.
3. Monitor the fetal heartbeat often. The normal range is 120 to 160 beats per minute, and changes in the baby's heart rate are sometimes the first warning of internal hemorrhage.
4. Pregnancy usually increases nausea, and so does trauma. Be prepared for vomiting and aspiration. Check for the presence of blood that could indicate gastrointestinal or respiratory trauma.
5. If you suspect spinal injury and have immobilized the mother on her back, place a small pillow or pad of towels under her right hip to shift the uterus away from the vena cava.
6. If there is significant bleeding from the vagina, suspect placenta previa, abruptio placenta, or uterine rupture. Have the patient lie supine with her feet and legs slightly elevated. Do not perform a vaginal examination. Try to determine the amount of bleeding by asking:
   - Have you had any aches or cramps that might be contractions?

- When did the bleeding begin?
- Was it associated with a specific event, such as intercourse, a vaginal examiantion, a fall, or an injury?
- Did it begin with spotting or with a gush?
- Is the blood dark or bright red?
- Did it contain any clots or tissues?
- How much did you bleed? A few tablespoons? How many pads have you used? Were they soaked or spotted? Is the bleeding heavy or light compared to your period? (Ask if a normal period is heavy or light.)

7. If possible, take the pads and any tissue or clots with you to the hospital for examination.

8. Be extremely alert for signs of shock: confusion, weakness, clammy skin, coldness, a rapid, weak pulse, etc.

9. In an accident where the mother is dead or dying, you have an excellent chance of saving the baby if you begin CPR immediately on the mother and continue until an emergency cesarean section can be performed by a physician. Chances of success are fair if CPR is delayed between five and ten minutes, dropping to unlikely if the interval is as long as twenty-five minutes. If you detect any fetal heartbeat, assume that a cesarean section is a possibility and maintain CPR until you can reach the hospital.

10. Be aware that a pregnant woman developing severe shock can compensate extremely well and then rapidly deteriorate. Use caution when treating this trauma patient.

chapter 35

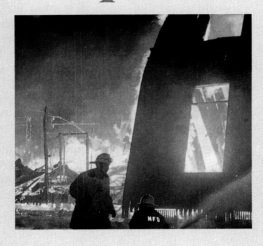

Burn Emergencies

✳ **OBJECTIVES**

- Describe the various burn classifications and how they relate to the anatomy of the skin.
- Identify the characteristics of first-, second-, and third-degree burns and be able to calculate the extent of burns using the Rule of Nines.
- Explain how to assess the severity of burns and describe appropriate burn management for thermal burns.
- Identify the signs and symptoms of inhalation injuries and describe appropriate emergency care.
- Recognize the various types of chemical burns and describe appropriate emergency care.
- Describe how electrical energy and lightning can injure the body and describe appropriate emergency care for electrical shock and lightning injuries.

□ TYPES OF BURN INJURIES

More than two million burn accidents occur each year in the United States. Of those who are burned (in fires, by chemicals, by the sun, in automobile accidents, or in other kinds of accidents), more than 12,000 die as a result of their burns, and almost one million require long-term hospitalization. Burns are a leading cause of accidental death in the United States, exceeded in numbers only by automobile accidents and falls. The number of productive years lost to burns is greater than those lost to cancer, heart disease, and strokes.

Burns can be complex injuries. In addition to the burn itself, a number of other functions may be affected. Since burns injure the skin, they impair the body's normal fluid/electrolyte balance, body temperature, body thermal regulation, joint function, manual dexterity, and physical appearance (Figure 35-1).

Children under the age of six receive more burns than people in any other age group. The most common kind of burn is a **scald.** Toddlers pull pans of boiling water off of stoves. People scurrying to get dinner on the table trip over an infant crawling across the floor and dump a steaming cauldron of soup all over the infant. People misjudging the temperature of bath water dip babies into steaming tubs and turn faucets of scalding water on soapy arms and legs. In terms of injury and death, scald burns are the most severe.

Second to scalds in this age group are **contact burns.** An eighteen-month-old who is just learning to walk needs to support his or her shaky steps, and he or she will lean against a radiator, oven door, woodburning stove, or other hot object as readily as he or she will lean against a sofa. There are other kinds of burns, too, as houses catch on fire and parents do not wake up. Small children sometimes chew on electrical cords, sustaining severe electrical burns.

Depending on the type of accident that caused the fire or burn, there is often associated trauma. Most frequently, you will see burn victims with internal injury, blunt trauma, head injury, multiple fractures, and serious lacerations.

The seriousness of a burn is determined by the following factors:

- Degree of the burn.
- Percentage of the body burned.
- Severity of the burn.
- Location of the burn.
- Accompanying complications (such as preexisting physical or mental conditions).
- Age of the patient.

FIGURE 35-1 Burns may cause shock by damaging surface tissue and dilating underlying blood vessels, which may lead to extensive loss of plasma.

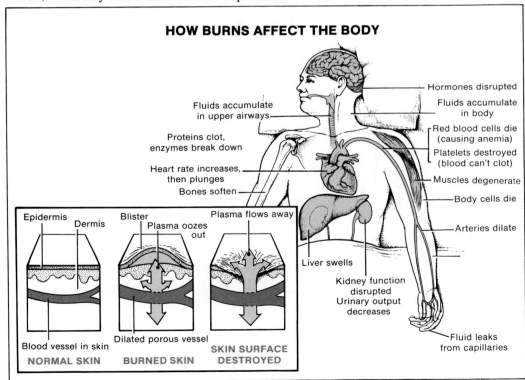

☐ DEGREE OF THE BURN

Burns are classified by degree of damage to the skin and underlying tissues. (See Figures 35-2–35-9 and Table 35-1.)

First-Degree Burns

First-degree burns can be caused by a flash, a flame, a scald, or the sun. They are the most common and the most minor of all burns. The skin looks pink and dry with *slight* swelling; no blisters occur. The skin is reddened and extremely painful, but the epidermal layer is the only one affected (Figure 35-10). The skin retains its elasticity and retains its ability to act as a barrier against bacteria, heat, and water. First-degree burns heal in two to five days with no scarring. Peeling of the outer epidermal layer usually occurs, and some temporary discoloration may result.

Second-Degree Burns

Second-degree burns result from contact with hot liquids or solids, flash or flame contact with clothing, direct flame from fires, contact with chemical substances, or the sun. The skin appears moist and mottled, and it ranges in color from white to cherry red. The burned area is blistered and extremely painful. The epidermis and **dermal** layers of skin are usually burned, and damage may result to some fat domes of the subcutaneous (fatty tissue just under the skin) layer (see Figure 35-10).

Second-degree burns heal spontaneously. The skin retains its elasticity, but loses its function as a barrier against bacteria, heat, and water. Second-degree burns are considered minor if they involve less than 15 percent of the body surface in adults and less than 10 percent in children. When 15 to 30 percent of an adult's body surface or 10 to 20 percent of a child's body surface is involved, a second-degree burn is considered moderate. The burn is considered severe if it involves the face, hands, feet, or genital area. A second-degree burn is considered critical if it involves more than 30 percent of the total body surface in an adult and 20 percent in a child.

Healing of a minor second-degree burn usually requires five to twenty-one days; if infection occurs, healing time usually takes longer.

Third-Degree Burns

Third-degree, or full-thickness **burns,** are the most serious, resulting from contact with hot liquids or solids, flame, chemicals, or electricity. The skin becomes dry and leathery; charred blood vessels are often visible. The skin is a mixture of colors: white (waxy-pearly), dark (khaki-mahogany), and charred. While a third-degree burn may be very painful, the patient often feels little or no pain, because the nerve endings have been destroyed (see Figure 35-10). The burn extends through all dermal layers and can involve subcutaneous layers, muscles, organs, and bone. The skin loses its elasticity and its function as a barrier against bacteria, heat, and water.

Third-degree burns are considered minor if they occur on less than 2 percent of the body surface. Moderate burns involve 2 to 10 percent of the body surface. Third-degree burns are classified as critical if they occur on more than 10 percent of the total body surface, if there is any involvement of the face, hands, feet, or genital area, or if the burns are caused by chemicals or electricity.

Third-degree burns that cover small areas require weeks to heal, while larger burns usually require skin **grafting** and take months or years to heal completely.

TABLE 35-1
Characteristics of Various Depths of Burns

	FIRST DEGREE	SECOND DEGREE	THIRD DEGREE
Cause	Sun or minor flash	Hot liquids, flashes, or flame	Chemicals, electricity, flame, hot metals
Skin color	Red	Mottled red	Pearly white and/or charred translucent and parchment-like
Skin surface	Dry with no blisters	Blisters with weeping	Dry with thrombosed blood vessels
Sensation	Painful	Painful	Anesthetic
Healing	3–6 days	2–4 weeks, depending on depth	Requires skin grafting

From Bryan E. Bledsoe et al., *Paramedic Emergency Care*, Prentice Hall, 1991, p. 517.

□ Types of Burns

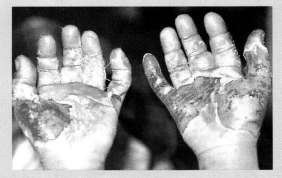

FIGURE 35-2 Second- and third-degree burns.

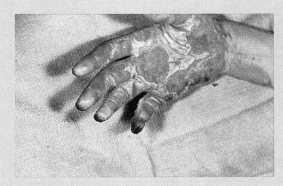

FIGURE 35-3 Third-degree flare burns.

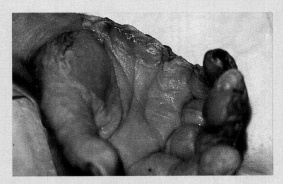

FIGURE 35-4 Second- and third-degree burns.

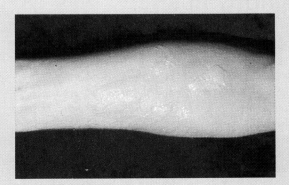

FIGURE 35-5 Second- and third-degree burns.

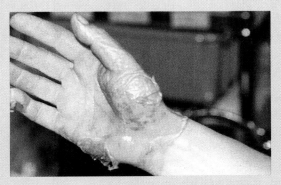

FIGURE 35-6 Second-degree burn.

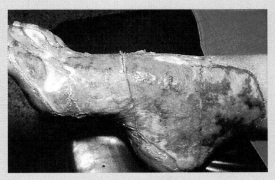

FIGURE 35-7 Second-degree burn.

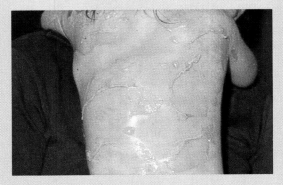

FIGURE 35-8 Second-degree burn.

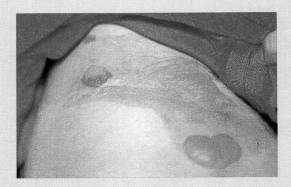

FIGURE 35-9 Second-degree burn.

BURNS CLASSIFICATION

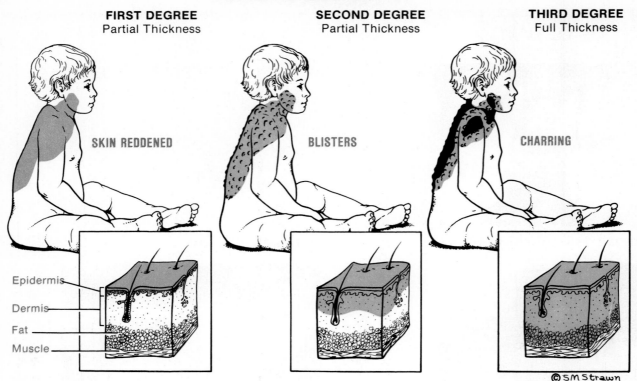

FIRST DEGREE
Partial Thickness

SKIN REDDENED

Epidermis
Dermis
Fat
Muscle

SECOND DEGREE
Partial Thickness

BLISTERS

THIRD DEGREE
Full Thickness

CHARRING

©SMStrawn

FIGURE 35-10

☐ PERCENTAGE OF BODY BURNED: THE RULE OF NINES

The **Rule of Nines** (Figure 35-11) can be used to calculate quickly the amount of skin surface that has received burns. It can help you quickly understand the severity of a burn, assist you in performing appropriate triage, and allow you to best prepare the hospital for patients who will be arriving.

An alternate method is the "palmar surface." The palm of the victim's hand is equal to approximately 1 percent of his body surface; this holds true regardless of the victim's age. You can use this as an estimate of the burned surface by mentally or physically making the measurement.

Consider estimates that a dispatcher receives over the telephone as just that — estimates. Often, a burn victim or a member of his family is too hysterical to give you an accurate evaluation, or he may exaggerate the extent of the burned area to inspire you to hurry.

☐ SEVERITY OF THE BURN

Most burn wounds are a combination of classifications; that is, part of the skin is burned to the first degree, part to the second degree, and maybe part to the third degree.

A **full-thickness burn** (third degree) is one that burns through all layers of skin into the subcutaneous tissues; first- and second-degree burns, going through only part of the skin, are referred to as **partial thickness burns.**

In general, the following burns are considered **critical** (Figure 35-12):

- Burns that are complicated by respiratory tract injuries or other major injuries or fractures.
- Third-degree burns involving the face, hands, feet, or genital area.
- Third-degree burns that cover more than 10 percent of an adult's body surface.
- Third-degree burns that cover more than 2 to 3 percent of a child's body surface.
- Any burns of the hands, feet, face, eyes, ears, or perineum.
- All inhalation injuries.
- Second-degree burns that cover more than 30 percent of an adult's body surface.
- Second-degree burns that cover more than 20 percent of a child's body surface.
- First-degree burns that cover more than 75 percent of the body surface.
- Most chemical burns.
- All electrical burns.

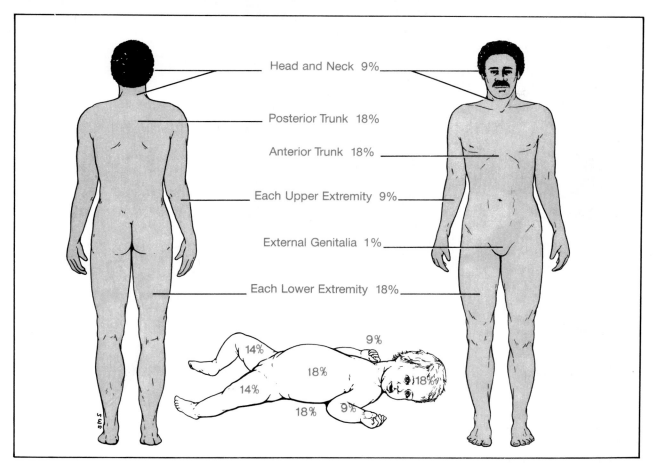

FIGURE 35-11 The Rule of Nines: A method for estimating percentage of body surface involved with burns. The body surface is divided into regions, each of which represents 9%, or a multiple of 9%, of the total surface, except in infants.

- Burns in patients who have serious underlying medical conditions, such as diabetes, seizure disorders, hypertension, or mental or psychiatric disorders.

When you reach the patient, quickly assess the *depth* of the burn as soon as you have determined the extent of body surface affected. The depth of the burn is almost impossible to determine from a verbal estimate alone. As a *very* rough rule, use the following guide to guess the depth of a burn described to you over the telephone or radio:

- If the burn is a scald on bare skin and the patient is an adolescent or adult, the burn is probably **superficial,** involving only the outer dermal layer, because the heat from such a burn dissipates rapidly. If the patient is an infant or an elderly person, the burn may involve additional dermal layers.
- If the burn is **thermal,** it may be partial or full thickness.

- If the burn was caused by hot grease, it is probably a full-thickness burn. Grease cools slowly and is difficult to remove; therefore, it may cause extensive and deep damage before it can be removed.
- Burns caused by electricity or chemicals are almost always full-thickness burns because of the extensive, unseen damage that accompanies even apparently minor skin injuries. Patients with such burns are almost always hospitalized so that physicians can monitor vital signs and functioning of major organs.

☐ LOCATION OF THE BURN

Certain areas of the body are more critically damaged by burns than others, and it is essential that you recognize which areas represent the greatest hazard.

Burns on the face or neck should be examined immediately because of possible burns to the eye area or respiratory complications. Check the eyes to make sure

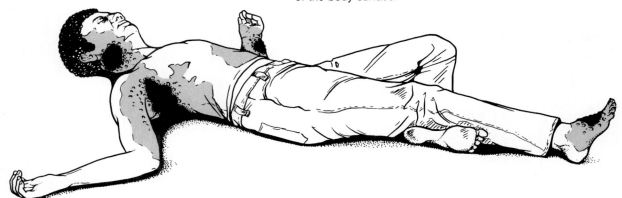

CRITICAL BURNS

NOTE: The general condition of the patient must also be considered. For example, a moderate burn in an aged or critically ill person might be serious.

CRITICAL BURNS are burns complicated by respiratory tract injury and other major injuries or fractures.

THIRD-DEGREE burns involving the critical areas of the face, hands, feet, or genitalia.

SECOND-DEGREE burns covering more than 30% of the body surface.

THIRD-DEGREE burns covering more than 10% of the body surface.

ELECTRICAL AND DEEP ACID BURNS

BURNS in patients with underlying physical or medical conditions.

FIGURE 35-12

that no injury has occurred. Then assess whether respiratory damage is present.

Other locations of burns that are particularly critical include the hands, feet, and external genitalia. Any burn to the upper body is more serious than a burn of similar extent and degree on the lower body. Patients with burns in any of these areas should be transported to the hospital or burn center immediately.

□ ACCOMPANYING COMPLICATIONS

Patients who have major diseases such as heart disease or diabetes or who have other injuries will always react more severely to a burn — even if it is a minor one. Try to determine the patient's medical history early in the course of care so that you will be aware of any underlying problems.

□ AGE OF THE PATIENT

Children under the age of five and adults over the age of sixty tolerate burns very poorly. In an elderly patient, a burn covering only 20 percent of the body can often be fatal.

Because the elderly and the very young have extremely thin skin, they will sustain much deeper burns from a much less severe source. The young and elderly also have a disproportionate fluid-to-surface-area ratio, so even a small fluid loss can result in serious problems. An additional problem is disease immunity — it is incomplete in the young child and is usually compromised in the elderly.

□ BURN MANAGEMENT

Don't attempt to rescue people trapped by fire unless you have been specially trained to do so; you could easily become a victim yourself. The first priority in the field is to prevent further injury. Make sure you are in an area remote from the fire, and remember that fire can rapidly spread. The problems most often associated with burns are:

- Airway or respiratory difficulties.
- Related musculoskeletal injuries.
- Loss of body fluids, contributing to shock.
- Pain contributing to shock.
- Anxiety contributing to shock.
- Swelling.
- Infection due to destruction of skin tissue.

Care of a burn and associated injuries must start immediately — preferably at the moment of burning. Unfortunately, this early emergency care is too often administered by terrified but well-meaning family, friends, or bystanders. Sometimes even the burn patient will attempt to care for the burn. One reason why burns are so often critically damaging or even fatal is that some individuals who administer early emergency care are poorly informed about methods of care. Instead of helping the patient, they hinder or even hurt the patient. Remember: an EMT does not *treat* a burn; he or she merely cares for the burn until the patient can be transported to a hospital or burn center for thorough treatment.

Emergency Care

Your first priority at the scene is to prevent further injury to the patient or injury to others. Emergency care for specific burns will be discussed later in this chapter. Regardless of the type of burn, use the following general guidelines in administering care (Figures 35-13–35-18):

1. Remove the patient from the source of the burn. This seems extremely simple — almost too simple to mention — but it is surprising how many fail to get the patient *away* from the source of the burn. If the patient was burned by a fire, take him or her as far away as possible without inflicting further injury. Get the patient far enough away so that he or she does not inhale smoke. If the burn resulted from the patient lying in a puddle of petroleum byproduct or strong chemical, take the patient out of the puddle. If he or she was struck by lightning, get the patient to shelter.

2. Eliminate the cause of the burn. Again, this is simple logic. Put out the fire. Wash away the chemicals. Immerse scald or grease burns in cold water to stop the burning (Figure 35-19). If the victim has been burned by hot tar, cool the tar with water but do *not* try to remove the tar. If the patient's clothes are on fire, roll him or her on the ground until the flames are extinguished, douse with water, and remove all clothing (including items) that tend to retain heat, such as jewelry and shoes). Do not remove clothing that is embedded in the burn. Never cover a burn with dirt in an attempt to extinguish flames unless it's the only available thing. If you sucessfully eliminate the cause of the burn, you can help prevent someone else at the scene from sustaining a burn injury.

3. Assess the patient's vital signs — airway, breathing, and circulation — as you would for any injury. Administer 100 percent oxygen, and maintain an open airway. Monitor vital signs continuously throughout treatment and transport — the victim's status can change suddenly. (For example, smoke inhalation causes progressive edema of the airway, and breathing can become progressively more labored.)

4. Determine the severity of the burn. Decide immediately how critical the burn is and how extensive the injury has become. Take into account the factors previously discussed: the extent of total body surface involved, the depth of the burn, the age of the patient, the location of the burn, and the possibility of preexistent disease or additional injury. Although it is critical that you determine the severity of the burn, do not delay treatment or transport while you do so.

5. Determine the history. How did the burn happen? What caused it? Did the patient fall from a window, or was he thrown by an electric current? Was he enclosed in a confined space or forced to inhale copious amounts of smoke? How long ago was the patient burned? What care has been given by bystanders (or by the patient himself)? If the burn involved chemicals, find out which chemical. If it was a scald, how did it happen? Does the mechanism of injury match the signs and symptoms — or could there be child abuse involved? All of this information will be vital in determining the method of emergency care.

6. Examine for respiratory/cardiac complications. Check the patient thoroughly to determine whether breathing or heartbeat has stopped. If the patient is still breathing, look for signs of injury to the respiratory system. Be especially alert for wheezing or coughing as the patient breathes, for a sooty or smoky smell on his or her breath, for particles of soot in his or her saliva, and for burns of the mucous membranes in the mouth and nostrils. If any of these signs are present, immediately assist breathing. Administer high-flow oxygen by nonrebreather mask. Use humidified oxygen if it is available. Even though the patient does not manifest actual breathing difficulty at the time he or she receives the burn, remember that respiratory injuries frequently do not manifest themselves until twelve to twenty-four hours after the actual injury. This patient requires hospitalization.

7. Cover the burn with a sterile, nonstick burn dressing or sheet; if less than 9 percent of the body surface is burned, if the skin is not broken, and if the patient is not in a cold environment, cover the burned area with cool, wet towels or compresses. Never use ice or ice packs on a burn.

☐ Care for Thermal Burns

TYPE OF BURN	TISSUE BURNED			COLOR CHANGES	PAIN	BLISTERS
	OUTER LAYER OF SKIN	SECOND LAYER OF SKIN	TISSUES BELOW SKIN			
1st Degree	Yes	No	No	Red	Yes	No
2nd Degree	Yes	Yes	No	Deep red	Yes	Yes
3rd Degree	Yes	Yes	Yes	Charred black or white	Yes/No	Yes/No

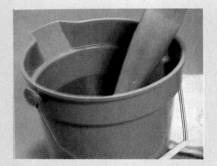

FIGURE 35-13

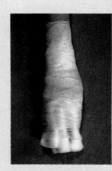

FIGURE 35-14

FIGURE 35-15

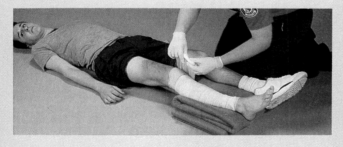

FIGURE 35-16

FIGURE 35-17

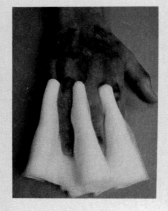

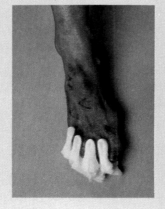

MINOR FIRST AND SECOND DEGREE:

- Have someone alert dispatch
- Immerse in cold water 2–5 minutes (Fig. 35–13)
- Cover entire burn with dry, sterile dressing (Fig. 35–14)
- Moisten — only if burn is less than 9% of skin surface

MAJOR BURNS:

- Stop burning process
- Have someone alert dispatch
- Maintain open airway
- Wrap area with clean, dry dressing (moisten if less than 9% of skin surface is affected)
- Provide care for shock (Fig. 35–15)

IF HANDS OR TOES ARE BURNED:

- Separate digits with sterile gauze pads (Fig. 35–16, 35–17)
- When appropriate, elevate the extremity

BURNS TO THE EYES:

- Do not open eyelids if burned
- Be certain burn is thermal, not chemical
- Apply moist, sterile gauze pads to both eyes (Fig. 35–18)

FIGURE 35-18

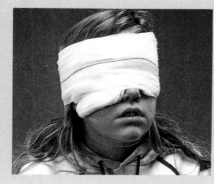

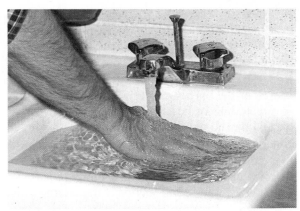

FIGURE 35-19 Cooling a burn by submerging in cold running water.

☐ INHALATION INJURIES

More than half of all fire-related deaths are caused by smoke inhalation; 80 percent of those who die in residential fires do so because they have inhaled heated air, smoke, or other toxic gases — not because they have been burned to death. Suspect inhalation injury in any victim of thermal burn, especially if the victim was confined in an enclosed space or was unconscious at any time during the fire.

Three causes of inhalation injury accompany burns:

- Heat inhalation.
- Inhalation of toxic chemicals or smoke.
- Inhalation of carbon monoxide gas (the most common burn-associated inhalation injury).

Heated air usually only burns the upper airway, since air is cooled as it progresses through the respiratory tract. Lower airway burns *can* be caused by steam, which has a higher heat capacity than air. Most of the damage done to the upper airway is a result of heat inhalation — mucous membranes and linings get scorched, and edema partially blocks the airway. The severity of the inhalation injury is determined by the products of combustion (what was burned), the degree of combustion (how completely the materials were burned), the duration of exposure (how long the victim was exposed to the smoke or gases), and whether the victim was in a confined space.

Because edema and other damage can be progressive, the inhalation injury may appear to be mild at first but may become more severe. Depending on the materials that were burned and the length of the victim's exposure to the fire, symptoms may occur within a few minutes but may not appear for many hours.

Specific signs and symptoms of **upper airway injuries** are (Figure 35-20):

- Singed nasal hairs.
- Facial burns.
- Burned specks of carbon in the sputum.
- A sooty or smoky smell on the breath.
- Respiratory distress accompanied by restriction of chest wall movement, restlessness, chest tightness, stridor, wheezing, difficulty in swallowing, hoarseness, coughing, and cyanosis.
- You may be able to see actual burns of the oral mucosa (Figure 35-21).

In the presence of these signs and symptoms, administer humidified oxygen to help minimize damage done by scorching heat. Assume respiratory injury if in doubt, especially if facial burns are present.

More critical respiratory injury results from the inhalation of agents such as noxious chemicals, carbon

FIGURE 35-20

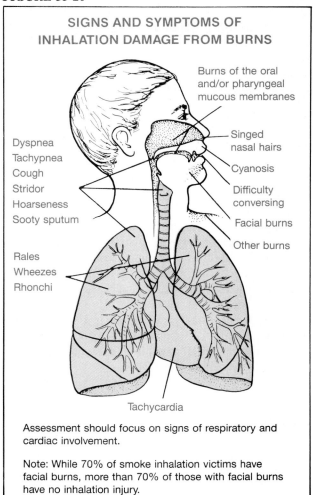

SIGNS AND SYMPTOMS OF INHALATION DAMAGE FROM BURNS

Burns of the oral and/or pharyngeal mucous membranes

Singed nasal hairs

Cyanosis

Difficulty conversing

Facial burns

Other burns

Dyspnea
Tachypnea
Cough
Stridor
Hoarseness
Sooty sputum

Rales
Wheezes
Rhonchi

Tachycardia

Assessment should focus on signs of respiratory and cardiac involvement.

Note: While 70% of smoke inhalation victims have facial burns, more than 70% of those with facial burns have no inhalation injury.

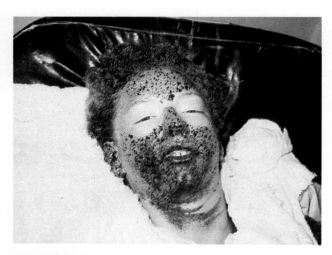

FIGURE 35-21 Facial inhalation burn.

monoxide fumes, or smoke. Noxious fumes can result from the burning of a number of ordinary household objects, such as carpets, draperies, wall coverings, floor coverings, upholstery, and lacquered wood veneer on furniture. Plastics, upholstery, and natural fabrics all emit cyanide fumes when burned. there are almost three hundred toxic substances that result from burning wood alone.

When noxious fumes are inhaled, mucosa in the lungs swell and break, leaking fluid into the nearby alveolar spaces and damaging the cilia. Mucus builds up and plugs the air passages. The final result is reduced oxygen exchange that can eventually lead to death if left untreated.

Carbon monoxide is released during the combustion of cellulose materials, such as wood, paper, and cotton. Carbon monoxide poisoning is the major cause of death at the scene of a fire. Even when carbon monoxide doesn't cause death, it can cause long-term neurological damage by depriving the brain of oxygen (while the damage will not be apparent for several days, its onset is usually rapid after that).

Almost everything gives off carbon monoxide when it burns. Carbon monoxide is colorless, odorless, and tasteless, making it extremely difficult to detect. Carbon monoxide is especially hazardous among sleeping victims, who simply never wake up.

Since burns usually do not alter levels of consciousness, assume that any burn patient who is unconscious is suffering from carbon monoxide poisoning (see Chapter 22, "Poisoning Emergencies").

Emergency Care

Start oxygen therapy immediately. Take the following measures to prevent further respiratory complications:

1. Place the patient in an upright position to allow for easier breathing if vital signs and injuries do not contraindicate it.

2. If respiratory distress occurs, insert an oropharyngeal or nasopharyngeal airway (if the patient will tolerate it) so that an adequate airway can be maintained.

3. Remove the patient as far as possible from the source of the burn — especially if it is a fire. Try to situate him or her so that he is breathing fresh air and has no danger of inhaling more smoke.

4. Mouth-to-mouth or mouth-to-mask ventilation may be required to help the patient initiate his or her own clear breathing. Clear all foreign particles from the airway, using suction if necessary.

5. Remove any clothing that may restrict chest movement or breathing. Remove neckties and necklaces if they have not burned and if they are not sticking to the skin.

6. If severe respiratory distress develops before you can transport the patient, administer 100 percent humidified oxygen by mask, and transport the patient *immediately* to the nearest hospital or burn center, where the patient can receive needed care (Figure 35-22).

7. Keep the hospital or burn center informed of the patient's status at all times so that if an emergency situation develops, you can be advised as to specific care. Give the hospital an estimate of the degree of burn, percentage of the skin involved, location of the burn, and age of the patient. When you arrive at the hospital or burn center, inform the attending physician what care you have administered and what you have been able to determine about the condition of the respiratory tract.

8. Similar measures should be taken in case of cardiac arrest. Inform the hospital or burn center, and request instructions for administering care. If cardiopulmonary resuscitation is necessary, take the appropriate precautions to prevent spinal injury.

FIGURE 35-22 Emergency care for smoke inhalation.

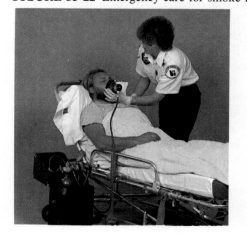

☐ THERMAL AND RADIANT BURNS

Thermal burns are caused by flame or radiant heat, including sunburn and scalding. Critical to the success of rescue work involving thermal burn patients is establishing an accurate history and assessing the extent of the injury.

Determine the following factors immediately:

- When did the burn occur? How much time elapsed before you arrived?
- What has been done to care for the burn?
- Was the patient trapped in a closed space with smoke, steam, or any other product of combustion? If so, for how long?
- Did the patient lose consciousness at any time?
- What caused the burn? (Was it open flame, hot liquids, or the sun?)
- Does the patient have any history of significant heart disease, pulmonary problems, diabetes, or any other major disease that might complicate **fluid therapy** or other aspects of treatment or that might increase the severity of the burn?
- Determine the depth and severity of burned tissue, and classify the burn according to first, second, or third degree.
- Was the patient exposed to an explosion or other mechanism of additional trauma?

Emergency Care

Field care prior to hospitalization differs with the degree of the burn, but always begin by removing the patient from the source of the burn or extinguishing the source itself. Unless specified as otherwise, do the following regardless of the degree of burn:

1. Put out the fire and extinguish burning clothing.
2. After assuring airway and breathing, remove any smoldering clothing that does not stick to the burned skin, and remove any shoes or jewelry that may retain heat. Be sure that they do not stick to the skin. If clothing adheres to the skin, cut carefully around it, but do not try to remove it forcefully.
3. First-degree burns should be immersed in cool water (see Figure 35-19); place a cool compress on burns located on the trunk or face. Whenever possible, make a moist compress with sterile gauze and saline; whatever you use, both water and dressings must be as clean as possible. Remoisten dressings periodically to keep them damp but not soaked. (Figure 35-23). *Note: Some EMS directors*

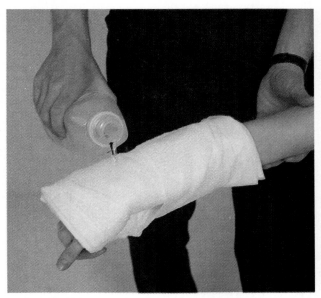

FIGURE 35-23 Remoistening a burn dressing.

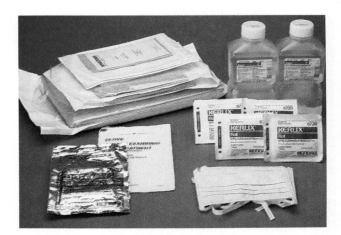

FIGURE 35-24 Burn care kit.

do not recommend wet burn dressings for any — type of burn — follow local protocol. Cover the burned area with a sterile dressing or other clean woven materials, such as sheets or towels; do not use material that might adhere or disintegrate (see Figure 35-24 for a burn care kit). Never use ice, ointments, or any other covering on any type of burn. For all but the most superficial first-degree burns, transport the patient to the hospital for observation and medical clearance; no further care is usually necessary.

4. Second-degree burns should be immersed in cool water and covered with cool compresses within thirty minutes of occurrence. Moderate and critical burns should be covered with a bulky, dry dressing and loosely bandaged in place (Figures 35-25 and 35-26). This treatment can substantially reduce swelling and provide significant pain relief.

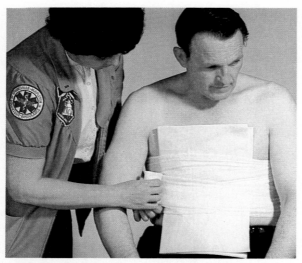

FIGURE 35-25 Application of bulky burn dressing for moderate and critical burns.

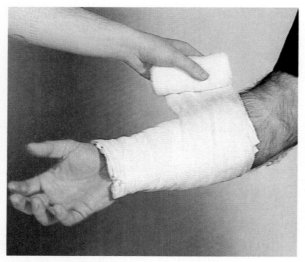

FIGURE 35-26 For moderate and critical burns, cover with a thick, clean, dry dressing and loosely bandage in place.

Never try to rupture blisters over the burn; if you accidentally break a blister, keep it as sterile as possible. If the eyelids are burned, cover them with sterile or clean pads moistened with sterile water. Insert sterile or clean pads between burned fingers and toes to prevent flesh from adhering. Elevate burned extremities slightly.

5. All patients with major burns require oxygen. If the patient is pregnant, regardless of the severity of burns, administer high-flow supplemental oxygen to protect the fetus.

6. Protect the patient from heat loss and possible hypothermia by covering him or her with a dry blanket, avoiding exposure to drafts, and turning up the heat in the rescue unit. Burn patients have had their body's normal thermal regulatory system disrupted, and they can lose heat rapidly.

7. Anticipate respiratory problems if burns are present around the face (especially if nasal hairs or openings are singed), if the patient has been unconscious in a burning area, or if the patient has been exposed to smoke or hot gases. Any burn patient can rapidly develop respiratory complications. *Assume that inhalation injury has occurred until proven otherwise.* Keep a suction unit available. Administer high-flow oxygen with a nonrebreather mask.

8. Take appropriate measures to prevent shock.

Once you have completed initial emergency care, examine the patient for any obscured damage. Especially examine the eyes for burns or other injury, the pulses in all extremities (since swelling can act as a tourniquet), and all limbs (to determine possible fractures or lacerations). Remove any other jewelry, belt buckles, or glasses that might constrict the body in the event of swelling. Transport the patient immediately to a hospital, trauma center, or burn center. Provide high-flow (100 percent) oxygen and ventilation as needed during transport.

Thermal burns in infants and small children pose a special problem, because their body surface is much larger in proportion to their total body mass. Therefore, potential fluid losses are massive, and the onset of shock is rapid. Wrap a burned baby in a moist, sterile sheet, and cover him or her with enough blankets to keep him or her warm. Transport to the nearest hospital *immediately* and maintain the airway during transport.

Scalding

Cover scald burns (Figures 35-27–35-29) with a cool, moist, sterile dressing, and transport the patient to a hospital. Do not apply ointment, grease, or butter to the scalded area.

☐ CHEMICAL BURNS

It is extremely difficult to assess the depth and severity of chemical burns in the field; therefore, the general guideline is to treat all chemical burns *aggressively*. *Every* victim of chemical burn needs to be transported. Speed is essential; the more quickly you are able to remove the source of the burn and initiate care, the less severe the burn will be. Any chemical burn is considered particularly severe if it involves the eyes, face, hands, feet, genital area, or large areas of tissue anywhere on the body (Figure 35-30).

☐ Scald Injuries

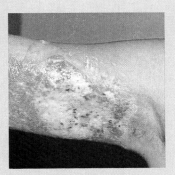

FIGURE 35-27 Scald burn.

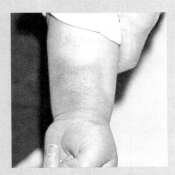

FIGURE 35-28 Scald burn.

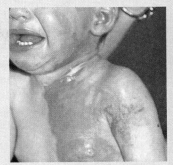

FIGURE 35-29 Third-degree scald burn.

Emergency Care

Prior to beginning emergency care, make sure that it is safe to approach the patient; if not, you should wait for trained rescue personnel to arrive. During each step of rescue, make sure that you protect yourself from contamination.

1. Immediately don gloves and begin to flush the burned area vigorously and forcefully with water; if the patient is at home, the shower or garden hose is ideal (Figure 35-31). Wear latex or rubber gloves to prevent injury to yourself. Irrigate the area continuously for at least *twenty minutes* under a steady stream of water, and make sure that no particles of chemical remain. There are three important exceptions to this rule:

   • Lime powder creates a corrosive substance when mixed with water; keep the lime powder dry, brush it off the patient's skin, and remove the patient's clothing if there is lime powder on it. Then flush with water (Figure 35-32).

   • Ideally phenol (carbolic acid) should be washed

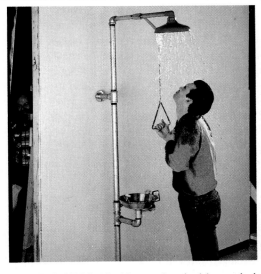

FIGURE 35-31 Flushing a chemical burn victim under an emergency wash/shower system at the worksite. (Courtesy of Lab Safety Supply.)

FIGURE 35-32 Lime powder should be brushed off the skin before flushing with water.

FIGURE 35-30 Chemical burn.

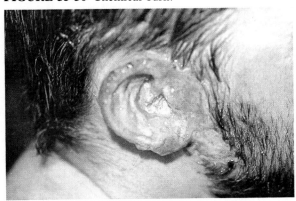

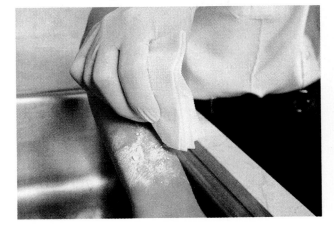

off with alcohol prior to irrigating the burn with water. If alcohol is not available, immediately irrigate with water. Follow local protocol.

- Concentrated sulfuric acid produces heat when mixed with water and may cause greater burn injuries, unless thoroughly flushed with a hose or in a shower. Follow local protocol.

2. While flushing, remove the patient's clothing, shoes, and stockings and any other items of jewelry or apparel that might be contaminated with the chemical. Take care not to contaminate your own skin, eyes, or clothing, with the substance.

3. After you remove the patient's clothing, continue flushing his entire body for about thirty minutes. Do not waste time trying to find a neutralizing agent — flushing with water is more effective and most available.

4. Make sure to flush the eyes if any chemicals splash into them (Figure 35-33). You must flush both eyes. Have the patient remove contact lenses if he or she is wearing them, because they prevent thorough irrigation of the eye. Use a faucet or hose running on low pressure; you might also use a rubber bulb syringe, a pan, a bucket, a cup, or a bottle. Be sure to irrigate well under the lids, and flush for at least twenty minutes; cover both eyes with moistened pads. Never use a chemical antidote in the eyes. See Chapter 17, "Injuries to the Eye."

5. When flushing is complete, cover the area with a sterile dressing and transport the patient to the hospital.

6. Do not make the mistake of trying to neutralize a burned area with alkali or acid solutions. You may guess wrong about the content of the chemical agent that caused the burn, and you may worsen the burn by attempting to neutralize it. You may also miscalculate the quantity needed to neutralize

FIGURE 35-33 Flushing a chemical burn of the eye.

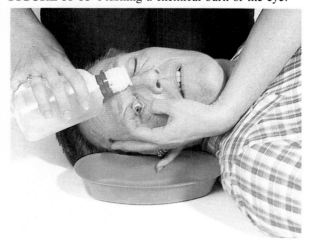

it. Worst of all, neutralization reactions generate heat that can extend the depth of tissue damage and intensify the injury.

The most common types of chemical injury result from acids and alkalis (e.g., lye). Oxidizing agents destroy tissue, reducing agents denature the body protein, and desiccants cause dehydration and excessive heat in bodily tissues. Depending on the chemical agent, burns from chemicals damage much more than just skin surface; underlying tissue damage is usually great and is intensified by failure to act quickly and irrigate properly. If possible, get the name of the chemical involved and bring the container to the hospital with you.

Hydrofluoric Acid

Hydrofluoric acid, widely used in industry to etch glass or in other manufacturing processes, is especially potent and dangerous. It will continue to burn through all layers of the skin and leave large ulcerations. It is readily absorbed by the skin layers and passed to the lymphatic system, where it can spread throughout the body with devastating results.

Hydrofluoric acid burns pose a hidden danger in that symptoms may not show up for hours. It is critical to take action in any *suspected* case of hydrofluoric acid burning, even if the patient manifests no obvious signs and symptoms.

Emergency Care

1. Immediately flush the burned area with generous amounts of cool water. Continue the flushing for at least ten minutes. Remove all affected clothing.

2. If the patient has inhaled hydrofluoric acid vapors, administer 100 percent humidified oxygen as quickly as possible. Administer oxygen throughout transport to any patient with respiratory distress. Administer oxygen even if you are unsure whether the patient inhaled the fumes — failure to do so can result in permanent damage and early death.

Ammonia

Ammonia is being used more frequently as an agent in fertilizers, pesticides, medications, and household products. Most common among ammonia burns are those that damage the eyes. Untreated, the burns cause a rapid rate of destruction, sometimes within thirty seconds. Ammonia fumes are almost always inhaled.

Emergency Care

In general, use the following steps in caring for ammonia burns of the eye:

1. Place the patient in a lying-down position, and turn his head to the side.

2. Lift the eyelid, and pour clean water into the inner corner of the eye. The patient probably will not be able to keep the eye open, so hold it open (and make sure that you do not get ammonia on your hands).

3. Irrigate the eye for at least thirty minutes. Use plenty of water, and make sure that it is flowing *across* the eye, not directly onto the pupil. If both eyes have not been burned, be especially careful that you do not contaminate the healthy eye by carelessly flushing the burned eye.

4. *Never use a chemical or neutralizing solution in the eye.* Keep vinegar, soda, and alcohol away from the eyes at all times. See Chapter 17, "Injuries to the Eye."

5. If particles of dry material are floating on the eye surface, use a sterile, moist piece of material to lift them off. Sterile gauze, a clean handkerchief, or a folded facial tissue work well. Attempt to remove all such particles so that you do not scratch the surface of the eye as you irrigate.

6. Apply a loose, dry dressing over both eyes. *Do not let the patient rub the eye*.

7. Transport the patient to a hospital. Continue irrigating the eye during transport if possible.

□ ELECTRICAL BURNS

Approximately 3,000 electrical injuries each year in the United States cause burns, and approximately 40 percent of all victims die as a result of their injuries. Low voltage can be just as dangerous and fatal as high voltage. While lightning accounts for approximately 25 percent of all electrical burn injuries, it only causes several hundred deaths per year in the United States. Approximately 3 percent of all serious burn injuries are caused by electrical accidents, and approximately 90 percent of the victims of electrical burns are male.

Understanding electrical burns is critical; it will not only help you to aid a patient, but it may also save your own life. (See Figures 35-34–35-36.)

Protecting Yourself and Your Patient

Follow these guidelines when approaching an accident that involves downed power lines or other electrical hazards:

- Look for downed wires whenever an accident has involved a vehicle that has struck a power pole.

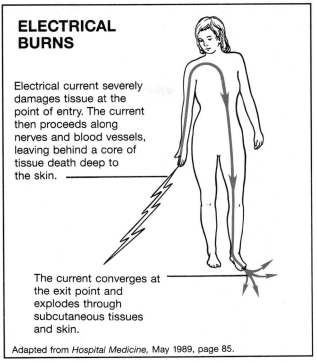

ELECTRICAL BURNS

Electrical current severely damages tissue at the point of entry. The current then proceeds along nerves and blood vessels, leaving behind a core of tissue death deep to the skin.

The current converges at the exit point and explodes through subcutaneous tissues and skin.

Adapted from *Hospital Medicine*, May 1989, page 85.

FIGURE 35-34

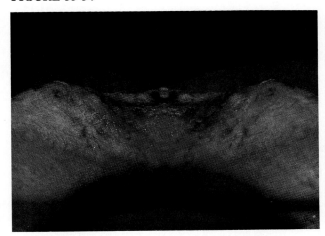

FIGURE 35-35 Deep third-degree electrical burn.

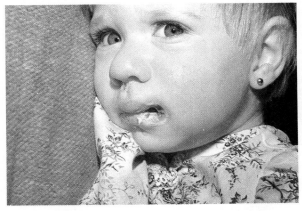

FIGURE 35-36 Electrical burn caused by chewing on an electrical cord.

How can you tell if a line might be downed and hidden in the grass or brush? Carefully look at the next pole down the line, and count the number of power lines at the top crossarm — there should be the same number of lines at the top crossarm of the damaged pole. If there aren't, watch out! If it is dark, use a flashlight or spotlight to inspect the poles and surrounding area.

- *Never* attempt to move downed wires! Only authorized repairmen from the power company should be allowed to touch a high-voltage wire; they have the skill and the proper equipment (including high-voltage rubber gloves and fiberglass rods).

- Radio for help from the power company *immediately* upon entering the scene of a downed power line.

- If a downed power line is lying across a wrecked vehicle, *do not touch the vehicle*, even if the victims inside are seriously injured. You will most likely die if you touch it. If the victims inside are conscious, shout to them and warn them not to leave the vehicle — if they touch the ground and the car at the same time, the current will kill them (Table 35-2).

- If the car begins to burn and the victims inside are at risk of dying in the fire, instruct them to open the car door and jump as far as they can away from the car. In any case, it is critical that they *not touch the car and the ground at the same time*.

- If a downed power line is in the area but is *not*

TABLE 35-2
Rules for Downed Power Lines

1. If any lines are suspected of being down, notify the power company and request an emergency crew. Then notify all rescue personnel of possible danger.
2. Inspect the emergency scene as you arrive. If there is a possibility of a downed line or weakened pole, do not proceed in your vehicle, and do not leave your vehicle until you have inspected the surrounding area.
3. If the vehicle is in contact with the line, stay inside and wait for the power company crew.
4. When entering an area, if the soles of your feet tingle, go no further. You are entering an energized area.
5. A downed power line should be assumed to be live unless the power company crew says otherwise.
6. Remember that vehicles, guardrails, metal fences, etc., conduct electricity.
7. If a vehicle is in contact with a live wire, maintain a safe distance, and tell victims to remain in the vehicle until the power company crews can assist. Never have a patient attempt to jump clear of a vehicle unless there is immediate danger of explosion or fire.
8. Remember that hurried actions in an emergency situation involving downed power lines can jeopardize the patient and the EMT.
9. Never attempt to move a high-voltage power line without instructions or power company assistance.

near or touching the vehicle, proceed as usual with extrication and emergency care.

Types of Electrical Burns

There are three kinds of electrical burns:

- **Contact burns** (when the current is most intense at the entrance and exit sites).
- **Flash burns** (when an extremity is close to an electrical flash or is struck by a flash of lightning).
- **Arcing injuries** (when a current jumps from one surface to another).

Severity of Electrical Shock

Severity of electrical shock is determined by the following factors:

- Voltage and amperage of the current (amperage kills).
- Amount of time the patient is exposed.
- Amount of moisture on the patient.
- Amount of body surface in contact with water.
- Amount of insulation worn by the patient.
- Area of the body through which the current passes.
- Type of current (AC or DC).

Signs and Symptoms of Electrocution

If you are unsure whether or not a person has been shocked, examine him or her for signs and symptoms of electrocution:

- Dazed and confused condition.
- Obvious and severe burns on the skin surface.
- Unconsciousness.
- Weak, irregular, or missing pulse.
- Shallow, irregular, or missing breathing.
- Possibility of multiple severe fractures due to intense muscle contractions.

Emergency Care

Do the following to care for an electrical shock patient:

1. Your first priority is to protect yourself while you get the patient away from the source of electrocution. Follow instructions given earlier in this chapter. Do *not* approach the patient if you cannot do so safely; instead, radio for appropriate help.
2. If possible, immobilize the patient's spine before you move the patient; he or she has probably suf-

fered spinal damage, since electrical injury usually throws a victim.

3. Check breathing and pulse; tissues of the airway may swell and obstruct breathing. Start CPR immediately if indicated (the patient has no carotid pulse), even if you are unsure about the extent of injury. Continue CPR during transport. Most electrical injury patients — even those in full arrest — can be successfully resuscitated with vigorous CPR. An electrocuted patient's heart may start up again on its own, but it is essential that you reduce the time when breathing is absent; therefore, begin CPR immediately.

4. Evaluate and treat any burns; cool burn sites and apply dry, sterile dressings. There will probably be entry and exit sites; look for wounds at both.

5. Treat the patient for shock and administer oxygen.

6. A patient sustaining electrical shock may become hysterical and start to run around in circles, behaving erratically. Force the patient to lie down and keep quiet; maintain his or her body temperature.

7. Transport immediately, splinting as necessary.

Note: If the patient is conscious and his or her condition is not urgent, provide basic burn care for entrance and exit wounds and splint fractures. *Never* delay transport for burn care in an unconscious or urgently injured patient.

Lightning Injuries

Lightning injures hundreds of Americans each year; approximately 200 people in the United States die from lightning strikes each year, usually because of cardiac or respiratory arrest. While approximately one-third of all those struck by lightning die as a result, approximately two-thirds can be revived.

It is very difficult to assess the damage from lightning injuries — there are almost always multisystem injuries. The longer the patient is in contact with the lightning, the more serious the injury. A patient who has been struck by lightning does *not* hold a charge, so it is safe to handle and treat this patient.

Always assume that a victim of lightning strike has sustained multiple injuries; the most immediate injuries involve the central nervous system and the heart. Most are knocked down or thrown, so also assume spinal injury. The three types of lightning injury are mechanical, electrical, and thermal; each does specific kinds of damage. In addition to related injuries, the victim of lightning strike generally has sustained injury to the following body systems:

- The nervous system: The nervous system is very sensitive to lightning injury, since nerves offer the pathway of least resistance to lightning. In almost all instances of lightning strike, the victim becomes unresponsive; few actually remember being struck. Even after consciousness returns, the nervous system is affected, and there may be a full spectrum of changes, including amnesia, disorientation, or seizures. Some patients suffer partial paralysis, and occasionally, paralysis of the respiratory system causes sudden death. Fixed and dilated pupils are a normal reaction and are not necessarily a signs of poor prognosis.

- The sensory system: Some patients experience a loss of sight or hearing. There may be damage to the cornea or retina; damage to the optic nerve; vitreous hemorrhage; or resulting cataracts. The bones and membranes of the ears may also be damaged. Some lose the ability to speak. Most patients regain their speech, hearing, and sight (usually to full capacity) within several days. A *little* blood coming from the ears is normal after a lightning strike, since the tympanic membranes are often ruptured. This does not necessarily indicate skull fracture or other head injury.

- The skin: Most victims of lightning strike sustain first- or second-degree burns; the entry and exit wounds are often third-degree burns. Lightning causes a burn that typically is mottled, feathery, or patchy, appearing in a scattered pattern over the skin and looking like tiny flowers. Called "ferning," this is not a true burn, but instead is an inflammatory reaction of the skin to the electrical currents. In some cases, the skin may be red, mottled, white, swollen, or blistered. The feathery burn usually fades and disappears within forty-eight to seventy-two hours (Figures 35-37 and 35-38).

- The heart: Half of all victims of lightning strike have cardiac complications. The heart is often in the line of current; the most serious injury occurs when the current crosses the heart. The lightning strike itself can disrupt the heart's rhythm, but ensuing complications are what generally lead to full

FIGURE 35-37 Lightning burn.

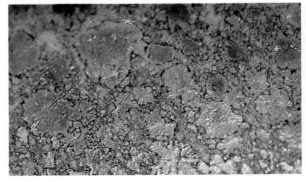

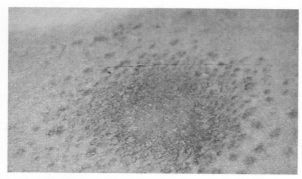

FIGURE 35-38 Lightning burn.

cardiac arrest or fibrillation. In some cases, the coronary arteries may undergo spasm.

• The vascular system: Within seconds following the lightning strike, the patient may become unresponsive, appear white and mottled, have cool arms and legs, and lose pulses. If the injury is moderate, the conditions will probably correct themselves quickly; in cases of severe injury, blood may coagulate, and tissues in the arms and legs may die, leading to amputation. Renal failure may result.

Emergency Care

The goal of management is to oxygenate the heart and brain until the heart regains its ability to function; you should always continue resuscitation of lightning victims longer than you would victims of other trauma. *Immediate* care consists of restoring and maintaining breathing and circulation. Victims of lightning strike have a greater chance of resuscitation than victims of cardiac or respiratory arrest due to other causes because all metabolism ceases, delaying tissue death. Resuscitation should be continued even if the patient appears lifeless — victims of lightning have been resuscitated as long as thirty minutes after the strike without any residual damage. If the strike occurred in an open area, quickly move the patient to a protected area to reduce the chance of a second strike. Most strikes involve multiple victims. If a group has been struck by lightning, reverse usual triage procedure — care for the apparently dead first. Those who display vital signs will probably recover spontaneously, even though burns will require further care. Transport all patients as soon as possible.

Initially, do the following:

1. Survey the entire scene. Assess what happened, and make sure that the patient is free from further injury. For example, remove any debris that has fallen on the patient, move him or her away from sources of electricity, and so on. Persons who are struck by lightning are safe to handle — it is impossible to get electrocuted by touching them.

2. Get a brief, accurate history if possible. If the patient is conscious, ask him or her what happened. Find out if he or she has any major medical problems that might be worsened by the lightning strike. If the patient is unconscious, look for characteristic lightning burns, find witnesses if possible, and ask them to provide you with the history.

3. Stabilize the victim's neck to prevent aggravating a possible cervical spine injury. If possible, move the victim to dry ground after stabilizing the neck.

4. Assess breathing and circulatory status. Begin artificial ventilation or CPR to maintain breathing and heartbeat. *The key to survival is early, vigorous, prolonged resuscitation efforts.* Make those efforts, even if the patient appears to be dead! Once breathing and circulation are initiated, monitor breathing and pulse continuously — the patient may arrest again. In administering artificial ventilation, do not tilt the head backward because of the possibility of spinal injury. Hold the head in a neutral position, and bring the jaw forward gently.

5. Check skin color.

6. If the patient is conscious, check movement in all the extremities.

7. Determine the patient's reaction to pain.

8. Examine the patient for open wounds or fractures and provide appropriate care.

☐ TRIAGE AND TRANSPORTATION OF BURN PATIENTS

1. In the case of an accident in which more than one person is involved, determine who should be transported first:

   • Send patients with facial and circumferential chest burns or with breathing or cardiac complications first.

   • Send patients with 60 to 80 percent burns before you send those with burns covering over 80 percent of the body area. Patients in the latter category usually die and often receive care last when there are multiple casualties. Measures should be taken first to save those who have a somewhat better chance of survival.

   • When patients' burns are equal in extent, send the ones first who do not complain of pain. In the most serious burns, nerve endings are destroyed, and the burns are painless; less serious burns hurt.

2. Decide quickly where you will transport the pa-

tient by communicating with your base hospital. If possible, take the patient to a burn center, where trained professionals have the knowledge and equipment necessary to most effectively care for burns of all degrees. Follow local protocol. If you are more than thirty minutes away from a burn center, transport the patient (in order of preference) to:

- A major teaching hospital with emergency facilities.
- A large community hospital with emergency facilities.
- The nearest community hospital with open emergency facilities.

3. Contact the facilities, and determine which has space to accommodate the patient. If possible, communicate directly to the physician who will care for the patient. Tell the physician everything that you have been able to learn about the burn — what caused it, how extensive it is, what complications (if any) have developed, and what care you have administered.

4. Prepare the patient for transport. If you have removed any clothing, bag it and take it with you —

it could be essential in determining long-range care, especially if it was burned. The physician can determine a great deal about the source of the burn itself by examining burned clothing.

5. Before you transport, make sure that the patient is well prepared and that you have done everything possible to stabilize his or her condition. Burn patients rarely improve during transport; in fact, they usually deteriorate.

6. Make sure that the patient's airway is clear and that associated injuries have been attended to before you begin transport.

7. If the patient needs to urinate or defecate during transport, assist him or her in any way that you can to make sure that the urine flow or feces do not contact the burn area and contaminate damaged tissues.

8. As soon as you arrive at your destination, consult with the attending physician. Describe in detail the care you have already administered and any care that the patient may have received before you arrived. Such information will determine how the physician should best proceed.

chapter 36

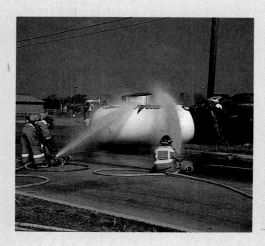

Hazardous Material Emergencies

✳ OBJECTIVES

- ■ Evaluate the complexity of dealing with hazardous materials, their risks, and related warning placards and labels.
- ■ Explain the general procedures and guidelines for managing a hazardous materials incident.
- ■ Describe treatment and decontamination procedures for patients and fellow rescuers who have been exposed to hazardous materials, including radiation.

The purpose of this brief chapter is to provide an overview of the complexity of hazardous material emergencies. EMTs should not attempt hazardous materials rescues unless they have had adequate training (as approved by local protocol) and have approval from their EMS director.

It is recommended that EMTs wear protective gloves whenever there is a possibility of coming in contact with a patient's blood, body fluids, mucous membranes, traumatic wounds, or sores. See Chapter 31.

A **hazardous material** is defined as one that, in any quantity, poses a threat or unreasonable risk to life, health, or property if not properly controlled during manufacture, processing, packaging, handling, storage, transportation, use, and disposal. More than 50 billion tons of hazardous materials are manufactured in the United States annually, and more than 4 billion tons of them are shipped in this country every year.

The government regulates the packaging, labeling, placarding, inspection, operation of facilities, containers, transporting vehicles, and training of personnel. But, despite all the regulations, hazardous materials can still be spilled or accidentally released because of equipment failure, vehicle accidents, container failure, environmental conditions, and human error. The result can be the loss of property and life.

The term "hazardous materials" includes hazardous chemicals, hazardous wastes, and other dangerous goods. They exist in every jurisdiction in the nation, especially because of interstate transport. Obviously, with the threat present, the primary concern is one of safety for the public, the patient, and the EMT who serves as rescuer.

Hazardous materials commonly shipped in the United States include explosives (materials that combust or detonate), compressed gases (pressurized flammable or nonflammable gas), flammable liquids (those with a flash point of less than 100 degrees Fahrenheit), flammable solids (nonexplosive solid material that burns vigorously and can be ignited readily), oxidizers (substances that give off oxygen and stimulate combustion of organic matter), poisonous gases, corrosives (materials that destroy skin), and radioactive materials. The principal dangers of hazardous materials are toxicity, flammability, and reactivity. Exposure can be limited to a few, or it may cause widespread destruction and loss of life.

The internal health problems caused by hazardous materials vary — the hazardous material can asphyxiate, irritate, act as a carcinogen, act as nerve or liver poisons, or cause loss of coordination or unconsciousness. External injury can include skin irritation, burns, respiratory distress (difficulty in breathing, coughing), nausea and vomiting, tingling and/or numbness of the extremities, and blurred and/or double vision. Whether it is internal or external, the amount of damage done depends on the dose, concentration, and amount of time the patient is exposed to the hazardous material.

Do not attempt a hazardous materials rescue unless you have had training. If you have had no training, radio immediately for help, and while you are waiting for help to arrive, protect yourself and bystanders by keeping away from the danger.

□ RESOURCES FOR HANDLING HAZARDOUS MATERIALS

Several resources can assist you in proper handling of hazardous material emergencies:

CHEMTREC

A public service, **CHEMTREC (Chemical Transportation Emergency Center)** is based in Washington, D.C., as a division of the Chemical Manufacturer's Association. You can reach officials at CHEMTREC twenty-four hours a day, seven days a week, by dialing their toll-free number, 1-800-424-9300. Officials at CHEMTREC can answer any questions and advise you on how to handle emergencies involving hazardous materials; CHEMTREC will even locate the shipper of the hazardous materials for appropriate follow-up.

In order to obtain help from CHEMTREC, you will need to provide the following information:

- The identification number or the name of the product.
- The nature of the problem.
- Your name and the number where you can be reached.
- The location of the incident.
- The product destination.
- The guide number you are using.
- The shipper or manufacturer of the product.
- The type of container.
- The rail car or truck number.
- The carrier's name.
- Local conditions (weather, terrain, and so on).
- Action that has already been taken.

Accidents involving hazardous materials often occur at inconvenient locations, making communication difficult. It is critical that you make every effort to keep a phone line open so that the shipper can reach you with guidance and assistance.

Printed Materials

One concise reference material is a guidebook published by the Department of Transportation called *Hazardous Materials: Emergency Response Guidebook* (DOT P5800.4, 1987). Compact enough to be carried with usual equipment and supplies, the book lists more than 1,000 hazardous materials with their identification numbers; it is cross-referenced so that you can quickly locate complete instructions for emergency procedures. Hazardous materials are listed both by identification number (in numerical order) and in alphabetical order. Other references are also available.

Government Agencies

State and local agencies, including the Department of Transportation, can help you identify hazardous materials and provide assistance in case of disaster.

☐ IDENTIFICATION

There are two ways to identify a hazardous material:

- **Placards:** The placard, a four-sided, diamond-shaped sign, will be displayed on the hazardous material container. Many placards are red or orange, while a few are white or green. The placard will contain a four-digit identification number as well as a legend that indicates whether the material is flammable, radioactive, explosive, or poisonous. See the accompanying hazardous materials placards and the United National Class Number System (Figures 36-1 and 36-2).

  The National Fire Protection Association has adopted an internationally recognized diamond-shaped symbol that is divided into four smaller diamonds. The NFPA system uses different background colors, as well as numbers ranging from 0 to 4, to indicate the dangers presented by a hazardous material. The blue diamond is a gauge of health hazard; the red, fire hazard; and the yellow, reactivity hazard. The white diamond is used for symbols that indicate additional information (such as radioactivity, oxidation, need for protective equipment, and so on). A symbol that has a 1 in the blue diamond and a 4 in the red diamond, for example, would present a relatively low health hazard but is extremely flammable.

- **Shipping paper:** If you can locate it, the shipping paper will have the name of the substance, the classification (such as flammable or explosive), and the four-digit identification number. With very few exceptions, the shipping papers identifying hazardous materials are required to be in the cab of a motor vehicle, in the possession of a train crew member in the engine or the caboose, in a holder on the bridge of a vessel, or in the aircraft pilot's possession.

A final, but less reliable, way to determine the presence of hazardous materials at the scene of an accident is to quickly scan the scene visually. A number of visual clues can indicate the probable presence of a hazardous material:

- Smoking or self-igniting materials.
- Extraordinary fire conditions.
- Boiling or spattering of material that has not been heated.
- Wavy or unusually colored vapors over a container of liquid material.
- Characteristically colored vapor clouds.
- Frost near a container leak (indicative of liquid coolants).
- Unusual condition of containers (peeling or discoloration of finishes, unexpected deterioration, deformity, or the unexpected operation of pressure-relief valves).

☐ GENERAL PROCEDURES

The goal of hazardous materials rescue is to avoid contact with any unidentified material, regardless of the level of protection offered by your clothing and equipment. In achieving that goal, there are three general priorities *whose order never changes:* first, protect the safety of all rescuers and victims; second, provide patient care; and, when those two priorities have been achieved, decontaminate clothing, equipment, and the vehicle.

The general rule of hazardous materials rescue is to *avoid risking your life or your health if the only threat is to the environment*. In other words, if victims are not involved, *do not enter the scene;* let specially trained environmental workers clean up the hazard. Simply cordon off the area and evacuate bystanders. Even if there are victims involved, this is one situation in which you should not automatically begin rescue work. Generally accepted guidelines call for weighing the situation according to your best judgment, determining whether the risk to rescuers is justified by the lives that can be saved. In making that kind of a difficult judgment, you should consider the risk to rescuers, the difficulty of the rescue, the flammability of materials, the possibility of explosion, any time or distance constraints, any available escape routes, and the probability of victim survival if they receive medical care.

If you decide to begin rescue operations, the general rule in working with hazardous materials is to *ACT QUICKLY* — time is critical! *But do not work so quickly that you endanger yourself and others at the scene and make patient injuries worse.*

As a first course of action, secure the scene and limit exposure to rescuers and bystanders. Then make sure there is enough additional equipment, personnel,

Hazardous Materials Warning Placards

DOMESTIC PLACARDING

Illustration numbers in each square ([1] through [18]) refer to TABLES 1 and 2 below.

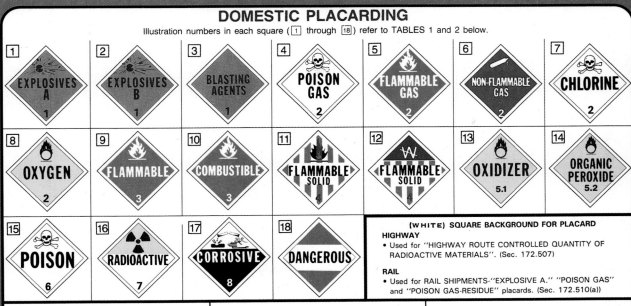

(WHITE) SQUARE BACKGROUND FOR PLACARD

HIGHWAY
- Used for "HIGHWAY ROUTE CONTROLLED QUANTITY OF RADIOACTIVE MATERIALS". (Sec. 172.507)

RAIL
- Used for RAIL SHIPMENTS-"EXPLOSIVE A." "POISON GAS" and "POISON GAS-RESIDUE" placards. (Sec. 172.510(a))

TABLE 1

HAZARD CLASSES	*NO.
Class A explosives	1
Class B explosives	2
Poison A	4
Flammable solid (DANGEROUS WHEN WET label only)	12
Radioactive material (YELLOW III label)	16
Radioactive material:	
Uranium hexafluoride fissile (containing more than 1.0% U^{235})	16 & 17
Uranium hexafluoride, low-specific activity (containing 1.0% or less U^{235}	16 & 17

NOTE: For details on the use of Tables 1 and 2, see Sec. 172.504 (See footnotes at bottom of tables.)

Guidelines
(CFR, Title 49, Transportation, Parts 100-177)

- Placard *motor vehicles, freight containers,* and *rail cars* containing *any quantity* of hazardous materials listed in TABLE 1.
- Placard *motor vehicles, freight containers* and *rail cars* containing 1,000 pounds or more gross weight of hazardous materials classes listed in TABLE 2.
- Placard *freight containers* 640 cubic feet or more containing *any quantity* of hazardous material classes listed in TABLES 1 and/or 2 when offered for transportation by air or water. Under 640 cubic feet see Sec. 172.512(b).

CAUTION

CHECK EACH SHIPMENT FOR COMPLIANCE WITH THE APPROPRIATE HAZARDOUS MATERIALS REGULATIONS:
Proper Classification   Marking   Placarding
Packaging   Labeling   Documentation
PRIOR TO OFFERING FOR SHIPMENT

TABLE 2

HAZARD CLASSES	*NO.
Class C explosives	18
Blasting agent	3
Nonflammable gas	6
Nonflammable gas (Chlorine)	7
Nonflammable gas (Fluorine)	15
Nonflammable gas (Oxygen, cryogenic liquid)	8
Flammable gas	5
Combustible liquid	10
Flammable liquid	9
Flammable solid	11
Oxidizer	13
Organic peroxide	14
Poison B	15
Corrosive material	17
Irritating material	18

INTERNATIONAL PLACARDING

- Most International placards are similar (color and pictorial symbol(s) to the Domestic placards illustrated above.
- International placards are enlarged ICAO or IMO labels (See International Labeling—Otherside).
- Placard MUST correspond to *hazard class* of material.

- Placard *ANY QUANTITY* of hazardous materials when loaded in FREIGHT CONTAINERS, PORTABLE TANKS, RAIL CARS and HIGHWAY VEHICLES.
- International placards *may* be used *in addition* to DOT placards for international shipments.

When required, *Subsidiary Risk placards* must be displayed in the same manner as *Primary Risk placards.* Class numbers are *not shown* on Subsidiary Risk placards.

- COMPATIBILITY GROUP DESIGNATORS *must* be displayed on EXPLOSIVES PLACARDS.
- UN CLASS NUMBERS and DIVISION NUMBERS *MUST* be displayed on hazard class placards when required.

UN and NA Identification Numbers

- The four digit UN or NA numbers must be displayed on all hazardous materials packages for which identification numbers are assigned. Example: ACETONE UN 1090.
- UN (United Nations) or NA (North American) numbers are found in the Hazardous Materials Tables, Sec. 172.101 and 172.102 (CFR, Title 49, Parts 100-199)
- Identification numbers may not be displayed on "POISON GAS," "RADIOACTIVE" or "EXPLOSIVE" placards. (Sec. 172.334)
- UN numbers are displayed in the same manner for both Domestic and International shipments.
- NA numbers are used only in the USA and Canada.

When hazardous materials are transported in Tank Cars, Cargo Tanks and Portable Tanks, UN or NA numbers *must* be displayed on:

PLACARDS OR ORANGE PANELS

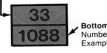

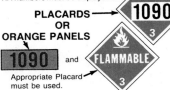

1090 and

Appropriate Placard must be used.

EUROPEAN NUMBERING SYSTEM—

Top Number—Hazard Index (Identification of Danger, 2 or 3 figures) Example: 33 = highly inflammable liquid.

33
1088

Bottom Number—UN Number of substance Example: 1088 ACETAL

For more complete details on identification Numbers see Sec. 172.300 through 172.338.

FIGURE 36-1

Hazardous Materials Warning Labels

DOMESTIC LABELING

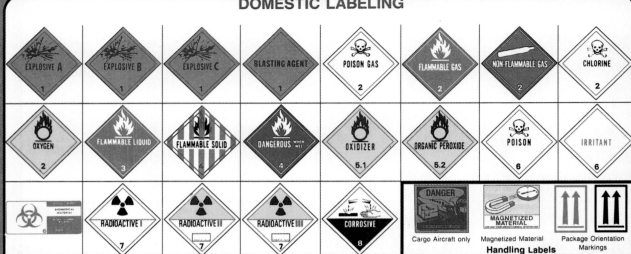

General Guidelines on Use of Labels

(CFR, Title 49, Transportation, Parts 100-177)

- Labels illustrated above are normally for *domestic shipments*. However, some air carriers *may* require the use of International Civil Aviation Organization (ICAO) labels.

- Domestic Warning Labels *may* display UN Class Number, Division Number (and Compatibility Group for Explosives only.) Sec. 172.407(g).

- Any person who offers a hazardous material for transportation MUST label the package, if required. [Sec. 172.400(a)].

- The Hazardous Materials Tables, Sec. 172.101 and 172.102, identify the proper label(s) for the hazardous materials listed.

- Label(s), when required, must be printed on or affixed to the surface of the package near the proper shipping name. [Sec. 172.406(a)].

- When two or more different labels are required, display them next to each other. [Sec. 172.406(c)].

- Labels may be affixed to packages (even when not required by regulations) provided each label represents a hazard of the material in the package. [Sec. 172-401].

Check the Appropriate Regulations

Domestic or International Shipment

UN Class Numbers

Class 1—Explosives

Class 2—Gases (compressed, liquified or dissolved under pressure)

Class 3—Flammable liquids

Class 4—Flammable solids or substances

Class 5—Oxidizing substances
    Division 5.1-Oxidizing substances or agents.
    Division 5.2-Organic peroxides.

Class 6— Poisonous and infectious substances

Class 7— Radioactive substances

Class 8—Corrosives

Class 9—Miscellaneous dangerous substances

INTERNATIONAL LABELING

Substance liable to Spontaneous Combustion

Poisonous Substance

Poisonous Substance

Infectious Substance

EXAMPLES OF INTERNATIONAL LABELS

- These are examples of International Labels not presently used for domestic shipments.

- Text, when used Internationally *may* be in the language of the country of origin.

   • Most of the domestic labels (illustrated above) *may* be used Internationally.

EXAMPLES OF EXPLOSIVE LABELS

- The NUMERICAL DESIGNATION represents the CLASS or DIVISION.

- ALPHABETICAL DESIGNATION represents the COMPATIBILITY GROUP (for Explosives Only)

- DIVISION NUMBERS and COMPATIBILITY GROUP combinations can result in over 30 different "Explosives" labels (see IMDG Code/ICAO).

For complete details, refer to one or more of the following:

- Code of Federal Regulations, Title 49, Transportation. Parts 100-199. [All Modes]

- International Civil Aviation Organization (ICAO) Technical Instructions for the Safe Transport of Dangerous Goods by air. [Air]

- International Maritime Organization (IMO) Dangerous Goods Code. [Water]

- "Transportation of Dangerous Goods Regulations" of Transport Canada. [All Modes]

U.S. Department of Transportation

Research and Special Programs Administration

Available from
American Labelmark Co.
5724 N. Pulaski Rd. • Chicago, IL 60646
Toll Free: 1-800-621-5808 • In Illinois: 312-478-0900

CHART 8
REV. FEBRUARY 1986
STYLE CU-F21

FIGURE 36-2

and whatever else you might need to handle the emergency effectively. Finally, make sure that every rescuer who enters the scene has adequate protective equipment: a positive-pressure, self-contained breathing apparatus and a full suit of protective clothing, including a coat and pants, at least two layers of gloves, boots, helmets, eye protection (preferably full-face protection), and lifelines. Use wide duct tape to seal off the protective suits at the wrists, ankles, neck, and other gaps or openings. Keep in mind that you'll need specialized suits if you are working in high temperatures or areas where you could be splashed with corrosive chemicals.

Preincident Planning

The most essential part of hazardous materials rescue is effective preincident planning. Before a hazardous materials incident ever occurs, all agencies that would probably be involved in a rescue need to know how forces will be mobilized to handle the emergency, much as in general disaster planning.

Generally, you should prepare for the worst possible scenario — that way, the community will be capable of handling any emergency that arises. Each plan should be specifically tailored to individual circumstances in the community, but the following should be part of any plan:

- There should be one command officer appointed; all rescuers should be aware of who the command officer is. That command officer, who is responsible for all decisions involving the rescue, should never hand the decision-making power to someone else without informing *all* rescuers of the change in command.
- There should be a clear chain of command from each rescuer to the command officer.
- There should be an established system of communications that will be used throughout the emergency. This, of course, can be an already-established system, as long as all rescuers are informed about it, know how to use it, and have access to it.
- Receiving facilities should be predesignated. Choose facilities that are capable of handling large numbers of patients, that have surgical capability, and, if possible, that have established decontamination procedures.

Implementing the Plan

The first priority in implementing a plan is to immediately establish a command post from which orders are given and to which information is directed. As quickly as possible, get the following information, which will help in formulating and implementing the best plan under the circumstances:

- The nature of the problem.
- What hazardous materials are involved.
- The kind and condition of the container.
- Existing weather conditions (wind or rain?).
- The presence of fire.
- The time that has elapsed since the incident occurred.
- What has already been done by people at the scene.
- How many victims are involved.
- The danger of victimizing more people.

As you make these assessments, summon help from fire personnel if you have not already done so or they are not already on the scene. All fires must be extinguished — not only do they threaten the safety of victims of rescuers, but toxins and particles of hazardous materials can be carried in the smoke, greatly widening the area of the hazardous material incident. *Unless you are a trained firefighter, do not attempt to extinguish the fires yourself:* hazardous materials often require special techniques (for example, many cannot be extinguished with — and are made worse with — water).

If you have hazardous materials training, work quickly to confine or contain the leak or the spill so that the smallest possible number of people will be exposed. You can quickly build a dam, dike, or berm, or cover the spill with dirt or plastic sheets to prevent vapors from permeating the area. If containers are leaking, seal the leaks but leave the material in the original container whenever possible for positive identification.

Establishing Safety Zones

As an early priority at the scene of any hazardous material contamination, you should establish zones that will clearly delineate where rescue operations will take place and define what procedures can be carried out in which areas (Figure 36-3). Some EMS areas use the circular model for depicting safety zones (Figure 36-4).

The **contamination zone** is where the contamination is actually present. It generally is the area that is immediately adjacent to the actual accident site and where contamination can still occur. (In Figure 36-3 of the nine-step decon procedure, areas 1 through 5 comprise the contamination zone.) Remember that you may not be able to see or smell the hazardous material: some are odorless and colorless, while others have anesthetic properties and will deaden your senses so you can't smell them. *Never* rely on your senses alone — sight,

DESCRIPTIONS OF ACTIONS

Description	Step
Personnel enter decon area and drop tools on contaminated side. Move to Step 2.	**1**
Remove as much contamination as possible. Dilution is conducted inside diked area. Personnel are in SCBA. Move to Step 3.	**2**
Remove SCBA to contaminated side and move to Step 4 or don new SCBA from clean side and re-enter work area. Move to Step 4.	**3**
Remove protective clothing and place on contaminated side. Move to Step 5 or transport personnel to a fixed decon facility.	**4**
Remove all personal clothing and isolate items on contaminated side. Bag personal items. Move to Step 6.	**5**
Personal showering using soap and sponges. Bag cleaning items for disposal. Move to Step 7.	**6**
Personnel dry off. Bag towels. Put on clean clothing. Move to Step 8.	**7**
Personnel receive medical evaluation and treatment as necessary. Move to Step 9.	**8**
Identify personnel. Complete field records. Transport personnel to hospital or to a fixed decon facility for steps 5-8.	**9**

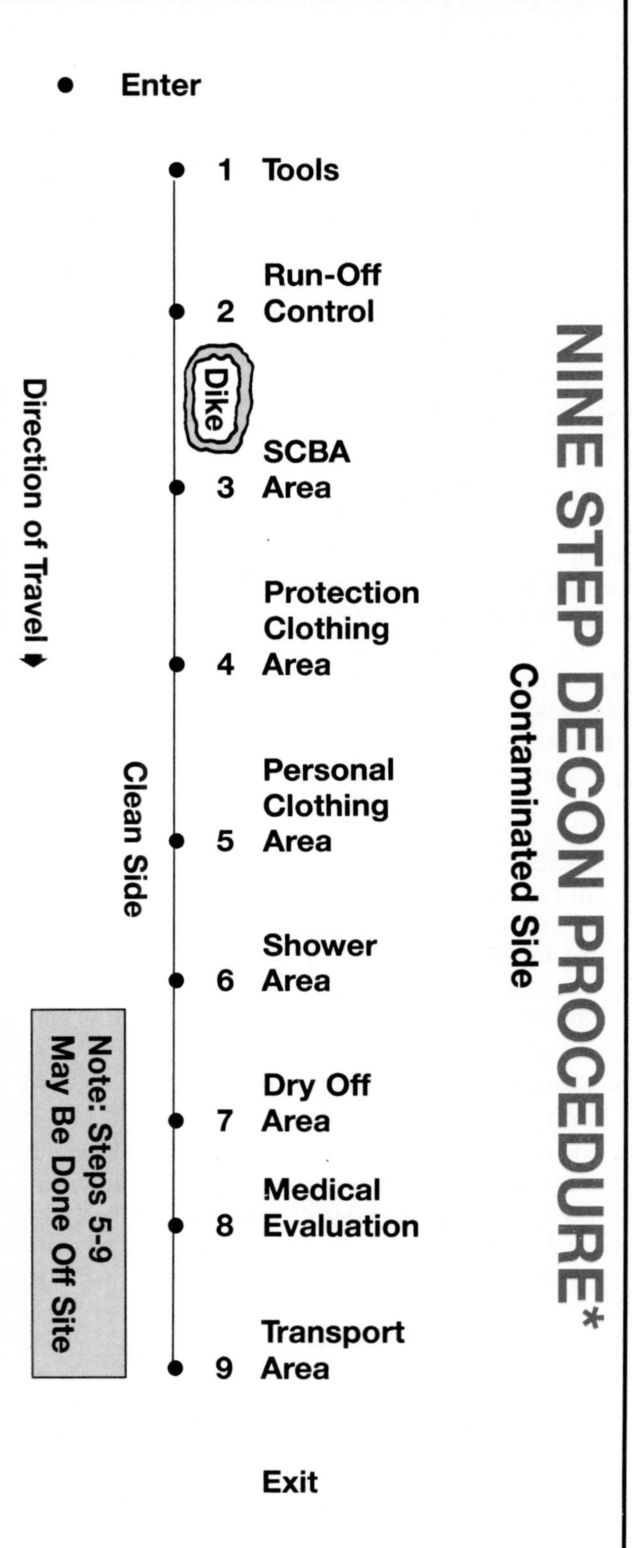

NINE STEP DECON PROCEDURE*

Contaminated Side

Clean Side

Direction of Travel ▶

- Enter
- 1 Tools
- 2 Run-Off Control
- Dike
- 3 SCBA Area
- 4 Protection Clothing Area
- 5 Personal Clothing Area
- 6 Shower Area
- 7 Dry Off Area
- 8 Medical Evaluation
- 9 Transport Area
- Exit

Note: Steps 5-9 May Be Done Off Site

* Decon procedure written by Kenneth J. Bouvier, NREMT-I, New Orleans Chapter President, Association of Nationally Registered EMTs.

FIGURE 36-3

ESTABLISHING SAFETY CONTROL ZONES AT SITE OF HAZARDOUS MATERIAL INCIDENT

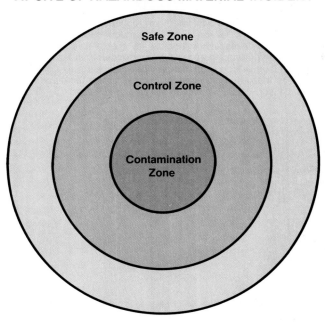

Contamination Zone

Contamination is actually present
Personnel must wear appropriate protective gear
Number of rescuers limited to those absolutely necessary
Bystanders never allowed

Control Zone

Area surrounding the contamination zone
Vital to preventing spread of contamination
Personnel must wear appropriate protective gear
Life-saving emergency care is performed

Safe Zone

Normal triage, stabilization, and treatment are performed
Rescuers must shed contaminated gear before entering the safe zone

FIGURE 36-4

smell, taste, or touch — to detect a hazardous material. *ALWAYS* assume that the area surrounding a spill or leak is dangerous, and *ALWAYS* wear protective gear.

Establish one entry and exit point into the contamination zone; all personnel should then enter and exit the zone at that point, limiting the possible spread of contamination. Designate one emergency exit to be used in case the scene deteriorates rapidly (in case there is an explosion, for example). *Never* smoke, eat, or drink in the contamination area — you will risk inhaling or ingesting the hazardous material.

Any personnel who enter the contamination zone should be wearing appropriate protective suits specially designed for hazardous materials work (Figures 36-5—36-9). The contamination zone should be strictly restricted; *only as many rescuers as absolutely necessary should enter the contamination zone.* In areas with a specialized **HazMat team,** only members of that team should enter the contamination zone. *Bystanders should never be allowed in the contamination zone.* If necessary, cordon off the area and appoint people to keep bystanders away.

The only work that should be done in the contamination zone is actual rescue, initial decontamination, and treatment for life-threatening conditions *by personnel who are wearing appropriate gear.*

The **control zone** is immediately adjacent to the contamination zone. (In the illustration of the nine-step decon procedure, areas 6 and 7 comprise the control zone.) While the hazardous material may not actually be in the control zone, there is still danger of contamination from the contaminated victims and rescue personnel who have come out of the contamination zone. For that reason, *all personnel in the control zone must wear appropriate protective gear.*

The control zone is vital in preventing the spread of contamination. All supplies used in the control zone must remain there until fully decontaminated; all water must also be contained in this area. Before rescuers enter the safe zone, all protective gear should be removed and left in the control zone.

Rescue work that should be performed in the control zone consists of life-saving emergency care, such as airway management and immobilization. A primary survey should be conducted in the control zone to determine the need for bleeding control, artificial ventilation, and other procedures.

The **safe zone** is immediately adjacent to the control zone where normal triage, stabilization, and treatment can take place. Rescuers should shed all contaminated protective gear before entering the safe zone, and patients should be as fully decontaminated as possible before being brought into the safe zone. Especially in cases of gross contamination, *some* contamination will still enter the safe zone; therefore, you should still exercise caution and take measures to protect your equipment and vehicle.

By the time patients enter the safe zone, life-threatening injuries should have been initially treated, and life-saving first aid should have been completed (or at least started). In the safe zone, you should triage patients to determine the order of care, perform necessary treatment, and stabilize patients prior to transport.

Keeping the three zones in mind, follow these general guidelines for hazardous materials emergencies:

1. Before entering the contamination zone, put on appropriate protective gear. Depending on the amount of contamination present, you may need anything from disposable surgical suits to specialized laminated suits. In case of gross contamina-

☐ HazMat Protective Suits

Special personnel and equipment are required at a hazardous materials incident. Several types of hazardous materials protective suits exist. The suits depicted below are encapsulated with a self-contained breathing apparatus worn underneath the suit. There are specialized suits that provide vapor and liquid protection as well as those that are used for working in high-temperature areas. Local protocol will dictate the type of suit used.

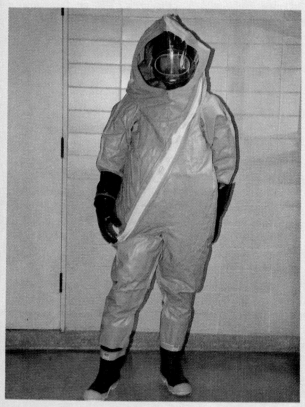

FIGURE 36-5

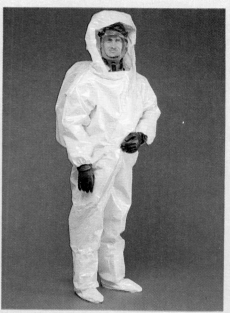

FIGURE 36-6
(Courtesy of Safety Lab Supply, Inc.
Janesville, WI)

FIGURE 36-7
(Courtesy of Safety Lab Supply, Inc.
Janesville, WI)

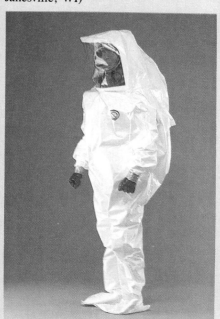

FIGURE 36-8
(Courtesy of Safety Lab Supply, Inc.
Janesville, WI)

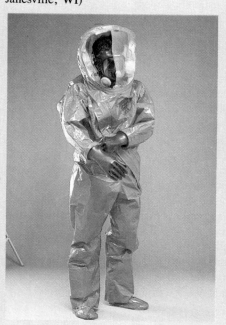

FIGURE 36-9
(Courtesy of Durafab, Inc.)

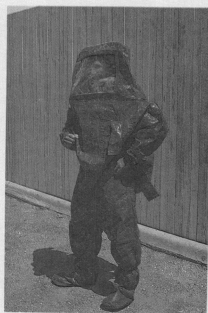

tion, you should wear a surgical hairnet, surgical gloves, and surgical shoe coverings. Over these, put on a laminated suit with a hood, and over that, wear a dust mask. Overlap the sleeves of the suit over neoprene rubber gloves and the pant legs of the suit over neoprene rubber boots; tape the sleeves to the gloves, and the pant legs to the boots.

2. Enter the contamination zone and begin to decontaminate the patient. At this point, attempt gross decontamination only. Before beginning, perform any necessary life-saving treatment to maintain vital functions. *Remove the patient from the actual accident site before treating or decontaminating,* but keep him or her within the contamination zone until you have performed initial decontamination.

3. To perform initial decontamination, use detergent soap and copious amounts of water to clean the victim; use sterile saline to irrigate the eyes. Do not rub the patient's skin. If you can, use a hose or other source of running water during this initial decontamination. *Make sure that all water, including water that runs off the patient, is contained in the contamination zone.* The patient's clothing, tools, and equipment should be removed and left in the contamination zone.

4. Even though you are wearing protective gear, keep as clean as possible. *Never* directly touch the hazardous material unless you have to in order to rescue the patient.

5. Before moving into the control zone, remove your neoprene rubber gloves and boots; leave them in the contamination zone.

6. *An obvious exception to the contamination zone procedures is the possibility of contamination with a hazardous material that reacts volatilely with water.* In such a case, do not wash the patient with water; instead, use dry cloths or sponges to wipe as much of the contaminant from his or her body as possible.

7. In the control zone, quickly perform a primary survey to determine the presence of life-threatening conditions, such as bleeding or respiratory problems. Perform life-saving emergency care to treat any life-threatening conditions, and stabilize the patient. *You should still be wearing protective clothing throughout treatment in the control zone.*

8. Once the patient is stabilized, perform complete decontamination. Thoroughly irrigate the eyes again with sterile saline. Using detergent soap and plenty of water, thoroughly wash the patient's hair, ear canals, underarm areas, pubic areas, and the creases at the neck, groin, elbows, and knees. Clean beneath the finger nails and toenails and between the toes. Clean out the umbilicus. Make sure that all water is contained in the control area.

9. Following thorough decontamination, treat any major injuries, such as fractures. Immobilize as appropriate, splint where needed, and move the patient to the safe zone.

10. At the edge of the control zone, remove your protective clothing and leave it in the control zone.

11. In the safe zone, perform a secondary survey including vital signs, and complete patient treatment for minor injuries. Prepare the patient for transport to the hospital.

12. Take precautions to protect your equipment and vehicle during transport, since there may still be some contamination on the patient.

13. Any clothing and equipment used in the contamination or control zones must be properly contained before being taken from the scene of the accident. Place any contaminated equipment or clothing in sealed plastic bags (Figure 36-10) or in metal containers with tight-fitting lids. Prior to transport, cover the benches, floor, and other exposed areas of your vehicle with thick, plastic sheeting; secure the sheeting with duct tape. Patients should be fully decontaminated before being placed into a helicopter for air transportation. A contaminated patient in such a closed, tight space could affect the breathing or vision of the air transportation team, resulting in an air crash.

14. Any corpses at the accident site need to be decontaminated fully before being transported to a morgue. Follow procedures as outlined above for patient care.

15. If you are accidentally exposed to hazardous materials during rescue operations, you need to decontaminate yourself thoroughly. Contamination occurs most easily in areas of your body where skin is thin or is usually moist (such as under the arms and in the groin). Wash with mild detergent or green soap and plenty of running water; irrigate exposed skin for at least twenty minutes. Seek medical attention, document the incident, and report the incident to your employer.

16. Following rescue, take measures to decontaminate your equipment and vehicle as outlined in the section, "Radiation Emergencies." If you fail to clean your equipment and vehicle thoroughly, you can suffer from chronic chemical exposure. Remember that the clothing under your protective gear also needs decontamination. Do not take clothing home to launder it — you can contaminate your family, and contaminants will be washed into the general sewer system.

17. All rescuers involved in the rescue should have thorough medical surveillance to treat any exposure-related injuries or illnesses; some don't mani-

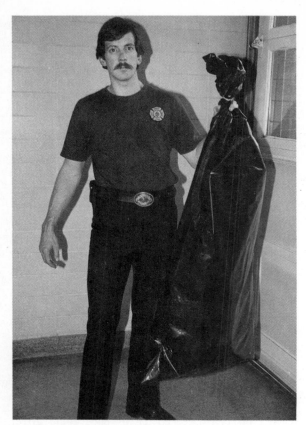

FIGURE 36-10 Contaminated equipment and clothing should be sealed in plastic bags.

fest themselves for hours, or even days, after exposure. Following any hazardous materials rescue, watch yourself for signs of exposure. Seek medical help immediately if you develop headache, nausea and/or vomiting, abdominal cramps and/or diarrhea, difficulty breathing, dizziness, lack of coordination, blurred vision, excessive salivation, or irritation of the skin, eyes, nose, throat, or respiratory tract.

18. Document the hazardous materials incident and report any possible exposure to your employer.

□ RADIATION EMERGENCIES

General Guidelines

Largely due to ignorance about radiation and to inexperience in dealing with radiation-related accidents, much fear has surrounded radiation, leading to a lack of widespread training. Radiation emergencies may be clean (meaning that the patient was exposed but not contaminated) or dirty (meaning that the patient was contaminated). Very few radiation accident victims are so contaminated that they pose a threat to rescuers.

You should remember two major principles about radiation-related accidents.

1. In most cases, the radioactive aspects of a radiation accident are not what require the most immediate care; the effects of radiation usually do not appear for several days, so don't assume that an asymptomatic victim has not been injured. *The first priority is to protect yourself and others from contamination.*

   • If you suspect radioactive contamination, approach the site from upwind.

   • If the wind is blowing or if you see smoke, wear protective clothing and a self-contained breathing apparatus even before entering the area so that you cannot inhale radioactive particles.

   • Until the police arrive, control traffic and keep bystanders away.

   • Before you enter the suspected area of contamination, don a positive-pressure, self-contained breathing apparatus plus protective clothing: two pairs of gloves, overalls, a hooded head covering, a surgical mask and gown, and shoe covers.

   • As you enter the area, carry a portable survey instrument to determine radioactivity.

   • Your second priority is now the patient — give top attention to breathing and circulatory problems, shock, hemorrhage, fracture, flail chest, and other emergencies. Medical emergencies have priority over radiation hazard assessment — never delay life-saving medical care to decontaminate a victim of a radiation accident.

2. No EMT should ever attempt to decontaminate a radiation victim. You have two choices if you suspect that a victim is contaminated.

   • You can wait for a **Radiation Safety Officer (RSO),** an expert specifically trained under federal government provisions to handle such situations. The RSO in your area is probably employed by the county or state health department and will respond to the scene when possible.

   • If an RSO cannot come to the site, you can transport the patient to the hospital for decontamination by experts there. To transport a contaminated patient, place him or her in a body bag up to the neck, cover the hair completely with a cap, and use disposable wipes to wipe off his or her face. (Put the disposable wipes in a plastic bag, seal it, and take it to the hospital with you.)

The Nature of Radiation

None of your five senses can detect radiation. We are always exposed to minute amounts of radiation, because cosmic rays that constantly bombard the earth contain radioactive rays. Some minerals that contain radiation have occurred naturally in the earth since its beginnings. But exposure to large amounts of radiation is a relatively new danger as people are exposed to x-rays or to accidental contamination from nuclear power plants and from radioactive transport vehicles.

Radiation is a general term that describes energy transmission. Radiation takes several different forms, including sound, light, and heat. Radiation can cause both internal and external damage, as well as incorporation of radioactive material into the cells and tissues of the body. Radiation *can* burn the eyes, sound can harm the ears, and heat can burn. However, **ionizing radiation** is the most harmful and cannot be detected without special equipment. Ionizing radiation has the unique property of being able to disrupt atoms and, therefore, to damage the cells of the body.

The three kinds of ionizing radiation are:

- **Alpha particles.** They do little damage if exposure is only external, because the particles are too large to penetrate the skin, and they travel only a few inches in the air. They can be prevented from penetrating the body by shielding with material as weak as clothing or a sheet of paper. Positively charged and consisting of two **protons** and two **neutrons,** they are considered to be the least dangerous of the ionizing radiation as long as they remain outside the body, but they cause the greatest internal damage. To protect against alpha particles, you must wear full protective clothing and a positive-pressure, self-contained breathing apparatus.

- **Beta particles** are higher in energy and are more dangerous and are 7,000 times smaller than alpha particles, but even they can be absorbed by heavy clothing. Beta particles have more penetrating power, and can penetrate the skin and the tissue below in large numbers. If they enter the body through respiration, ingestion, or damaged skin, they can cause as much damage as alpha particles. Thick aluminum can act as an effective shield.

- **Gamma rays** are extremely dangerous. High-energy light similar to x-rays, they are stopped by several inches of lead but can pass completely through the body as they inflict damage to the cells. Gamma rays have 10,000 times the penetrating power of alpha particles, and protective clothing does not stop them. A radioactive substance emits gamma rays spontaneously; the rays contain large amounts of energy and are capable of inflicting damage, including localized skin burns and extensive internal damage.

Gamma rays are measured in **roentgens** (designated by the initial R). One roentgen (R) is the amount of radiation that will produce one unit of ionization in one cubic centimeter of dry air under normal pressure and temperature conditions. Roentgens can be measured as the amount of radiation that is being delivered at a given surface. Radiation that has been absorbed is measured in **rads** (radiation-absorbed dose), a measurement that considers both the amount of ionized radiation that is being emitted at the surface and the amount that has been absorbed and is active within the tissues.

- **Neutrons** are a form of ionizing radiation that is caused by radioactive decay or the chain reaction in a nuclear power plant. These have the greatest penetrating power of all, and can be shielded only with very thick concrete or lead.

There are three general kinds of radiation problems. *Radiation sickness* is caused by exposure to large amounts of radiation; it starts the day after exposure to the radiation, and can last anywhere from a few days to seven or eight weeks, depending on the dose. Common signs and symptoms include nausea and vomiting, diarrhea, hemorrhage, weight loss, appetite loss, malaise, fever, and sores in the throat and mouth. Radiation sickness also affects the immune system, lowering resistance to disease and infection.

Radiation injury is a local injury that is generally caused by exposure to large amounts of less penetrating particles, such as alpha particles. General signs and symptoms include hair loss, skin burns, and generalized skin lesions (Figure 36-11).

Radiation poisoning occurs when the victim has been exposed to dangerous amounts of internal radiation. The result is a host of serious diseases, including cancer and anemia.

While a victim of a radiation accident is *not* "contagious" or infectious and generally will not endanger a rescuer, you *are* at risk of becoming contaminated if the victim still has radiation particles on his or her skin.

Types of Radiation Patients

There are four general types of radiation patients:

- The patient who has received partial or whole body exposure from external radiation, such as from an accelerator, an x-ray machine, or a radioactive object. Even if the patient has received a lethal dose, he or she poses no danger to EMTs and should be handled routinely.

- The patient who has been contaminated internally by breathing in radiation particles or by eating contaminated food. An EMT is in no danger of handling this kind of a patient, either, but certain safeguards should be taken. If the patient has ingested or inhaled a gross amount of contaminated

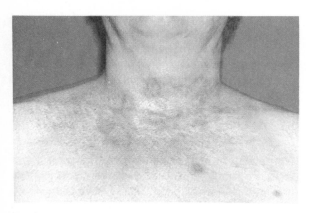

FIGURE 36-11 Radiation burn.

material, any excreta — blood, vomitus, feces, or urine — should be collected and saved so that the type and amount of radiation absorbed (a factor that is critical in some types of care) can be determined.

- The patient who has been externally contaminated by radioactive liquid or dirt particles (contamination can involve either the skin, hair, or clothing). EMTs should protect themselves by covering the stretcher (including the pillow) with a blanket and wrapping the patient in a blanket to contain the contamination. Of course, some patients will have injuries that cannot be cared for if the patient is wrapped in a blanket, and you should take whatever steps necessary to care for life-threatening injuries.

- The patient who has external contamination *and* an open body wound. In these cases, prevent contaminated particles of dirt or other materials from getting into the wound.

Protection from Radiation

As you approach the scene of an accident, protect yourself and other EMTs if you know ahead of time that radiation sources may be involved. Immediately involve the Radiation Safety Officer with your federal, state, or county government.

The following factors determine the amount of radiation damage that you may sustain during a rescue if an unshielded radiation source is present in the vicinity:

- The amount and type of shielding that you can use as an individual.
- The strength of the radiation source.
- Your distance from the radiation source.
- The type of radiation (gamma, alpha, or beta).
- How long you are exposed.
- How much of your body is exposed.

If you are a member of a rescue team, try to reduce your danger by considering the above factors. Some will be out of the question — shielding yourself with a lead apron, for instance, is impossible both because the lead apron is not usually on hand and because it would make your rescue attempts too cumbersome.

You can, however, reduce your risk in other ways. The best approach is to divide the rescue work among many EMTs, with teams composed of as few EMTs as possible. The Federal Nuclear Regulatory Commission recommends that an individual in an emergency situation be exposed to no more than a one-time whole body dose of twenty-five roentgens. This means that if the **geiger counter** at the patient's location indicates fifty roentgens per hour, then a new team of EMTs should move in and relieve the first team after thirty minutes.

The second best method is to shield the radiation source itself (*not* the EMTs or the patients). The best protection against gamma rays is lead, preferably one to two inches thick. If lead is not available, use any material that has thick mass (such as bricks, dirt, or concrete). If you use dirt, make sure that it is deep enough — two to three feet — to adequately cover the source.

If you have reason to suspect that radiation particles may be in the air or in smoke (has an explosion or fire occurred?), wear a closed rescue breathing system, known as **SCBAs (Self-Contained Breathing Apparatus).**

Never smoke in an area where radiation has contaminated the air, and do not eat food that comes from a contamination site. Smoking and eating are the two most common ways of becoming internally contaminated.

Emergency Procedures

Time is the critical factor in managing radiation emergencies. Your first priority is to protect yourself and then remove the patient from the source of radiation as quickly as possible, before beginning emergency care. Never delay advanced life-saving rescue while assessing a victim's contamination status. Other priorities are to create a shield between you and the patient, and the radiation source (the denser the material, the better the shield), and to increase the distance from the source of radiation. Keeping those priorities in mind, follow these general guidelines:

1. As you approach the accident scene, visually survey the area to determine the location of the radiation source. (If you only suspect that radiation may be involved, look for the radiation symbol on the sides of vehicles or machinery involved.) (See Figure 36-12.) Be alert for the presence of other chemicals or hazardous materials, since they are often present at the site of a radiation emergency.

If you determine that radiation is a possibility, park your vehicle upwind of the accident to reduce the chance of radiation particles being blown to your location. Do not park near any liquid spills or near any transport vehicles that may be leaking. Do not park near any containers that might have been cracked or damaged in an accident.

2. As you approach the accident on foot, be alert for any danger of explosion or fire. If you can, quickly remove those dangers before you begin rescue efforts with the patients. If patients are seriously hurt and require immediate care, assign someone else (a bystander, another EMT, or a patient who is not seriously hurt) to remedy any situations that may lead to explosion or fire.

3. If the radiation level is hazardous, quickly remove the patient from the area, even if some of the rules of initial emergency care are violated. Move the patient away from direct hazards, but stay within the controlled area.

4. If you can, find out immediately what **isotope** was involved in the accident. In many cases, this information is listed on identification tags or labels on the containers, the material itself, or on the transport vehicle. The management personnel at a facility or manufacturing plant will probably be able to give you this information. The driver of a transport vehicle probably also knows the nature of the material. If it is possible that someone might become contaminated in a search for the isotope information, *do not* instigate such a search. Have police directly dispatch the manufacturer or owner to determine the identity.

5. Limit the time you spend in a contaminated area to as little as possible; keep as far away from the source as you can. (Exposure to radiation is cumulative and is determined by an inverse square relationship: if you are twice as close, you will receive

FIGURE 36-12 Radiation hazard labels.

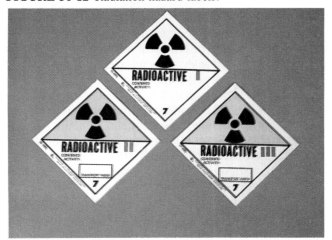

four times the exposure; if you move twice as far away, you cut your exposure by four times.)

6. Wear clothing that will offer the greatest amount of protection. Leave no skin or hair exposed. Wear several layers of clothing if you can, with an outer layer of tightly woven protective clothing; seal all openings with duct tape. Your collar, cuffs, and buttonholes should be closed and sealed with duct tape. Wear two pairs of rubber examining gloves under a pair of heavy work gloves. Wear a pair of shoes covered by two pairs of paper shoe covers under a pair of heavy rubber boots. Wear a cloth hair cover under a cloth hood and/or helmet.

7. If metal containers are available, carry them to the scene to contain contaminated articles. If no metal containers are available, use plastic bags. Always label containers, marking them for contents, source of the material, and time of bagging.

8. If you have one, use a Geiger counter (or similar device) to determine the presence and amount of radiation. Once you get a clear picture of where the radiation is the strongest, you can choose the safest area for administering emergency care to patients.

9. Approach the patients from upwind. Stay clear of dust clouds or smoke if you can. When you reach the patients, disentangle them and remove them as quickly as possible. Speed is of the essence in performing a rescue near a radiation source. If removal will take too much time, do it in shifts to limit exposure to any one rescuer. In most cases, a good rescue technique is to splint a patient and care for injuries where he or she lies, mainly to avoid the possibility of causing further injury. Radiation, however, poses a life-threatening environmental hazard, and patients should be removed to protect both themselves and you. Move the patient away from the accident scene upwind. Use the minimum number of rescuers possible.

10. As you assess the patient's condition, first care for conditions that pose a threat to life: artificial ventilation and circulation are of primary concern, as are hemorrhage, shock, and fracture. Use a Geiger counter to determine whether the patient is contaminated; hold the gauge one inch from the patient's body, and move it slowly along the entire length of the body. If the patient is contaminated, remove and bag his or her clothing; removing clothing can reduce contamination by as much as 70 percent. Remove all jewelry, but bag valuables separately. If the contamination is from radioactive but not chemical sources, do not try to decontaminate the patient — you can spread the radioactivity. If the contamination is chemical, remove it as indicated in Chapter 35.

11. If the patient has sustained an open wound, remove the clothing that surrounds the wound, cover the wound with a clean dressing, and secure the dressing with an elastic bandage. (Do *not* use adhesive tape on a patient who has been exposed to radiation).

12. Once the patient has been treated for all injuries and his or her condition has stabilized, prepare to transport the patient by covering the stretcher (including the pillow) with a blanket.

13. Notify personnel at the hospital or medical center that you will be transporting a patient of possible radiation contamination. If you can, tell personnel at the receiving facility the kind of radiation to which the patient was exposed and the probable amount of dosage.

14. Before you transport the patient, perform the following decontamination procedures:

    • Remove as much of the patient's clothing as possible, including jewelry and shoes. Place it in a properly labeled protective container (ideally, a heavy-gauge plastic bag sealed and placed in a container — preferably metal — that has a tight-fitting lid, such as a galvanized garbage can).

    • Remove the outermost layer of your clothing (including your boots and breathing mask), and place it in the same or another protective container. Leave the containers at the edge of the contamination zone, and have someone guard them so that bystanders will not open or remove them.

    • Use a plastic bag for all contaminated personal items and equipment, such as bandages, blood pressure cuff, eyeglasses, jewelry, etc. Follow the procedure outlined above.

    • Clean any wounds and cover them, and immobilize fractures.

    • Do not wash the patient or yourself. Runoff of contaminated water can enter wounds, can be absorbed by the ground, or can enter other water sources, causing widespread contamination.

    • Wrap the patient in a blanket or several sheets or use a zip-front body bag; never wrap a radiation-exposure victim in plastic, since it can cause shock. Use a towel to wrap the patient's head so that only his or her face is exposed; you must contain any contamination that may be in the hair.

    • Spread a sheet or blanket over the floor of the ambulance to help control contamination and make clean-up easier. If there is gross contamination, remove any nonessential equipment from the ambulance prior to transport. All ambulance personnel should wear gloves, eye protection,

and surgical masks to reduce the chance of infection.

    • Notify the hospital that you are transporting a patient who might be contaminated. Radio the estimated type of radiation, time of exposure, and approximate level of contamination. You might want to radio this information early on in the management of the patient so that the hospital will have additional time to prepare for isolation and contamination control. You can also attach a triage tag to the patient that contains the necessary information.

Personal Decontamination

Because you are transporting the patient to a hospital or medical center, you should leave decontamination of the patient to the medical personnel at the receiving facility. However, you should be concerned with your own decontamination and with that of the vehicle in which you transported the patient. Remember — all personnel and equipment must remain at the hospital until cleared to do otherwise by the responsible agency.

1. Remove all of your clothing; remove outer protective clothing first, bag it, and then remove personal clothing and bag it. If you cannot launder it separately in a machine that can also be decontaminated, throw your clothing away. Leather cannot be decontaminated even with washing and drying; it should be discarded, because it will cause continued exposure and contamination if you continue to wear it. (Clothing that has been contaminated should be disposed of under authority of the state and federal government; regular disposal sites have been designated and are subject to certain specifications.)

2. After you have removed and bagged your clothing, remove your self-contained breathing apparatus; do not remove it if you are still in the wind or there is still fire at the site. Do not handle your face, nose, mouth, or genital area until you have been decontaminated.

3. Carefully wash your entire body in a shower of running water (a tub bath will not adequately remove the particles of contamination). Use warm water with a moderately forceful spray (too much pressure from spray can inject contaminants into the skin) — hot water will increase circulation to the skin, possibly carrying contamination into the system, while cold water will close your pores, trapping the particles in your skin. Pay special attention to your hair, under your fingernails, your body openings, and any body parts that rub together (upper arms and chest, thighs, between fingers and toes, and the buttocks). Use mild nonabrasive or surgical soap (green soap is best);

scrub with a surgical sponge or soft brush, but avoid vigorous scrubbing. Shampoo your hair several times, and rinse thoroughly; avoid getting water from your hair in your eyes, ears, mouth, or nose. Avoid shaving, since you could nick or abrade your skin, possibly introducing contamination. Stay in the shower long enough to wash yourself thoroughly and for the rinse water to completely remove all traces of soap from your body.

4. After you finish showering, let the water run for some time; you need to wash the particles of radiation deep into the hospital's sanitary system. (Some hospitals will not allow this unless they have a separate holding tank. Follow local protocol.) Use clean disposable towels to dry off, and dispose of the towels according to protocol. Dress in clean clothes.

5. You may need more than one shower to remove contamination. Make sure that you use clean towels after each shower.

Vehicle/Equipment Decontamination

Any equipment that you used to care for the patient — including blankets, towels, bandages, cots, stretchers, or equipment used in transportation — must be checked for radiation contamination before it can be used again. Authorities at the hospital or medical center can arrange for an equipment check.

The vehicle used to transport the patient needs to be washed inside and out before it is placed back in service. Any radioactive dust must be removed from the vehicle. Pay special attention to the tires and other contact points. You may need to use a commercial decontamination solution; follow local protocol. (Never use these commercial preparations on the skin.)

If equipment or tools cannot be completely decontaminated, they will need to be disposed of. Signs of incomplete decontamination include debris adhering to the equipment, discoloration, corrosion, or stains.

chapter 37

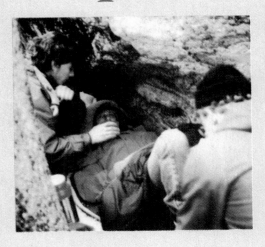

Heat and Cold Emergencies

✳ OBJECTIVES

- Describe how the body attempts to maintain normal temperature and how the body can lose heat.
- Recognize the causes, signs, and symptoms of heat stroke, heat exhaustion, and heat cramps.
- Describe appropriate emergency care for heat stroke, heat exhaustion, and heat cramps.
- Identify the causes, signs, and symptoms of hypothermia and frostbite.
- Describe the appropriate emergency care for hypothermia or frostbite.

It is recommended that EMTs wear protective gloves whenever there is a possibility of coming in contact with a patient's blood, body fluids, mucous membranes, traumatic wounds, or sores. See Chapter 31.

Heat and cold produce a number of different injuries. Critical to your ability to care for those injuries is a basic understanding of the way in which the body maintains its temperature and how it physiologically adjusts to extremes in heat and cold.

□ HOW THE BODY ADJUSTS

The human body stubbornly defends its constant core temperature of 98.6° F. Obviously, if this temperature is to be maintained, heat loss must equal heat production. This equilibrium is maintained by variations in the blood flow to the outer part of the body: when the core temperature rises, vessels near the skin dilate, and the blood brings increased heat to the skin, where it is dissipated by radiation and convection (Figure 37-1). This works only as long as the skin temperature is lower than the temperature of the outside environment. What happens when the temperature of the air approaches or exceeds the temperature of the skin? Heat loss by radiation or convection is impossible, and the body relies on dissipation through evaporation of sweat. But the sweat mechanism also has its limits. The normal adult can sweat only about one liter per hour and can sweat at that rate for only a few hours at a time. In addition, sweating only works if the relative air humidity is low; sweat evaporation ceases entirely when the relative humidity reaches 75 percent.

Since body temperature is actually a measure of heat content or storage, a fall in temperature indicates a decrease, while a rise denotes an increase in the total heat content of the body. A normal-sized, unclothed man can reach and maintain thermal equilibrium in a room with a temperature of 86° F. He retains only that amount of heat generated by his basic metabolic processes and does not need to utilize any of his reserve mechanisms of heat loss. For persons wearing normal indoor clothing, the optimum comfort range is considered to be 70° to 80° F., with relatively humidity between 40 and 60 percent.

How the Body Loses Heat

The body loses heat through radiation, conduction, convection, and evaporation of moisture (Figure 37-2).

Radiation

Radiation, the most significant method of heat loss, involves the transfer of heat from the surface of one object

FIGURE 37-1

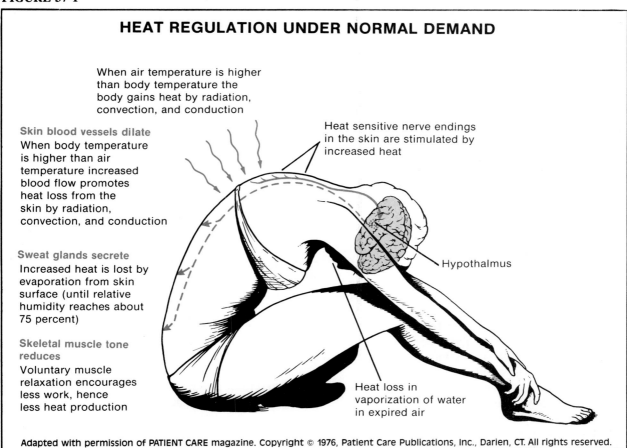

HEAT REGULATION UNDER NORMAL DEMAND

When air temperature is higher than body temperature the body gains heat by radiation, convection, and conduction

Skin blood vessels dilate
When body temperature is higher than air temperature increased blood flow promotes heat loss from the skin by radiation, convection, and conduction

Sweat glands secrete
Increased heat is lost by evaporation from skin surface (until relative humidity reaches about 75 percent)

Skeletal muscle tone reduces
Voluntary muscle relaxation encourages less work, hence less heat production

Heat sensitive nerve endings in the skin are stimulated by increased heat

Hypothalmus

Heat loss in vaporization of water in expired air

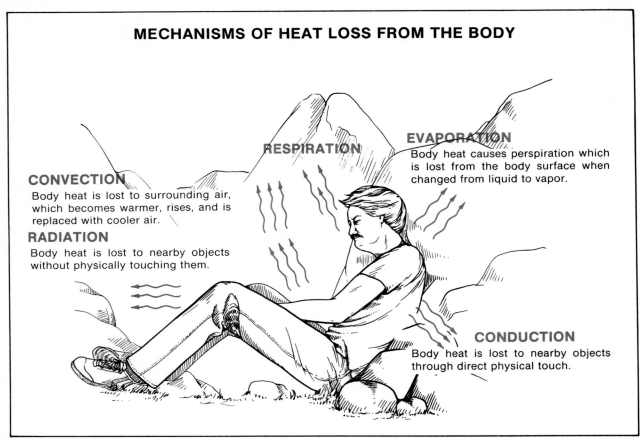

MECHANISMS OF HEAT LOSS FROM THE BODY

RESPIRATION

EVAPORATION
Body heat causes perspiration which is lost from the body surface when changed from liquid to vapor.

CONVECTION
Body heat is lost to surrounding air, which becomes warmer, rises, and is replaced with cooler air.

RADIATION
Body heat is lost to nearby objects without physically touching them.

CONDUCTION
Body heat is lost to nearby objects through direct physical touch.

FIGURE 37-2 The illustration assumes that a wet, poorly dressed climber has taken shelter in a crevasse or among cold, wet rocks.

to the surface of another without physical contact. Heat loss from radiation varies considerably with environmental conditions. In a temperate climate and under normal conditions, a person loses about 60 percent of his or her heat production by radiation. Most heat loss is from the head (approximately 50 percent), hands, and feet. At temperatures of 90 degrees F., however, radiation loss will probably drop to zero; in subzero temperatures, loss of heat through radiation will skyrocket.

Conduction and Convection

Conduction and convection, less important methods of heat loss in temperature climates, are major considerations in cold regions. By convection, the cold air in immediate contact with the skin is warmed. The heated molecules move away, and cooler ones take their place. Those, in turn, are warmed, and the process starts all over again. Any process that speeds movement of the air — such as wind — also speeds the cooling process.

The phenomenon of convection has been incorporated into the concept of **windchill** (Figure 37-3). A unit of windchill is defined as the amount of heat that would be lost in an hour from a square meter of exposed skin surface with a normal temperature of 91.4 de-

grees F. In essence, the windchill factor combines the effects of the speed of the wind and the temperature of the environment into a number that indicates the danger of exposure. When the windchill factor is −10, the temperature is bitterly cold; at −20, exposed flesh may freeze; at −70, exposed flesh will freeze in less than one minute; and at −95, exposed flesh will freeze in less than thirty seconds. For instance, flesh will freeze in less than one minute in only ten-mile-per-hour winds if the temperature is forty degrees below zero.

Conduction is the method of heat loss in **waterchill.** Water conducts heat 240 times more quickly than air. This means that wet clothing conducts heat away from the body at a much higher rate than dry clothing. A person whose clothing is wet, then, is in exceptional danger of losing heat. The wet clothing pulls heat away from the body more rapidly than the body can produce it.

Heat loss by conduction also occurs when heat is transferred to **tidal air** as it is warmed in the respiratory passages and lungs (a person inhales cold air and exhales warm air), when water and food are taken into the digestive tract, and when waste materials (urine and feces) are eliminated.

WIND CHILL INDEX

WIND SPEED MPH	WHAT THE THERMOMETER READS (degrees F.)											
	50	40	30	20	10	0	−10	−20	−30	−40	−50	−60
	WHAT IT EQUALS IN ITS EFFECT ON EXPOSED FLESH											
CALM	50	40	30	20	10	0	−10	−20	−30	−40	−50	−60
5	48	37	27	16	6	−5	−15	−26	−36	−47	−57	−68
10	40	28	16	4	−9	−21	−33	−46	−58	−70	−83	−95
15	36	22	9	−5	−18	−36	−45	−58	−72	−85	−99	−112
20	32	18	4	−10	−25	−39	−53	−67	−82	−96	−110	−121
25	30	16	0	−15	−29	−44	−59	−74	−88	−104	−118	−133
30	28	13	−2	−18	−33	−48	−63	−79	−94	−109	−125	−140
35	27	11	−4	−20	−35	−49	−67	−82	−98	−113	−129	−145
40	26	10	−6	−21	−37	−53	−69	−85	−100	−116	−132	−148

Little danger if properly clothed	Danger of freezing exposed flesh	Great danger of freezing exposed flesh

FIGURE 37-3

Evaporation

Loss of heat by vaporization (evaporation) of perspiration is usually more massive in hot weather; it slows down when the air is humid. In cold climates, the only loss from perspiration is due to wearing improper clothing. When the temperature of the air equals or exceeds the temperature of the skin, body heat must be eliminated through vaporization.

How the Body Conserves Heat

How does the human body conserve body heat? Since approximately 80 to 85 percent of all heat loss occurs from the body surface, any reduction in skin temperature should conserve body heat. The skin is heated in four ways: (1) blood rushes to the surface of the skin from internal organs; (2) hair erects, thickening the layer of warm air trapped immediately next to the skin; (3) little or no perspiration is released to the skin surface for evaporation; and (4) the body produces more heat (through shivering and certain hormones, such as epinephrine) (Figure 37-4). Therefore, the ways in which humans remain cool are restricting blood flow to the skin, limiting the amount of body hair, and wearing only one layer of clothing.

Blood flow is also increased to the skin surface when the body becomes overheated. When vessels at the skin surface dilate, the heat in the blood is taken to the skin surface, where it is lost through radiation and convection. Additional heat is lost through perspiration and respiration.

☐ HYPERTHERMIA (HEAT-RELATED INJURY)

Hyperthermia is an increase in body temperature that results from a hot environment. Heat-related injuries fall into three major categories: heatstroke, heat exhaustion, and heat cramps. Heat emergencies are most frequent on days when the temperature is 95 to 100 degrees F., when the humidity is high, and when there is little or no breeze (Figure 37-5).

Most heat injuries occur early in the summer season, before people have acclimated themselves to the higher temperatures. The heat and humidity risk scale (Figure 37-6) indicates when problems are most likely to occur.

Heat Stroke

Heat stroke, a true life-threatening emergency, has a mortality ranging from 20 to 70 percent. Heat stroke is sometimes called **sunstroke,** although the sun is not required for its onset. The condition results when the heat-regulating mechanisms of the body break down and fail to cool the body sufficiently. The body becomes overheated, the body temperature rises to between 105 and 110 degrees F., and no sweating occurs in about half the victims. Because no cooling takes place, the body stores increasingly more heat, the heat-producing mechanisms speed up, and eventually the brain cells are damaged, causing permanent disability or death.

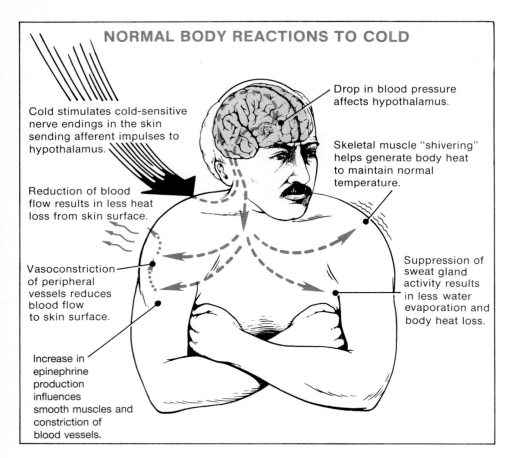

NORMAL BODY REACTIONS TO COLD

Cold stimulates cold-sensitive nerve endings in the skin sending afferent impulses to hypothalamus.

Reduction of blood flow results in less heat loss from skin surface.

Vasoconstriction of peripheral vessels reduces blood flow to skin surface.

Increase in epinephrine production influences smooth muscles and constriction of blood vessels.

Drop in blood pressure affects hypothalamus.

Skeletal muscle "shivering" helps generate body heat to maintain normal temperature.

Suppression of sweat gland activity results in less water evaporation and body heat loss.

FIGURE 37-4

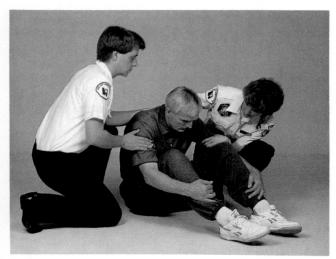

FIGURE 37-5 Heat injury victim.

There are two basic kinds of heat stroke. Classic heat stroke, in which people lose the ability to sweat, generally affects the elderly or the chronically ill during a heat wave. Exertional heat stroke, in which victims retain the ability to sweat, is accompanied by physical exertion and muscle stress (Figure 37-7).

Heat stroke most seriously affects the aged; infants and children (who sweat less, generate more heat, and have a smaller body surface); debilitated, malnourished,

and inexperienced athletes; those who have a prior history of heat stroke; or those who are short, stocky, and heavily muscled. It is more apt to affect those who have had recent fever or those with chronic diseases, such as renal (kidney) disease, cerebrovascular disease, mental retardation, **Parkinson's disease,** diabetes, alcoholism, obesity, and dermatological (skin) diseases such as **eczema, scleroderma,** and healed burns. Drug abusers are especially susceptible, especially those who use barbiturates and hallucinogens. Even healthy individuals, when overexerted, can fall victim. Young people who suffer from heat stroke may not completely lose the ability to sweat, and their skin may be moist and hot instead of characteristically dry.

Heat stroke commonly occurs during times of high temperatures combined with high humidity and low wind velocity. It may be due to other factors: fever that will not respond to therapy, consumption of alcohol, use of diuretics, or use of some kinds of drugs that act either to promote internal body heat or to hamper sweating.

Signs and Symptoms

Heat stroke is indicated by the following signs and symptoms (Figure 37-8):

- Temperature of 105° F. or higher.

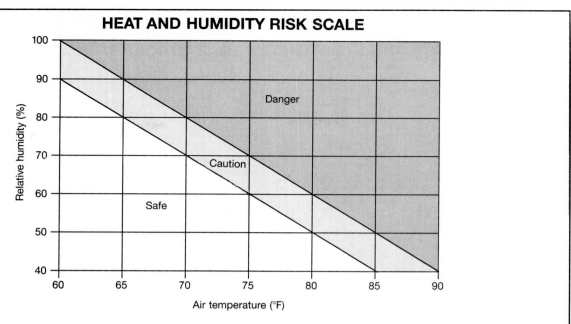

HEAT AND HUMIDITY RISK SCALE

Danger

Caution

Safe

Relative humidity (%)

Air temperature (°F)

FIGURE 37-6 The risk of illness is increased when heat and humidity produce dangerous conditions. Lower temperatures with high humidity can also cause the body's temperature to rise.

FIGURE 37-7

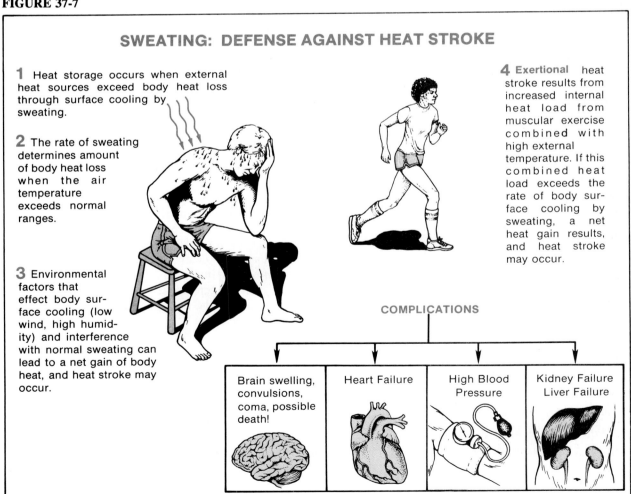

SWEATING: DEFENSE AGAINST HEAT STROKE

1 Heat storage occurs when external heat sources exceed body heat loss through surface cooling by sweating.

2 The rate of sweating determines amount of body heat loss when the air temperature exceeds normal ranges.

3 Environmental factors that effect body surface cooling (low wind, high humidity) and interference with normal sweating can lead to a net gain of body heat, and heat stroke may occur.

4 Exertional heat stroke results from increased internal heat load from muscular exercise combined with high external temperature. If this combined heat load exceeds the rate of body surface cooling by sweating, a net heat gain results, and heat stroke may occur.

COMPLICATIONS

Brain swelling, convulsions, coma, possible death!

Heart Failure

High Blood Pressure

Kidney Failure Liver Failure

551

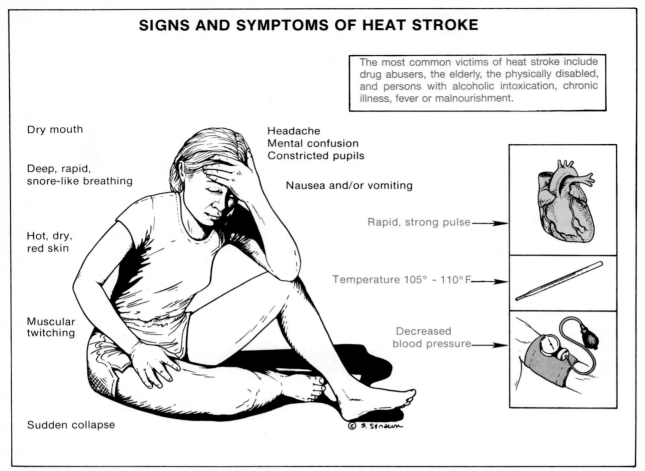

SIGNS AND SYMPTOMS OF HEAT STROKE

The most common victims of heat stroke include drug abusers, the elderly, the physically disabled, and persons with alcoholic intoxication, chronic illness, fever or malnourishment.

Dry mouth

Deep, rapid, snore-like breathing

Hot, dry, red skin

Muscular twitching

Sudden collapse

Headache
Mental confusion
Constricted pupils

Nausea and/or vomiting

Rapid, strong pulse →

Temperature 105° - 110° F →

Decreased blood pressure →

© S. Strauss

FIGURE 37-8

- Hot, reddish skin; skin can be wet or dry, since approximately half of all heat stroke victims sweat profusely.
- An initially rapid, strong pulse of 160 or more, continuing rapid but becoming weak as damage progresses.
- Initially constricted pupils, later becoming dilated.
- Tremors.
- Mental confusion and anxiety; victims may show unusual irritability, aggression, combative agitation, or — in the extreme — psychotic or hysterical behavior.
- Initially deep, rapid breathing that sounds like snoring; breathing becomes shallow and weak as damage progresses.
- Headache.
- Dry mouth.
- Shortness of breath.
- Loss of appetite, nausea, or vomiting.
- Increasing dizziness and weakness.
- Decreased blood pressure.

- Convulsions, sudden collapse, and possible unconsciousness; *all* heat stroke victims have compromised levels of consciousness, ranging from disorientation to coma.
- Decreased urinary output.

Patients may lapse into a coma, become delirious, and die. About 4,000 Americans die of heat stroke each year; 80 percent of those deaths occur among people over the age of fifty. Heat stroke is the second most common cause of death among high school athletes (second only to spinal cord injury). Untreated, all patients die. The longer care is delayed, the more permanent and disabling the damage, particularly to the central nervous system.

Emergency Care

Emergency care of heat stroke is aimed at *immediate* cooling of the body and adequate hydration. *Act fast*; do whatever is necessary to cool the body. Cooling can and should be accomplished during transport so that transport is not delayed. The priority of treatment is to remove the patient from the source of heat when possible;

other top priorities include airway, ventilation, oxygenation, circulation, and transport. To treat:

1. Remove the patient when possible from the source of heat, establish an airway, and administer high-concentration oxygen.

2. Remove as much of the patient's clothing as possible or reasonable, pour cool water over his or her body (avoiding the nose and mouth), fan the patient briskly, and shade him or her from the sun if still outdoors. Place cold packs or wrapped ice bags in the patient's armpits, in the groin, at each side of the neck, behind each knee, around the wrists, and around the ankles to cool the large surface blood vessels (Figure 37-9). Simple ice packs or hyperthermia blankets will not effectively lower temperature when used alone; use a variety of methods. Wrapping a wet sheet that has been soaked in ice water around the patient's body and then directing an electric fan at the patient are also good ways of cooling (Figure 37-10). Use slower cooling if the patient starts to shiver, since shivering produces heat. Continue until the patient's temperature falls to 102° F., and transport as soon as possible. Continue cooling measures during transport. If transport must be delayed, submerge the patient up to the face in a tub of cool water. Administer high-concentration oxygen and treat for shock.

3. Because heat stroke involves the entire body, a number of complications may result from the ailment itself or from necessary care. Be prepared to care for the following complications as cooling proceeds:

   • Convulsions. Tremors and convulsions tend to accompany rapid cooling and, because convulsions produce great body heat, they can impair

FIGURE 37-9 Use cold applications on the head and body to cool a heat stroke patient.

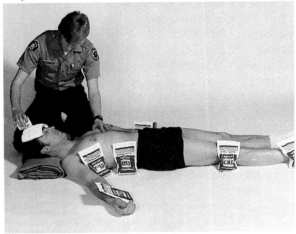

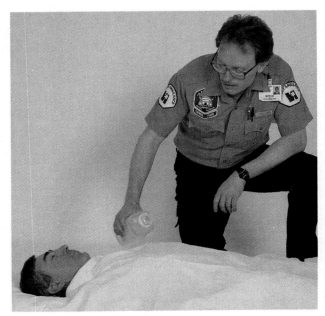

FIGURE 37-10 Wrapping a heat stroke victim in a wet sheet and directing a fan at the patient are good ways of cooling.

treatment. Convulsions are most likely to occur once the body cools to 104° F.

   • Aspiration of vomitus. Vomiting commonly accompanies convulsions caused by cooling techniques. Position the patient for easy drainage and suctioning.

4. During transport, run the vehicle's air-conditioning system at maximum capacity if possible. If that is not possible, wrap the patient in wet sheets and direct a fan at him.

5. *Always* transport a victim of heat stroke, even if you are able to lower the body temperature; a victim of heat stroke always needs hospital care.

Heat Exhaustion

Heat exhaustion, the most common heat injury, occurs in an otherwise fit person who is involved in extreme physical exertion in a hot, humid environment. It results from a serious disturbance of the blood flow, similar to circulatory disturbance of shock. Heat exhaustion is, in fact, a mild state of shock brought on by the pooling of blood in the vessels just below the skin, causing blood to flow away from the major organs of the body. Due to prolonged and profuse sweating, the body loses large quantities of salt and water. Heat exhaustion can also occur among the elderly or the infirm, who have too little salt even without activity. When the water is not adequately replaced, blood circulation diminishes, affecting brain, heart, and lung functions. Heat exhaustion is sometimes, though not always, accompanied by **heat cramps** due to salt loss.

There are two basic kinds of heat exhaustion:

- Salt-depletion (sodium depletion), in which unacclimatized individuals exert themselves and drink enough water but do not replace the sodium.
- Water-depletion, which usually occurs among the elderly or chronically ill who do not drink enough water during extreme heat. This type of heat exhaustion is characterized by extreme anxiety and agitation, intense thirst, headache, weakness, fever, muscle incoordination, and decreased sweating.

Signs and Symptoms

Primary signs and symptoms of heat exhaustion are much like flu symptoms. They can include the following:

- Headache, giddiness, and extreme weakness.
- Nausea and possible vomiting.
- Dizziness and faintness.
- Profuse sweating.
- Loss of appetite.
- Fatigue.
- Diarrhea.
- Collapse and unconsciousness (usually brief).
- Thirst.
- Below-normal body temperature or normal body temperature; in occasional cases, body temperature may be slightly elevated.
- Dilated pupils.
- Weak and rapid pulse.
- Rapid, shallow breathing.
- Pale, cool, sweaty skin, usually ashen gray in color.
- Possible heat cramps or muscle aches.
- Inelastic skin.
- Difficulty in walking.

Heat Exhaustion Versus Heat Stroke

While the signs and symptoms of heat exhaustion may seem similar to those of heat stroke to the casual observer or to an uninformed patient, there are some distinct differences that will help you make the correct evaluation (Figure 37-11).

The two most reliable and distinct differences are the condition of the skin and the body temperature. In heat stroke, the skin is flushed and hot to the touch; patients experiencing heat exhaustion usually have wet or clammy, pale, cool skin. Body temperature in a patient with heat stroke can soar to above 106° F.; in a victim of heat exhaustion, it usually stays at normal or sometimes even dips below normal.

Emergency Care

To treat a patient of heat exhaustion:

1. Move the patient to a cool place away from the source of heat, but make sure that he or she does not become chilled. Apply cold, wet compresses to the skin, and fan him or her lightly.
2. Have the patient lie down. Keep him or her at rest, and administer oxygen if needed. Raise the patient's feet eight to twelve inches, and lower the head to help increase blood circulation to the brain. Remove as much of the patient's clothing as possible, and loosen what you cannot remove. Help make the patient as comfortable as possible (Figure 37-12).
3. If the patient is fully conscious, administer cool water at the rate of one-half glassful every fifteen minutes for one hour (Figure 37-13).
4. If the patient is unconscious, remove his or her clothing and sponge off with cool water.
5. If the patient vomits, stop giving fluids and transport immediately to a hospital, where he or she can receive intravenous fluids. (This is usually the only instance in which a heat exhaustion patient will require hospitalization.)
6. Take the patient's temperature every ten or fifteen minutes; transport as soon as possible. If the patient's temperature is above 101° F. or rising, there are other injuries, there is a history of medical problems, the patient fails to respond, or the patient is unconscious, transport immediately.

Heat Cramps

Heat cramps are the least serious heat injury. They are muscular spasms that occur when the body loses too much salt during profuse sweating, when not enough salt is taken into the body, when calcium levels are low, and when too much water is consumed. Occasionally, heat cramps can also be caused by overexertion of muscles, inadequate stretching or warmup, and **lactic acid** buildup in poorly conditioned muscles. Heat cramps can be mild or extremely painful. When the body becomes low on salt and water, the patient interprets it as thirst. To quench thirst, one consumes large quantities of water without replacing the salt. Heat cramps usually occur in the arms, legs or abdomen (the major complaint may be severe abdominal pain) and are often a signal of approaching heat exhaustion.

Hot weather is not necessarily requisite to heat cramps. A person who exercises strenuously in cold weather and perspires may develop heat cramps if he or

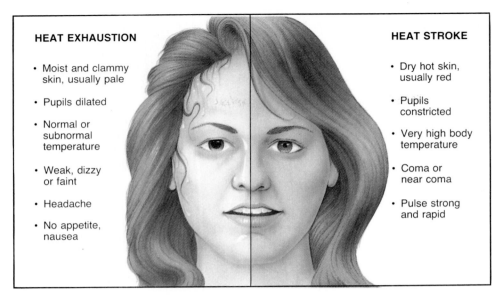

HEAT EXHAUSTION

- Moist and clammy skin, usually pale
- Pupils dilated
- Normal or subnormal temperature
- Weak, dizzy or faint
- Headache
- No appetite, nausea

HEAT STROKE

- Dry hot skin, usually red
- Pupils constricted
- Very high body temperature
- Coma or near coma
- Pulse strong and rapid

FIGURE 37-11

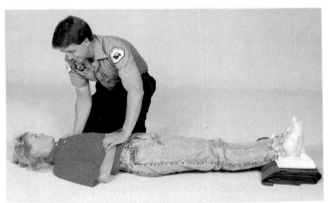

FIGURE 37-12 Have the heat exhaustion patient lie down with feet elevated.

she drinks water but does not replace salt. Heat cramps result when blood calcium levels are too high in proportion to blood sodium levels. In order to function properly, the muscles need a strict balance of water, calcium, and sodium; whenever that balance is disrupted, regardless of temperature, muscular contraction malfunctions, and heat cramps may result. Cramping occurs when the muscle contracts without relaxing again; the muscle remains firm in a knotted configuration, leaving a cavity at its origin.

Signs and Symptoms

Signs and symptoms of heat cramps can include (Figure 37-14):

- Severe muscular cramps and pain, especially of the arms, fingers, legs, calves, and abdomen.
- Hot, sweaty skin.
- Normal body temperature.

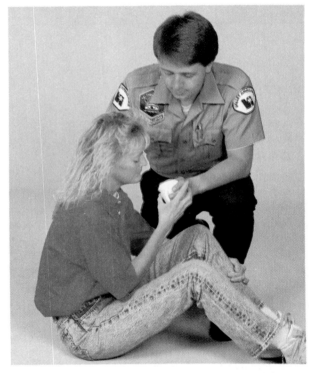

FIGURE 37-13 If the heat exhaustion patient is fully conscious, administer cool water.

- Normal blood pressure.
- Rapid heartbeat.
- Faintness and dizziness.
- Exhaustion or fatigue.
- A stiff, board-like abdomen.
- Possible nausea and vomiting.
- Normal mental status and consciousness level.

Heat and Cold Emergencies   **555**

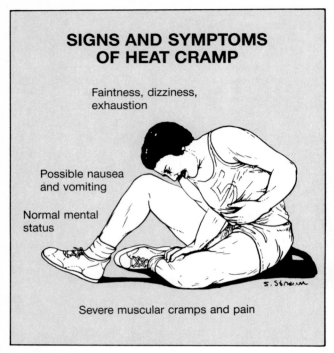

**SIGNS AND SYMPTOMS
OF HEAT CRAMP**

Faintness, dizziness,
exhaustion

Possible nausea
and vomiting

Normal mental
status

Severe muscular cramps and pain

S. Strom

FIGURE 37-14

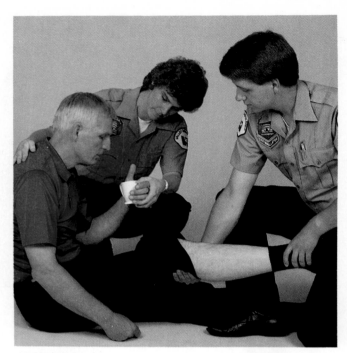

FIGURE 37-15 A patient with heat cramps can be given sips of cool saltwater.

Emergency Care

To care for a patient with heat cramps:

1. If the patient is in a hot environment, remove him or her from the heat immediately.

2. Administer sips of saltwater to the patient at the rate of one-half glassful every fifteen minutes (Figure 37-15). Dilute one teaspoon of salt or one boullion cube in one quart of water, or use a commercial product with a low glucose content. Do *not* give the patient salt tablets.

3. Apply moist towels to the patient's forehead and over the cramping muscles. Massage the cramping muscles unless massage increases the pain. To relieve pain, try gently stretching the involved muscle groups. Manipulate or push the knotted muscle mass back to its normal position. (*Note*: The use of massage is somewhat controversial. Some systems do not advocate the use of massage, while others recommend massage as long as it does not increase pain or discomfort; follow local protocol.)

4. Explain to the patient what happened to him or her — and why — so that he or she can avoid a recurrence. Assure the patient that nothing is critically wrong with him or her; some individuals fear a blood clot or muscle tear. Help the patient remain calm and relaxed, since relaxation will speed recovery of the muscle spasm. The patient should avoid exertion of any kind for twelve hours.

A victim of heat cramps is prone to recurrence; if the patient resists restricted activity, you may have to transport him or her to prevent heat stroke or heat exhaustion. Finally, advise the patient to salt food more heavily and to increase fluid intake until all cramping stops.

5. Follow local protocol regarding transport. Generally, you should transport if the patient has other injuries or illnesses, if other symptoms develop, or if the patient worsens and/or does not respond to care. The patient may need an intravenous solution of sodium.

See Figures 37-16–37-18 for a summary of signs and symptoms and emergency care procedures for all three types of heat-related emergencies.

☐ HYPOTHERMIA (COLD-RELATED INJURY)

Major injuries related to extreme cold temperatures are general hypothermia, **immersion hypothermia,** and frostbite.

General Hypothermia

General hypothermia is due to an increase in heat loss, a decrease in heat production, or both. The most life-threatening cold injury, hypothermia affects the entire body with generalized severe cooling. Mortality from general hypothermia is as high as 87 percent. Hypothermia can be either acute (occurring suddenly, as when someone falls through ice) or chronic (developing gradually from prolonged exposure to wind, cold, or cool water).

There are three categories of general hypothermia that are determined by core body temperature:

- Mild hypothermia (90 to 95° F.).
- Moderate hypothermia (82 to 89.9° F.).
- Severe hypothermia (less than 82° F.).

Cases have been documented in which patients have survived with a core temperature as low as 64.4° F. In general, thermal control is lost once the body temperature is lowered to 95° F. and the body is no longer in thermal balance. Coma occurs when the body's core temperature reaches approximately 79° F.

General hypothermia is usually due to exposure without ensuing frostbite. However, it can happen indoors, and it does not necessarily require cold weather. Extremely low temperatures are not necessary to induce hypothermia — it can occur in temperatures as high as 65° F., depending on the windchill factor, and at temperatures well above freezing. Most cases result when the temperature is about 60° F. or less. Wetness — either from water or perspiration — always compounds the problem; exhaustion also affects any case of hypothermia. Always consider hypothermia in any victim of trauma in cold weather.

Some of the contributing factors to hypothermia, even in the absence of thermal stress, include the following:

- Use of drugs.
- Surgery.
- Water activities.
- Disease.
- Trauma.
- Extremes of age.
- Immobility.

Basically, hypothermia occurs when the body loses more heat than it produces. Death can occur within two hours of the first signs and symptoms (Figure 37-19).

Hypothermia can occur with little warning. Initial reactions to cold, of course, are shivering and "goosebumps," but in hypothermia, these are not enough to maintain body temperature. As the core temperature drops, the body's thermal-regulating mechanism becomes confused. A patient, even though he or she is dangerously cold, may undress because he or she *thinks* he or she is too warm.

Signs and Symptoms

It is possible to measure core body temperature only with a specialized thermometer, and it can't normally be done in the field. You must rely on signs and symptoms, not body temperature measurement, to determine the severity of hypothermia. Signs and symptoms of hypothermia are vague and mimic other disorders, often causing misdiagnosis; hypothermia, in fact, is often mistaken for stroke. General signs and symptoms of hypothermia include (Figure 37-20):

- Skin that is cold to the touch (especially on the abdomen).
- Uncontrollable fits of shivering.
- Vague, slow, slurred, and thick speech.
- Amnesia, memory lapses, and incoherence.
- Poor judgment.
- Staggering gait.
- Postural dizziness.
- Muscular rigidity in later stages.
- Skin color ranging from cyanosis to waxen; skin often appears gray and bloodless.
- Disorientation and mental confusion.
- Sluggish pupils.
- Apathy.
- Semi-rigid skin.
- Bloated face.
- Increased blood pressure, heart, and respiratory rates at first; decreased heart and respiratory rates, irregular heartbeat, weak, shallow, or absent pulse and respiration as hypothermia progresses.
- Dehydration.
- Low blood pressure.
- Drowsiness and/or stupor; unresponsiveness to verbal or painful stimuli.
- Apparent exhaustion; inability to get up after rest.
- Unconsciousness, deep coma with severe hypothermia.

Note: The above symptoms are not in any order of progression; for a progressive list of symptoms, see Figure 37-21.

How the patient looks and acts depends in part on the severity of the hypothermia. If the core temperature is above 90° F., the patient will probably shiver violently and complain of being very cold. While the patient will be able to answer questions and will have almost normal thinking abilities, he or she may be slower than normal in responding to questions and commands. He or she will most likely be oriented as to where and who the patient is and what day and time it is. The pa-

CONDITION	MUSCLE CRAMPS	BREATHING	PULSE	WEAKNESS	SKIN	PERSPIRATION	LOSS OF CONSCIOUSNESS
Heat cramps	Yes	Varies	Varies	Yes	Moist-warm No change	Heavy	Seldom
Heat exhaustion	No	Rapid Shallow	Weak	Yes	Cold Clammy	Heavy	Sometimes
Heat stroke	No	Deep, then shallow	Full Rapid	Yes	Dry-hot	Little or none	Often

HEAT CRAMPS

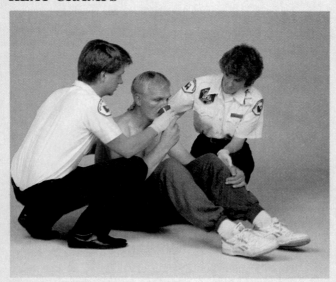

FIGURE 37-16

HEAT EXHAUSTION

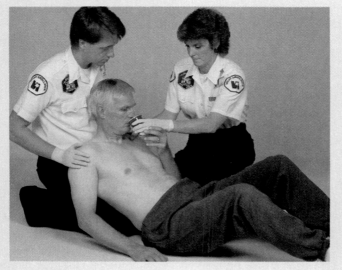

FIGURE 37-17

SYMPTOMS AND SIGNS:

Severe muscle cramps (usually in the legs and abdomen), exhaustion, sometimes dizziness or periods of faintness.

EMERGENCY CARE PROCEDURES:

- Move patient to a nearby cool place.
- Give patient salted water to drink or half-strength commercial electrolyte fluids.
- Massage the "cramped" muscle to help ease the patient's discomfort; massaging with pressure will be more effective than light rubbing actions. (Optional in some EMS systems.) Follow local protocol.
- Apply moist towels to the patient's forehead and over cramped muscles for added relief.
- If cramps persist, or if more serious signs and symptoms develop, ready the patient and transport.

SYMPTOMS AND SIGNS:

Rapid and shallow breathing, weak pulse, cold and clammy skin, heavy perspiration, total body weakness, and dizziness that sometimes leads to unconsciousness.

EMERGENCY CARE PROCEDURES:

- Move the patient to a nearby cool place.
- Keep the patient at rest.
- Remove enough clothing to cool the patient without chilling him (watch for shivering).
- Fan the patient's skin.
- Give the patient salted water or half-strength commercial electrolyte fluids. Do not try to administer fluids to an unconscious patient.

- Treat for shock, but do not cover to the point of overheating the patient.
- Provide oxygen if needed.
- If unconscious, fails to recover rapidly, has other injuries, or has a history of medical problems, transport as soon as possible.

HEAT STROKE

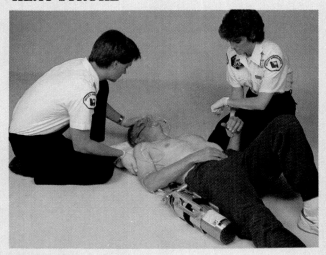

FIGURE 37-18

SYMPTOMS AND SIGNS:

Deep breaths, then shallow breathing; rapid strong pulse, then rapid, weak pulse; dry, hot skin; dilated pupils; loss of consciousness (possible coma); seizures or muscular twitching may be seen.

EMERGENCY CARE PROCEDURES:

- Cool the patient — in any manner — rapidly move the patient out of the sun or away from the heat source. Remove patient's clothing and wrap him or her in wet towels and sheets. Pour cool water over these wrappings. Body heat must be lowered rapidly or brain cells will die!
- Treat for shock and administer a high concentration of oxygen.
- If cold packs or ice bags are available, wrap them and place one bag or pack under each of the patient's armpits, one behind each knee, one in the groin, one on each wrist and ankle, and one on each side of the patient's neck.
- Transport as soon as possible.
- Should transport be delayed, find a tub or container — immerse patient up to the face in cooled water. Constantly monitor to prevent drowning.
- Monitor vital signs throughout process.

tient will probably be able to move around quite normally but may be slightly uncoordinated and unable to perform simple tasks requiring manual dexterity, such as unzipping a zipper or tying shoes.

When core temperature drops below 90° F., the patient will be quite disoriented about who he or she is, where he or she is, and what day it is. His or her speech may not make much sense; he or she may become confused and withdrawn. The patient may not be able to care for himself or herself, and may even do senseless or wrong things in confusion. The muscles may be quite stiff, even resembling rigor mortis; he or she may be uncoordinated, unable to perform physical tasks, and stumble when trying to walk. When the core temperature reaches the low 80s, he or she will probably drift into unconsciousness, and the heart may fibrillate.

Most patients with a core temperature above 90° F. will survive with emergency care; those with a lower core temperature require extreme care in handling and rapid transport.

Emergency Care

The basic principles of emergency care for hypothermia include preventing heat loss, rewarming the patient as quickly and safely as possible if transport is delayed, and remaining alert for complications (see Figure 37-19). Remember — hypothermia is an emergency.

Some general guidelines apply to emergency care for hypothermia victims, whether they are wet or dry, on land or in water. Patients in seemingly unlikely situations can be hypothermic. Hypothermia can be a complication even when the weather is warm and the patient is dry. Remember to check temperature!

The most basic guideline and top priority is to *never allow the patient to stay in a cold environment.* Insulate the patient from the cold however you can: use wool blankets, plastic sheets, newspapers, plastic air-bubble packing material, or a sleeping bag; prewarm a sleeping bag by lying in it. Insulate the patient from the ground up; get something underneath him or her as quickly as possible. In general, do *not* try to rewarm a patient if you can transport him or her immediately. Rewarming is best done in the hospital. Initiate rewarming only if transport is delayed.

Do everything possible to prevent further heat loss. If possible, warm instruments and use warm, humidified oxygen. If it is needed, however, use oxygen even if it is not warmed.

Whenever possible, keep the patient in a horizontal position; it helps prevent shock and increases blood flow to the brain. If you are transporting a hypothermia victim out of the mountains, injuries should be directed uphill. Elevate the patient's head if he or she has sustained head or chest injuries, if he or she has shortness of breath, if he or she has symptoms of myocardial infarction, or if the terrain is extremely steep.

STAGES OF HYPOTHERMIA
(General Body Cooling)

1. **Shivering** (a response by the body which generates heat) does not occur below a body temperature of 90°F.

2. **Apathy** and decreased muscle function, first fine motor and then gross motor functions.

3. **Decreased level of consciousness** with a glassy stare and possible freezing of the extremities.

4. **Decreased vital signs** with slow pulse and slow respiration rate.

5. **Death**

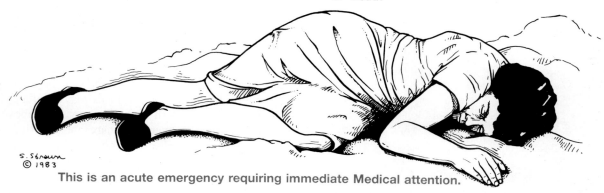

S. Sörauer © 1983

This is an acute emergency requiring immediate Medical attention.

EMERGENCY CARE

- Keep the patient dry and remove wet clothing.
- Apply external heat to both sides of the patient using whatever heat sources are available including the body heat of rescuers.
- If the patient is conscious and in a warm place have him breathe warm, moist air or oxygen if available.
- Monitor respirations and pulse and provide pulmonary and cardio-pulmonary resuscitation as required. No one is dead until warm and dead.
- Do not give hot liquids by mouth.
- Do not allow patient to exercise.
- Handle the patient gently.

If less than 30 minutes from medical facility:	If more than 30 minutes from a medical facility:
1. Prevent further heat loss	1. Prevent further heat loss
2. Handle with care.	2. Handle with care.
3. Administer oxygen.	3. Administer oxygen.
4. Transport.	4. Follow rewarming techniques
	5. Prepare for CPR.
	6. Transport.

There is disagreement among some experts regarding the temperature used for rewarming cold injuries. It is important that you follow local protocol.

FIGURE 37-19

To treat, follow these general guidelines:

1. Handle the patient *very* gently and do not allow the patient to exert himself or herself. Jostling a hypothermia victim can cause ventricular fibrillation. Keep the patient in a horizontal position to help provide adequate perfusion to the brain.

2. Check the vital signs.

   - Vital signs are slowed in hypothermia victims, so measure for one full minute to make an accurate assessment.
   - Open the airway, and restore breathing and circulation if necessary by administering CPR. Be prepared for lengthy resuscitation: a severely hy-

SIGNS AND SYMPTOMS OF HYPOTHERMIA

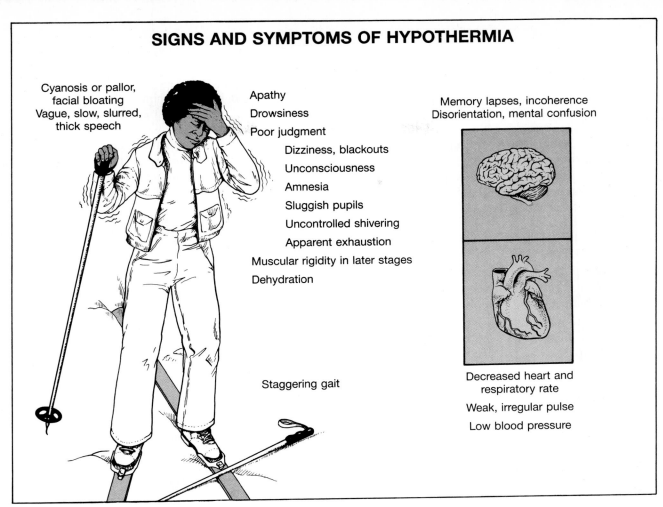

Cyanosis or pallor, facial bloating
Vague, slow, slurred, thick speech

Apathy
Drowsiness
Poor judgment
Dizziness, blackouts
Unconsciousness
Amnesia
Sluggish pupils
Uncontrolled shivering
Apparent exhaustion
Muscular rigidity in later stages
Dehydration

Staggering gait

Memory lapses, incoherence
Disorientation, mental confusion

Decreased heart and respiratory rate
Weak, irregular pulse
Low blood pressure

FIGURE 37-20

SIGNS AND SYMPTOMS OF A SINKING CORE TEMPERATURE

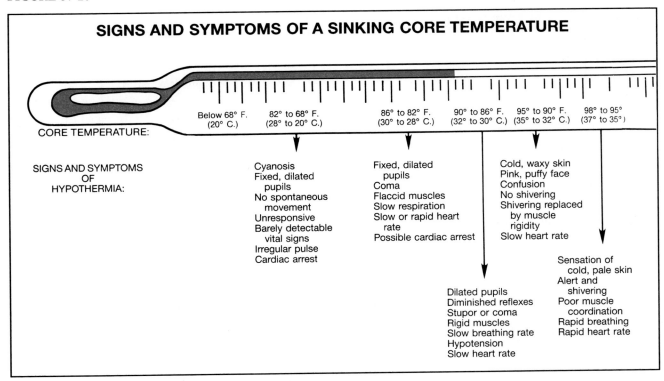

CORE TEMPERATURE:

| Below 68° F. (20° C.) | 82° to 68° F. (28° to 20° C.) | 86° to 82° F. (30° to 28° C.) | 90° to 86° F. (32° to 30° C.) | 95° to 90° F. (35° to 32° C.) | 98° to 95° (37° to 35°) |

SIGNS AND SYMPTOMS OF HYPOTHERMIA:

Cyanosis
Fixed, dilated pupils
No spontaneous movement
Unresponsive
Barely detectable vital signs
Irregular pulse
Cardiac arrest

Fixed, dilated pupils
Coma
Flaccid muscles
Slow respiration
Slow or rapid heart rate
Possible cardiac arrest

Cold, waxy skin
Pink, puffy face
Confusion
No shivering
Shivering replaced by muscle rigidity
Slow heart rate

Dilated pupils
Diminished reflexes
Stupor or coma
Rigid muscles
Slow breathing rate
Hypotension
Slow heart rate

Sensation of cold, pale skin
Alert and shivering
Poor muscle coordination
Rapid breathing
Rapid heart rate

FIGURE 37-21

pothermic patient may require as much as four hours of CPR before resuscitation is successful. Administer warmed, high-concentration oxygen. Take care not to hyperventilate the patient.

- *Before* you begin CPR, make sure that there is *no* pulse. In severe hypothermia, a patient may breathe only three or four times a minute; a heartbeat of only five to ten beats per minute is enough to sustain life in a hypothermic patient. A slow pulse is tolerable if breathing is also slow. If you cannot detect pulse or respiration, but an unconscious patient shows any movement at all, assume that there is some cardiac activity, and do not perform CPR.

3. If possible, place the patient in a warm, draft-free environment. Prevent further heat loss by insulating the patient:

   - Insulate the head as well, since as much as 70 percent of the body's heat can be lost this way.

   - Do not allow the patient's skin to be exposed to wind, cold air, or water spray.

   - If the patient can be sheltered in a warm, windless place, *gently* remove wet clothing and replace it with dry. Wrap the patient in dry blankets. The vigorous movement of removing many wet clothes, however, can cause ventricular fibrillation. If the patient cannot be sheltered or might be in danger from removal of wet clothing, do not remove them. Instead, layer dry clothing and coverings on top of the wet.

   - If dry clothing or coverings are not available, press as much water as possible out of the wet clothes and cover them with plastic sheeting to insulate.

   - If the patient is wearing a coat or jacket, have him put his arms next to his body instead of in the sleeves.

4. If a patient is *not* shivering, do not try to rewarm him or her; instead, transport immediately, keeping the head lower than the feet; perform CPR during transport if necessary. if the patient is conscious and shivering and transport will be delayed, begin rewarming. *Add heat gradually and gently*; the slower, the safer. Body temperature should not raise more than 1° F. per hour. Check every fifteen minutes to make sure that you are not rewarming too rapidly. As a general rule, keep the patient's extremities protected against the cold and frostbite, but do not warm the extremities. During rewarming, insulate the skin against direct contact with heated objects; hypothermic skin burns easily. General methods of rewarming include the following:

- Passive external rewarming, for patients with mild to moderate hypothermia, consists of simply removing the patient from the cold environment and insulating him or her against further heat loss. Wrap him in dry blankets or sleeping bags. In most cases, the body will begin to rewarm itself. Monitor the patient carefully. *Passive external rewarming is all you should do in the field if you can transport the patient within a reasonable amount of time.*

- Active external rewarming can be dangerous to the patient and should be done in the field *only* if you cannot transport immediately. *Follow local protocol.* It is essential that you monitor the patient closely, watching for cardiac complications. To rewarm, apply heat packs, hot water bottles, or an electric blanket to the patient to *add* heat. Heat packs should be applied to the groin, neck, and lateral chest and should not exceed 110° F. Protect the skin from burns. *Never* immerse the patient in a tub of hot water or in a hot shower in the field.

- Internal rewarming is generally used only in a hospital where constant monitoring is available and life-saving equipment is on hand. Basic EMTs should never attempt internal rewarming. Internal rewarming consists of using warmed oxygen, warm **enemas,** heated intravenous fluids, warm gastric lavage, and other methods.

5. Have the patient breathe 100 percent, warmed, humidified oxygen.

6. *Never* rub or manipulate the extremities; you can force cold venous blood into the heart, resulting in cardiac arrest.

7. Never give the patient tobacco, coffee, or alcohol.

8. Administer fluids to the patient only after uncontrollable shivering stops and the patient has a clear level of consciousness; he or she should be able to swallow and cough.

9. Examine the patient for other injuries, such as frostbite and fracture. Treat accordingly.

10. Try to keep the temperature of the room and/or the vehicle constant throughout treatment and transport. Continue to monitor vital signs carefully.

12. Transport as quickly as possible. Do not waste time in the field; transport is the most important factor. If there will be a long delay in transport, provide rescuer heat: wrap a rescuer with the patient in a sleeping bag or blanket. Use rescuer heat with caution and only in emergency — it can cause ventricular fibrillation.

Severe Hypothermia

Signs and Symptoms

Signs and symptoms of severe hypothermia are a little different, as is treatment. The signs and symptoms of severe hypothermia include:

- Core temperature less than 82° F. (oral temperature less than 90° F.).
- Extremely low respiration, heart rate, and blood pressure, progressing to apnea and pulselessness.
- Absence of shivering, even though the patient is extremely cold.
- Fruity, acetone odor on the breath.
- Gross errors of judgment.
- Fixed, dilated pupils.
- Deep coma.
- Death-like appearance.

Severe, life-threatening hypothermia can make a patient appear clinically dead. He or she may be in a coma, be cold to the touch, have fixed and dilated pupils, be in shock, have slow or no reflexes, breathe only once or twice per minute, be stiff (like rigor mortis), and assume a fetal position. The key in hypothermia is that *a person is not dead until he or she is warm and dead. Always* assume that the patient is still alive.

Emergency Care

Initiate the following treatment for severe hypothermia:

1. *Do not* allow any physical exertion; the patient should not move at all. Any movement can cause sudden death.
2. *Never* try to rewarm a severely hypothermic patient. Wrap him or her in blankets to insulate against heat loss, but do not apply any heat source, such as hot water bottles or electric blankets.
3. Handle the patient with great care.
4. Assess vital signs over a two-minute period. Avoid usual advanced cardiac life support, such as defibrillation, since a cold heart does not respond normally. If there is no heartbeat after two minutes, initiate CPR. *Note:* There is controversy about the use and rate of CPR for severe hypothermia; follow local protocol.
5. Use gentle mouth-to-mouth or mouth-to-nose ventilation if the patient is not breathing. Rapid mouth-to-mouth or forceful bag/mask breathing can trigger ventricular fibrillation.
6. If you are less than fifteen to thirty minutes from a medical facility, do not take time to treat in the field; treat during transport.
7. Do not administer drugs: drugs do not metabolize normally in a cold body.
8. Transport as quickly as possible. Maintain the ambulance at an optimal temperature, continually monitor vital signs, and handle the patient with extreme caution.

Hypothermia in the Elderly

The elderly probably account for nearly half of all victims of hypothermia. The likeliest patients are the very old, the poor who are unable to afford adequate housing or heating, and those whose bodies do not respond normally to cold. The greatest risk is to the aged whose temperature regulation is defective; they may not shiver, and therefore cannot conserve body heat when they need it the most. The elderly are also more likely to be taking medication, and they typically already have a lower core temperature. They cannot feel temperature changes as easily, often have chronic illness, and are usually on a fixed income. They tend to have less body fat and an inadequate diet and lead a sedentary lifestyle.

Signs and symptoms of hypothermia in the elderly include:

- Facial bloating; skin color pale and waxy, at other times oddly pink.
- Absence of shivering, but skin feels cold to the touch.
- Irregular, slow heartbeat; slurred speech; shallow, very slow breathing that may be barely discernible.
- Low blood pressure.
- Drowsiness, perhaps lapsing into coma. The lower the body temperature, the more likely the patient will be unconscious.

Always consider the possibility of hypothermia in an unconscious elderly patient. In addition to other treatment guidelines already mentioned, *never* use a hot bath with an elderly patient.

Immersion Hypothermia

Immersion hypothermia — a lowering of the body temperature that occurs as a result of immersion in cold water — should be considered in all cases of accidental immersion. Immersion in cold water can cause breathing abnormalities and muscle dysfunction.

Body temperature drops to equal the water temperature within ten minutes; body temperature drops twenty-five to thirty times faster in water than in air of the same temperature. When the water is 50° F. or lower, death can occur within a few minutes. Therefore, emergency care is vital and consists of getting the patient out of the water immediately. Most deaths in cold water (75° F. or less) are due to rapid loss of body heat, leading to unconsciousness and, in some cases, drowning and heart failure. Hypothermia in this instance is likely to become fatal when body temperature drops to 94° F. (See Figure 37-22.)

The shock of sudden immersion in cold water can cause **immersion syndrome,** resulting in immediate ventricular fibrillation. The body preserves the core temperature for the first fifteen to twenty minutes, even though there are signs of hypothermia; after that, the core temperature drops rapidly. Immersion hypothermia can creep up unnoticed on divers and swimmers as body temperature drops. Extra fat layers tend to insulate individuals from cooling. Pound per pound, adult women have greater heat loss resistance in cold water than men. Similarly, adults last longer than children, and girls have more resistance than boys. Insulating layers of clothing are important, too, so *never* remove clothing from a person in the water.

Victims who have been in the water for some time should be lifted in a horizontal position because of the likelihood of vascular collapse. Do not allow the patient any rapid activity in the water; turbulence and activity decrease survival time by 75 percent. Instruct the patient to make as little effort as possible to keep afloat until you can reach him or her.

Once the patient is out of the water, follow these guidelines:

1. Keep the patient still and quiet. The coldest blood is in the extremities; if the patient walks, moves, or struggles, the coldest blood will circulate rapidly to the heart, dropping core temperature by as much as 6° F. If the patient must be moved, use a stretcher. Determine if near-drowning has occurred.

2. Remove the patient's wet clothing carefully and gently if he or she can be sheltered in a warm place out of the wind. Do not let the patient struggle to help you.

3. Handle the patient very gently; never rub or massage him or her. Rough handling or abrupt movement can cause ventricular fibrillation.

4. Protect the patient from cold air or water spray. Dress in dry clothing, the arms next to the body instead of in sleeves. If no dry clothing is available, use any insulation material — even dry newspapers. Cover the insulation with a waterproof material, such as plastic sheeting. Insulate the patient from the ground up.

5. Protect the patient from the wind. If no shelter is available, position rescuers' bodies around him to keep him or her sheltered. If the patient is to be transported by helicopter, shelter him or her from the rotor wash.

6. Never give hot liquids by mouth, and never give alcoholic beverages.

7. Follow rewarming techniques described under general hypothermia.

8. Transport immediately.

If a patient in the water cannot be rescued immediately, instruct him or her verbally to limit exertion as

FIGURE 37-22 Survival in cold water.

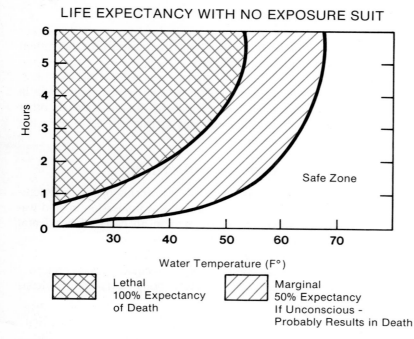

LIFE EXPECTANCY WITH NO EXPOSURE SUIT

Hours / Water Temperature (F°)

Safe Zone

Lethal
100% Expectancy
of Death

Marginal
50% Expectancy
If Unconscious -
Probably Results in Death

much as possible. The patient should keep his or her head and face out of the water, cross his or her legs under water to decrease heat loss, and do as little as necessary to stay afloat. If there are several in the water, have them form a tight circle with their chests together to maintain heat.

Frostbite (Local Cooling)

Frostbite, the literal freezing of body tissue, often accompanies hypothermia. In those cases, care of the hypothermia always takes precedence. Frostbite — which most commonly affects the hands, feet, ears, nose, and cheeks — occurs when ice crystals form between the cells of the skin, and then grow by extracting fluid from the cells. Circulation is obstructed, causing additional damage to the tissue affected.

Factors that increase the likelihood of frostbite include:

- Any kind of trauma; always check for frostbite in trauma victims who are injured in cold weather.
- Age: the elderly and the newborn are most susceptible.
- Tight or tightly laced footwear.
- Use of alcohol during exposure to cold (alcohol acts as a vasodilator and lowers the ability to conserve heat.)
- Wet clothing.
- High altitudes.
- Loss of blood.
- Race: blacks are three to six times more likely to get frostbite.

Stages of Frostbite

There are three general stages of frostbite (Figure 37-23).

INCIPIENT Sometimes called "frost nip," incipient frostbite usually only involves the tips of the ears, the nose, the cheeks (over the cheekbones), the tips of the toes or fingers, and the chin. The patient is usually unaware that he or she has frost nip and will not realize it until someone mentions that his or her skin looks blanched or white. Incipient frostbite comes on slowly and is painless while developing; at first the skin is reddened; then it becomes white. Incipient frostbite develops after direct contact with a cold object, cold air, or cold water. Nipped fingers can be rewarmed by holding them in the armpits or on someone's abdomen. The skin should *not* be rubbed. The area will tingle slightly as it thaws and as circulation improves.

SUPERFICIAL Superficial frostbite involves the skin and the tissue just beneath the skin. While the skin itself is firm, white, and waxy in appearance, the tissue beneath it is usually soft. While you may palpate gently, never "poke" or probe excessively to determine the softness of underlying tissue, and never rub the skin. As the area thaws, it may become purple or mottled blue and may tingle and burn after initially becoming numb. The area usually swells during thawing, and there may be blisters filled with clear or straw-colored fluid (see Figure 37-24).

DEEP In deep frostbite, the tissue beneath the skin is solid to the touch; it may involve the entire hand or foot. The skin is mottled or blotchy and ranges in color from white to grayish-blue. Deep frostbite is an extreme emergency and can result in permanent tissue loss (Figure 37-25).

Assessing Frostbite

Frostbite is difficult to assess. While still frozen, even severely frostbitten tissue may appear almost normal; it is usually pale and firm to the touch, with a gray or waxy white color. Some purplish tinge and sensitivity may be present. The tissue may be completely numb, but it is usually very painful, burning, and stinging before it becomes frozen. After freezing it is numb, and as it thaws, there is a feeling of burning and throbbing.

It is difficult to assess the actual extent of damage from looking at frostbite, particularly if the tissue has not thawed. Find out how long the patient was exposed, estimate the temperature and wind velocity at the time of exposure if you can, and find out the kind of clothing that was protecting the tissue. Also determine the preinjury condition of the patient.

During thawing, the skin turns pink, then purplish blue or violet, becomes extremely painful, and develops large blisters. Within seven to ten days, black scabs form where blisters were present; the scabs can limit mobility, and require surgical repair. Gangrene may result. The possibility of permanent damage depends on the temperature and the duration of freezing; amputation may be required. Frostbite is always worse if the patient's skin is wet or if it is exposed to cold metal and then torn when separated from the metal.

Emergency Care

The key to emergency care for frostbite is to *never* thaw the tissue if there is any possibility of refreezing. General guidelines for care include the following (*follow local protocol*):

1. Remove the patient immediately, if possible, from the cold environment.
2. If the tissue is still frozen, keep it frozen until you can initiate care. *Never* initiate thawing procedures if there is any danger of refreezing — keeping the tissue frozen is less dangerous than submitting it to refreezing.

STAGES OF FROSTBITE

1. INCIPIENT (Frost Nip)
Affects tips of ears, nose, cheeks, fingers, toes, chin - skin blanched white, painless

FROSTBITE is localized cooling of the body.
- 70% of the body is composed of water.
- When the body is subjected to excessive cold, the water in the cells can freeze; resulting ice crystals may even destroy the cell.
- Never rub the skin of a patient with frostbite; rubbing can result in permanent tissue damage.

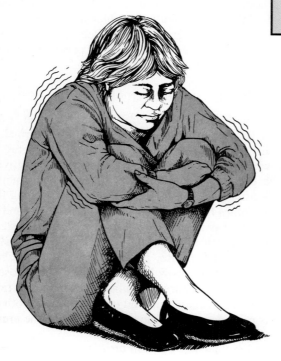

2. SUPERFICIAL
Affects skin and tissue just beneath skin; skin is firm and waxy, tissue beneath is soft, numb, then turns purple during thawing.

3. DEEP
Affects entire tissue depth; tissue beneath skin is solid, waxy white with purplish tinge.

1. Emergency care for Incipient Frostbite:
The skin can be warmed by applying firm pressure with a hand (no rubbing) or other warm body part, by blowing warm breath on the spot or by submerging in warm water.

2. Emergency care for Superficial Frostbite:
Treatment includes providing dry coverage and steady warmth. Submerging in warm water is also helpful.

3. Emergency care for Deep Frostbite:
This patient needs immediate hospital care. Dry clothing over the frostbite will help prevent further injury. Submerging in warm water can help thaw. Rewarm by immersion in water heated to 100°-110° F, administer oxygen and maintain body core temperature. The frostbitten part should not be rubbed or chaffed in any way. The part should not be thawed if the patient must walk on it to get to the medical facility. Do not delay transport for rewarming. *Follow local protocol.*

FIGURE 37-23

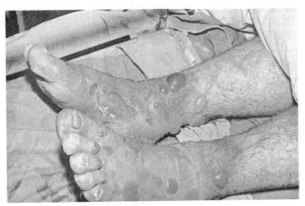

FIGURE 37-24 Superficial frostbite.

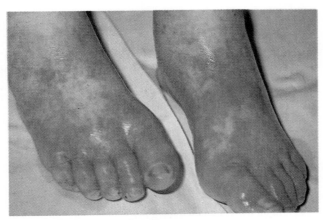

FIGURE 37-25 Deep frostbite.

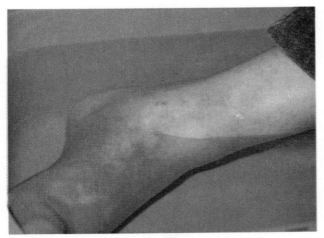

FIGURE 37-26 Thaw the frostbitten part rapidly in water just above body temperature (100°–110° F.).

3. Protect the injured area from friction or pressure. Remove any constricting clothing or jewelry. If clothing is frozen to the skin, leave it; remove it after thawing.

4. It is a mistake to thaw frostbitten tissue gradually; thaw the tissue *rapidly* in water just above body temperature (approximately 38°–44°C. or 100°–110° F.) (Figure 37-26). Check the water temperature with a thermometer and keep the water warm by adding warm water; never heat the cooled water with any type of flame or electric unit. The heat must be evenly distributed and kept constant. *Never use dry heat* — it is too difficult to control the temperature. Slow rewarming leads to tissue loss, and water that is too hot may add burn injury to the frostbite. *Follow local protocol.*

5. Rewarming is extremely painful; the patient may want to take analgesics (aspirin or nonaspirin products) to help relieve pain during rewarming. *Follow local protocol.*

6. Keep rewarming until the color no longer improves. The affected area should turn deep red or bluish, and the skin should be soft and pliable. *Never* attempt to rewarm the area by rubbing or massaging, and never rub a frostbitten area with snow or alcohol. Do not delay transportation for rewarming. *Follow local protocol.*

7. Once the skin is thawed, any solution that comes in contact with it must be sterile. Cover thawed parts with loosely applied dry, sterile dressings. Elevate the affected extremities.

8. Transport the patient as quickly as possible, preferably while continuing the rewarming process. *All* victims of frostbite require hospitalization.

9. During transport, monitor vital signs, keep the patient warm, and elevate affected parts. Protect affected tissue from further injury or irritation. Cover the affected part with a blanket for warmth, but do not allow direct contact with the injured tissue. Place sterile cotton or gauze between affected toes and fingers; do not break blisters or treat them with salve, ointment, or bandages.

10. If feet are involved, do not allow the patient to walk.

chapter 38

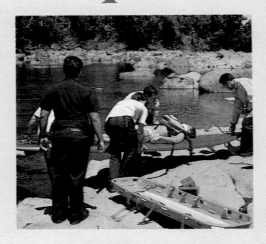

Water Emergencies

✳ OBJECTIVES

- Explain how drowning and near-drowning occur and identify the mechanism of injury that occurs with different types of drowning.
- Describe appropriate emergency care for near-drowning victims.
- Describe proper handling and stabilization techniques for water emergencies.
- Recognize the common types of diving emergencies.
- Describe appropriate emergency care for the common types of diving emergencies.

Nearly 9,000 people die each year in the United States from water accidents. While drownings are most commonly associated with water emergencies, drownings are actually responsible for only about one in twenty water-related deaths. The rest are mostly caused by diving and deep-water exploration, boating, and water skiing. Water-related deaths may also result from motor vehicle accidents. In addition to drowning and near-drowning, water-related accidents can cause bleeding, soft-tissue injuries, and fractures.

Drownings and near-drownings don't always occur in large bodies of water: an adult can drown in a just a few inches of water, and an infant in even less. Recent studies indicate that one-fourth of all infants who drown do so in five-gallon buckets; others drown in bathtubs and toilets.

The statistics regarding water emergencies are especially tragic, because a number of the deaths could be prevented with prompt and proper care (see Figure 38-1). Certain deep-water accidents require specialized equipment to correct medical complications, but many victims of water-related emergencies can be saved by some of the simple essentials of basic life support, such as removing them from the water and suctioning their airway.

Unless a water emergency occurs in open, shallow water that has a stable, uniform bottom, *never go out into the water unless you 1) are a good swimmer, 2) are specially trained, 3) are wearing a personal flotation device, and 4) are accompanied by other rescuers.* Failure to follow these guidelines can result in becoming a victim yourself.

☐ DROWNING AND NEAR-DROWNING

Drowning is defined as death from suffocation due to submersion; **near-drowning** is survival, at least temporarily (twenty-four hours), from near-suffocation due to submersion. Drowning is the third leading cause of accidental deaths in the United States. Among adults,

FIGURE 38-1

PREVENTING NEAR-DROWNING ACCIDENTS

Three caveats apply to the vast majority of drowning and near-drowning incidents (see table).
- *Children should be under constant supervision if a lake, pool, or pail of water of any size is nearby.*
- *Water sports and alcoholic beverages never mix.*
- *Life preservers or life jackets should always be worn when boating.*

Where people drown

Type of water or site	Drownings (%)	
Salt water	1-2	
Fresh water	98-99	
Swimming pools		
Private		50
Public		3
Lakes, rivers, streams, storm drains		20
Bathtubs		15
Buckets of water		4
Fish ponds or tanks		4
Toilets		4
Washing machines		1

Adapted with permission from Orlowski JP: Drowning, near-drowning, and ice-water submersions. *Pediatr Clin North Am* 1987;34(1):77.

These and other standard water safety precautions for swimming, diving, and boating should be made clear and repeated frequently.

Effective prevention in children requires constant supervision and common sense. A young child can find and fall into water in just a minute or two — less time than anyone would realize he or she is gone unless attention is continuous — and fences are not always effective in keeping children out of places where they should not go. A fence may appear to enclose a pool completely, but the gate may not be self-closing or the lock may be broken. The vast majority of children who drown in swimming pools do so in the backyards of their own homes, usually in the later afternoon on summer weekends. And isn't it sensible to require that baby sitters know CPR?

Programs that claim to "drown-proof" or teach young children to swim are controversial, and many experts feel they provide a false sense of security. The American Academy of Pediatrics does not recommend teaching children younger than 3 years of age to swim, although some regional programs take children as young as 6 months. Drown-proofing programs fail — studies indicate that a significant number of children have submersion accidents despite their training — because the sequential patterning approach used to teach the very young child in a structured environment engenders, in effect, learned helplessness. The cues a child learns in the class or pool setting are missing in the real-life crisis.

A large number of adult drowning victims have detectable levels of blood alcohol. Swimmers should be warned about diving in shallow or unexplored water. Boating precautions should be heeded by all boaters. Seizure disorders are an important but easily overlooked risk factor in persons of all ages.

alcohol intoxication is a factor in approximately 45 percent of all drownings. Five times as many males drown as females; male drowning mortality peaks at fifteen to nineteen years of age, with the highest female mortality appearing at the preschool ages of one to four. In addition, approximately 80,000 near-drowning incidents occur each year in the United States.

The poorest prognosis for drowning victims is among the older, those who struggle in the water, those who suffer associated injuries, those who have prolonged submersion time, and those who are in warm, dirty, or brackish water. Panic on the part of a swimmer can often contribute to a drowning death (Figure 38-2).

The major causes of drowning are:

- Becoming exhausted while swimming, skin diving, or attempting a rescue.
- Losing control and getting swept into water that is too deep.
- Losing a support (sinking or capsizing of a boat).
- Getting trapped or entangled while in the water.
- Using drugs or alcohol prior to entering the water.
- Suffering seizures while in the water.
- Using poor judgment while in the water.

- Suffering hypothermia.
- Suffering trauma.
- Suffering a diving accident.

"Wet" Versus "Dry" Drowning

"Wet" drowning occurs when fluid is aspirated into the lungs; "dry" drowning occurs when severe laryngospasm cuts off respiration but does not allow aspiration of a significant amount of fluid into the lungs. Approximately 10 to 40 percent of all drownings are estimated to be "dry" — and autopsies reveal that only about 15 percent of all drowning victims aspirate a significant amount of water (Figure 38-3).

Warm-Water Versus Cold-Water Drowning

There is a significant difference between warm-water and cold-water drownings. The concept of developing brain death after four to six minutes without oxygen is not applicable in cases of near-drowning in cold water. Some patients in cold water (below 68° F.) can be resuscitated after thirty minutes or more in cardiac arrest. However, persons under water sixty minutes or longer usually cannot be resuscitated. A possible contribution

FIGURE 38-2 The effect of panic in water accidents, where panic can often contribute to the death of the person who loses self-control.

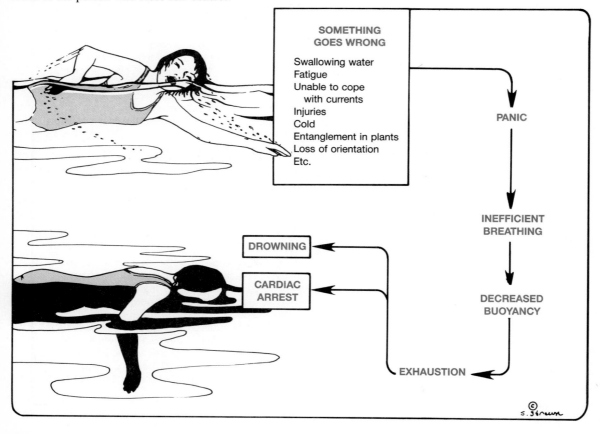

DROWNING

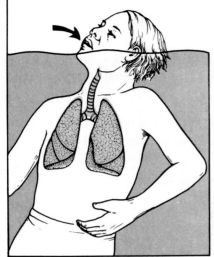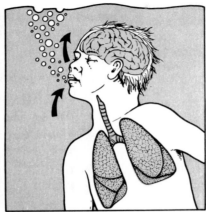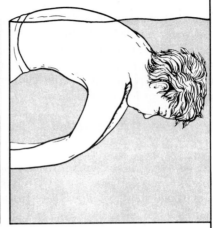

Drowning is a major source of accidental death and can be a result of cold, fatigue, injury, disorientation, intoxication, etc., or of the victim's own limited swimming ability.

The drowning victim struggles to inhale air as long as possible, but eventually he goes beneath the water where he must exhale air and inhale water.

Loss of consciousness, convulsions, cardiac arrest and death follow.

In about 10% of all drownings, a muscle spasm of the larynx closes the victim's airway, causing him to die of asphyxiation without ever inhaling water.

FIGURE 38-3

to survival may be the **mammalian diving reflex.** When a person dives into cold water, he or she reacts to the submersion of the face. Breathing is inhibited, the heart rate decreases, and vasoconstriction develops in tissues relatively resistant to asphyxia, while cerebral and cardiac blood flow is maintained. In this way, oxygen is sent and used only where it is needed to immediately sustain life. The colder the water, the more oxygen is diverted to the heart and brain.

The diving reflex can also be precipitated by fear. The diving reflex is more pronounced, and cooling is more rapid, in the young. However, in water at or below 68° F., the body's metabolic requirements are only about half of normal.

Reaching the Victim

You need to reach the victim, but you must do it with due concern for your own safety. As mentioned earlier, *never go in the water unless you can swim, have been trained in water-rescue techniques, are wearing a per-*

sonal flotation device, and are accompanied by other rescuers.

If the victim is conscious and is close to shore, hold out an object for the victim to grab. The best thing to use is a rope; you can also use an oar, branch, fishing pole, towel, shirt, or other strong object that will not break. Before you hold out the object for the swimmer to grab, make sure you have solid, firm footing and will not slip into the water yourself. Once the swimmer has grabbed the object, pull him or her to shore.

If the victim is conscious but too far away from shore to reach, toss out a line. Tie a rope to an object that floats, toss the object to the swimmer, and pull on the rope to tow the swimmer in. You can use anything that will float and is heavy enough to throw: an automobile tire, inflatable ball or toy, log, thermos jug, picnic cooler, or capped empty milk jugs. Again, be sure of your own footing and stability before attempting to tow in a swimmer.

If the victim is unconscious or too far from you to reach with a line, you will need to go to him or her *if you have been trained in water-rescue techniques, are a good swimmer, and are wearing a personal flotation device.* If at all possible, go to the victim in a boat.

Always provide resuscitative care to a drowning victim, even if he or she has been in the water for a prolonged period — especially if the water is cold. All mammals, including humans, have a "mammalian diving reflex" that slows body systems and preserves life when cold water hits the face. Infants and children survive even longer than adults, and the colder the water, the better the chances for survival. Some victims have been successfully resuscitated after being submerged (and not breathing) for as long as an hour.

Treating Patients without Neck or Spinal Injury

Always assume that an unconscious victim has sustained neck or spinal injury. If you are relatively sure there is no neck or spinal injury, follow these treatment guidelines:

1. Remove the patient from the water. If you do not suspect neck or spinal injuries, remove the patient from the water as quickly as you can and by any method that is safely possible.

2. *As rapidly as you can,* establish an airway and initiate ventilations; if necessary, begin ventilations while the patient is still in the water. Use mouth-to-mouth or mouth-to-nose ventilations. You might encounter more resistance to ventilations than you expect because of water in the airway. Once you have determined that there are no foreign objects in the airway, apply ventilations with more force; adjust ventilations until you see the patient's chest rise and fall but not until you see gastric distention. *Do not attempt to remove water from the patient's lungs or stomach.*

3. If there is no pulse, begin CPR. If you can feel the carotid pulse within sixty seconds, do not begin CPR.

4. Administer high-flow supplemental oxygen; suction as needed.

5. Once the patient is breathing and has a pulse, assess for hemorrhage; control any serious bleeding that you find.

6. Cover the patient to conserve body heat. If the patient can be moved, take him to a warm place; do not allow the patient to walk.

7. Handle the patient very gently.

8. Transport the patient as quickly as possible, continuing resuscitative measures during transport. *Always transport a near-drowning victim,* even if you think the danger has passed. A near-drowning victim can develop secondary complications (such

as pulmonary edema) and die up to seventy-two hours after the incident. (Approximately 15 percent of all drowning deaths are due to secondary complications.)

Treating Head- and Spinal-Injured Patients

In general, there are four basic rules you should follow if you are *not specially trained* in water rescue (see Figure 38-4):

1. Do not remove the injured person from the water.

2. Keep the injured person afloat on his or her back.

3. Wait for help.

4. Always support the head and neck level with the back.

5. Maintain the airway and support ventilation in the water.

If an unconscious person is found in shallow, warm water, don't try to remove the victim. If he or she is breathing, keep the victim in a face-up position, supporting the back and stabilizing the head and neck.

If the water is unsafe (too deep, too cold, or containing tides or currents) or if the patient needs CPR, you will need to remove him or her from the water to prevent further injury.

It is important that you properly stabilize the patient in the water and remove the patient carefully. The American National Red Cross suggests that the patient not be removed from the water until a backboard or other rigid support can be used as a splint. Many water accident victims may be found floating face-down and must be rolled onto their backs. To turn a patient, see Figure 38-4.

Once the patient is out of the water, begin serious attempts at resuscitation. If necessary, begin CPR; use the jaw-thrust technique to avoid further injury to the neck or spine.

Continue treatment as for a non-spine-injured patient; maintain immobilization of the neck and spine throughout treatment and transport.

☐ DIVING EMERGENCIES

Diving emergencies can result either from diving board accidents or scuba diving accidents.

Diving board accidents aren't limited to those who dive into water from a diving board — they can also occur among those who dive from a shore, poolside, boat, or dock. The most common injuries that result are to the head and neck; fractures of the extremities and ribs are also common.

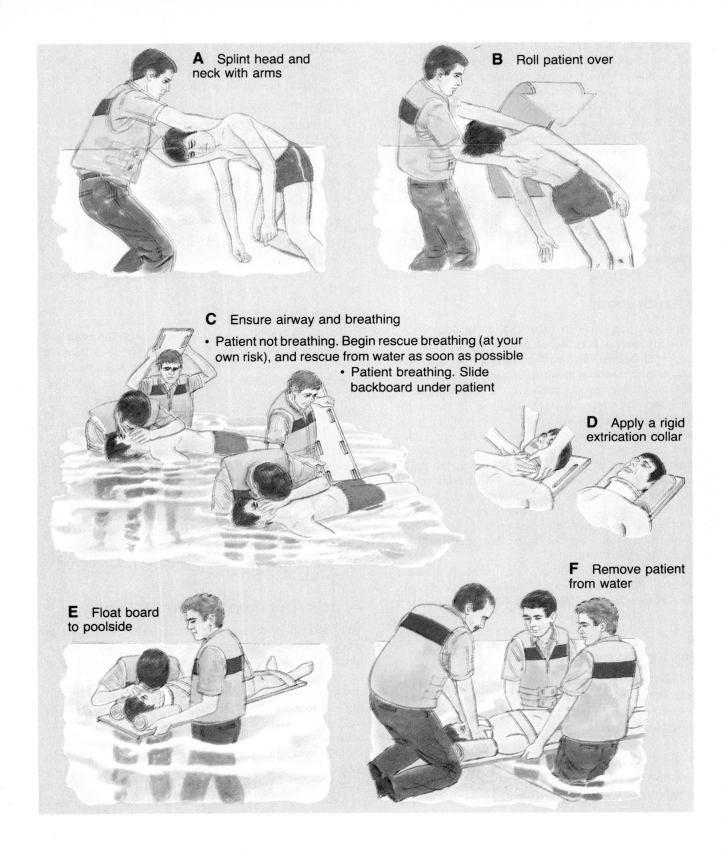

A Splint head and neck with arms

B Roll patient over

C Ensure airway and breathing

• Patient not breathing. Begin rescue breathing (at your own risk), and rescue from water as soon as possible

• Patient breathing. Slide backboard under patient

D Apply a rigid extrication collar

E Float board to poolside

F Remove patient from water

FIGURE 38-4 Water rescue — possible spinal injury.

In treating a diving board accident victim, always assess for medical problems that may have caused the diving accident. *Always assume that the diver has sustained neck and spinal injuries,* even if still conscious. If the victim is still in the water, treat as for swimming accidents. If the victim has left the water. assess and treat as for any other injury.

A major complication of scuba or deep-water diving emergencies is coma, which may result from asphyxiation, head injury, heart attack, air tank contamination, intoxication, aspiration, decompression sickness, and embolism. In addition to the necessity for resuscitation, two ascent problems — air embolism and decompression sickness — require recompression. A third, **barotrauma,** may require special medical facility treatment.

Air Embolism

Air embolism can occur in either shallow or deep water, and usually occurs because of breath-holding during a dive. Air embolism (also called arterial gas embolism) can occur whenever the pressure exerted on the body by its environment is rapidly reduced: the air in the lungs expands rapidly, rupturing the alveoli and damaging the adjacent blood vessels. As a result, air bubbles travel through the heart and are dumped into the aorta. Air bubbles then leave the injured lung and enter the bloodstream. They can be circulated anywhere in the body, but most often go through the carotid arteries to the brain. The blood vessels that contain the air bubbles then become unable to perfuse the tissue with oxygen and nutrients. Obviously, the most critical places for an air embolism to lodge are the heart, the brain, the brain stem, or the spinal cord.

When assessing a diver who manifests unusual symptoms, don't automatically assume air embolism without considering the possibility of head injury or a stroke.

Signs and Symptoms

The signs and symptoms of air embolism have rapid onset; the victim may appear to be drunk. Signs and symptoms of air embolism include the following, which occur within fifteen minutes of surfacing:

- Blotching or itching of the skin.
- Frothy blood in the nose and mouth.
- Pain in the muscles, joints, and tendons, or pain in the chest or abdomen.
- Numbness or tingling in the extremities.
- Difficulty breathing (due to chest injury).
- Dizziness and possible convulsions.
- Vomiting.

- Blurred or distorted vision.
- Possible coma.
- General weakness or paralysis.
- Distorted senses.
- Swelling and crepitus in the neck.
- Loss or distortion of memory.
- Slurred speech, lack of coordination.
- Cardiac arrest.
- Respiratory arrest.
- Behavioral changes — sometimes the only sign.

Emergency Care

To care for a patient with air embolism, act rapidly as follows:

1. If there is no sign of neck or spinal injury, position the patient on the left side, with the head and chest lower than his feet (see Figure 38-5). Such a position may help force any air bubbles (air emboli) to remain in the lower abdomen and legs, preventing them from reaching the lungs, heart, or brain.

2. Administer oxygen, preferably 100 percent.

3. If the patient requires CPR, place the patient flat on the back with the head and chest lower than the feet, and initiate CPR.

4. Once the patient has been stabilized, transport immediately, keeping the head and chest lower than the feet during transport. Continue administering oxygen during transport. *The patient must have recompression treatment immediately,* so transport is vital.

Bends (Decompression Sickness)

The "bends," or decompression sickness, usually occurs when a diver comes up too quickly from a deep, prolonged dive. It can also occur among sports enthusiasts or those in the military, industry, or space travel — anyone who is exposed to increasing pressure while breathing compressed air. Decompression sickness can be mild ("pain-only" sickness) or severe (involving the central nervous system).

More common than air embolism, decompression sickness — often called the **bends** — occurs when gases (usually nitrogen) breathed by the diver are absorbed into the bloodstream. Over a period of time, a high concentration of nitrogen is absorbed; when the diver ascends, the nitrogen becomes transformed into tiny bubbles, which lodge in tissues of all types and locations. Bubbles get bigger, causing pain and interference with circulation. Gas bubbles eventually enter the bloodstream; the worst injuries result when bubbles lodge in

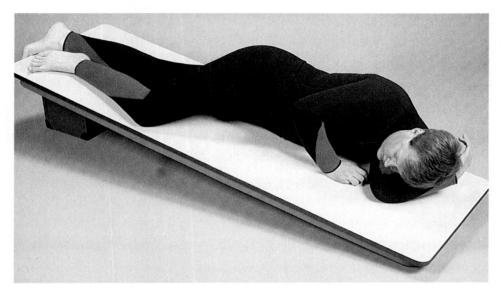

FIGURE 38-5 Positioning the patient after a scuba diving accident.

the brain, lungs, heart, or spinal cord. The most dire injury associated with decompression sickness is a burst lung.

The risk of decompression sickness is increased if the diver flies within twelve hours of the dive.

Signs and Symptoms

The signs and symptoms of decompression sickness are gradual in onset, usually occurring twelve to twenty-four hours (but as long as forty-eight hours) after the dive. Because of the gradual onset of symptoms, the diver may not associate them with the dive.

The most common signs and symptoms include the following:

- Minor skin rash with itchy and mottled skin; the rash often continues to change appearance.
- Pitting edema.
- Migraine-like headache.
- Difficulty breathing.
- Fatigue.
- Dizziness.
- Choking or coughing.
- Chest pain.
- Severe central nervous system complaints.
- Blurred vision.
- Tinnitus or partial deafness.
- Nausea and vomiting accompanied by colicky-like abdominal pain.
- Severe, deep, aching pain in the joints and muscles (the "bends").
- Numbness or paralysis.

- Inability to void the bladder.
- Staggering gait.
- Collapse, sometimes leading to unconsciousness.
- Hallucinations.

Emergency Care

To treat a patient with decompression sickness:

1. Provide basic life support; administer 100 percent oxygen by mask, and initiate CPR if needed
2. If the patient is fully conscious, give fluids by mouth.
3. If there is no sign of neck or spinal injury, position the patient on the left side with the head down; slant the entire body 15 degrees. This prevents gas bubbles from injuring the brain.
4. Transport immediately to a facility with a recompression chamber; recompression treatment must be performed rapidly.

Barotrauma

Sometimes called "the squeeze," barotrauma can involve any part of the body that is filled with air. When divers descend or ascend, air pressure must be equalized to maintain proper pressure in the body's air cavities, such as the sinuses and the middle ear. If proper pressure is not maintained, barotrauma — injury to the tissues of the air cavities — results, leading to ruptured sinuses and eardrum. If there is an air pocket in a tooth (due to decay or a defective filling), the tooth may rupture.

Divers are at increased risk of barotrauma if they have an upper respiratory infection of allergy.

Signs and Symptoms

Signs and symptoms of barotrauma include the following:

- Mild to severe pain in the affected area.
- A bloody or fluid discharge from the nose or ears.
- Extreme dizziness.
- Nausea.
- Disorientation.
- Hemorrhage from the tiny blood vessels in the eyes.
- Tinnitus and possible deafness

Emergency Care

Barotrauma should be cared for immediately at a medical facility to prevent permanent blindness, deafness, residual dizziness, or inability to dive in the future.

1. Suction the airway and administer oxygen if needed.
2. Transport the patient immediately on the left side with the upper torso lowered.
3. Keep the patient calm and quiet during transport to lessen the chance of further injury.

chapter 39

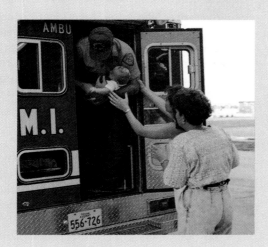

Psychological Emergencies and Special Communication Needs

✳ OBJECTIVES

- ■ Explain the principles of psychological emergency care.
- ■ Recognize common emotional responses to physical illness and injury of patients, family, friends, and bystanders.
- ■ Describe and demonstrate assessment and management of a psychological emergency.
- ■ Recognize common physical disorders that may resemble a psychological emergency.
- ■ Identify the special communication needs of geriatric, pediatric, deaf, blind, non-English-speaking, and confused and/or developmentally disabled patients.
- ■ Recognize the common signs and symptoms of burnout and describe recommended prevention techniques.
- ■ Describe the role of the critical incident stress debriefing and describe its stages.

It is recommended that EMTs wear protective gloves whenever there is a possibility of coming in contact with a patient's blood, body fluids, mucous membranes, traumatic wounds, or sores. See Chapter 31.

Effective emergency care requires not only an understanding of the nature and care of psychological emergencies, but also of the normal emotional responses to illness and injury experienced by your patients. Everyone involved in a critical illness or injury — the patient, the family, bystanders, and even health professionals — responds to stresses that occur naturally in such emergencies. You can deal effectively with these responses, both in others and in yourself, only if you understand and anticipate the reactions.

□ PRINCIPLES OF PSYCHOLOGICAL EMERGENCY CARE

Physical emergency care is tangible — it is bandaging wounds, splinting bones, or restoring breathing. You can physically perform emergency care, and you can immediately see the results of your efforts.

Psychological emergency care is different. You cannot readily see the comfort that you provide to a husband who loses his wife in a fire. It is hard to immediately gauge the results of caring for a child who is depressed because a flood destroyed his home. Remember, too, that you may offer assistance to your patient, but it may not necessarily be accepted. In most psychological emergencies a patient has to *want* to be helped. Even the most skilled rescuer cannot make a difference when a patient does not want to help himself or to receive help from others.

It is important that you understand the following basic principles for psychological emergency care:

- Every person has limitations. In psychological crises, every person there — including yourself — is susceptible to emotional injury. Each person has a different **threshold.** You may be able to cope with more than someone else, but each person has limitations.

- Each person has a right to his or her feelings. Each person reacts individually to the environment and to the way in which the environment acts on him or her. Each person has a *right* to feel the way that he or she does. A person who is emotionally or mentally disturbed does not want to feel that way, but at that particular time, those feelings are valid and real. Those suffering an emotional crisis simply need help to pull themselves together. Psychological care means that you are accepting and helpful, not critical or judgmental.

- Each person has more ability to cope with crisis

than he or she might think. A person who is under severe emotional stress will probably manifest actions that lead you to believe he or she has lost total control. For every manifestation of crazed emotion, some strength is probably left within.

- Everyone feels some emotional disturbance when involved in a disaster or when injured. However, you do not know what a particular physical injury may mean to a given individual. A relatively minor hand injury may seem of little consequence to you, but it could ruin the career of a concert violinist. Often, a person becomes anxious and afraid about the future effects of the injury, not the immediate pain and inconvenience.

- Emotional injury is just as real as physical injury. Unfortunately, physical injury is often visual, so people accept it more readily as being real. You would not expect a person to walk one month after having a leg amputated in an industrial accident; yet too many times, the patient suffering emotional trauma is expected to act normally immediately.

- Remember that people who have been through a crisis don't just "get better." They will probably suffer from their pain and loss for a long time, sometimes for months or even years. Don't expect automatic results; the patient probably won't realize the extent of the event until long after you leave. You are the first on the scene, and your role is not to heal, but to be a positive beginning to a long, difficult healing process.

- Remember that you will encounter people of all races and cultural backgrounds. You will be called on to give help to people whose religion, language, skin color, customs, and economic level vary from yours. Your patient might have strong cultural or personal views that medical treatment is a private matter, and he or she might be unnerved at the prospect of being treated for angina in front of dinner guests. You know that you must attempt resuscitation in every case, but you need to respect the heartache of a weathered farmer who wants to let his wife die peacefully — and you need to consider him as well while you work perhaps in a different way to help his wife. Every patient needs to be given considerate care, whether a battered child, a police officer with a bullet in the chest, or an inebriated, unbathed person in a gutter. Cultural differences have special meaning when you are called to intervene in psychological emergencies. Come to terms with your own feelings as you approach a situation, and take the time to understand where your patient is coming from.

☐ EMOTIONAL RESPONSES OF PATIENTS TO ILLNESS AND INJURY

Although patient's reactions to critical illness or injury are largely determined by mechanisms that they have already developed, most of these reactions follow common patterns. Patients usually become aware of painful or unpleasant sensations, and sometimes of decreased energy and strength, when they become ill. The common response to this awareness is anxiety.

Feelings of loss of control are common among ill or injured patients. They may feel helpless in knowing that they are completely dependent on someone else, often a stranger, whose experience in medical care and whose ability they cannot easily evaluate. Patients whose self-esteem depends on their being active, independent, and aggressive are particularly prone to anxiety in these situations.

Patients often respond to discomfort or limitation of activity by becoming resentful and suspicious. They may vent this anger on you by becoming impatient, irritable, or excessively demanding. Remember that the patient's anger stems from fear and discomfort, not from anything you have done. Once patients begin to see themselves as ill or injured, the signs and symptoms depicted in Figure 39-1 may occur.

In addition, patients usually have uncomfortable feelings about being examined by a stranger; some may

FIGURE 39-1

SIGNS AND SYMPTOMS OF PSYCHOLOGICAL EMERGENCIES

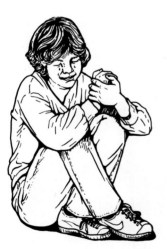

FEAR
May be afraid of a person or persons, activity or place.

ANXIETY
Not related to any specific person, place or situation.

CONFUSION
May be preoccupied with fears or imaginary attacks.

BEHAVIORAL DEVIANCE
Radical changes in lifestyle, values, relationships, etc.

ANGER
Inappropriate anger directed at an inappropriate source usually brief but destructive.

MANIA
Unrealistically optimistic — unwarranted risks and poor judgement.

DEPRESSION
May range from crying to inability to function to threatened suicide. Often has feelings of hopelessness, helplessness, unworthiness, and guilt.

WITHDRAWAL
Loses interest in people or things that were previously considered important.

LOSS OF CONTACT WITH REALITY
Has trouble distinguishing or identifying smells, sounds, and sights in the real world from those in an imaginary world.

One or more of the above symptoms may indicate a psychological emergency. These may also be accompanied by physical signs and symptoms such as sleeplessness, loss of appetite, loss of sex drive, constipation, crying, tension, irritability.

consider the physical assessment a humiliating invasion of privacy. Therefore, try to establish a relationship with the patient during an initial interview, and then conduct the physical assessment. Furthermore, always be aware of the unclothed patient's probable embarrassment, and make sure that he or she is properly draped or shielded from the stares of curious onlookers. Conduct the examination in an efficient, businesslike manner, and continue talking with the patient during the entire procedure. Both the patient and bystanders will be very aware of your actions, even those that are very subtle. Exercise great care in how you treat the patient and in the things you say.

□ RESPONSES OF FAMILY, FRIENDS, OR BYSTANDERS

Those at the scene with the patient also may show many of the responses just described. Family members may be anxious, panicky, or angry. Their anger often results from their feelings of guilt. As a means of coping with their own anxiety, they may demand immediate action, or they may pressure you to move the patient to the hospital before appropriate assessment and stabilization have been completed. They may state or imply that you are not competent to handle the situation ("Get him to the hospital so he can be seen by a doctor.") No matter how upsetting this may be, you must realize that the patient's family and friends are concerned and that their behavior, however irritating, arises from distress. Remember that you must remain in control of the scene. Remain calm and sympathetic, and explain emergency care procedures to friends and family members. They should be reassured that emergency medical assistance has been requested.

In some situations, you will need to control a gathering crowd of bystanders or onlookers. Ask bystanders to enforce the boundaries that you set around the rescue scene; ask others to keep pathways cleared between patients and rescue vehicles. You can also help control the crowd by asking family members or bystanders to retrieve supplies, hold IV lines, direct traffic, help with stretchers, and so on.

□ PATIENT ASSESSMENT IN PSYCHOLOGICAL EMERGENCIES

Assessment should begin as soon as you approach the scene. Observe the patient's general appearance and clothing; note whether he is neat or disheveled. Observe the patient's rate of speech. If it is slow, he may be de-

pressed or intoxicated, and if it is rapid, he may be manic or under the influence of stimulants (such as amphetamines).

Keep the following questions in mind when assessing patients in psychological distress (Figure 39-2):

- Is the patient expressing rage or hostility?
- Is the patient alert and able to communicate coherently; oriented to time, place and person?
- Are the patient's responses appropriate?
- Is the patient's memory intact?
- What is the patient's mood? Depressed?
- Does the patient seem abnormally elated or agitated?
- Does the patient appear fearful or worried?
- Does the patient show evidence of disturbances in judgment, delusions, disordered thoughts, or hallucinations?
- Has the patient tried to hurt himself or herself or others?
- Is the patient withdrawn? (Generally, patients in psychological distress do not want to help themselves, nor do they want help from others.)

Initial questions should be direct and specific to establish whether the patient is alert, oriented, and able to communicate. Only information that is crucial to immediate management should be obtained.

In general, seriously disturbed patients should be seen by a physician, who can decide whether they need to be hospitalized. In most cases, patients who are alert,

FIGURE 39-2 Patients in psychological distress may be withdrawn and not want to help themselves, nor want help from others.

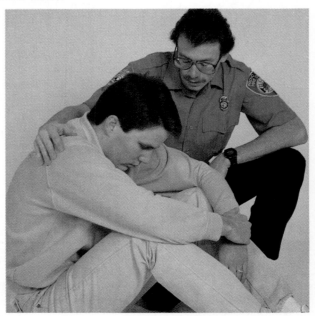

oriented, and conscious can be taken to the hospital only with their consent. If they do not consent, they can be taken against their will only at the request of the police. The same applies to forceful restraint. When these measures are necessary, law enforcement officers *must* be called (unless, of course, they are already present). Follow local protocol.

☐ PHYSICAL DISORDERS THAT RESEMBLE PSYCHOLOGICAL DISTURBANCES

As obvious as this sounds, a key part of assessment is to make *sure* that you are dealing with a psychological, and not a *physical,* emergency. Diabetes, seizure, severe infections, hypoxia, metabolic disorders, head injuries, hypertension, stroke, alcohol, depressants, stimulants, psychedelics, and narcotics can all cause disturbed behavior.

What initially appears to be a psychological disturbance may, upon closer examination, prove to be physical in nature. For example, fever can cause delirium. A brain tumor can cause personality changes and confusion. Hypoglycemia can cause delirium, confusion, and even hallucinations. It is *critical* that you examine each patient, because ignoring a life-threatening problem or serious illness could cause the patient to die while you are trying to care for a nonexistent psychological disorder.

Just because you smell alcohol on a patient's breath, do not automatically assume that he is intoxicated. Persons in diabetic coma or insulin shock may appear to be intoxicated, and you may indeed smell alcohol on their breath. A patient who appears to be drunk (and who has alcohol on his breath) may have hit his head on something. He will appear confused, not because he is drunk, but because he has suffered a brain injury. **Antabuse,** a drug used by alcoholics to assist in decreasing alcohol dependency, can also produce a breath odor similar to that of alcohol.

It is critical that you determine a patient's physical well-being before you begin the long and sometimes tedious procedure of handling the psychological emergency.

Some clues that the problem is probably physical (organic) include:

- The onset of symptoms was relatively sudden; most psychiatric disorders develop over many months.
- If the patient has hallucinations, they are visual but not auditory (a psychiatric patient is more likely to "hear voices").

- The patient has memory loss or impairment; in most psychiatric disorders, the memory remains intact and the patient is usually oriented as to time, location, and events.
- The patient's pupils are dilated, constricted, or uneven, or they respond differently to light (many pupillary changes are indicative either of drug use or head injury, but not of psychiatric disorders).
- The patient has excessive salivation.
- The patient is incontinent.
- The patient has unusual odors on his breath ("fruity," acetone, or like alcohol).

Finally, remember that psychological trauma often *follows* (or is a result of) physical trauma or illness. Even if all the clues point to strictly a psychological emergency, probe deeply enough before ruling out a physical cause.

☐ GENERAL GUIDELINES FOR MANAGEMENT OF PSYCHOLOGICAL EMERGENCIES

EMTs are frequently called to transport or care for patients experiencing psychological disorders. Because the situation presented by such a patient can be difficult, you are usually able to perform in a way that would be unacceptable if you were dealing with more "normal" patients. But remember that even "normal" people are not used to dealing with crisis, and any kind of emergency can bring up an entire flood of "abnormal" emotions. In addition to the specific management techniques already discussed under specific disorders, the following are general guidelines in dealing with the emotionally disturbed (Figure 39-3):

- Act *promptly*. Just as in physical trauma, seconds count; delay can worsen the situation.
- Become an acute observer. As you approach a scene, look for clues as to what is happening. Note the condition, cleanliness, and temperature of the house; the presence of alcohol or medicine bottles; how the patient is dressed; the patient's shoes; the presence of medical equipment; and so on. Be aware of potentially dangerous situations. Determine whether the situation is safe; if it is not, stay in a safe place until help arrives.
- Be prepared to spend time with the patient. It is often impossible to evaluate these patients properly without investing time. Some psychological disorders, such as paranoia, stem from suspicion or mistrust of others; if you are hurried, the pa-

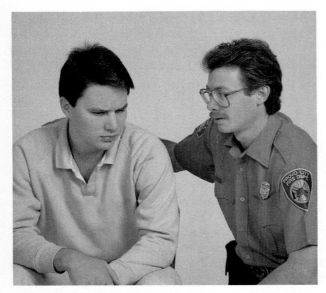

FIGURE 39-3 When dealing with a psychological emergency, be calm and show through your actions that you have confidence in the patient's ability to maintain self-control.

tient may think that you are trying to hurt him or her.

- Be as calm as possible. Stay polite, use good manners, show respect, and make no assumptions or judgments. Use a calm tone of voice, and eliminate as much noise and chaos as possible.
- Most emotionally disturbed people are terrified of losing self-control. You will elicit the best cooperation if you show the patient through your actions that you have confidence in his ability to maintain control of himself and the situation. If you are anxious or panicky, you will only further convince the patient that the situation is overwhelming or hopeless.
- Do not rush to the hospital immediately unless a medical emergency dictates the need for life-saving care. Instead, spend time at the scene to gain important clues from the environment and to avoid panicking the patient.
- Interview the patient alone (or with a partner if you fear violence) in a quiet room, even if you know that later you will have to get details from others. Ask family members and friends to go to another room. Guarantee that the patient has privacy. A patient might hesitate to talk in front of friends or family members because he or she is ashamed of his problems and does not want to lose respect in their eyes. They might even be the source of the problem.
- The EMT should never allow himself or herself to be left alone with an emotionally disturbed patient, especially one of the opposite sex.

- Ask specific questions that will help you measure the patient's level of consciousness and contact with reality.
- Avoid asking questions that can be answered with a simple "yes" or "no." Give the patient a chance to explain his situation; the method of explanation may help *you* during the assessment (for example, does the patient seem paranoid or depressed in explaining the problem?).
- Communicate confidence in yourself throughout the interview; move with assurance. The patient will be more open if he or she senses that you have control.
- Make the interview brief; do not spend a lengthy amount of time trying to sift through details. Once the patient has told you his or her story, briefly go over it again to make sure that you understand. Clear up any points that are vague, and ask questions that you could not ask while the patient was talking.
- Look at the patient's eyes throughout the interview; they can often tell you what is going on in the mind. A patient's eyes can reflect emotions and tell you whether he or she is terrified, confused, struggling, in pain, or dying.
- Be interested in the patient's story, but do not oversympathize. If you overwhelm the patient with pity, he or she may decide that his situation is indeed hopeless. Treat the patient as though you expect improvement and recovery.
- Never be judgmental. The patient is convinced that his or her feelings are accurate, and they are real to him, no matter how ridiculous they may appear to you.
- Be genuine and honest. Give the patient supportive information that is truthful. Tell the patient what you expect from him and what he can expect from you. Make sure that you follow through; do not make promises that you cannot keep.
- Make a definite plan of action.
- Do not force the patient to make decisions, because he or she may have lost the ability to cope effectively. Remember, though, that some patients may want to maintain control and therefore make their own decisions or at least contribute to the decision-making process.
- Encourage the patient to participate in a motor activity; it helps to reduce anxiety. Let the patient do as many things as he can. Encourage him or her.
- Consider all psychiatric patients to be escape risks; stay with the patient at all times. Once you have responded to the emergency, the patient's safety is legally your responsibility. Even if the patient

pleads to be left alone for just a few minutes, firmly explain that you realize he or she is capable of handling things but that you could get fired if you leave a patient alone. If the need is to go to the bathroom, allow the patient to go, but leave the door open and be discreet as you watch. If he or she tries to get away, use minimal force to detain the patient. Follow local protocol.

- Never assume that it is impossible to communicate with a patient until you have tried, even if friends or family members insist it cannot be done.

- If a patient is extremely fearful or violent, skip the physical assessment unless you have serious suspicions of a physical problem that requires immediate medical attention. Wait until you have developed a rapport before you begin the physical assessment.

- Do not be afraid of silences. They may seem intolerably long, but maintain an attentive and relaxed attitude. If the patient stops talking because he or she is overwhelmed by emotion, it is especially critical that you refrain from speaking.

- As you talk to the patient, encourage him or her to communicate. Use gestures such as a nod of the head or verbal responses such as "I see," or "Go on." Remain interested, and let the patient see that you would like to learn more.

- Do not foster unrealistic expectations. Instead of saying, "You have nothing to worry about," say something like, "Despite all the problems you have had, you seem to have done very well at work."

- Maintain a respectful distance between you and the patient. After you have established a rapport, ask the patient if it is okay to touch him or her.

- Do not abuse or threaten the patient. If you do, the patient may become convinced that you are going to hurt him or her. At that point, the patient will resist help or try to prevent you from approaching, usually by violence.

- Do not allow the patient to get you angry. Many patients with a psychological disorder are adept at picking out your weaknesses; they may feel threatened themselves and try to improve their situation by belittling you. Remain kind and calm. You may be upset by what the patient says to you, but do not react in any way. He is ill, and his comments are not directed against you personally. Help the patient through his problems, and help him or her regain his self-confidence.

- Often you will be called to a situation where the patient has attracted a crowd — he or she may be threatening someone in a store or teetering on the edge of a tall building with an anxious crowd on the sidewalk below. The excitement of the crowd can encourage the patient, and the patient may do things that he or she would otherwise not consider. If you arrive at the scene and a crowd has assembled, do what you can to disperse it so that you can deal with the patient on a one-to-one basis. If no crowd has gathered, take every precaution to prevent one from forming. Try to avoid bringing in fire or riot control equipment.

- If the patient is severely disturbed and has become violent, it will be necessary to restrain him or her. Never attempt physical restraint alone; wait until assistants have arrived. Do not be ashamed to call for help. A violently disturbed individual can be capable of inflicting great harm.

- If the environment or the scene of the accident is especially hectic, remove the patient from the scene before you try to question or calm him or her. The patient will probably remain disturbed as long as the environment is chaotic.

- Once you have determined the patient's problem, make every effort to explain it fully to him or her. Explain that he can be helped and what the probable outcome will be. Do not try to frighten the patient, but be honest in explaining what will be done to help him or her. A patient may be more anxious and fearful because of uncertainty about what is going to happen to him or her now that you have arrived.

- Find out if the patient has been given psychiatric care prior to the present emergency. If so, suggest that the family contact the therapist and ask him to meet you at the emergency room. Find out, too, whether the patient is taking any medications.

- Make detailed notes on what you have learned about the patient, recording patient statements word-for-word in quotation marks — for medical as well as legal reasons. Note carefully what you did for the patient.

☐ COMMUNICATING IN PSYCHOLOGICAL EMERGENCIES

In any psychological emergency, you need to get information quickly. You can't risk holding back or being shy. In such situations, your communication not only gathers information, but protects your personal safety and provides reassurance to a troubled patient.

While your medical skills are of utmost importance in most calls, your ability to communicate clearly and effectively is the key to dealing with psychologically disturbed patients. Each patient is unique and will react differently, but use the following general guidelines to develop a rapport with a patient:

- Identify yourself clearly to establish contact with the patient.
- Immediately establish good eye contact; look into the patient's eyes. Never wear sunglasses when you are dealing with a patient.
- Use touch to help communicate. Squeeze the patient's shoulder, or hold the patient's hand to communicate that you care what happens to him or her.
- Avoid the temptation to start out with your mind made up. Remain open, and genuinely listen to what the patient is telling you.
- Express your desire to help; let the patient know that you will be responsible for his or her care.
- Communicate on the patient's level, using easily understandable terms.
- Use the patient's proper name, if invited to do so, or call the patient "Mr.," "Mrs.," or "Ms." Never use a nickname, such as "Gramps."
- Be aware of your own body language.
- Speak slowly, clearly, and distinctly.
- Tell the patient what you are doing every step of the way and explain your reason and the probable outcome; you will help diffuse suspicion and will help establish trust.
- Do not rush the patient; allow sufficient time for your questions to be answered.
- Listen intently; hear the patient's feelings as well as words. Wait for answers. Pay attention and listen to the patient's message, not just the words. Use body language to let the patient know you are listening.
- Act interested and concerned.
- Give calm and warm reassurance.
- Never use physical force unless the patient poses a danger to self, to you, or to others.
- Never lie to or mislead the patient.
- Avoid stock phrases such as "Everything will be okay."
- Carefully explain the situation to the patient, and explain your plan of action step by step to avoid apprehension or fear; make it clear that you are in control.
- Verbalize even if the patient is unconscious. Hearing is the last of the senses to go and the first to return, and you may be able to communicate with someone who appears to be in a coma. Your talking to the patient will also calm and ease any by-standers who are anxious about what you are doing.

☐ HELPING PATIENTS WITH SPECIAL COMMUNICATION NEEDS

Just as in a medical emergency, you will be called to help patients with special communications needs. The number-one rule is to *avoid* **stereotyping.** Regardless of the patient's communication difficulties, use the patient's name (first or last) in addressing him.

Geriatric Patients

In dealing with geriatric patients, use these guidelines:

- Carefully identify yourself to avoid confusion.
- Do not assume senility or lack of understanding.
- Check for hearing deficiency; speak into the patient's ear if you need to be heard, but do not shout. (Shouting can distort the audibility of a hearing aid user.)
- Allow extra time for patient response.
- Ask the patient what makes him the most comfortable.
- Maintain eye contact.
- Allow the patient to control the pace of the interview unless a life-threatening medical emergency dictates that you set the pace.
- Include the patient's spouse if he or she is present.

Pediatric Patients

When a child is involved in a psychological emergency, you will need to revise your procedure slightly. A child is not merely a "miniature adult." You need to keep in mind, too, that you'll have two patients: the child and the parent.

A child in crisis will probably regress to behavior typical of a much younger child. The primary emotion for an ill or injured child is fear, and you'll have to work quickly to diffuse it. A child may be unable to talk about problems directly; you might be able to work around the problem by using techniques such as storytelling, game-playing, or picture-drawing, which help to establish rapport. If the child refuses to talk, watch as he or she interacts with others, and try to ascertain the extent of the problem. Use the following guidelines (Figure 39-4):

- Make the interview short; a child has a short attention span.

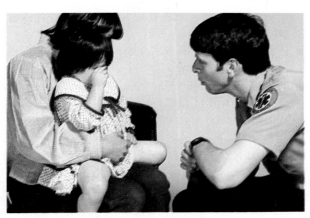

FIGURE 39-4 When children are victims, one of the most difficult emotions to deal with is panic caused by fear of the unknown. It is important to communicate strength, control, and friendliness. If possible, gain the assistance of others whom the child knows and trusts.

- Even though you want to protect the child or shield him or her from unpleasant facts, do not lie. If you have to tell a child something unpleasant, do it gently and gradually.

- Assume authority in the situation; you will have to make sure the parent understands that you have to make decisions for the child.

- As mentioned, a child may regress; a common situation is a child who refuses to stop crying. Be patient, and don't belittle the child. Don't let anyone tell the child to stop crying. And, above all, remember that the child's crying is not a sign of your failure.

- Unless absolutely necessary, don't separate the child from the parents — you may cause greater trauma.

- Get the child's parents or other responsible adults to help you *if* you do not suspect that they have abused the child and if they themselves are in control.

- You might need to suggest some possible feelings before the child will be able to tell you exactly how he or she feels.

- Do not think that the capacity for violence is absent just because you are working with a child. Children can be especially prone to suicide and homicide; many adults mistakenly brush off a child's destructive tendencies.

- Modify the rule for confidentiality. Because the child cannot be responsible for his or her own care or actions, you need to confide in the parents or other responsible adult authorities if the child's psychological condition warrants it.

- Remember that a child, more than any other patient, is likely to be frightened, not only by the or-

deal itself but by the appearance of strangers in uniform and unfamiliar medical equipment.

- Protect a child's modesty.

- Move slowly, and carefully explain what you are doing in simple terms that a child can understand. Move in reverse order, toe to head, so that you can build a level of confidence before examining more threatening areas (Figure 39-5).

- Take the child's age group into consideration. Children aged one to three will suffer special anxiety from being separated from parents; be especially gentle, and allow the child to keep a favorite toy or blanket during the examination if possible. Children aged three to six tend to become especially upset over injury; you should cover even slight external wounds with dressings or bandages so that the child cannot see them. Children of elementary school age are particularly concerned about modesty; take extra measures to help them remain modest and covered at all times during the exam. Children of this age are naturally curious and want to know what is going on; if you can, you might let the child touch the equipment as you explain how you are going to use it.

- Teenagers are very anxious about the possibility of disfigurement; they may become hysterical and overemotional.

- Be honest about any pain that might be caused by a procedure.

- With small children use dolls when appropriate to explain a procedure.

- Use a friendly tone of voice.

- If the child seems comforted by their presence, let parents or siblings remain with the child throughout the assessment and interview.

FIGURE 39-5 A confused child is likely to be frightened. Progress slowly and allow the child to tell you how he or she feels.

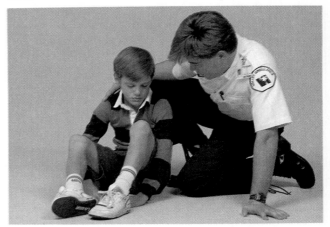

Deaf Patients

In working with patients who you know or assume to be deaf, do the following:

- Get the patient's attention before you speak by gently tapping the shoulder or waving your hand where it can be seen.
- Maintain eye contact.
- Be especially courteous.
- Determine if the patient can read lips. If so, he will probably understand only 30 to 40 percent of the conversation (or even less, since the patient is going through an emergency). Lipreading is more difficult for the patient if you have serious orthodontic problems, a foreign accent, or a beard or mustache.
- Face the patient while you are speaking.
- Speak slowly and clearly. Even if you determine

that the patient cannot read lips, speak as you gesture or use signs.
- If possible, use an interpreter who can communicate in sign language.
- Try pantomiming, using broad gestures.
- Use common signs for sick, hurt, help, and so on (Figure 39-6).
- Do **not** shout; if the patient has even partial hearing and is wearing a hearing aid, you could distort his or her hearing.
- Use written messages. If deaf since birth, the patient may not understand some grammatical combinations; therefore, keep it simple.

Blind Patients

In working with a blind patient, use the following guidelines:

FIGURE 39-6 Communicating with a deaf patient.

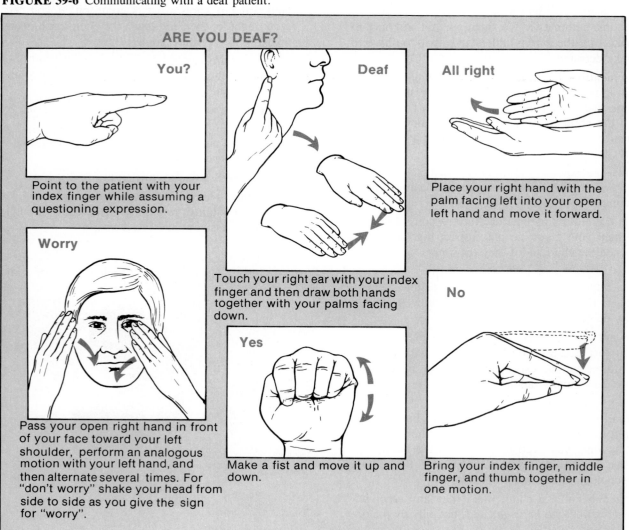

ARE YOU DEAF?

You?
Point to the patient with your index finger while assuming a questioning expression.

Deaf
Touch your right ear with your index finger and then draw both hands together with your palms facing down.

All right
Place your right hand with the palm facing left into your open left hand and move it forward.

Worry
Pass your open right hand in front of your face toward your left shoulder, perform an analogous motion with your left hand, and then alternate several times. For "don't worry" shake your head from side to side as you give the sign for "worry".

Yes
Make a fist and move it up and down.

No
Bring your index finger, middle finger, and thumb together in one motion.

- Determine whether the patient also has a hearing impairment.
- Do *not* shout.
- Maintain touch contact by lightly resting your hand on the patient's forearm.
- Explain procedures in detail before you do them.
- If the patient is **ambulatory,** lead him or her by standing one step ahead and one step to the side, letting the patient rest his hand at the inside of your bent elbow. Walk forward slowly, alerting the patient to any obstacles.
- Identify the source of any strange noises.

Non—English-Speaking Patients

Use the following guidelines in working with non—English-speaking patients:

- Try communicating in English first.
- Show the patient your badge or patch to establish your identity.
- Use an interpreter if one is available.
- Try to find a common language; if you speak a language other than English, try using it.
- Use gestures and signs.
- Speak slowly and clearly in English throughout the assessment and treatment. The patient will probably know some words and phrases, and many medical terms will be familiar, since many have roots in another language.
- Point to the part of the body you need to examine before you begin any examination.
- Do not shout.

Confused and/or Developmentally Disabled Patients

In speaking with patients who are especially confused or who have some kind of developmental disability (such as mental retardation), use the following guidelines:

- Determine the patient's level of understanding by asking questions.
- Speak at an appropriate level.
- Wait for a delayed response when it is the patient's turn to answer or respond; have patience.
- Speak as you would to any adult.
- Evaluate the patient's understanding by asking a few questions, and re-explain something if necessary.
- Listen carefully.
- Display caring concern.

- Do not hesitate to ask the patient about his disability.
- Speak slowly and distinctly.
- Use the word "disability" instead of a slang word to describe the patient's condition.

☐ STRESS RESPONSES OF EMTS

Stress is any change in the body's internal balance; stress occurs when the external demands become greater than your personal resources.

EMTs are not immune to the stresses of emergency situations. You may suffer both good (eustress) and bad (distress) reactions; eustress may occur, for example, as a result of successfully responding to a challenging emergency situation. Distress — or "bad" stress — is not a sign of weakness. When dealing with the critically ill and injured, you may experience a wide range of feelings, some of which are unpleasant. You may feel irritated by the family or the patient's demands, be anxious when faced with life-threatening injuries, become defensive at implications that you are not competent to handle emergencies, and become sad in response to tragedy. You are forced to "depersonalize" during an emergency — to emotionally "estrange" yourself from the patients and the situation. Although these feelings are natural, it is best not to express them during an emergency. Furthermore, if you give an outward appearance of calmness and confidence, it will help to relieve the anxiety of those on the scene. Helping others to remain calm is part of your therapeutic role.

Another common reaction among EMTs is irritation with the patient who does not appear particularly ill. This reaction can be a special problem for those who are prepared to deal with life-threatening problems and may regard minor complaints as burdensome and annoying. Patients may be worried about injuries, pain, disturbing feelings, or bodily functions that they think are abnormal. It is not your duty to judge whether such complaints are real or imagined. These complaints are always real to the patient. Although it is more dramatic to rescue the multiple-trauma patient than to reassure the patient with a minor cold, both have indicated that they are distressed and want help. In both cases, you must be supportive and nonjudgmental and render whatever care is needed.

Top sources of stress for EMTs include long hours, too much work, being on call and having to respond suddenly, being responsible for someone's life, having to make life-and-death decisions, making a serious error, dealing with dying people and grieving survivors, watching a child die, demanding physical labor, little recognition, not knowing what is expected, little decision-making ability, poor pay, and boredom.

Dealing with Stress

One increasingly popular way of helping EMTs and other emergency personnel to defuse stress is a procedure known as "stress debriefing," usually used under the guidance of trained professionals following particularly serious incidents (see page 591). Stress debriefing can be used after any incident that creates especially strong emotions for the responder — a situation in which a colleague dies, a responder's own life is seriously endangered, a child dies, or a situation in which the victims are close in age or circumstance to the responder's own family.

In stress debriefing, responders are helped to realize that their emotions and reactions are normal and that they can mobilize their own responses in coping with a situation. While different programs use different specific techniques, most help workers to sort out the facts of the incident, how they feel about what happened, and how they reacted to the incident. They are then helped to explore symptoms that may have developed in response to an incident and to mobilize coping mechanisms for overcoming the stress associated with the incident.

Special stress can be encountered in a disaster or multiple-victim incident, and specific techniques can help you avoid the results of that stress. Experts with the Department of Health and Human Services suggest, among others, that you try these techniques:

- Develop a "buddy" system with a co-worker; keep an eye on each other, and suggest when breaks are advisable.

- Encourage and support your co-workers; make positive remarks, and avoid the temptation to criticize.

- Periodically take a break to get some exercise.

- If you can, eat frequently but in small amounts.

- Use tasteful humor to break the tension and provide relief; use extreme care not to make patients feel as though they are the "brunt" of the humor.

- Use relaxation techniques; for example, take a deep breath, hold it, and blow it out forcefully.

- Use positive "self-talk"; remember that you are doing the things you have been trained to do, and that your work is making a difference.

- When you find your effectiveness diminishing, take a brief break.

Following a disaster, seek professional help; attend stress debriefing sessions if they are offered. A professional can help you sort out your thoughts and reactions to the disaster, assume an appropriate pace, and work yourself smoothly back into a professional situation.

Burnout

Burnout is defined as emotional exhaustion and cynicism that result from chronic stress and tension. EMTs, responding in varying roles to emergencies and disasters, expose themselves to overwhelming personal stress in their desire to help meet the needs of patients. Many feel completely responsible for everything that happens on a run (even things clearly out of their control), and some become so involved with their jobs that their entire self-image is based on their jobs. One possible result is the burnout syndrome — a state of exhaustion, irritability, and fatigue that can markedly decrease your effectiveness. The chief signs of burnout are a growing disinterest in patient welfare and a desire to distance yourself from patients. Burnout can result from personal difficulties and is the result of long-term chronic stress brought about by work-related problems involving an emotionally charged environment, stressful situations, and erratic hours. The best way to prevent burnout is to expect it, to be alert to its early signs, and to act in relieving the stress. Five areas of symptoms have been identified:

- Thinking: mental confusion, inability to concentrate, slowness of thought, inability to make judgments and decisions, loss of ability to recognize alternatives or to prioritize tasks, loss of objectivity in evaluating and functioning, loss of motivation for job, attempts to block change, failure to make contributions, chronic forgetfulness, and distraction.

- Psychological: depression, irritability, anxiety, hyperexcitability, negative "self-talk" (using negative labels to describe yourself), excessive anger reactions, negativism, feelings of not being appreciated, hostility, defensiveness, hypochondria, mood swings, and feelings of worthlessness.

- Bodily complaints: persistent physical exhaustion, headaches, loss of emotional and physical energy, gastrointestinal distress, loss of sexual drive and/or interest, appetite disturbances, hypochondria, sleep disorders (insomnia and nightmares are common), tremors. In one study it was estimated that 40 to 80 percent of all illness that causes EMTs to miss work is stress-related. Other physical manifestations include chronic fatigue, menstrual cycle disturbances, profuse sweating, chronic diarrhea, frequent urination, muscle twitching, dizzy spells, chest pain, and pounding heart.

- Behavioral: hyperactivity, overeating, excessive fatigue, inability to express self verbally or in writing, increased alcohol or drug use, stuttering, grinding teeth, nightmares, absenteeism, and lack of energy.

- Social: decrease in ability to relate to patients as individuals, especially in a constructive, friendly, caring manner. Decrease in social activities, increased interpersonal conflicts with co-workers, chronic feelings of decreased worth.

Management of Burnout

Before you consider management of burnout, remember — there is a spectrum for burnout. Not all EMTs are in terrible condition when they seek help. Some need only a little diversion, while others need aggressive management (such as extended time off the job).

The first step is to be aware of the symptoms when they appear. The earlier they are recognized, the better. All EMTs need to be able to recognize early symptoms, not only in themselves, but also in their fellow workers. Any such observations should be reported to supervisors. Supervisors also must be alert to any early symptoms in their staff so that they can intervene. It is important that the EMT's feelings be acknowledged and that co-workers support him or her.

The supervisor should talk to the individual and point out the symptoms. The supervisor should relieve the person from his or her duties for a short period of time or reassign that person to a different work environment. Guilt over leaving the activity is relieved by giving "official" permission to stop and by pointing out how the EMT is no longer helping because of the loss of effectiveness. The EMT can be reassured that he or she can return and will have improved greatly as a result of a short recuperation.

It is important that the time off not be viewed as a form of weakness or failure. Time off may best be accomplished by a change of assignment.

In-service training can be an important tool in helping avoid burnout. Improving skills and techniques can definitely help reduce the stresses often associated with the EMT lifestyle, as well as increase confidence. The following suggestions may be helpful to the EMT dealing with stresses, crises, and burnout in his or her own life (see Figure 39-7 for a Burnout Index).

- Decide what is causing the problem. Look toward, not away from, your problems and feelings. You cannot work out a solution until you identify a cause. This seems frightening, but you will find that knowledge often kills fear. Once you find out more about what is causing your feelings, you can get a grip on them. Remember to look at the broad picture — many cases of burnout are due to accumulated stress over a period of months or years.
- Learn to accept what you cannot change. Realize that you are the only person over whom you have total control. You have no control over most things and never will; you cannot right every injustice, nor can you make people over. You must come to the realization that you cannot change many situations — you can only learn to cope with them and adjust to them. Learn your own limitations, and learn to say no when you know something will exceed your limitations.
- Accept the fact that you will occasionally make mistakes — and honestly admit that no person is right all of the time. Understand that a mistake does not reduce your value. You do not have to be perfect to do a good job.
- Share your worries with someone else. Verbalizing your problems and fears to someone who you love, trust, or respect helps to relieve the stress and often helps you to discover alternatives that otherwise might have escaped your eye. A good confidante will listen empathetically and will often ask questions that will help you to explore your feelings honestly.
- Get enough exercise. Exercise has all sorts of benefits: one of the greatest is that it provides a physical release for the pent-up rage and hostility that accompany many crises. Choose any kind of exercise that will relieve your boredom, excite your senses, and provide you with fun and relaxation — jogging, tennis, swimming, handball, or walking are good ones to try. As you concentrate on your exercise, your mind will be diverted from your problems, and you will be refreshed enough later to tackle them with new vigor.
- Avoid self-medication. Reaching for a bottle — whether it is filled with alcohol or pills — does not teach you to cope with a crisis. Your problems are still there when you come out of the stupor, and sometimes they have become even worse because you did not act on them immediately. Your crisis may be causing you pain, but do not add the extra pain of dependence on alcohol or drugs.
- Serve others. Avoid self-pity; do something for someone else, and you will find yourself thinking of their problems instead of your own. Learn to love people and use things, not to love things and use people.
- Avoid loneliness. You will undoubtedly need some time alone to collect your thoughts and sort out your feelings, but the difference between aloneness and loneliness is vast. Withdrawing will not solve crises. Keep yourself in touch with those around you who have offered a helping hand.
- Try a temporary diversion. If your well is empty — if you have tried everything and you are at the end of your rope — try a brief diversion to refresh yourself. Go see a funny movie, read a book that you have always wanted to read, or go to a concert with a friend. Cut loose a little bit.

SYMPTOM	HOW LONG?				HOW OFTEN?			HOW INTENSE?			
PHYSICAL	One month	Six months	One year	Several years	Monthly	Weekly	Daily	Constantly	Mild	Moderate	Severe	Alarming
Fatigue												
Depression												
Insomnia												
Headaches												
Gastrointestinal problems												
Lingering cold												
Weight loss or gain												
Shortness of breath												
INTERPERSONAL and BEHAVIORAL												
Bored												
Restless												
Discouraged												
Resentful												
Irritable												
Fault-finding												
Moody												
Resistant to change												
Work harder/enjoy less												
Pass up breaks												
Live for breaks												
Make "little" mistakes												
Defensive												
Obsessive												
ESCAPE												
Dependence on alcohol												
Dependence on drugs												

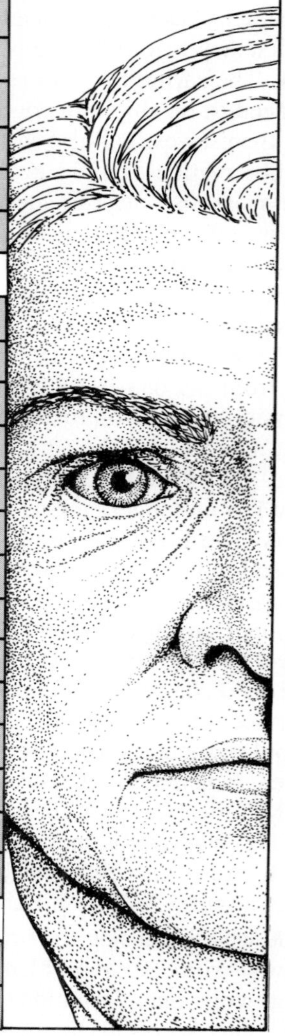

Developed by Edwina A. McConnell, RN, MS, reprinted with permission of RN Magazine.

FIGURE 39-7 The burnout index.

- Take active management steps. Create a plan of action for solving the problem. Keep your options open, and be creative in solving your problems. Your solution might not be the one you originally thought of, but try it anyway.
- Assess your priorities. Uncertainty runs rampant during a crisis. As a result, you may find yourself running around like a chicken with its head cut off. During a crisis, it is hard to decide what to do first. Take a few minutes to list on paper your priorities. Decide what is the most important thing you need to do; write that down first. Order the rest of your activities the same way; listing the most important first. Then tackle them in that

same order, and do not move down the list to an easier task until you have completed the ones ahead of it.

- Have a physical checkup to eliminate the possibility of physical illness.
- Get the support of your family and friends. Help them understand the nature of your work, and let them share your experiences and successes.
- Learn to love — and appreciate — yourself for your unique contributions and abilities!

☐ CRITICAL INCIDENT STRESS DEBRIEFING

One of the best ways of dealing with burnout is a form of support called **critical incident stress debriefing,** or CISD, a tool first developed at the University of Maryland that helps prevent and alleviate the unique kinds of stress caused by a "critical incident."

A critical incident is any situation that causes an EMT to experience unusually strong emotional reactions — and that interferes with the ability to function, either during the critical incident or later. Common critical incidents include the following:

- The death of an emergency team member in the line of duty.
- Serious injury to an emergency team member in the line of duty.
- The suicide of an emergency team member.
- Injury or death involving friends or family members of the rescuer.

- The death of a patient under particularly tragic or emotional circumstances.
- The death of a patient after prolonged or intense rescue procedures.
- The sudden death of an infant or child.
- Injuries to children that are caused by child abuse.
- Injuries or death to civilians that are caused by emergency service personnel (a civilian killed when an ambulance collides with a car, for example).
- An event that threatens the life of a responder.
- An event that attracts unusual media attention.
- An event that has distressing sights, sounds, or smells.
- A mass-casualty event.

Rescuers who suffer critical incident stress develop many of the signs and symptoms of stress and burnout; in addition, they may suffer from repeated mental images of the stressfull scene, fear of continuing in EMT work, and inability to function at the scene of subsequent emergencies.

The Debriefing Process

The goal of the debriefing process is to help rescuers deal with the stress caused by a critical incident; in the process, other feelings associated with job stress and burnout are generally resolved (Figure 39-8). The debriefing itself is a seven-step process that is often mandatory for emergency personnel involved in a critical incident.

Brief CISD is sometimes initiated at the scene of a

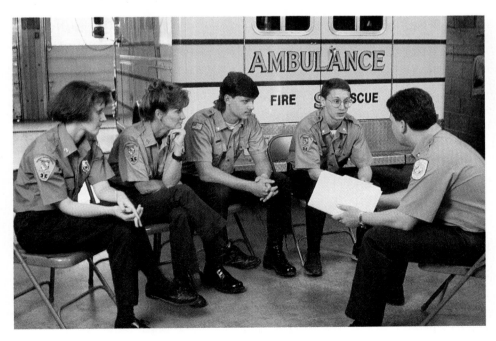

FIGURE 39-8 Informal discussions with colleagues concerning your feelings and frustrations are helpful and should be encouraged. Following particularly stressful incidents, a critical incident stress debriefing may be warranted.

disaster or within a few hours after the critical incident, but formal CISD is almost always delayed for at least twenty-four to forty-eight hours after the critical incident is over. That brief interval allows involved emergency personnel to sort through feelings and work through the denial process that is almost always a part of critical incidents.

During the seven stages of CISD, skilled professionals work with emergency services personnel in the following phases:

- The introductory phase, during which confidentiality is assured and participants are guaranteed that what they say will in no way affect their job status.

- The fact phase, in which participants review the details of what happened during the critical incident; participants stick to the facts, trying to vividly recall what happened.

- The feeling phase, during which participants explore how they feel about what happened; participants are helped to talk about guilt, anxiety, fear, and anger about the incident.

- The symptom phase, during which participants are urged to explore any physical, mental, or emotional symptoms they may be experiencing that could be related to the critical incident; participants are also urged to explore what may be going on at home or on the job as a result of the critical incident.

- The teaching phase, during which skilled professionals help participants sort through the array of emotions and symptoms; the professional emphasizes that these are *normal* reactions to what happened.

- The re-entry phase, during which skilled professionals give participants a specific plan of action for returning to the job; the participants may also set some goals or plan some activities that help to further diffuse the stress.

- The follow-up phase, which is held several weeks or months after the initial CISD, helps resolve any issues that may still be present.

In conducting critical incident stress debriefing, make sure that the debriefing includes anyone involved in the incident, including law enforcement personnel, firefighters, emergency medical personnel, dispatch operators, first responders and emergency room personnel. In some cases, the debriefing may even include family members, who are inevitably affected by the stress.

In cases of mass-casualty incidents, such as earthquakes or tornadoes, a number of debriefings involving hundreds of people may need to be conducted.

chapter 40

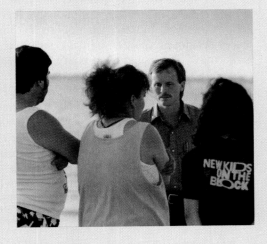

Crisis Intervention

✷ OBJECTIVES

- Describe the common behavioral emergencies that may precipitate a crisis.
- Recognize suicidal behavior and describe appropriate management.
- Outline how to assess the potential for violence in an aggressive and disruptive patient.
- Describe techniques for managing an assaultive or violent patient.
- Recognize the common indicators of spouse abuse.
- Recognize the characteristics of the rape trauma syndrome and describe appropriate emergency care.
- Describe appropriate management of a dying patient and his family and friends.

It is recommended that EMTs wear protective gloves whenever there is a possibility of coming in contact with a patient's blood, body fluids, mucous membranes, traumatic wounds, or sores. See Chapter 31.

Simply stated, a **crisis** is any serious interruption in the equilibrium of a person, family, or group. It is a state of emotional turmoil that acts as a turning point — for better or worse — in a person's life. **Distress** is generally regarded as acute physical or mental suffering and can arise from anything that causes pain, anxiety, strain, or sorrow.

Crisis intervention is a specific form of psychological emergency care for helping people handle emotional distress. When emotional pressure becomes too great for an individual or his or her support system to handle, a crisis may occur. The individual may experience impaired function, anxiety, excess loss of psychic energy, and even mental illness or self-destructive behavior. *Every emergency patient is in a potential crisis situation.*

☐ ANXIETY DISORDERS AND PHOBIAS

Anxiety is a state of painful uneasiness about impending problems. It is characterized by agitation and restlessness and is one of the most common emotions; in fact, anxiety disorders are thought to be the most common form of mental illness. According to estimates, anxiety disorders affect approximately 13.1 million Americans, or about one in every ten American adults. Most clinicians feel that approximately three-fourths of the cases are never correctly diagnosed because they so closely mimic other disorders.

Phobias, which are closely related, are irrational fears of specific things, places, or situations. One of the most disabling is **agoraphobia,** or "fear of the marketplace," which renders its victims terrified of leaving the safety of their own homes.

Patients having anxiety attacks may show evidence of intense fear. Tense and restless, they often wring their hands and pace. They frequently suffer from tremors, tachycardia, irregular heartbeat, dyspnea, sweating, and diarrhea; if severe, anxiety has been known to cause sudden cardiac death.

These patients feel overwhelmed and cannot concentrate. Sometimes they will hyperventilate and develop all the symptoms of that syndrome, including dizziness, tingling around the mouth and fingers, and carpopedal spasms (spasms of the hands and feet). They are often troubled by depression; the suicide rate is significantly higher among victims of anxiety disorders. They are also more prone to abuse alcohol. Their behavior creates anxiety in those around them as well, and they may be surrounded by a crowd of anxious and excited people when the EMS team arrives.

To manage a patient with an anxiety disorder, first separate the patient from the excited people around him. Identify yourself and tell him or her clearly and confidently — being firm but supportive — that effective treatment is available for this problem. Explain what you are doing, and do not leave the patient alone. En route to the hospital, continue to reassure the patient.

A patient with a phobia focuses all his or her anxiety in the form of intense, unreasonable fear. Phobic reactions include intense fear of such things as high places, enclosed spaces, animals, weapons, and public gatherings. The patient's anxiety becomes unbearable when confronted with the feared situation.

When dealing with a phobic patient, explain carefully and in detail each step involved in transporting the patient to the hospital ("Then we will walk down the stairs, and I will hold your arm; then we will get into the back of the ambulance. You will sit on a bench in the ambulance, and I will be beside you."). Repeat each description as the action occurs ("now we are going down the stairs"). Such explanations can lessen the patient's fears.

☐ DEPRESSION

Depression, one of the most common psychiatric conditions, is a factor in approximately 50 percent of all suicides. Many researchers feel that some people have a hereditary tendency or predisposition to depression. Depression can lead to a psychiatric emergency such as suicide and may cause other psychological disorders.

Depressed patients have a sad appearance, crying spells, and listless or apathetic behavior. They feel worthless, helpless, hopeless, withdrawn, and pessimistic; they often suffer appetite loss, fatigue, despondence, and severe restlessness. Believing that no one understands or cares about them or that their problems cannot be solved, they often express the desire to be left alone. Their speech may be halting and retarded, as if they hardly have enough energy to talk. If able to give a history, they may report that they awaken at 3 or 4 a.m. and cannot go back to sleep; depression can either increase or decrease both eating and sleeping habits. Some say that they feel bad in the morning but improve during the day.

Some depressed patients do not feel like talking. In such cases, you might confront a patient with your own observation, such as "you look very sad." Such a comment might encourage the patient to talk about depressed feelings. The patient might burst into tears. Do not discourage crying; maintain a sympathetic silence, and let the patient "cry himself out."

While not common, **bipolar disorder** — sometimes called **manic-depressive disorder** — causes a patient to swing to opposite sides of the spectrum. During one phase, he has an inflated view of himself; he may feel deliriously happy, elated, and almost superpowerful. The manic phase alternates between normal moods and a depressive state, in which the patient loses interest, feels worthless, worries, and may contemplate suicide. In either the manic or depressive stage, the patient may suffer delusions and hallucinations. Sometimes the phase may last for months; at other times, the patient may swing from one "mood" to another rather quickly (sometimes within a matter of hours).

Every depressed patient should be questioned directly about suicidal thoughts. You might ask, for example, "Have you ever wished that you were dead or thought about killing yourself?" If the response is yes, ask the patient how he or she would commit suicide, and determine whether he has made concrete plans. *Any patient who expresses suicidal thoughts should be transported for further help.* If in doubt, always consult a base physician and follow local protocol.

Depressed patients need sympathetic attention and reassurance. They need to know that you are concerned about them. It is usually best to interview a depressed patient in a quiet room with only a couple of staff members present, since the presence of many people may make him uncomfortable. Patients should be told that although many people experience unhappiness, they *can* be helped to feel better.

□ SUICIDE

Suicide is any willful act designed to end one's own life. Men are more often successful at suicide, but women make three times as many attempts. More than half of all suicides are committed with firearms; among nonsuccessful attempts, the most common methods are drug ingestion and wrist slashing. Suicide is now the tenth leading cause of death in the United States among all ages and the second leading cause of death among college-age students. Even with these staggering statistics, many researchers believe that suicide is vastly underreported due to the stigma surrounding it (see Figure 40-1).

Most suicides occur during April and May, while the least number occur in December. The suicide rate is highest on Monday between noon and 6 p.m. It is highest among divorced people and lowest among married people with children. More suicides occur in the west and in urban areas of more than 100,000 people than in the south and rural areas. Suicide classified by profession is highest among psychiatrists, physicians, dentists, and attorneys. At least half of all people who succeed at suicide have attempted it previously, and 75 percent give clear warning that they intend to kill themselves. The most common methods, in order, are: firearms, hanging, poisoning by ingestion, and carbon monoxide poisoning.

Typically, a suicide attempt occurs when a person's close emotional attachments are in danger, when he or she loses a significant family member or friend, or when he or she is seriously ill. Suicidal people often feel unable to manage their lives, and they frequently lack self-esteem. *Every suicidal act or gesture should be taken seriously, and the patient should be evaluated by a psychiatrist.* Always alert the police to a suicide or attempted suicide.

Many suicide victims make last-minute attempts to communicate their intentions; most do not really want to die but use the suicidal attempt as a way to get attention, receive help, or punish someone. Commonly, family members and friends will note a complete turnaround in the patient's mood. Such a change commonly occurs for a person who has decided on suicide, because it represents a solution to the person's problems. Regard this kind of turn-around as ominous — and be wary! When an individual phones to threaten suicide, someone should stay on the line until the rescue squad reaches the scene. When the EMS team arrives, the area should be surveyed quickly for instruments that a patient might use to cause self-injury. Discreetly remove any dangerous articles, and then consider the following management techniques. When patients attempt suicide, their medical treatment has priority.

Management

In managing a suicide emergency, your primary concern is to ensure the patient's safety and prevent further self-injury. The following techniques can be of help:

- Listen carefully to anything that the patient wants to tell you. Often a suicidal individual is simply lonely. Try to understand what the patient is telling you, and let him or her know that you understand.

- Assess the seriousness of the patient's thoughts and feelings. Always take a suicide threat seriously; if the patient has devised a concrete way to attempt suicide, the problem is more serious than if he or she has simply considered it but has not figured out *how*.

- Accept all of the patient's complaints and feelings. Do not underestimate what the patient might be feeling, and do not dismiss what *you* consider to be a minor complaint — it might be of great importance in reconstructing the events that precipitated the suicide attempt.

- Do not be afraid to ask the patient directly about suicidal thoughts. If you suspect that he or she might be suicidal, ask if he or she has considered suicide.

- Do not trust rapid recoveries. The patient might express initial relief following the incident and express confidence that all has returned to normal. Talking about feelings can cause a sense of relief,

IS YOUR PATIENT SUICIDAL?

MISCONCEPTION	FACT
People who talk about suicide don't commit suicide	Eight out of ten people who commit suicide have given definite warnings of their intentions. Almost no one commits suicide without first letting others know how he feels.
You can't stop a person who is suicidal. He's fully intent on dying.	Most people who are suicidal can't decide whether to live or die. Neither wish is necessarily stronger.
Once a person is suicidal, he's suicidal forever	People who want to kill themselves are only suicidal for a limited time. If they're saved from feelings of self-destruction, they often can go on to lead normal lives.
Improvement after severe depression means that the suicidal risk is over.	Most persons commit suicide within about 3 months after the beginning of "improvement," when they have the energy to carry out suicidal intentions. They also can show signs of apparent improvement because their uncertainty is gone — they've made the decision to kill themselves.
If a person has attempted suicide, he won't do it again.	More than 50% of those who commit suicide have previously attempted to do so.

ASSESSING LETHALITY

Age and sex: incidence of suicide is highest in adolescents (ages 15 to 24) and in persons age 50 and over. Men succeed at suicide more often than women.

Plan: Remember these points:
Does the patient have a plan? Is it well thought out?
Is it easy to carry out (and be successful)?
Are the means available? (For example, does the patient have pills collected, or a gun?
A detailed plan with availability of means carries maximum lethality potential.

Symptoms: What is the patient thinking and feeling?
Is he in control of his behavior? (Being out of control carries higher risk.)
Alcoholics and psychotics are at higher risk.
Depressed people are most at risk at the onset and at decline of depression.

Relationships with significant others: Does the patient have any positive supports?
Family, friends, therapist? Has he suffered any recent losses? Is he still in contact with people? Is he telling his family he's made his will? Is he giving away prized possessions?

Medical history: People with chronic illnesses are more likely to commit suicide than those with terminal illnesses. Incidence of suicide rises whenever a patient's body image is severely threatened — for example, after surgery or childbirth.

The goal is to shift the intensity of a suicidal act from a desire to commit suicide to conflict over the need to commit suicide. The following guidelines can help:

- Specifically talk to the patient about his intent.
- Ask the patient how serious he/she is about killing himself.
- Ask what his concerns are about taking his life. He will probably have some conflict.
- Ask why he thinks suicide is the answer to his problems.
- Ask what other alternatives the patient has considered and what problems block the choice of the other alternatives.
- Ask what hope the patient has - even if it seems remote or blocked.
- By this time you may have helped decrease the intensity of the patient's need to commit suicide, even though it may be temporary.
- Always transport a suicidal patient to the hospital for evaluation even though he says everything is okay. Police assistance may be necessary.

Source: **Assessment**, Nurses Reference Library, Intermed Communications, Inc. Springhouse, PA. Copyright © 1982, p. 116. Reprinted with permission. All rights reserved.

FIGURE 40-1

but the suicidal thoughts will most likely recur later. Relapses are frequent; you should transport the patient even if he seems to believe that he is "better."

- Be specific in your actions. Do something tangible for the patient. Arrange for his clergyman to meet him at the hospital. It is frustrating for the patient to feel that nothing of value was gained by the intervention, and it may actually contribute to suicide intentions.

- Never show disgust or horror when you care for the person. Chances are good that a feeling of rejection caused, in part, the contemplation of suicide. The patient needs to know that he or she is acceptable to other people, especially after what was attempted.

- Do not try to deny that the suicide attempt occurred. Your denial might specifically condemn the patient's feelings, which are very real to the patient.

- Never try to shock the patient out of a suicidal act. Never challenge the patient to go ahead. Do not try to argue him or her out of it. Remain calm. Point out that if the choice is to die, that choice is irreversible. As long as the patient remains alive, he or she has a chance of working out his or her problems. Remind the patient that although the depressed feeling is very real, it will pass. Tell the patient that matters are sure to get better if he or she decides to live and work things out.

- Never leave the patient alone during a suicidal crisis — isolation might precipitate a violent act.

- If it is necessary to protect the patient from harming himself, use restraints. Never use restraints as a substitute for observations, and never use metal handcuffs. Use restraints *only* if treatment would be dangerous or impossible without them.

- Transport the patient to a hospital for further care. *Every* patient who expresses suicidal thoughts or who attempts suicide should be transported.

☐ PARANOIA

Paranoia is a highly exaggerated or unwarranted mistrust or suspiciousness without cause. Paranoid patients are often hostile and uncooperative and suffer from the firmly held, but untrue, belief that someone is "out to get them." Most paranoid patients have elaborate delusions, mostly of persecution. They tend to brood over real or imagined injustices, carry grudges, and recall wrongs done to them years before. They seem cold, aloof, antagonistic, hypersensitive, defensive, and argumentative. They cannot accept fault or blame, avoid in-

timacy, and are excitable and unpredictable, displaying outbursts of bizarre or aggressive behavior. Their personalities often provoke dislike and anger in others.

Less common is the **paranoid schizophrenic,** who suffers debilitating distortions of speech and thought, bizarre delusions, hallucinations, social withdrawal, and lack of emotional expressiveness.

Management

To manage the paranoid patient:

- Explain all of your actions carefully and clearly (Figure 40-2). Let the patient ask questions, and answer them fully and clearly, even if they seem trivial or obvious to you. Avoid becoming angry at the patient's anger.

- Before you start the interview, make sure that the patient is unarmed. Arrange beforehand for law enforcement personnel to stand by in case the patient becomes suddenly violent or combative or suddenly produces a weapon.

- Do not try to be friendly or informal, but behave consistently. Paranoid individuals often misinterpret attempts at friendliness as an effort to deceive them. Maintain some distance, and act in a businesslike manner. Do not grant the patient special consideration or privileges — this will be misunderstood, and you will be suspected of trying to win the patient over so that you can harm him or her more easily. There is one exception to this rule: you may offer a special service if the patient

FIGURE 40-2 The paranoid patient should be dealt with in a quiet, formal manner. Explain all actions carefully and clearly.

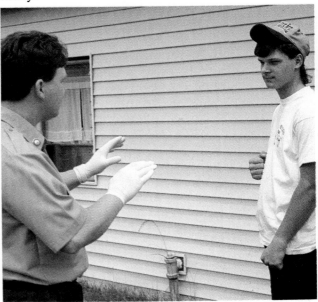

clearly requests it and fully explains why it is necessary.

- If the patient becomes suddenly hostile and it is necessary for you to overcome him or her with force, do so firmly. A hostile paranoid may be extremely dangerous, and it is important that he not think he can overcome you. If you make it clear that he or she cannot win, the patient will usually give up without a struggle.
- Do not go along with the delusions of such patients in order to pacify them.
- Interview family or friends in the patient's presence. Taking a relative aside and speaking in hushed tones only reinforces the paranoid's delusions that people are plotting against him or her.
- Use tact and firmness to persuade the patient to go to the hospital. Often, paranoid patients will go to the hospital willingly and will need no persuasion.

□ RAGE, HOSTILITY, AND VIOLENCE

Violence is generally an attempt to gain security or control; 60 to 75 percent of all psychiatric emergency patients will become assaultive or violent. The angry, violent patient may be ready to fight with anyone who approaches, and he or she may be difficult to control. The anger may be a response to illness, and the aggressive behavior may be the patient's way of coping with feelings of helplessness. Violence can be precipitated by patient mismanagement (real or perceived), psychosis, alcohol or drug intoxication, fear, panic, or head injury.

In approaching any psychiatric emergency scene, visually locate the patient before you physically approach. Determine whether the patient is disoriented, whether drugs or alcohol are involved, whether the patient has a gun or other weapon, whether the situation involves a hostage, and whether others are involved. *Early* in your assessment, *before* you physically approach the patient, determine whether you and your partner can handle the situation alone. Even a small person who is sufficiently agitated can be very difficult to handle. *If you doubt that you can handle the patient alone, summon the police and wait for their arrival.*

Early signs that a person may have lost control and may become violent include pacing nervously, shouting, threatening, cursing, throwing things, or having clenched teeth and/or fists. In any situation, *follow your intuition* — if you suspect that a person may become violent, prepare for violence.

Management

To manage an assaultive or violent patient, do the following:

- *Your first priority is to protect yourself.* Never go into a potentially violent situation by yourself.
- While you are en route to a call where violence might be involved, check to see whether police are also en route to the scene.
- While you are still a few blocks from the area, stop the siren and turn off the lightbar.
- Routinely park two or three houses away from the address, or safely outside the **killing zone:** if someone inside the house has a gun, an area about 120 degrees in front of the house is at least partially exposed to fire.
- Walk on the grass, not the sidewalk.
- If you are using a flashlight, hold it beside — not in front of — your body.
- If you are walking with a partner, walk single-file; the last person in line should carry the life kit. Only the first person in line should carry a flashlight; anyone behind the first person will backlight the ones in front.
- As you approach the scene, make a mental map of all possible concealment (objects that will hide you, such as shrubbery) and cover (objects that will both hide you and stop bullets, such as trees). Keep scanning the darkness for movement.
- Stand to the side of a door when you knock on it; never stand in front of it. Take a half-second look at windows and corners. If you need to take a longer look, change positions.
- As soon as the door is open, assess the situation before you decide whether to retreat and call for reinforcement or to have your partner move the unit up in front of the building. Never appear to block the patient's route of escape.
- Negotiate with the patient from a safe distance (at least six feet away) and position (facing patient); never turn your back on the patient.
- Keep the door to the room open, and identify as many exits as possible. *Regardless of the situation, make absolutely sure that you have at least one certain route of escape.*
- Have other rescuers remove other people slowly from the room. You may need to use a predesignated signal to let them know they should start taking people to a safe place.
- Approach the patient slowly and quietly; don't rush. Let the patient clearly see that you are not going to make a sudden move. Stay at least six feet away from him as you talk, and stand at a "friendly angle" of 45 degrees.
- Talk quietly, and use a nonconfrontational tone of voice. Encourage the patient to think — ask for detailed responses to questions. Doing this will di-

vert his attention to the situation instead of to the patient's anger.

- Use a calm, soothing manner when dealing with the patient; avoid reacting with anger and defensiveness.
- If you are going up a stairway, keep your back to it and your downhill side against the wall. That way, you only need to make a ninety-degree turn to move out.
- Scan the area for possible weapons, such as scissors, knives, and firearms.
- Have trouble codes. On emergency calls, have the dispatcher make routine checks every ten minutes. If you fail to respond with the correct code, it means that you need help.
- Have emergency plans with your partner so that you have a personal safety procedure just as you have a medical emergency procedure.
- Help the patient maintain a sense of dignity.
- Show your concern, and actively show the patient that you are listening. Nod your head, and repeat some of the things he or she is saying in your own words to show that you understand.
- Use the words "we" and "us" to inspire a feeling of cooperation.
- Don't disturb the patient any more than necessary. If he or she becomes too edgy, abandon your efforts to provide examination and treatment until calm is restored.
- Do not take the patient's anger personally, and avoid overreacting to anything said.
- Explain what you are doing carefully, step by step. Do not lie. If trust in you is not established, the patient may become violent.
- Acknowledge the patient's fear and upset.
- *Never* ignore or disregard a weapon. In a calm and nonconfrontational way, tell the patient that you want to help, but you cannot do so until the weapon is released. Ask the patient to put the weapon in a neutral place.
- Give the patient instructions regarding his or her behavior. Clearly state the consequences of an aggressive behavior *before* it happens.
- Tell the patient briefly and honestly what he or she can expect from you.
- If the patient becomes too agitated or increasingly violent, back off. Discontinue touching the patient, and wait for reinforcements to arrive.

Barroom Calls

If you are called to a barroom:

- If the call occurs in the daytime, wear sunglasses en route if you can; they will cut down on the length of time your eyes will need to adjust to the darkness of the barroom.
- Enter the room slowly. Have your partner stand and survey the crowd at all times. Do not turn your back on the crowd. If the situation becomes tense, retreat temporarily and call for support.

Calls to Car Passengers

If you are called to a person in a car:

- Park at least one car-length behind the patient's vehicle with your wheels turned slightly to the left. If you have to back up, you will not go any deeper into the shoulder of the road.
- Align your headlights in the middle of the trunk of the patient's car, and turn them to high beam. Try to reflect your beams off the rear-view mirror, illuminating the car's interior and also making your approach more difficult for the patient to see.
- While still in your vehicle, write down the patient's license number and leave it at the radio. Note how many people are in the car, their positions, and the driver's apparent condition.
- As you pass the trunk, check to see if it is locked; look on the rear seat and the floor as you pass.
- Have your partner open the passenger door a split second before you open the driver's door; if you are alone, wait for help to arrive.
- Keep your eyes on the victim's hands. If there are any sudden movements, retreat.
- Keep behind the center post. Carry an object, such as a report book or bag, that you can throw at the occupant's face if he or she becomes violent.
- If you have to retreat, immediately get into your vehicle and back up rapidly; move 100 to 150 yards to clear the killing zone.

Use of Restraints

A more difficult situation arises when a patient is out of control. If no one is able to communicate with him and you believe that he may be dangerous to himself or others, you must notify the police. Never leave a violent patient alone; watch him constantly, and remain alert.

If you are called to help transport a violent patient against his or her will, you may need to use restraints. *Even if a violent patient comes with you voluntarily, be prepared to use restraints — the situation may change at any time during transport. Restraints may require police authorization; follow local protocol. Do nothing unless it is authorized by law.* It is critical that you protect yourself legally; if you are not authorized in your state to use restraints, wait until someone with authority arrives.

Restraints should be padded so that they will not injure a patient who struggles against them; use soft leather or cloth restraints, but never metal handcuffs (Figures 40-3 and 40-4). When applying restraints, explain what you are doing (for the benefit of both the patient and any bystanders). Tell the patient that the restraints are to protect him or her and others from injury.

Remember that a violent physical struggle is usually brief: most people cannot sustain the intensity needed. If you still feel the need for restraints, follow these steps (Figures 40-5–40-21 on pages 602–606):

1. Gather enough people to clearly overpower the patient *before* you try to restrain him or her. Effective teamwork is more important than the strength of any individual team member.

2. If not physically injured, place the patient in a supine position.

3. Apply a restraint strap to each wrist and ankle, or use improvised restraints with a girth hitch. You can use a sheet as a girth hitch to fasten both ankles to the main frame of the cot.

4. For the most effective restraint, fasten the patient's arms across the chest, with wrists fastened to the main frame of the cot.

5. Secure the tails of the restraints to opposite sides of the stretcher frame.

6. Secure the patient's body with two or three straps around the chest, waist, and thighs. Make sure that none of the straps are unduly tight and that none will impair the patient's breathing.

7. Never inflict pain or use unwarranted force in restraining a patient.

8. Once you have applied restraints, do not remove them en route to the hospital.

9. Never bargain with the patient, and *do not* agree to remove the restraints upon a promise to behave well.

10. It is always preferable to restrain a violent patient, but if you have to transport a violent patient without restraints, have the patient lie down. Watch him or her at all times. Position yourself between the patient and the door in case you need to exit rapidly. If the patient becomes dangerous, restrain the patient en route.

11. If possible, leave any kind of restraining to the police.

Management of a Crime Scene

At times, you may need to handle a patient at a crime scene. To avoid disturbing crucial evidence and to keep your treatment priorities intact, use the following guidelines:

• Your first priority is to protect yourself; your sec-

□ Examples of Commercial Wrist and Ankle Restraining Straps

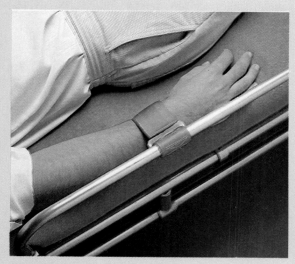

FIGURE 40-3

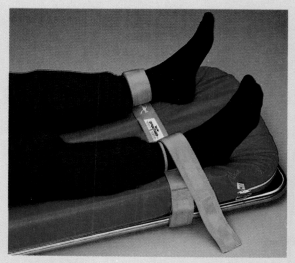

FIGURE 40-4

ond priority is to treat and protect your patient. If the crime perpetrator is still on the scene, notify police and wait for their arrival before attempting treatment. Follow local protocol.

- Secure the crime scene; do not allow bystanders through.

- Introduce yourself to the patient carefully and state your purpose (that you are there to help he or she) so he doesn't become confused and think you are another aspect of the crime.

- Where appropriate, assist police in collecting and recording anything on the patient, such as blood, hair, seminal fluid, gunpowder residue, or clothing fibers, that may indicate a crime. *Follow local protocol.*

- Take extreme care not to disturb any evidence that is not directly on the patient's body (footprints, soil, broken glass, tire tracks, and so on).

- Never touch or move suspected weapons unless it is absolutely necessary for treating the patient's injuries. If you do touch a weapon, do not disturb any fingerprints that may be on the weapon. Pick up a gun by the edge of the grip, and use gauze pads to pick up a knife at the very edge of the blade.

- Wear surgical gloves throughout treatment to avoid leaving your own fingerprints at the crime scene.

- If you need to tear or cut away clothing to expose a wound, make sure that you do not cut through a bullet hole or knife slash in the clothing. Keep the clothing and submit it as evidence to the police.

- If the patient was strangled and still has the rope or cord around the neck, cut it instead of untying it — the knot can be used as evidence and may identify the perpetrator.

- If the patient is conscious, do not burden him or her with questions about the crime. Treat injuries and transport.

- Realize that the patient will probably show extremes of emotion, and be prepared to handle them.

- Document in writing who is at the crime scene when you arrive.

- If the patient is obviously dead when you arrive, do nothing and disturb nothing. Summon the police, if they have not already been called, and wait for their arrival.

□ SPOUSE ABUSE

Spouse abuse is violent behavior between two people who are involved in an intimate relationship. Either the man or the woman may be the abuser, but the largest percentage of cases involve the man beating his female partner. An estimated 1.8 million women are victims of batterings from their husbands or live-in boyfriends. While spouse abuse (as with all other forms of abuse) is probably grossly underreported, it is estimated that one-fourth of all women experience beatings at some time in their marriage, and that one-sixth of all couples have at least one episode of violence each year of their marriage. Pregnancy can increase the stress that leads to abuse, and it is estimated that approximately one-fourth of all women who are battered are pregnant at the time of the beating. Spouse abuse is estimated to be the single major cause of injury to women.

Abuse of a spouse may be physical, emotional, financial, or sexual. In about one-fifth of all wife abuse cases, the children are also abused — and half of all child abuse cases occur in conjunction with spouse abuse.

The typical female victim of spouse abuse was abused herself as a child, is depressed, may have suicidal ideas, abuses drugs, was married as a teenager, and was pregnant before marriage. She may have a variety of physical complaints, the most common being gastrointestinal symptoms, persistent headache, chest pain, insomnia, and anxiety.

Suspect spouse abuse in the following situations:

- The woman has multiple injuries.

- There are injuries to the face or head (especially the areas covered by hair), back, chest (especially the breasts), stomach, and/or buttocks. Accidental injuries usually involve the extremities.

- The patient's story of how she was injured is not consistent with her injuries, or her explanation is vague or simplistic. She may even refuse to tell you how she was injured.

- The partner is extremely oversolicitous (an incident of battering is almost always followed by a period of remorse and courtesy as the partner feels sorry about the beating).

- The partner does not want to be separated from the injured spouse during your interview, assessment, or treatment.

- The partner answers all the questions on behalf of the injured spouse.

- There are injuries in various stages of healing, indicating repeated battering incidents.

- The patient is experiencing an abortion, miscarriage, or premature delivery that cannot be explained by usual medical cause or that seems to be associated with blows to the abdomen.

In managing a spouse abuse situation, provide calm, gentle reassurance to the patient. Treat injuries as you would for any other patient, provide the patient

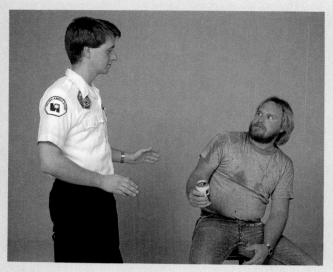

FIGURE 40-5 The angry, combative patient is ready to fight with anyone who approaches. Convey a sense of helpfulness rather than of hostility or frustration. Present a comfortable, confident, and professional manner.

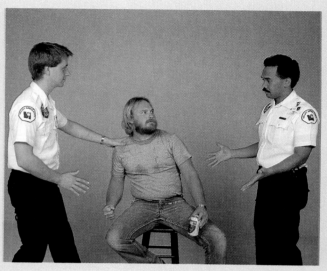

FIGURE 40-6 If a possibility of danger exists, the patient should be interviewed with another EMT present. Identify yourself and let the patient know what you expect.

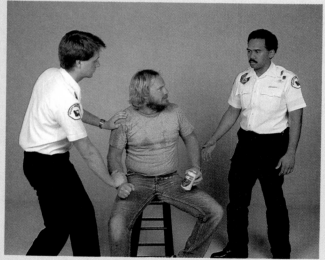

FIGURE 40-7 EMTs should avoid reacting with anger and defensiveness and should not threaten or make physical gestures until sufficient help is available to safely restrain the patient.

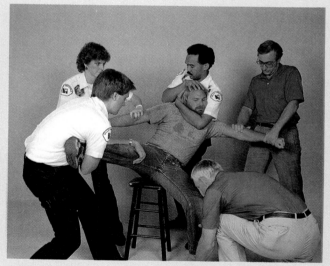

FIGURE 40-8 Never try to restrain a patient until you have sufficient help and an appropriate plan. If necessary, create a safe zone and wait for police. *Follow local protocol.*

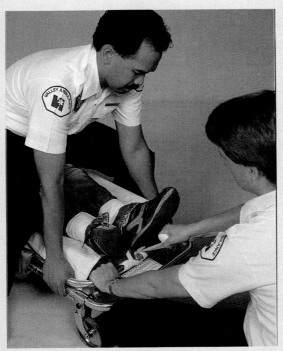

FIGURE 40-9 Place patient on ambulance stretcher and apply ankle and wrist restraints.

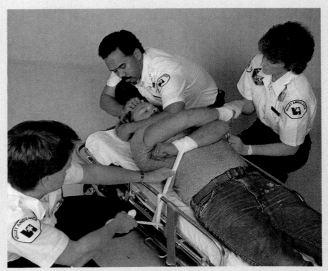

FIGURE 40-10 Pull arms tightly across patient's chest and tie on opposite sides of stretcher frame.

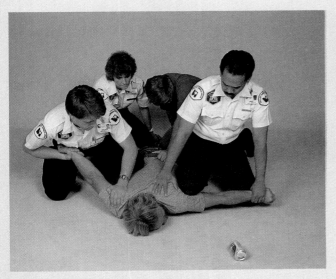

FIGURE 40-11 Never use more force than is necessary to restrain a patient.

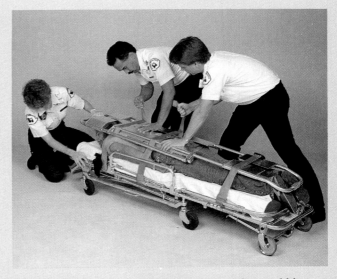

FIGURE 40-12 If necessary, a scoop stretcher could be secured over a combative patient for extra protection.

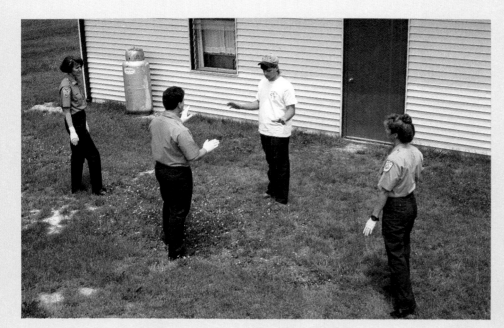

FIGURE 40-13 If it is necessary to restrain the patient, make sure you have adequate assistance.

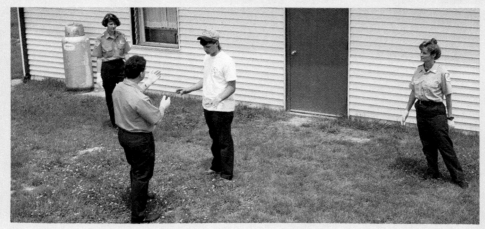

FIGURE 40-14 Offer the patient a final opportunity to cooperate and encircle the patient.

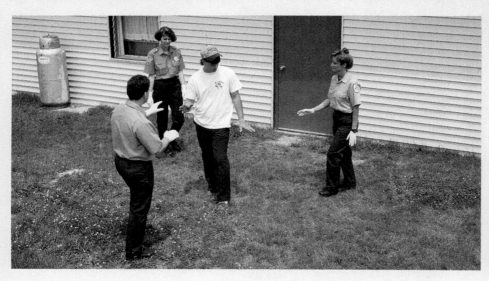

FIGURE 40-15 The patient cannot keep his eye on more than one person at a time. Two of the EMTs should rush the patient at the same time.

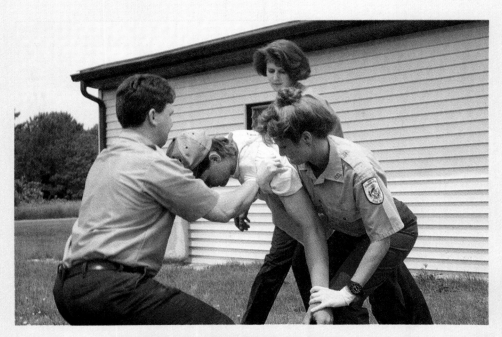

FIGURE 40-16 If necessary, "take down" the patient by placing a leg in front of the patient's leg and bringing the patient forward.

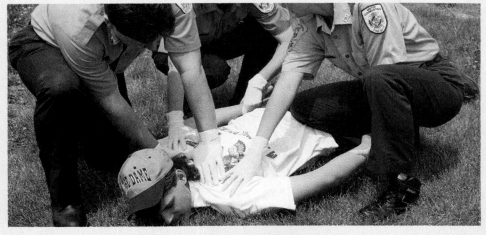

FIGURE 40-17 Maintain the patient on his or her stomach so that he or she cannot kick.

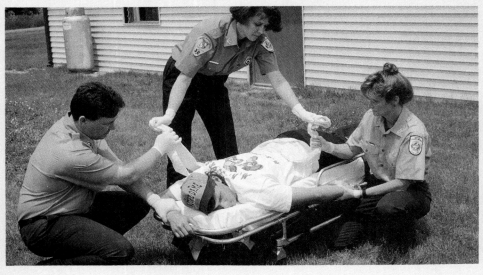

FIGURE 40-18 Place the patient on the stretcher face down and restrain as directed.

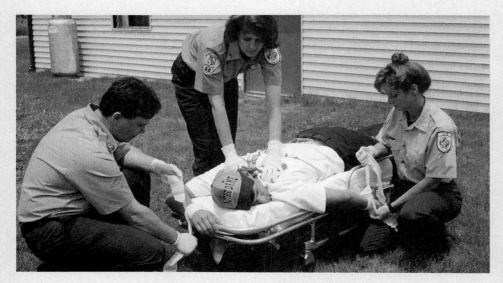

FIGURE 40-19 Secure the arms and legs.

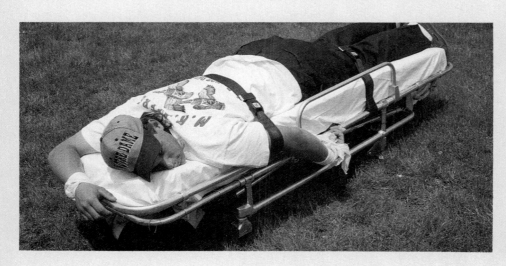

FIGURE 40-20 Prepared patient for transport.

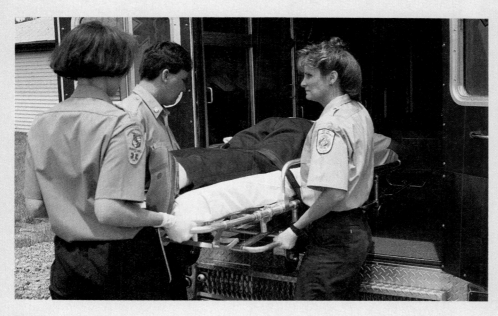

FIGURE 40-21 Transport with adequate assistance.

with privacy. Have the woman's spouse wait in another room or a separate area until you have ruled out the possibility of abuse. Ask the woman in a calm, nonjudgmental way if she was battered. Once separated from the perpetrator, many women will freely admit that they were abused — but many won't even when separated from the abuser. Even if injuries are not that severe, explain that she needs to be transported to the hospital for further observation by a physician. *Always* report your suspicions to the receiving physician, and provide the patient with information on available shelters and programs where she can get help.

□ RAPE AND SEXUAL ASSAULT

Forcible rape is the fastest-growing crime in the United States; according to FBI statistics, a woman is sexually assaulted every seven minutes in this country. The crime of rape rose 54 percent in just one decade, and an estimated one in thirty American women will be raped at some time in their lifetime. In addition, countless children and men are raped or sexually assaulted each year. Even with these frightening figures, the FBI estimates that only about 10 percent of all rapes are reported.

Rape is one of the most devastating life crises that can occur. It involves both emotional and physical trauma. Legally, rape is defined as the carnal knowledge of one person by another without consent by compulsion through force, threat, or fraud. Sexual assault is defined as any touch that the victim did not initiate or agree to and that is imposed by coercion, threat, deception, or threats of physical violence. The rapist can be a stranger, but more often is someone that the victim knows, at least slightly. Rape is often committed by a relative, friend, boyfriend, date, neighbor, mother's boyfriend, or classmate.

Rape Trauma Syndrome

The commission of an intensely personal experience under forced or terrifying circumstances can disintegrate a person's defense structure. Most rape victims go into acute emotional shock during or shortly after the attack. Common physical reactions to rape include:

- Struggling and screaming to avoid penetration.
- Physical and psychological paralysis.
- Pain and shock from penetration or physical abuse.
- Choking, gagging, nausea, vomiting.
- Urinating.
- Hyperventilating.

- Loss of consciousness.
- Seizure, especially if the victim has epilepsy.
- Dazed state.

Following rape, most patients experience a great deal of disorganization in their lives. This emotional trauma follows a pattern described as "rape trauma syndrome," which involves four general sequences:

1. Acute (impact) reaction: taking effect immediately after the rape and continuing for several days.
2. Outward adjustment: lasting weeks or months after the rape.
3. Depression: intermittent and recurring for days and months after the rape.
4. Acceptance and resolution: taking months or years to resolve.

Your major concern as an EMT is to provide medical care, not to act as judge and jury in convicting someone of rape. As an EMT, you will be concerned with the acute (impact) reaction phase.

Rape is a difficult and complex problem involving potential physical and emotional trauma as well as significant legal ramifications. Supportive handling of the rape patient is of critical importance, especially during the acute phase. The patient's coping system has already been stressed to the limit by the attack itself. Yet, the patient must face your care and interview, the family, and the interview with police, and must undergo medical examination for injuries and possible care for pregnancy or sexually transmitted disease. Later, the patient may face the trauma of a courtroom trial or have to handle unresolved emotion if the rapist is not brought to trial or is found not guilty.

Rape patients react to this life-threatening situation individually. Their behavior varies in sequence and time element as they are affected by their own ego strength, social support network, family up-bringing, number and punitive behavior of assailants, and so on. The tortured, beaten, and brutally assaulted patient may encounter greater problems.

Too often, however, the seriousness of a rape is equated with the amount of physical damage suffered by the patient. This is deceptive, for regardless of whether physical injury occurs, the patient suffers profound emotional trauma. Because of current social and legal traditions, the patient who sustains external physical injury as evidence of the assault is more readily believed and often fares better than the patient who is not beaten or physically marked. Long after physical wounds have healed, the world still appears as a traumatic environment to the rape patient trying to relearn trust in the presence of hurt and fear.

Management

EMTs, and particularly police, are often called to respond to a report of rape. The following are essential considerations:

- Your immediate reaction is important. Do not impose your feelings on the patient. Try to determine the patient's emotional state. Get the facts with empathy, not sympathy.
- Action can minimize the helplessness that the patient may be feeling. Tell the patient what can and should be done immediately.
- While the gender of a rescuer has less impact than

FIGURE 40-22 Assist the rape patient with calming and supportive reassurance. While assisting the rape patient, speak softly, ask and answer questions simply and directly, and do not be judgmental. Encourage the patient to report the rape.

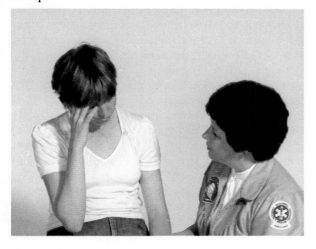

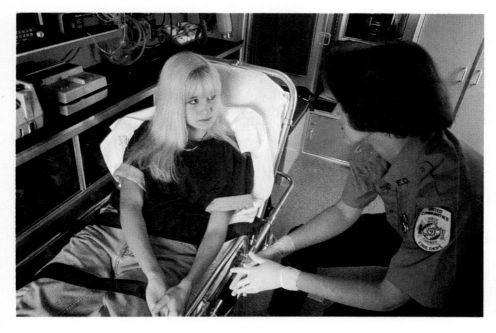

the rescuer's ability to relate well, a female patient might be comforted if a female EMT or police officer is available to talk to her (Figure 40-22) and to accompany her to the hospital after initial treatment in the field (Figure 40-23).

- Call the police to the scene, and encourage the patient to cooperate with the police. Stress that it is the patient's prerogative to answer questions — and remember that a refusal to report the incident or prosecute the rapist does not mean the rape did not occur.
- If you are informed that the victim is not injured or if the victim is obviously uninjured, postpone the patient survey to avoid further violation of the victim.
- In assessing the patient, do the primary survey as for any other patient. Treat any life-threatening injuries as appropriate. Check for trauma, especially around the thighs, lower abdomen, and buttocks. If vaginal bleeding is significant, give appropriate care.
- Provide normal physical care for existing injuries.
- Once life-threatening injuries have been corrected, slow down — conduct further surveys and treatment slowly and calmly.
- Do not cleanse the patient.
- Keep the patient from cleansing, douching, or urinating; doing so will destroy important evidence.
- Once you have cared for the patient's injuries, check the surroundings for evidence. Bag each piece separately and transport it with the patient; use paper bags instead of plastic bags; the latter encourage overgrowth of bacteria. If you had to

FIGURE 40-23 If possible, have a female EMT or paramedic accompany the victim of alleged sexual assault to the hospital.

remove any of the patient's clothing during treatment, place it in a paper bag and transport it with the patient. *Collect evidence even if the victim of the rape does not intend to prosecute the rapist.*

- Transport the patient. Be supportive and calming; help the patient feel safe.

- Do not surround the patient with silence or reproach. Alienation promotes guilt and shame, as if the patient has done something wrong.

- Notify the receiving facility that you are transporting a rape patient. The hospital can thus receive the patient calmly and efficiently, easing the patient's emotional state considerably.

- In your report to the emergency department, state only what the patient said, not what you observed. Your opinion as to whether the rape occurred should not be included in the report. Every rape is a potential court case, and your report is a legal document. Be thorough and accurate. Follow local protocol.

- As an emergency responder, your role in helping the patient deal with the attack is vital. You can be the first to help the patient begin to overcome the stigma of the attack and readjust to a normal life. Do not be callous or judgmental; speak softly and explain everything you can to the patient. Do not be surprised if the patient seems angry or uncooperative — this is a normal response under the circumstances, and you should not take it personally. Do not force emergency care on a patient who is resisting due to fear or embarrassment. Care for the patient as you would any critically ill or injured person.

- If any members of the patient's family are present when you arrive, treat them with sensitivity. Let them know that the patient will be cared for. Help alleviate their fears by explaining the procedures that will be followed. Try to remain completely nonjudgmental with the family as well as with the patient.

☐ DEATH AND DYING

Most of the dying patients who you see as an EMT will be slipping in and out of consciousness. Occasionally, however, you will encounter a dying person who is alert and in touch with what is about to happen.

A person who is faced with the prospect of dying is clearly experiencing a psychological emergency. Your first consideration should be the patient's feelings. Provide reassurance, and do what you can to calm any fears. Make sure that the patient understands that you are doing everything possible, and that you will see that

he or she gets to a hospital as quickly as possible for further help.

Of course, you should continue to care for the patient's physical injuries and illnesses, but you should devote prime consideration to his or her emotional needs. Many dying people will want messages delivered to survivors. Make yourself available and take notes on what the dying person is telling you — something that will help make the individual feel more at ease. Your notes should be precise, because some of them may have legal implications.

Occasionally, you may be caring for two patients at the same time — one who is dying, and one who is not. The idea of a patient dying may be very disturbing to the survivor, and you should reassure him that you are doing everything possible to save the person.

It is difficult for anyone to deal with death, so come to terms with your own feelings about what is happening. Everyone has a hard time dealing with death, and your own feelings are completely normal — do not let them interfere with your ability to administer care.

Help a Dying Patient

To help lessen a dying patient's emotional burden:

- Tell the patient who you are, what you are doing, what others are doing, and where you are going to take him or her.

- Avoid negative statements about the patient's condition. Even a semiconscious patient can hear what you say and can read fear into your words.

- Assure the patient that you will locate and notify his or her family of what has happened. He or she may or may not be able to help you, but make a concerted effort to find the family. They will not only be of great comfort, but they will want to talk to the patient before he or she dies. Tell the family briefly who you are, what has happened, and where they can meet you and the patient. Make sure that they understand the urgency and seriousness of the situation, and encourage them to have someone else drive them.

- Unless the family lives a great distance away, do not tell them over the phone that the patient is dying. Say something like, "Your relative is seriously ill, and you need to come immediately." This type of notification is usually done by hospital personnel. Follow local protocol.

- Allow family members (except, of course, young children) to stay with the patient during resuscitation efforts.

- Help the patient become oriented to his or her surroundings. Explain again what has happened and where he or she is.

- Be honest with the patient. State the facts about what is happening to his or her body, but be tactful.

- Allow for some hope. The patient may ask if he is dying; do not confirm this. Patients who do the most poorly are often the ones left in a black-and-white situation. Instead, say something like, "I don't know that for sure. You and I are going to fight this thing out together. I won't give up on you, and don't you give up on yourself." If the patient insists that he or she is going to die, say something like, "That might be possible. But we can still try the best we can, can't we?"

- If other family members were present during the accident, make sure that they are stable before you tell them the details of the death. Will and desire to survive are often derived from a person's desire to be reunited with loved ones. Knowledge of the death of a significant other may seriously impede recovery, especially during the first critical hours. Do not volunteer information unless you are asked. Follow local protocol.

Responding to the Patient's Family and Friends

People facing the sudden death of a loved one will react to that death much as they would if they were facing their own death. In responding to the needs of family and friends of a patient who is dying or has died:

- Offer help to family members who might have been at the scene of the accident. Your first concern upon arriving at the scene is the injured person, but members of the patient's family may themselves be slightly injured or in a state of shock after having witnessed the accident or injury. Do not ignore them in your concern for the injured patient.

- Involve family members during resuscitation; they can help retrieve equipment, direct traffic, and so on.

- Communicate with family members throughout resuscitation; give straightforward answers to questions. Report what you know to be true, but do *not* guess or make assumptions.

- If a family member asks to accompany the patient in the ambulance, if possible make necessary arrangements for this family member to do so. Both the patient and the relative benefit. The patient feels somewhat reassured if he can see a familiar face and can ask questions and have them answered. The relative benefits from the knowledge that someone is with the patient to lend support and reassurance. It is a mistake not to allow the relative to ride in the ambulance with the patient, because by the time the relative arrives at the hospital, the patient has often been taken to surgery or intensive care, or has died.

- Even though your team may be working frantically to save the patient's life, the family may want to see the patient. Stay with the family, if possible, and keep them constantly informed of the patient's condition. If possible, arrange for a specific time when they *can* see the patient.

- Family members may react with extreme anger, lashing out at you or other medical personnel who attended the patient. There is nothing personal in this kind of attack, it is a normal part of the grieving process, and it is healthy for the family members to vent their frustrations and anger so that they can move on to the next step in the grieving process. Try to understand their feelings. Do not become hostile or angry in retaliation.

- Be cautious with people who do not express any emotion or who react only slightly. These individuals should be treated with great concern. People who cry and scream after a sudden death are able to express their grief; those who are unable to — or who do not — express emotion may eventually experience pathological grieving.

- If relatives arrive at the scene before the patient dies — even if death is imminent — arrange for family members and relatives to see the patient. It is important that they be allowed to express their love once more — whether it is verbal or nonverbal. You might provide them with the chance to ask forgiveness for some wrongdoing or to answer some unfinished business before it is too late. Some, however, may simply need reassurance that everything possible is being done to save the patient.

- Some may want to touch or hold the body after death. Let them do so if it does not compromise your care and local protocol. There are things that you can do to improve the appearance of the body. Wash the face and hands to remove blood, vomitus, and foul odors. Cover any severely mutilated part of the body with clean linen, or bandage the injured part. If necessary, elevate the head for a few minutes to clear out some of the facial orifices. Make sure that the family knows in advance that the patient is mutilated and that you have covered the mutilated parts. Do not rush around trying to get the relatives away if it is not interfering with your tasks at hand.

- Show utmost respect for the patient, especially when death is imminent. Families in the stressful situation of having a relative die soon will be extra sensitive to how the dying relative is treated; even attitudes and unspoken messages are perceived. Show the greatest respect possible for the patient's dignity; even if in a coma, talk to the patient as if he or she were fully conscious. Explain what you are going to do before you do it.

- Encourage the family to talk to a comatose patient; they gain relief from this, especially if they arrived after the patient lost consciousness. Tell them that the patient still may be able to hear and understand, even though he or she is unable to respond. This may give the family some hope of communicating with the patient one last time and may help immensely in their adjustment to the death.

- Carefully explain (without wasting time in giving care) to the family any procedures that you need to carry out — they are concerned about what you are doing and what their loved one is being put through.

- Allow family members to express themselves. Acknowledge that it is all right. They should be able to scream, cry, or act in any way they wish without risk of being censored. Have someone stay with them. Eveyone reacts to grief in a different way.

- Help family members in any way you can. If they ask you to pray with them, do so. Families are often receptive to advice given them when it is done in the form of a prayer.

- If you know the cause of death, explain it gently and kindly in terms the family can understand. Stay at the family's eye level. Outline completely what was done to save the patient's life so that the family will know everything possible was done.

- Stay with the family until the medical examiner or coroner arrives. Follow local protocol.

chapter 41

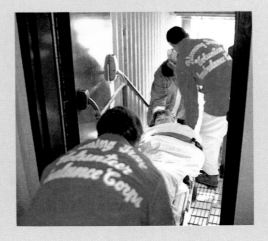

Patient Packaging, Moving, and Triage

✳ OBJECTIVES

- ■ Outline the principles of patient packaging and moving, including special concerns for moving infants, toddlers, obstetric patients, the elderly, and the handicapped.

- ■ Recognize the circumstances and types of moves that can be used in an emergency.

- ■ Explain the basic guidelines for moving patients, including the advantages and disadvantages of common equipment.

- ■ Describe and demonstrate how to use the various lifts, carries, and equipment in moving patients.

- ■ Outline the principles of triage and describe a three-level triage system.

This chapter was written in conjunction with Thom Dick, EMS author, teacher, and full-time paramedic in La Mesa, California.

It is recommended that EMTs wear protective gloves whenever there is a possibility of coming in contact with a patient's blood, body fluids, mucous membranes, traumatic wounds, or sores. See Chapter 31.

Securing the safety of an accident scene, gaining access to the patient, and assessing, treating, packaging, and transporting the patient are the basic elements of pre-hospital emergency care. The field care that you render as an EMT is temporary care, meant to stabilize the patient until definitive medical care can be given at a hospital or other facility. After initiating emergency treatment, you must "package" the patient — simply stated, get him or her ready for transport. As difficult as it may seem, you need to continue emergency care throughout the packaging process and during transport for the best possible results.

Some texts on rescue offer more "rules" than information on how to package patients — but few "rules" apply across the board when it comes to preparing patients for transport. As a rescuer, you will face many different kinds of problems and will quickly find out that there is more than one "right way" to package and move a patient. It is important to analyze the advantages and disadvantages of each method and become proficient in the use of each one. Then, when you are confronted with a situation, you will need to judge which will work best. Choosing the best equipment for moving a patient depends on early observations about a patient's condition and environment. Your first responsibility is to detect safety hazards in the environment — both for yourself and for your patient.

☐ WHEN TO MAKE AN EMERGENCY MOVE

Normally, top priorities during a rescue call include maintaining the patient's airway, breathing, circulation, and spinal status and controlling hemorrhage. Under normal conditions, you should do all of those things before you move a patient. In fact, the rule of thumb is to make sure you have controlled any life-threatening problems and stabilized the patient before beginning transport.

But when the scene of the accident is unstable, threatening your life as well as that of your patient, your priority changes — you must first move the patient. Under life-threatening conditions, you need to move the patient without taking normal precautions, like splinting. You may have to risk injury to the patient in order to save his or her life. *You should make an emergency move only when no other options are available.*

Obviously, there are several situations in which you should not enter the scene at all until law enforcement personnel have secured it. You must avoid increasing the size or scope of an emergency by becoming a victim yourself, especially when other rescuers will need to risk their lives in order to help you.

Consider an emergency move under the following conditions:

- Uncontrolled traffic: If you do not have the immediate resources to direct traffic away from the accident victim, move the victim to safety as quickly as possible.
- Physically unstable surroundings: Immediately move a patient out of an environment that poses an immediate threat to life, such as a vehicle that you cannot stabilize and is in danger of toppling off an embankment.
- Exposure to hazardous materials: When a patient is directly exposed to substances that can cause grave injury or death, move him or her immediately. A common example is a patient who is lying in gasoline spilled from an overturned vehicle.
- Fire: Fire should always be considered a grave threat, not only to the victims, but to the rescuers.
- Hostile crowds: Crowds are at the very least a nuisance — but when you sense that onlookers are becoming unruly or hostile, move the patient to a safer place immediately. This applies especially to accidents that occur in bars, where people may behave unpredictably.
- Repositioning: There will be times when you need to reposition a patient in order to provide life-saving treatment. You may need to move a patient in order to control hemorrhage, for example; or a patient who needs CPR may not be on a firm, flat surface where you can effectively perform it.
- Access: In cases where more than one patient has been injured, you may need to move one patient in order to gain access to another. This may especially apply if you need to move a moderately injured person in order to gain access to one who has life-threatening injuries.
- Weather conditions: Move a patient immediately if you cannot minimize or control his or her exposure to dangerous weather in any other way. Generally, the patient is in a dangerous situation if the weather is very cold (especially if the patient is wet), very hot (especially if the patient is lying on asphalt), or windy enough to turn objects into projectiles.
- Patient demand: The patient may demand to be moved. You should always try to convince a patient that it's in his or her best interest *not* to be moved, but he or she may insist on it because of an unpleasant smell, sight, or sound — or just because he or she wants it. It's illegal to restrain a patient against his or her will unless you are a law enforcement officer; in these cases, you must move a patient if you can't convince the patient otherwise.

When you need to move a patient immediately —

such as when he or she is in danger of an explosion, collision, fall, fire, or hazardous material spill — applying a cervical collar and immobilizing the spine waste precious time. However, there are several safe ways to move a patient even under emergency conditions. They include the blanket drag, the shirt drag, the sheet drag, and the fireman's carry.

□ EMERGENCY MOVES

The Blanket Drag

The **blanket drag** is an effective way for a single rescuer to move a patient to safety. Follow these techniques (Figure 41-1):

1. Spread a blanket alongside the patient; gather about half the blanket into lengthwise pleats.
2. Roll the patient away from you onto his or her side, and tuck the pleated part of the blanket beneath the patient as far as you can.
3. Roll the patient back onto the center of the blanket, preferably on his or her back; wrap the blanket securely around the patient.
4. Grab the part of the blanket that is beneath the patient's head, and drag the patient toward you. If you need to traverse a stairway, keep the body parallel to the overall angle of the stairway and keep the patient's body from bouncing on the steps.
5. If you do not have a blanket, roll the patient onto a coat and drag him to safety.

The Shirt Drag

If the patient is wearing a shirt, use it to support his head and to pull him or her. Follow these guidelines (Figure 41-2):

1. Fasten the patient's hands or wrists loosely to-

FIGURE 41-1 Blanket drag.

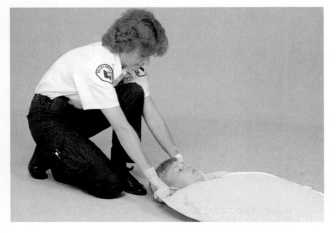

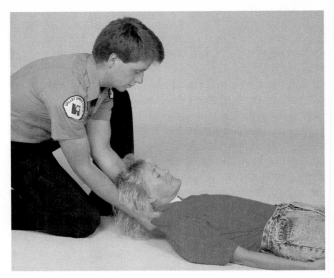

FIGURE 41-2 Shirt drag.

gether, and link them to his or her belt or pants; use a small Velcro strap or rubber tourniquet. You need to prevent the patient's arms from flopping toward you or slipping out of the shirt.
2. Grasp the shoulders of the patient's shirt under the head to form a support.
3. Using the shirt as a "handle," pull the patient toward you. Be careful not to strangle the patient; the pulling power should engage the axillas, not the patient's neck.
4. The **shirt drag** cannot be used if the patient is wearing only a tee-shirt.

The Sheet Drag

Sheets can be used in many ways to move patients; one of the easiest is the **sheet drag,** or the fashioning of a drag harness out of a sheet. Follow these guidelines (Figure 41-3):

FIGURE 41-3 Sheet drag.

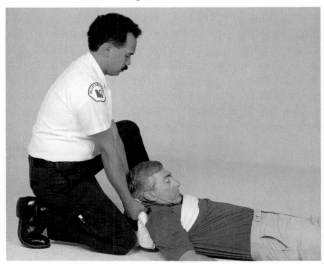

1. Fold a sheet several times lengthwise to form a narrow, long "harness."

2. Lie the folded sheet centered across the patient's chest at the nipple line.

3. Pull the ends of the sheet under the patient's arms at the axillas and behind the patient's head; twist the ends of the sheet together to form a triangular support for the head, being careful not to pull the patient's hair.

4. Grasping the loose ends of the sheet, pull the patient toward you.

5. The sheet drag can also work well to slide a patient out of a car and onto a board when you need to move him or her head-first.

The Fireman's Carry

The **fireman's carry** is not as safe as most ground-level moves because it places the patient's center of mass high — usually at the rescuer's shoulder level — and because it requires a fair amount of strength. If you need to move the patient over irregular terrain, however, it can be a better choice than a drag. Unless it is a life-or-death situation, do not attempt a fireman's carry if the patient has fractures of the extremities or suspected spinal injury.

To perform the fireman's carry, follow these steps (Figures 41-4–41-6):

1. Position the patient on his or her back, with both knees bent and raised. Grasp the back sides of the patient's wrists.

2. Stand on the toes of both of the patient's feet. Lean backward, pulling the patient up and toward you. As the patient nears a standing position, crouch slightly and pull him or her over your shoulder.

3. Stand upright.

4. Pass your arm between the patient's legs and grasp the patient's arm that is nearest your body.

5. The fireman's carry can also be accomplished with an assisting EMT. See Figures 41-7 through 41-9.

Other Emergency Moves

Other emergency moves include the **piggyback carry** (Figures 41-10–41-11), the **packstrap** (Figure 41-12), the **one-rescuer crutch** (Figure 41-13), the **one-rescuer cradle carry** (Figure 41-14), the **fireman's drag** (Figure 41-15), the **shoulder drag** (Figure 41-16), and the **foot drag** (Figure 41-17).

□ The Fireman's Carry

FIGURE 41-4

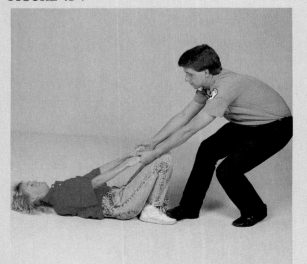

FIGURE 41-5

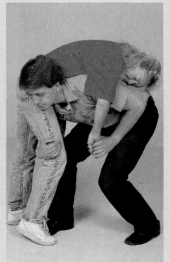

FIGURE 41-6

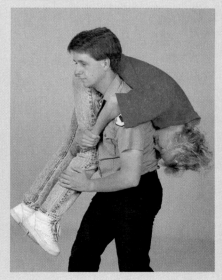

☐ Fireman's Carry with Assisting EMT

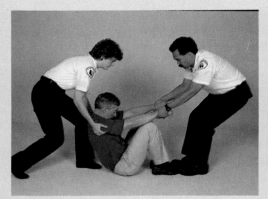

FIGURE 41-7

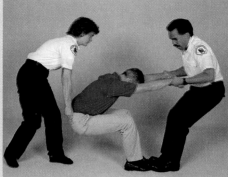

FIGURE 41-8

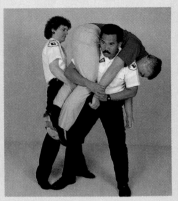

FIGURE 41-9

☐ BASIC GUIDELINES FOR MOVING PATIENTS

Once you have decided that the scene is safe, assessed the patient, administered life-saving treatment, and stabilized all injuries, you need to determine the best way to move the patient. Base your decision on the patient's injuries or medical condition, the patient's status, the environmental surroundings, and your resources — available manpower and equipment to assist in the move.

Generally, the best way to move a patient is the easiest way that will not cause injury or pain. That in-

☐ Piggyback Carry

FIGURE 41-10

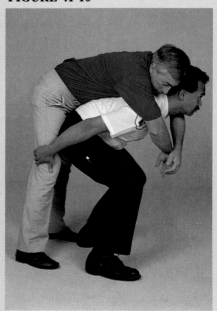

FIGURE 41-11

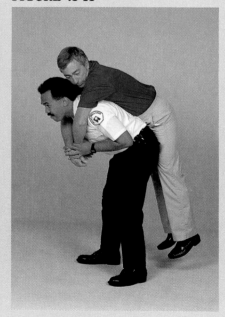

FIGURE 41-12 The packstrap.

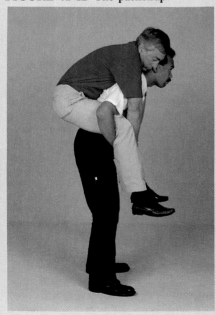

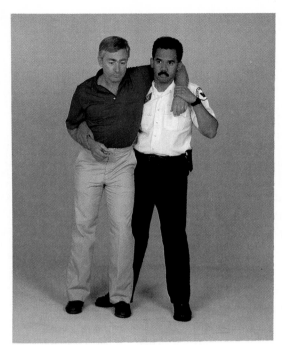

FIGURE 41-13 One-rescuer crutch.

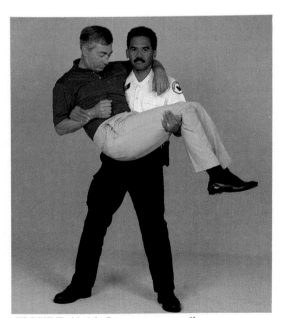

FIGURE 41-14 One-rescuer cradle carry.

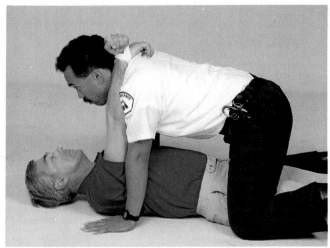

FIGURE 41-15 Fireman's drag.

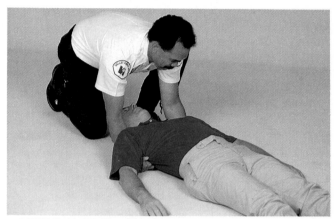

FIGURE 41-16 Shoulder drag.

FIGURE 41-17 Foot drag.

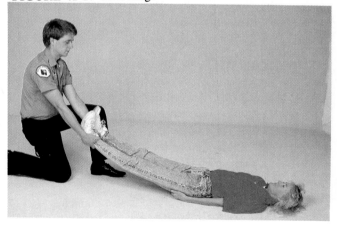

cludes "walking" a patient if he or she is able, giving support as he or she walks to the cot. *Never* walk a patient who is having cardiac problems, who has a fracture of the lower extremity, or who has respiratory problems; always bring the cot to the patient in those cases.

Let your equipment do the work — especially your wheels. First, get the ambulance as close to the patient as you can; then move the cot as close to the patient as you can.

Whenever possible, drag or slide the patient instead of lifting him or her. If you must lift a patient, do it only with a device designed for the job unless you are faced with making an emergency move to save the patient's life. As a rule, carry a patient only as far as absolutely necessary — and get help if you can. If you think that sounds too conservative, remember that you may perform as many as 20,000 lifts in a ten-year period and that you risk a fall or back injury with every one.

Patient Packaging, Moving, and Triage   **617**

□ UNDERSTANDING YOUR EQUIPMENT

Understanding the sometimes-complex application of various equipment, as well as the advantages and disadvantages of each piece you carry, will help you make educated decisions about which equipment to use when packaging and moving a patient (Table 41-1).

Ambulance Cots

The **ambulance cot** is one of the most frequently used pieces of equipment carried on any ambulance. It can be your best friend or your worst enemy, depending on how you use it. Ambulance cots are designed to accommodate patients weighing up to 400 pounds and can adapt to almost any imaginable patient condition. For the safety of the patient and the EMTs, ambulance cots should always be handled by at least two EMTs. An EMT should be at each end of the cot during any lifting or moving of the patient. A patient should *never* be left alone on an ambulance cot.

A thorough understanding of the ambulance cot is essential to the patient's safety and comfort as well as to the safety and health of the EMTs. There are two basic styles of ambulance cots currently available in North America. The lift-in cot (Models 30 and 30SC) requires two attendants to lift the cot from each side when loading and unloading it from the ambulance (Figure 41-18). The roll-in style cot (Models 28, 29M, and 35A) utilizes special loading wheels at the head-end of the cot to simplify the loading and unloading procedure (Figure 41-19). These cots significantly reduce the amount of lifting and twisting required by the EMTs. These cots weigh between 65 to 78 pounds and are constructed of aluminum alloys.

An ambulance cot has several unique capabilities:

- It can be wheeled from one point to another and seldom requires carrying.
- It can serve as a means of carrying various prehospital care equipment to the location of the patient.
- It is the safest and most comfortable means of transferring a patient.
- Each type of ambulance cot is mechanically reliable, and each can be lifted in a variety of ways depending on the space and personnel available and the weight of the patient.
- Some can be adjusted to provide various positions of comfort, as well as for specific treatment such as shock.

The Scoop Stretcher

Designed for patients weighing up to 300 hundred pounds, the **scoop stretcher** (Figure 41-20) is made to be assembled (or dissembled) "around the patient." It can be used in confined areas where other conventional stretchers can't fit. An advantage of the scoop stretcher is that it can be used to transport a patient vertically for short distances; a disadvantage is that it is all metal and, as such, picks up the temperature of the environment.

To use a scoop stretcher (Figures 41-21–41-29):

1. Adjust the stretcher to the length of the patient.
2. Separate the stretcher halves, and place one-half on either side of the patient. Rock the patient's body slightly away from you, and slide one-half of the scoop underneath the patient. If you suspect that the patient might have spinal injury, position another rescuer at his or her head to maintain it in a neutral position during the entire procedure.
3. If you have not been able to examine the patient's back before, do it now. Then return the patient to a supine position.
4. Assemble the head end of the scoop.
5. Roll the patient's body toward you while the rescuer at his or her feet swings the remaining half of the scoop into a closed (assembled) position; latch the foot end of the stretcher.
6. Pad the patient's head with a pillow; if spinal precautions are in effect, use a folded sheet. (When the scoop stretcher is placed on a hard surface, it can cause a blow to the head.)
7. Use at least three body straps to fasten the patient securely to the stretcher.

To move a patient vertically, use the following technique:

1. Using two sheets, form a "doughnut" out of each that makes a ring through the patient's crotch at the bottom and continues through a shoulder-level hand-hole at the top.
2. Secure the ends of each sheet in a square knot.
3. Secure the patient to the scoop with straps and transport normally, raising the head to a vertical position as needed.

Because the scoop stretcher is designed to accommodate the posterior shape of the pelvis and thorax, you can use the stretcher to immobilize both of these areas. To stabilize the chest, fold a sheet lengthwise into a ten- to twelve-inch binder. Fasten the binder tightly around the chest and the scoop stretcher; tie the ends of the

TABLE 41-1
Equipment Comparison Chart:

DEVICE	ADVANTAGES	DISADVANTAGES
Backboard (long)	Good spinal immobilizer Good lifting device Floatable Good CPR surface Mechanical simplicity X-ray translucency Low cost Consumes little space Can be lifted from sides or from ends Lightweight Usable for shoring, chuting, various extrication purposes Usable for walkway surface Can be used as a dog- or knife-shield Ohio-style will fit into a basket stretcher Easily cleaned via contact cleaner Can be carried or loaded from ends or sides	Normally must be left with patient Slippery; not a good litter Unstable for inclined moves Uncomfortable May develop splinters May weaken with time

Backboard (Short)	Doubles as CPR board
	Valuable for shoring
	Can be used as cervical immobilizer during
	   extrication
	Low cost
	Can be used as a shield
	Easily cleaned via contact cleaner
	X-ray translucency
		Vastly outperformed by
		   Corset-type immobilizers

Basket Stretcher	Good for traversing rough terrain Can be fitted with flotation harness for water rescue Easily cleaned Extremely durable Easily cleaned via hose or contact cleaner A good CPR surface Poly version: X-ray translucency Fairly good comfort Can be carried from sides or ends	Bulky High cost Usually must be left with patient Metal style interferes with some X-rays

Emergency Blanket	Low cost
	Lightweight
	Compact size
	Can be used as a stretcher
	Can be used as a shield against heat, dogs,
	   insects, broken glass, or powdered
	Comfort
	Can be used for drags
	Can be used as padding in various applications
	Can be used to shield patient from public
	   view during some procedures
	Can be used as a sling for removal of
	   patient from bathtub
	Can be used to restrain small patients
	Will fit into a basket stretcher
	X-ray translucency
	Can be loaded from sides or ends
		When used as a stretcher, normally
		   requires several carriers
		Can be heavy when wet
		Out of service for a prolonged time
		   when wet or soiled
		Can only be carried from sides
		   chemicals

Pole Stretcher	Lightweight Low cost Compact size Comfort Will accommodate other stretchers Good carrying device Easily cleaned via contact cleaner X-ray translucency	Provides little immobilization Profile too high around perimeter for slides Will not fit into a basket stretcher Not a good CPR surface Can be carried only from ends

(continued)

TABLE 41-1 *(continued)*

DEVICE	ADVANTAGES	DISADVANTAGES
Corset Immobilizers (Ferno KED)	Good extrication tools Lightweight Durable Reliable Can be used as stair-chairs Good immobilizers for flail chest, C-spine X-ray translucency Simplicity Can be removed from patient on arrival in E.D. Comfort Integrates well with other devices Easily cleaned via contact cleaner	Dependence of Velcro limits value in bad weather Some small portions lost easily in emergency departments
Cot (Model 28)	Capable of chair position, and can be carried that way Can be carried by sides or ends Enables movement without carrying Comfort	Little height variation possible (2 levels) Difficult to maneuver when lowered X-ray opacity
Cot (Model 29)	Loading does not require great strength if vehicle parked — then, considerable upper body strength required Easy on rescuer's lumbar spine under normal circumstances Can be lifted or loaded from sides or ends Enables movement without carrying Comfort	Cumbersome on stairs Will not shorten for cornering in lower positions Mechanical complexity Balkiness in cold weather Limited height variation possible (4 levels) Difficult to maneuver when lowered X-ray opacity
Cot (Model 30)	Good height variation (8 levels) Enables movement without carrying Accommodates variety of positions Safe traversal of stairways and curbs Will shorten for cornering at any level Durability Mechanical simplicity Can be lifted or lowered from ends or sides	Difficulty of loading or unloading by 2 rescuers X-ray opacity
Cot (Model 35)	Benefits of a multi-level cot with roll-in style feature Designing for a variety of ambulance floor heights Works with station wagons, vans, and modular ambulances Has 8 height positions Can be shortened 14 inches for easy manevering	Difficulty of loading or unloading by 2 rescuers X-ray opacity
Drawsheet	Good for movement of patient off of a raised surface Appropriate mostly to lateral moves	Depends on strength of a sheet — an unknown factor Requires considerable space, including for ingress and egress of ambulance cot Often results in loss of linen
Scoop Stretcher	Facilitates movement of almost any patient encountered on a ground-level surface Good CPR surface Integrates well with various other equipment items Allows easy application of restraint Good general immobilizer Good carrying device, if fitted with straps Allows efficient movement of CPR patient Can be used in brief vertical moves, if fitted with simple pelvic support harness	Requires occipital padding, although more comfortable than a backboard Consumes space of 2 backboards Must be pre-warmed if ambient temperature is cold

TABLE 41-1 *(continued)*

DEVICE	ADVANTAGES	DISADVANTAGES
Stair-Chairs	Good for use on compound stairways Series 107 accommodates C-spine patients, can be made into a stretcher	Series 40 has fairly limited range of applications, does not accommodate trauma patients Fairly complex and consume considerable space

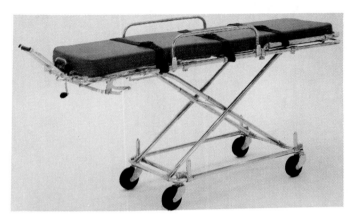

FIGURE 41-18 Model 30SC.

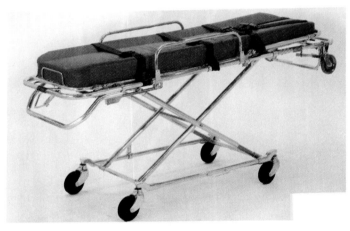

FIGURE 41-19 Model 35A.

FIGURE 41-20 Scoop stretcher.

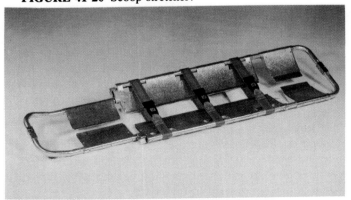

sheet together in an unaffected area (beneath the scoop, if necessary). To stabilize the pelvis, apply a blanket stabilizer and secure it in place with a sheet binder, as described.

Pole Stretchers/Canvas Litters

Pole stretchers/canvas litters (Figure 41-30) have been used by armies worldwide for at least two centuries. The modern tubular-framed, vinyl-coated nylon version accommodates patients weighing up to three hundred and fifty pounds.

The pole stretcher is comfortable to lie on, especially if the head is padded. It is lightweight, folds compactly, and is easy to clean. It is valuable in situations where there is not enough space for an ambulance cot or when a multiple-casualty incident calls for more cots than are available.

Pole stretchers work well when a patient can be log-rolled, but do not work as well when the patient has to be moved lengthwise. They generally should not be used when spinal immobilization is necessary unless they are used with a long backboard.

Loading a patient into the ambulance is easier if you place the pole stretcher on the cot, load the cot into the ambulance, then transfer the patient on the pole stretcher to a hanger or bench seat. This results in less jostling of the patient.

The Flat Stretcher (Folding Emergency Stretcher)

The flat stretcher is a standard piece of equipment on most all ambulances in North America. Similar to a pole stretcher but designed with a continuous frame around the edge, these stretchers are simple to use and compact to store. Flat stretchers come in three basic styles: the basic flat, a flat stretcher with folding wheels and posts, or the breakaway flat. Flat stretchers are used as an auxilliary stretcher that can be placed on the squad bench or suspended from hanging hardware inside the ambulance. They also work well in multiple-casualty incidents, because they can be easily loaded onto an ambulance cot and easily off-loaded once inside the ambulance. Flat stretchers weigh between 8 and 15 pounds and have a load capacity of 350 pounds. They are usually folded in half for storage, except for the breakaway

☐ Moving a Patient with a Scoop Stretcher

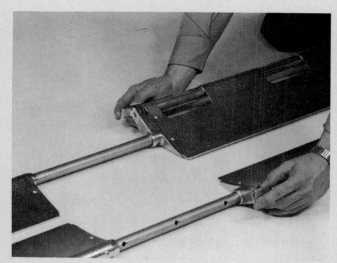

FIGURE 41-21 Adjust length of stretcher.

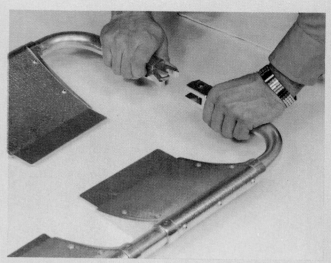

FIGURE 41-22 Separate the stretcher halves.

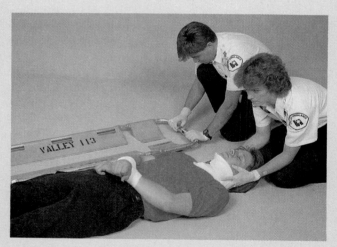

FIGURE 41-23 Carefully support patient's head while stretcher halves are separated.

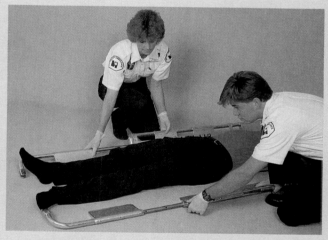

FIGURE 41-24 Slide the stretcher halves under the patient, one at a time.

flat which is usually left on top of the cot mattress at all times.

The Backboard

Backboards (Figures 41-31 and 41-32) are some of the rescuer's most versatile tools. Two major styles are commonly in use: the Farrington type is rectangular with rounded corners, and the Ohio style is shaped more like a coffin lid, featuring mitered corners at the head and gradually tapering sides. Some of the plastic backboards have runners molded into the underside, as well as strap systems that are built into the board so the straps can't be separated from the backboard at the hospital. While their use is largely based on rescuer preference, the Ohio fits into most basket stretchers and can be more easily maneuvered through many car door openings. Backboards are useful as spinal immobilizers, can be used virtually any time to pick up a recumbent patient, and are excellent carrying devices when the patient is firmly strapped to the board.

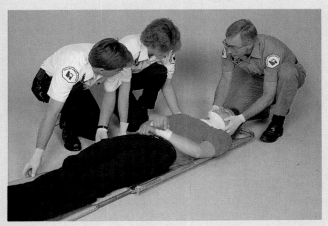

FIGURE 41-25 Head support is maintained while stretcher halves are put in position.

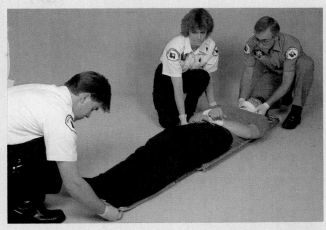

FIGURE 41-26 The stretcher halves are locked together while head is properly positioned.

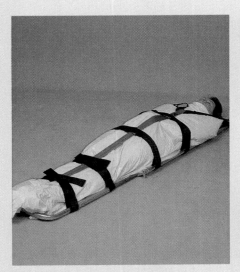

FIGURE 41-27 Patient is properly positioned, covered, and secured to stretcher.

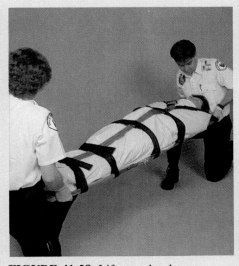

FIGURE 41-28 Lift stretcher by the end–carry method.

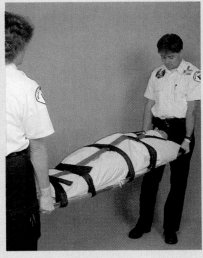

FIGURE 41-29 Move patient to a long backboard as soon as possible.

FIGURE 41-30 Pole stretcher.

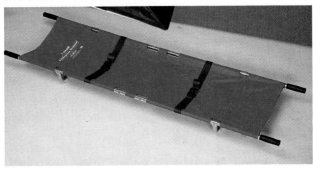

The Emergency Blanket

You can use an **emergency blanket** (Figure 41-33) as a stretcher when space is limited, you need to traverse stairs or cramped corners, there is an equipment shortage, or you need to get a patient in or out of a basket stretcher. Depending on how you support it, you could also use an emergency blanket as a stair-chair. Use a blanket only if the patient has no suspected neck, back, or pelvic injuries.

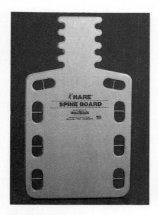

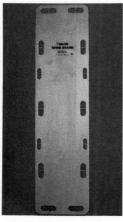

FIGURE 41-31
Short backboard.

FIGURE 41-32
Long backboard.

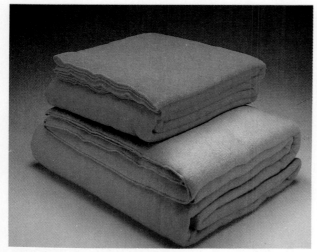

FIGURE 41-33 Emergency blankets.

Any blanket used as a stretcher should be strong, free of holes, and in good condition. It must be large enough to support the patient's entire body; if you are not sure, test it by trying it out on a rescuer. If the weather is cold, you might use two blankets instead of one, wrapping alternating folds of the blankets around the patient for warmth.

To use a blanket as a stretcher (Figures 41-34–41-36):

1. Log-roll or slide the patient onto the center of the blanket.
2. Tightly roll the side edges of the blanket toward the patient; these rolled edges will form handholds.
3. Position as many rescuers around the patient as needed to distribute the hands evenly. Lift and carry the patient smoothly and evenly.

Blankets can also be folded and rolled to immobi-

lize the head or other body parts, be wrapped around a patient and secured with cloth tape as a restraint, and be used to protect you from hazards (such as broken glass) on the ground. *If you use a blanket to drag a patient, always pull rather than push.*

The Basket Stretcher

Most commonly called the **Stokes litter, a basket stretcher** (Figure 41-37) is shaped like a basket and comes in two basic styles. The first has a welded metal frame fitted with a contoured chicken-wire web that may include a partition separating the legs. The second style has a tubular aluminum frame riveted to a molded polyethylene shell; it has no leg partition.

A basket stretcher has the advantage of enabling you to completely immobilize a patient who is already on a backboard and to move him or her over any kind of terrain. The lightweight polyethylene style slides easily and smoothly over rough terrain while protecting the patient from branches and twigs (Figure 41-38). Either version without the partition will accommodate a scoop stretcher, blanket stretcher, or Ohio-type backboard. You can also place the mattress from an ambulance cot in the basket stretcher increasing patient comfort and insulation from the cold. If you do not use a cot mattress, be sure to pad the patient's head. If you anticipate especially rough transport, pad the edges of the patient's body with rolled blankets and strap him or her securely into place with nylon webbing.

Both kinds of basket stretchers will fit onto an ambulance cot, and both will work with any vehicle large enough to accommodate them.

☐ THE MECHANICS OF LIFTING

One of the most important things to remember when lifting a patient is to *protect your own safety* — if you injure yourself during the move, you will be unable to help the patient and will become a victim yourself.

A first step is to protect your back. Whenever you can, keep your back straight throughout the entire lift; if you have to flex your back, straighten it again as quickly as you can. *Never* twist or turn at the waist while you're lifting; instead, shift your feet and turn your entire body. Use the large muscles of your thighs to provide the strength for the lift, not the muscles of your back.

Before you begin a lift, assess the available equipment. Know how to use your equipment, and respect the equipment's limitations. *Don't try to make a lift that your equipment is not designed for*; unless it's a dire emergency, you're better off waiting for better equipment to arrive. Inspect your equipment before you begin

☐ Blanket Lift and Carry

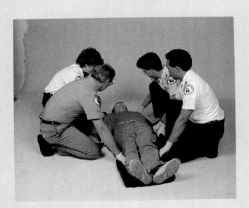

FIGURE 41-34

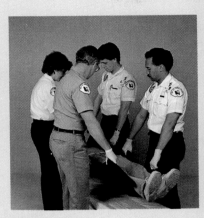

FIGURE 41-35

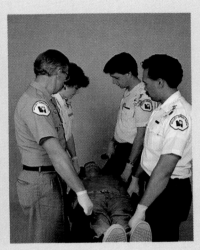

FIGURE 41-36

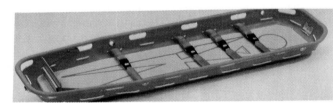

FIGURE 41-37 Basket stretcher.

FIGURE 41-38 Using a basket stretcher to move a patient over rough terrain.

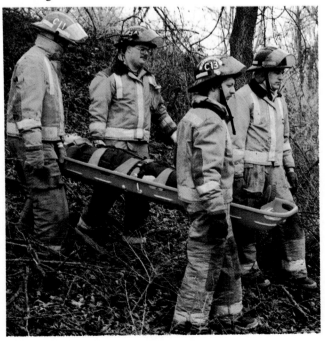

each lift — briefly check nuts, bolts, pins, and aluminum welds. Make sure the wheels of stretchers are clean.

Take the time to mentally rehearse the lift before you get started. Go through each step in your mind, deciding how you'll handle it. Decide *with your partner* the sequence, and decide ahead of time the verbal signals you'll use to communicate with each other during the move.

To begin the actual move, follow this sequence:

1. Tell the patient what you are going to do before you do it. You will avoid surprising the patient, and he or she will be less likely to upset your balance if he or she is not startled.

2. Realistically size up your load. The most important thing to remember when lifting a patient is *not to overestimate your strength.* When you see that your attempts to move a patient may result in injury to you or the patient, *stop* and call for help. Consider using bystanders; if they do not meet your needs, call your communications center for help. If you use more than one EMT or bystander, make sure that someone is in charge to give the signal to move at the same time. The person at the head, who is managing the airway or keeping the head and neck stable, is the most logical person to give the commands.

3. Stand with your feet apart, and be sure of your footing. Wear sturdy, laced boots that extend well over your ankles for protection during load-bearing. Boots should have thick, nonskid soles

for walking on debris and broken glass or for getting up and down slopes. If you have to work in deep mud, protect yourself and other rescuers by lying down several backboards to serve as a walking surface, even if you have to call for additional units to get them. They can easily be hosed off by an engine company on the scene. It is important that you have a strong base on which to stand. If you need to lift the patient from the ground, log-roll him onto the board, then lift the board.

4. Use the large muscles in your arms and legs to do the lifting. Lift the board to your chest, then raise yourself to a standing position. Support the patient as close to your body as you can, keeping your back straight. Dorsoflexing your back — arching it backward — will place the weight more squarely on your lumbar vertebrae, causing less strain.

5. If the lift does not feel right, *stop lifting* and get help — or choose a different method. If the lifting feels right, it generally is right. Whatever method you choose, have plenty of help — lifting is the motion that places you at the greatest risk of injury.

You can move a heavy patient more easily with an accessory stretcher, such as a scoop stretcher, but sometimes it is necessary to lift him or her without the accessory stretcher. If you have no other choice, and if the patient's weight allows it, cradle the patient in the arms of two or three rescuers.

When the Patient Is in a Sitting Position

There are at least four ways to move a patient in a sitting position: manually (as a last choice), with a Ferno KED (Figure 41-39), with a stair-chair, or on a chair.

Ferno KED or XP-1

If the patient is a potential trauma victim and you cannot lie him or her down (because of space or because of a medical condition, such as respiratory/cardiac problems), apply a collar and a corset-type immobilizer like the KED or XP-1. Transfer the patient to a long backboard on a cot, and transport him in the appropriate position (including sitting, if necessary). See pages Chapter 16 for application procedures.

Stair-Chair

If the patient has not sustained trauma and you need to traverse a number of stairs, manually lift him or her to a **stair-chair** (Figures 41-40–41-42). Use the stair-chair to move the patient to the cot, and chair-lift the patient to the cot. Stair-chairs should not be used for patients with suspected spinal injury or fractures of the lower extremities, or those who are unconscious or disoriented.

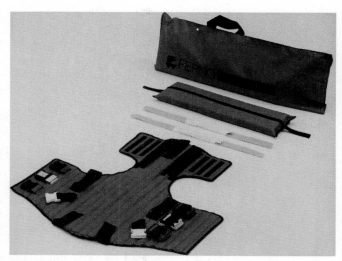

FIGURE 41-39 Ferno KED.

Chair-Lift

If the patient has probably not sustained trauma and you do not have a stair-chair, chair-lift him or her onto an ordinary chair. Strap the patient to the chair, and carry the chair to the cot. A serious disadvantage is that this method depends on the structural strength of the chair — if it fails, you bear the responsibility. Once you have moved the patient to the cot, chair-lift him or her onto the cot.

□ LIFTS AND CARRIES

Draw-Sheet

The **draw-sheet** enables you to move a patient who is lying on a sheet. It requires a minimum of three people (more for an obese patient), enough space for EMTs to stand at each side and at the foot, and enough room for the cot to be positioned near the patient. Draw-sheeting is normally used only for patients who have not been traumatized. It is quick and comfortable for the patient and is relatively safe for both the patient and the EMTs. It is generally used to move a patient from a slightly higher surface to one that is slightly lower. The sheet should be strong enough to bear the patient's weight.

Follow these guidelines (Figures 41-43–41-47):

1. Tell the patient in which direction he or she will be moved. Ask him or her to "hug" himself or herself and to let the EMTs do the work.

2. Position the weakest EMT at the patient's feet; two other EMTs are positioned on each side near the patient's shoulders.

3. The EMT at the end grasps the bottom of the sheet, forming a sling for the ankles. The EMTs at the top grasp the sheet with one hand at about the

☐ Using a Stair-Chair

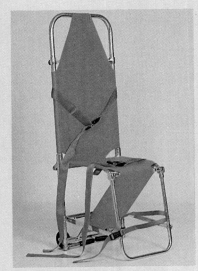

FIGURE 41-40 Stair-chair.

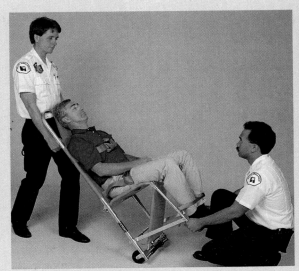

FIGURE 41-41 Moving a properly secured patient on a stair-chair.

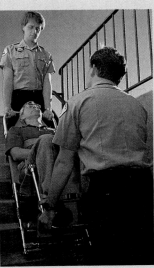

FIGURE 41-42 Moving a stair-chair down steps.

level of the patient's ear, and with the other hand at about the level of the patient's flank.

4. If the patient is obese, add two more EMTs at the patient's hip level.

5. Using a count of three to make sure all move at once, drag the patient toward the cot.

Ground-Level Patient

When transferring a ground-level patient to a stretcher (two rescuers), use the method shown in Figures 41-48–41-50.

Flat Lift (Two Rescuers)

The **flat lift** is valuable when the patient cannot sit in a chair and when neither a cot nor an accessory stretcher can be brought close to the patient. It is difficult for two rescuers to lift a patient who weighs more than 180 pounds; it is dangerous if the patient is on the ground (or some other low surface) or is uncooperative.

To perform the flat lift, follow these guidelines (Figures 41-51–41-53):

1. Position the cot as close to the patient as possible; it should be where it can be reached in as straight a

☐ Two-Rescuer Draw-Sheet Method #1

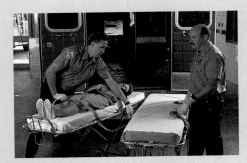

FIGURE 41-43

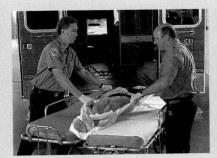

FIGURE 41-44

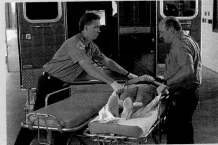

FIGURE 41-45

☐ Two-Rescuer Draw-Sheet Method #2

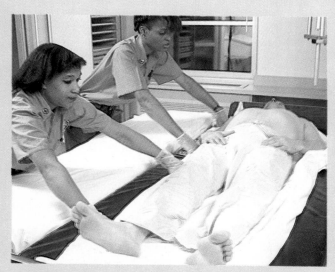

FIGURE 41-46 Bottom sheet of bed is rolled from both sides of bed toward patient. The stretcher, with its rails lowered, is placed parallel to bed, touching side of bed.

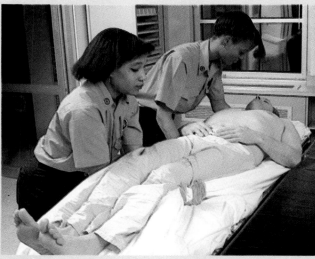

FIGURE 41-47 EMTs pull on draw-sheet to move patient to side of bed. They each use one hand to support patient while they reach underneath to grasp draw-sheet. EMTs simultaneously draw patient onto stretcher.

line as possible. Undo the straps, lower the railings, and clear any equipment off the mattress.

2. Tell the patient what you are going to do; ask him or her to "hug" himself or herself and to remain very still throughout the move. Warn that his or her stillness is essential to your balance.

3. Kneel or bend alongside the patient.

4. Grasp the patient's forearm closest to you and lie it across the patient's chest. Grasp the elbow of the same arm. At the same time, your partner grasps the trouser leg of the patient's knee on the

☐ Transferring the Ground-Level Patient

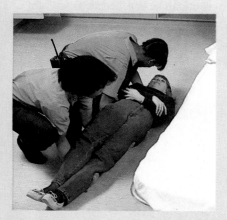

FIGURE 41-48 Stretcher is set in its lowest position and placed on opposite side of patient. EMTs drop to one knee, facing patient. Rescuers' arms are positioned as they are for a direct carry.

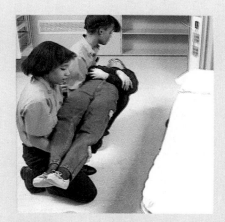

FIGURE 41-49 EMTs lift patient to their knees.

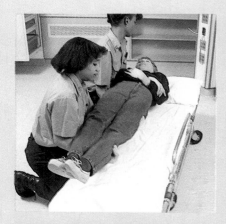

FIGURE 41-50 They stand and carry patient to stretcher, drop to one knee, and roll forward to place patient onto mattress.

☐ Flat-Lift Method

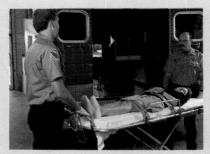

FIGURE 41-51

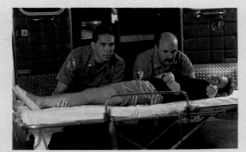

FIGURE 41-52

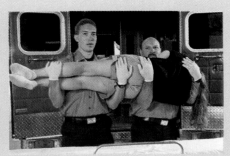

FIGURE 41-53

same side, or grasps the knee itself, bringing the knee into a raised position.

5. Holding the patient's elbow and knee, roll the patient away from you as a unit. With the patient lying on his side, place your arms underneath him or her. Your left arm grasps the shoulder on which the patient is lying; your right arm grasps the hip on which the patient is lying. Your partner's left arm is placed against your right arm, also grasping the patient's hip, and his or her right hand grasps the ankle on which the patient is lying.

6. Rock the patient slightly so that he or she rolls toward you and onto your forearms. When the patient is supine, continue rocking him or her until cradled in the bends of your elbows. Tuck his or her head in toward your chests. Stand, move toward the cot, and place the patient on the cot.

7. To remove your arms, withdraw your left arm first, then use it to roll the patient's pelvis slightly so that both of you can withdraw your arms from beneath the hips. Finally, your partner can let go of the patient's ankle.

If the patient is slightly heavier, have a third person carry the patient's feet. That frees your partner's ankle-arm for added support at the hips and enables you to move your right arm slightly toward the patient's head. If the patient is lying on the floor and you have no other options, have a third person lift opposite you at the patient's hips.

If you think that the patient might be incontinent, place your right arm and your partner's left arm inside a heavy-duty 20- or 30-gallon trash bag before you slide your arms underneath the patient's pelvis. When you withdraw your arms after the patient is on the cot, leave the bag beneath the patient to protect the linen on the cot.

Seat Carries (Two Rescuers)

Follow these guidelines:

1. Raise the patient to a sitting position.
2. Each EMT steadies the patient by positioning an arm around his or her back.
3. Each EMT slips his other arm underneath the patient's thighs, then clasps the wrist of the other EMT. One pair of arms should make a seat, the other pair a backrest.
4. Slowly raise the patient from the ground. Make sure that you move in unison.

In another method, the EMTs form a seat with four hands and the victim supports himself or herself by placing his or her arms around the EMT's necks. (Figures 41-54–41-56).

Extremity Lift (Two Rescuers)

Never use the **extremity lift** when the patient has back injuries. If you do not suspect an injury of this type, proceed as follows (Figures 41-57 and 41-58):

1. One EMT kneels at the patient's head; the other kneels beside the patient's knees.
2. The EMT at the patient's head places one hand under each of the patient's shoulders; the second EMT grasps the patient's wrists.
3. The EMT at the patient's knees pulls the patient to a sitting position by pulling on the patient's wrists; the EMT at the patient's head assists by pushing the patient's shoulders and supporting the patient's back.
4. The EMT at the patient's head slips his or her hands under the arms and grasps the patient's wrists.

Patient Packaging, Moving, and Triage **629**

☐ Seat Carry

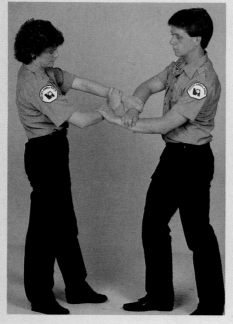

FIGURE 41-54

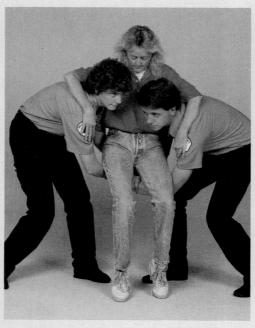

FIGURE 41-55

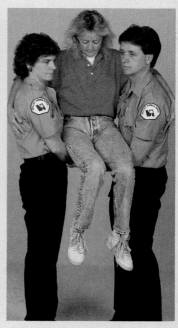

FIGURE 41-56

☐ Extremity Lift

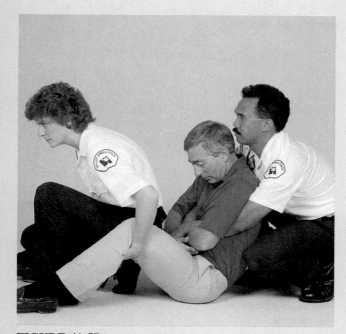

FIGURE 41-57

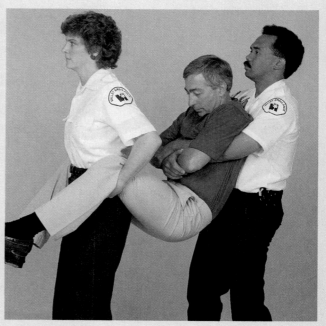

FIGURE 41-58

5. The EMT at the patient's knees slips his or her hands beneath the patient's knees.

6. Both EMTs crouch on their feet.

7. Both EMTs simultaneously stand in one fluid motion, moving with the patient to the stretcher.

Chair Litter Carry

If the patient does not have contraindicating injuries, and if a chair is available, sit the patient in the chair and tie him or her securely to it. One EMT then carries the back of the chair while the other carries the legs; the chair itself is used as a litter (Figures 41-59–41-60).

Flat Lift and Carry (Three Rescuers)

The three-rescuer flat lift and carry is an effective way to move a severely injured patient. Be careful of backstrain, however. If there is no spine injury, use the following technique (Figures 41-61–41-64):

1. Three EMTs line up on one side of the patient. The tallest stands at the patient's shoulders, another stands at his hips, and another at his knees.

2. Each EMT kneels on the knee closest to the patient's feet.

3. The EMT at the patient's shoulders works his or her hands underneath the patient's neck and shoulders; the EMT at the hips works his or her hands underneath the patient's hips and pelvis; the EMT at the knees works his or her hands underneath the patient's knees and ankles.

4. In unison, raise the patient to knee level and slowly turn the patient toward all three EMTs until the patient rests on the bends of their elbows. *Follow local protocol.*

5. In unison, all three rise to a standing position. Walk with the patient to a place of safety or to the stretcher.

6. To deposit the patient on the stretcher, simply reverse the procedure.

One of the great advantages of the three-rescuer flat lift and carry is that it enables you to move the patient through narrow passages and down stairs. The procedure can also be done with four rescuers, positioning EMTs at the patient's head, chest, hips, and knees. Support is then given to the head, chest, hips, pelvis, knees, and ankles.

□ Chair Carry

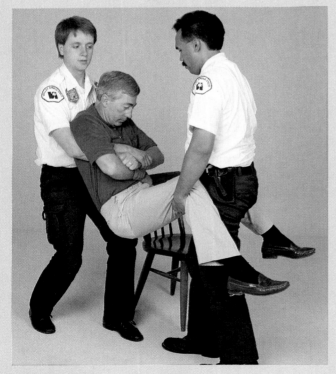

FIGURE 41-59

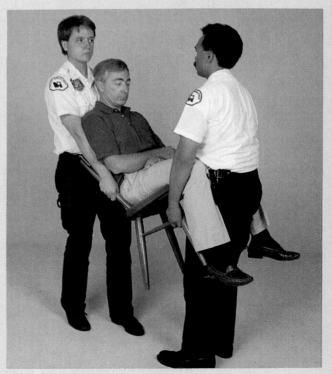

FIGURE 41-60

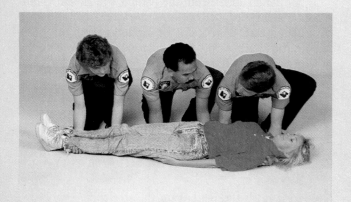

FIGURE 41-61

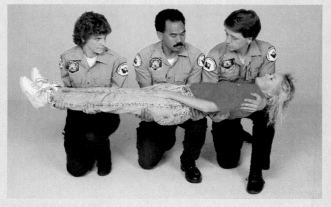

FIGURE 41-62

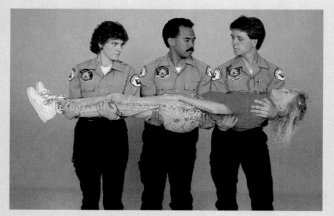

FIGURE 41-63

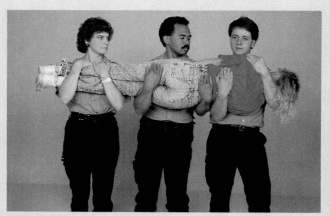

FIGURE 41-64

Chair-Lift (Two Rescuers)

When you use either a chair or a stair-chair to move a patient, you need to move him or her in a sitting position. If the patient's upper extremities are sound, use this technique.

1. Inform the patient that you are going to pick him or her up.
2. Stand behind the patient's back, reach beneath his or her shoulders, and grasp the left wrist with your right hand and the right wrist with your left hand.
3. Have your partner grasp both of the patient's knees with one forearm.
4. Lift.

If the patient's upper extremities are not sound, you can still perform a chair-lift, but it will take more upper-body strength on your part and you will need space at the patient's sides. Follow this technique:

1. Tell the patient that you are going to pick him or her up.
2. Position yourself at the patient's side, with your partner on his or her opposite side.
3. Slip one of your forearms beneath the patient's knees, upward to about the mid-thighs; have your partner do the same.
4. With your other arm, reach around and support the patient's back; have your partner do the same.
5. Tell the patient to sit back and use you like a chair.
6. Lift.

Because the chair-lift places a tremendous strain

on your back, it is best not to use it without a stair-chair or some other device for more than about thirty to forty feet. It is also not recommended for trauma victims.

□ MOVING A COT

Standard guidelines for moving an ambulance cot include the following (see Figures 41-65–41-82 on pp 634–637 for loading, unloading, and moving the cot):

- Keep the cot clean and ready to use at all times. Blood, vomitus, other body fluids, and other debris must be wiped up and the cot cleaned after each use.

- Plan all movements in advance; having to retrace your steps and go about a move in a different direction is a waste of time and energy. If the route between the cot and the ambulance is complex, involving stairways and multiple corners, it might be worthwhile to take an empty cot on a trial run first to eliminate guesswork.

- If you are moving the cot in its fully raised position (which is the most common position used), keep both hands on the cot at all times to maintain firm control.

- Tell the patient to keep his or her head on the pillow. Unless injuries prevent it, fold the patient's arms across his or her chest. Cover the patient to preserve body warmth, and secure him or her with straps.

- Whenever possible, move the cot foot-first, and if the patient can tolerate it, elevate the head slightly. That way, the patient can see where he or she is going and will not be as anxious.

- If you have to traverse unlevel ground, lower the cot to its lowest position and situate it perpendicular to the grade. Position the cot so that the head end is downhill, but keep the patient's head elevated.

- Where possible, use at least six people to carry the stretcher; you'll have a "margin of safety" in case one rescuer trips or stumbles.

- If rough terrain or debris makes it literally impossible to walk with the stretcher, use a "passing" technique. Have two rescuers go to the other side of the debris; the remaining rescuers then pass the stretcher to the waiting rescuers. Keep the stretcher at shoulder level while passing to provide the greatest stability and the least strain on rescuers. This "passing" technique can also be used to traverse extremely rough terrain: as the stretcher is passed to the two empty-handed rescuers, the two rescuers at the head of the stretcher then move to its foot. This procedure is repeated as the stretcher is slowly moved along the rough terrain, passed from hand to hand.

- For greatest convenience, stow on the cot the items you usually use in conjunction with the cot. These might include a rain cover, a CPR board, a sheet, a disposable diaper, a large plastic trash bag, a wrist strap, and at least two heavy blankets if the weather is cold.

"Curbing" a Cot

Most calls will require you to traverse at least one curb with a loaded cot. When you can, use a wheelchair ramp or driveway apron; even single steps are dangerous, because they affect your balance and impair your vision when you are carrying a loaded cot.

Instead of carrying a loaded cot over the curb, you can cantilever it. Follow these guidelines (Figure 41-75):

1. Explain to the patient that the cot will be tilted at a slight incline.
2. When you approach the curb, step onto or off of it; have your partner push down on his or her end of the cot, minimizing the weight you will need to bear.
3. Once you are firmly past the curb, push down on your end of the cot while your partner lifts his wheels past the curb.
4. With the entire load stable, your partner can now step past the curb.

□ TRAVERSING STAIRWAYS

Often the only route to the ambulance includes a stairway Stairs pose a complication, but they can be negotiated safely. Before moving down any stairs, lower the cot to its lowest position and make sure that the patient is strapped in securely.

Follow these general guidelines:

- The most desirable position for a patient to be carried up or down a flight of stairs is with his or her head and shoulders elevated. However, you also need to move the cot so that the head end points down the stairs. With the patient's head at the uphill end of the stairway, his or her center of mass is about 30 percent higher, making the cot much more unstable and difficult to control. Losing control of a cot on a stairway causes it to topple end-over-end, resulting in serious injury.

- A spine board is the first possible choice for traversing stairs.

□ Unloading the Ambulance Cot

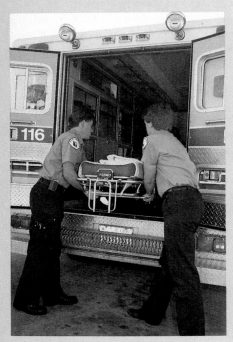

FIGURE 41-65

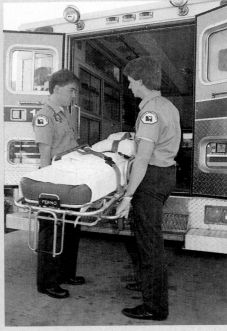

FIGURE 41-66

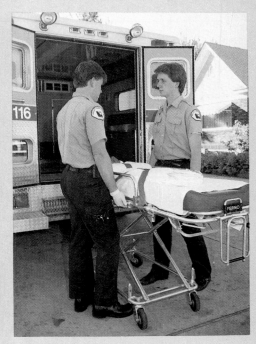

FIGURE 41-67

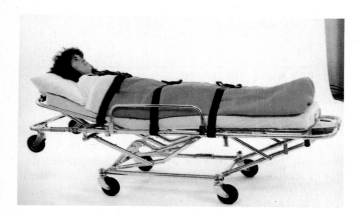

FIGURE 41-68 Patient covered, secured and ready for moving.

- You can also use a scoop stretcher, but use it with a pelvic harness fashioned out of a pair of sheets, as described earlier. Since the head end of a scoop cannot be raised, you normally will carry the patient with the foot end of the scoop downward. A scoop stretcher with a pelvic support harness or a stair-chair can be used to traverse compound stairways (stairs with more than one flight), especially those joined by a corner.

- If you have no other option, you can strap the patient to an ordinary chair and use it to move him down the stairs.

- During any stairway move, try to have a bystander or a third EMT provide support on the downward end of the stretcher. If a third person is not available, the downstairs-end rescuer should stay close to the wall and use it for stability between steps.

- One rescuer calls out a cadence, such as "step, step, step," to keep the rescuers moving smoothly as a unit.

- If either EMT begins to lose his or her balance, he or she should immediately instruct the partner to "set it down." The EMT at the uphill end of the stairway can then simply sit down on the stairs. A cot that is resting on stair treads can easily be kept from sliding down the stairs, even by a single EMT.

□ SPECIAL CONCERNS IN MOVING PATIENTS

Keep in mind the following suggestions when moving patients with special needs.

☐ Moving the Ambulance Cot

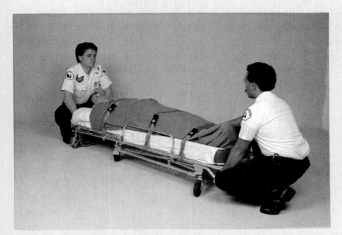

FIGURE 41-69 Preparing to lift patient secured to a stretcher.

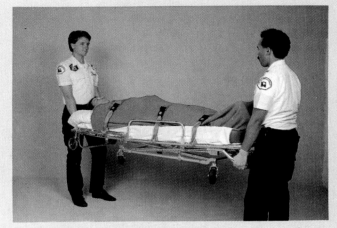

FIGURE 41-70 Secured patient is lifted for end-to-end carry.

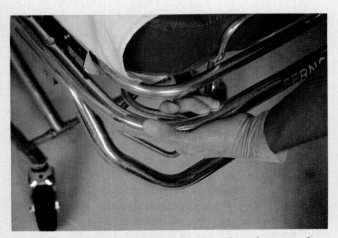

FIGURE 41-71 Release mechanism is activated to extend stretcher legs.

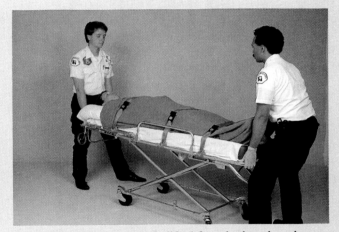

FIGURE 41-72 Stretcher is lifted from both ends as legs extend.

FIGURE 41-73 Rolling is the preferred method with a wheeled stretcher.

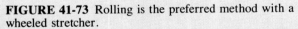

FIGURE 41-74 Side-carry and lift.

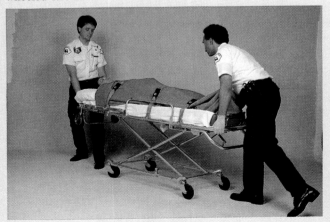

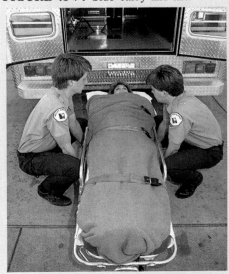

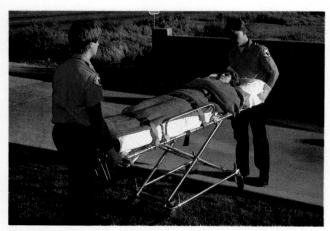

FIGURE 41-75 "Curbing" a cot.

Infants and Toddlers

An infant or toddler can usually be carried with ease in an infant car seat. When possible, use the child's own car seat to reduce the child's fear of being in an unfamiliar environment. Fasten the car seat to an ambulance cot with a standard body strap, and regulate its position with the head-end part of the cot.

You can also use a car seat as an immobilizer. Simply pack the space around the child with rolled towels or folded sheets that are taped in as padding.

Obstetric Patients

An obstetric patient will probably feel more comfortable lying on her side. That position takes the weight of the fetus off the great vessels and some of the nerve trunks in the abdominal cavity. If you suspect placenta previa, place the patient in shock position; if you suspect prolapsed cord, place the patient in a supine position with hips elevated on a pillow. *Follow local protocol.*

Elderly Patients

Some elderly people are extremely deliberate in their movements, and many are vision- or hearing-impaired. If the nature of the emergency allows for it, take a little extra time in helping the patient understand what is happening and where you are moving him or her. Speak clearly and directly to the patient in a voice loud enough to be heard.

A possible limitation in an elderly patient is osteoporosis, a loss of bone more common in women that makes the bones extremely brittle and prone to fracture. In these cases, exercise extra care in handling the patient to avoid accidental injury.

Handicapped Patients

Use common sense in handling patients who are handicapped; the nature of the handicap will let you know how to compensate. If a patient is blind, for example,

reduce his or her anxiety by describing what you are doing and where you are going with each step. If the patient cannot hear, use sign language if you know it; if not, signal with pantomime or write brief messages to let the patient know what is happening.

If the patient has fused joints, twisted limbs, or other obvious deformities, position to provide the greatest amount of comfort and take extra care in strapping. Whenever possible, use a rolled towel or other padding to support areas of deformity and to enhance patient comfort.

□ TRIAGE

All the medical knowledge in the world, and all the finest care, is of no avail if priorities are not ordered properly. It is critical that you know which patients of a multiple-victim accident or disaster require treatment first. Your ability to save lives depends upon your evaluation of the patients and upon **triage** — the ability to classify which patients require attention and treatment the most desperately, and which patients can wait without being endangered.

Triage, a French term meaning "picking" or "sorting," is a process of sorting and classifying sick and injured patients. The triage system was first developed by the military; its effectiveness resulted in a striking improvement in survival of the injured during the Korean and Vietnam wars. Under the original interpretation, triage is a procedure by which the sick and wounded are classified as to type and urgency of condition and are then routed under the assigned priorities to any installation available for care.

Triage should be used at the scene of any disaster or multiple-victim accident where there are more victims than rescuers. (If you arrive at a scene alone and there are two victims, you need to perform triage to determine your priorities.) Triage dictates priorities for both treatment *and* transport, and helps to maximize the number of victims who survive an incident.

Under triage, care is dedicated to the patients who are most "salvageable" so that valuable and limited time and resources are not spent on patients who are mortally wounded (and who will die even with excellent care). Triage often requires judgments on the part of rescuers: you may be faced with deciding which of two patients will receive care, and which may not.

Emergency Care of Patients in Triage

In general, treatment of patients in a triage situation follows this order:

1. Airway patency (an open airway), with control of cervical spine.

☐ Loading the Ambulance Cot

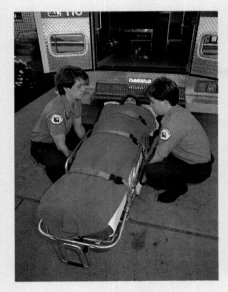

FIGURE 41-76 Preparing to lift with proper hand and back positioning.

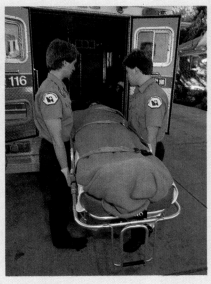

FIGURE 41-77 Lifting stretcher to standing position.

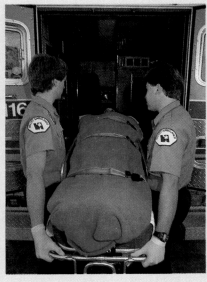

FIGURE 41-78 Moving patient into ambulance.

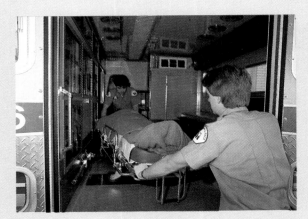

FIGURE 41-79 Moving front of stretcher into securing device.

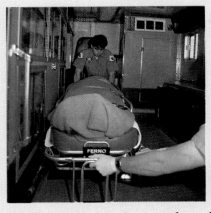

FIGURE 41-80 Securing rear of stretcher into place.

FIGURE 41-81 Make certain both front and rear catches are engaged and secure stretcher.

FIGURE 41-82 Use additional personnel to lift if necessary.

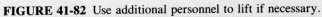

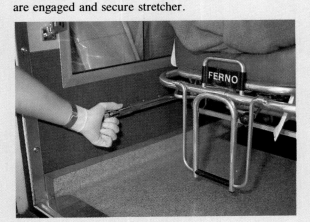

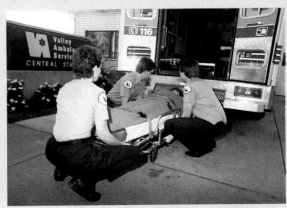

2. Breathing to ensure adequate ventilation.

3. Circulation support, including assessment of the patient, control of bleeding, and providing CPR when adequate manpower is available.

4. Wound management.

5. Fracture management.

Triage Techniques

The most critical but *salvageable* victims are treated and transported first. Unfortunately, the distinction between categories can sometimes be subtle, and some practice is usually required before triage becomes really effective.

The most widely accepted international code for triage uses colors. Red indicates the highest priority (the most urgent), yellow the second priority, and green the third priority; black is used to designate the dead (Figure 41-83).

A variety of tags and other marking systems are used, and triage categories vary slightly from one system to another. Make sure you learn and follow the system used by your local department, and always follow local protocol in sorting, tagging, and transporting.

Three-Level Systems

Among the most common of triage techniques are the three-level systems, by which patients are sorted according to their priority for emergency care.

DEAD The lowest priority is assigned to individuals who show obvious signs of death; they are given black tags. Injuries considered certain to cause death include lack of a pulse for more than twenty minutes, falls from high places resulting in multiple injuries, decapitation, severed trunk, and total incineration. Also in this category are those who are unresponsive and who have no circulation. Patients who have experienced cardiac arrest should be treated as dead in triaging unless there are sufficient personnel to care for both them and other patients.

LOWEST PRIORITY OR DELAYED Lowest priority, or those whose treatment will be delayed, are patients whose wounds are localized and are not life-threatening *and* those who will require a minimum of care without deteriorating while waiting for treatment. These are given a green tag according to the international code. Injuries in this category include minor fractures, extremely minor burns, small abrasions, sprains, or lacerations that do not involve significant blood loss. The lowest priority also includes people whose wounds are so severe that they have little chance to survive, even with aggressive care (a patient with a head wound and exposed brain tissue, for example).

SECOND PRIORITY Second priority — or yellow tagging — is assigned to patients who have life-threatening injuries but who are not yet in shock and who can withstand a one-hour wait for treatment with no risk to their lives. It also includes patients with catastrophic injuries who have a poor chance of survival; they are treated and transported *after* those whose chances for recovery are better (and who are tagged highest priority).

Second-priority patients may include those with back injuries (with or without spinal cord damage), with asthma not accompanied by severe respiratory distress, and with pain accompanied by normal vital signs. Also in this category are medical conditions and injuries such as seizures, emergency childbirth, moderate blood loss (less than two pints of blood), stable abdominal injuries, stable drug overdoses, stable poisoning victims, head-injured patients who are still conscious, eye injuries, moderate to minor burns, or major or multiple fractures. These patients are treated and transported after the most seriously injured *but salvageable* have received care, but before those who have minor injuries or are dying.

HIGHEST PRIORITY Patients to be treated and transported first are given a red tag and must meet three criteria:

- Injuries are life-threatening, and risk of asphyxiation or shock is imminent or present.

- The patient can be stabilized without requiring constant care.

- The patient has high probability of survival *if* he or she is treated and transported immediately.

Those with catastrophic injuries of the head or chest are not included in this category because of the bleak chance of recovery. The high-priority category does include victims with severe uncontrolled bleeding, respiratory arrest, witnessed cardiac arrest (only if sufficient personnel are available, otherwise these are given lowest priority), major burns, respiratory tract burns, cervical spine fractures, open abdominal wounds, open or closed chest wounds, severe (but not catastrophic) head injuries, open eye wounds, fractures without a distal pulse, severe shock, hyperthermia, hypothermia, those who are unconscious in the absence of head injury, and those who are suffering from medical complications (of diabetes, heart disease, and so on).

Also in the highest priority are those with burns over more than 25 percent but less than 50 percent of the body.

Triage Tags

After victims are sorted and assessed in the triage process, they must be tagged for rapid identification. Triage tags, which come in a variety of sizes, shapes, and colors, provide the necessary identification regarding

TRIAGE SUMMARY

Triage means sorting multiple casualties into priorities for emergency care or for transportation to definitive care. Priorities are usually given in three levels as follows: In a two-level system, the Lowest and Second Priorities would be in the delayed category and the Highest Priority maintains that immediate status.

LOWEST PRIORITY

- Fractures or other injuries of a minor nature
- Obviously mortal wounds where death appears reasonably certain
- Obvious dead
- Cardiac arrest (if sufficient personnel are not available to care for numerous other patients)
- Follow local protocol

SECOND PRIORITY

- Burns
- Major or multiple fractures
- Back injuries with or without spinal cord damage

HIGHEST PRIORITY

- Airway and breathing difficulties
- Cardiac arrest if sufficient personnel available
- Uncontrolled or suspected severe bleeding
- Severe head injuries
- Severe medical problems: poisoning, diabetic and cardiac emergencies, etc.
- Open chest or abdominal wounds
- Shock

PROCEDURES

1. The most knowledgeable EMT arriving in the first ambulance must become triage officer. One of the first units should establish a command post and communications center.

2. Primary survey should be completed on all patients first. Correct immediate life-threatening problems.

3. Call for additional assistance if needed.

4. Assign available manpower and equipment to priority-one patients.

5. Transport priority-one patients and those that are stabilized first.

6. Notify hospital(s) of number and severity of injuries.

7. Triage officer remains at scene to assign and coordinate manpower, supplies and vehicles.

8. Patients must be reassessed regularly for changes in condition.

FIGURE 41-83

which category the patient has been assigned to. Generally, use triage tags only if more than ten victims are involved in a single incident.

Once a patient has been tagged, do not remove the original tag. If the patient changes status before he has been treated, draw a bold line through the original tag, note the time, and put a new tag on the patient that reflects the new status. This procedure enables EMTs to know that the patient has had a change in status.

One of the most popular and recommended triage tags is the Mettag (Figure 41-84). It uses symbols in lieu of written words, making identification rapid and uncomplicated. It is also bright and colorful, so it is highly visible. With perforated divisions, it contains a strip for each of the categories: green (an ambulance with an X through it) for the noninjured or those not needing transport, yellow (turtle) for second priority, red (rabbit) for highest priority, and black (a shovel and cross) for the dead. EMTs simply tear off the strips not needed so that the applicable strip is on the outside edge. The Mettag also enables EMTs to change a patient's status without assigning a new tag.

In performing triage, avoid tags that require a ballpoint pen, that use carbons, that are too detailed, or that require too much information.

Conducting the Triage

Triage should be completed by the most experienced personnel as soon as the scene is secured. Triage personnel must become so familiar with the classification levels that the knowledge becomes second nature. *It is also imperative that the various rescue agencies in a community use the same type of tag system.*

At the accident site, the triage EMTs can move from patient to patient, performing very limited, life-saving treatment and applying tag cards for later treatment. The key is for the triage EMT to not stop at one patient and become preoccupied with a bloody wound or shock, but to move through the patients to complete the triage. This sets the stage for the next arriving rescuers, who can focus on treating salvageable patients.

Many patients experience an injury (such as a blunt trauma injury) that does not show on the surface but that is more devastating to life than many observable injuries. Patients who are in cardiopulmonary arrest should not be treated during multiple-injury triage but should be tagged as apparently dead. EMTs must learn the limits of triage care, or they will be unable to complete the job, since they will waste valuable time and equipment on the unsalvageable.

The triage EMTs quickly evaluate each patient's condition, categorizing and prioritizing for care and applying the ABCs on a limited basis (depending on the availability of triage and emergency care personnel) un-

til triage is completed. The following evaluation order should be followed:

1. During primary survival scan, if a patient is conscious and talking, with no major bleeding, he or she should be reassured and the EMT should move on. During the secondary triage, the EMT should quickly tag the patient according to priority and may ask questions for tagging purposes. Ask a *conscious patient* the following questions:

   • Where do you hurt? A response may indicate if the patient can hear and understand and may reveal the condition of his or her thought processes.

   • Are you allergic to anything, and have you had any serious illness recently? This tests the patient's recall and thinking processes.

   • Were you unconscious at any time? This question may reveal possible head injuries and help to recall the immediate past.

   • Do you have any medical illnesses, such as diabetes? Have you taken any medication or drugs/alcohol within the past six hours? Do you hurt anywhere specifically? Are you experiencing any vision, hearing, balance, or other abnormal problems? Do you have feeling in your arms and legs? (Pinch each limb prior to asking.) How long since you last ate?

2. The *unconscious patient* needs the following specific priority examination. Perform it within thirty seconds.

   • Open the airway by tilting back the head (with careful attention to the cervical spine) or lifting the chin and supporting the neck.

   • Listen for breathing and any possible airway obstruction.

   • If airway obstruction is present, perform the manual thrust (Heimlich maneuver) with the patient lying on his or her back.

   • Check chest movement and the mouth for breathing.

   • If breathing is absent, perform mouth-to-mouth resuscitation. *Note:* In some areas, patients who do not breathe after the airway has been opened are triaged as dead, and mouth-to-mouth resuscitation is not performed. *Follow local protocol.*

   • Check the carotid pulse for heartbeat and circulation. If you find no pulse, tag the patient and move on to the next triage patient unless other triage personnel are available.

   • Hemorrhage should be controlled quickly by direct pressure or a dressing/pressure bandage and

THE METTAG

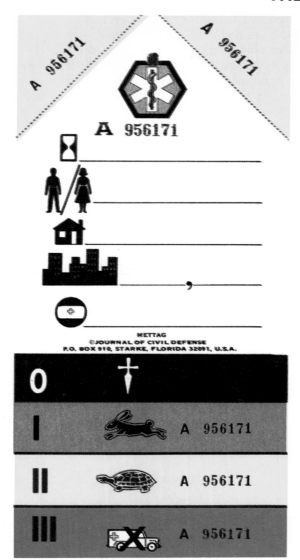

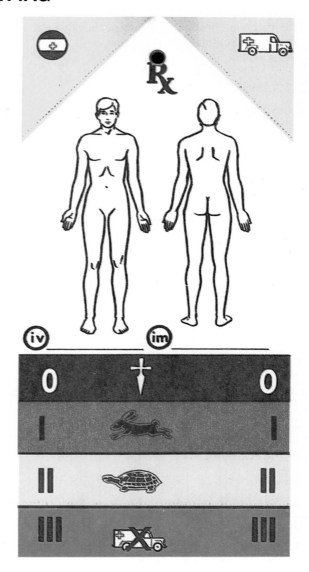

FIGURE 41-84

elevation. You give only limited treatment. You cannot afford to wait six to seven minutes for the blood to clot.

- The patient now needs to be marked or tagged according to the seriousness and kinds of injuries involved.

3. Patients considered to have a poor salvage rate include those with open skull fracture and exposed brain tissue, gross deformity of the head, cardiogenic shock, cardiac tamponade, sucking wounds of the chest, severe abdominal evisceration, catastrophic head or chest injuries, crushed trachea,

lost airway that cannot be quickly corrected with conventional methods (such as suctioning or the Heimlich maneuver), catastrophic injury of the trunk, massive subcutaneous emphysema, major facial burns with inhalation of hot air/gas, cervical spine fracture with quadriplegia, or second- or third-degree burns covering 40 percent or more of the body.

4. To protect other patients and avoid contamination at the hospital, isolate victims with obvious infection. Generally, suspect infection if the patient has a fever of more than 103° F. (with or without a rash), purulent sputum, an open draining wound,

purulent drainage from a body opening, a rash, or if the victim is known to be carrying an infectious disease. Communications should make sure that the receiving hospital is aware of the situation before an infectious patient arrives.

Triage Log

If sufficient help is available, keep a triage log. The completeness of the log will depend on the amount of help available and on the condition of the patient and others who need to provide information. A sample log is provided in Figure 41-85.

Other Factors Affecting Triage

Several additional factors figure into the classification that you will use during triage. Depending on the nature of the crisis and the available staffing, you may not always be able to take these into consideration. The urgency of treatment and the extent of the injury are the most important considerations. If enough staff is available, other factors that should be considered include age (you would be willing to take more chances on reviving a young person than an old one), general physical condition (someone who is obviously in poor physical condition might not recover anyway), and medical history (obtained only from conscious victims).

FIGURE 41-85 Triage Log.

EMT TRIAGE LOG

Victim Number	Age	Sex	Vital Signs			Description of Injuries	Triage Priority	Field Care	Transported
			Blood Pressure	Pulse	Respirations				
1									By_____ To_____
2									By_____ To_____
3									By_____ To_____
4									By_____ To_____
5									By_____ To_____

Date: _____ Time: _____

Rescuer Completing Log: _____

chapter 42

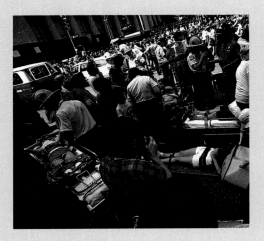

Multiple-Casualty Incidents and Disaster Management

✱ OBJECTIVES

- Outline the phases of a disaster and requirements of effective disaster management.
- Describe the problems of disaster plans.
- Describe the general procedures of a disaster/multiple–casualty incident plan.
- Identify the appropriate steps for disaster prewarning and evacuation.
- Explain how to set up communications in a disaster.
- Describe various approaches for reducing rescue personnel stress during disaster situations.

> It is important that you are familiar with your local disaster plan and your assigned role in the event of a disaster.

> It is recommended that EMTs wear protective gloves whenever there is a possibility of coming in contact with a patient's blood, body fluids, mucous membranes, traumatic wounds, or sores. See Chapter 31.

□ WHAT IS A DISASTER?

In general, a disaster is a sudden catastrophic event that overwhelms natural order and causes great loss of property and/or life. It is a disparity between casualties and resources. It exceeds the capabilities of available management resources and may disrupt the community, the medical establishment, or both. It may be defined a "disaster" because of the overwhelming number of victims involved, or because just a few victims are so severely injured.

Disasters may be natural, such as those caused by hurricanes, earthquakes, floods, and tornadoes, or man-made, such as airline crashes, fires, toxic gas leaks, and nuclear accidents.

□ PHASES OF A DISASTER

In general, disasters occur in five phases. The *anticipatory phase* consists of long-range planning and prevention measures; in essence, it's the realization that a disaster could sometime occur. It entails drawing up a disaster plan, for instance, or using earthquake-proof building codes in an area where earthquake may happen.

The *preimpact phase* is the period immediately before the disaster occurs. During this time, an imminent threat is perceived, and an official warning may or may not be issued. During the preimpact phase, people are much more likely to respond to emergency directives if they can see some evidence of the impending emergency (such as the darkening skies and increased winds associated with an approaching hurricane).

During the *impact phase,* the disaster actually occurs. Depending on the disaster, this period may be extremely brief (such as the minute of an isolated explosion), or it may last several hours (such as a severe hurricane) or several weeks (such as continued flooding).

In the *recoil phase,* victims — including rescuers — assess the surroundings and make a preliminary estimate of damages. During this phase, assistance from the outside arrives, and victims are rescued. Within a minute or so of the initial impact, many of the victims themselves will extricate themselves and begin to help others. In some disasters, as many as 75 percent of the victims act as rescuers.

During the *postimpact phase,* or rehabilitation phase, which may last for weeks or months, victims grieve and develop coping mechanisms as the reality of the loss becomes evident. Rebuilding takes place.

□ REQUIREMENTS OF EFFECTIVE DISASTER ASSISTANCE

In general, effective disaster assistance requires:

- Preparation of the entire community; community members at large need to be trained in basic life-supporting first aid and simple rescue procedures.
- Careful preplanning.
- The ability to quickly implement a plan.
- The application of triage skills.
- The ability to organize quickly and utilize fully all emergency personnel.
- The ability to adapt the plan to meet special conditions, such as inclement weather or isolated locations.
- A contingency plan that provides for shelter and transportation of an area, such as an entire community or county.
- The ability to do the greatest good for the greatest number.
- A plan that avoids simply relocating the incident from the scene to the local hospital.

□ GENERAL PROCEDURES OF A DISASTER PLAN

In any disaster/multiple–casualty, *call for plenty of help early in the disaster*. Be realistic about what kind of help you'll need, but it's better to call too many teams than not enough. Make sure you call plenty of rescuers who have advanced life-saving skills.

A disaster/multiple–casualty plan should include the following general procedures:

1. Make absolutely clear from the beginning who is in charge, and establish that person in a command post located in a safe area near or at the patient collection area. An **incident command system** should already be organized. The system is a management program that should be designed to control, direct, and coordinate emergency response resources (see Figure 42-1).

2. If the disaster/incident is weather-related, take measures to protect all rescuers during the impact phase. It is best to wait to begin actual rescue work until the storm has settled.

3. The first uniformed responder to arrive at the

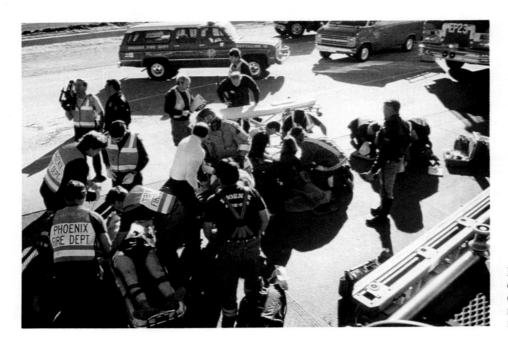

FIGURE 42-1 The incident command system assists in controlling and coordinating resources at a multiple-casualty incident (MCI).

scene rapidly assesses the scene for possible hazards to victims or to the surrounding public.

4. The first EMT or medically trained individual who reaches the scene locates and reassures victims. If the disaster is small-scale, the responder quickly assesses victims, performs triage, and radios for help as he or she begins life-saving treatment. Any first responder also instructs conscious victims about what they can do for themselves, such as applying direct pressure to stop bleeding, and stresses that help is on the way. If there is immediate and obvious danger to the victims, the responder immediately begins moving people, regardless of their injuries. Those who can walk are instructed to do so, and passersby can help evacuate others.

5. The first responder radios for help. He or she gives the exact location of the disaster/incident, the estimated number of victims, and the best routes of approach for other responders.

6. Those at headquarters who receive confirmation of the disaster immediately confirm it on all frequencies (ambulance, police, and fire), including exact location and routing instructions. All transmissions are brief, precise, and in clear, normal language. No codes are used during transmission. If the disaster/incident is large enough to warrant it, a communications headquarters is established, and a full, region-wide communication is dispatched.

7. Communications personnel contact all nearby hospitals to confirm the disaster/incident and report the estimated number of victims. Hospital personnel begin activating their disaster plans.

8. The community should have a list of ambulances and EMS squads that are *predesignated* to respond in disasters/incidents. Communications headquarters contact the ambulances and EMS squads on the call-up list, informing them of the exact location, routing instructions, and estimated number of victims. Predesignated units are told to respond with double crews and mass-casualty equipment. Fire and police departments are then radioed and sent to the scene. The plan should also designate which ambulances should stay on standby to cover normal EMT calls during the disaster; not all available ambulances should be dispatched to the scene of the disaster.

9. The first fire officer to arrive at the scene assesses the site for fire hazards. He or she quickly plans what to do in case of fire and decides how the fire will be handled. He or she determines how incoming equipment should be routed and enlists the help of a police officer to direct incoming trucks. He or she positions a truck at each end of the disaster site and places rescue equipment as close as possible to the victims.

10. As fire and rescue personnel arrive, they are briefed by the fire officer who has made the plans; once the area is safe for fire personnel to proceed, the plan is carried out and the equipment is placed. Rescue personnel immediately assess the scene and render it safe for rescue work.

11. Once the site is safe for rescue work, the rescue workers move quickly to the victims.

12. The first ambulance that arrives is positioned a safe distance from the disaster itself but near the patient collection area and is used as headquarters. The EMT establishes direct radio contact with area hospitals and uses the vehicle as a field emergency surgical center if necessary.

13. The senior EMT arriving assumes responsibility as the EMT control officer until the predesignated officer arrives. This EMT is responsible for seeing that the EMS portion of the disaster/incident is set up in a controlled and orderly way and that all responsibilities are carried out.

14. The second EMT who arrives becomes the primary triage officer. The goals of triage are to assess the victim's condition, determine the urgency of his or her condition, assign a priority to his or her treatment and transport, and determine his or her disposition. The EMT performs a primary scan on each patient, checking for airway, breathing, and bleeding. If an airway is not open, he opens the airway and inserts a mechanical airway if appropriate. He checks for a pulse; if there is no pulse, he or she moves on. If a pulse is felt, he or she checks for major hemorrhage. If hemorrhage is found, he quickly applies a cravat to the wound and moves on. If there are others still waiting to be triaged, the only initial treatment that should be done is airway management and control of severe hemorrhage.

15. As more EMTs arrive, one is designated as the secondary triage officer, responsible for tagging the patients in order of priority. If the primary triage officer completes the survival scan before other EMTs arrive, *he or she* tags patients for priority treatment. (Figure 42-2).

Remember that triage is ongoing — many victims' categories will change as their conditions deteriorate.

Designate a treatment site that is close to the area where ambulances arrive. It should be on high ground, and, if possible, should be covered and lighted. It should be safe from falling debris, and a safe distance from the incident. Put all equipment in this one area, and strip all incoming ambulances of their equipment. Clearly mark the treatment area — use a tall flag if you have one.

16. As each EMT arrives, he or she reports to the command post and is assigned tasks by the control officer. Victims are moved to the patient collection area *in order of their priority*. In some systems, the primary triage officer tags as he or she goes, and there is no secondary officer.

17. An EMT is designated as loading officer. This person ensures that ambulances are accessible and that transportation does not occur without the direction of the EMS control officer and the triage master. The loading officer coordinates patient transportation with the triage master and communicates with the hospitals involved.

18. The triage master should be a *predesignated* individual who has special training in triage. He or she is responsible for monitoring the patient collection area, ensuring that equipment is placed near the area for patient use, coordinating care of the patients with other EMTs, and updating or changing the priority of the patients. He or she

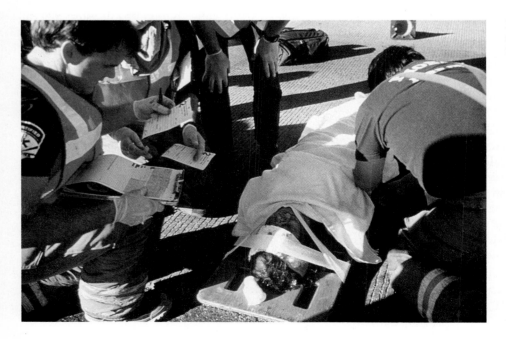

FIGURE 42-2 Triage tagging is essential in multiple-casualty incidents.

also coordinates transportation of patients by priority with the loading officer.

19. As soon as the chief of police arrives, he or she joins the disaster control chief at headquarters and is briefed. The chief of police confers with the disaster control chief to determine the best routes of entry for additional arriving rescue vehicles. The two decide how transport vehicles should most smoothly leave the scene. The chief of police is then designated as the alternate disaster control chief. All incoming rescue personnel now report either to the disaster control chief or the alternate (the chief of police) for instructions.

20. Victims are now moved to triage stations according to injuries. Immobilize all victims before moving them, and place them in rows according to their triage category. *The priority is to save life and limb; treat only salvageable patients.* If color-coded triage tags or cards are used, the same colors should be used on color-coded flags that are erected at the triage stations. Victims are positioned in rows as they await treatment. Since the dead are the last to be transported, a morgue should be set up in a separate, out of-sight area.

21. As incoming equipment arrives, it is moved to the central equipment area, and rescue equipment is stashed in orderly piles (all cervical collars together, all spine boards together). Additional personnel are utilized where needed.

22. As the highest priority victims are stabilized, transport begins. Before and during transport, one or two triage officers (depending on the number of victims) move along the rows constantly, monitoring the victims in case there is a change in status.

23. Before leaving the disaster/incident, EMTs receive specific instructions from the transportation officer or the disaster control chief (*follow local protocol*) on how to leave the area (preferred route) and to which hospital to take the victims. High-priority victims are transported first, immediately after stabilization; the disaster control chief attempts to distribute these serious victims evenly among available hospitals.

24. Once the highest-priority victims have been stabilized, rescue workers move to the second-priority triage station and begin treatment. The head triage officer remains in constant communication with the transportation office or disaster/incident control chief regarding transport availability and needs. Follow local protocol.

25. Take shortcuts with non–life-threatening injuries. For example, immobilize victims to a long board instead of trying to splint each individual fracture.

26. If the routing in the area is complex, the loading officer and his or her assistant provide EMTs with marked maps to the appropriate hospital.

27. As each ambulance leaves, the transportation officer appointed by the EMS control officer or the loading officer (follow local protocol) radios the hospital that the ambulance is en route and briefly describes the injuries involved. An estimated time of arrival is given. Individual EMTs should *not* try to communicate with the hospital unless an emergency develops during transport.

28. As soon as the town's chief executive arrives, he or she is briefed by the disaster/incident control chief. Communications are set up with city hall, and personnel at city hall work to locate additional help and supplies, evacuate neighborhoods, or contact relatives of the victims, as assigned by the town's chief executive.

29. When the only victims left at the site are ambulatory, they are loaded onto a bus that has been brought to the site for this purpose. Five to ten rescue personnel carrying rescue equipment (oxygen masks, suction equipment, crash kits, and portable radio) board the bus, and a fully equipped ambulance with its crew leads the bus slowly and safely to an outlying hospital that has little or no load. If a victim on the bus suddenly deteriorates during the trip to the hospital, EMTs can handle the situation.

30. When all victims have been moved from the disaster/incident scene, emergency personnel go to hospitals to assist hospital personnel. The disaster/incident control chief and his assistant remain at the scene to supervise clean-up and complete restoration.

31. Psychological stress is acute at the scene of a disaster or multiple–casualty incident. Any rescuer who breaks down or becomes hysterical during the disaster operation should be removed immediately to a hospital; a rescuer who is injured or becomes ill during rescue operations should be treated immediately and transported so that other rescuers can continue their work.

32. Emergency care will probably be needed for days or weeks following impact, depending on the size and scope of the disaster/incident. Measures should be taken to prevent stress and burnout among rescue personnel.

☐ PREWARNING AND EVACUATION

In some cases, you may learn that a disaster is approaching and may have time to evacuate local residents. If you can conduct an orderly evacuation, you can prevent further injury, preserve life, and protect property.

Relocation should, as much as possible, keep people in their natural social groupings. Make every effort to provide home-based relocation instead of relocating people to hospitals and clinics if they are not injured.

Alerts for the evacuation must be repeated often and with clarity. You must convince people that a disaster is really about to occur and that there is a substantial threat to their safety. At a minimum, the evacuation and warning message *must* contain the following information:

- The nature of the disaster and its estimated time of impact on the area; if possible, relate the expected severity.
- Safe routes to take out of the area.
- Appropriate destinations for those who evacuate, indicating where food and shelter will be available.

Use whatever means you have available to spread the message with frequent urgency — radio, television, roving police cars with loudspeakers, public address systems in buildings, and short-wave radios. Make sure that *each* message contains all pertinent details concerning the nature and impact of the disaster, how people should evacuate, which routes are safest, and where people should meet for assistance after evacuation.

□ SETTING UP COMMUNICATIONS

Critical to any successful rescue effort is an efficient communications system that includes a back-up system to be used in case the primary system fails. The specific system that you choose will depend on your area and requirements, but the following apply to any disaster/incident communications system:

- Establish details of the system ahead of time. The communications network should be apart of your disaster drill — decide what kind of system you want, who will be responsible for operating it, and what equipment will be used.
- Appoint *one person only* at the scene of the disaster/incident who will communicate to those outside the disaster area. It is usually best to use the disaster control chief: he or she should be aware at all times of what is going on and can be a source of reliable information to the outside.
- The person who is designated to communicate should stay in touch with local hospitals and rescue units who may be called upon to respond to the disaster. Make sure ahead of time that the per-

son will have access to appropriate equipment to keep in touch with the outside.

- Area-wide communications are vital — they give people warning of an impending disaster as well as help people receive information regarding the status of family members, friends, and the community as a whole.
- Since it may be impossible to restore telephone service to an area immediately, establish a central location where people can register concerning their whereabouts, safety, health status, and so on.
- Make sure that information regarding road conditions, alternate routes, and closed roads is constantly monitored and communicated, especially in the case of a weather-related disaster.
- Constantly monitor and link all hospitals, trauma centers, and clinics in the area so that you can determine which can receive more patients and when those patients can be transported to a specific facility. The status of hospitals will change constantly throughout the recoil and post-impact phases of the disaster; therefore, keep communications open.
- Do *not* allow ambulance drivers or EMTs who are en route to the hospital to communicate via radio to the hospital *unless* an emergency occurs en route. The person designated to take care of communications will contact the appropriate hospital as the ambulance leaves the disaster/incident scene; individual ambulance communication will jam lines and create confusion.
- If the disaster/incident area is large, individual rescue workers should be equipped with walkie-talkie units or radios so that they can communicate with their commands.
- You should include a recorder or some other device that will allow you to record crucial communications.

Many communities are now using the HEAR network (Hospital Emergency Administration Radio), a network that links hospitals together for communication purposes. If your community opts to use the HEAR system, you will need to make some adjustments to correct for the difficulty when all hospitals are attempting to use the same frequency.

□ PSYCHOLOGICAL IMPACT OF DISASTERS

Faced with the grim physical injuries that can accompany a disaster, it is difficult to remember that the psychological injuries can be severe — even among those not physically injured. The overwhelming reaction to disaster is a reaction to the loss of either life or property (see Figure 42-3). Almost all people experience fear; many also feel shaky, perspire profusely, become confused, and suffer irritability, anxiety, restlessness, fatigue, sleep disturbances, nightmares, difficulty concentrating, moodiness, suspiciousness, depression, nausea, vomiting, and diarrhea. Survivors of a disaster often experience fear, anxiety, anger, guilt, shock, depression, denial, feelings of isolation, and vulnerability. All these reactions are normal. As soon as people begin working to remedy the disaster situation, their physical responses usually become less exaggerated, and they are able to work with less tension and fear.

At high risk for severe emotional reactions include children, the elderly, those in poor physical or emotional health, the handicapped, and those who have an unresolved past loss or crisis.

The reactions of children depend on their age, individual disposition, family support, and community support. Generally, preschoolers cry, lose control of bowel and/or bladder, become confused, and suck their thumbs. Elementary-age children suffer extreme fears about their safety and show confusion, depression, headache, inability to concentrate, withdrawal, poor performance, and the tendency to fight with their peers. Preadolescents and adolescents may show the same reaction as elementary-age children coupled with extreme aggression and stress that is severe enough to disrupt their lives.

Rescuers, too, react, often the same way as victims do. Common are fears regarding personal safety, crying, anger, guilt, numbness, preoccupation with death, frustration, fatigue, and burnout; approximately two-thirds of all rescuers suffer long-term reactions. Most rescuer reactions peak within about one week and then diminish. Approximately half have recurrent dreams and repeated recollections of the disaster for weeks or months afterward. In some cases, the rescuer may not react for weeks or months.

□ GENERAL GUIDELINES FOR DISASTER RESCUERS

While each disaster presents individual problems, the following guidelines apply to any disaster to which you may be called (see Figure 42-4).

- Do not let yourself become overwhelmed by the immensity of the disaster. Administer care to those who need it. Carefully evaluate the injuries and determine which patients should be cared for

first. Then set about administering the aid, caring for patients one by one. This will help you maintain some calm and feel that you are making progress.

- The chief town executive, the public relations officer, or the incident commander obtains and distributes information about the disaster and the victims. The families of victims deserve accurate information. This is too often overlooked in the rush to begin emergency care. As soon as possible, assign several rescue workers to gather information and disseminate it to local radio and television stations so that psychological stress to other family members may be lessened.

- Reunite the victim with his family as soon as possible. Emotional stress will be lessened once the victim is with family members, and family members may be able to provide you with critical medical history that may increase your ability to care for the patient.

- Encourage victims to do necessary chores. Work can be therapeutic and should be used to help the victims get over their own problems. You might think that the victim is unable to do any work because his or her condition appears to render him unfit, but many victims simply do not know what to do first and are generally overwhelmed.

- If the disaster has involved a large number of people, group the victims with their families and neighbors. This will help reduce feelings of fear and alienation.

- Provide a structure for the emotionally injured, and let them know your expectations. Tell the victim exactly what is happening; tell him or her that he or she is suffering a temporary setback, that he or she is likely to recover rapidly, and that meanwhile, you expect certain minimal tasks to be performed. Explain those tasks clearly and simply, then follow up to make sure that he or she is performing them.

- Help the victims confront the reality of the disaster. Help them work through their feelings. Encourage them to talk about the disaster and its long-term effects. If you sense that they are not facing reality or that expectations are much worse than reality, help them adjust their views.

- Try not to use sedatives or drugs. Some victims will need a tranquilizer to help them over the initial shock, but it is dangerous to continue their use, because the victim will not be able to resolve the situation as long as he or she is sedated.

- Do not give false assurances. The victim needs help in facing problems and deciding how he or she will react to them. The victim needs to face

EMOTIONAL REACTIONS IN MASS CASUALTIES AND DISASTERS

Reaction	Signs and Symptoms	Do's	Don'ts
Normal	Fear and anxiety Muscular tension followed by trembling and weakness Confusion Profuse perspiration Nausea, vomiting Mild diarrhea Frequent urination Shortness of breath Pounding heart These reactions usually dissipate with activity as the person organizes himself	Normal reactions usually require little emergency care Calm reassurance may be all that is necessary to help a person pull himself together Watch to see that the individual is gaining composure, not losing it Provide meaningful activity Talk with the person	Don't show extreme sympathy
Panic (blind flight of hysteria)	Unreasoning attempt to Loss of judgment — blindness to reality Uncontrolled weeping or hysteria often to the point of exhaustion Aimless running about with little regard for safety Panic is contagious when not controlled. Normally calm persons may become panicked by others during moments when they are temporarily disorganized	Begin with firmness Give something warm to eat or drink Firmly, but gently, isolate him from the group. Get help if necessary Show empathy and encourage him to talk Monitor your own feelings Keep calm and know your limitations	Don't brutally restrain him Don't strike him Don't douse him with water Don't give sedatives
Overactive	Explodes into flurry of senseless activity Argumentative Overconfident of abilities Talks rapidly — will not listen Tells silly jokes Makes endless suggestions Demanding of others Does more harm than good by interfering with organized leadership Like panic, overactivity is contagious if not controlled	Let him talk and ventilate his feelings Assign and supervise a job that requires physical activity Give something warm to eat or drink	Don't tell him he is acting abnormally Don't give sedatives Don't argue with him Don't tell him he shouldn't act or feel the way he does
Underactive (daze, shock, depression)	Cannot recover from original shock and numbness Stands or sits without talking or moving Vacant expression Emotionless "Don't care" attitude Helpless, unaware of surroundings Moves aimlessly, slowly Little or no response to questioning Pulls within self to protect from further stress Puzzled, confused Cannot take responsibility without supervision	Gently establish contact and rapport Get him to ventilate his feelings and let you know what happened Show empathy Be aware of feelings of resentment in yourself and others Give him warm food or drink Give and supervise a simple, routine job	Don't tell him to "snap out of it" Don't give extreme pity Don't give sedatives Don't show resentment
Severe physical reaction (conversion hysteria)	Severe nausea Conversion hysteria — the victim converts his anxiety into a strong belief that a part of his body is not functioning (paralysis, loss of sight, etc.). The disability is just as real as if he had been physically injured	Show interest Find a small job for him to take his mind off the injury Make him comfortable and summon medical aid Monitor your own feelings	Don't say, "There's nothing wrong with you" or, "It's all in your head" Don't blame or ridicule Don't call undue attention to the injury Don't openly ignore the injury

Source: American Psychiatric Association

FIGURE 42-3

GENERAL GUIDELINES FOR DISASTER MANAGEMENT

While each disaster presents individual problems, there are some guidelines that are general and that will usually apply to any disaster you may be called to respond to:

1 Don't let yourself become overwhelmed by the immensity of the disaster. Administer aid to those who need it. Carefully evaluate the injuries, and determine which victims should be treated first. Then set about administering the aid, treating victims one by one. This will help you maintain some calm and feel that you are making progress, despite the immensity of the disaster.

2 Obtain and distribute information about the disaster and the victims. The families of victims deserve accurate information about both the disaster and the victims themselves.

3 Reunite the victim with his family as soon as possible. There are two benefits of this: first, emotional stress will be lessened once the victim is with family members. Second, family members may be able to provide you with critical medical history that may affect your ability to treat the victim.

4 Encourage victims who are able to do necessary chores. Work can be therapeutic, and should be used to help the victim get over his own problems. Help the victim devise a schedule to perform his own daily routines like he did before the disaster.

FIGURE 42-4

facts sooner or later; if he or she finds that you have lied, he or she may resist any further outside help, and recovery period will probably be extensive. Honestly appraise the situation for the victim, then offer your help in areas where it's needed. Express your confidence in his or her ability to overcome the crisis and handle the situation.

- Permit the victim limited dependency. There are many reasons why a victim may refuse offers of help. It may be against his or her cultural upbringing, it may compromise his or her self-image, or the victim may not have an accurate concept of the seriousness of the situation. Explain that by accepting help no one is in any way admitting weakness. Make sure it is understood that the help (and, therefore, his or her dependency) is only temporary and that as soon as things are under control he or she may be needed to help someone else.
- Identify high-risk victims: the elderly, children, the bereaved, those with prior psychiatric illness, those with multiple stresses, those with low or no support systems, those from low socioeconomic backgrounds, and those with severe injuries. Target these people for immediate crisis intervention care.
- Arrange for a group discussion where victims can exchange ideas as soon as physical needs are taken care of.
- Identify people who are in a unique position to help people in need, and recruit and train them in psychological emergency care.
- Arrange for all those involved in the disaster — including rescuers — to get good follow-up care and support; let each one talk about his or her feelings.

□ REDUCING STRESS ON RESCUE PERSONNEL

Once the rescue operation is underway, a new danger arises: rescue workers may begin to suffer from stress. If measures are not taken immediately, rescue workers can become inefficient and, at worst, can become victims themselves.

To help reduce stress on rescuers from the beginning of the rescue operations, follow these guidelines:

- As each rescue worker reports to the staffing area for assignment, he or she should be instructed to rest at regular intervals — perhaps once every one to two hours; follow local protocol. During rest periods, which may last as long as you decide on, the worker should return to the staffing area (preferably an area that is away from the hub of the disaster), sit or lie down, have something to eat or drink, and relax as much as possible. If rest periods are effectively rotated, there will always be enough rescue workers to carry on disaster assistance, and the entire team will be rested and relieved periodically.

- Make sure that each rescue worker is fully aware of his or her exact assignment. Have a well-designed plan that enables you to fully utilize your personnel, and fully explain to each worker what his or her responsibility is. It will help reduce stress if a worker has well-defined limits, and you will eliminate the problem of workers wandering aimlessly around wondering what to do.

- Several workers in the staffing area should circulate among the rescue workers and watch for signs of physical exhaustion or stress. If one of the workers appears to be having problems, he or she should immediately be required to return to the staffing area and rest for a longer period than usual. After resting, if possible, a less stressful task should be assigned, possibly in another area of the disaster site.

- Make sure that rescue workers are assigned to tasks according to their skills and experience. If there is a question about whether a certain worker can handle a task, do not gamble — give him or her the task that you are *sure* he can handle.

- Provide plenty of nourishing drinks and food; encourage rescue workers to eat and drink whenever necessary to keep up their strength.

- Encourage rescue workers to talk among themselves; talking helps relieve stress. Discourage lighthearted conversation and joking, however — some victims as well as workers may be offended by it, increasing the stress level at the disaster scene.

- Do whatever is necessary to keep the disaster scene well organized and running smoothly.

- Make sure that rescuers have the opportunity to talk with trained counselors after the incident. See section on Critical Incident Stress Debriefing in Chapter 39. Counselors can help minimize long-term effects of the disaster. If your team has access to critical incident stress debriefing, make sure all rescuers who worked on the disaster take advantage of this help.

chapter 43

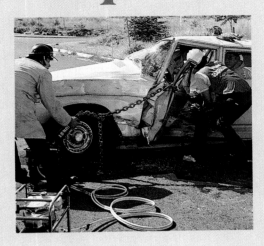

Vehicle Stabilization and Patient Extrication

✳ OBJECTIVES

- List the proper protective clothing and what rescue tools are appropriate and standard.
- Define the major principles of extrication.
- Discuss extrication techniques and tools.
- List the hazards and dangers involved in extrication.
- Demonstrate how to stabilize a vehicle, gain access to a patient, stabilize and disentangle him, and properly prepare him for removal or transfer.
- Demonstrate how to operate in specialized extrication situations, such as snow, ice, water, buildings, and underground.

It is recommended that EMTs wear protective gloves whenever there is a possibility of coming in contact with a patient's blood, body fluids, mucous membranes, traumatic wounds, or sores. See Chapter 31.

As an emergency medical technician, you will encounter patients who are located in difficult-to-reach places that may be dangerous both to you and to the patients. These individuals must be **extricated** carefully so that they can be transported for more intensive care. The movement should be orderly, planned, and unhurried (unless, of course, the situation is dangerous), so that the patients are not injured further. In many cases, you will also need to immobilize the patients before you can begin extrication.

Situations calling for extrication include:

- Household accidents, where the patient has fallen or become jammed in an unusual position.
- Natural calamities like floods, cave-ins, hurricanes, landslides, or avalanches, where the environment has created an extrication problem.
- Fires.
- Automobile accidents, where highway and street conditions, traffic density, location of other vehicles involved in the accident, location of official and public safety vehicles, and weather affect the time you have to extricate a patient and impact your procedure.

This chapter discusses the most common extrication situation: an automobile accident.

□ IMPORTANCE OF PROTECTIVE CLOTHING

At a minimum, rescue workers should wear the following OSHA-approved protective clothing (Figure 43-1):

- Impact-resistant protective helmet with ear protection and a strap under the chin. A construction

hard hat is also compact and lightweight. Be sure you choose a model with full suspension and secure chin strap. Be sure that, regardless of type, the helmet is brightly colored with reflective stripes and EMT identification.

- Safety goggles (specified for work with power equipment) with an elastic strap and vents to prevent fogging. If you wear glasses, get goggles that will fit over them. Ordinary glasses and fire helmet face shields do not provide side protection.
- Turn-out coat to prevent puncturing (light in weight).
- Slip-resistant, waterproof gloves, or leather gloves as the situation warrants.
- Rubber boots with steel insoles and toes, or high-top work shoes that have ankle protection. Be sure that your pants cover the boot tops so that debris cannot fall inside.
- Long underwear and a warm hat or stocking cap in cool weather to protect against hypothermia.
- A strobe light that can be hand-held or hooked to the upper arm or belt for EMT identification and traffic safety in the dark.
- A dust respirator is helpful in accidents involving cement, grain, or similar accidents.
- A good quality, versatile pocket knife.

Your protective clothing should be lightweight and flexible enough to allow you full range of motion. Some protective clothing offers excellent protection but is too cumbersome to be practical in rescue situations.

□ RESCUE TOOLS

Basic rescue tools should be standard equipment in every ambulance, and every EMT must be well trained in their use (Figure 43-2—43-3). Rescue tools may be carried in the rescue vehicle if it accompanies an ambulance on every call. This is the only permissible exception to having the tools in the ambulance itself. Time is so critical in life-threatening situation that delays

FIGURE 43-1 Good tools and proper protective clothing are necessary.

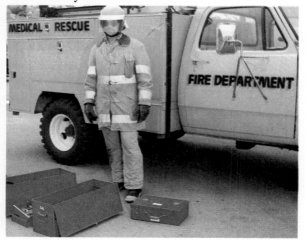

FIGURE 43-2 Porta-power tool set for extrication.

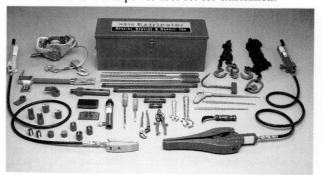

in waiting for tools and equipment cannot be tolerated. (If a separate rescue vehicle is used, it should be equipped strictly for rescue and not for a dual rescue/transportation vehicle.) For a complete list of rescue tools, see Table 43-1.

TABLE 43-1
Rescue Equipment List

Road warning devices
Hammer
Sheet-metal — cutting tool

- Tin snips
- Cold chisels
- Webbing cutter
- Baling hook
- Shovel
- Pry bar, crow bar, or wrecking bar
- Safety blankets
- Can-opener cutting tools

Tool kit including

- Assorted screwdrivers
- Assorted pliers
- Hacksaw with carbon blades
- Spring-loaded center punch
- Linoleum knife or equivalent

20 lb ABC chemical fire extinguisher
Hand-held lights
Wheel chocks
Rescue helmet with full-face shield/goggles
Protective gloves
Rope — 1 length 50/100 foot, min. 1/2″

Porta-power (4-ton with accessories)
Come-along (1-ton)
Rescue chain set
36-inch bolt cutter
Forcible entry tool
Flat-head fire axe
Long-handled sledgehammer
Air chisels and air packs and blades
Reciprocating power saws
Hydraulic spreader cutters

Assorted open/box wrench (3/8″ through 1″)
Socket set with sockets (3/8″ through 1″)
Wood cribbing
Hardwood wedges — min. 6
Jack (2-ton or larger)
Rope — 4 lengths 50/100 ft. min. xia 5/8″

Self-contained breathing apparatus with spare cylinder (to be used only with adequate training)
Stokes rescue basket or equivalent
Block and tackle
Snatch hook
Rescue harness

☐ PRINCIPLES OF EXTRICATION

Although accidents that require extrication can differ vastly, the following principles apply to all rescue situations:

1. Identify your position on the extrication team.
2. Size up the situation.
3. Find all of the victims.
4. Control the scene.
5. Stabilize the vehicle.
6. Gain access to the patient.
7. Determine the patient's status.
8. Stabilize the patient.
9. Disentangle the patient.
10. Prepare the patient for transfer.

Extrication is best handled by trained professionals who have the correct tools. Proper patient extrication requires a basic knowledge of mechanics, correct extrication tools, hard work, ingenuity, and continued training and practice.

Identifying Your Position on the Extrication Team

If a Rescue Team Is Present

If a rescue team is working on extrication, meet with the individual who is in command of the rescue activities and ask if you should begin emergency care for the victims involved. Stand by until the rescue team has finished its work.

Cooperate with the rescue team in all ways, but remember — you are responsible for the patient's welfare. If you see the rescue team operating in a way that could impair the patient's health or cause further injuries, do all you can to insure that proper emergency care is administered. Use diplomacy and tact.

The police are responsible for documenting the accident, establishing responsibility, handling crowd control and civil order, and providing for legal follow-through. This function usually will not interfere with your job. Anyone injured badly enough to need immediate care and transport will be available to the police later at the hospital.

If You Are the Rescue Team

Follow these procedures if you are the rescue team. *Have due regard for your own safety:*

1. Assess the situation. How many patients do you

have? If there are more patients than you and your partner can promptly assist, radio immediately for help.

2. Monitor the scene for any potential hazards to the rescuer and take appropriate precautions. Is the accident scene itself life-threatening? For example, a car hits a tanker that is now leaking an unknown substance. Since you are dealing with an unknown, the patient should immediately be removed a safe distance from the leak regardless of his condition. It is vital, however, to immobilize the patient's head and neck during movement.

3. If the accident scene is not immediately life-threatening, assess the patient's condition and manage critical situations first: establish an airway, control hemorrhage, and treat for shock.

4. Suspect spinal or cervical injuries if your patient is unconscious or has face/skull injuries. Immobilize, then move the patient with extreme care.

Size Up the Situation

Immediately upon arrival, survey the accident scene quickly but thoroughly. It may be difficult to locate all victims at first, but it is critical during the first minutes that you find out how many victims were involved, locate them, and decide whether or not medical help is needed. When this has been accomplished, determine whether surrounding people or property are in danger as a result of the accident (downed electrical wires, fires, and so on).

Armed with basic information about injuries and the threat of danger, determine whether enough rescue personnel are on hand to deal with the situation; if not, send for more help immediately.

Continuously evaluate the situation for the most efficient, least dangerous ways to aid the injured patients and protect the rescue team.

Control the Scene

The accident scene can be a combination of environmental hazards (downed electrical wires), traffic problems, and confusion and frustration. You will generally have help from law enforcement and fire department personnel to control these potential hazards, or to secure the scene. Your main job is to aid and assist these personnel or to begin scene control if support personnel have not yet arrived.

The accident victims — and any potential new victims to the hazards present — are your first concern. Quickly deal with bystanders by having them carefully move out of the danger zone. Try to avoid confrontation, and do not argue with a bystander who wants to be involved. A bystander who wants a "piece of the action" and is difficult to manage can be given an assignment that will not interfere with patient care. If necessary,

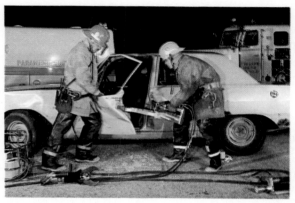

FIGURE 43-3 Access to modern extrication equipment is essential for a fast, efficient rescue.

the police will be able to assist in keeping bystanders out of the way and securing or removing unruly bystanders. Others should be asked to move on or to stay well back of the accident scene.

Flammable Material

Often, spilled gasoline is present. *Allow no smoking.* Turn all vehicle ignitions off. Any flammable materials should be washed down at the scene. A fire crew with hoses should stand by during the rescue.

Vehicles on Fire

If the car is on fire and fire-fighting personnel have not yet arrived, decide if you can remove the passengers quickly enough or whether you should fight the fire. If the passengers are not trapped, move them first. If they cannot be extricated quickly, deal with the fire.

Do not waste time trying to disconnect the battery. (Follow local protocol here. If your training protocol advises battery disconnection, remove the negative battery cable first.) The main cause of most vehicle fires after a crash is from a ruptured fuel tank or fuel lines that have been ignited by internal or external sources. The most common ignition point, however, is under the hood, which rarely presents a serious hazard to vehicle occupants unless combustion is enhanced by gasoline. Most underhood fires will not spread unless fueled by an external source.

The best fire-suppression agent for ambulance vehicles is a multi-rated (ABC type) dry chemical extinguisher. Any fire-suppression substance will cause some side effects, however, especially to the sick and injured when used in a confined space. Halon 1301, which contains bromotri-fluoromethane, is usually safer to use in an enclosed environment. It is of limited use on open, unconfined fires.

If the fire is in the engine compartment and the hood is open, try to stand with your back to the wind and close to an A-pillar of the vehicle (Figure 43-4). Use short bursts and no more than is necessary to extin-

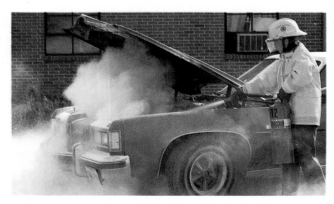

FIGURE 43-4 Extinguishing a fire in the engine compartment when the hood is fully open.

guish the fire. If there is a flare-up, you will need what is left.

If the hood is open to the safety latch, leave it. It will help restrict the flow of oxygen. Direct the nozzle of the fire extinguisher through the crack, through an opening around the grill, or under a wheel well.

If the hood is closed tight, quickly punch two or three holes through the hood and direct the nozzle through one of them. If the fire is in the passenger compartment or under the dash, carefully and sparingly apply the extinguisher directly to the flames.

If the fire is in the trunk, don't unlock and raise the trunk lid. The oxygen will intensify the flames and you may be struck by exploding material. Jab a hole through one of the light wells (preferable) or through the lid with a forcible entry tool and direct the nozzle through the opening.

Electrical Hazards

En route to the accident, watch for unlit houses, darkened advertising signs, unlit street lights, or inoperable traffic signals. These could point to a possible power-line involvement at the crash site. Assume that all downed lines are live, and call for expert assistance as soon as you arrive at the scene.

When you arrive, park your vehicle at a safe distance from any downed power line. If bystanders are present, use your public address system to warn them to stay clear and to tell victims to stay inside their vehicle. Persons inside a vehicle with an electrical line contacting it are safe, as the tires provide insulation. Quickly contact the electric company to shut off power and handle downed lines, etc. Wait until the scene is secure to proceed with rescue.

Chemical or Radiation Hazards

American railroads and over-the-road trucks annually move thousands of tons of chemicals and radioactive materials. You should carry in your glove box the cur-

rent edition of *Hazardous Materials — Emergency Action Guide*, available from the National Highway Traffic Safety Administration, General Service Division (NAD-42), 400 7th Street SW, Washington, D.C. 20590.

If the chemical in question is not listed in this guide, or if you are not sure of the chemical involved, ask your dispatcher to call CHEMTREC at (800) 424-9300 and ask for details about the load being carried. You will need to provide the name of the trucking company, the vehicle number, and the license number. CHEMTREC monitors the shipments of hazardous materials and can tell you what action to take.

Chemical hazards and radioactive materials are discussed in Chapter 36.

Traffic Control

The major goals of traffic control at the scene of an accident are:

- To clear the scene so that other emergency vehicles can have speedy access.
- To monitor the flow of regular traffic around the accident scene so that no further accidents or injuries occur.
- To monitor traffic so that passing vehicles have a minimum of inconvenience (Figure 43-5).

Unless a distinct hazard merits the stopping of all traffic, keep traffic moving around the scene. If the roadway is blocked, try to route traffic to an alternate road.

Whatever you choose to do, make sure that motorists and pedestrians in the area know *exactly* what you want them to do. Keep rescue personnel well-positioned along the roadway, and use clear visual signals coupled with attention-getting devices, such as road flares. It is a good idea to outfit rescue personnel

FIGURE 43-5 EMTs may need to direct traffic until police help arrives.

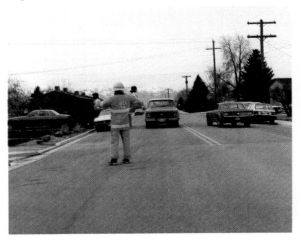

with fluorescent or reflective clothing (a lightweight vest is effective and usually not bulky enough to interfere with rescue operations) so that they can be easily seen, even at night.

Use flares, cones, or chemical lights to give approaching traffic adequate warning.

Use of Fusees (Flares)

One aid to the safe emergency control of traffic is the highway fusee or "flare." Many EMS systems are recommending the use of high intensity light sticks in place of fuses. Fusees can produce thermal burns if used improperly, but fusee smoke should not be particularly toxic in unconfined spaces. The greatest threat of injury seems to occur during the lightning process. Learn how to light and handle fusees properly (Figure 43-6). When you arrive at the accident scene, determine if fusees are needed and if it is safe to use them. *Do not* use them if flammable or explosive materials are present.

Ignite the fusees this way, to avoid being struck by molten sulphur:

1. Grasp the fusee near the base with one hand. Pull the tear strip away from the plastic cap with the other. You will see the scratching surface.

2. Pull the cap away from the body of the fusee. You will see the ignitor. Hold the cap with the scratching surface against the ignitor.

3. Hold the cap station and move the fusee quickly away from your body so that the ignitor rubs against the scratching surface. Repeat, if necessary.

4. Hold the lighted fusee away from your body as you position it on the wire stand on the ground in its plastic holder.

FIGURE 43-6 Properly igniting a traffic fusee.

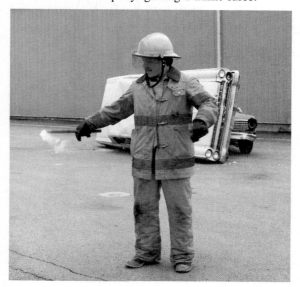

Set out the proper amount of fusees ten to fifteen feet apart, extending them to about fifty to one hundred feet toward the traffic. The fusee pattern should lead traffic *around* the emergency site and keep traffic moving. Try to reduce as much as possible the decision-making requirements of the motorists. A specific fusee pattern will be contingent upon motorists' visibility (hills, curves, weather, etc.) and the traffic pattern (number and speed of vehicles).

Use this basic rule for positioning fusees: the farthest fusee should be placed at a distance from the edge of the danger zone equal to the stopping distance for the road's posted speed plus the distance in feet equal to the posted speed. Thus, even though a motorist does not see the first fusee until he is even with it, he or she will still be able to stop in time.

The danger zone includes a fifty-foot radius or more around the wrecked vehicles. When the accident occurs on a curve, consider the start of the curve as the edge of the danger zone. On a hill, one edge of the danger zone should be the crest of the hill. If the highway is two-lane, position flares in both directions. If heavy trucks use the highway, extend the flare string. Trucks take much longer to stop than cars.

As you are setting out the flares, have someone watch for oncoming traffic and check your flare pattern. Do not expose yourself to the roadway any longer than necessary. One way to do this is to "daisy-chain," or stack, the needed number of flares so that a lighted one will ignite another one just before it burns out.

Do not throw away end caps. Place them on the nonburning end of the tube, which will help keep the flares in the right position on the road. If possible, allow flares to burn out.

Find All of the Victims

During extrication and emergency care, treat all patients who can be located immediately, then scour the area (ditches, bushes, etc.) for any victim who may be hidden. Use a systematic approach so that no victims are missed.

- If a passenger is conscious and coherent, ask how many people were in the car.
- Question witnesses about whether someone left the site or whether a passerby took a patient away.
- In cases of high impact, search the area carefully, especially in ditches and tall weeds.
- Look for tracks in the earth or snow. A victim who can free himself or herself from the vehicle may leave to get help, or wander aimlessly.
- Search the vehicle itself carefully, including under dashboards.
- Look quickly for items, such as children's lunch

boxes, a diaper bag, or extra jackets, that may be clues to unaccounted-for children.

Stabilize the Vehicle

Suspect any vehicle of being unstable until you have made it stable, regardless of how it may have come to rest after the collision. Suspect that a vehicle is *not* stable if it is on a tilted surface (such as a hill), if part of it is stacked on top of another vehicle, or if it is on a slippery surface such as ice, snow, or spilled oil. Vehicles that have come to rest on their side or roof should also be considered unstable. Even when the vehicle is upright and appears to be stable, use blocks or wedges at wheels to prevent unexpected rolling. Chock wheels tightly against the curb when possible (Figure 43-7).

Cribbing

Probably the most basic of all extrication tools are blocks of wood referred to as **cribbing,** in which the wood is stacked in box-like squares and wedges are used to keep the pressure uniform. The cribbing is arranged in such a fashion that it is diagonal to the vehicle frame, rather than over the middle of one piece of wood (Figure 43-8). This arrangement creates a more stable envi-

ronment. You should not crib under wheels or tires, because the vehicle will tend to roll.

Cribbing should never be stacked higher than its own length, and there should be no more than one to two inches between the cribbing and the vehicle being lifted.

Overturned Vehicle

To stabilize an overturned vehicle, place a solid object — such as a wheel chock, spare tire, cribbing, or timer — between the roof and the roadway (Figures 43-9 and 43-10). If necessary, use the vehicle's bumper jack to angle the vehicle against the solid object until the vehicle is stable. Hook a chain to the vehicle's axle, then loop the chain around a tree or post. Never use your ambulance as the securing post. Any vehicle that can be moved easily during extrication or patient care needs to be stabilized by the placement of cribbing or step-blocks under the frame, and by clipping the valve stems of the tires. Excess motion of the vehicle could prove fatal for a patient with severe spinal injuries and may injure the rescue team.

FIGURE 43-9 Spare wheels can be used when cribbing is not available.

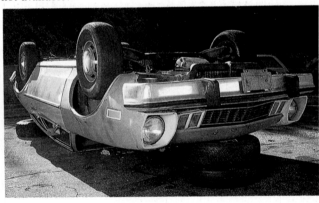

FIGURE 43-7 A wheel chock has been positioned to prevent forward movement.

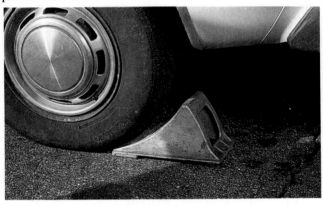

FIGURE 43-10 Stabilizing the overturned vehicle with cribbing.

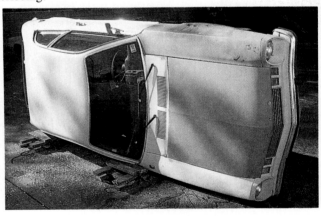

FIGURE 43-8 The proper use of cribbing.

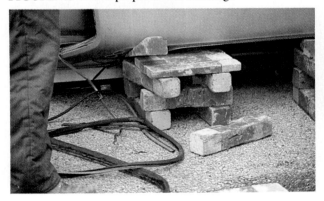

Upright Vehicles

One of the first steps in stabilizing a vehicle that rests on all four wheels is to simply place the gear selector in park or, on a standard shift, into reverse. Another immediate stabilization technique is to cut the valve stems so that the car rests on the tire rims, thus reducing the amount of vehicle movement even with the use of power tools.

Air Bags

If the air bag has deployed, you may use standard rescue techniques. There may be some cornstarch residue present. This cornstarch is used as a lubricant and is not harmful. It can be washed off later.

If the air bag was not triggered by the crash, disconnect the negative side of the battery and the yellow air bag connector found where the base of the steering column meets the dashboard. Do not cut the connector or its wires; they will keep the shorting bar activated, preventing accidental triggering.

Gain Access to the Patient

Remember that a door is always the access of choice because it is the largest uncomplicated opening in the vehicle. Always start out by testing the door handle to see if you can simply open it. Use the following procedures if you need to use force in gaining access.

Doors

1. Attempt to open the door nearest the patient by using the door handle. If the doors are locked, try to open the lock by either having a person in the car do so, or by using a coat hanger or other device between the door frame and window. Routinely unlock all other doors when you gain entrance to the vehicle to allow access by other EMTs. If the doors cannot be opened, determine the best point of entry and proceed accordingly. See Figures 43-11–43-20 for specific instructions on how to open undamaged and damaged doors. The car may have powered door locks. Look at the inside door panels and arm rests for toggle switches. If the doors are locked, break a side window, reach in, and unlock the doors with these switches. Also operate the control switches to lower the powered windows.

2. If access must be gained via a door that cannot be opened without cutting, again determine the best entry point and proceed. You can open the door without removing it completely by using a hand tool to cut the sheet metal around the door handle, then reaching inside to trip the lock release (Figures 43-21–43-23). If the lock release will not trip, insert a power chisel on the lock mechanism where it attaches to the vehicle, and cut through

☐ Opening an Undamaged Door

FIGURE 43-11 An undamaged door may be unlocked by prying the frame away from the vehicle body, then inserting the "thief's" tool.

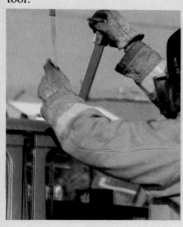

FIGURE 43-12 Pull up on the tool and reinsert until the lock opens.

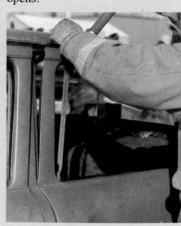

FIGURE 43-13 An unframed window can be pried open enough to insert a screwdriver for lifting up the lock button.

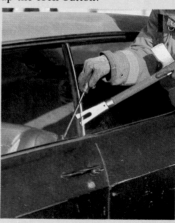

☐ Using a Noose Tool

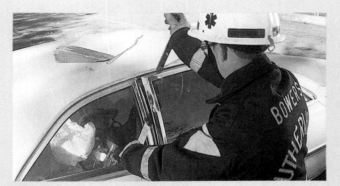

FIGURE 43-14 An opening is made with pry bars.

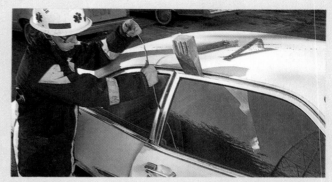

FIGURE 43-15 While a wedge maintains the opening, the lock button is captured with the noose.

☐ Opening a Damaged Door

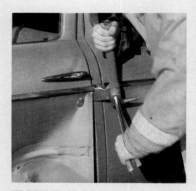

FIGURE 43-16 Use prying tool to widen opening between door edge and frame.

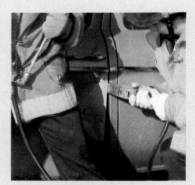

FIGURE 43-17 Insert smaller porta-power tool into opening.

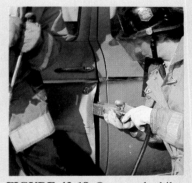

FIGURE 43-18 Open tool while partner leans against door to prevent it from springing open.

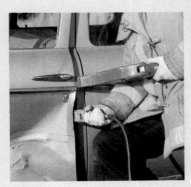

FIGURE 43-19 When opening is wide enough, insert spreader or large porta-power tool.

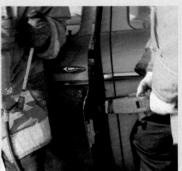

FIGURE 43-20 Continue opening spreader until door latches separate or are pulled away.

□ Exposing a Locking Mechanism

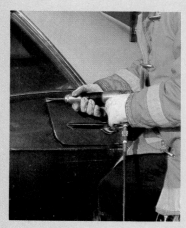

FIGURE 43-21 Cut around handle and lock with an air chisel, panel cutter, or screwdriver, and sledge hammer.

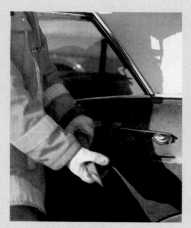

FIGURE 43-22 Pry open the cut area to expose locking mechanism.

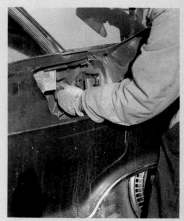

FIGURE 43-23 Unlock door by operating rods and levers to pop open lock. Push on plate behind push button.

the steel supporting post. Bend the door backward to create an opening.

In cars manufactured after 1983, a collision beam inside the door supplies extra protection to the passengers by reducing the ease with which a door may be caved in. This beam may buckle under the impact of an accident, and the sharp end may protrude into the passenger compartment. As you apply compression or prying pressure in gaining access through a door, be sure that the angle of force does not propel the beam further into the vehicle.

Windows

Windows of vehicles are usually made of tempered glass (Figures 43-24 and 43-25); rear and side windows are designed to break into small granules. Cover the patient with a heavy safety blanket at the earliest opportunity (Figure 43-26).

It is preferable to remove the window without breaking it. Finely divided particles can remain unnoticed deep in a wound, continuing to cause damage even after the wound closes. If the fixed windows are installed in a U-shaped black plastic or rubber, remove the trim, insert the point of a linoleum knife or similar tool into the molding at the midpoint of the glass, keep the blade as flat against the glass as possible, and draw the knife across the top and down the side. Repeat the process on the other side. Soapy water from a squirt bottle will keep the blade moving easily. Work the end of a

short pry bar behind the glass and pry it loose from the top. The window will pivot on its bottom edge.

If you must break a window, locate the window farthest from the victim, and give a quick hard thrust in the lower corner with a spring-loaded punch, screwdriver, or other sharp object. If you have time and the correct materials, put strips of broad tape or a sheet of contact paper over the glass to prevent the broken pieces from spraying onto the patient.

Powdered glass can travel as much as twenty feet in a breeze. Coat the glass with adhesive spray in two layers, the second at right angles to the first with a minute's drying time in between. Or use tape if you are using an ax blade. If you are on a window next to a pa-

FIGURE 43-24 Tempered glass should be shattered with a sharp tool. Strike tool with a hammer in a lower corner close to the door.

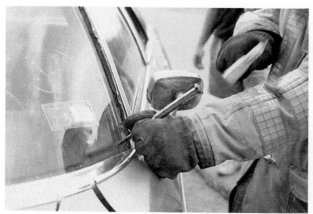

662   *Chapter 43*

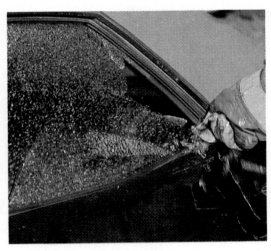

FIGURE 43-25 Tempered glass — usually found in side and rear windows.

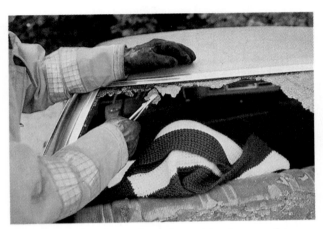

FIGURE 43-26 Cover the patient with a heavy safety blanket.

tient, overlap the strips to cover the entire window. Pieces of glass will still fall inside, but they will drop straight down instead of being propelled forward. Use your gloved hand to carefully pull the glass outside the vehicle. Clear all glass away from the window opening.

Before you crawl in, drape a heavy tarp or blanket over the door edge and the interior of the car just below the window.

Windshield

Windshields are usually made of laminated safety glass, which cannot be broken safely. If the windshield is largely intact, pry up the chrome trim at the joints, using a baling hook, pry bar, or screwdriver.

Determine how the windshield was set in the car: models before 1969 will have a soft rubber seal, while those after 1969 will be set with **mastic**. To remove the rubber seal, use a linoleum knife to slice the rubber bead. Drive the point into the channel and keep the blade flat against the glass. Then force a screwdriver be-

hind the glass and simply pop out the windshield (Figures 43-27—43-33), then carefully remove it. For a mastic-set windshield, remove the molding, then use a mastic cutter to free the windshield (Figures 43-34—43-35). The mastic cutter may be obtained from an auto parts store or an auto windshield business.

Removal of a broken mastic-set windshield may cause a great deal of splintering. Therefore, as with any extrication problem, the EMT and the patient must be protected properly. Cover the patient with a safety blanket, and make sure that each rescue technician has full facial protection and wears a long-sleeved shirt and gloves. Always consider using an alternate entry method before breaking or cutting glass.

To use an ax to remove the windshield, apply duct tape to the glass and make cuts with the ax, as shown in Figures 43-36—43-37.

Roof

Sometimes the easiest way to reach a patient in a vehicle that rests on its side is through the roof. With an air chisel or a manual device such as the K-Bar-T, you can open the entire roof with a three-sided cut (Figures 43-38—43-40). This cut will allow the top to be folded down to the ground, thus avoiding a razor-sharp edge over which the patient must be removed. When practical, leave the pillars or roof support intact to keep the vehicle stable.

In an upright vehicle, remove the entire roof by cutting through all four pillars with either a pneumatic chisel, power saw, or hydraulic cutter (Figures 43-41—43-43). Cut through the front two posts and any other rolled or reinforced metal. Avoid cutting where the seat belt anchors are fastened, as these are reinforced with heavy-gauge metal. Then score (or crease) the metal roof, and fold it back along the fold line. Cover the sharp edges of cut posts with short lengths of scrap fire hose.

If the roof has been severely crushed, you may need to use a hydraulic jack to lift the roof as far from the body of the car as possible, then cut the posts.

If no power tools are available, pry the metal trim away from the posts with pry bars or screwdrivers and attempt to cut through the posts with a hacksaw. This can be a difficult and time-consuming procedure.

Stabilize the Patient

As soon as you are able to gain access to the patient, do the following:

1. Conduct a quick but thorough primary survey to determine the extent of injuries.
2. If more than one victim is involved, complete triage.
3. Perform the ABCs.

□ Removing a Windshield

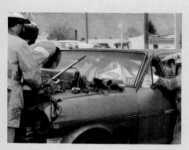
FIGURE 43-27 Patient should be protected with a rescue blanket before windshield removal occurs.

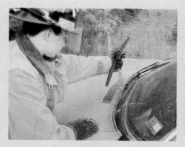
FIGURE 43-28 When removing a windshield, first pry off or bend back the wipers.

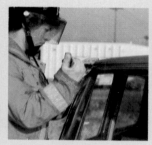
FIGURE 43-29 Start removal of chrome trim by prying up a joint or corner of trim.

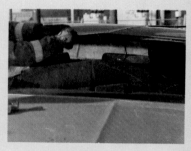
FIGURE 43-30 Remove chrome trim with baling hook, pry bar, or screwdriver.

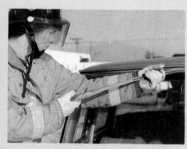
FIGURE 43-31 Much of trim can be pulled off by hand.

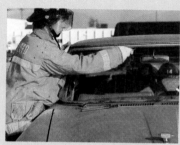
FIGURE 43-32 To remove a molding-mounted windshield, use a linoleum or other hooked knife to cut the rubber. Drive the point into the channel and keep the blade flat against the glass.

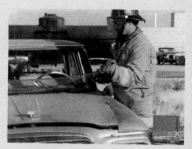
FIGURE 43-33 Force a screwdriver behind the glass to force the windshield out; carefully remove it.

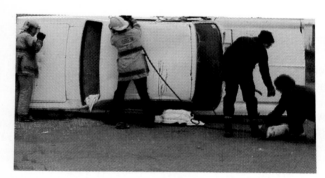
FIGURE 43-38 The roof is cut on three sides by an air chisel or other metal-cutting tool.

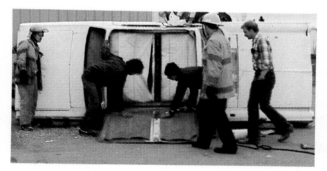
FIGURE 43-39 Observe the cribbing for vehicle stabilization.

4. Correct life-threatening problems (Figure 43-44).
5. Provide other emergency care as needed.
6. On occasion, you may need to move the patient quickly and immediately, such as when the vehicle is on fire, before you can immobilize him or her

with a spine board. Cut any jammed seat belts (Figure 43-45). If there is any possibility of a cervical spine injury, immobilize the patient's spine using one of the following methods:

• The **horse-collar technique** is one of the easier

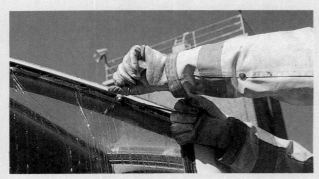

FIGURE 43-34 To remove a mastic-mounted window, the knife is pushed into the mastic, turned ninety degrees, and drawn across the top and down each side of the glass.

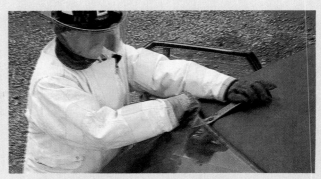

FIGURE 43-35 The window is pried from the frame with a bar.

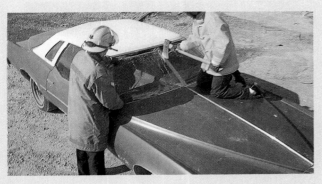

FIGURE 43-36 Duct tape is applied to the glass to minimize debris, and four cuts are made with an ax.

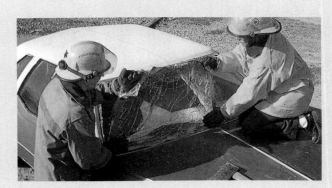

FIGURE 43-37 The cut section of windshield is removed from the frame. Use the same procedure to remove the entire windshield.

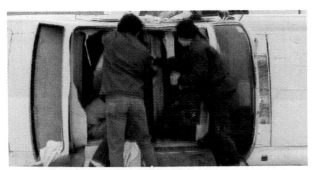

FIGURE 43-40 An air-operated chisel will quickly cut open a roof. The roof is then folded down.

methods of one-person rescue in a life-and-death situation. Used when the patient is sitting, take a standard blanket and roll it lengthwise until it is approximately four to six inches across. Reach in with one hand and provide gentle immobilization while placing the blanket behind the pa-

tient's head, allowing both long ends to fall across his chest. Pass the blanket across his chest from one side to the other. Place gentle tension on both long ends, then pass the ends under opposite arms. Gather the blanket behind the patient, and rotate him or her from the seat into your arms. The horse collar also provides support of the head and neck without taking the time to place a cervical collar on the patient (Figure 43-46).

- Another technique, especially useful when speed of removal is important, involves three or four EMTs (Figures 43-47–43-52). While you perform a primary survey, have your partner hold the patient's head in-line with the body from the back seat. Apply a cervical collar. Remove the driver's door or force it open beyond its normal range of movement. If possible, place the long spine board on an ambulance cot next to the pa-

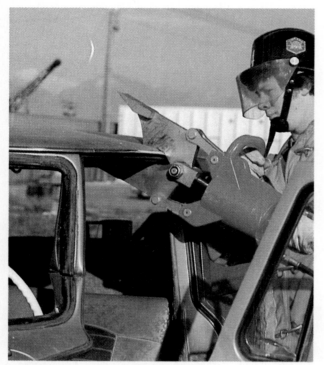

FIGURE 43-41 A roof may be removed by making peripheral cuts with a hydraulic extrication device or a hacksaw. See also Figure 43-42.

FIGURE 43-42 Cut through the front two posts with a hydraulic cutter.

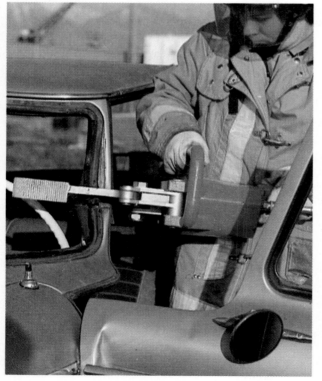

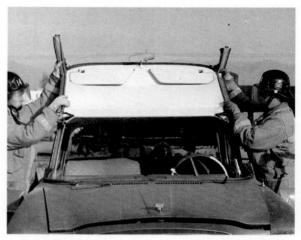

FIGURE 43-43 A bumper jack is helpful in moving the roof upward. Two EMTs can fold the roof backward.

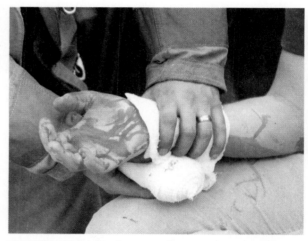

FIGURE 43-44 Perform a patient assessment and give needed emergency care in the car.

FIGURE 43-45 Cut jammed seat belts. Support your patient against the sudden loss of support.

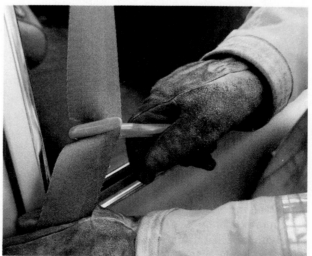

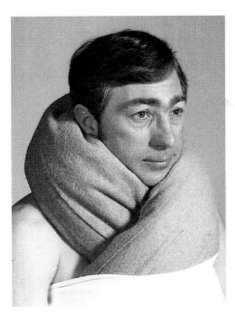

FIGURE 43-46 Improvised cervical collar or horse-collar.

tient's seat with the board actually under the patient's buttocks. If possible, have a third EMT steady the board. Take over head immobilization from the EMT in the back seat, standing as flat against the car as you can, while he or she moves to the front seat and takes the patient's legs just under the knees. The fourth EMT slips one hand under the patient's armpit and puts his or her other hand flat on the patient's thorax. Moving on the count of the lead EMT, gently rotate the patient so that the knees come up on the seat, still in a sitting position, with the patient's back positioned toward the spine board. On a slow count, and when everyone is ready, lift the patient's knees and move him or her from a sitting to a lying position. Slide the patient gently onto the backboard, moving six to twelve inches at a time, being sure that you do not pull on his or her head. Once he or she is on the backboard, you can resuscitate, immobilize, and prepare for transport. This procedure can still be safely performed with three EMTs, using a competent bystander to steady the cot and backboard. If the driver's door is jammed and there is not time to completely remove it, simply reverse the maneuver and take the patient out of the passenger door.

7. When the situation is not a life-threatening emergency, stabilize the spine and neck with the proper devices, and instruct the patient to remain still during extrication. A soft cervical collar is ineffective in immobilizing the neck. Rigid collars, such as the Stifneck® (which has enlarged openings in front to allow for pulse examination, and observa-

tion of tracheal deviation are more effective (Figure 43-53). Still, tests of several devices show that they are all less effective at immobilization than a long spine board with foam bags or styrofoam and blanket rolls and tape. Until you can get your patient on a spine board, remind him or her to be still, or have someone immobilize the head and neck during extrication. Commercial extrication devices, such as the KED, XP-1 Green Splint, and CID, are discussed later in this chapter.

8. During a long extrication procedure, shock combined with temperature extremes can be fatal. If it is cold, maintain your patient's body temperature with blankets, large-wattage lights, and tarps. Provide shade during the summer. (Be aware that equipment such as BP cuffs and stethoscopes can malfunction in extreme cold.)

9. Place one EMT in the vehicle with the patient, if possible, to treat and comfort the patient during extrication. Remember that rescuer safety is as important as patient safety and treatment. Cover the patient with a safety blanket as soon as practical. Predict the consequences of each procedure before it is initiated, then check the EMT and patient inside the vehicle to ensure that no debris is being forced down on either. The goal of collision extrication is to remove wreckage from the patient, rather than to remove the patient from the wreckage.

10. During each step of access and extrication, keep evaluating the possibility of further injury. Practice good safety procedures at all times. It is critical that no additional injuries be inflicted.

Disentangle the Patient

To determine your disentanglement priorities, note the mechanism(s) of injury (bent steering wheel, star on windshield, etc.). For example, if the patient is sustaining ongoing injury from the steering column, remove the steering column first. Pay attention to broken glass, sheared metal, and crushing objects. Explain what procedures and tools you will use and what the patient can expect. Try to lessen the patient's fears, and work carefully to protect him or her from further injury.

Move Seats Back

If the seats are jammed or you need more space, use a **come-along.** Pass the steel cable through the rear window, attach it to the frame around the bumper, and lock it around the base of the seat. Then apply pressure from the rear to pull the seat free of its attachments toward the rear of the car.

In some cases, you can use the seat lever or latch to manually move the seat backward, away from the victims in the front seat.

"RAPID ROLLOUT"

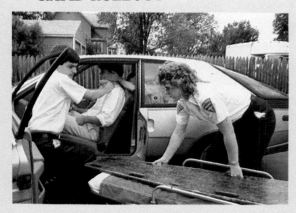

FIGURE 43-47 While you perform a primary survey, have your partner hold the patient's head in-line with the body, from the back seat. Apply a cervical collar.

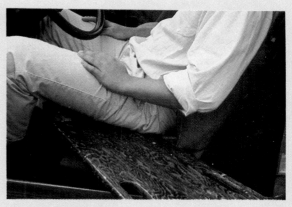

FIGURE 43-48 Place the long spine board on an ambulance cot next to the patient's seat with the board actually under the patient's buttocks.

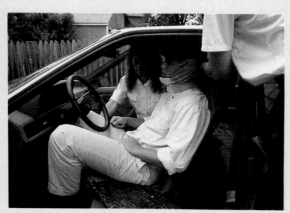

FIGURE 43-49 Take over head immobilization from the EMT in the back seat, standing as flat against the car as you can, while he or she moves to the front seat and takes the patient's legs just under the knees.

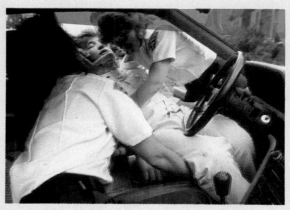

FIGURE 43-50 Rotate the patient so that the knees come up on the seat, still in a sitting position, with the patient's back positioned toward the spine board.

FIGURE 43-51 On a slow count, and when everyone is ready, lift the patient's knees and move him on her from a sitting to a lying position.

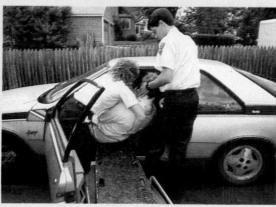

FIGURE 43-52 Once the patient is on the backboard, you can resuscitate, immobilize, and prepare for transport.

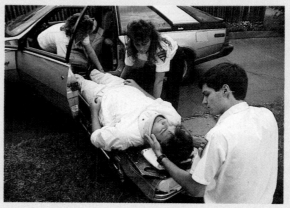

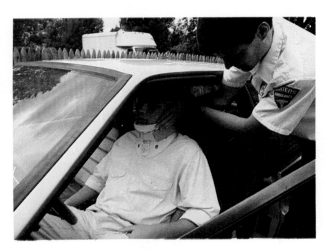

FIGURE 43-53 Application of a rigid cervical collar.

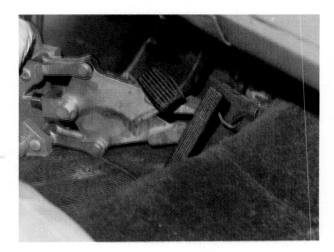

FIGURE 43-54 Using an extrication device to force a floor pedal out of the way.

Stabilize the patient by placing a short spine board between him or her and the seat back. The patient's entire weight may be supported by the seat. If the legs are fractured, a sudden jerk of the seat will cause pain.

Displace the Steering Wheel and Column

Attach a come-along to chains looped around the steering column and on the frame of the car. Put blocks on the hood for the cable to lift against. Be careful when attaching the chains to the steering column itself and when placing blocks at the junction of the windscreen and hood. If the chains are not properly placed, the steering column may slip and hit the patient, causing further injury. The patient should be protected by a short backboard and blanket.

Do not remove the chains or relax the tension of the steel cable until the patient has been completely removed from the steering column area.

Caution: Do not use this technique on front-wheel drive and tilt-wheel vehicles, as the steering column can separate at the knuckle of the firewall.

In the past, the steering wheel and column was the major cause of victim entrapment. Today, the dashboard and fire wall are more likely to be responsible, because the modern-mounted column brackets are designed to separate from the dash.

Displace Pedals

If a patient's foot has been trapped between a floor pedal and the floor (common in head-on collisions), use an extrication device (Hurst Tool) to force the pedal out of the way (Figure 43-54).

If you do not have an extrication device, tie a firm slip-knot around the pedal with a manila rope and pull it taut. Holding the rope taut, loop it several times around the door handle or window frame of the door that is in the direction in which you want to pull the pedal. With

two rescue personnel working side by side, jerk firmly on the door; the pedal should displace easily.

If manual removal does not work, use portapower hydraulic tools, a jack, or a hand winch.

Prepare the Patient for Removal or Transfer

While preparing your patient for removal to an ambulance, maintain cervical stabilization, care for other injuries that you have not been able to reach, and use a spine board. (Refer to specific chapters for patient stabilization techniques.)

Immobilizing the Patient with a Backboard

The traditional short backboard works well in large-size automobiles but not in small cars and trucks. New backboards are now available to correct the difficulties in patient extrication from small cars and trucks or cars with bucket seats. These boards have support pads on the side of the head and tapered lower portions to allow insertion of the boards into bucket seats; there is also adequate space for padding.

The tapered end of the board is placed toward the bottom of the seat. The patient's thorax is secured to the board by two diagonally placed straps with one transverse strap at the bottom for the pelvis.

Follow these procedures for immobilizing a spinal-injured victim in a vehicle:

1. You should be behind the patient, and your partner should be to the patient's side.
2. Gently move the cervical spine into a neutral position by axial or in-line traction of the head. **Warning:** If the patient shows resistance or com-

plains of pain, leave the neck in its current position and splint it with the horse-collar technique discussed in this chapter.

3. With the tapered or narrow end down, slip the backboard between the patient and the seat, and push it down until the lower edge is resting on the bottom of the car seat. Position this lower end of the board close to the patient's lower back.

4. Bring the patient's back flush to the backboard. Place padding behind the head and neck as indicated. Place a blanket (folded lengthwise) over the top of the patient's head in a horseshoe shape. Then secure his body to the backboard with two chest straps (over the blankets) and a waist strap.

5. Secure the patient's head to the board with wide cravats (four inches), making sure that the head and neck are in an in-line neutral position and not secured too tightly. (Note: In the absence of triangular bandages, use a four-inch elastic wrap or two-inch adhesive tape, but *do not* secure the head too tightly.) Then secure the arms and legs to the board with tape or cravats to prevent further injury.

6. *Before* extricating the patient, check all ties, paddings, and straps one last time. *At least two* rescuers are needed to move the patient from the vehicle. Lift the patient and the backboard together. When lowering the patient onto the longboard, keep the legs at a ninety-degree angle or in a sitting position.

7. As rapidly as possible, move the patient to the long spine board. The amount of leg mobility allowed on the short board may compromise an already injured spinal column. You can simply immobilize the patient, shortboard and all, to the long board.

Patient Lodged under the Dashboard

If your patient is lodged under the dashboard or lying on the floor between the front and back seats:

1. Remove the front seat or move it as far back as you can. If this provides enough room, you can slide the spine board under the patient with no problems.

2. If you cannot remove or move the seat, force both front doors open beyond their normal range or remove them so that you will have a clear working area.

3. Place a long spine board on the front seat.

4. Maintain a clear airway and slight traction while you apply a cervical collar to the patient.

5. One EMT remains at the patient's head, while another positions himself or herself at the patient's feet. Two more crawl behind the front seat.

6. While one EMT supports the head and the other supports the feet, the two EMTs in the car lean over the seat and grab the patient's clothes at his or her shoulder, chest, waist, and thighs. If the patient is wearing loose clothing, the EMTs place their hands underneath the patient's body. On signal, they lift the patient, keeping him or her parallel to the seat, and place the patient on the long spine board. The spine board can then be slid from the car.

7. The patient should be straight on the spine board with hands and arms at his or her side.

8. Since tucking a blanket around a patient on a narrow spine board can push his or her spine out of alignment, wait until the spine board is on a wheeled stretcher before you cover the patient.

9. Use a minimum of three straps to secure the patient to the long spine board — one across the shoulder girdle, one across the hips, and one at mid-femur, just above the knees. If you think that the patient might have a spinal injury, use foam bags, pillows, rolled blankets, or commercial head immobilization devices such as the Bashaw CID to stabilize him further.

10. Move the patient to a wheeled ambulance stretcher as soon as he is stabilized.

11. Treat for shock and transport.

Difficulties with Short Backboards

Disadvantages of many short backboards in current use include the following:

- Those with wide bases are difficult to maneuver into compact cars or bucket seats.
- The straps on the backboards are difficult to position around the patient's legs, especially when he or she has to be lifted vertically out of the vehicle. Without proper placement of the leg straps, the patient is not secured well enough to the backboard.
- The metal buckles on most commercial spine boards are difficult to maneuver underneath a patient. Some rescue personnel have suffered lacerations when broken glass was trapped under the victim.
- While the major function of the backboard is to stabilize the cervical spine, it is extremely difficult to stabilize the head to the backboard. Chin straps may not be used.
- Most backboards result in the legs being held at a ninety-degree angle to the body, which decreases flexibility and makes extrication difficult.

Corset-Type Extrication Devices

Extrication devices are flexible commercial devices useful in auto extrications for patients who need to be immobilized in a sitting position or in confined spaces. They function much like a short spine board.

As for any spinal immobilization, you must first apply and maintain manual stabilization of the head and neck, then check the ABCs. The other EMT assesses pulse, movement, and sensation to upper and lower extremities prior to proceeding. After these have been noted, apply the extrication device (Figures 43-55–43-64):

1. Apply a cervical collar.
2. Position the extrication device behind the sitting patient; with the smooth side toward the patient, slide the body part of the extrication device far enough so that the patient is centered on the device and the board clears the top of the car doorway.
3. Pull the leg straps down so that they are clear of the extrication device.
4. Position the extrication device snugly under the patient's armpits; as the patient is lifted, the weight should be borne on his or her armpits, and there should be no sagging.
5. Fasten and snug up the bottom and middle chest straps.
6. Pass the leg straps under the patient's legs, cross the straps at the crotch (check local protocol here), and connect each strap to the fastener on the opposite side. Prior to securing the leg straps across the groin, fold the storage case into a square and place it over the groin area, then secure each leg strap. This will provide sufficient padding in most cases.
7. Use the Velcro head straps to secure the patient's head against the extrication device; fasten and snug up the top chest strap. Check all straps to make sure that they are secure and that the patient can still breathe properly.
8. Two EMTs then grasp the handles on opposite sides of the extrication device while passing their other arm under the patient's legs and grasping (locking) their arms together. As the patient is removed, his or her legs must be kept in a forty-five-degree angle (the same as when the patient was sitting) at the hip.
9. Once the patient has been placed and secured on the long spine board, you must reassess pulse, movement, and sensation.
10. Loosen the leg straps and lower them until they are flat.

☐ OTHER EXTRICATION SITUATIONS

Rope-Sling Extrication

The rope-sling extrication is used (1) if a patient is wedged under wreckage or collapsed material, (2) if the patient has no cervical injuries, and (3) if it is necessary to remove the patient quickly. Use an eight-foot length of low-stretch, high-strength nylon rope.

Attach a metal ring sliding connector. *Do not attempt to use this technique without the connector.* Then splice or tie the rope into a loop.

Place the loop over the patient's chest below the breasts, under the armpits, and under the shoulder blades so that the two ropes of the loop exit, one on each side of the patient's head.

Slide the connector down tight between the patient's shoulder blades at the base of the neck. These precautions will keep the loop from pressing on the nerves and vessels in the armpits and causing injury. Then, pull evenly on both ropes of the loop and drag the patient out.

Vehicles in Water

Check with local diving clubs, a sheriff's underwater rescue team, or a local military unit with dive rescue capabilities to determine in advance what support is available and how they can be activated. Do not attempt underwater rescue or extrication operations unless you are properly trained and equipped.

Accidents in which a car is completely or partially submerged can show all of the complications of any motor vehicle accident but with the added complexities of instability, the threat of drowning, and hypothermia.

To attempt a water rescue, you *must* be a good swimmer and be trained in water rescue. You must also be prepared for the cold of immersion by wearing a wetsuit or having a rewarming system readily available. Otherwise, the risks of *your* becoming a victim are too great.

Extrication in Buildings and Underground

When a building is seriously damaged or collapses due to earthquake, structural defect, explosion, or fire, or when a mine caves in or someone is injured in a cave-in at the side of a hill or underground, you *must* let the emergency crews that are prepared to handle volatile situations do their job (Figures 43-65 and 43-66). You cannot help a patient by interfering with specially trained rescuers. Also, the extrication equipment in your ambulance is not designed for heavy duty. You should be familiar with local disaster operating procedures. Specially trained personnel such as heavy equipment op-

☐ Applying an Extrication Device

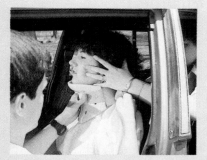

FIGURE 43-55 Apply a cervical collar.

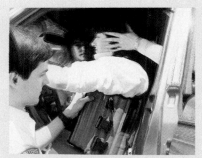

FIGURE 43-56 Position and center extrication device behind patient.

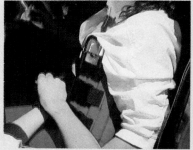

FIGURE 43-57 After pulling the leg straps down, fasten and snug up the bottom and middle chest straps.

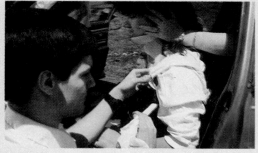

FIGURE 43-58 Make sure that the extrication device fits snugly under the patient's armpits.

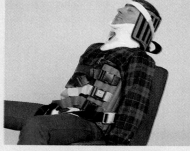

FIGURE 43-59 Secure each leg strap.

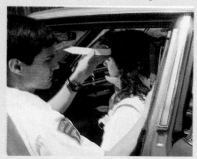

FIGURE 43-60 Secure the patient's head with the velcro head straps. Fasten and snug the top chest strap.

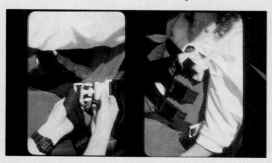

FIGURE 43-61 Another view of an extrication device in the proper position.

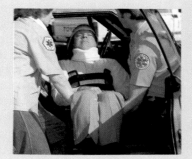

FIGURE 43-62 Grabbing a handle under each armpit and one leg, remove the patient from the vehicle.

FIGURE 43-63

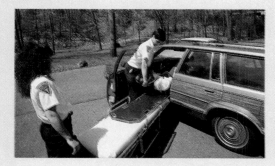

FIGURE 43-64 The patient immobilized and secured to the stretcher.

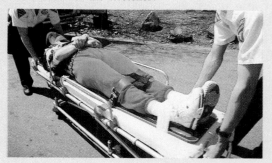

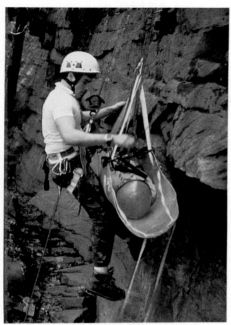

FIGURE 43-65 High-rise extrication. (Courtesy of Skedco.)

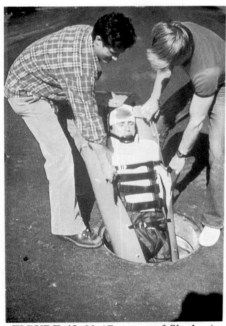

FIGURE 43-66 (Courtesy of Skedco.)

erators or construction foremen may be in charge of the extrication operation; however, competent medical command must come into the overall operation to ensure that patient care is not compromised during extrication. This may require you to place yourself in an extremely hazardous situation to initiate patient care while the heavy extrication begins or continues.

Follow local protocol in the division of labor. It is essential that leadership on the accident scene be in the hands of someone who is medically trained so that cor-

rect judgments will be made about patient care. A good system is to have the EMTs reach the patient to provide life support while the trained rescue squad with heavier equipment and specialized rigs begins the task of removal and extrication.

Unlike triage protocol, which requires treating the most serious but saveable victims first, you should first remove the victims that are easiest to reach, then those whose rescue will take an extended period of time. Last would be those who have died, unless the bodies must be removed so that you can continue to reach those who are still living.

General procedures for building collapses or underground accidents include the following:

1. Assure the stability of the material over or through which you will be crawling.

2. Wear appropriate protective clothing.

3. If you are going to be working a considerable distance from your ambulance, carry all of the tools, supplies, and equipment that you feel reasonably sure you will need. Do you have adequate lighting? Designate your partner as liaison to keep you supplied as the extent of patient care becomes more clear.

4. Is there new, continued, or continuing danger of fire or explosion?

5. Do you know how many patients are involved?

6. Once you have reached the patient, assess his or her condition, ensure a patent airway, ensure circulation, and manage life-threatening injuries.

7. You have more flexibility in beginning rescue breathing than you do in commencing CPR. Even though a patient is not lying flat on his or her back, you can still inflate the patient's lungs two or three times to "buy time." But if his or her heart has stopped beating, you cannot perform effective CPR unless the patient is lying on his or her back on a hard surface. In such cases, extrication — or at least repositioning onsite — becomes the high priority.

8. Another useful device is the SKED, a device that resembles a full-body, lace-up sled that will accommodate an adult on a spine board. After a patient with suspected neck or spinal injury is immobilized with a short board, he or she can be log-rolled onto a SKED, stabilized with foam blocks or a horseshoe blanket roll, then "packaged" with the SKED straps securely enough that he or she can be lifted vertically. This device is sufficiently space-thrifty so that a patient can be evacuated upright through a manhole cover or a relatively narrow crevice without compromising the spine excessively.

chapter 44

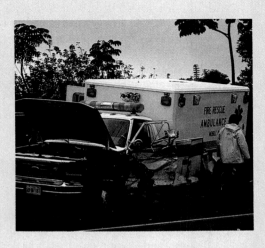

Ambulance Operations

✳ OBJECTIVES

- ■ Demonstrate how to drive an ambulance safely and skillfully.
- ■ Discuss the laws, regulations, and ordinances that apply to ambulance operations.
- ■ List factors contributing to unsafe driving conditions.
- ■ Discuss the skills for controlling the ambulance.
- ■ Discuss how and when to use the ambulance warning devices properly.
- ■ Identify all vehicle systems and equipment requiring daily inspection.
- ■ Discuss how to prevent carbon monoxide build-up in the ambulance and what to do in case of fire.
- ■ List and discuss the seven major phases of the ambulance run.
- ■ Know safety guidelines for air helicopters.

It is recommended that EMTs wear protective gloves whenever there is a possibility of coming in contact with a patient's blood, body fluids, mucous membranes, traumatic wounds, or sores. See Chapter 31.

☐ DRIVING SAFETY

Few people think of an ambulance as a hazardous place, except for the patient who is already suffering from a life-threatening situation. But statistics tell a different story. According to national data, about 10 percent of all ambulances are involved in an accident each year. Ironically, only about 3 to 5 percent of all ambulance runs are true life-and-death situations. Haste in transporting patients is unnecessary in about 95 percent of all cases.

It takes time to learn how to drive an ambulance safely and skillfully. However, you can learn the regulations and guidelines *before* you get behind the wheel.

☐ AMBULANCE COLORS AND MARKINGS

While anyone from a traffic officer to a school child can instantly recognize ambulances, their colors and markings are an aid to traffic safety and reduce the need for excessive dependence on lights and sirens. An early DOT/EMS study, "Ambulance Design Criteria" by the National Academy of Sciences, recommended a nationwide system of specific colors and markings. Later, the General Services Administration and DOT developed and published federal specifications for ambulances (1974:KKK-1822).

The standard color is white; the markings are an orange stripe running around the body, blue lettering, and the "Star of Life" symbol (Figures 44-1–44-3). It is recommended that any added lettering be kept below the orange stripe so as not to distract from the basic markings. For maximum effectiveness, these standard colors and markings must not be duplicated on nonambulances.

☐ LAWS, REGULATIONS, ORDINANCES

As an ambulance operator, you should be familiar with the laws and regulations that apply on both the state and local levels and *consistently obey them.* You have certain privileges under the law as the operator of an emergency vehicle, as do the operators of police cars and fire engines. *At no time* is it justified to operate an ambulance in a method that jeopardizes anyone else. Remember that your first duty to your patient is to arrive at the scene — safely! After that, you must get your patient to definitive care carefully and safely.

While statutes in each state vary slightly, most states give you the privilege, with proper precautions, to:

- Exceed the speed limit posted for the area as long as you are not endangering lives or property.
- Drive the wrong way down a one-way street or drive down the opposite side of the street.
- Turn in any direction at any intersection.
- Park anywhere as long as you do not endanger lives or property.
- Leave the ambulance standing in the middle of a street or intersection.
- *Cautiously* proceed through a red light or red flashing signal.
- Pass other vehicles in no-passing zones.

In executing the above, you must first signal, ensure that the way is clear, and avoid endangering life and property.

By law, you must meet several qualifications before you can exercise these privileges:

- You must have a valid driver's license and have completed a formal training program in defensive driving and emergency vehicle operation.
- You must be involved in a "true emergency" in which a life is at risk. A broken arm is not a true emergency; cardiac arrest is. If you are involved in an accident while operating under emergency conditions at a red light or driving the wrong way down the street, you will need to satisfy the police and possibly a court that you were responding to a call in which human life was threatened.
- You must use warning devices — red lights, horns, and sirens — so that other vehicles on the road will be aware of you and will have a chance to yield. You must use these devices in the manner prescribed by law.
- You must exercise due regard for the safety of others. This means that you may cautiously move through a red light, but you must slow down while entering the intersection so that all traffic can stop to allow you to pass. It means that you may park your ambulance anywhere to care for a patient, but you must not park it just over the crest of a hill on a busy highway unless you post flares and get a police officer or a volunteer to divert traffic out of your line. The law states that if you do not exercise due regard for the safety of others, you are liable for the consequences.
- Many companies provide additional guidance. For instance, some specify that your top speed cannot be more than ten miles over the speed of *traffic,* which may or may not be the *posted* speed. This allows the emergency vehicle to overtake other moving traffic but promotes safer driving. In some

□ Types of Ambulances

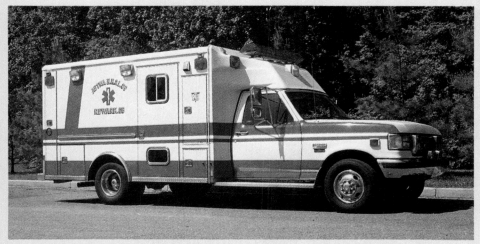

FIGURE 44-1 Type I ambulance.

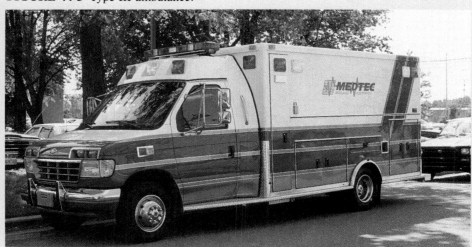

FIGURE 44-2 Type II ambulance.

FIGURE 44-3 Type III ambulance.

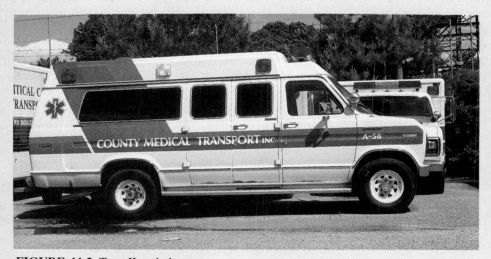

areas, ambulances entering an intersection against the light must come to a complete stop before proceeding.

Be sure that you know the general vehicle code, the regulations for emergency vehicles, and your agency code. Also, know the qualifications in your state for ambulance drivers and be sure that you can qualify. Several states require special licenses and/or special training for ambulance drivers. Sample regulations include the following:

- The vehicle operator or driver shall possess a valid Special Chauffeur's License, issued by the State Department of Safety and/or such special class licenses as required by another state of residence.
- No person under the age of nineteen years shall drive any ambulance authorized for operation in (state), and each ambulance driver shall have at least three years of licensed driver or operator experience.
- Ambulance services shall assure that at least 80 percent of ambulance drivers employed by the service have completed a course in emergency vehicle operations, including at least six hours of classroom instruction and two hours of personal behind-the-wheel instruction.

☐ FACTORS LEADING TO UNSAFE DRIVING

Five factors may contribute to unsafe driving for an EMT:

- Lack of expertise in the dispatcher: The dispatcher should have enough experience to judge quickly and accurately the urgency of an emergency.
- Inadequate equipment in the ambulance: When adequate equipment is available in the ambulance, you can take the time to stabilize the patient before transport. However, remember the "Golden Hour" of trauma support: transport a trauma patient as quickly as possible. If you do not have enough equipment or the proper type, you may need to rush the patient to a hospital.
- Inadequate training of the EMT: If you are not trained adequately, you will not be able to stabilize the patient at the scene; instead, you will try to get to the hospital as quickly as possible. A trained EMT will be better able to judge whether the patient should be referred to a more advanced unit for emergency care and transport. A well-trained and experienced EMT will know when to take the time to fully stabilize and when to "scoop and

run." If delay of full stabilization will compromise the patient, stabilize as much as possible and then transport immediately.

- Inadequate driving ability: Just because you can drive a car does not make you qualified to drive an ambulance. You need specialized training and experience in emergency driving.
- Inadequate job definition: The vehicle operator's first job is to operate the vehicle safely. The second job is to transfer the patient safely to the hospital. Usually you cannot do your second job if your first job is not being done properly.

Typical Driving Mistakes

Ambulance drivers can get themselves in trouble by:

- Having a poor attitude about safe, careful driving. Drivers who are too confident, frustrated, fatigued, or overly excited may commit critical driving mistakes.
- Believing in their enhanced visibility. Driving with lights and siren activated may produce unfounded confidence that other drivers can hear or see you; that is often not the case, especially when a radio or air-conditioner is in operation.
- Not paying attention to blind spots. Changing lanes too fast, backing up too fast, and not knowing how to use mirrors may all lead to an accident.
- Driving at excessive speed. Traveling too fast reduces your reaction time and does not permit you to maintain a safe distance between vehicles. It also increases stress on you and on the vehicle.
- Having tunnel vision. Staring at the "tunnel" in front of you is almost hypnotizing and does not allow you to see the wider "scene." As a result, you do not react well to forthcoming situations.

☐ DRIVING EXCELLENCE

An excellent ambulance driver understands the capabilities and limitations of his vehicle, evaluates weather and road conditions quickly and accurately, appraises and responds to traffic conditions quickly and appropriately, and minimizes risk and discomfort to other members of the crew and to the patient. Notice that fast, dramatic driving is not part of the definition.

The Five P's

The following are the "Five P's" or basic principles for effective driving:[1]

---

[1] Adapted from William Heim, "EMS Training: Don't Leave the Driver Behind," *Emergency Medical Services*, June 1988.

- **Perception:** Perceive the complete picture of what is ahead by rotating your eyes 180 degrees, looking to the horizon, and scanning from side to side. That way you will see what is developing before it becomes a problem.

- **Planning:** Go through various driving situations in your mind and think through "escape route" options to prepare yourself beforehand for unexpected hazards.

- **Prevention:** Practice defensive driving and be ready to adjust to the other person's mistakes. Give yourself time to react so that you can remove yourself from another driver's folly.

- **Publicity:** Broadcast your driving intentions early enough so that other drivers have time to react to you. Make eye contact when possible. Avoid sudden movements, and be as visible as the situation requires by using available lights, sirens, turn signals, flashing headlights, etc.

- **Professionalism:** Proper attitude is very important in safe driving. Many accidents are caused by bad decisions influenced by anger, speed, and frustration. When emotions run high, recognize and neutralize any tendency to forego safe driving practices.

Hold the steering wheel with both hands at all times. One hand should be in the nine o'clock and the other in the three o'clock position. In turning, one hand pulls while the other slides, paralleling the pulling hand's position. Neither hand should pass the twelve or six o'clock positions to prevent them from becoming tangled. When you reach these limits, the opposite hand begins to grip the wheel and the first hand slides.

You also need to practice enough with your ambulance that you are familiar with how it accelerates and decelerates, the kind of space it requires for its fenders and bumpers, how it brakes, and how it corners.

Driving at Night

While only about one-third of all accidents occur at night, more than half of the fatalities from accidents stem from night-time driving. In fact, based on miles driven, there are two and a half times more fatal accidents at night than during the day. This is because less light is available and vision is restricted. Night vision varies considerably among people. Older people generally cannot see well in the dark, and eyestrain can substantially reduce night vision. Bright light, such as lightning or high-beam headlights, can cause temporary blindness at night.

Headlights on low beams illuminate the roadside for about 150 feet. On high beam, visibility will be 350 to 400 feet. At fifty-five miles per hour, it takes 4.5 seconds to cover 350 feet. For night driving, control speed so that your stopping range is within headlight range.

To improve your visibility and the ability of others to see you, do the following:

- Make sure that your ambulance has quartz-halogen headlights, which provide much more light to the road.

- Turn your headlights on at dusk, and leave them on until full daylight.

- Keep your headlights clean and properly aimed. Check them each day before your shift begins. If the weather is bad, especially if there is sleet or snow, stop as necessary during your shift to clean debris off your headlights.

- Replace burned-out headlights immediately.

- Dim your high beams within 500 feet of an approaching vehicle or within 300 feet of a vehicle in front of you.

- Never stare into the high beams of another car; guide your ambulance by watching the right edge of the road.

- Do not flick your high beams up and down to remind another driver to dim his brights — it can blind him temporarily.

- Never use high beams when going into a curve.

- Keep your windshield clean, inside and out. Keep a bottle of windshield or glass cleaner in the cab for mirrors and interior windshields.

- Keep your instrument panels dim.

- Keep your eyes moving; avoid focusing on any one object.

- If the washing solution under your hood does not leave the glass clean after ten wiper cycles, replace the blades and/or use a stronger concentration of washing fluid.

- Be sure that you are rested before you begin a night driving shift.

- Between 11 p.m. and 3 a.m., be particularly alert for drunk or drowsy drivers. If you notice erratic speeds, weaving across lines, or delayed starts at intersections, use extreme care in passing. Avoid using your siren, since the combination of confusion and delayed reaction time may make the driver jam on the brakes or swerve into your path.

Driving in Bad Weather

Bad weather affects your ability to control your ambulance. Stopping on wet pavement takes approximately twice the distance as stopping on dry pavement. On ice or sleet, it takes you five times the distance to stop. Leave adequate space between you and the vehicle in front of you in any kind of weather. Despite myths to the contrary, 66 percent of ambulance accidents occur in clear or cloudy weather, and 70 percent occur in daylight. Furthermore, 63 percent of ambulance accidents occur on dry roads. Follow these precautions for specific weather situations:

Rainy or Wet Weather

About six times more people are killed on wet roads than on snowy and icy roads combined. Roads are slipperiest when it just starts to rain. When the road is wet, your vehicle **hydroplanes** — the front tires literally lift so that the vehicle is riding on a film of water rather than the actual pavement. Hydroplaning begins at speeds as low as thirty-five miles per hour if the tires are worn. Do the following when driving on wet roads:

- Keep your mirrors cleared of water.
- Avoid sudden braking and sudden moves of the steering wheel.
- If you are about to go through a large standing pool of water, slow down and turn on your wipers before you hit the water. As you leave the water, tap the brake lightly a few times to dry it out. If the ambulance pulls to one side, pump the brake slowly and smoothly to dry the brake out.
- If you begin to hydroplane, hold the wheel steady, take your foot from the accelerator, and *gently* pump the brake. If you turn the wheel from side to side to try and get down through the water, or if you jam on the brake, you will probably skid.

Winter Driving

Sleet, freezing rain, packed snow, and ice decrease visibility and increase skidding. Powder snow and gusty winds can create a total white-out with zero visibility for several hundred yards. To ensure safety, do the following:

- Make sure that your engine is tuned, your heater and defroster are in good working order, and your battery is charged.
- Carry emergency weather equipment — chains, a shovel, sand, booster cables, and a towing device.
- Equip the ambulance with studded snow tires if you can; chains are the best insurance against skidding.
- Stay aware of the temperature. Wet ice and freezing rain, the most hazardous road conditions, occur between 28° and 40° F. Bridges and overpasses freeze sooner than road surfaces.
- Avoid sudden movements of the steering wheel and sudden braking.

Fog, Mist, Dust Storms, Smog

When visibility is poor, do the following:

- Slow down but avoid decelerating suddenly.
- Watch the road ahead and behind carefully for other cars that are traveling slowly.
- Turn on your lights, regardless of the time of day, and use your wipers. Never use the high beam on your headlights. The reflection of the beams from the fog will actually reduce your visibility. Even if the lights do not improve your own visibility (as in daylight), they will make it possible for other motorists to see you better.
- If you are traveling fifteen miles per hour below the speed limit or lower, use four-way flashers (may not be legal in some states). Use the four-way flashers if you pull off the road and stop.
- Use the defroster to keep as much fog as possible off the inside of the windshield.
- If you need to slow down, tap your brake pedal several times so that the flash of your brake lights will warn motorists behind you.
- Fog can occur suddenly, and patches of greater density may appear. Vehicles in front may brake suddenly or come to a complete stop when encountering a thicker patch of fog. Be alert for vehicles in front of you.

Animals in the Road

If you encounter an animal running into the road, do the following:

- Gauge your reaction by the size of the animal and your vehicle speed.
- Try to avoid the animal by slowing or swerving, but remember that it is better to hit a small animal (dog, cat, rabbit) than to risk losing control of the vehicle.
- Hitting a large animal (horse, deer, cow) will have an impact equal to hitting another vehicle. Remove your foot from the accelerator, steer the vehicle in the opposite direction from the one in which the animal is running, and be prepared for the animal to stop suddenly. Do not jam on the brake. Keep all steering wheel and brake motions smooth.
- In urban areas, be alert for children who may run after the animal.

Objects on the Road

If you see an object on the road and cannot stop before reaching it, follow these guidelines:

- Decelerate and steer to the right. If you can pass the object safely, do so. Do not drive onto the shoulder of the road unless absolutely necessary and then reduce your speed as much as possible before hitting the shoulder. It if is soft, you may skid or roll over.

- Do not steer to the left. You may enter the lane of opposing traffic.
- Do not try to straddle the object unless you are absolutely certain that you can do so safely. If it hits the underside of the ambulance or ricochets from a wheel, it could damage the steering mechanism and/or drive shaft, puncture the gas tank, or dislodge the oil pan.

Tire Blowout

Front tire blowouts are most dangerous, because loss of a front tire dangerously interferes with the steering of the ambulance. You may hear an explosive boom, and the vehicle will veer suddenly to the side of the blown-out tire. To regain control, follow these steps:

1. Take your foot off the accelerator, giving the ambulance a chance to slow down.
2. Hold the steering wheel firmly with both hands — expect it to be difficult to steer.
3. When you have gained control of the steering, put on the brake slowly; avoid locking the wheels.
4. Come to a gradual and complete stop, if you can, off the roadway so that you can change the tire safely.

Brake Failure

Signs of brake failure include a warning light or drastically reduced resistance when you press the brake pedal.

1. If the ambulance has an automatic transmission (most common), allow the vehicle to slow to forty miles per hour, then increase the engine speed and downshift to a lower drive range. When the speed has dropped to about twenty miles per hour, increase the engine speed and downshift to low. At a very low speed, use the soft shoulder of the road or rub against the curb to bring the ambulance to a stop. While you risk blowing your transmission or engine with this technique, engines are cheaper than lives and ambulances.
2. Gently apply your parking brake. You cannot pump an emergency brake. Remember that this is a cable brake. The rear wheels may lock if you apply too much force and the vehicle will probably pull to one side.
3. Pump the brake pedal rapidly. It may build up pressure in the brake lines and restore some braking force.

4. If neither of these slow the vehicle, honk your horn to alert traffic, and activate all your emergency lights.
5. If you have to collide with something, choose an impact-absorbing object, such as a clump of shrubs or a chain-link fence. Avoid head-on collisions — sideswipe whatever you hit.
6. At slow speeds, simply turn off the engine and let the ambulance coast to a stop.
7. If the ambulance has slowed down enough, select an off-road stopping place. If the road is going uphill, wait until the natural hill slows the vehicle, then pull off the road. If no upgrade is in sight, select the path of exit that will result in the least amount of damage and injury.
8. Notify your dispatcher as soon as you are stopped. Under no circumstances try to move your ambulance again after you have come to a full stop.

Steering Failure

Steering failure most often occurs in ambulances with power steering. The most common cause is when the belt that drives the power steering unit breaks. Check the belt often for wearing and cracks.

If your steering fails, do the following:

1. Grasp the wheel firmly with both hands, and anticipate difficulty in steering.
2. Immediately take your foot off the accelerator and apply force to the steering wheel to move to the side of the road. Find a safe spot, and pull off the road.
3. If there is a total steering failure, immediately take your foot from the accelerator, turn on your warning lights and siren, and prepare for a skid or rollover. If the steering has been disengaged completely, there is nothing to hold your front wheels in a straight line. A bump, the shaping of the road, or a pothole could make your wheels change direction suddenly. *Do not* apply the brake, since the brakes may pull the ambulance to one side and throw you in the path of other vehicles. Coast until you are moving slowly enough to stop the ambulance with a pumping motion.

Stuck Accelerator

If your accelerator gets stuck to the floor and there are *no vehicles ahead of you*, do the following:

1. Try to release the pedal by slipping the toe of your shoe between the pedal and the floor. *Never try to release the pedal with your hand while you are*

moving. When you lose your vision of the roadway ahead and are simultaneously moving your body sideways, it is very difficult to steer your ambulance straight.

2. If you cannot release the pedal with the toe of your shoe, shift the vehicle into neutral. This will cut acceleration but allow the brakes and steering systems to work under power and eliminate the dangers of locking the steering column. If you have power brakes, apply steady pressure; if you do not have power brakes, pump them.

3. Select a safe off-road stopping place, and pull off the road. If the engine is still running, turn it off.

4. If you lose accelerating power, coast to the side of the road and call your dispatcher. If necessary, creep along on the shoulder at idle speed until you reach a safe place.

5. Activate your flashers to warn motorists.

Wheels Off the Road

Avoid the shoulder of the road. Stay in the left-hand lane if there is one; the exception to this rule is if you are traveling over a road with many curves. In that case, stay in the right-hand lane of a four-lane roadway and the middle of a six-lane roadway. You will run less risk of getting hit by someone who wanders into your lane from the opposite direction, and you will run less risk of losing control and jutting into the line of opposing traffic. If you are on a single-lane road, do not let your right wheel dip into the shoulder. You may lose control (especially if you are going at a high speed), and you may overreact by wrenching your steering wheel to the left to correct for the error.

If one or more of your wheels suddenly hit the shoulder, recover control of the ambulance by following these steps:

1. Hold the steering wheel firmly with both hands; the ambulance will be hard to steer.

2. Check for traffic ahead and to the rear.

3. Ease off the accelerator to reduce your speed.

4. If you must use your brakes to reduce your speed, do so *very* gradually. If the shoulder of the road is graveled or muddy, expect to skid.

5. Center the ambulance over the edge of the road.

6. Turn on the left turn signal.

7. Turn the wheel gradually and steer back on the road. As soon as your front right wheel touches the road surface, correct steering to stay in the lane. If you have to avoid a collision with an obstacle before getting back into the road surface, accelerate slightly while turning the wheel.

Pulling Off the Road

If you need to pull off the road due to adverse weather or some other problem, you need to protect yourself and the ambulance and provide early, visible warning to other motorists. Pull the ambulance as far off of the road as you can.

The most effective warning devices are triangular reflectors, flares, or chemical light sticks. (Reflectors are best because they pose no fire hazard, as with flares.) The second best alternative is to use your overhead beacon, four-way flashers (if acceptable in your state), and cab lights. Cab lights alone are ineffective, but they increase safety when used at night with the overhead flashers, and they provide good warning to vehicles approaching from behind. Do not use headlights or parking lights.

If it is likely that the ambulance may be hit by another vehicle, remove any patients, leave the ambulance, and wait a safe distance away.

To place warning devices:

1. Start your four-way flashers before you leave the ambulance.

2. Put one device on the traffic side of the ambulance, right next to the ambulance.

3. Place a second device 100 to 200 feet to the rear of the ambulance on the edge of the road. If the ambulance is on the road, put the device in the middle of the lane.

4. Place a third device approximately 300 feet behind the ambulance on the edge of the road (or in the lane, if the ambulance is on the road). To gauge your distance, a normal stride is a little more than two feet.

5. If there is two-way traffic on the road, place another device about 200 feet in front of the ambulance on the edge of the road.

6. Do not light a fusee until you are ready to put it down. Pull the tab near the top of the fusee to free the cap; strike the matchlike head of the flare against the strike surface on the inside of the cap, and point the fusee *away* from your body while you strike it. Push the fusee between slabs of concrete or simply lay it on the road. If you can find one, use a rock or other anchoring device to keep the fusee from rolling. *Never* use a fusee (or other warning device with a flame) if:

• You can smell gasoline.

• Any fluid is leaking from the ambulance.

• There is any possibility of fire.

Selecting Alternate Routes

During transport, select the route best suited for safe travel — this is not necessarily the shortest route. Avoid schools, railroad crossings, detours, construction sites, bridges, tunnels, and similar trouble areas whenever you can, even if it means driving a few extra miles. If you are unfamiliar with the roads in your city, get a good, detailed city map and study it. Patrolling will help you get a feel for topography. Keep posted about roads undergoing repair or new building sites, and avoid them when you can. Select an alternate route during rush-hour traffic. If you are responding to a traffic accident that can back up traffic on a busy highway, select an alternate route by which to approach the accident.

□ CONTROLLING THE VEHICLE

For vehicle control, remember the rule about speed: go the posted limit unless the situation is critical. Speed can complicate patient care, decrease ambulance stability, and be a greater risk to your life and others in the ambulance.

A number of factors other than speed affect your ability to control the ambulance, and you need to keep them in mind so that you can correct the situation.

Braking

Sudden braking may result in loss of control. The brakes will cause wheels to lock, and you may skid dangerously. Pump your brakes slowly and smoothly. (Newer ambulances may have an antilock braking system.) Never brake on a curve. Brake when going into the curve and gradually accelerate when going out. When decelerating, rest your foot slightly on the brake. Your stopping distance is the time it takes you to react plus your braking time.

Railroads

You may encounter a railroad crossing and have to wait for a long train to crawl along the tracks. Keep calm, and monitor the patient. If there is simply no way that you can get around the train, such as an underpass or overpass within a reasonable distance, wait it out instead of trying inappropriate stunts. Plan an alternate route when you can.

Bridges and Tunnels

There is little room for passing on bridges or in tunnels. If you are in heavily congested traffic near a bridge or tunnel, consider an alternate route. If there is none, try to get control of the situation *before* you enter the bridge or tunnel. Remember that you probably will not be able to pass, so go with the flow of traffic at a safe speed until you emerge.

Day of the Week

You can expect less traffic on weekends than on workdays in most areas of the country. Traffic around shopping centers is heaviest on Saturdays, and traffic is most congested Monday through Friday on commuter routes or in urban or industrialized areas. Keep in mind what kind of traffic you are most likely to encounter.

Time of Day

Rush-hour traffic is more congested in most urban centers than in the country, so plan accordingly. Watch for school zones and industrial plant shift changes.

Road Surface

Always be on the lookout for potholes and bumps. Your goal is to give your patient the smoothest ride possible. The two inner lanes on a four-lane highway are generally the smoothest.

Backing Up

Many ambulance accidents occur when the ambulance is backing up. Use all resources (mirrors, EMT in the rear of the ambulance, etc.) and back up slowly and carefully.

Parking

Park in front of or behind an accident, but never alongside it. On a narrow, no-parking road, take up the entire road so that no one will try to squeeze past you. Park in a driveway or on the shoulder of the road whenever possible. Turn off headlights so that you do not blind oncoming traffic. Stay a minimum of 10 feet from a burning vehicle, and 2,000 feet from a hazardous materials spill, ideally uphill and upwind.

Higher Speeds

At higher speeds, be cognizant of the following:

- Be especially careful on curves that lead into a population pocket (a town or school), curves that lead to intersections, and curves that crest hills. Practice negotiating curves in the ambulance during the early mornings when there is little traffic. Get a good idea of what speed you need to get around the curve safely.
- Brake to the proper speed *before* you enter a curve. Enter the curve on the outside (or the

"high" part), and start turning as early as possible. Go only as fast as feels comfortable while in the curve. Do not accelerate or brake in the curve — the scrubbing action of the tires will slow the ambulance down sufficiently. It is dangerous to brake after you have entered the curve, so make sure that you decelerate to a safe speed before entering.

- Accelerate carefully and gradually as you leave the curve. Too quick an acceleration can cause you to lose control.
- Keep your exit from the curve slow and steady.
- When going down a long hill, use a lower gear instead of riding your brake to maintain control.
- Always use a smooth braking motion. Your stopping distance increases dramatically as your speed increases; allow for it.

Intersection Accidents

The most common accidents in which ambulances are involved are those at intersections. There are three main causes of intersection accidents:

- A motorist approaches the intersection just as the light is changing; he does not want to sit through the red light, so he sails through the intersection. Always slow down at each intersection to make sure that it is clear, especially if you are crossing against the light.
- There are two emergency vehicles when motorists expect only one. Maintain a safe distance between your vehicle and the emergency vehicle in front of you, but follow closely enough so that the motorist can see both of you in the same glance. Do not use the same siren mode on both vehicles. Whenever you are using the emergency privileges that allow you to suspend traffic regulations, always use your flashers and siren for the fullest possible warning to the public. In some states, use of your siren when you are driving in the emergency mode is mandated by law.
- Vehicles waiting at an intersection may block your view of pedestrians in the crosswalk. Again, slow down.

☐ WARNING DEVICES

Warning Lights

Activate emergency lights on the ambulance at all times when responding to an emergency call. Lights should be used even when you are not using the siren. You should also turn on your headlights during the daytime — in some situations, the warning lights on top of the vehicle are not noticeable because they blend in with traffic lights, signs, Christmas decorations, building colors, and tail lights of vehicles traveling in the opposite direction.

Emergency Lights

Placement of the ambulance emergency lights on the vehicle is very important. They should be high enough to cast a beam *above* the traffic. Lower lights are needed to be visible in the rear-view mirror of the car ahead of you.

When an ambulance has strobe lights, use them with emergency lights that flash or revolve with a longer duration. White lights can be seen from a longer distance than red or blue, especially at sunrise or sunset. They can also be seen more effectively when wet streets are reflecting.

Headlights are a part of the emergency lighting system and should be on whenever you are traveling in an emergency. Specially wired headlights that flash alternately are also effective in gaining attention. (These are not legal in some states — check local protocol.) A spotlight can be used to get a driver's attention who has not noticed you, but do not panic him. Flash the light across the driver's rear-view mirror so that it gets his attention but is gone before he looks in the mirror. The glare could blind him or oncoming traffic, so be careful.

Use only minimal lighting during heavy fog or when you are parked. Use your emergency lights only when needed, such as when the patient's condition requires rapid transport.

Be aware of the siren's effect on you. Even if you can normally drive your own car or the ambulance flawlessly, the siren can have a bizarre effect on your ability to drive the ambulance safely. Studies have shown that ambulance drivers tend to increase their speed about fifteen miles per hour when the siren is going — an increase that sometimes takes them out of the limits of safe speeds. Some drivers are easily hypnotized by the siren and are unable to negotiate curves, turns, and obstacles; this hypnotic trance makes it seem as though the siren itself were controlling the vehicle. The siren can also mask your own hearing so that you cannot hear sirens or horns of other emergency vehicles responding to the same or other incidents.

Using Your Siren

Even if you are operating your flashing lights and sirens, do not assume that drivers are aware of you unless they look up to check their interior rear-view mirror, look to the left to check the exterior rear-view mirror, pull over, or stop.

The insulation in newer automobiles can reduce the interior decibel level of an approaching siren by 35 to 40 percent when parked. In motion, the noise of the motor, air-conditioner/heater, and/or radio in the automobile may make the siren completely inaudible. (This also applies to you in the ambulance!) Other obstacles are conversation, pelting rain, dense shrubbery or trees, buildings, and thunder. If the driver is wearing headphones, talking on a phone, inattentive, or partially/totally hearing-disabled, your problem is even more severe. Some drivers may not even recognize a two-tone klaxon as a siren.

Never pull directly behind a car and blast your siren. The driver may panic and slam on the brakes or swerve into another lane. Also, be prepared for the irrational maneuvers of inexperienced, drunk, or disoriented drivers.

Since the siren signals "emergency," it can create emotional stress (as well as physical stress from the noise level) for your patient. This is another reason for using your siren sparingly. Always let your patient know before you activate the siren.

Using Your Horn

Avoid overuse of the horn, but consider it when you need to clear traffic quickly. You can use the horn with or without a siren. Do not honk your horn when you are close to other vehicles — it may frighten a driver and cause him to slam on the brakes. (The horn may, however, be used safely much closer to other cars than may your siren.) Do not assume that other drivers can hear your horn or that they will heed it — proceed with caution.

Escorts

Using a police or other emergency vehicle escort en route to the accident or the hospital should be a last resort. It is dangerous, not only to the escort, but also to the EMT driver, to the patient in the ambulance, and to others on the road. All hazards associated with ambulance driving are doubled when an escort is involved, because you are the second car through an intersection and motorists may only expect one.

Use an escort *only* if you are unfamiliar with how to get to the hospital or if you do not think that you can find the victim's location. Allow for a safe distance between the escort vehicle and your ambulance.

☐ AMBULANCE EQUIPMENT

Your ambulance must contain supplies for handling medical emergencies, injuries, extrications, and childbirth. Table 44-1 is an equipment standards checklist, or rig checksheet developed by the state of New Jersey, Emergency Medical Services.

TABLE 44-1
Ambulance Check List

Registration
Insurance card
Light and siren permit
All red lights
Nonflashing headlights

Oxygen Equipment - on board — all cylinders coded green, meet current hydro test
- Capacity min. 1200 L with regulator meets Fed Specs
- Flow meter 0 to 15 LPM
- Universal 15/22 mm fittings
- Positive-pressure - 35/55 mm pressure
- Adult bag-valve mask - 1700 cc vol/rate 25/min
- Mask, transparent adult large min 1
- Mask, transparent adult medium min 1
- Child bag-valve mask - 750 cc vol/rate 40/min
- Mask, transparent, child
- Mask, transparent, infant
- Capability for humidified oxygen
- Nasal cannula - adult min 2
- Nasal cannula - child min 2
- Simple face mask - adult min 2
- Simple face mask - child min 2
- Non-rebreathing mask - adult min 2
- Non-rebreathing mask - child min 2
- Oropharyngeal airways - min 1 set
- Spare oxygen cylinder - min 300 L
- Pocket mask with valve and O_2

Portable oxygen system
- Minimum of 300 L capacity
- Flow meter 0 to 15 LPM
- Universal 15/22 fittings
- Positive-pressure - 35 to 55 mm pressure
- Nasal cannula - adult min 1
- Nasal cannula - child min 1
- Simple face mask - adult min 1
- Simple face mask - child min 1
- Non-rebreathing mask - adult min 1
- Non-rebreathing mask - child min 1
- Oropharyngeal airways - 1 complete set

Aspirator/suction devices (on board): Located to permit aspiration of stretcher patient and meets current specs flow/vacuum
- Wide bore, thick wall, non-kink tubing
- Non-breakable collection bottle
- Rinsing water bottle with water
- Catheters - Rigid min 2
- Catheters - Semi-rigid min 2

Suction (portable): meets current specs flow/vacuum
- Wide-bore, thick wall, non-kink tubing
- Non-breakable collection bottle
- Rinsing water bottle with water
- Catheters - Rigid min 1
- Catheters - Semi-rigid min 1

Communications Equipment
- 2-way radio rig/dispatch & rig/hospital
- Portable radio - optional

Patient litter
- Wheeled litter with patient securing devices, adjustable from flat to semi-seated position

The following items may be combined:
- Portable stretcher with securing devices
- Stair chair with securing devices
- Orthopedic litter with securing devices
- Long spine board with appropriate holes
- CPR board
- Reeves-type stretcher or equivalent

Splinting equipment
- Splints - assorted sizes
- Traction splint - adult
- Head immobilizer and/or sandbags
- Short spine board with straps or equivalent
- Rigid extrication collars - 1 each child through adult

Wound dressing and burn treatment
- Cravats - min 24
- 4 × 4's sterile - min 24
- Kling or equivalent gauze rolls - 12 rolls assorted
- Multi-trauma dressings 9" × 30" (or equivalent)
- Occlusive dressings sufficient for 4 app.
- Sterile burn sheets - min 2 individual wrapped
- Saline - sterile - min 2 liters
- Adhesive tape - assorted sizes

Miscellaneous patient care equipment - inside rig
- OB kit - sterile - min 1
- Stethoscope - min 1
- Sphygmomanometer - adult min 1
- Sphygmomanometer - child min 1
- Hot and cold packs - min 6
- Sugar - min 4 packets or 1 oz. glucose
- Paper bags - min 2
- Syrup of Ipecac - min 4 oz.
- Activated charcoal - min 1 packet
- Penlight or flashlight
- Ring cutter
- Bandage scissors
- Sheets
- Blankets
- Pillow and pillow cases
- Towels
- Disposable latex gloves
- Surgical masks
- Eye protector
- Disinfectant
- Bee sting swabs - min 6
- Sterilized aluminum foil in separate packets for use as occlusive dressing and for newborn warming
- Band-aids
- Large safety pins for securing bandages, slings, and swathes

First aid kit (jump kit)
- Assorted wound dressings
- Kling or equivalent - assorted
- Cravats
- Bandage scissors

- Stethoscope
- Spygmomanometer - adult min 1
- Spygmomanometer - child min 1
- Sugar - min 4 packets or 1 oz. glucose
- Paper bags - min 2
- Syrup of Ipecac - min 4 oz.
- Activated charcoal - min 1 packet
- Penlight or flashlight
- Disposable gloves
- Surgical masks

Basic extrication equipment
- Road warning devices
- Hammer
- Sheet metal cutting tool
- Tool kit including
  a. Assorted screwdrivers
  b. Assorted pliers
  c. Hacksaw with blades
  d. Spring loaded center punch
  e. Linoleum knife or equivalent
- 20 lb A:B:C chemical fire extinguisher
- Hand-held lights
- Wheel chocks
- Rescue helmet with full face shield/goggles
- Protective gloves
- Rope - 1 length 50/100 foot, min 1/2"

Optional supplies and extrication equipment suggested if possible
Supplies
- Traction splint - child
- Rigid extrication collars
- Unpadded board splints
- Various size wound dressings
- Burn kit
- Snakebite kit
- Ammonia inhalants
- Partial rebreathing masks - adult min 2
- Partial rebreathing masks - child min 2

Extrication equipment
- Porta-power (4 ton with accessories)
- Come-along (1 ton)
- Rescue chain set
- 36 inch bolt cutter
- Forcible entry tool
- Flat head fire axe
- Long-handled sledgehammer
- Assorted open/box wrench (3/8" through 1")
- Socket set with sockets (3/8" through 1")
- Wood cribbing
- Hardwood wedges - min 6
- Jack - (2 ton or larger)
- Rope - 4 lengths 50/100 ft min xia 5/8"
- Self contained breathing apparatus with spare cylinder
- Stokes rescue basket or equivalent
- Block and fall
- Snatch hook
- Rescue harness

If your area has an industrial plant that makes certain accidents probable, you may also want to handle special kits, such as chemical detection devices, a self-contained breathing apparatus, decontamination supplies, or special burn supplies.

☐ VEHICLE MAINTENANCE

Basic Maintenance

Basic ambulance maintenance should include oil and filter changes, transmissions and differential check, wheel bearing check, and tie rod end inspection.

Daily Inspection of Vehicle

Inspect the following vehicle systems daily. Most ambulance systems have a checklist of these items (Figures 44-4–44-8:

- Fuel: The tank should be full of gasoline. Refuel as needed. Never let the tank get below half full.
- Oil: Keep oil levels at their maximum; check daily and change as appropriate.
- Fluid circulation system: Check transmission fluid, power steering fluid if applicable, and water levels in the radiator and battery, if applicable. Do not overfill pre-shift transmission and power-steering fluids, since they expand when heated and can cause serious damage, including fires. Also check windshield washer fluid. This can be a life-saver on slushy winter trips.
- Battery: Most ambulances use a two-battery system, and both are used all the time to keep each one fully charged. If one battery dies, the switch can be dialed to both to charge it back up. Check the water level, if applicable. Some batteries are sealed. Make sure that battery cables are clean and tight. The battery voltage meter should be no lower than 9 or 10 when starting and show about 14 when running. The ammeter should come back to zero a few minutes after the engine is started. If it does not, there may be a problem.
- Brakes: Test brakes for pressure, pedal travel, and hold.
- Tires: Keep a tire pressure gauge and a tire-inflation device in the ambulance, and check daily to make sure that they work. Carefully check the tires, including the spare tire, each day for signs of damage, unusual wear, or bulging spots. Change tires as soon as you spot potential trouble. Check tire pressure daily, and inflate as needed. If your area has snow and ice in the winter, check daily to make sure that snow tires, chains, and other winter driving devices are in good condition.

- If your service uses shoreline power connectors, check the condition of the cord, receptacle, receptacle weather cover, and plug. You should have a quick disconnect about twelve inches from the vehicle receptacle. It should be loose enough to separate the cord from the ambulance if you fail to unplug it when responding to an emergency call.
- Headlights: Make sure that headlights, including high beams, are in good working condition; if headlights seem weak, change bulbs; keep glass clean.
- Brake lights: Check daily to make sure that they are working; change bulbs as needed. Keep glass clean.
- Turn signals: Check to see that each operates correctly.
- Emergency lights: Check to see that they operate effectively.
- Wipers: Make sure that wipers are in good condition and are able to keep the windshield clean; change wiper blades as necessary.
- Horn: Check to see that it operates effectively.
- Siren: Check to see that it operates effectively.
- Windows: They should be clean.
- Door closing and latching devices: All doors should open and close properly and should completely latch when closed; check the rubber stripping around the door interior for worn or cracked spots.
- Power systems: Check the shore line connection operation and on-board recharger circuits.
- Air-conditioning, heating, and ventilation systems: Make sure that they work properly.
- Radiator hoses and fan belts: Check before you make your first run; if there are any weak spots or cracks in the belt, replace it.
- Seat belts: Check for webbing damage, for correct fastening and unfastening, and for correct winding on the spool. Make sure that every passenger in the ambulance is belted.
- Seat: Adjust the seat to your specifications.
- Dash lights: Check each dash light to be sure that it is working.
- After you start the engine, check the gas indicators, test the brakes and parking brake, turn the steering wheel, turn on the wipers and washers, and have your partner check the warning lights, headlights, turn signals, four-way flashers, brake lights, back-up lights, ICC marker lights, and side and rear spots.
- Test your radio for send and transmit.
- Keep a close inventory of needed supplies, and

□ Daily Vehicle Inspection

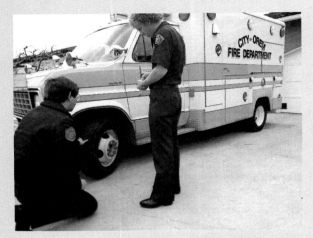

FIGURE 44-4 Check tires for inflation, wear, or danger spots.

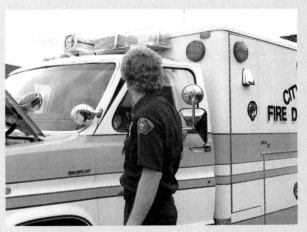

FIGURE 44-5 Make sure all lights are functional.

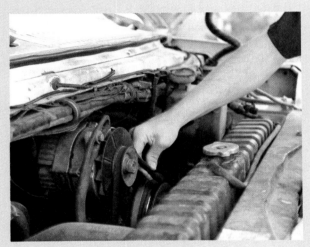

FIGURE 44-6 Check all belts and hoses.

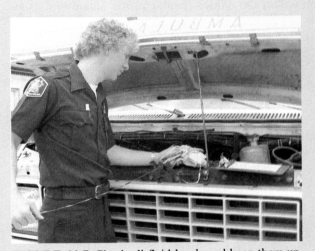

FIGURE 44-7 Check all fluid levels and keep them up.

FIGURE 44-8 Make sure all reports are complete and properly filed.

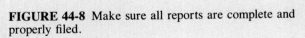

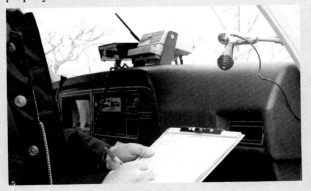

check it daily to make sure that your equipment is complete.

- Check the interior and exterior of the vehicle before you start your run to make sure that it is completely clean and decontaminated.
- Wheels: Check for any cracks, deformities, loose lug nuts, etc.

If your service does not have a clear protocol for reporting problems with vehicles, taking them out of service if they are deemed unsafe, and performing regular service and maintenance, work locally to insure such procedures. Legally, you may be within your rights to refuse to use a vehicle which you have reason to believe is unsafe; and correspondingly, you may be legally liable for damage caused by a malfunctioning machine if you are aware of the deficiency.

Ambulance Winter Maintenance[2]

If your area experiences snow and cold temperatures routinely in the winter, winterize the ambulance properly:

- Use proper-weight multipurpose oil (check with the fleet operator).
- Install rubber-surfaced wiper blades that do not allow ice and snow build up. Place a strong wind shield solvent in the washer fluid.
- Flush the radiator and test the thermostat.
- Make sure that the radiator solution is good down to $-40°$ F.
- Check and repair the exhaust system for possible leaks and faulty parts. Have the interior of the rig checked for carbon monoxide levels.
- Check doors for adequate weather stripping.
- Check and adjust transmission bands so that the vehicle will give high performance in heavy snow.
- Check all belts, hoses, battery, and wiring. Carry an extra fan, alternator belt, and power steering belt.
- Carry de-icer and add it to a full tank of gas periodically.
- Carry lock de-icer and use it periodically on all locks.
- Radial all-weather tires work well on snow and ice. Follow local protocol on studs and chains.
- Keep appropriate winter equipment on hand, such as:

— Heavy blankets.

— Snow shovel or scoops.
— Tow rope or chain.
— Jumper cables.
— Extra clothing.

☐ CARBON MONOXIDE IN AMBULANCES

Carbon monoxide (CO) is colorless, odorless, tasteless, and deadly. If an ambulance is not properly cared for, a CO level that is harmful to stressed patients and even to emergency personnel may build up. Any amount of CO over 10 ppm above the ambient CO level in the air may be dangerous.

Excessive amounts of CO may come from:

- The vehicle's own exhaust gases.
- Supplemental gasoline or LPG-powered equipment.
- The exhaust gases of vehicles parked next to or traveling by the ambulance.
- Greater outside air pressure, which forces the CO into the ambulance.

Be aware of the symptoms of low concentrations:

- Yawning.
- Dizziness.
- Dimmed vision.
- Headaches.
- Irregular heart rhythms.
- Vomiting.

Be aware of these symptoms of higher concentrations:

- Skin is warm and turns a cherry color (a very late sign).
- Dilated pupils.
- Erratic breathing.
- Coma.
- Twitching.
- Respiratory and cardiac arrest.

If any of these symptoms or signs occur, remove the patient from the ambulance and administer oxygen. Perform CPR if necessary.

Prevention

Prevent CO poisoning by:

- Having frequent engine tune-ups.

---

[2] Clarence H. Olson, Division of Emergency Health Services, North Dakota State Department of Health, State Capitol, Bismarck, North Dakota 58505.

- Having an adequate exhaust system that discharges beyond the side of the vehicle.
- Keeping rear windows shut.
- Making sure that doors shut tightly with proper gaskets and adjustments.
- Covering any opening to the outside.
- *Not* using ventilation exhaust fans or static roof vents.
- Keeping the heater or air-conditioner on. They create continuous positive interior pressure.
- *Not* using supplemental gasoline or LPG-powered equipment inside the ambulance.

A bright light or water spray under pressure will help you identify possible spots where CO can enter. CO testers for the inside of ambulances are available. There are also color-change CO monitors that stick to the sun visor, dash, etc.

□ PHASES OF AN AMBULANCE RUN

There are seven major phases of an ambulance run:

- Daily pre-run inspection.
- En route to the scene.
- At the scene.
- En route to the hospital.
- At the hospital.
- En route to the station.
- After the run.

En Route to the Scene

Follow these guidelines en route to the scene:

- Be sure that you leave the station with everything you will need.
- Have the dispatcher's message on a notepad so that you can refer to the address en route. Confirm the location of the call with your dispatcher, ask if there are further details, and listen for other units on the radio and also for the exterior sound of sirens. Also listen for status reports from other units on the scene.
- Picture in your mind the location of the equipment you think you will need at the scene.
- Drive responsibly, *using emergency privileges only if the need exists.*
- Assign each of the team members specific responsibilities at the scene, and assign projected equipment needs to each.

- Make sure that their responsibilities are clear.

At the Scene

Follow these guidelines while at the scene:

- Carefully observe the *complete* accident scene as you approach it. Be on the lookout for children, curiosity-seekers, or victims who may have wandered away. Closely observe possible mechanisms of injury. Park the ambulance in the safest and most convenient place to load the patients, taking into consideration the traffic, the roadway, and any known hazards. Come to a complete stop before putting the ambulance in "Park." "Hot stops" can damage the transmission and contribute to drive-line failures. The locking mechanism is relatively fragile, and the entire weight of the vehicle rests on it. If this weight is multiplied by the vehicle's forward velocity, these rolling stops will eventually wear out the parking mechanism (see Figure 44-9).
- Identify and control hazards, such as damaged utility poles and downed electrical wires, hazardous materials or explosives, or burning vehicles. If a hazard exists, establish a danger zone and park the ambulance outside this zone. Guard against further injury of patients or EMTs. If some accident or mechanical failure occurs or you need backup equipment or personnel to help, call the dispatcher immediately.
- Once you have parked the ambulance and controlled hazards, carefully gain access to the victims. Guard against injury. Make sure that the vehicle wreckage is stabilized before you enter, and use the simplest method to enter (i.e., try *all* doors first). See Chapter 43 on patient stabilization and extrication. As soon as you reach the victims, apply the ABCs and give appropriate care.
- If the accident involves a vehicle, stabilize your patient using appropriate extrication and splinting principals. "Unwrap" the wreckage from the patient. Carefully prepare your patient for transport. Take the time needed to properly splint the injured patient (long, short backboard, KED, etc.) *before* you move him or her. If the patient has experienced severe multiple trauma and time is precious, perform the ABCs, give the necessary emergency care, quickly splint the patient to a longboard, and transport.
- Once the patient is properly packaged, carefully and slowly remove him from the wreckage, and transfer him or her to the waiting ambulance. Make sure that the patient is securely strapped on the wheeled stretcher and properly loaded, and that the stretcher locks securely into place.

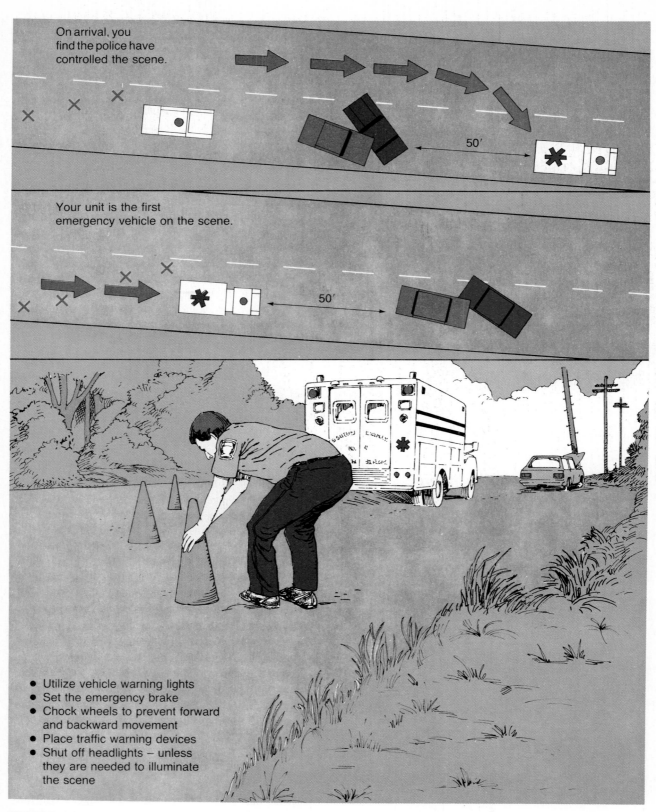

On arrival, you find the police have controlled the scene.

50'

Your unit is the first emergency vehicle on the scene.

50'

- Utilize vehicle warning lights
- Set the emergency brake
- Chock wheels to prevent forward and backward movement
- Place traffic warning devices
- Shut off headlights – unless they are needed to illuminate the scene

FIGURE 44-9

En Route to the Hospital

Follow these guidelines en route to the hospital (Figures 44-10–44-18):

- Make sure that the patient is stabilized and settled before moving the ambulance. Place unconscious non-trauma patients in the coma position to allow proper drainage. Place a conscious patient in the most comfortable position for him or her (e.g., semi-reclining position for a heart attack patient). Adjust stretcher straps so that they are tight but not binding. Loosen any clothing that may interfere with breathing and circulation. Check bandages. Give psychological support to the patient.

- If a patient's relative or friend accompanies him or her, follow local guidelines as to where the friend should sit. Allow the companion in the patient compartment only if local protocols allow it and if the relative or friend is in emotional control. If the patient is a child, it is often helpful to have a parent with you.

- Focus on the patient. Smile and reassure him or her as often as you can. Take advantage of brief stops (such as stop lights) to monitor blood pressure. Treat each patient like an individual, not like a "case." Gentleness, listening, answering questions honestly, and providing as much explanation as the patient wants will make a world of emotional difference — for them and for you.

- The driver should drive prudently, only use the necessary speed, and obey all regulations. Keep the patient as comfortable as possible during the trip. Continue to monitor the patient and give any needed additional care. Continually reassure the patient.

- If you are the EMT with the patient, you should keep the driver informed of the patient's condition. Instruct him or her to slow down or take a different route if the patient is suffering from speed and bounces. If the patient's condition suddenly worsens and it become urgent to reach the hospital immediately, tell him or her so that he or she can proceed as quickly as possible.

- Notify the hospital that you are bringing the patient in and give the necessary patient information. This usually involves:
  - The hospital identification.
  - The ambulance identification.
  - A brief description of the situation.
  - A description of any information you have gathered, subjective and objective, and a report of the vital signs.
  - Your opinion of the suspected problem or injuries.

  - The emergency care being given.
  - The estimated arrival time at the hospital.
- This complete call should take less than a minute.

At the Hospital

Follow these guidelines while at the hospital:

- The patient is usually presented to emergency room nurses at the emergency department of the hospital. As you make the HAND OFF (switching the patient from prehospital to hospital emergency care), continue to concentrate on the care of your patient. Give a verbal report on the patient's vital information to the receiving emergency room personnel. If the emergency department is crowded, continue to care for your patient in the ambulance until you can transfer him or her to the emergency room. Never leave the patient unattended! Participate in emergency care at the hospital if requested.

- When you are able, transfer all records and information that you have about the patient, both verbally and by written report, if possible. Be specific about vital signs, any change in condition, and emergency care given.

- Make sure that any valuables or personal effects of the patient are also transferred, and indicate this on your report.

- The patient report should be completed before you leave the hospital, and a written copy of the information on the patient's condition should be left at the emergency room. You may consider leaving a copy of the run sheet with the patient in the emergency room. Follow local protocol.

- After the disposition of the patient, exchange any linens, spine boards, and other equipment that you may have to leave at the hospital.

- Before you leave, ask hospital personnel if you are needed further. If you leave without a release, you may be recalled to transfer the patient to another medical facility or to return the patient to his or her home if his or her condition is not serious enough to warrant admission.

- Quickly check and clean the ambulance. You may receive a call before you return to base!

En Route to the Station

Follow these guidelines en route to the station (Figure 44-19):

- Radio the dispatcher that you are returning to the station, then proceed in a safe, cautious manner.
- Buckle your seat belt.

☐ Responding to a Call

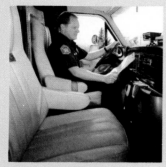

FIGURE 44-10 Keep necessary information close at hand when responding to a call.

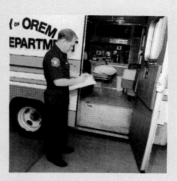

FIGURE 44-11 Complete, concise records are essential.

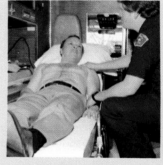

FIGURE 44-12 Give calming reassurance. Make sure that the patient is stabilized and settled.

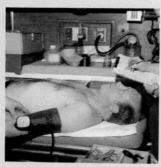

FIGURE 44-13 Collect patient information with a standard report form while your partner checks vital signs.

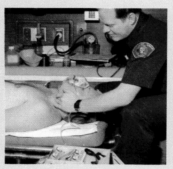

FIGURE 44-14 Continue monitoring vital signs.

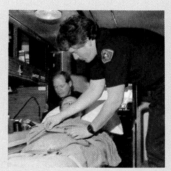

FIGURE 44-15 Make sure that stretcher and patient are secure. Check straps and adjust any that may be too tight.

FIGURE 44-16 Continually monitor vital signs.

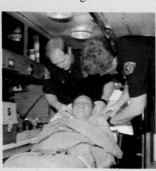

FIGURE 44-17 The driver should drive prudently. Advise driver of any changing conditions in patient.

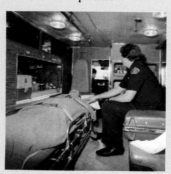

FIGURE 44-18 Notify the hospital that you are bringing the patient in.

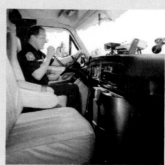

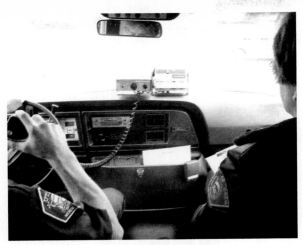

FIGURE 44-19 Advise base station that you are returning and buckle your seat belt. Fill out reports.

- Refuel according to local protocol.
- If a team member is in the patient compartment, he or she can "straighten up" the compartment as needed from a buckled seat position. (A good teaching experience is to have the driver ride on the gurney as a patient on the way back from the call. This will sensitize the EMT to how various accelerations affect the patient.)

Post-Run

Follow these guidelines after the run (Figures 44-20–44-23):

- Fill out and file reports as required by local protocol. *Do not* postpone this activity. See Chapter 45 on how to fill out reports and why. Then ready yourself for the next call.
- After each run, check fuel; if the tank is approaching half empty, fill it.
- Complete an inventory of equipment and supplies. Replace what you used during the run, and clean and decontaminate the nondisposable equipment used.
- Wash blood, vomitus, and other contaminants from the inside of the ambulance. Use hot, soapy water, disinfectant, and hot rinse water to completely wash down the floors, ceilings, and walls.
- At the end of each run, wash the exterior of the ambulance if you were driving in rain or snow or over muddy roads, or were in an area of radioactive fallout.
- Change soiled uniforms.

Post-Run Critique

If the call qualifies for stress debriefing (multiple casualties, overloaded capacities, or emotional trauma from the involvement of a child), is an appropriate support system in place for crisis counseling? Refer team members and seek assistance.

What did the run show about competencies and skills? Where do you need more practice? How much time in each workshift is devoted to training and skills development? Make each run a learning experience. The most helpful attitude is that it doesn't matter *who* is right or wrong. What matters is *what* was right or wrong. It is helpful to use a basic outline to be sure that there is a standard way of covering key points.

☐ AIR AMBULANCES

Many medical personnel involved in helicopter rescue consider a helicopter to be not just transport but an extension of the emergency room. Industry statistics show that many of those transported by helicopter would have died without the accompanying aeromedical support.

If your agency cooperates with air ambulances in transporting patients over long distances or in difficult access areas, keep these guidelines in mind:

- Make sure that the landing area is clear of obstructions. This area should be a square with 60-foot sides by day for a small helicopter, but larger — about 100-foot sides — by night. If the helicopter is medium-sized or large, it will need about double that area. Pick up loose debris that might blow up into the rotor system. Choose a landing site at least 50 yards from accident vehicles, if possible, so that noise and rotor wash will not be a problem for rescuers.
- If the landing site is a divided highway, stop the traffic going in both directions, even though the aircraft will land on only one side of the highway.
- Consider the wind direction. Helicopters take off and land into the wind by preference, rather than making vertical descents and ascents. Warn the crew by radio of power lines, poles, antennas, and trees.
- Mark each corner of the landing area with a highly visible device: a flag or surveyor's tapes by day and a flashing or rotating light at night. Use flares either by day or night but only if there is no danger of fire.
- Put a fifth warning device on the upwind side to designate the wind direction.
- If conditions are dusty or dry enough to create a fire hazard, have the area wetted down, if possible.
- Keep the patient and crew clear of the air downwash area. Spectators should be at least 200 feet away. EMT personnel should be at least 100 feet away during landing.

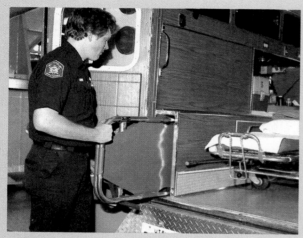

FIGURE 44-20 Put all equipment in proper place.

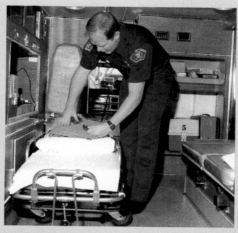

FIGURE 44-21 Make up wheeled stretcher and lock in place.

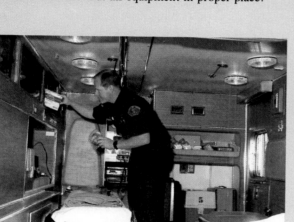

FIGURE 44-22 Complete an inventory of equipment and supplies. Replace necessary equipment so that ambulance is fully stocked.

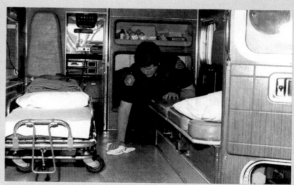

FIGURE 44-23 Wash blood, vomitus, etc. Clean ambulance interior as needed.

- Assign one person to guide the pilot in. He or she should wear eye and ear protection and should stand near the wind direction marker with his or her back to the wind, facing the touchdown area, arms raised overhead to indicate the landing direction (Figure 44-24).

- Give primary care to the patient and follow the instructions of the pilot or crew members *exactly* when those instructions relate to the craft's operation. Never try to open a door, for instance, without instructions.

- Be extremely cautious about the rotor-blade pattern. Remember that the tips can dip to as low as four feet above the ground. Always crouch when approaching or leaving the helicopter (Figure 44-25).

- Never approach a helicopter from behind the pilot. The pilot cannot see behind the craft, the tail rotor is spinning very quickly, and the pilot sometimes needs to move the tail boom without warning. If you have to go from one side to another, always cross in front of the craft, never behind it or underneath it.

- Secure all loose items so that nothing will blow into the rotor blades when you are approaching or leaving a helicopter.

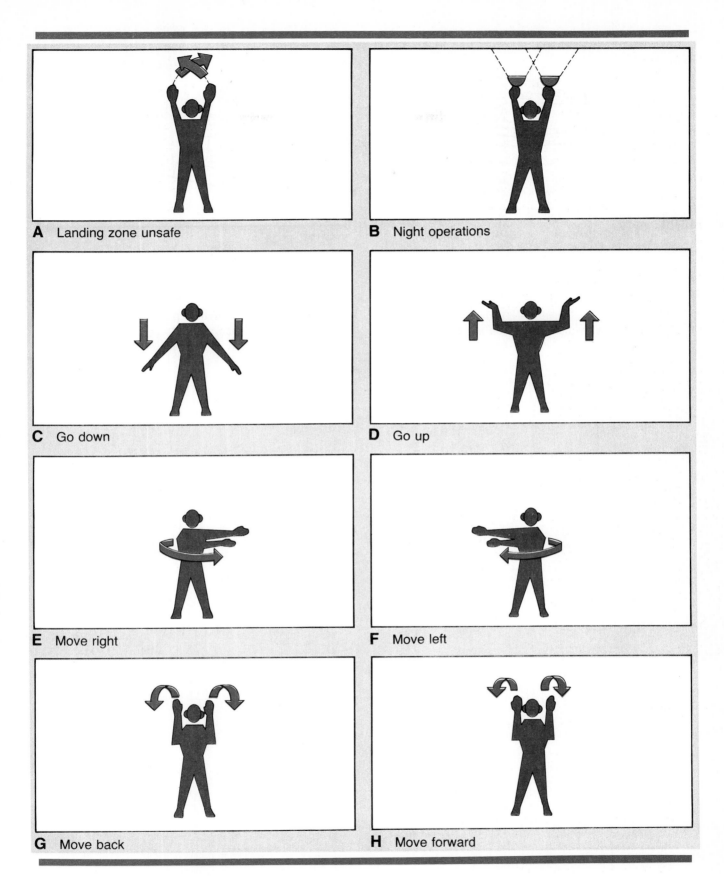

A Landing zone unsafe

B Night operations

C Go down

D Go up

E Move right

F Move left

G Move back

H Move forward

FIGURE 44-24

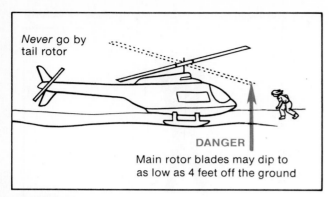

FIGURE 44-25

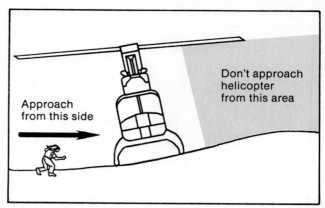

FIGURE 44-26

- No one should smoke within 50 feet of the aircraft.
- If the helicopter has to land on an incline, always approach from the downhill side, never from the uphill side (Figure 44-26).
- Never point spotlights up at a helicopter that is on its final approach at night.

chapter 45

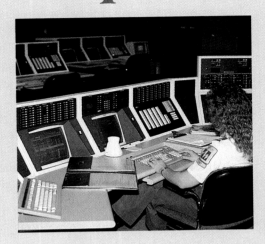

Communications, Records, and Reports

✱ OBJECTIVES

- List the skills of effective communication.
- Define the basic functions of communications in an EMS system.
- Discuss the components of an emergency medical communications system and list correct radio procedures.
- Discuss the functions of the emergency medical dispatcher.
- Demonstrate how to use radio communications equipment.
- Explain why efficient record keeping and reporting are essential.
- Demonstrate how to fill out the ambulance report properly.

It is recommended that EMTs wear protective gloves whenever there is a possibility of coming in contact with a patient's blood, body fluids, mucous membranes, traumatic wounds, or sores. See Chapter 31.

IMPORTANCE OF COMMUNICATIONS

Telephone and radio communications are what connect the components of an EMS system. Members of emergency health care teams function best when they can communicate effectively over long distances. It is vital that every EMT be able to use and understand the limitations of his EMS communications system. You must be able to understand and appreciate the role of the EMS dispatcher, conditions that you find at an emergency site, and the conditions and emergency care given to patients. You also must be able to report the status of your ambulance accurately. The *Standard Operating Procedure Manual,* developed by the Associated Public Safety Communication Officers (APSCO), has contributed much toward standardizing EMS communications.

Emergency care communication also includes talking with bystanders at the scene to gain information about the patient and the mechanism of injury. A valuable part of a patient assessment is asking the patient the right questions in a proper way, and listening carefully to the answers. A successful emergency care provider is able to communicate trust and confidence.

It is essential that you communicate effectively and properly with other members of the EMS system (fellow EMTs, dispatcher, first responders, ER staff). It is also important that you listen carefully to others so that you understand what they are saying. The successful EMT communicator is able to:

- Use common sense and good judgment in verbal and telemetry communication.
- Listen carefully.
- Follow instructions and protocols.
- Communicate so that he is completely understood.
- Be familiar with all the communication tools available, including radio and telephone, P.A. system, written reports, and ambulance lights and siren.

And do not forget that reading and writing reports are important, though less exciting, parts of being an EMT. Read reports and documents that pertain to you carefully. If you do not understand something, discuss it with someone who does. Write your reports in a clear, accurate format, using correct terminology.

BASIC FUNCTIONS OF EMERGENCY COMMUNICATIONS

Any communications system used by EMTs should coordinate the various agencies involved in emergency care and follow-up medical care. Seven basic functions are served by emergency communications:

- Detecting and reporting accident or sudden illness incidents.
- Assigning emergency personnel to respond to specific incidents.
- Maintaining contact between personnel, especially those in the ambulance and at the hospital.
- Alerting other emergency personnel if needed.
- Relaying information about the patient's condition and receiving suggestions on how to care for the patient at the scene.
- Determining the hospital to which a patient should be taken, and distributing the patients of a multiple-patient accident to various hospitals.
- Informing emergency room personnel about the kinds of patients being brought in and the kinds of injuries they should prepare for.

COMPONENTS OF AN EMERGENCY COMMUNICATIONS SYSTEM

While emergency prehospital care systems vary considerably, many of the systems serving moderate to large population densities employ the following radio communications components.

Base Station

The base station serves as a dispatch and coordination area and ideally is in contact with all other elements of the system. The base should be located in a suitable terrain, preferably a hill, and be in proximity to the hospital that serves as medical command center. Base stations generally use relatively higher power output (80 to 150 watts) and should be equipped with a suitable antenna within a short distance. The antenna plays a critical part in transmission and reception efficiency. Transmission power levels are limited by the FCC, and the minimum usable signal level for reception is limited by man-made noise. A good antenna system can compensate to some degree for these limitations.

Mobile Transmitter/Receivers

Mobile, vehicle-based transmitter/receivers come in a variety of power ranges, and the power output determines the distance over which the signal can be transmitted effectively. A transmitter in the seventy-five-watt range with V.H.F. will transmit for distances of ten to twelve miles over slightly hilly terrain to base. Transmission distances are greater over water or flat terrain and are reduced in mountainous areas or where there are many tall buildings. Mobile transmitters with higher outputs have proportionally greater transmission ranges.

Portable Transmitter/Receivers

Portable, hand-carried transmitter/receivers are useful when you must work at a distance from your vehicle but must stay in communication with the base or with one another. Such portable units may also be used by physician consultants when they are stationed at a hospital that has no radio. Portable units usually have power outputs up to five watts and thus have limited range, although the signal of a hand-held transmitter may be boosted by retransmission through a repeater.

Cellular Phones

Some EMS communications systems are turning to cellular phones. The concept is as follows: A particular geographical service area is divided into a network of slightly overlapping goegraphical cells that range from two to forty square miles in size. Telephone transmission cannot be received outside of the cell. Benefits of a cellular phone service include excellent sound quality, availability of channels, easy maintenance, and private communications. Disadvantages include the limitations of the cell, which can be overwhelmed during multiple casualty disasters. Cellular communication should not be considered the primary means of providing medical control.

□ PERMITTED AND RECOMMENDED COMMUNICATIONS

The Federal Communications Commission (FCC) has jurisdiction over all radio operations in the United States, including those used by EMT systems. In 1974, it created a block of ten UHF "MED" channels to be used for EMT services. The FCC licenses individual base station operations, assigns radio call signs, approves equipment for use, establishes limitations for transmitter power output, and monitors field operations.

Several services have reported serious communications difficulties with interruptions coming from licensed emergency and nonemergency uses. Electronic pagers both inside and outside of hospitals sometimes interrupt emergency radio communications. The ten MED channels are used with hospital administrative offices, medical schools, and national and state physician organizations.

Radio Codes

Some EMS systems use radio codes, either alone or in combination with English. Radio codes can shorten radio air time and provide clear and concise information. They can also allow transmission of information in a format not understood by the patient, family members,

or bystanders. There are, however, some disadvantages. First, the codes are useless unless everyone in the system understands them. Second, medical information is often too complex for codes. Third, several codes are infrequently used, so valuable time may be wasted looking up a code's meaning.

Some systems still use the **Ten-Code system.** Published by the Associated Public Safety Communications Officers (APCO), it is used primarily for dispatch, occasionally in EMS. Many EMS systems, however, have abandoned all codes in favor of standard English.

Times

Times (A.M. and P.M.) are not confused if military time is used. It is a very simple system and goes as follows:

- □ 1 AM–12 NOON = 0100–1200 hours
- □ 1 PM–MIDNIGHT = 1300–2400 hours

Examples of this time system are:

- 1427 hours is 2:27 P.M.
- 0030 hours is thirty minutes after midnight.

Radio Terms

Conversation can be shortened by use of one- or two-word phrases that are used universally. The following is a list of frequently used radio terms:

- □ Clear — end of transmission.
- □ Come in — requesting acknowledgment of transmission.
- □ ETA — estimated time of arrival.
- □ Go ahead — proceed with your message.
- □ Landline — refers to telephone communications.
- □ Over — end of message, awaiting base station reply.
- □ Repeat/say again — did not understand message.
- □ 10-4 — acknowledging that message is received and understood.
- □ Stand by — please wait.
- □ Spell out — asking sender to spell out phonetically words that are unclear.
- □ Break — afford a "pause" so that the hospital can respond or interrupt if needed.

□ RELAYING INFORMATION TO THE PHYSICIAN

Radio communications between EMTs in the field and their medical director should also be to the point and accurate. For this purpose, it is helpful to have a standard format for communicating patient information over the radio. This assures that the significant information is relayed in a consistent manner and that nothing is omitted. The format should include:

- Patient's age and sex.
- Patient's chief complaint.
- A brief, pertinent history of the present illness, including scene assessment and the mechanism of injury.
- State of consciousness.
- Vital signs.
- Pertinent physical findings.
- Emergency care given.
- Patient's response to the treatment or emergency care.
- Estimated time of arrival.

As you communicate with other medical personnel over the air waves, remember to:

- Speak calmly and slowly enough to be completely understood. Identify yourself.
- Use complete sentences and language that you know and understand, but be brief.
- Use correct terminology when it is appropriate. Speak as a professional; no joking, singing, profanity, etc.
- Do not use individual's names. Use unit, dispatch, and hospital identifications.
- Always monitor the channel before speaking so that you do not interfere with another unit's transmission.
- Speak distinctly but do not shout. Hold the microphone about two inches from your mouth.
- Always acknowledge a transmission promptly. If you cannot take a long incoming message, simply acknowledge the call with "Stand by."
- *Never* pretend to understand a communication if you do not. Ask for a repeat in other terms.
- Be certain of the message received; if you are unsure, ask for repetition of the message.
- Do not cut off the sender until you have received the complete message.
- Be brief and concise, and know what you are going to say beforehand.
- Do not try to transmit if other EMS personnel are using the channel or the dispatcher is sending to you.
- Sign off at the end of the transmission.

- Always check in and out of service with the dispatcher.

During a call, you must report verbally at these points:

1. To acknowledge the dispatch information.
2. To estimate your time of arrival at the scene while en route and to report any special road conditions, unusual delays, and so on.
3. To announce the unit's arrival on the scene and to request additional EMTs or public safety assistance, then help coordinate the reply.
4. To announce the unit's departure and the destination hospital, number of patients transported (if more than one), and estimated time of arrival at the hospital.
5. To announce your arrival at the hospital or another facility.
6. To announce that you are "clear" and available for another assignment.
7. To announce your arrival back at base.

☐ COMMUNICATIONS CONTROL CENTER

The communications control center (Figure 45-1) is at the heart of any EMS system. Sophistication can range from a simple radio base station run by one communications operator to a large staff of communication specialists involved with complex electronics systems and computers. The control center monitors and coordinates all other communication components, including base stations, mobile units, telephone sets, hand-held portables, and remote consoles.

FIGURE 45-1 An EMS communications control center.

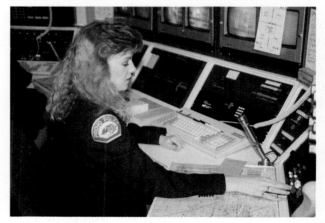

□ PATIENT ENTRY INTO THE EMS SYSTEM

The first important duty of an EMS communication system is to promote easy and quick patient access into the EMS system. The logical means of public access is the public telephone. EMS telephone numbers should be easy to remember and quick to dial. The 911 universal emergency telephone number, which gives access to public safety services including EMS, satisfies these criteria.

The most technologically advanced 911 system, available in all communities whose telephone companies have electronic switching equipment, is the Enhanced 911 System, or E911. Improved public use is provided by automatic number identification, automatic call location identification, and automatic ringback. This advanced system allows the dispatcher a digital display of the phone number being used by the caller and the address of that particular phone. So often, a caller hangs up prematurely. The E911 system can prevent disconnection of the call and automatically rings back the number.

Some communities still have seven-digit telephone numbers, or may use CBs, ham radios, highway call boxes, governmental, or mutual aid radio systems. Whatever system is used, become familiar with it. Be sure that calls are promptly received, properly screened, and acted upon efficiently by the EMS dispatcher.

□ DISPATCH

It is the job of the dispatcher to obtain as much information as possible about the emergency, to direct the appropriate vehicle to the scene, and to provide the caller with whatever advice may be needed to manage the situation until help arrives. The dispatcher also monitors and coordinates communications with the field.

The dispatcher is the first component of the EMS team. Dispatchers often handle fire and police traffic as well and may have little EMS training. Turnover among dispatchers is often high, which reduces long-term training and quality of dispatchers. Encourage your dispatcher to obtain EMT training and help him or her feel an important part of the EMS team.

Information Gathering

The method used to gather information is most often a series of short questions asked by the dispatcher. When the call for an ambulance is received, the caller may volunteer most of the information, and the dispatcher must record that information as rapidly as possible. If tape-recording equipment is available, record each call to serve as a back-up.

Information that should be obtained includes the following:

- The exact location of the patient, including the street name and number. Be sure to obtain the proper geographic designation (e.g., if the street is East Maple or West Maple) and the name of the community, since adjacent towns may have streets by the same name. If the call comes from a rural area, try to establish landmarks, such as the nearest crossroad or business establishment, a water tower, antenna, or any other readily identifiable landmark by which the rescue team can orient themselves. Obtain the address quickly, as the caller may hang up!

- Phone number and name of the caller, in case the caller needs to be contacted for more information (e.g., if the rescue team cannot find the address and needs better directions). It also helps to minimize nuisance calls, since false callers are generally reluctant to give their phone numbers. The telephone exchange may also help you to pinpoint the caller's location if he is unfamiliar with the region, as in the case of a traveller calling from the road.

- The caller's perception of the nature of the patient's problem.

- Specific information concerning the patient's condition. Is he or she conscious? Is he or she breathing? Is he or she bleeding badly? Is he or she in severe pain?

- If the emergency is a vehicular accident, additional information should be sought:

    — The kinds of vehicles involved (cars, trucks, motorcycles, buses). If trucks are involved, it is useful to know what they are carrying, since a truck carrying dynamite will require a different approach than one carrying bananas.

    — The number of persons involved and the extent of the injuries. Even if the caller can only guess, you will get some idea of the magnitude of the problem.

    — Known hazards, including traffic hazards, downed electrical wires, fire, submerged vehicles, and so forth. Information about hazards enables the dispatcher to contact other agencies that may have to be involved.

A special, pre-printed form can help the dispatcher obtain all the necessary information and will also provide a lasting record of the call.

Upon receiving the information, the dispatcher should ask the caller to wait on the line. The dispatcher then must determine, assuming that the call is a medical emergency within his or her service's jurisdiction, which crew(s) and vehicle(s) will be dispatched. This will be governed by the nature and location of the call as well as by the availability of various units at the time. The appropriate crew, which should be the closest unit, is then contacted. This will help obtain the important goal of a shortened response time.

Importance of Training for the Emergency Medical Dispatcher

Just as the control center is the cornerstone of the EMS communications system, the emergency medical dispatcher is the key to the functioning of the communications system.

The EMS program, Emergency Medical Services, has undergone a tremendous change from basic mortuary services two decades ago to highly trained and efficient EMTs and paramedics covering all aspects of basic to advanced life support. At the center of this well-trained specialization is the emergency dispatcher, deciding if a response is needed, who should respond, and how they should respond. Too many emergency dispatchers have little, if any, specialized training for interaction with the EMS team and are often the weakest link of the EMS chain.

The EMS-D program expands the training of the existing dispatcher protocols by teaching the dispatchers to correctly interrogate a caller, compute and carry out a response, and guide an untrained caller through the first few minutes after trauma or sudden illness occurs, and while the EMS team is traveling to the scene. The dispatcher has thirty-two dispatch medical protocol cards containing key questions that dictate prearrival instructions for the caller and then suggest an appropriate ambulance response mode (Figure 45-2). More specifically, the EMS-D system is a department-approved reference system used by a local dispatch agency to dispatch aid to medical emergencies which includes:

A. Systemized caller interrogation questions.

B. Systemized pre-arrival instructions (e.g., giving the caller step-by-step instructions for performing CPR).

C. "Protocols matching the dispatcher's evaluation of injury or illness severity with vehicle response mode and configuration."[1]

---

[1] Karen Uber, "Emergency Dispatch Training," *JEMS*, June 1986, p. 23.

The advantages of such a system are:

1. Consistency of dispatch. Every dispatcher handles every type of call in the same way.

2. Increased professionalism. Standard questions let dispatchers relax and concentrate on obtaining significant information, rather than trying to remember what to ask.

3. Increased quality of dispatch. Medically significant questions allow the dispatcher to gather pertinent information only. Responding units can be better prepared when they arrive at the scene.

4. Improved patient care. The dispatcher becomes the first professional on the scene but nothing is left to chance or individual memory.

5. Dispatcher stress reduction. Standard questions and prearrival instructions reduce anxiety.

6. Training is short and flexible.

7. Increased teamwork.

Strong medical control is built into the key questions, which emphasize the importance of obtaining symptoms rather than diagnosing, in addition to obtaining the patient's age, state of consciousness, and breathing status. The "Four Commandments" of medical dispatch (chief complaint, age, state of consciousness, and breathing) are reinforced as an absolute baseline of information obtained and relayed on every call. Priority dispatching can send out the type of unit needed, which is a system of tiered response. As a consequence, fewer unnecessary emergency responses (lights and sirens) are made, which in turn reduces the time spent on hazardous emergency responses, lessens stress to personnel, and cuts down on wear-and-tear of emergency vehicles and equipment.

This program allows trained dispatchers to operate from sound guidelines and protocols. It safely activates the caller, transforming him or her from a passing watcher to a type of first responder who, in those first minutes, can save lives.

☐ USING RADIO COMMUNICATIONS EQUIPMENT

Because radio communications equipment varies among manufacturers, the directions in this section are general, rather than specific. The directions must be supplemented with more specific instructions for the equipment in use.

CHEST PAIN

KEY QUESTIONS	PRE-ARRIVAL INSTRUCTIONS

KEY QUESTIONS

1. Breathing normally?
2. Turning blue?
3. Alert?
4. Location of pain?
5. Sharp or dull pain?
6. Cardiac history?
7. Fever or cough?

PRE-ARRIVAL INSTRUCTIONS

a. Lay victim down (semi-reclining).

b. Treat as specific symptoms indicate.

c. Stay on phone with potential rescuer. Consider beginning discussion of CPR.

List all current medications or place all medications in a paper bag for the paramedics. Write down name and phone # of doctor.

DISPATCH PRIORITIES

Determinant		Response

A. Chest pain **WITH** normal breathing (age < 35)

B. Chest pain **WITH** difficulty breathing (age < 35)

C. Chest pain (age ≥ 35) **OR** Not alert

D. Chest pain (age ≥ 35) **WITH** prior cardiac history **OR** turning blue

CHILDBIRTH SEQUENCE

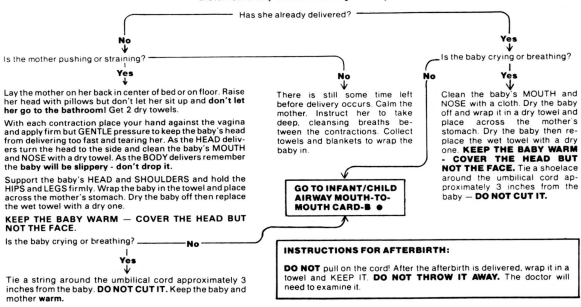

Help is on the way — you must be calm, OK?! Listen carefully and do **exactly** as I say.

Has she already delivered?

No → Is the mother pushing or straining? → **Yes**

Lay the mother on her back in center of bed or on floor. Raise her head with pillows but don't let her sit up and **don't let her go to the bathroom!** Get 2 dry towels.

With each contraction place your hand against the vagina and apply firm but GENTLE pressure to keep the baby's head from delivering too fast and tearing her. As the HEAD delivers turn the head to the side and clean the baby's MOUTH and NOSE with a dry towel. As the BODY delivers remember the **baby will be slippery - don't drop it.**

Support the baby's HEAD and SHOULDERS and hold the HIPS and LEGS firmly. Wrap the baby in the towel and place across the mother's stomach. Dry the baby off then replace the wet towel with a dry one.

KEEP THE BABY WARM — COVER THE HEAD BUT NOT THE FACE.

Is the baby crying or breathing? — **No** —

Yes

Tie a string around the umbilical cord approximately 3 inches from the baby. **DO NOT CUT IT.** Keep the baby and mother **warm.**

No

There is still some time left before delivery occurs. Calm the mother. Instruct her to take deep, cleansing breaths between the contractions. Collect towels and blankets to wrap the baby in.

GO TO INFANT/CHILD AIRWAY MOUTH-TO-MOUTH CARD-B ●

Yes → Is the baby crying or breathing? → **No** / **Yes**

Clean the baby's MOUTH and NOSE with a cloth. Dry the baby off and wrap it in a dry towel and place across the mother's stomach. Dry the baby then replace the wet towel with a dry one. **KEEP THE BABY WARM - COVER THE HEAD BUT NOT THE FACE.** Tie a shoelace around the umbilical cord approximately 3 inches from the baby — **DO NOT CUT IT.**

INSTRUCTIONS FOR AFTERBIRTH:

DO NOT pull on the cord! After the afterbirth is delivered, wrap it in a towel and KEEP IT. **DO NOT THROW IT AWAY.** The doctor will need to examine it.

H CHILDBIRTH SEQUENCE (Bottom Card)

Reprinted with permission of Medical Priority Consultants, Inc.

FIGURE 45-2 Dispatch medical control cards. (1) Chest Pain; (2) Childbirth

Mobile Transmitter/Receiver

To use a mobile transmitter/receiver:

1. Turn the unit on.
2. Adjust the squelch.
3. Listen before transmitting to be sure that airways are free of other communications.
4. Hold the microphone far enough from your mouth to avoid air noise made by exhaling.
5. Push the push-to-talk button, and pause before speaking. Talk across the mike, not into it.
6. When calling another unit, use its call letters first and yours second.
7. Follow these guidelines when using the radio:
   - Use an understandable rate of speed.
   - Articulate clearly.
   - Speak with good voice quality.
   - Avoid dialect or slang.
   - Do not show emotion.
   - Avoid vocalized pauses (such as "um," "uh," or "hmm").
   - Use proper English.
   - Avoid excessive transmission.
8. Use the call sign to let others know that the transmission has been completed.

Portable Transmitter/Receiver

Using a portable transmitter/receiver is similar to using a mobile transmitter/receiver. However, the antenna on the portable unit is not fixed in place and must be kept vertical while in use so that the signal can be transmitted property to the vehicle. From the vehicle, the signal can be transmitted to the base station.

Digital Encoder

To use a digital encoder:

1. Turn the unit on.
2. Adjust the squelch.
3. Listen before transmitting to be sure that the airways are free of other communication.
4. Select the address code to be dialed.
5. Dial the address code.
6. Hold the microphone far enough from your mouth to avoid air noise made by exhaling.
7. Push the push-to-talk button and pause before speaking.
8. Call the dialed unit.

9. Use the call sign to let others know that the transmission has been completed.

☐ RECORDS AND REPORTS

Efficient record keeping and reporting (both orally and in writing) are essential for continuity and quality of patient care. You must learn to observe and question carefully while caring for the patient so that proper information is gathered for medical, legal, administrative, community health, and evaluation purposes. A key point is that the emergency department staff often uses information from ambulance reports as a back-up in their emergency care decisions.

Information must be obtained and records maintained for the following reasons:

- To provide for continuity of patient care.
- To enable evaluation of quality of care.
- To provide data for analysis of illness and injury.
- To furnish legal evidence that will protect the EMT and answer civic questions.
- To provide administrative and billing records.

While these records are extremely important, they *never* take precedence over emergency care. Never stop rendering life-saving care to make reports.

In most states, it is common that ambulance services are required to produce:

- Personnel records, including training and assignments.
- Dispatch records — a written log of runs with specified data.
- Maintenance inspection records for all vehicles.
- Run reports with specified data elements.
- Incident reports of untoward situations or unusual circumstances.

EMTs in field functions may not be required to complete reports in all of these areas, but they should recognize the purpose of the documentation.

Written reports may include: patient assessment and care forms (also called field or street forms), special assessment forms (for example, neurologic), ambulance run reports, release forms when consent for treatment is not granted, and vehicle inspection forms. Customarily, two or more of these functions are combined with each other in the run sheet.

Run Sheet

One of the most critical reports is the run sheet or ambulance report. While the form differs with organizations, the following information is generally included:

- The date and time the ambulance run occurred.
- Whether the run was an emergency.
- The names of the EMTs who made the run.
- Time of departure from quarters, arrival time at the scene, and location of the scene.
- All critical information concerning evaluation of the accident scene, assessment of the patient or patients, all emergency care given, and any change in the patient's condition.
- Time of departure from the scene, destination, and time of arrival.
- Official transfer of patient to other EMS personnel (e.g., physician or nurse at hospital emergency room).
- Time back in quarters.

Although notes can be taken during the run, the report itself may be completed at the hospital so the emergency department can retain a copy. Do not procrastinate report writing, as you may forget or lose important information. The report should be written correctly with no spelling mistakes. It should be accurate and complete.

Follow these specific guidelines in completing the report:

- Use black ink. It makes the record possible to photocopy and is required if the chart is to be microfilmed.
- Print. It takes a little longer but it makes for a more legible record, particularly in carboned multiforms.
- Draw a line through blank spaces.
- If you fill in some information at a later time, note "late entry" with the date and time.
- If you make an error in charting, draw a line through it and initial the line. Note "incorrect entry."
- Anyone who performs procedures on the patient or writes on part of the record should also sign it — first name, middle initial, last name, and license/certification.

You should be as meticulous in documenting "routine" calls and patient refusals as serious medical emergencies. You may need to justify why you downgraded what the patient thought was an emergency or why the patient didn't require emergency treatment.

Litigation and the Run Sheet

A realistic concern for EMS personnel is litigation. The threat of litigation should not intimidate you, but rather motivate you to take every precautionary step possible. In a court of law, it is the written proof that is closely examined. A professional, organized, well-written document of a one- or two-year-old run may literally save you from devastating litigation.

A consistent form helps to capture details (see Figure 45-3 for a good example). One possibility is the SOAP method, which stands for:

S: Subjective — the patient's verbal history of the injury or illness.

O: Objective — physical findings of the examination.

A: Acute history — the facts relating to the injury or illness prior to the EMS team's arrival, including patient condition and level of consciousness.

P: Plan — treatment.

The history should include all pertinent information relating to events that occurred prior to the squad's arrival — past history, aggravation and alleviation of symptoms, and the patient's activity at the time of the incident. This should be written using as much of the patient's terminology as is practical (use quotation marks to distinguish the patient's terminology from that of the writer).

Subjective history is an in-depth, precise summary of what is bothering the patient when the squad arrives. Sometimes these facts overlap the acute history.

All of your findings are described in the objective category — pupils, lung sounds, swelling or discoloration at the fracture site. A head-to-toe survey can serve as a good outline for this category. Vital signs may be included here, as well as in the space provided on the run sheet, at the writer's discretion.

Finally, the plan should detail any emergency care given to the patient — oxygen, monitor, IV, or splinting, for instance. Also, any changes in patient condition should be noted.

The system used needs to accommodate reporting of the slightly injured patient (typical patient) and must address the critically injured patient who needs a cervical collar, rapid extrication, MAST in the ambulance, IVs started en route, and rapid transport. Common abbreviations can be used to conserve time and space. It is important to report on what was *not* done and why, as well as what *was* done. An important last statement is. "If it isn't recorded, it wasn't done!"

After you have completed your record, follow local protocol in turning it in. Records must be handled with care and stored appropriately. They are confidential documents of potential legal importance.

PROVO CITY FIRE DEPARTMENT EMS REPORT

Date _____

LOCATION	(Street)	(City)	INCIDENT #	DISPATCH CODE	EMS # 2505L	SECTION 1 2 3 4 5 6 7 8 9	Incident Time

Dispatched
Unit Enroute
Arrived Scene

PATIENT NAME (Last)	(First)	(MI)	Patient's Phone

Left Scene
Arrived Hospital

PATIENT ADDRESS	(Street)	(City/State)	(Zip)	Parent/Guardian/Kin

In Quarters

MAILING ADDRESS	(Street)	(City/State)	(Zip)	Date of Birth

Ending Miles
Begining Miles

AGE	SEX	OTHER INSURANCE	MEDICARE #	MEDICAID #

Miles Driven

PATIENT HISTORY OF PROBLEMS

1 ( ) Hypertension
2 ( ) Diabetes
3 ( ) Heart Disease
4 ( ) Convulsives Disorders
5 ( ) Allergies
6 ( ) Other Serious Illness
7 ( ) Unknown specify
( ) None
( ) _____

CHIEF COMPLAINT

History of Present Injury/Illness

MEDICATIONS USED BY PATIENT | **DOSE**

PULSE		BLOOD PRESSURE		RESPIRATION		SKIN CONDITIONS	NEUROLOGICAL		CRAMS	GLASCOW

Time | Rate | Sys / Dias | Rate

Cap Refill
( ) absent
( ) delayed
( ) normal

Motor Function
Right   Left
( ) moves arms ( )
( ) moves legs ( )

Pupils
Right   Left
( ) unreactive ( )
( ) reactive ( )

CIRCULATION
2 norm cap refill
1 delayed cap refill
0 no cap refill

OPEN EYES
1 none
2 to pain
3 to speech
4 spontaneously

Condition

Sensory present
distal to injury
( ) yes   ( ) no

( ) dilated ( )
( ) midrange ( )
( ) pinpoint ( )

RESPIRATION
2 normal
1 abnormal/labored
0 absent

VERBAL RESPONSE
1 none
2 incomprehensible
3 inappropiate
4 confused
5 oriented

Radial Pulse | Neck Veins | Respiratory Effort
( ) regular
( ) irregular
( ) weak
( ) absent
( ) distended
( ) flat
( ) normal
( ) absent
( ) shallow
( ) retractive
( ) air hunger
( ) normal

( ) moist ( ) pale
( ) dry ( ) cyan
( ) warm ( ) red
( ) cool ( ) normal

Pulse present
distal to injury
( ) yes   ( ) no

ABDOMEN/THORAX
2 abd/thor nontender
1 abd/thor tender
0 abd rigid, flail
impaled object

Physician		Time	EKG Rhythm	Code

MOTOR
2 norm on command
1 responds to pain
0 no response

MOTOR RESPONSE
1 flacid
2 extends to pain
3 flexes to pain
4 withdraws
5 localizes pain
6 obeys commands

Time	Repeat	Drug or Solution	Code	Dose	Route

SPEECH
2 norm oriented
1 confused
0 no sounds

SCORE ___ | SCORE ___

NARRATIVE:

FRONT   BACK

Patient Refusal of Care / Treatment

I authorize the release of medical information necessary to process the claim and request payment of MEDICARE benifits either to myself or to the party who accepts assignment below

SIGNATURE _____ DATE _____

TREATMENT CODES (Circle all that apply)

000	Assess and Release		
520	VS/Assessed Mon.	260	IV
020	Airway Inserted	280	MAST Inflated
040	Assisted Ventilation	300	MAST Not Inflated

01	Abdominal Pain/Prob.s	09	Cardiac/Resp. Arrest	18	Headache	25	Psych/Behavior Prob.s	060	Bleeding Controlled	320	NG Tube
02	Allergies/Hives/Med. Reactions/Stings	10	Chest Pain	19	Heart Problems	26	Specific Dx as Chief Comp.(sick pers.)	080	Blood Tubes Drawn	340	OB Care
		11	Choking	20	Heat/Cold Problems			100	Burn Care	360	Oxygen Mask
03	Animal Bites	12	Convulsions/Seizures	21	Hemorrhage	27	Stab/GSW	120	Cervical Immobilization	380	Oxygen Cannula
04	Assault/Rape	13	Diabetic Problems	22	Industrial/Mach. Accident	28	Stroke/CVA	140	CPR	400	Pneumo Tube
05	Back Pain	14	Drown (Near Drown/ Diving Accident)	23	Overdose/Poisoning Ingestion	29	Traffic Inj Accident	160	Defibrillation	420	Spinal Immobilization
06	Breathing Problems					30	Traumatic Inj Specific	180	Endotrachial Intub	440	Splinted
07	Burns	15	Electrocution			31	Unconcious/Fainting	200	Esophageal Obturator	460	Suctioned
08	Carbon Monoxide Poisoning/Inhalation	16	Eye Problems	24	Pregnancy/Childbirth/ Miscarriage	32	Unknown Problem	220	Extrication Equipment	480	Turned on Side
		17	Falls			99	Routine Transfer	240	Heimlich Maneuver	500	No Treatment Given

Medical Control Hospital	Medical Control Phys.	Medical Control Nurse	Advanced Unit	Basic Unit
Transport Unit	Transported ( ) yes ( ) no	Contacted Resource Hosp ( ) from scene	PM/EMT	PM/EMT
Hospital Delivered		Code	( ) in transit ( ) used standing orders	PM/EMT	PM/EMT

1 ( ) transport without paramedics
2 ( ) transport single paramedic aboard
3 ( ) transport double paramedics aboard
4 ( ) transport by helicopter
5 ( ) cancelled before arrival
6 ( ) cancelled after arrival
7 ( ) DOA at scene

12/88

FIGURE 45-3 The Ambulance Run Report. This report form documents patient identification and history, physical findings, the rescuer's diagnostic impressions, and the emergency care or treatment given.

appendix 1

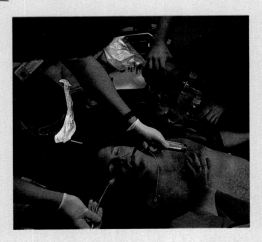

Advanced Airway Management

✳ OBJECTIVES

- Identify the importance of an open airway in the patient primary assessment.
- Describe proper information, equipment, and skills for advanced airway management using endotracheal intubation (ET).
- Describe proper information, equipment, and skills for advanced airway management using an esophageal obturator airway (EOA).
- Describe proper information, equipment, and skills for advanced airway management using the pharyngeo-tracheal-lumen airway (PTLA).

It is recommended that EMTs wear protective gloves whenever there is a possibility of coming in contact with a patient's blood, body fluids, mucous membranes, traumatic wounds, or sores. See Chapter 31.

Advanced airway control is used only for patients who cannot adequately ventilate and for whom the simple noninvasive airway management techniques found in Chapter 4 have been unsuccessful. These advanced airway techniques require excellent initial training, periodic refresher training, and consistent manikin practice. You also must be allowed to use these skills through your state medical protocols. You must also complete specific training and be certified to practice these skills. Check your local protocols on airway management!

□ PATIENT ASSESSMENT

Even though the more dramatic sight of blood and soft tissue injuries will naturally attract your attention, the primary assessment of an open and functioning airway, adequate breathing, and adequate circulation are of paramount importance. The first critical aspect of prehospital emergency care is an open airway.

If a conscious patient's airway is open, assess the breathing, provide any needed supplementary oxygen, and continue to monitor breathing. If the patient's airway is not open, it must be established and maintained. A semiconscious patient may need an oral or nasal airway and suctioning. Unconscious patients whose airways have not successfully been maintained by the noninvasive techniques may need the more advanced airway control that this section discusses.

Emergency advanced airway management maintains an open airway, allows more efficient oxygen administration, and frees you or your co-worker to attend to other aspects of prehospital care.

Advanced airway management is generally accomplished with either the **endotracheal tube** (ET), the **esophageal obturator airway** (EOA), or the **pharyngeo-tracheal-lumen airway** (PTLA).

□ ENDOTRACHEAL INTUBATION

Endotracheal intubation, performed either orally or nasally, is used for short-term and long-term airway control. It maintains an open airway and protects the patient from aspiration. The endotracheal tube (ET), open at both ends, is usually placed through the mouth (in prehospital emergency care) and directly through the larynx between the vocal cords into the trachea. The ET tube (Figure A1-1) comes in varying lengths and widths. It is a flexible tube that has an inflatable balloon cuff on the tracheal end to keep the tube in place. (Uncuffed tubes are used in infants and small children, however). There is a fifteen-millimeter adapter on the distal end for placement of a bag-valve device.

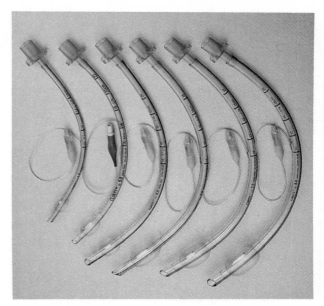

FIGURE A1-1 An assortment of different-sized endotracheal tubes.

Advantages of the ET-tube are the following:

- It offers complete airway control.
- It prevents aspiration.
- It allows for positive-pressure ventilation.
- Tracheal suctioning is possible.
- It prevents gastric distention.
- You may provide high-volume, high-concentration oxygen and ventilation.

Disadvantages of the ET-tube are the following:

- It often requires direct visualization of the vocal cords for proper placement.
- It may damage tissue.
- There is a possibility of esophageal or bronchial intubation.
- Laryngospasm (an involuntary constriction) may occur during an intubation attempt, causing the airway to close.
- It may delay oxygenation of the patient prior to a successful intubation, and may cause a reflex bradycardia.
- It may lose its effectiveness with cuff puncture.

The numbers, identifying sizes of endotracheal tubes, reflect the outside diameter of the tubes in millimeters. Children ten years and older may take tubes of sizes 5.0 and up, while the average adult can be fitted with a size 8.0 tube.

Method of Placement
for Oral Intubation

If other simpler methods to keep the unconscious patient's airway open have failed, and *you have the necessary training and equipment*, prepare to insert an ET tube. You will need a laryngoscope with either a curved or straight blade (the curved blade is recommended because it causes less trauma), a proper size tube, water-soluble lubricant, a 5- to 10-ml syringe for inflating the cuff (be sure that the cuff will inflate beforehand), and suction equipment. Proper preparation should allow you to intubate within fifteen to twenty seconds. Prepare the ET tube by checking the cuff, then leaving the syringe attached. Then follow these steps (Figures A1-2–A1-3):

1. Adequately ventilate the patient with manual ventilation (e.g., bag-valve-mask) and high oxygen concentration. (CPR should not be interrupted for more than fifteen seconds.)

2. In the *nontrauma* patient, position the head in the "sniff" position (head/neck slightly extended). In the *trauma* patient, have a partner maintain inline stabilization by holding the patient's head in a neutral position. Only the mandible and tongue should be moved during oral intubation. You may lie prone or straddle the patient's head, superiorly, during the intubation (Figure A1-4).

3. Remove the bag-valve-mask.

4. Insert the blade of the laryngoscope into the patient's mouth from the right, gradually sweeping the tongue to the left (Figure A1-5). Follow the natural contour of the mouth. Do *not* force the low lip or the blade against the teeth (you can break the teeth by using the blade as a lever).

5. Pass the *curved* blade through the mouth and pharynx until the blade tip slips into the vallecula, the small space just above the epiglottis at the base of the tongue. The *straight* blade is inserted in the same way, but the tip of the blade is advanced *over* the epiglottis and used to lift it. Now lift the tongue and mandible with the laryngoscope/blade (at a forty-five-degree angle), but be gentle with pressure. This should fully expose the glottis and the vocal cords.

6. Insert the endotracheal tube from the side with your right hand, down the right side of the oral cavity toward the vocal cords. Keep the cords visible throughout the tube insertion. Now insert the ET-tube between or through the vocal cords and into the trachea. Be sure that you see the tube slip through the cords. The cuff should rest just below the vocal cords (Figure A1-6).

7. Remove the laryngoscope/blade.

8. Check for air sounds in both lungs and the stomach.

9. Inflate the cuff to not greater than ten cc's, and place an oral airway into the patient's mouth to keep him or her from biting the tube. Then tape the ET-tube in place.

10. If you find that
    - the ET-tube is in the esophagus
    - no breath sounds are ausculated during ventilations
    - air is ausculated in the stomach during ventilation
    - you are unable to properly place the ET-tube

    you should return to bag-valve-mask ventilation. After the patient is well-ventilated, make a second attempt to intubate. A wire stylet may be helpful here.

11. Connect a bag-valve device or a demand valve to the ET-tube adapter and ventilate the lungs. Assure adequate ventilations by watching for both sides of the chest to rise evenly, and auscultate for breath sounds.

12. If you hear breath sounds on the right side only, listen to the left chest and withdraw the tube slowly until you can hear breath sounds in the left lung field. *Note:* Cuffed tubes generally require 5 to 10 ml of air in adults and 3 to 5 ml of air in children over eight. Do not overinflate, and use only uncuffed tubes in infants and small children.

If the patient has a short neck, it is very difficult to position the ET-tube. One practitioner suggests straightening the tube when you lubricate it, then putting a three-inch kink, like a bird's foot, in the end before insertion.[1]

Transillumination (Lighted Stylet) Intubation

This alternative method of ET intubation is based on the assumption that a bright light, introduced into the larynx or trachea, can be seen shining through the soft tissues of a patient's neck. This allows the EMT to pass an endotracheal tube through the glottic opening without having to directly visualize the structures. Endotracheal intubation can be performed in this way without manipulating the head and neck. The transillumination technique calls for a special device, known as a lighted stylet. This stylet is a malleable, plastic-coated wire that features a small, high-intensity bulb at its distal end. Power for the device is supplied by a small battery housed at the proximal end, and is controlled by an on-off switch. This method works best in a darkened room or, if in sunlight, shield the neck.

---

[1] Thom Dick, "Tubular Tricks: Fool-Proofing Your Field Intubations," *JEMS*, May 1990, p. 26.)

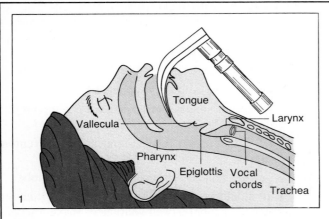

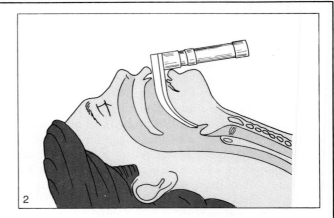

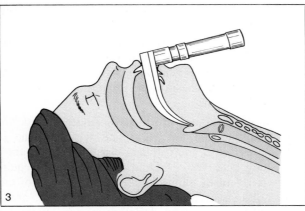

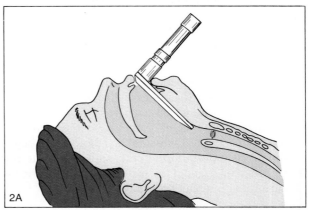

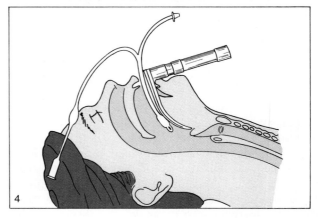

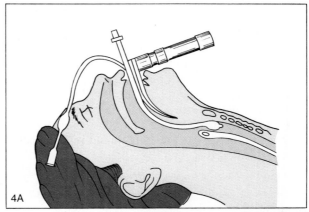

1. **Insert the blade** of the laryngoscope into the patient's mouth from the right, gradually pushing the tongue to the left. Follow the natural contour of the mouth, as indicated by the arrow, making sure not to force the lower lip against the teeth, or the blade against the teeth.

2. **If using a curved blade**, pass it through the mouth and pharynx until the tip of the blade slips into the vallecula, the small space just above the epiglottis at the base of the tongue. Be careful to avoid pressure damage or the blade against the teeth. If using a straight blade, insert it in the same way, but advance the tip of the blade over the epiglottis, as shown in 2A.

3. **The curved blade** is designed to fit into the vallecula. When the handle is lifted anteriorly, it elevates the tongue and indirectly elevates the epiglottis, allowing the medic to see the glottic opening. Because the curved blade does not touch the larynx itself, it should not traumatize or accidentally stimulate the very sensitive gag receptors located on the posterior surface of the epiglottis. The curved blade also permits more room for viewing and tube insertion. The straight blade, on the other hand, is designed to fit under the epiglottis. When its handle is lifted anteriorly, it directly lifts the epiglottis up and out of the way. A straight blade is preferred in treating infants, since it provides greater displacement of the tongue and better visualization of the glottis.

4. **Insert the endotracheal tube** from the side, with your right hand (keeping the blade positioned as in step 3), down the right side of the oral cavity toward the vocal cords. Make sure you see the cords throughout insertion; they should be visible from about eight inches away from the patient's face. Pass the tube through the vocal cords and into the trachea, so that the cuff rests just below the vocal cords (see 4A). Remove the laryngoscope, to avoid passing the tube into the right mainstem bronchus.

FIGURE A1-2

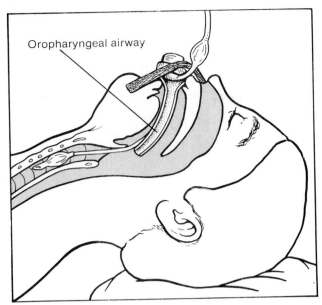

FIGURE A1-3 After you have assured the proper positioning of the ET, tape it in place. Insert an oropharyngeal airway to prevent the patient from biting the ET.

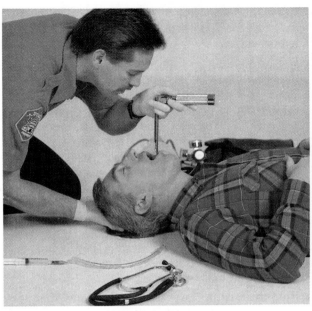

FIGURE A1-5 Insert the blade of the laryngoscope into the patients' mouth from the right, sweeping the tongue to the left.

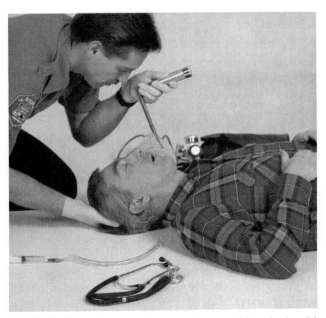
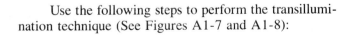

FIGURE A1-4 In a nontrauma patient, position the head in a "sniff" position.

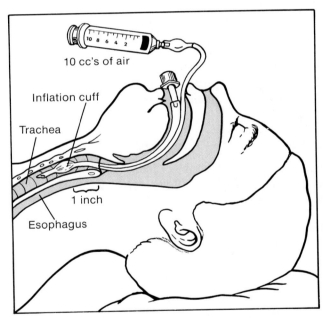

FIGURE A1-6 The upper edge of the balloon should lie approximately one inch below the level of the vocal cords.

Use the following steps to perform the transillumination technique (See Figures A1-7 and A1-8):

1. While maintaining ventilatory support, hyperventilate the patient with 100 percent oxygen.
2. Assemble and check your equipment. The endotracheal tube should be 7.5 to 8.5 i.d., and will need to be cut to 25–27 cm in order to accommodate the stylet. Place the stylet into the tube and bend it just proximal to the cuff.
3. Kneel on either side of the patient, facing his or her head.
4. Turn on the stylet light.
5. With your index and middle fingers inserted deeply into the patient's mouth and your thumb on the chin, lift the patient's tongue and jaw forward.

6. Insert the tube/stylet combination into the mouth and advance it through the oropharynx into the hypopharynx.

7. Use a "hocking" action with the tube/stylet to lift the epiglottis out of the way.

8. When you see a circle of light at the level of the patient's Adam's apple, hold the stylet stationary. Advance the tube off the stylet into the larynx approximately one-half to one full inch. A diffuse, dim, or hard-to-see light indicates that the tube/stylet combination is in the esophagus. (See Figure 11-49.) A bright light that appears laterally to the upper aspect of the laryngeal prominence indicates that it has moved into the right or left pyriform fossa. Both of these situations can be corrected by withdrawing the tube and reattempting intubation after the patient has been ventilated with 100 percent oxygen for several minutes.

9. Hold the tube in place with one hand and then remove the stylet. Attach a bag-valve device to the 15/22 mm adapter of the endotracheal tube and deliver several breaths.

10. Check for proper tube placement by observing breath sounds, chest rise, and the absence of sounds in the epigastrium when ventilations are delivered.

11. Inflate the distal cuff with 5 to 10 mL of air.

12. Recheck for proper tube placement and continue delivering ventilations while securing the tube in place.

Removal of the ET-tube

Removal of the ET-tube is not indicated in the field unless the patient develops intolerance to the tube and/or has a gag reflex, even while unconscious.

FIGURE A1-7 Lighted stylet/endotracheal tube in position.

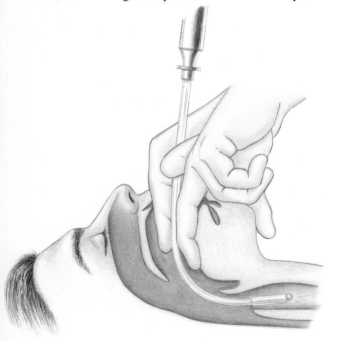

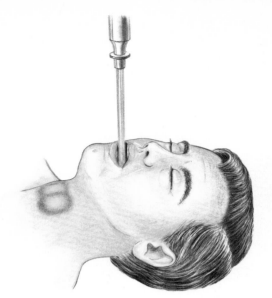

FIGURE A1-8 The properly positioned stylet should be visible on the front of the patient's neck.

To remove the ET-tube:

1. Have suction available.
2. Deflate the cuff completely.
3. Withdraw on inspiration.
4. Assess respiratory status.
5. Oxygenate.

□ THE ESOPHAGEAL OBTURATOR AIRWAY

The esophageal obturator airway (EOA) is also used for advanced airway management, especially with CPR. Its effectiveness does remain controversial. While the properly placed endotracheal tube is the most efficient airway for oxygen administration, the EOA takes less practice and skill to use effectively. It was devised to help eliminate gastric distention.

The esophageal obturator airway (Figure A1-9) is 34-cm (15-inch), flexible plastic tube with a face and nose mask adapter at the proximal end; it is closed at the distal end. The top third of the tube has sixteen perforations to allow the flow of oxygen in the airway. When the EOA is properly placed, these perforations are positioned at the pharynx level where oxygen-enriched air can flow to the lungs. The other two-thirds of the tube lie in the esophagus. A balloon situated at the end of the tube is inflated to block the esophagus and prevent potential vomitus from coming up into the airway.

Certain EOAs are modified to include a gastric decompression tube, which is referred to as an esophageal gastric tube airway. This tube vents stomach gas to the outside, thereby decreasing gastric distention, a potential problem during mouth-to-mouth resuscitation and CPR.

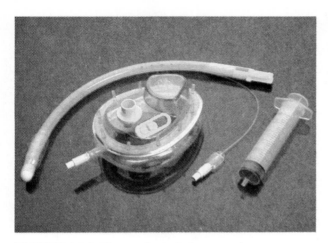

FIGURE A1-9 The esophageal obturator airway.

To use an EOA properly, the following equipment is necessary:

- A 35-cc syringe.
- Lubricant.
- Bag-valve or demand valve mask.
- Oxygen with connecting tube.
- Suction equipment.
- Stethoscope.
- Oral airway.

Advantages of the EOA are the following:

- It affords rapid insertion.
- It prevents regurgitation and aspiration.
- It provides for delivery of high concentrations of oxygen.
- Blind insertion is possible.
- It allows for ET-tube placement.
- It requires less training than ET-tube intubation.
- It inserts without neck flexion or hyperextension.

Disadvantages of the EOA are the following:

- It requires the patient to be unresponsive without a gag reflex.
- It must be removed when the patient becomes responsive or agitated.
- It can possibly lacerate the esophagus.
- You may intubate the trachea, which would prevent oxygenation to the patient.
- It may be used for short periods of time only.
- It requires a tight seal of the mask to adequately oxygenate the patient.

- It does not prevent blood and secretions from the face/head from entering the lungs.

The EOA should *not* be attempted under the following conditions:

- Known or suspected esophageal disease of the patient.
- Caustic poisoning ingestion.
- Gag reflex present.
- The patient is under five feet tall or over seven feet tall.
- The patient is younger than sixteen.

Inserting an Esophageal Obturator Airway

If you have the proper skills and equipment and decide that your patient will benefit from the use of an EOA, proceed in the following manner (Figure A1-10).

1. Prepare suction equipment, then test the balloon cuff by attaching a 35-cc syringe of air to the proper valve; inflate the balloon with 20 cc of air, and check for leaks. Leave the syringe attached, but deflate the balloon. Also, check the inlet port integrity.
2. Assemble the mask and tube by attaching the mask to the tube and locking the mask in place with a snap.
3. Lubricate the lower two-thirds of the tube with a water-soluble gel.
4. Place the patient's head in a neutral position and oxygenate him or her with a bag-valve-mask device or mouth-to-mouth resuscitation if necessary.
5. Keep your patient's head in a neutral or flexed position (flexed only if the patient is not suspected of having a neck injury). Grasp the patient's chin and lower jaw with your index and middle fingers while using your thumb to depress the base of his or her tongue. Pull the tongue and lower jaw upward and forward. Avoid hyperextension of the neck, which can easily lead to accidental tracheal intubation.
6. Grasp the EOA with the attached mask in your right hand and, following the curve of the airway, pass the tube through the mouth and into the esophagus. Use light to moderate pressure, and insert the tube until the mask makes good contact with the face. The bite block should lie at the level of the incisor teeth. If the tube does not slip into place easily, it may inadvertently have gone into the trachea. Withdraw the tube slightly, then readvance it.

Advanced Airway Management **713**

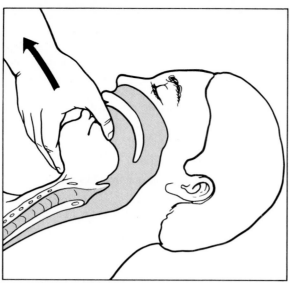

1. Grasp the patient's chin and lower jaw with your index and middle fingers while depressing the base of his tongue with your thumb. Pull the tongue and lower jaw upward and forward, being careful to avoid hyperextension of the neck (which can easily lead to inadvertent intubation of the trachea).

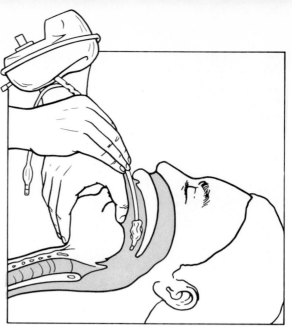

2. Pass the EOA, with mask attached, through the mouth and into the esophagus, following the curve of the natural airway. If the tube does not readily slip into place, withdraw it slightly and then readvance it. *Make sure that the tube does not accidentally enter the trachea.*

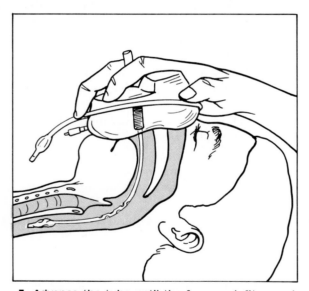

3. Advance the tube until the face mask fits snugly over the patient's nose and mouth. If the mask does not fit well, check to be sure that it is properly positioned. As when using a bag-valve-mask device, a good seal and hyperextension of the neck are essential for ventilation to be accomplished.

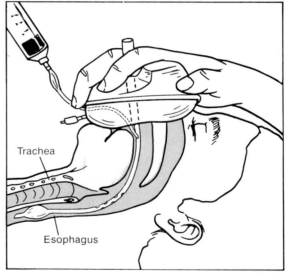

Trachea

Esophagus

4. Check the positioning of the EOA by hooking an oxygen line to it or blowing air into it, watching for bilateral expansion of the chest and auscultating for bilateral breath sounds. If the chest does not rise on both sides and breath sounds are not heard, withdraw the tube and reinsert it. When the tube is correctly positioned, the cuff will lie below the carina of the trachea. To avert possible esophageal rupture, inflate the cuff. Use no more than 35 ml air.

The EOA will now allow oxygen-enriched air to pass from the side holes into the trachea.

FIGURE A1-10 The EOA will now allow oxygen–enriched air to pass from the side holes into the trachea.

7. Hold the mask in place with both hands to create a tight seal, then test the airway by using a bag mask or a demand valve. Watch for the patient's chest to rise. If it does not, remove and reinsert the tube. Then retest the EOA. Your partner can listen for breath sounds over both lung fields with a stethoscope. If the EOA is properly placed in the esophagus, breath sounds should be heard over both lung fields. If no breath sounds are heard, the EOA is most likely in the trachea. If the EOA is in the right mainstream bronchus, breath sounds will only be heard on the left side. In either case, remove the EOA, ventilate the patient, and properly place the EOA.

8. When your partner can hear good breath sounds over both lung fields, inflate the esophageal balloon with 20–35 cc of air, then remove the syringe to keep the balloon inflated.

9. As you continue to kneel at the patient's head, establish a good mask-face seal by using your index finger and thumb to hold the mask to the face and the other three fingers to hold the mandible against the mask. Attach a thumb-triggered, oxygen-powered, positive-pressure device to the opening in the face mask for ventilation.

Method of Removal

Remove the EOA only if the patient is intubated, regains consciousness, or has a gag reflex. Be alert for vomiting. Do not deflate the cuff or remove the EOA until an endotracheal tube has been inserted with its cuff inflated in the trachea, or the patient has resumed breathing. The procedure is as follows:

1. Have suction available.
2. Turn the patient on his side if not intubated.
3. Detach the mask from the tube.
4. Deflate the cuff.
5. Gently and quickly remove the tube.
6. Be prepared for vomiting.
7. Assess the respiratory status.
8. Oxygenate.

□ ESOPHAGEAL GASTRIC TUBE AIRWAY (EGTA)

Essentially, the esophageal gastric tube airway (Figure A1-11) is the same as, and an alternative to, the

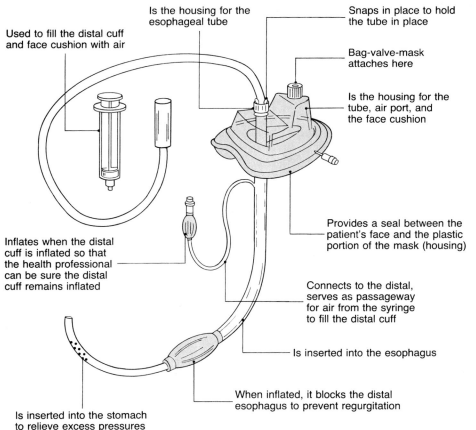

Used to fill the distal cuff and face cushion with air

Is the housing for the esophageal tube

Snaps in place to hold the tube in place

Bag-valve-mask attaches here

Is the housing for the tube, air port, and the face cushion

FIGURE A1-11 The esophogeal/gastric tube airway (EGTA).

Inflates when the distal cuff is inflated so that the health professional can be sure the distal cuff remains inflated

Provides a seal between the patient's face and the plastic portion of the mask (housing)

Connects to the distal, serves as passageway for air from the syringe to fill the distal cuff

Is inserted into the esophagus

When inflated, it blocks the distal esophagus to prevent regurgitation

Is inserted into the stomach to relieve excess pressures and unwanted substances

E.O.A. The esophageal gastric tube allows for the passage of a nasogastric (NG) tube for the decompression of the stomach, which reduces the chance of regurgitation and allows for suctioning of the patient's stomach contents.

The EGTA consists of an inflatable face mask and a tube, which is open throughout its length to permit passage of a gastric (Levine) tube necessary for decompression of the stomach. The transparent face mask has two ports: one for attachment of the esophageal tube, and the other—a standard 15 mm connector—which serves as the ventilation port. During ventilation, air is blown into the upper port of the mask. With the esophagus blocked, air has nowhere to go but into the trachea and lungs. Insertion is the same as with the EOA except for the measurement and placement of the NG-tube. To measure the NG-tube, extend the tubing from the tip of the nose, then to the earlobe, and then to the xiphoid process.

□ THE PHARYNGEO-TRACHEAL-LUMEN AIRWAY

The pharyngeo-tracheal-lumen airway (PTL) (Figure A1-12) is a dual-lumen airway adjunct, designed to be inserted into the patient's airway only *once*. Actually, the PTL airway is a tube within a tube. A long, endotracheal-type tube is located within a short tube with a larger diameter. The distal end of the long tube opens into either the trachea or esophagus, while the short tube opens just above the level of the glottis. Both tubes have low-pressure balloons at their distal ends. On the long tube, the balloon provides a seal for either the trachea or esophagus, depending on placement. On the short tube, the larger-volume balloon seals off the oropharynx when the balloon is fully inflated.

When the PTL airway is placed in the esophageal position, the large cuff diverts air delivered through the short tube into the trachea. Both tubes are fitted with 15-mm adapters to allow universal connection to ventilatory devices. Inflation lines are provided in order that each cuff may be inflated simultaneously or separately. A stylet facilitates insertion, and a plastic bite block prevents the teeth from occluding the airway. The following equipment is necessary for insertion:

- A water-soluble lubricant.
- Bag-valve-mask or demand valve mask.
- Oxygen and connecting tube.
- Suction equipment.
- Stethoscope.

Advantages of the PTL are the following:

- The PTL airway cannot be improperly placed.
- No reliance on a mask seal is required.
- It requires little skill training or skill maintenance.
- It requires minimal C-spine movement for insertion.
- Patients with short necks make endotracheal tube

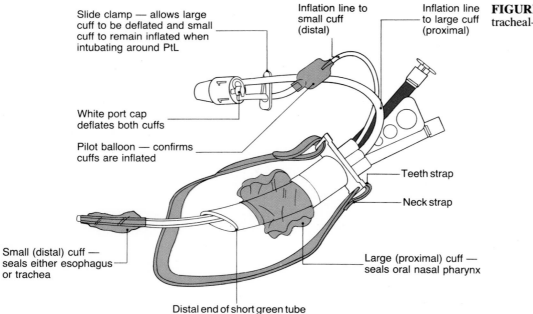

Slide clamp — allows large cuff to be deflated and small cuff to remain inflated when intubating around PtL

Inflation line to small cuff (distal)

Inflation line to large cuff (proximal)

FIGURE A1-12 The pharyngeo-tracheal–lumen airway (PTL).

White port cap deflates both cuffs

Pilot balloon — confirms cuffs are inflated

Teeth strap

Neck strap

Small (distal) cuff — seals either esophagus or trachea

Large (proximal) cuff — seals oral nasal pharynx

Distal end of short green tube

placement impossible. The PTL airway can be inserted in such cases.

- Protects the airway from secretions from the head/neck.

Disadvantages of the PTL are the following:

- It requires the patient to be unresponsive without a gag reflex.
- It must be removed when the patient becomes responsive or agitated.
- It should be replaced with an endotracheal tube as soon as possible in cases of facial burns, inhalation of heat, and airway or facial trauma with the possibility of the development of upper airway edema.
- The PTL may lose its effectiveness with cuff malfunction.

The PTL should *not* be used if:

- A patient is under five feet or over seven feet tall or younger than fourteen–sixteen years of age, depending on size.
- Caustic ingestion has occurred.
- Esophageal disease is present.
- The patient has a gag reflex.

Inserting a PTL Airway

The major steps in inserting a PTL are to lubricate the tube, insert it, then pressurize the two cuffs and ventilate. Follow these steps:

1. Hyperextend the patient's head unless you suspect a C-spine injury (in this case, your partner would stabilize the head and neck in a neutral position while you perform the jaw thrust).

2. Insert your thumb deep into the supine patient's mouth, grasping the tongue and lower jaw between the thumb and index finger, and pull the jaw forward.

3. While holding the jaw in one hand, take the PTL airway so that it curves in the same direction as the natural curvature of the oral pharynx.

4. Insert the tip into the patient's mouth and advance it carefully behind the tongue until the teeth strap touches the patient's teeth. There will be modest resistance in passing the tube when making the right-angle bend at the oral pharynx. *Do not use force.* If the tube does not advance, either redirect it or withdraw it and start over.

5. When the flange meets the teeth, the tube is in proper position.

6. Flip the neck strap over the patient's head and tighten it with the hook tape closures on both sides.

7. Inflate both cuffs simultaneously by blowing into the main inflation valve with a sustained breath. By using pressure against the patient's cheek's, the seal may be improved.

8. Ventilate the lungs by first blowing forcefully into the number 2 short green tube. If the chest rises, the long, clear tube number 3 is in the esophagus (Figure A1-13) and you may continue to ventilate

FIGURE A1-13 The PTL airway in place.

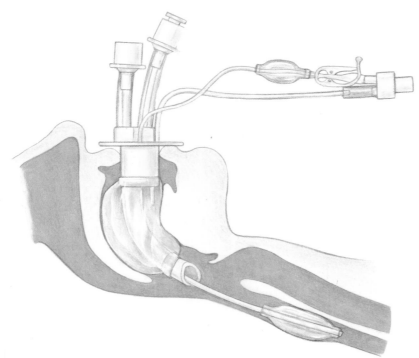

through the number 2 tube (use a bag-valve with a reservoir to achieve approximately 100 percent concentration of oxygen).

9. If the chest does not rise, the number 3 tube may be in the trachea. In this case, remove the stylet from tube number 3 and ventilate through it. During lung inflation, listen for breath sounds bilaterally and over the stomach with a stethoscope.

Method of Removal

Remove if the patient regains consciousness, if the protective airway reflexes return, or if endotracheal intubation is to be attempted. In some cases, you may be able to intubate while the PTL airway is in place.

1. If there is no spinal injury, turn the patient on his or her side.

2. Evaluate for stomach decompression to reduce the possibility of emesis.

3. Open the white port on the number 1 inflation valve to deflate both cuffs and remove.

appendix 2

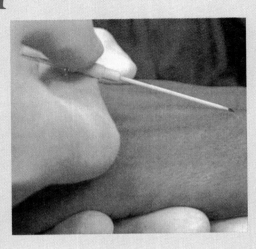

Intravenous Fluid Therapy

✱ OBJECTIVES

- Explain what IV therapy is and why it is used in prehospital medicine.
- Describe the equipment and supplies needed to provide IV therapy.
- Learn the steps of and demonstrate proficiency in starting an IV infusion.
- Discuss the importance of proper maintenance and monitoring of the IV patient.
- Demonstrate how to transport the IV patient properly.
- Describe the possible complications of IV therapy.

It is recommended that EMTs wear protective gloves whenever there is a possibility of coming in contact with a patient's blood, body fluids, mucous membranes, traumatic wounds, or sores. See Chapter 31.

In many states, EMTs are being taught the basics of **venipuncture** and **intravenous (IV) therapy** for use in the field to expand the level of life support care given. IV therapy should only be administered by IV-certified EMTs; follow local protocol.

□ WHAT IS INTRAVENOUS INFUSION?

Intravenous therapy, commonly called IV, refers to the administration of fluids, drugs, or blood directly into the circulatory system by way of a vein. When blood is administered, the technique is called **transfusion.** When sterile fluids other than blood or blood products are administered through a line injected into the venous system, the technique is called **infusion.**

An IV is a lifeline through which fluids and medications are administered to a patient. The fluid container can empty its reserve in minutes. A dropcock, or drip chamber, placed below the container, regulates the flow of the fluid.

□ BODY FLUID COMPOSITION

Body fluids bathe each cell and are involved in all bodily chemical reactions. Without the proper amounts of body fluids, cells dehydrate and die. Body fluid consists of water (60 percent of the volume of adult bodies and 75 percent of infant bodies) and electrolytes (sodium and potassium). These fluids are found both inside and outside the cell. Extracellular fluid includes the interstitial fluid between the cells and the capillary walls, and blood plasma within the vascular system.

□ WHY INFUSION?

IVs are started in the field for four major reasons:

- To add fluid volume to the circulatory system when there is an imbalance or depletion of normal body fluids, as in hemorrhage, burns, and dehydration.
- To establish and maintain a life support or access line for fluid or medication in a patient whose condition is questionable. It is difficult to get into a vein and start an IV after hypovolemia or circulatory collapse.
- To provide access for the administration of medications in a myocardial infarction or cardiac arrest, diabetic emergencies, drug overdose, etc.

- To maintain electrolyte, fluid, and nutrient balances for those unable to eat or with problems of severe nausea, vomiting, and/or diarrhea.

Be sure to get specific instructions from the physician and document the orders.

□ ADDING FLUID VOLUME

A significant decrease in fluid volume must be countered rapidly, or shock may result. The body may also go into chemical imbalance and negatively affect the functioning of vital organs. The types of solutions used for field IVs include **crystalloids** and **colloids.**

Colloids and crystalloids are volume expanders given to patients whose condition results in compromised circulation of blood to body tissues. They do not carry oxygen or replace blood but can provide electrolytes, protein, and volume expansion to help maintain blood pressure.

Crystalloid solutions quickly expand plasma, are rich in electrolytes, and take effect more quickly than colloids. However, they last only a short time. Colloids take effect more slowly than crystalloids but last longer in the plasma. They are particularly helpful for patients with hypovolemic or cardiogenic shock. Examples of colloids are **dextran** and **hetastarch (serum albumin** is a natural colloid). Examples of crystalloids are: (Table A2-1)

- **N.S.,** or **normal saline,** which is 0.9 percent sodium chloride in sterile water.
- **Lactated Ringer's,** an isotonic, buffered solution of electrolytes (sodium, chloride, potassium, calcium, and lactate) that closely approximates normal blood electrolyte contents (Figure A2-1).
- **D_5W,** which is 5 percent dextrose and sterile water. It is used in cases where an IV is established as a lifeline or a medication route.

□ SETTING UP AN IV

The equipment used by EMTs is usually disposable. Some medical facilities provide reusable, sterile infusion sets. In any case, the equipment will basically be the same, consisting of:

- The fluid to be infused.
- The IV set (Figure A2-2 shows micro drip and macro drip sets), consisting of the connector (to the fluid bottle or bag), drip chamber, screw clamp or flow adjustment valve, Y injection site (for medications), needle adapter, and needle and catheter.

TABLE A2-1
Common Intravenous Fluids

SOLUTION	ABBREVIATION	COMPONENT ELECTROLYTES
Lactated Ringer's	LR	NaCl, potassium chloride (KCL), calcium chloride (CaCl), sodium lactate
Quarter-normal saline	1/4 NS	0.2 NaCl
Half-normal saline	1/2 NS	0.45% NaCl
Normal saline	NS	0.9% sodium chloride (NaCl)
5% dextrose	D5W	5% dextrose
10% dextrose	D10W	10% dextrose

Note: D5 or D10 as a prefix indicates the solution is made containing dextrose. For example, Lactated Ringer's in 5% dextrose would be abbreviated D5LR.

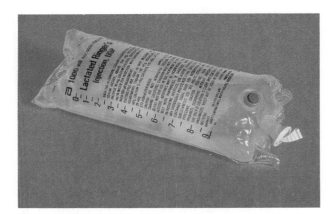

FIGURE A2-1 Lactated Ringer's, a solution commonly used in IV administration.

- Auxiliary equipment (Figure A2-3), such as an arm board, antiseptic solution, tape to secure the IV tubing to the patient's arm and the arm to the board, a tourniquet to aid in selection of the insertion site, gauze pads or a sterile dressing such as Opsite to cover the insertion site, materials to log or write down any necessary records concerning the procedure, and IV extension tubing to give added length to the IV while transporting.
- Several gloves and possibly a face mask and eye protector to be worn by the EMT.

It is important that all equipment be sterile. If the equipment is contaminated, germs may be introduced into the body and cause infection. If you do not *know* that the equipment is sterile, consider it *contaminated*. A sterile object remains sterile only if touched by another sterile object. It is very important that you be honest and make it known if a piece of equipment becomes contaminated — it needs to be replaced.

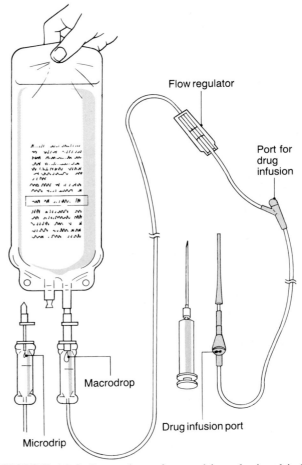

FIGURE A2-2 Comparison of macrodrip and microdrip IV administration sets.

Choosing the IV Set, Needles, and Catheters

Two types of IV sets are commonly used — **macro drip** and **micro drip.** The macro drip sets are used for rapid fluid replacement by large drops of fluid through a large-bore tube. This macro drip, or standard, infusion set is typically used for adults to give large amounts of

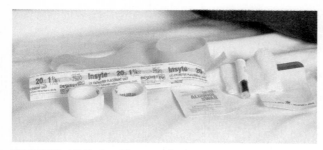

FIGURE A2-3 Auxiliary equipment.

fluid. The micro drip set has a small-bore tube, allowing a smaller drop, and is used for children, for maintaining a lifeline, or for other situations where control of the IV rate is critical.

The primary type of needle used to enter the vein in the field is an over-the-needle catheter (a plastic catheter inserted over a hollow needle). Other types of needles are a butterfly or winged hollow needle, or a plastic catheter inserted through a hollow needle. (Figure A2-4). In general, a short, large-bore needle is best for IV therapy. One- or-two-inch-length catheters are the most commonly used in the field, with needle sizes of 14, 16, and 18 gauge (the lower the gauge, the larger the bore of the needle) for fluid replacement. An 18 gauge is generally the smallest used in any adult and most children, but a 20 gauge may be used for small children or older adults with fragile veins that will not accommodate a lot of fluid.

The other variable that should be considered when selecting an intravenous cannula is its length. The longer the cannula, the less the flow rate will be. The flow rate through a 14 gauge, 5 cm catheter (approximately 125 mL/minute), is twice the flow rate through a longer, 16 gauge, 20 cm catheter. For cannulation of a peripheral vein, a needle and catheter length of 5 cm is adequate while the cannulation of a central line requires a needle length of 6–7 cm and catheter length of at least 15–20 cm.

Other needed equipment includes alcohol swabs, povidone-iodine solution, tape, and sterile dressings.

FIGURE A2-4 The IV needles most commonly used to administer IV fluids in the prehospital setting.

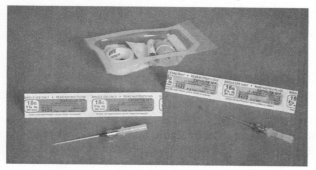

Assembling the Equipment

Following these procedures, and using only the type of fluid ordered by the physician, perform the following steps.

1. Check the container to make sure that the expiration date has not passed.

2. Plastic bag infusion sets are preferable to glass in the field. If a glass bottle is used, inspect it for cracks.

3. Remove the sterile seal from the end of the tubing closest to the drip chamber and insert the tubing into the container. The tubing also has a sterile seal on it. You may have to loosen this seal to allow the liquid to flow, but you should not remove it.

4. With either container, check for seal leakage, cloudiness, discoloration, or contamination. Do not use any fluid that is colored or cloudy or that contains floating particles. Save the bag and report the problem to your equipment manager so that he or she can inspect other supplies in the same lot.

5. As you open the packages to assemble the infusion set, keep all necessary items sterile by *not* touching areas that will come in contact with the fluid. Do *not* use your teeth to rip open the coverings on the bags and tubes. It is a good idea to have extra alcohol wipes and a spare catheter near. Tear the tape to the right size for securing the catheter and tubing.

6. Connect the infusion set to the fluid container by holding the drip chamber, removing any protective coverings (do not touch the spike tip), then inserting the piercing pin into the fluid container with a twisting motion (Figure A2-5).

7. Attach the extension tubing, then squeeze and release the drip chamber or reservoir on the infusion set until it is about half full.

8. Remove the protective cover from the needle adapter. Inspect the needle and cannula for irregularities. If the needle is not sharp and without burrs and if the cannula is not smooth, discard them.

9. Open wide the flow adjustment valve, and flush any air from the tubing. No air should be left in the line, or it may enter the patient's vein, causing an air embolus or blockage. Some EMTs save time and eliminate this step by prehanging IV fluids. If you use this procedure, label the bag with the time, date, and your initials. Fluids and tubing should be discarded after a maximum of twelve hours.

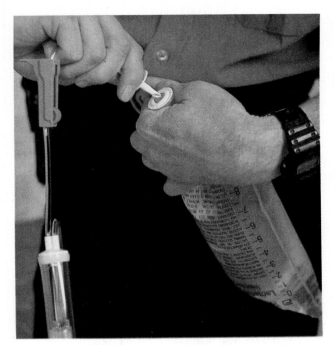

FIGURE A2-5 Hold the drip chamber and insert the piercing pin into the fluid container with a twisting motion. (Apply protective gloves before initiation of an intravenous line.)

10. Adjust the flow valve until the flow stops, then replace the protective cover over the needle adapter and protect it from contamination.

11. Select the needle or IV catheter best suited to the patient (18 gauge is normally used). The needle should be large enough that it will enter the vein easily but without tearing it.

12. Select an appropriate infusion set. Is it for fluid replacement? Micro or macro?

   • Be familiar with the type of IV fluid — always use the same type of fluid if hanging a new container.

   • Be aware of any additives in hanging a new bottle or in the original container of the IV field.

   • Keep the container three feet above the insertion site at all times.

   • Time-label the IV solution container. Tape the side of the container with date, time hung, and rate of solution per hour.

These points are discussed with ideal conditions in mind, but often in the field, they are not, and time is at a premium. Documentation is often left until you reach the emergency department, where the flow rate and possibly the fluid may be changed. It is very helpful to hospital personnel if, on a piece of tape over the insertion site, you write the gauge of the needle, the date, the time the IV was started, and the initials of the EMT who started the IV.

☐ THE IV PROCEDURE

Follow these steps in administering an IV:

1. Explain the procedure to your patient and why you are doing it. Be professional and calm, allowing the patient to have confidence in you. Ask the patient about any possible allergies to tape, fluids, iodine, etc.

2. Prepare yourself properly to prevent any possibility of the patient's blood coming into contact with you. Wear surgical gloves and possibly a face mask and eye protection (see Chapter 31).

3. Select a proper site.

   • Unless the patient's arms have been severely traumatized, use arms rather than legs for placing IVs. The arms have a lower risk of phlebitis than legs.

   • Have the patient hang his or her arm for a couple of minutes. Apply the tourniquet three or four inches (adult) above the antecubital fossa (Figure A2-6). The tourniquet should occlude the venous pressure but not the arterial. If a blood pressure cuff is used as a tourniquet (sometimes good for better control), inflate it to 15 to 20 mmHg below the systolic blood pressure. The distal pulse should still be present.

FIGURE A2-6 Place a constricting band above the site for the venipuncture.

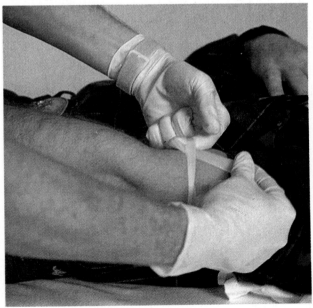

- If it is not, loosen the tourniquet until the arterial pulse returns.
- Look on the forearm or back of the hand for a fairly straight vein that lies on a flat surface. The vein should feel springy when you palpate it. Usually the forearm is the first choice. Creation of a **pulse wave** helps in locating a good vein (Figure A2-7). (The American Heart Association's Advanced Cardiac Life Support Text recommends using the antecubital vein in cases of cardiac arrest. This vein can also be used in cases of severe circulatory collapse.)
- Choose the top side of the arm above the wrist or the back of the hand.
- It is a good idea to start the IV as low as possible on the limb. If a problem arises, the next IV will need to be inserted above the heart in relation to the first site. The **basilic, cephalic,** or **median veins** are common sites for IVs.
- Avoid sites where veins are near injured areas, or where arterial pulsations are found close to the vein being considered.
- Stay away from joints.
- Because the needle must enter the vein lengthwise, know the direction of the vein. Track the direction for one to one and one-half inches (or at least the length of the catheter used).

4. Prepare the IV site. You should scrub and disinfect the site in two separate steps. Use an alcohol scrub to remove dirt, dead skin, blood, mucous, and other contaminants from the surface.
   - Cleanse the selected site with an iodine or alcohol swab. Sponge the antiseptic directly over the selected vein, then rub in a circle until an area one to three inches is covered. Rub in a circular motion, starting at the puncture site and going out. Never go back over the area just cleaned with the same wipe.
   - If a povidone-iodine solution is used, follow with an alcohol wipe in a circular motion, starting at the venipuncture site. This reduces the risk of a reaction. If you have scrubbed and disinfected with alcohol in both steps, be sure to prep for at least sixty seconds using at least two or three wipes. Do not rush this step. It takes time for alcohol to act on the skin microorganisms.

5. If the patient is responsive, briefly explain the purpose of the IV and the procedure for initiating it.

6. Have the patient clench and unclench his or her fist several times. This will improve venous distention. Now select a distended vein that appears straight and that lies on a flat surface. Do not palpate the vein with your bare fingers or soiled

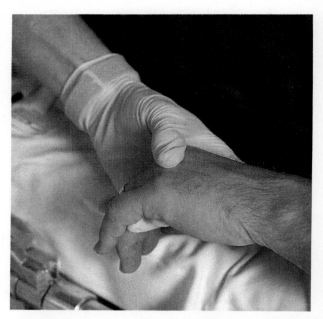

FIGURE A2-7 Hold the patient's hand and press downward with your thumb. This will create a pulse wave that will help your select a good vein.

gloves after disinfection. Put on a pair of fresh, clean gloves immediately before starting the IV.

7. Stabilize the vein by gently applying pressure on it an inch below the point where the needle will enter. (If you feel a pulse, *do not* use this site. It is an artery! Select another site.)

8. Press the vein downward, toward the wrist, so that the vein does not roll.

9. With the bevel (the slanted end of the needle) up, align the needle so that it will enter the skin at a twenty- to forty-degree angle and in the direction of the venous flow. Remember — the needle must enter the vein lengthwise (Figure A2-8). Some services use a bevel-down technique in cases of difficult or rolling veins.

10. Pierce the skin and insert the needle into the vein (Figure A2-9). Smooth movement of one-fourth to one-half inch hurts the patient much less than small, apparently insignificant movement as the IV is started. You should feel some resistance, then a "pop" when the vein is punctured. A confirmation that the needle is in the vein is when the blood appears in the **flash chamber** at the end of the needle (Figure A2-10).

11. A difficult IV start may be enhanced by using a syringe. A syringe may mean the difference between success or failure. To perform this procedure:
    - Insert the needle about 5 mm, but no more.
    - Slide the catheter into the vein by pushing the hub until the catheter is fully in the vein (Figure A2-11). *Do not* advance the needle and catheter

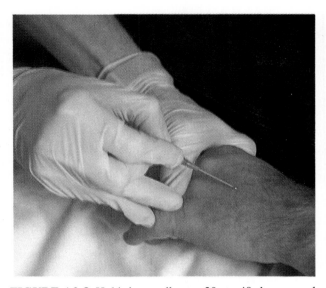

FIGURE A2-8 Hold the needle at a 20- to 40-degree angle in the direction of the venous flow, bevel up!

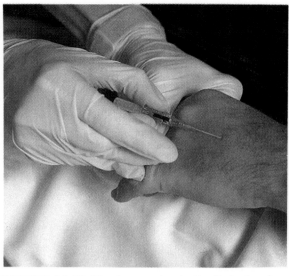

FIGURE A2-10 Blood appearing in the flash chamber is confirmation that the needle is in the vein.

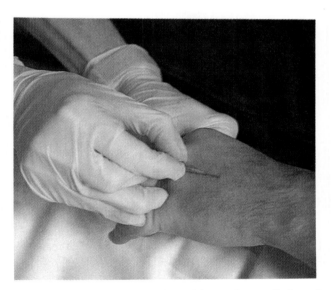

FIGURE A2-9 Pierce the skin and insert the needle into the vein.

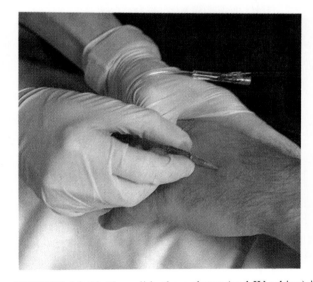

FIGURE A2-11 Now slide the catheter (and IV tubing) into the vein.

together, and *do not push the catheter back over the needle or push the needle back into the catheter.* This action may cause the catheter to be sheared off by the needle.

- While holding the catheter hub in place, carefully withdraw the needle.

12. Maintain firm pressure on the vein above the catheter and make a quick, visual check to see that all is ready.

13. Remove the protective cap from the end of the infusion set, then attach the needle adapter by twisting it securely into the hub. The area around the infusion site should be clean and dry.

- Remove the tourniquet (Figure A2-12).
- Blood loss through the catheter can be stopped by compressing the vein near the tip of the catheter with a finger or thumb.

14. Open the flow adjustment valve.

15. The fluid should drip steadily into the drip chamber. If it does not, gently pull the catheter out 2 to 3 mm only. The drip should now flow steadily.

16. Apply povidone-iodine solution and cover the infusion site with a small gauze pad (follow local protocol; some use a clear cover for the IV site, such as **opsite**). Be aware of **radine** allergy (swelling and redness).

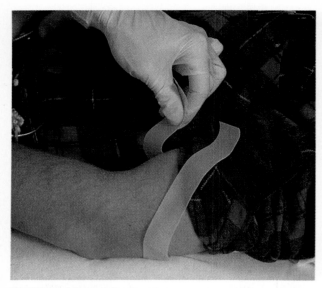

FIGURE A2-12 After holding the catheter hub in place and withdrawing the needle, remove the tourniquet.

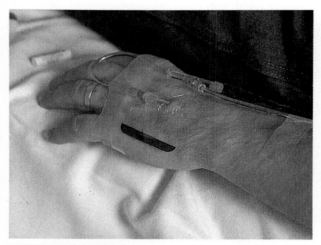

FIGURE A2-13 Tape the catheter securely in place and tape the looped IV tubing to the arm.

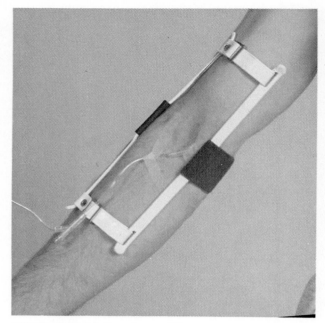

FIGURE A2-14 Securing an IV.

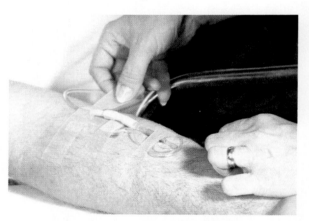

FIGURE A2-15 A butterfly catheter may also be used in the field. Loop the IV tubing and securely tape it to the arm.

17. Tape the catheter securely in place (Figure A2-13). Taping is critical in maintaining the IV. However, do not apply tape completely around the extremity. This could cause a tourniquet effect, decreasing circulation to the distal portion of the extremity.

18. Loop the IV tubing and tape it to the arm with generous, secure taping (Figure A2-14). Attachments such as a T-tube and IV loop can reduce the problem of pinching off a large loop of IV. *Do not* tape the point of connection between the catheter and the infusion set, however. Apply an arm board if it is necessary to minimize arm motion. (See also Figure A2-15).

19. Write with ink on the tape the type of cannula used, the needle gauge, the catheter length, the time and date, and the initials or signature of the EMT who performed the procedure (Figure A2-16).

20. Adjust the infusion to the flow rate (ml/hour) ordered by the physician. It is essential that the proper flow rate be monitored and maintained (Figure A2-17). Too much IV fluid can be dangerous to the patient, especially to children. To adjust the infusion to the ordered flow rate, you must know the volume to be infused and the amount of time that the volume is to be infused. The following formula will allow you to calculate the proper flow rate:

$$\text{flow rate in drops per minute} = \frac{\text{volume to be infused} \times \text{drops per ml that the set delivers}}{\text{Infusion time in minutes}}$$

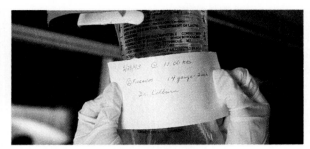

FIGURE A2-16 Label the bag.

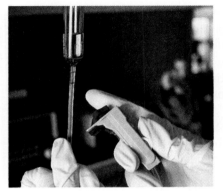

FIGURE A2-17 Turn on the IV and check the flow.

If the physician orders an infusion of 1 liter (1,000 ml) of normal saline in four hours, and the infusion set is capable of providing 10 drops per minute is calculated thus:

$$\frac{1000 \text{ ml} \times 10 \text{ (drops per ml)}}{240 \text{ minutes}} = 42 \text{ drops per minute}$$

The greater the pressure, the greater the flow. However, pressures greater than 250 mmHG to 300 mmHG may cause rupturing.

☐ MAINTAINING THE IV

The IV is fragile and must be handled with care. Carefully monitor the flow rate and make sure that the flow adjustment valve is working properly. Occasionally reposition the arm and inspect the tubing for kinks. Check fluid levels to make sure that you do not run out. Palpate the area around the IV to confirm that the IV is infiltrating the vein and not the tissues surrounding the vein.

If the IV stops dripping:

1. Check the tourniquet to make sure that you have released it.
2. Check the level of fluid in the bottle or container, and increase its height. The IV bottle should always be at least three feet above the insertion site.
3. Reposition the arm.

4. Check the tubing.
5. Check the catheter by pinching off the tubing a few inches ahead, then pinch and release the tubing between the kink and the catheter. You should see a reddish tinge of blood enter the line. If the catheter is plugged, radio the hospital and follow the physician's instructions. He will probably have you begin an IV at another location.
6. Check to see that the flow adjustment valve has not been accidentally closed.

☐ SIGNS TO LOOK FOR AT THE SITE

1. Check that the tape is holding the catheter secure and is not wet.
2. Ask the patient if there is any pain or burning at the IV site.
3. Check the skin to see if it is cool to touch around the site. If it is warm to the touch, there is probably or infiltration.
4. Make sure that the connection between the catheter and tubing is secure.

An infected IV site could cause complications. Signs of infection include:

1. A red line coming from the site (a hard red vein, indicating **phlebitis**) or *any* redness.
2. Any discharge at the site.
3. Any swelling around or above the site. This probably means that the IV catheter is out of the vein and that the fluid is escaping into the tissues. You must discontinue the IV immediately.

☐ TRANSPORTING THE IV PATIENT

When the stabilized patient is ready to be moved, elevate the fluid container well above the level of the heart via an IV pole or a well-instructed helper. If the fluid is in a bag rather than a bottle, the bag may be placed under the patient's head or shoulder until it can be hung up. The helper carrying the IV needs to stay at the infusion site as the patient is moved. Watch the IV continuously for complications.

Moving down a staircase or over rough terrain can dislodge an IV, so take steps to guard against accidental dislodging. You can safely stop the IV drip for two to three minutes if necessary and strap the fluid container to the patient to move over rough terrain. Do not exceed this limit, however, as the blood will clot and the IV will need to be restarted.

When the ambulance is reached, the IV carrier enters the compartment *before* the patient. Place the container on the hanger when possible. A quick check of the IV equipment and the patient should take place before the ambulance proceeds. Continually monitor vital signs during transport. When you arrive at the hospital, the IV helper takes the IV off of the holder. *Then* the patient can be unloaded, with the helper again at the infusion site.

It is necessary to transport a patient with an IV, make sure that all information about the patient and the fluid has been given to the ambulance team and that an IV-trained EMT is on the ambulance. Know what the physician wants you to do if the fluid runs out before the ambulance reaches its destination.

☐ PATIENT ASSESSMENT PRIOR TO TRANSPORTATION[1]

Before transporting an IV patient to another facility, obtain a report about the patient from the nurse in charge. Also do a quick evaluation with the nurse present. It is of prime importance that you have as much information as possible regarding that patient, since any problem that may occur from then on is your responsibility. Be aware of and plan for the problems that can occur if the patient is anxious or confused. A confused patient can try to pull out the IV.

Figure A2-18 is the recommended documentation form that you need to fill out along with the nurse. This is another precaution. If, during the examination, you find something wrong, draw it to the attention of the nurse and tactfully ask the nurse to correct the problem. The documentation form is necessary and helpful for the following reasons:

- It provides a complete checklist for IV and other body tubings.
- You are able to use this checklist as a quick patient assessment.
- It validates any abnormalities that may be present.
- It provides continuity for health-care workers.
- The form filled out accurately is important for insurance claims and for verification of the health-care facility.
- It provides patient protection for optimum care.

---

[1] These sections were prepared with the help of Dave Dodds.

☐ IV MEDICATION

Before transporting a patient with an IV infusing, make sure that you have the following information:

- Patient's name.
- Physician's name.
- The diagnosis.
- Allergies.
- List of medications previously administered.
- The name, dosage, drip rate, and amount of time over which the medication should be infused.
- The reason why the patient is receiving this medication (certain drugs can be administered for different reasons).
- The kind of solution and number of milliliters the container holds. The label on the solution is usually bright-colored. The label should contain the name of the patient, the name of the medication, the dosage, the date, and the time administration was started.
- Do not forget to check at the IV site and make a quick assessment of the body area for any rash that could be the beginning of an allergic reaction to the medication, along with a change in vital signs.

It is extremely important to know the following information about medications:

- The generic and chemical name.
- The classification.
- Indications for use.
- Adverse reactions.
- Normal dosage.
- Signs and symptoms of a reaction.
- What to do if a reaction occurs.

Important tip: At the time you obtain the medication information, write the facts on index cards and file them in an accessible place in your ambulance. You can then refer to them in the future (they are also handy for studying purposes). The dispatcher should have a current Physician's Drug Reference.

☐ IV COMPLICATIONS

Three major complications that can result from infusion are infection, **pyrogenic reactions,** and phlebitis. These risks can be minimized with proper attention to technique.

CHECK OFF PRIOR TO TRANSFER WITH NURSE

Patient's Name _____

Diagnosis _____

Reason for Transfer _____

IV MAINTENANCE

Solution _____

Kind _____

Labeled with patient's name _____

Labeled if there are additives _____

Drip rate _____

Is solution time labeled _____

How many ml in bag or bottle _____

Need another bag or bottle _____

    Label check with bag that is hanging _____

Is IV patent _____

Clamp on tubing correct _____

IV secure to extremity — armboard _____

IV site

    Redness _____

    Swelling _____

    Any wetness _____

Patient complaining of IV burning _____

_____

Signature, EMT and Nurse

BODY TUBINGS

Does patient have any of the following tubings

Nasogastric _____

Feeding _____

Tracheostomy _____

Gastrostomy _____

Colostomy _____

Urostomy _____

Foley catheter _____

Rectal tube _____

Are tubes secured correctly? _____

Are tubes patent — no kinks? _____

Are colostomy or other stoma bags
   intact and empty? _____

Is foley bag empty? _____

_____

Signature, EMT and Nurse

FIGURE A2-18

Infection usually results from poor aseptic techniques. Being careful to *prevent contamination* is the key. A patient who has an IV in his or her vein has an open entry into his or her circulatory system.

To prevent contamination when working with an IV:

- Keep all possible equipment sterile.
- Use sterile or unsterile but clean gloves. Use of a surgical mask is also suggested.
- Examine equipment, solutions, and tubing for flaws.
- Always use aseptic or sterile technique.
- Remove rings and watches from the patient. The watch may act as a tourniquet.
- Always maintain sterility when opening packages or any IV equipment.
- Examine all packages and equipment for flaws.
- Inform the patient of the reasons for your precautions.

Pyrogens (foreign proteins) enter the body by way of contaminated fluid. If fluid shows leakage or cloudiness, *do not use it*. Pyrogenic reactions usually begin one-half hour after the IV is begun and present with the following:

- Abrupt fever.
- Severe chills.
- Backache, headache.
- Nausea, vomiting.
- Malaise.
- Shock, with a possibility of vascular collapse.

If these reactions occur, *stop the infusion immediately!* Begin a new IV with new equipment in the other arm. Treat for shock, and advise the physician by radio.

A misplaced needle (misses the vein or tears through it) will cause fluid to leak into the surrounding tissues. Visible and palpable swelling will occur, and the patient will experience a painful, burning sensation. Stop the IV and begin a new one in the other arm. Inform the physician of your actions.

Phlebitis

Phlebitis is the localized inflammation of a vein that leads to the formation of a small clot. As the clot grows, inflammation increases, partially or completely blocking the vessel, or detaching from the vessel and lodging elsewhere in the body. Phlebitis greatly increases the patient's risk of sepsis, as bacteria tends to accumulate at the site. Trauma, diabetes mellitus, age, or immunodeficiency can foster such an accumulation, rapidly leading to septic shock and death.

Patients in emergency departments have almost twice the risk of complications from IV therapy as patients whose IVs were initiated in other parts of the hospital. And patients whose IVs were begun in the field have over four and one-half times as much phlebitis than patients whose IVs were begun in the emergency room. Twenty-two percent also developed fevers — five and one-half times the percentage of those whose IVs were started in the emergency room. Even more alarming, symptoms of phlebitis can continue to develop even after the catheter has been removed and may not appear for days.[2]

The causes for these higher rates of complication seem to be incomplete decontamination, catheters that are too large, and rough insertions. In a field setting involving trauma, there must necessarily be trade-offs between ideal circumstances and speed. With trauma patients, using smaller catheters is not an option because of the need for rapid fluid infusion. But experts recommend that there be no attempt to speed up decontamination and that all IVs started in the field be removed and replaced in the hospital.

☐ OTHER IV THERAPY COMPLICATIONS

Other complications may arise from an IV that is not started or tended to properly. Always check to see if the IV is positioned properly, and if the tourniquet is still on.

Plastic Embolus

A plastic embolus may be caused by withdrawing the needle from the catheter, then reinserting the needle, causing the sharp, beveled tip of the needle to cut off a small piece of the plastic catheter. Radio-opaque catheters are better than radiolucent for finding catheters that have been sheared off. However, the opaque catheters are more difficult to "slide" into the skin.

Air Embolus

An air embolus may result from a malfunction of the infusion line, or from allowing the fluid to run out completely, thus drawing air into the line via the air vent. The victim of an air embolus will rapidly develop shock and cyanosis and may possibly become unconscious. If an air embolus is suspected, use a hemostat to clamp the tubing close to the body. Place your patient on his left side, with legs elevated and head down. Inform the base physician. Lower the head of the stretcher or bed. Give oxygen and transport to the nearest emergency room.

---

[2] David Lawrence, "Prehospital IV Therapy," *JEMS*, January 1990, pp. 51–52.

Circulatory Overload

Circulatory overload, or too much fluid in the circulatory system, can be caused by a "runaway" IV, or by an IV that provides too much fluid. This may force fluid into the lungs, causing pulmonary edema. Signs of circulatory overload are:

- Venous distention.
- Raise in blood pressure.
- Shortness of breath.
- Coughing.
- Increased respiratory rate.
- Dyspnea.
- Frothy sputum resulting from fluid buildup in the lungs.
- Cyanosis.

If these signs are present:

1. Use a microdrip.
2. Elevate the patient's head.
3. Turn the IV to **TKO** (to keep open). Leave the IV inserted, as the patient will probably need it for IV medications such as **Lasix,** which is used to rid the body of fluid.
4. Notify the physician immediately. Monitor the patient closely, be prepared to give emergency care, and document the entire procedure.

Allergic Reactions

If your patient has an IV medication infusing or has an additive to his or her IV, be alert to a possible allergic reaction. Watch for the following signs:

- Itching.
- Rash.
- Shortness of breath.
- Anaphylactic shock can develop.

If there is a medication infusing:

1. Clamp off.
2. *Do not discontinue the IV,* but slow down to TKO.
3. Monitor the patient closely.
4. Be prepared to give emergency care.
5. Transport to the nearest emergency room.
6. Document the entire procedure.
7. A medical doctor may order fluid or a medication change.

Infiltration

Infiltration means the escape of IV fluids into the surrounding tissues, which can cause tissue damage and **necrosis.** If the IV solution contains a drug toxic to subcutaneous tissue, it can be disastrous; it could require reconstructive surgery.

It is of utmost importance to monitor the IV site for edema, pain, and temperature. The area above the IV site may feel cooler or warmer. Look for leakage of fluid around the site. Another sign could be a sluggish flow rate.

Stabilize the extremity with the IV. It is important for the extremity with the IV to be still. Use of the catheter over the needle rather than the butterfly will reduce the occurrence of damage with movement. If infiltration occurs, stop the IV and begin a new one in the other arm. Inform your base physician of your actions.

Blood Back-up In Tubing

During your observation, you may notice blood beginning to back up in the tubing and/or possibly a clot at the end of the catheter. Look for the obvious first, remembering that a blood back-up or clotting usually occurs due to a slow or absent flow rate or improper placement of the IV solution container. Also, if you forget to flush the IV, the blood will run up the tubing. If this happens, the tube must be unhooked from the IV, flushed, then reconnected.

Start at the top. Check to see that the IV container is not empty. Is it elevated enough? How is the flow rate? If the purpose of the IV is TKO (to keep open), that can be a factor. Do not forget that a TKO drip rate needs to be wide open for one to two seconds, every one-half to one hour. Is the drip chamber half full? Check the flow clamp for position. Observe if the tubing in kinked, or if the tubing is dangling and preventing the solution from reaching the patient.

Next, check the IV site. Are any signs present that might explain the problem, such as the catheter being lodged against the vein wall? Gently move the catheter slightly. You may have to attempt to aspirate the clot out of the catheter with a sterile syringe. Never irrigate IV if you cannot aspirate a clot, for this could cause an embolus. Remove the IV and start a new one.

Cold

IV solutions can freeze in the tubing or container very rapidly. You may want to start an IV in the ambulance or in a heated building, if possible. Protect the tubing and container from cold during transport. If a patient in hypovolemic shock is receiving large volume of fluid, warm them to body temperature or you may cause the patient's core temperature to drop, triggering hypothermia.

□ BLOOD TRANSFUSIONS

As an EMT, you do not normally transport blood transfusion patients. If you feel uncomfortable or if the medication maintenance does not fall within the realm of your duty, ask the facility to send a nurse or physician to perform those duties/skills.

□ IV DISCONTINUATION

It is important to evaluate the circumstances before you decide to discontinue the IV. Use the following guidelines:

- Discontinue an IV immediately if the fluid is going into the tissues, not the vein.
- With a clotted-off IV, it is possible (if your arrival to the other facility is within five minutes) to wait for another opinion before you discontinue.
- If your patient has thrombophlebitis (signs include sluggish flow rate, edema around the IV site, and a vein that looks like a red line; the vein will be hard, warm, and sore), you *must* discontinue the IV.

To discontinue an IV:

1. Explain to the patient why his or her IV needs to be discontinued. Also, explain that he or she will probably need to have another one inserted upon arrival at the other facility.
2. Gather all equipment: two 2 × 2s or 4 × 4s and tape.
3. Whenever blood or body fluids are being handled, wear protective clothing.
4. Open your packages and prepare two pieces of tape about three inches long.
5. Clamp off the IV.
6. Loosen all the tape on the IV site.
7. Stabilize the extremity and hub.
8. Gently pull out the catheter and apply pressure immediately upon removal.
9. Place a 2 × 2 on the IV site and hold pressure for

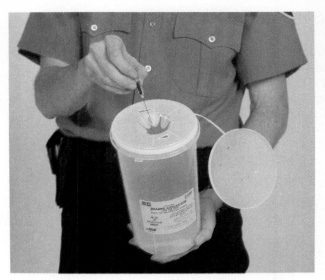

FIGURE A2-19 Dispose of used needles in a Sharps container.

two minutes to prevent a hematoma from forming. (Be aware of patients with clotting problems — you may have to apply a pressure dressing.)

10. Apply a 2 × 2, and tape.
11. If infiltration is present, elevate the extremity on a pillow.
12. Apply a warm, moist pack when possible.
13. Document and record:
    - Amount of fluid left in the bag.
    - Amount of fluid the patient received.
    - Time of discontinuation of the IV.
    - Any other problems.
14. Dispose of used needles in a Sharps container (Figure A2-19).

□ COMMUNICATION WITH THE EMERGENCY DEPARTMENT

During IV therapy, it is essential that you communicate effectively with personnel in the emergency department. Repeat all orders verbally to the emergency department so that everyone understands what has been ordered.

appendix 3

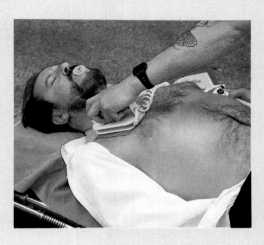

EMT-D
Prehospital
Defibrillation

✳ OBJECTIVES

- ■ Define defibrillation as it relates to EMTs.
- ■ Discuss and understand cardiac structure and function, including the electrical system of the heart.
- ■ Review the signs, symptoms, assessment, and management of the sudden cardiac death patient.
- ■ Discuss the principles of defibrillation and demonstrate the skills of defibrillation.
- ■ Discuss the hazards, problems, and safety steps of defibrillation.

NOTE: The details of this section are consistent with the National Standards for EMT-Defibrillation developed by the National Council for State-Emergency Medical Services Training Coordinators.

It is recommended that EMTs wear protective gloves whenever there is a possibility of coming in contact with a patient's blood, body fluids, mucous membranes, traumatic wounds, or sores. See Chapter 31.

□ INTRODUCTION

One of the very exciting developments in EMS today is EMT defibrillation. As CPR and defibrillation work in tandem, a high percentage of cardiac arrest victims in ventricular fribrillation can be saved.

To be authorized to defibrillate patients in the field, you must be part of a formal program. Though programs may differ in specific requirements, they all must meet and follow the national guidelines for EMT-D:

- EMTs must be certified in the state where they practice and must maintain all basic life support skills; in addition, their defibrillation program must be authorized by the state emergency medical systems organization.
- There must be a medical director who is a physician. This person assumes legal responsibility for EMT-defibrillation treatment given to patients.
- EMTs must adhere to the standing orders of their medical director. These orders authorize specific action to occur without delay in the event of cardiac arrest.
- Regular skills review, usually every three months, must occur through an EMS continuing education class. This class emphasizes ability to perform the skill of defibrillating a cardiac arrest patient within ninety seconds of arriving at the patient's side.
- Portable defibrillators with a dual channel recorder must be used to record the electocardiograph and to make a voice record to the events at the scene.
- Each cardiac arrest incident must be reviewed later by the medical director or his designated representative.

Prerequisites for entry into a defibrillation class should be based upon recent certification in CPR. You should also possess satisfactory skills in basic life support, airway management, and patient assessment. EMT-defibrillation is a *separate* skill beyond basic EMT training and, as such, requires special training, including:

- An understanding of cardiac structure and function (including the electrical system).
- A clear understanding of ventricular fibrillation and cardiac death.

This appendix has been adapted from Judith Graves and Richard Cummins, "Defibrillation by Emergency Medical Technicians: A Review," Hafen and Karren (eds.), *ETC Review Manual*, Morton Publishing, 1987, and Weigel, Atkins, and Taylor, *Automated Defibrillation*, Morton Publishing, 1988.

- Knowledge and practical skills development of defibrillation.
- An understanding of the potential problems in defibrillation.

□ CARDIAC STRUCTURE AND FUNCTION

Structure

The heart is located in the chest, behind and slightly to the left of the sternum. It sits in front of the spine and rests on the diaphragm (see Chapter 6).

As a pump, the heart is extremely efficient and durable. At rest, it usually beats 60 to 90 times per minute; when exercising, up to 180 to 200, depending upon the person's size, sex, general health, and level of activity. Each day, the normal heart beats up to 100,000 times and pumps 4,000 gallons of blood.

The heart is a muscle about the size of your fist. Its primary job is to pump blood through the body in a closed loop — the arteries and veins. It is composed of four separate, hollow chambers. The right side of the heart, composed of the right atria and right ventricle, receives unoxygenated blood from the veins of the body and pumps it through the lungs, where carbon dioxide is given off and oxygen is picked up. The left side of the heart, which includes the left atria and left ventricle, receives this oxygenated blood from the lungs and pumps it out of the heart through arteries, where it is sent to various parts of the body. This cycle is repeated with each contraction of the heart.

Function

Like any pump, the heart needs a "stimulus," or electrical system, to tell it when to contract. This is performed by a specialized group of cells, called **pacemaker cells,** located throughout the heart.

A group of these special pacemaker cells, called the sinus or **SA node,** located near the top of the right atria (Figure A3-1) is responsible for starting the pumping action of the heart. When this happens, the SA node sends a tiny electrical signal to the atrium, causing it to contract. This then forces blood into the ventricles (Figure A3-2). This same signal is received and delayed at the atrioventricular or **AV node,** allowing the ventricles time to fill with the blood from the atria. This delayed electrical signal is then passed from the AV node to the muscle cells surrounding the ventricles, causing them to contract and force blood out of the ventricles (Figure A3-3). This electrical signal from the AV node to the ventricles generates a mechanical contraction of the heart. Figure A3-4 depicts an ECG tracing of a normal, functioning heart.

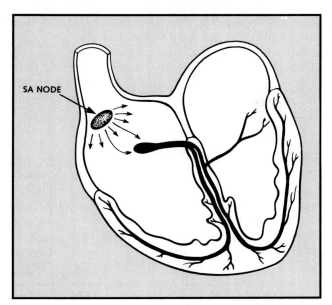

FIGURE A3-1 Location of the "pacemaker cells" in the heart.

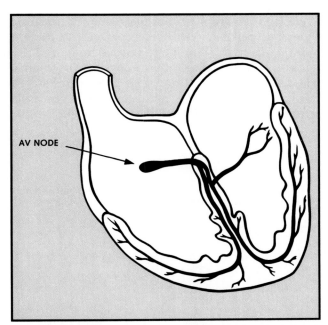

FIGURE A3-2 Normal flow of the heart's electrical signal.

The body times the normal conduction of the electrical signal described above so that the chambers of the heart contract and relax in a coordinated way. An electrical impulse may not always result in a muscular contraction of the heart. That is why EMS personnel should always *manually* check for a pulse instead of depending upon the electrical signal on a monitor.

☐ FAST HEART RHYTHMS

Seventy percent of the time when cardiac arrest occurs, the heart is in a state of rapid quivering called **ventricu-**

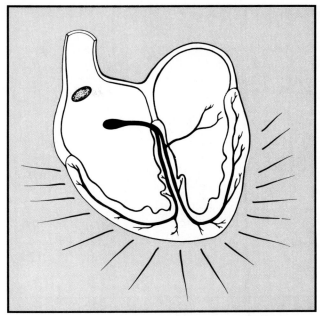

FIGURE A3-3 Coordination of the heart's electrical signal and mechanical contraction.

FIGURE A3-4 An ECG tracing of the normal, functioning heart.

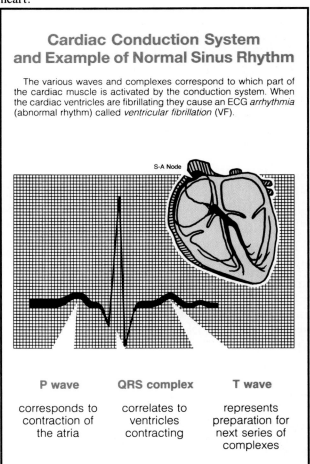

Cardiac Conduction System and Example of Normal Sinus Rhythm

The various waves and complexes correspond to which part of the cardiac muscle is activated by the conduction system. When the cardiac ventricles are fibrillating they cause an ECG *arrhythmia* (abnormal rhythm) called *ventricular fibrillation* (VF).

P wave	QRS complex	T wave
corresponds to contraction of the atria	correlates to ventricles contracting	represents preparation for next series of complexes

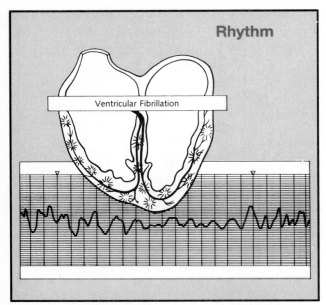

FIGURE A3-5 Ventricular fibrillation (VF) is shown as it occurs in the heart. This same VF is also seen as it would appear on an ECG tracing.

lar fibrillation or **ventricular tachycardia** (Figure A3-5). In this situation, the pacemaker cells are sending electrical signals faster than the heart can respond.

Between 50 and 60 percent of all cardiac arrest victims will be experiencing ventricular fibrillation (VF) by the time you arrive. The heart has plenty of electrical energy, but the energy is chaotic. The heart muscle is jumping and quivering erratically and cannot pump normally. Ventricular tachycardia is very unusual and is observed in less than 10 percent of all out-of-hospital cases. The heart's chambers are not filling with enough blood between contractions to perfuse the brain adequately. In both conditions, the heart can only be restored to normal beating by means of defibrillation. (Some protocols do not allow defibrillation for pulseless ventricular tachycardia. Know and follow your local protocol.)

In 15 to 20 percent of cardiac arrest victims, the heart muscle itself fails, even though the electrical rhythm is relatively normal. This condition is called electromechanical dissociation, because the electrical activity has become separated from the mechanical, or pumping, activity. Defibrillation will not help these people.

In the remaining 20 to 25 percent of cardiac arrest victims, the heart has stopped generator electrical impulses altogether. As a result, there is no pulse, no blood flow, and no electrical impulse. Defibrillation is, of course, useless; and only CPR has any effect.

Defibrillation is also not effective when the heart is beating regularly but too slowly (**bradycardia**).

Defibrillation is the delivery of an external elec-

trical current into the heart muscle. Just as the heart normally responds to internal electrical impulses, it will also respond to external electrical impulses. If successful, this "shock" stops the uncontrolled electrical activity and allows the heart's normal pacer to take over. CPR will not effectively restore the heart's normal beating during these two states of cardiac arrest.

You may not be able to tell the difference between ventricular fibrillation and ventricular tachycardia. In both cases, the heart is usually not able to pump blood; therefore, no pulse is present. The victim will not be breathing, will have no blood pressure, and will be unconscious. CPR should be started immediately if there is no pulse, and defibrillation should occur as quickly as possible. Only defibrillation will return the heart to its normal rhythm.

□ SLOW HEART RHYTHMS

In 30 percent of cardiac arrest cases, the heart is either beating critically slow (**bradycardia**) or has stopped (**asystole** — Figure A3-6), or there is an electrical signal with no pumping (**electromechanical dissociation**). In EMD, the heart is unable to respond to the electrical signals which are being sent. In asystole (no contractions), no impulses are being sent. These cases are different from ventricular fibrillation and ventricular tachycardia in that defibrillation will not help.

FIGURE A3-6 Asystole is shown as it would occur in the heart. The straight line on the ECG tracing shows the electrical signal physically displayed.

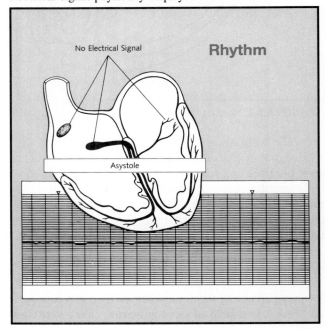

☐ AUTOMATED VERSUS MANUAL DEFIBRILLATION

The two major ways in which you can defibrillate a cardiac arrest patient are automated defibrillation (automatic and semiautomatic) and manual defibrillation. The choice is usually determined by the program medical director. Either choice requires close review by physicians who oversee the EMT-D field performance.

Manual defibrillators require that you recognize lethal cardiac rhythms, whereas automated defibrillators recognize the rhythm for you. Therefore, the automated defibrillation program requires less training and is less time-consuming. Studies show that either choice is equally effective in saving lives. The operation and use of automated defibrillators is discussed in the next section of this appendix.

☐ MANAGEMENT OF THE SUDDEN CARDIAC DEATH PATIENT

In general, the EMT-D protocol for treatment of prehospital sudden cardiac death is:

1. Arrive quickly; identify the presence of cardiac arrest; take control of the scene.
2. One EMT begins basic life support.
3. Another EMT operates the defibrillator as soon as possible (this should occur within ninety seconds of arrival at the patient's side).
4. Transport the patient to more advanced life support.

These standing orders allow for a total of six shocks of ventricular fibrillation, at energy levels between 200 and 360 joules. The standing orders are signed by the program medical director and act as a legal order to perform these specific skills without delay. Each EMT-D program's standing orders will vary slightly.

Automated Defibrillation

Automated defibrillators are becoming increasingly popular and more widely available despite a base price of about $4,600. Landmark studies in the last five years show that trained laypersons who treat individuals in ventricular fibrillation have long-term "saves," meaning that the heart attack victim survives not only to hospital admission but to discharge. In one study of 120 lay trainees, 96 percent operated the device successfully with a mannequin and kept their skills for up to twelve months without review. Another study on a small sample (fifteen patients) who had witnessed cardiac arrests at work, recreation, and commercial sites showed that five lived to be discharged from the hospital after lay defibrillation on the scene. This rate of long-term saves was as high as any reported for professional rescuers for witnessed out-of-hospital ventricular fibrillation.

Automatic defibrillators are far from being as common as fire extinguishers, and their price is still prohibitive for widespread placement. Still, their community acceptance, sensitivity in diagnosis, and ease of use means that they have some strong advantages for EMTs.

A majority of EMT-D training programs are moving to automated defibrillators. For this reason, the following step-by-step approach will detail the use of this equipment.

STEP 1: Anticipation and Planning

1. Analyze dispatch information.
2. Decide on team leader and defibrillator operator.
3. Outline duties.
4. Prepare and check equipment. Remember to carry spare batteries.
5. *Anticipate* the upcoming cardiac arrest, mentally "visualizing" your roles and actions.
6. Assume that "patient collapse" means cardiac arrest.
7. If the patient is experiencing cardiac symptoms (chest pain, sweating, syncope, etc.), anticipate a witnessed arrest in your presence and be prepared to defibrillate immediately!

STEP 2: Scene Entry and Placement

1. Pinpoint the exact location of the patient at the scene.
2. Transport all equipment needed to manage cardiac arrest to the patient's side.
3. Position the patient for effective CPR and defibrillation.
4. Position team members and the defibrillator based on assessment of available space, layout, and work "room."

Ideally, place the automated external defibrillation (AED) device close to the patient's head. Perform defibrillation from the *left side of the patient*. This position provides better access to the defibrillator controls and placement of the electrode pads on the chest.

*Both the AED and operator should be on the **left***

TYPICAL DEFIBRILLATION "CODE" LAYOUT SHOWING POSITION OF TEAM MEMBERS AND AUTOMATED DEFIBRILLATOR

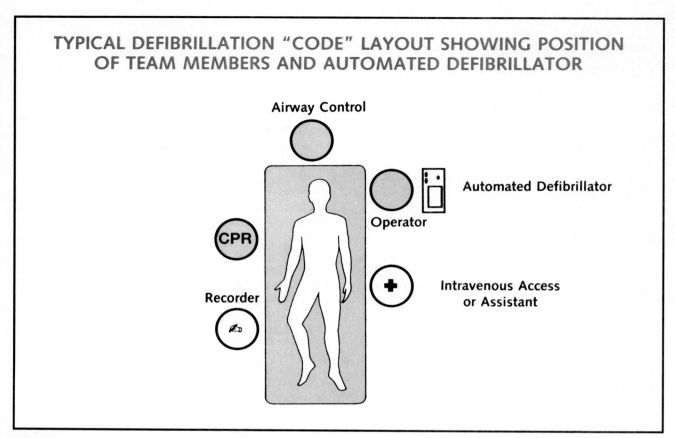

FIGURE A3-7

side. Typical positions for the operator, device, and team members are depicted in Figure A3-7. This layout may not be possible in all field situations. Alternative arrangements should be tried and practiced.

STEP 3: Check Patient and Start CPR

1. A — Airway:
   - Assess patient (determine unresponsiveness).
   - Open airway (head-tilt/chin-lift).
   - Assume appropriate positions for patient/rescuer.
2. B — Breathing:
   - Breathing normally?
   - Blow in two breaths (1 to 1.5 seconds each).
3. C — Circulation:
   - Check for carotid pulse.
   - Call for ALS backup (if available).
   - Compress the chest.

As team leader, it is the defib operator's responsibility to see that adequate CPR is being performed.

STEP 4: Prepare Patient and Attach Electrodes

Expose the patient's chest by removing clothing. Wipe the chest dry if necessary.

Note: Improper pad placement and poor adhesive contact are one of the most common errors in prehospital defibrillation.

Take the necessary time to carefully:

1. Open the packaging for the self-adhesive pads and remove both electrodes.
2. Peel off the adhesive backing.
3. Position each pad correctly on the chest.
4. Secure the pads firmly to the chest wall (Figures A3-8 and A3-9).
   - *Sternum pad* should be on the right upper border of the sternum, with the top edge just touching the bottom of the clavicle.
   - *Apex pad* should be on the left lower ribs, at the anterior axillary line (below and to the left of the nipple).

The person doing CPR must briefly move his or

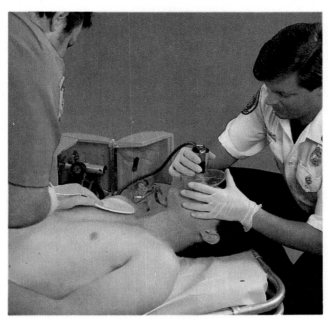

FIGURE A3-8 The plastic backing is removed from the first pad and the pad is placed on the chest.

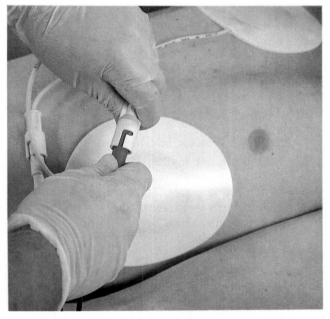

FIGURE A3-9 The second pad is placed on the patient's chest and the cables are connected.

her hands while the pads are being positioned and placed.

Attach defibrillator cables to the adhesive pads (according to manufacturer's instructions). Some manufacturers recommend connecting the defibrillator cables to the adhesive pads *prior* to placement on the patient's chest.

Although *either pad may be attached to either ca-*

ble, it is recommended for consistency that units employing color-coded cables or pads be placed as follows:

- The red color (cable or pad, depending on manufacturer) should be applied over the apex area.
- The white color (cable or pad) should be applied over the right border of the sternum.

This placement ensures correct "positioning" of the patient's ECG signal into the monitor circuitry.

Taking the additional time to shave excessive chest hair at the pad sites is *not* worth the effort, as every second counts, unless there is too much hair to get an acceptable tracing.

Note: Improper positioning or connection of the pads and cables will result in either:

- An error message or "NO CONTACT" signal from the AED.
- Less energy delivered to the dying heart muscle, lowering the chances for a successful defibrillation.

STEP 5: Turn Power On and Analyze Rhythm

Some units may be turned on at this time. Others cannot be turned on until it is time to shock. For units that can be turned on before shocks, narration is helpful as described below.

NARRATION   The team leader should:

1. Call out time ("Device on at 04:00 hours").
2. Identify himself or herself and the responding EMS unit.
3. Briefly describe the history of the present episode and current clinical situation ("60-year-old male patient witnessed collapsing 5 minutes prior to our arrival by spouse — currently pulseless and apneic").
4. Report each step while proceeding through the standing orders.
5. State whether shocks are delivered: call out when ("2nd shock delivered at 200 joules").
6. Explain important actions, events at the scene, decisions, problems, time of transport, etc.
7. Keep verbal reports brief and to the point. Overly long reports delay action at the scene and detract from overall performance of the code.

Note: The exact details of rhythm analysis vary considerably with the type and brand of AED. Consult machine protocols for specifics.

For fully automatic devices, rhythm analysis is activated automatically as soon as the power switch is turned on. For semiautomatic units there is a separate control switch for rhythm analysis. It may be labeled "Analyze," "Press To Analyze," "Automatic/Manual Mode," etc.

GETTING CLEAR As soon as the correct switch is tripped and rhythm analysis is activated, *everyone should be clear of the patient!* The AED will also advise you to clear with voice prompts or message delays. However, it is a good practice to clear everyone away from the patient *before* rhythm analysis starts.

If the device has separate controls for the tape or chart recorder, make sure that they are on and running.

Semiautomatic AEDs require that several "YES" or "NO" questions appearing on an LCD display be answered by the operator. These questions must be answered before the device will continue with rhythm interpretation and assessment.

Assessment: All those present must remain clear during the duration of the assessment. Rhythm assessment takes between 7 to 20 seconds depending on the brand and model of AED.

Operators should count to 15 slowly out loud ("1:1000, 2:1000, etc.") during the assessment period. If by the count of 15 the device has not delivered a shock or has indicated that a shock was *not* advised,

- Check pulse and respirations.
- If no pulse, either re-analyze by pressing switch or resume CPR *per local protocol.*

Charging: The devices will indicate that charging is underway with a tone, voice message, or light indicators. Make doubly sure that everyone is clear of the patient.

Note: Physical motion of the patient, the defibrillator, or both (in a moving ambulance) may cause interference and false rhythm interpretation. Some models of AEDs are more motion-sensitive than others. Semiautomatic devices may indicate that motion is interfering by means of a visual or voice message.

STEP 6: Defibrillation

SEMIAUTOMATIC In semiautomatic defibrillation, the operator activates the "Shock" button or a voice synthesizer when informed to do so by the device. The commands "shock now" or "shock advised" will appear on the LCD device.

Successive cycles of rhythm analysis, charging, and "clear and shock" must be repeated through constant interaction between the operator and the semiautomatic defibrillator. The operator must promptly react both to the signals and messages given by the device *and* to the patient's responses to each defibrillation.

AUTOMATIC Fully automatic AEDs will deliver successive countershocks without additional actions by the operator. These automatic devices are programmed to shock the patient up to three, four, or more times until the power is automatically switched off, ending a cycle of defibrillation. This cycle usually lasts sixty to ninety seconds.

However, the power may be switched off or to monitoring mode at any time during use. This will stop the cycle whenever the operator chooses to do so. Turning the power back on or back to the assessing mode will restart the cycle.

Standing orders for delivery of countershocks will vary among EMS systems. As a general rule, ACLS standards should be used as the basis for setting the number of shocks and their energy levels in local protocols.

The ACLS protocols for ventricular fibrillation (VF) and pulseless ventricular tachycardia (VT) call for delivery of three consecutive shocks followed by a pulse check as follows:

Perform CPR until a defibrillator is ready.

If **VF** or pulseless **VT**

1. Defibrillate at 200 joules.
2. Defibrillate at 200 to 300 joules.
3. Defibrillate with up to 360 joules.

Check Pulse → Continue CPR if no pulse.

1. Pulseless VT should be treated identically to VF.
2. Check pulse and rhythm after each shock. If VT recurs after converting to a perfusing rhythm (with palpable pulse), use whatever energy level has previously been successful for defibrillation. After the first shock is given, fully automatic devices will give a voice prompt "shock delivered." If a second shock is required, these devices will repeat the process up to three times before shutting off.

Many localities now specify a second round of shocks after resuming CPR.
Resume CPR.
Perform one to four cycles of compressions and ventilations, depending on local standing orders.
To do so may require:

- Turning the power off or to a monitoring mode in automatic devices.
- Switching from the "analysis" to a standby or "monitoring" mode in semiautomatic devices.

Repeat rhythm assessment and shock delivery.

Local protocols will vary on the number of repeat countershocks and rhythm assessment periods.

Various standards recommend:

- Three consecutive shocks.
- Fifteen to sixty seconds of CPR (1 to 4 cycles).
- Three more shocks.

OUTCOMES OF USE OF AEDS   An AED will only shock ventricular fibrillation or occasionally ventricular tachycardia. Depending on the response time of the system and the percentage of witnessed arrests, only 40 to 70 percent of the patients have a shockable rhythm. Hence, the device will frequently say "No Shock" advised or "Resume CPR."

When the AED advises shock or automatically analyzes and discharges a shock, about half the time the rhythm will change with the first shock and you will get a "No Shock" or "Resume CPR" message. If you get the "No Shock" or "Resume CPR" message, proceed as in the following paragraph. In the remainder of the cases, the rhythm will remain in ventricular fibrillation. After each shock, follow the procedure for the device and analyze the rhythm again (some devices will automatically reanalyze; in others, the analysis button will have to be pushed).

Local protocols may require a pulse check between each shock. If a pulse check is required, turn off the fully automatic types of machines. If unsuccessful after three shocks, it is usually advisable to do CPR for one to two minutes before analyzing again. If the responders must transport the patient, it is advisable to start transport after the third shock.

If you get a "No Shock" or "Resume CPR" message, check for a pulse. If no pulse is present, resume CPR. If a pulse is present, check for breathing. If there is no breathing, perform rescue breathing. If patient is breathing, observe him or her closely for loss of pulse and breathing. If the patient again loses his or her pulse, analyze the rhythm or turn on the AED.

The four most common sequences found with the use of the device in the order of occurrence are as follows:

- No shock advised (resume CPR message).
- Shock — No shock advised.
- Shock — Shock — No shock advised.
- Shock — Shock — Shock — No shock advised.

Rarely have four or more shocks been required with these devices.

STEP 7: Patient Stabilization and Maintenance

If a palpable pulse (BP>60mm) and respirations return, maintain a good airway and provide 100 percent oxygen and assist ventilations, if necessary, per local protocol. Carefully lift and move the patient to the ambulance in a gentle but expedient manner.

Be prepared for the possibility of return to cardiac arrest and refibrillation at any point. To date, available evidence shows that refibrillation is likely to occur in about 25 percent of patients.

Check pulse and blood pressure at frequent intervals — e.g., every two to three minutes. Vital signs that are stable now were not even there moments ago!

STEP 8: Family Notification and Spectators

Even though the primary concern of the EMS defibrillation team is the patient, it is both necessary and appropriate to communicate effectively with the other people at the scene: family, friends, and spectators.

- Keep spectators out. Honor and respect the patient's and family's right to privacy. This is especially true in defibrillation, where shocking the patient's bare chest is high drama.
- Inform the family of the patient's status and condition prior to and after resuscitation/defibrillation. It is important to identify the patient, establish the relationship of those present, accurately restate the events leading up to cardiac arrest, briefly outline resuscitation efforts by the EMS team (CPR and whether or not the patient was defibrillated), and portray the patient's present condition — briefly and objectively.

STEP 9: Transport

As soon as the patient is safely secured and stabilized in the ambulance, transport without delay. Monitor vital signs en route to the hospital. Keep your guard up and anticipate that vital signs may deteriorate any second. Keep team attention acute.

Be prepared to run another code at a moment's notice. Stop the ambulance for rhythm analysis and defibrillation if arrest recurs. Notify receiving hospital medical control of the patient's status and ETA.

STEP 10: Transfer of Care to Hospital/ALS

Assure an orderly transfer of patient care to the hospital or prehospital ALS or paramedic team.

Provide a *brief* report of clinical information (e.g., "Unwitnessed arrest, patient responded to second defibrillation at 200 joules, and regained consciousness in ambulance, latest vital signs are pulse 60 and regular BP 100/80, patient responds to verbal stimulus").

Do not dwell on presenting information that is not vital for further patient care (e.g., how the AED performed).

STEP 11: Critique

1. Prepare a report as soon as possible after the call while information is fresh.
2. Give tape and "medical control/command chips" for transcribing by receiving hospital medical control physician or official.

Hospital medical control should give feedback both to the EMS service and the personnel on the code. Initially, members of the EMS defibrillation team should be briefly informed of the patient's outcome and disposition at the hospital.

The emergency department staff can simply restate the patient's:

- Vital signs — stable or unstable?
- Cardiac rhythm — perfusing or not?
- Disposition (e.g., transferred to CCU).
- Level of consciousness.
- Death and decision to terminate code.

At a later time, hospital medical control can formally critique the code and performance of the EMS team. This critique will be enhanced by review of written reports and transcriptions provided from information stored on the device's cassette tapes or "electronic memory" modules.

□ MAINTENANCE CHECKLIST

The Food and Drug Administration Defibrillator Working Group issued a report on defibrillator failure and recommended actions for improvement. Table A3-1 lists activities that you should perform every shift, not only to be sure that the equipment is performing adequately but also to review mentally how to operate it.

□ MANUAL DEFIBRILLATION

Manual defibrillation must accurately record the heart rhythm and display that rhythm in a clear, understandable way. That display allows the EMT-D to interpret for ventricular fibrillation.

TABLE A3-1
Defibrillator Maintenance*

☐ Ensure that the unit is clean, with no signs of fluid spills and nothing stored on the unit.

☐ Check that two sets of defibrillator electrodes, in sealed packets, are available.

☐ Verify the presence and proper condition of all disposable supplies (conductive medium, monitor electrodes, recorder paper, recorder cassette, alcohol swabs, and razors).

☐ Check that defibrillator and monitor are plugged into a "life" outlet and that batteries are charging (where applicable).

☐ Turn on power to defibrillator and to monitor (if separate) and inspect all indicators, including charge light, energy display, power on, and monitor screen. (This check may require attachment to brand-specific simulators.)

☐ Where applicable, check that electrocardiographic recorder advances paper and that paper is present in sufficient amount.

☐ Verify that change/discharge cycle functions correctly and that rhythm analysis is operable by attaching electrodes to appropriate simulator. Check against normal sinus rhythm, ventricular fibrillation, asystole, and loose electrodes.

☐ For ventricular fibrillation, allow device to charge to lowest energy level and discharge into the test simulator. Check that all indicators are appropriate to each rhythm.

☐ Confirm presence of event documentation mechanism (depending on manufacturer, this may be tape cassette, solid-state memory module, or card), properly inserted, and that a spare is available. Check that tape recorder functions.

☐ Correct, when possible, simple problem (e.g., unplugged charger cord) or supply shortages.

☐ Report problems with an out-of-service unit to the individual responsible.

☐ Sign that unit is ready for clinical use.

Emergency Services Newsletter, September 1990, p. 3.

Cardiac monitor electrodes attached to the patient's chest record the heart rhythm and display it on a paper rhythm strip or a cardiac monitor screen. When the EMT-D observes the rhythm as ventricular fibrillation, the "charge" switch on the defibrillator is pressed to allow the power source to charge the capacitors. The EMT-D then presses the appropriate "discharge" or "shock" switches, which deliver the electrical countershock across the chest. The following defibrillation steps below should be followed:

1. Place the defibrillator near the patient's head when possible. This allows best access to the device controls and the patient.
2. Turn on the power control switch. The power switch activates the voice/ECG tape recorder.
3. Begin a verbal report of events. Identify yourself, describe the situation, and report each treatment step as it occurs. Do not delay treatment to give this report, however.
4. Attach the three monitor leads to the patient (Figure A3-10).
5. Clear the patient of all human contact. Stop CPR.

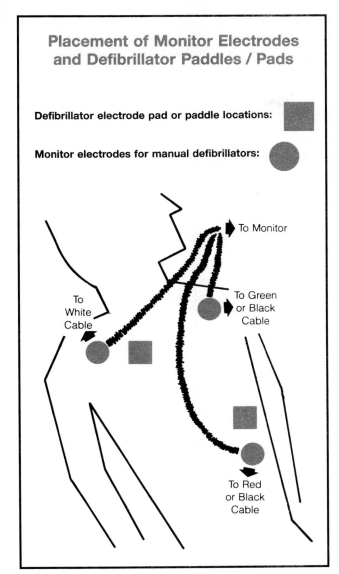

Placement of Monitor Electrodes and Defibrillator Paddles / Pads

Defibrillator electrode pad or paddle locations:

Monitor electrodes for manual defibrillators:

To Monitor

To White Cable

To Green or Black Cable

To Red or Black Cable

FIGURE A3-10

6. Review the ECG rhythm displayed on the monitor screen or the paper strip. Do *not* assess the ECG rhythm in a moving vehicle or while anyone is touching the patient.

7. Apply gel to the paddles, select the proper energy level, and charge the defibrillator. Make sure that no one is touching the patient by loudly and distinctively saying, CLEAR!.

8. Apply the defibrillator paddles to the chest in the proper position and press the shock delivery controls.

9. Identify that a shock has been delivered.

Continue CPR at all times, except during the assessment and treatment cycles.

☐ TROUBLESHOOTING

Defibrillation team members must learn to recognize the most common problems that can occur when treating cardiac arrest patients with a defibrillator. These include:

- Poor electrode contact on patient's chest. Sweaty (diaphoretic) patients need to be dried off with whatever is available. Extra sets of adhesive pads should be close at hand. Excessively hairy chests may need to be shaved with a small, disposable safety razor. Before placing electrodes, always be sure to remove anything on the surface of the patient's chest. This includes bandages, nitro paste patches, and other objects that will interfere with the placement or operation of the electrodes on the patient's skin surface. Place electrode pads away from nitro patches. Remove paste with a gauze pad or whatever works. A known pacemaker (see section blow) implanted in the patient's skin requires you to move the pad four to six inches away from the pacemaker site.

- Loose cable-electrode connections. Check to see that connectors are properly snapped into place. Always carry spare cables and electrodes.

- Monitor/cable movement. Excessive motion may be caused by patient movement during lifting, moving, and transport. Always stop the ambulance for rhythm analysis and defibrillation. This goes for all forms of patient transport, whether by stretcher, backboard, or gurney.

- Audio tape recorder. The cassette unit is the most frequent operational problem in everyday use of automated defibrillators using audiotape storage. Always check the tape drive (motor) operation and speed, and tape loading and unloading before the call.

- Error messages. Each AED will send specific error messages if problems arise or procedures are not being followed closely. These messages may be audio or visual signals, or both, depending on the device and the problem. Get to know the error messages unique to your AED, and learn how to react to them quickly and decisively through repeated practice and "problem" simulation.

- Cold. Battery-operated defibrillators are designed to operate within a defined temperature range — usually between 32° and 130° F. A defibrillator will typically deliver less than half of the total number of consecutive shocks at 32° F. than it would at 80° F.

- Wetness. The electrical charge used in the defibrillation is potentially lethal to anyone who interrupts the electrical pathway. Because of the risk of electrical shock to the operator or bystanders, defibrillators cannot be safely used near such obvious hazards as bathtubs, jacuzzis, pools, and flammable liquids and gases.

- Small, bony, or irregular chest preventing close contact with the monitor patches. Quickly move the leads to the arms or another portion of the chest.

- Dry or defective monitor patches. Monitor patches should be replaced when they become outdated, but in the meantime, apply a small amount of electrode gel under them.

- Muscle tremors. Dying patients often gasp irregularly (agonal respirations) or have involuntary muscle twitching. Sometimes you can assess rhythm between such respirations; if not, continue CPR untill the agonal respirations cease.

- Excessive electrical interference. You may need to unplug nearby appliances like electrical blankets, televisions, clocks, and radios. Fluorescent lights can also cause interference.

□ AICDS

Since 1982, more than 3,000 Americans have received Automatic Implantable Cardioverter Defibrillators (AICDs). The Food and Drug Administration approved implantation of these devices for those who have survived a sudden cardiac death episode resulting from ventricular tachycardia and/or ventricular fibrillation and those who have inducible ventricular dysrhythmias that cannot be controlled by medication.

The AICD monitors heart activity and countershocks a heart in fibrillation or tachycardia with the surgically implanted electrodes. The monitor is set to a specific cut-off rate; for example, 155 beats per minute for a predetermined period of time. Most devices are programmed to deliver the first shock at 25 to 30 joules within 10 to 35 seconds of recognizing the abnormal rhythm and rate. Most can deliver four to five shocks, monitoring the heart for normal sequences between hearts.

During your preliminary assessment, look for surgical scars on the chest. Also check the upper left quadrant of the abdomen for an AICD pulse generator and an implant scar. Check the patient's wrist for a Medic Alert bracelet. The patient should also be carrying in a wallet or purse a patient identification card which contains such important information as device cut-off rate, model, energy levels, physician's name and phone num-

ber, and the manufacturer's twenty-four-hour technical assistance number.

If the patient is conscious, allow the device to operate, stabilize the patient, and prepare him or her for transport. If the patient is unconscious, treat him or her as if he or she did not have the AICD, begin CPR, and prepare the patient for transport.

You should be aware that the AICD has an insulated backing that will deflect the current from your paddles. If your countershock is not successful, adjust the paddles slightly.

Your ECG unit will not show any visible sign of the AICD during its monitoring or charging modes; but when the AICD delivers a shock, it will overwhelm the ECG amplifiers and make the tracing move off the baseline.

No injury to anyone who is touching a patient with an AICD during the shock has ever been reported, but you may feel a slight buzzing sensation. Wearing rubber gloves may insulate you.

You should follow your local protocols. When in doubt, proceed as if the patient did not have an AICD.[1]

□ PRECAUTIONS

Defib team members must learn to recognize situations where it is *not* safe or appropriate to use the AED, or defibrillate.

The AED should *never* be used on a:

- Child less than twelve years old, or seventy-five to eighty pounds (approximately 30 kg). If this information is not known, follow your best judgment for approximating a child's age or weight, then consult medical control. Defibrillation is rarely required for small children in the prehospital setting, as they have a relatively low incidence of ventricular arrhythmias (rhythm disturbances).
- Conscious patient.
- Patient with an obstructed airway.
- Respiratory arrest patient (check pulse).

Sometimes local protocols will preclude defibrillation of trauma victim victims. Follow your local protocols regarding defibrillation of the trauma patient in cardiac arrest. This may depend on whether the cardiac arrest was the primary cause for the trauma in the first place, whether it was a result of the injury process, or whether this information can even be determined at the scene. Always check with medical control if in doubt.

---

[1] Rosemary Ziga, "Keeping pace," *Emergency*, February 1991, pp. 41–43.

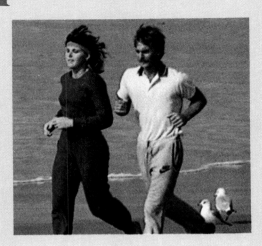

Maintaining a Healthy Lifestyle

✳ OBJECTIVES

- Define health and wellness.
- Discuss what a good health and wellness program is.
- List the health risks for EMTs.
- List and discuss the guidelines for a healthy lifestyle.

It is recommended that EMTs wear protective gloves whenever there is a possibility of coming in contact with a patient's blood, body fluids, mucous membranes, traumatic wounds, or sores. See Chapter 31.

☐ HEALTH AND WELLNESS

According to one estimate, life styles are responsible for 51 percent of reported health problems (Elswick et al., 1988.). As an EMT, your demanding profession exposes you to physically strenuous activities, emotional stress, and the risk of illness and/or injuries. Safeguarding your own health is an important part of your professional responsibility (Figure A4-1).

Wellness is more than the absence of illness. It's a positive state of "mental health, emotional health, physical health, social health, occupational health, and spiritual health in no order of priority" (Bruess and Richardson, 1989.). A healthy body that is strong, fit, and well nourished can resist disease and overcome injury. A positive attitude and the ability to deal realistically with daily demands — neither overreacting nor suppressing normal reactions — helps you combat stress and tension.

Tom Healey, Deputy Chief, Phoenix FD, and one of the major developers of the Health Center, discusses his feelings about the importance of wellness among EMS personnel:

The lifestyles of firefighters, paramedics, and EMTs are truly different than most people's lifestyles. Health problems, either mental or physical, tend to take their toll after a few years. I have seen positive, life-loving people, excited about their new career in pre-hospital care; in a few years, they can be very negative about

FIGURE A4-1 Certain occupations, such as firefighting and prehospital emergency care, involve tremendous physical stress.

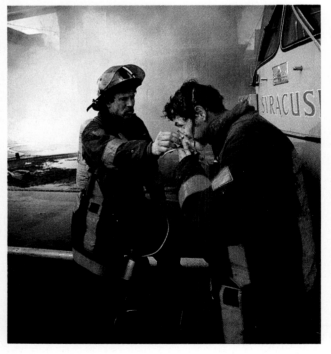

life. For years, emergency services have treated the victims, and being ordinary people, we become victims also.

Our department feels from the Fire Chief on down that health maintenance is as important to protecting life as a firefighter's self-contained breathing apparatus or protective clothing.

Health maintenance is a personal thing. People will not maintain their health if they don't want to. Stress tends to lower self-esteem and bring on depression. We have found fundamental health maintenance, education and motivation causes most of our members to want healthy lifestyles. This is the foundation of our program. (Healey).

A good wellness program emphasizes a total balance of lifestyle. Its purpose should be to promote good health and encourage self-competition, not to weed out personnel.

EMS personnel are often mandated by OSHA to have an annual physical exam. This has lead to the idea that physical fitness is all important. Physical fitness is one of only five dimensions of health, the others being social, mental, emotional and spiritual. The key is to develop the concept and practice of *total* health, not a mandatory fitness program.

EMS personnel learn to care so much for the *other* people that we often don't care enough for ourselves. We are intelligent decision makers, so education can become a motivator to pursue wellness and health maintenance. Stress management, safety practices, a strengthened immune system for greater disease resistance, and a more positive, aware personality are all results of a good wellness program.

Little research has been done on the health of EMTs, and much more needs to be done before we have accurate nationwide profiles and warning patterns. However, the results of one survey administered in November 1987 in Salt Lake City at the Eleventh Annual Prehospital Emergency Care and Crisis Intervention Conference to 346 area EMTs are worth sharing (Hawks, Hafen, and Karren, 1989). Although the results cannot safely be generalized outside the Utah-Idaho region, they provided interesting and informative results.

Fifty-three percent of the respondents were male and 47 percent were female; the average age for both sexes was thirty-six. Eighty-five percent were between the ages of twenty-five and forty-five. Eighty-two percent were EMTs, 10 percent were nurses, 4 percent were paramedics, and 4 percent had other professions. They had averaged 5.7 years as EMTs. Part of the survey focused on heart disease, assessing the respondent's risk for heart disease through a combination of such uncontrollable factors as sex, race, age, and family history, and such controllable factors as hypertension (about 140/80), cholesterol over 220, smoking, obesity, diabetes, and body type. No respondent was in the extremely high-risk group, and only one was high risk; 13 percent were in the lowest group, 31 percent were low risk, and the remaining 56 percent were average risk. These statistics showed that EMTs were knowledgeable and aggressive about lowering their risk of heart disease. Furthermore, 90 percent reported that they did not smoke, only 16 percent reported high blood pressure, and only 40 percent indicated that they possessed Type-A personalities. Significantly, since nearly half of all accidental deaths, suicides, and homicides are alcohol-related, 83 percent of the EMT respondents had one drink a week or less.

However, some warning signs also appeared. Thirty-one percent reported high-cholesterol diets, and 53 percent had blood cholesterol levels above 220. Forty-seven percent were fifteen pounds or more overweight; a full 10 percent were more than fifty pounds overweight. Only 20 percent indicated regular aerobic exercise. Breaking down the responses by gender shows that women reported more weight problems and men higher blood cholesterol levels, but there were no significant differences by gender in exercise or smoking.

Clearly, the EMTs in this this survey were aware of health-related issues; but equally clearly, they were far from being ideal models of good health habits.

☐ HEALTH RISKS FOR EMTS

Injury

Although little data exists on the rate of injury among EMTs, studies of firefighters may be illuminating. The number-one injury they suffer is lower back strain, with other musculoskeletal injuries like dislocations, fractures, shin splints, tendonitis, and joint/muscle soreness occurring less frequently (Phoenix, 1988). It seems reasonable that EMTs are susceptible to the same type of risk. They, like firefighters, must make physical exertions quickly in high-stress situations with little or no warm-up period. (Figure A4-2).

All EMTs have to lift — lift equipment, lift patients, lift debris out of the way, and so on. It is important that you function in a way that will make full use of your body's strength but minimize the risk of injuring your back. Back pain is the most common disability among adults under age forty-five; about 70 percent of the population in general will have back trouble; and the costs, according to the American Academy of Orthopedic Surgeons, may be as high as $16 billion annually. Over 200,000 people annually will have surgery, although it will fail completely in 20 percent of the cases; and in 40 percent of the "successful" cases, the patient will still have back pain (Schatz, 1988).

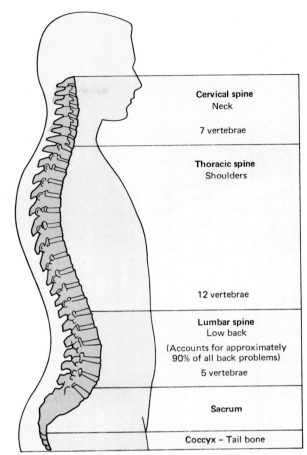

FIGURE A4-2 The number-one injury firefighters, and presumably EMTs, suffer from is lower back strain. Major regions of the spinal column are shown here. The lumbar spine is the area where pain is usually experienced.

Here are some simple guidelines for avoiding the most obvious causes of back trauma:

1. When you are lifting something, squat down rather than lean over, and then use the strength in your legs as you stand up. Do not twist. (Figures A4-3 and A4-4.)
2. Build flexibility and strength exercises into your physical fitness program so that you will not overestimate your ability to tackle physically strenuous jobs. If you have a tendency toward back problems, work with a physical therapist on a program of daily exercises that will keep your back limber and strong.
3. Whenever possible, warm up before working the muscles in your back hard.
4. Rest your back muscles when sitting by getting up to stretch or walk around. Also, sitting with your knees higher than your hips can reduce the pressure on your spinal discs. Other "resting" exercises are standing with one foot higher than the

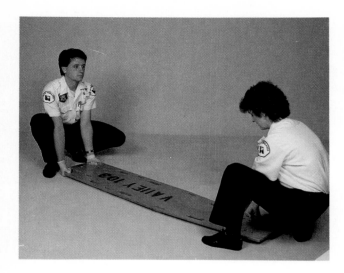

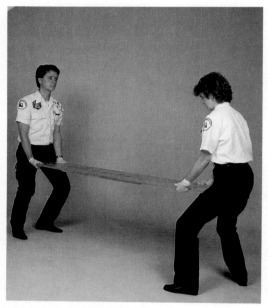

FIGURE A4-4 Use the strength in your legs as you stand up.

other (the "bar-rail" position) and shifting your weight frequently, or lying with pillows propped under your knees and your head to reduce the pressure on your lower back.

5. Be aware of your posture. Pull in your buttocks, tighten your abdominal muscles, keep your shoulders back, and keep your rib cage up. Don't arch your back.

See Figure A4-5 for a fifteen-minute exercise program to help keep limber.

The physical conditions of work often make it im-

possible to pace yourself. Interruptions to eating and sleeping can bring additional complications.

Working with others whom you respect and trust can provide a great emotional support; but difficulties with superiors or colleagues on the job can sometimes feel like the straw that breaks the camel's back.

For suggestions on dealing with emotional stress, see the section called "Learn to Manage Stress."

□ GUIDELINES FOR A HEALTHY LIFESTYLE

A recent report (Breslow and Enstrom, 1980) pinpoints health habits, rather than health status, as the keys to long life. The seven health habits that made the difference were never smoking, regular physical activity, moderate to no use of alcohol, seven to eight hours of sleep regularly, maintaining proper weight, eating breakfast, and not eating between meals.

At every age level between twenty and seventy, the study continues, people who had all seven habits lived "significantly longer" than those who followed only six. Men who were sixty or older and had followed all seven habits had better health than men of thirty who followed none to three of them.

The study also showed that men aged forty-five who practiced none to three of these habits could expect to live about sixty-six and one-half years. Those at forty-five who followed four or five could anticipate living to be seventy-three, and those who followed six or seven could expect to live to be seventy-five. (See Figure A4-7.)

Maintain a Fitness Program

An increasing number of EMS departments in major United States cities are making physical fitness programs a mandatory part of their training. They have discovered that the payoff in lower injury rates, less sick leave, and better morale make these programs worth the time they take.

Physical conditioning usually falls in three areas: cardiovascular conditioning, strength, and flexibility. Exercise that helps in one area will not necessarily increase ability in the other two areas, so it is wise to include a range of activities. (Figure A4-8)

1. Cardiovascular conditioning: The increased public attention given to cardiovascular conditioning in the past twenty years has made jogging a leading recreation in the United States and has generated literally hundreds of books on proper exercise. Although experts are far from having total consensus on ideal programs, most agree that conditioning requires at least thirty minutes of exercise three or

YOUR 15-MINUTE WORKOUT

By doing your 15-minute workout 3–5 times a week, you can condition the muscles and joints that support your back and keep it in healthy balance throughout the day. Strengthening exercises help build strong muscles, while stretching exercises increase flexibility. Begin each group of exercises from the starting position indicated, and follow the sequence shown. Try not to rush or strain. Relax and enjoy the feeling!

Before beginning a new exercise program, it's wise to check with your health care professional. (If you have back problems, you may need a medical evaluation). Don't do any exercise that causes pain.

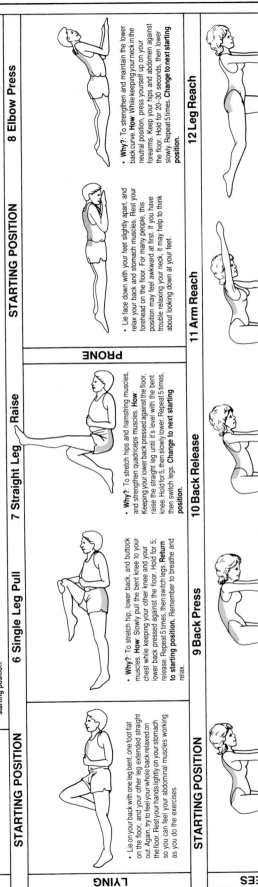

LYING

STARTING POSITION

- Lie on your back with your knees bent and feet flat on the floor. Try to feel your whole back on the floor. Breathe deeply, expand your lungs, and rest your hands on your pelvis. You should feel comfortable and relaxed.

1 Pelvic Tilt

- **Why?**: To stretch back muscles and strengthen stomach muscles. **How**: Tighten your abdomen and buttocks. Keep your abdomen and buttocks, pressing your lower back onto the floor (a small, subtle movement). Hold for a count of 5; release. Repeat 5 times. **Return to starting position.**

2 Lower Back Rotation

- **Why?**: To stretch and strengthen back rotation muscles. **How**: Drop both knees to one side while rotating your head to the opposite side. Hold for a count of 5. Repeat 10 times slowly alternating sides. **Return to starting position.**

3 Double Leg Pull

- **Why?**: To stretch your lower back and buttocks. **How**: Gently pull both knees to your chest. Hold for a count of 5. Repeat 5 times at first; gradually work up to 20 repetitions. **Return to starting position.**

4 Hip Lift

- **Why?**: To strengthen your buttocks. **How**: Without arching your back, slowly raise your hips upward. Keep a straight line from knees to shoulders. Hold for 5; lower. Repeat 5 times. **Return to starting position.**

5 Partial Curl-Ups

- **Why?**: To strengthen abdominal muscles. **How**: Cross your arms loosely, and tuck your chin in. Tighten your abdomen and curl halfway up directly in front of you. Hold for 5; curl down. Repeat 5 times. **Change to next starting position.**

LYING

STARTING POSITION

- Lie on your back with one leg bent, one foot flat on the floor, and your other leg extended straight out. Again, try to feel your whole back relaxed on the floor. Rest your hands lightly on your stomach so you can feel your abdominal muscles working as you do the exercises.

6 Single Leg Pull

- **Why?**: To stretch hip, lower back, and buttock muscles. **How**: Slowly pull the bent knee to your chest while keeping your other knee and your lower back pressed against the floor. Hold for 5; release. Repeat 5 times, then switch legs. **Return to starting position.** Remember to breathe and relax.

7 Straight Leg Raise

- **Why?**: To stretch hips and hamstring muscles, and strengthen quadriceps muscles. **How**: Keeping your lower back pressed against the floor, raise the straight leg until it's level with the bent knee. Hold for 5, then slowly lower. Repeat 5 times, then switch legs. **Change to next starting position.**

PRONE

STARTING POSITION

- Lie face down with your feet slightly apart, and relax your back and stomach muscles. Rest your forehead on the floor. For many people, this position may feel awkward at first. If you have trouble relaxing your neck, it may help to think about looking down at your feet.

8 Elbow Press

- **Why?**: To strengthen and maintain the lower back curve. **How**: While keeping your neck in the neutral position, press yourself up on your forearms. Keep your hips and abdomen against the floor. Hold for 20–30 seconds, then lower slowly. Repeat 5 times. **Change to next starting position.**

HANDS & KNEES

STARTING POSITION

- Switch to your hands and knees, keeping your knees directly under your hips and your hands directly under your shoulders. Keep your abdomen slightly firm, so that your spine stays in neutral. Allow your head to drop slightly keeping hands and knees still. Keep your neck relaxed in its natural curve so that your ears are aligned with your shoulders.

9 Back Press

- **Why?**: To strengthen abdominals and buttocks and stretch your back. **How**: Press your back upward by tightening your abdominal and buttock muscles. Allow your head to drop slightly keeping hands and knees still. Hold for a count of 5; return to starting position. Repeat 5 times. **Return to starting position.**

10 Back Release

- **Why?**: To stretch your back muscles. **How**: Allow your stomach and the muscles of your buttocks to relax and let your back sag. Be sure to keep your weight evenly distributed; don't sit back on your hips. Hold for a count of 5, then return to starting position. Repeat 5 times. **Return to starting position.**

11 Arm Reach

- **Why?**: To strengthen your shoulders and your upper back. **How**: Stretch one arm straight out in front of you. Don't raise your head, and be sure not to "sink" into your supporting arm. Hold for a count of 5; return to starting position. Repeat 5 times, then switch arms. **Return to starting position.**

12 Leg Reach

- **Why?**: To strengthen the muscles of your buttocks. **How**: Extend one leg straight out behind you and hold it parallel to the floor for a count of 5. Don't let your back, head, or stomach sag, and try not to arch your back. Return to starting position. Repeat 5 times, then switch legs. **Change to next starting position.**

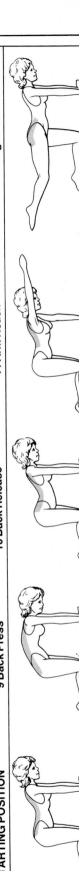
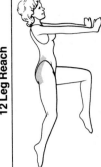

FIGURE A4-5

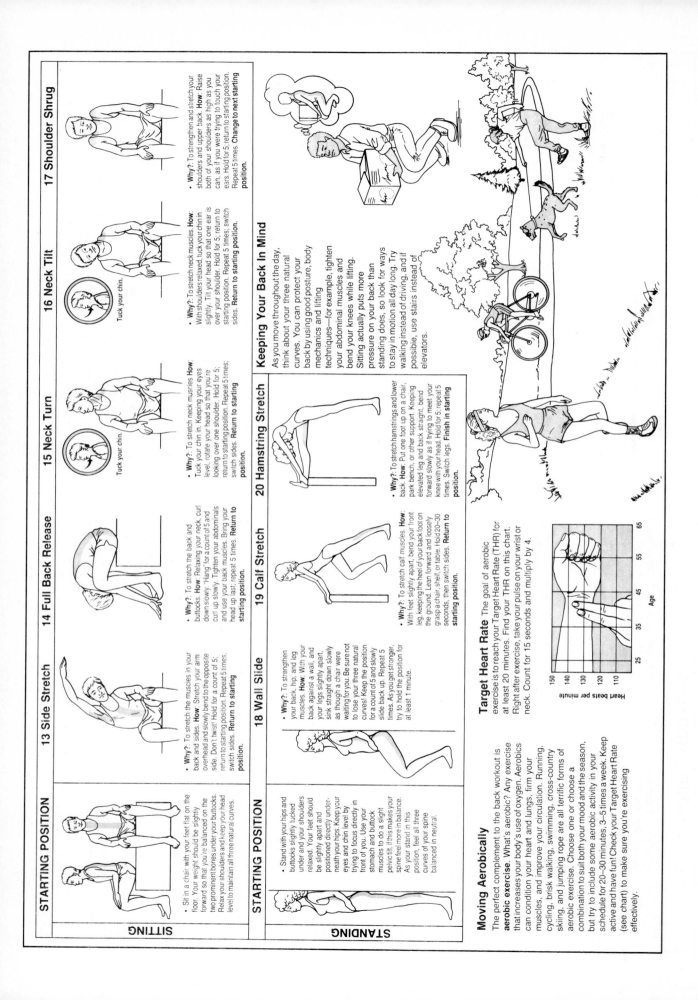

SITTING

STARTING POSITION

Sit in a chair with your feet flat on the floor. Your weight should be slightly forward so that you're balanced on the two prominent bones under your buttocks. Relax your shoulders and keep your head level to maintain all three natural curves.

13 Side Stretch

- **Why?**: To stretch the muscles in your back and sides. **How**: Stretch your arm overhead and slowly bend to the opposite side. Don't twist! Hold for a count of 5; return to starting position. Repeat 5 times. switch sides. **Return to starting position.**

14 Full Back Release

- **Why?**: To stretch the back and buttocks. **How**: Relaxing your neck, curl down slowly. "Hang" for a count of 5 and curl up slowly. Tighten your abdominals and use your back muscles. Bring your head up last; repeat 5 times. **Return to starting position.**

15 Neck Turn

Tuck your chin.

- **Why?**: To stretch neck muscles **How**: Tuck your chin in. Keeping your eyes level, rotate your head so that you're looking over one shoulder. Hold for 5; return to starting position. Repeat 5 times; switch sides. **Return to starting position.**

16 Neck Tilt

Tuck your chin.

- **Why?**: To stretch neck muscles. **How**: With shoulders relaxed, tuck your chin in slightly. Tilt your head so that one ear is over your shoulder. Hold for 5; return to starting position. Repeat 5 times; switch sides. **Return to starting position.**

17 Shoulder Shrug

- **Why?**: To strengthen and stretch your shoulders and upper back. **How**: Raise both of your shoulders as high as you can, as if you were trying to touch your ears. Hold for 5; return to starting position. Repeat 5 times. **Change to next starting position.**

STANDING

STARTING POSITION

Stand with your hips and buttocks slightly tucked under and your shoulders relaxed. Your feet should be slightly apart and positioned directly underneath your hips. Keep your eyes and chin level by trying to focus directly in front of you. Use your stomach and buttock muscles to do a slight pelvic tilt, if this makes your spine feel more in balance. As your stand in this position, feel all three curves of your spine balanced in neutral.

18 Wall Slide

- **Why?**: To strengthen your back, hip, and leg muscles. **How**: With your back against a wall, and your legs slightly apart, sink straight down slowly as though a chair were waiting for you. Be sure not to lose your three natural curves! Keep the position for a count of 5 and slowly slide back up. Repeat 5 times. As you get stronger, try to hold the position for at least 1 minute.

19 Calf Stretch

- **Why?**: To stretch calf muscles. **How**: With feet slightly apart, bend your front leg, keeping the heel of your back foot on the ground. Lean forward and loosely grasp a chair, shelf, or table. Hold 20–30 seconds, then switch sides. **Return to starting position.**

20 Hamstring Stretch

- **Why?**: To stretch hamstrings and lower back. **How**: Put one foot up on a chair, park bench, or other support. Keeping elevated leg and back straight, bend forward slowly as if trying to meet your knee with your head. Hold for 5; repeat 5 times. Switch legs. **Finish in starting position.**

Keeping Your Back In Mind

As you move throughout the day, think about your three natural curves. You can protect your back by using good posture, body mechanics and lifting techniques—for example, tighten your abdominal muscles and bend your knees while lifting. Sitting actually puts more pressure on your back than standing does, so look for ways to stay in motion all day long. Try walking instead of driving, and if possible, use stairs instead of elevators.

Moving Aerobically

The perfect complement to the back workout is **aerobic exercise**. What's aerobic? Any exercise that increases your body's use of oxygen. Aerobics can condition your heart and lungs, firm your muscles, and improve your circulation. Running, cycling, brisk walking, swimming, cross-country skiing, and jumping rope are all terrific forms of aerobic exercise. Choose one or choose a combination to suit both your mood and the season, but try to include some aerobic activity in your schedule for 20–30 minutes, 3–5 times a week. Keep active and have fun! Check your Target Heart Rate (see chart) to make sure you're exercising effectively.

Target Heart Rate

The goal of aerobic exercise is to reach your Target Heart Rate (THR) for at least 20 minutes. Find your THR on this chart. Right after exercise, take your pulse on your wrist or neck. Count for 15 seconds and multiply by 4.

Heart beats per minute

150 140 130 120 110

Age

25 35 45 55 65

Prevention of Cancer

Primary prevention refers to steps that might be taken to avoid those factors that might lead to the development of cancer

Smoking	Cigarette smoking is responsible for 85 percent of lung cancer cases among men and 75 percent among women—about 83 percent overall. Smoking accounts for about 30 percent of all cancer deaths. Those who smoke two or more packs of cigarettes a day have lung cancer mortality rates 15 to 25 times greater than nonsmokers.
Sunlight	Almost all of the more than 600,000 cases of nonmelanoma skin cancer diagnosed each year in the United States are considered to be sun-related. Recent epidemiologic evidence shows that sun exposure is a major factor in the development of melanoma and that the incidence increases for those living near the equator.
Alcohol	Oral cancer and cancers of the larynx, throat, esophagus, and liver occur more frequently among heavy drinkers of alcohol.
Smokeless tobacco	Use of chewing tobacco or snuff increases risk of cancer of the mouth, larynx, throat, and esophagus and is highly habit-forming.
Estrogen	For mature women, estrogen treatment to control menopausal symptoms increases risk of endometrial cancer. Use of estrogen by menopausal women needs careful discussion between the woman and her physician.
Radiation	Excessive exposure to ionizing radiation can increase cancer risk. Most medical and dental X-rays are adjusted to deliver the lowest dose possible without sacrificing image quality. Excessive radon exposure in homes may increase risk of lung cancer, especially in cigarette smokers. If levels are found to be too high, remedial actions should be taken.
Occupational hazards	Exposure to several different industrial agents (nickel, chromate, asbestos, vinyl chloride, etc.) increases risk of various cancers. Risk from asbestos is greatly increased when combined with cigarette smoking.
Nutrition	Risk for colon, breast, and uterine cancers increases in obese people. High-fat diets may contribute to the development of cancers of the breast, colon, and prostate. High-fiber foods may help reduce risk of colon cancer. A varied diet containing plenty of vegetables and fruits rich in vitamins A and C may reduce risk for a wide range of cancers. Salt-cured, smoked, and nitrite-cured foods have been linked to esophageal and stomach cancer. The heavy use of alcohol, especially when accompanied by cigarette smoking or chewing tobacco, increases risk of cancers of the mouth, larynx, throat, esophagus, and liver.

Source: *Cancer Facts and Figures*, 1990, p. 18.

FIGURE A4-6

four times a week that raises your pulse and breathing to a conditioning point. This point is determined by this formula: 220 minus your age times 60 percent. The resulting figure should be the minimum heart rate you want to achieve during exercise. Recommended forms of aerobic exercises include brisk walking (two to five miles daily), swimming (a good all-round exercise with little injury potential), jogging (be sure you warm up and cool down and have proper shoes to prevent injury), and bicycling. (This can also have the advantage of cutting down on some driving time. Be sure to use protective headgear and have proper reflectors and safely equipment on your bicycle.) Noncontact recreational sports such as handball, racquetball, basketball, and tennis are also good for aerobic conditioning.

2. Strength: Increased strength depends on increasing the power of a particular muscle group to overcome resistance. A weight-lifting program is the most specific and efficient way to concentrate on increasing your strength. To avoid straining or overtraining, conservative guidelines recommend exercising each major muscle group no more than three times a week and not on consecutive days, performing exercises slowly and deliberately with

HEALTH FACTORS
YOU CAN CONTROL

DIET
Eating sensible amounts of nutritious foods can improve your health and control weight.

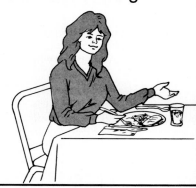

EXERCISE
The right kind and amount of exercise promotes healthy heart, lungs, and muscles; helps control weight and relieve stress.

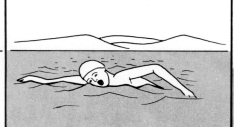

REST
Many physicians recommend 7 to 8 hours of sleep each night for good health.

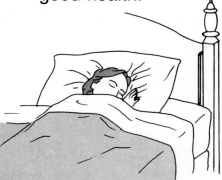

STRESS
Stress can cause physical and emotional problems, but it can be managed and its effects controlled.

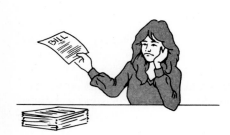

BAD HABITS
Avoiding both smoking and drug and alcohol abuse can help prevent serious illness.

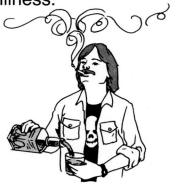

ATTITUDE
An optimistic outlook can be the first step toward lasting wellness.

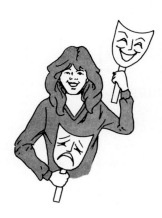

FIGURE A4-7

Table 15.2 Activities Comparison

Although no single activity gives you complete fitness benefits, most exercises provide benefits in the areas of strength, flexibility, and aerobic capacity. This table provides a quick comparison between 16 popular activities in these areas. If your favorite activity provides lower-than-average benefits in one or more areas, you will have to supplement your program with exercises or programs designed to improve fitness in the areas your activity lacks.

Activity	Aerobic Capacity	Upper Body Strength	Lower Body Strength	Flexibility
Aerobic dancing	♡ ♡ ♡ ♡ ♡	●—●	●—●—●	🌿🌿🌿
Basketball	♡ ♡ ♡	●—●	●—●—●	🌿🌿
Bicycling	♡ ♡ ♡ ♡ ♡	●—●—●	●—●—●—●	🌿🌿
Brisk walking	♡ ♡ ♡ ♡	●—●	●—●—●	🌿🌿
Cross-country skiing	♡ ♡ ♡ ♡ ♡	●—●—●—●—●	●—●—●—●—●	🌿🌿🌿
Downhill skiing	♡ ♡ ♡	●—●—●	●—●—●—●	🌿🌿🌿
Gymnastics	♡ ♡ ♡	●—●—●—●	●—●—●—●	🌿🌿🌿🌿🌿
Jazz dancing	♡ ♡ ♡	●—●	●—●—●	🌿🌿🌿
Jogging	♡ ♡ ♡ ♡ ♡	●—●	●—●—●	🌿🌿
Marital arts (Aikido/ Tai Chi)	♡ ♡ ♡ ♡	●—●—●—●	●—●—●—●	🌿🌿🌿
Racquetball/handball	♡ ♡ ♡ ♡	●—●—●—●	●—●—●—●	🌿🌿
Soccer	♡ ♡ ♡ ♡ ♡	●—●	●—●—●	🌿🌿
Softball	♡	●—●	●—●	🌿🌿
Swimming	♡ ♡ ♡ ♡ ♡	●—●—●—●—●	●—●—●—●—●	🌿🌿🌿🌿🌿
Tennis	♡ ♡ ♡ ♡	●—●—●—●	●—●—●	🌿🌿
Volleyball	♡	●—●—●	●—●—●	🌿

5 = superior benefits; 4 = above-average benefits; 3 = average benefits
2 = below-average benefits; 1 = poor or no benefits

Your fitness program should provide average or above-average benefits in two or more areas. Remember that to obtain aerobic benefits, you must be able to sustain your target heart rate continuously for 20 to 25 minutes.

SOURCES: Charles B. Corbin and Ruth Lindsey, *Fitness for Life* (Dallas: Scott, Foresman, 1979); and Charles B. Corbin, Linus J. Dowell, Ruth Lindsey, and Homer Tolson, *Concepts in Physical Education*, 3rd ed. (Dubuque, IA: Wm. C. Brown, 1978).

FIGURE A4-8

ample recovery time between each, and performing all exercises through a full range of motion to maintain flexibility and prevent soreness. It is also important to breathe in while lifting and breathe out while lowering to avoid creating excessive pressures in the chest cavity and hampering the flow of blood back to the heart (Phoenix, 1989). (See Figure A4-9.)

Although strength-training equipment such as Nautilus and Universal has the advantage of providing structure and sequence to a program, it is also quite possible to carry on a full program without weights by using your own body weight to provide the resistance. Activities would include stepping up a stair or onto a box or sturdy chair twelve or fifteen inches high, jumping as high as possible from a standing position, push-ups, sit-ups, leg curls, pull-ups, pushing yourself away from a wall, and so on. (Hoeger, 1986).

3. Flexibility is the ease with which your joints and muscles can move through a range of motion. Being properly warmed up can increase your flexibility by as much as 20 percent (Hoeger, 1986). During warm-up and cooling-down periods, exercises that stress flexibility will help prevent strain and rupture. There are many books, exercise programs, and physical therapies to increase flexibility, but they all rely on the basic technique of stretching a particular muscle group to a point just short of pain and holding it for ten seconds or so. Do not bounce, jerk, or hyperextend. Our muscles have a built-in protective reflex that causes them to contract when they reach the point of extending dangerously far, and bouncing will actually cause a muscle to contract, sometimes so vigorously that it can spasm. It is important to build flexibility exercises into your fitness program for another reason, as the Phoenix Fire Department manual

Maintaining a Healthy Lifestyle

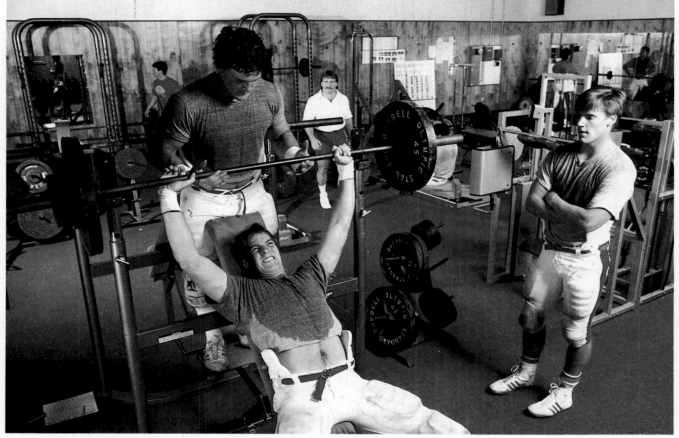

FIGURE A4-9 Weight training, which is now practiced by people in many fields, is an effective way to increase muscular strength.

notes: "We normally will not have time to warm up before an emergency. The fact is we need to be in better condition than the professional athlete." (See Figure A4-10.)

Manage Your Nutrition and Weight

Nutrition

A healthy diet consists of sensible amounts of nutritious foods. You feel better, stay in charge of your weight, resist illness, and heal more quickly from injuries. According to the U.S. Department of Agriculture's "Dietary Guidelines for Americans," the ideal is "to maintain a balanced and varied diet that provides the nutrients essential to good health, and to increase consumption of complex carbohydrates and fiber while decrease consumption of fat, sugar, sodium, and alcohol" (Hawks, Hafen, and Karren, 1989). No one food or food group supplies all of the nutrients you need, so select a variety of foods.

Disease

It is significant that cardiovascular disease is currently the leading cause of on-the-job deaths among firefighters (Phoenix, 1988).

It is also surprising to learn that the cancer rate for firefighters soared from 18 percent in 1950 to 38 percent in 1980. Since 1950, the average age of death from cancer for firefighters dropped from age forty-nine to forty-four (Phoenix, 1988). Since the three leading cancers were throat, mouth, and lung (all about 200 times the normal rate), it seems reasonable that exposure to carcinogens in the firefighting environment may have something to do with these diseases, and that EMTs who are not firefighters may not be at higher risk than the general population. For information on cancer prevention, see Figure A4-6.

EMTs are also at higher risk than the general population of contracting infectious diseases. Patients who cough or sneeze toward you pose a risk of infecting you. In fact, so does contact with any body fluid — saliva, sputum, blood, urine, vomit, and fecal matter. A punc-

Rate Your Fitness Level

This short group of fitness tests can be completed in 30 minutes or less. If you are over 40 or have chronic medical disorders such as diabetes or obesity, check with your physician before taking this or any other test. You will need a stopwatch, a 12-inch bench or stepladder, a horizontally hung bar for the arm-hang test, a yardstick, some adhesive tape, and another person to monitor your test and keep time.

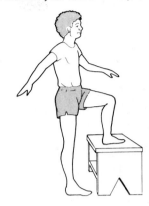

Aerobic capacity: 3-minute step test

Equipment: 12-inch bench, crate, or stepladder stopwatch (metronome if possible).

Procedure: Face bench. Step 24 steps per minute (metronome set at 96) up, up, down, down, for 3 minutes. (Up, up, down, down = 1 step). After finishing, sit down, find pulse within 5 seconds. Take pulse for 1 minute.

Score: pulse rate for 1 minute.

Scoring Standards (heart rate for 1 minute)

Age	18–29		30–39		40–49		50–59		60 +	
Sex	F	M	F	M	F	M	F	M	F	M
Excellent	<80	<75	<84	<78	<88	<80	<92	<85	<95	<90
Good	80–110	75–100	84–115	78–109	88–118	80–112	92–123	85–115	95–127	90–118
Average	>110	>100	>115.	>109	>118	>112	>123	>115	>127	>118

Abdominal and low back strength

Equipment: stopwatch.

Procedure: Lie flat on upper back, knees bent, shoulders touching the floor, and arms extended completely at sides, palms down. Mark a line at the ends of the fingertips. Mark another line 3 inches forward (toward the feet) of the first mark. Bend knees so that feet are flat and 12 inches from the buttocks. Curl up by lifting head and shoulders off the floor, sliding hands toward second mark. Keep hands of floor. Curl down and repeat.

Score: number of curls in 1 minute. (Partner holds feet).

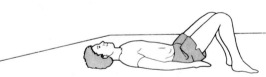 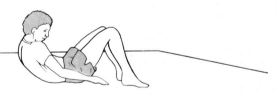

FIGURE A4-10

ture wound from a needle contaminated by the patient's blood or other body fluid constitutes a "*significant exposure* risk to treatment personnel" (City of Phoenix, 1988).

It makes sense to wear gloves, masks, and eye protection when appropriate and wash hands for ten seconds (minimum) after dealing with each patient (City of Phoenix, 1988). At least one fire department routinely vaccinates its personnel with Heptavax vaccine against hepatitis-B (Pedrotti, 1986).

Emotional Stress

There is no question that stress can jeopardize your health. A partial list of stress-related symptoms range from life-threatening to minor irritants, including can-

Scoring Standards

Age	18–29		30–39		40–49		50–59		60+	
Sex	F	M	F	M	F	M	F	M	F	M
Excellent	>45	>50	>40	>45	>35	>40	>30	>35	>25	>30
Good	25–45	30–50	20–40	22–45	16–35	21–40	12–30	18–35	11–25	15–30
Average	<25	<30	<20	<22	<16	<21	<12	<18	<11	<15

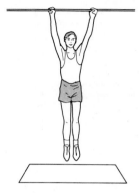

Upper body strength: arm hang

Equipment: horizontal bar hung high enough so your feet don't touch the floor, stopwatch.

Procedure: Hang with straight arms, palms facing away from you. Start watch when in position. Stop timing when person drops.

Score: number of minutes and seconds.

Scoring Standards (minutes and seconds)

Age	18–29		30–39		40–49		50–59		60+	
Sex	F	M	F	M	F	M	F	M	F	M
Excellent	>1:30	>2:00	>1:20	>1:50	>1:10	>1:35	>1:00	>1:20	>:50	>1:10
Good	:46–1:30	1:00–2:00	:40–1:20	:50–1:50	:30–1:10	:45–1:35	:30–1:00	:75–1:20	:21–:50	:30–1:10
Average	<:46	<1:00	<:40	<:50	<:30	<:45	<:30	<:35	<:21	<:30

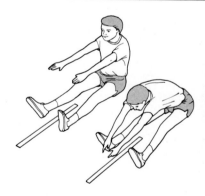

Hamstring flexibility: Sit and reach

Equipment: yardstick, adhesive tape.

Procedure: Sit with legs straight and heels about 5 inches apart. Tape yardstick to floor so that the 15-inch mark is even with heels. Slowly stretch forward, stretching fingertips on yardstick.

Score: number of inches.

FIGURE A4-10 *continued*

cer, heart attacks, high blood pressure, adult diabetes, tension headaches, muscle tension, sleeplessness, stomach disturbances, skin eruptions, virus infections, blurred vision, chronic fatigue, confusion, inability to concentrate, irritability, and explosive anger.

Emotional stress for EMTs comes from a variety of sources. Each call has the potential of bringing you in contact with people who are in pain and whose lives are often at risk. The conscientious attempt to meet those needs in a professional way and to communicate with the patient in an empathic manner without being overwhelmed by fear and pain is stressful. As a human being, you carry away the images of people like yourself, of children like your own, of older people like your parents who are sometimes trapped, helpless, wounded, or dying.

Sit and Reach Scoring Standards (inches)

Age	18–29		30–39		40–49		50–59		60 +	
Sex	F	M	F	M	F	M	F	M	F	M
Excellent	>22	>21	>22	>21	>21	>20	>20	>19	>20	>19
Good	17–22	13–21	17–22	13–21	15–21	13–20	14–20	12–19	14–20	12–19
Average	<17	<13	<17	<13	<15	<13	<14	<12	<14	<12

Upper body strength: push-ups (men)

Equipment: stopwatch.

Procedure: Assume a front-leaning position. Lower body until chest touches floor. Raise and time; repeat 1 minute.

Score: number of pushups in 1 minute.

Upper body strength: push-ups (women)

Equipment: stopwatch.

Procedure: Assume a front-leaning position with knees bent, hands under shoulders. Lower chest to floor, raise, and repeat.

Score: number of pushups in 1 minute.

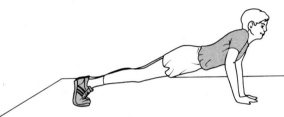

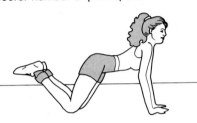

Scoring Standards (number in 1 minute)

Age	18–29	30–39	40–49	50–59	60 +
Excellent	>50	>45	>40	>35	>30
Good	25–50	22–45	19–40	15–35	10–30
Average	<25	<22	<19	<15	<10

Scoring Standards (number in 1 minute)

Age	18–29	30–39	40–49	50–59	60 +
Excellent	>45	>40	>35	>30	>25
Good	17–45	12–40	8–35	6–30	5–25
Average	<17	<12	<8	<6	<5

FIGURE A4-10 *continued*

Our 1987 survey of Utah-Idaho EMTs had mixed results in the category of nutrition and diets — with almost 65 percent showing room for significant improvement. On the positive side, over 75 percent trimmed visible fat from meat products; 85 percent drank low-fat or skim milk; 50 percent reported three or more servings daily of complex carbodydrates (although 53 percent ate white bread, rather than whole-grain bread); more than 80 percent regularly ate green cabbage-family vegetables and foods rich in vitamin A; and two thirds passed up cake-and-ice-cream desserts in favor of something with lower calories. However, 50 percent regularly ate deep-fried foods; 75 percent ate butter, cream cheese, or margarine; 35 percent ate the skin of chicken; nearly 64 percent chose snacks that were high in sodium, sugar, or fat (chips, nuts, or cookies); and 61 percent failed to eat an adequate breakfast (Hawks, Hafen, and Karren, 1989).

Here are some general guidelines for sensible nutrition. If you have specialized needs — such as low fat, high fiber, or low cholesterol — consult your physician. (See Figure A4-11.)

1. Choose daily from the four basic food groups:
   - Milk: Low-fat or non-fat milk products will still give you needed protein and calcium but less fat. Two servings per day are recommended for adults.
   - Vegetables and fruits: Daily choose a citrus fruit or juice, a raw vegetable or fleshy fruit like apples or pears, and a cooked green or yellow veg-

Maintaining a Healthy Lifestyle **757**

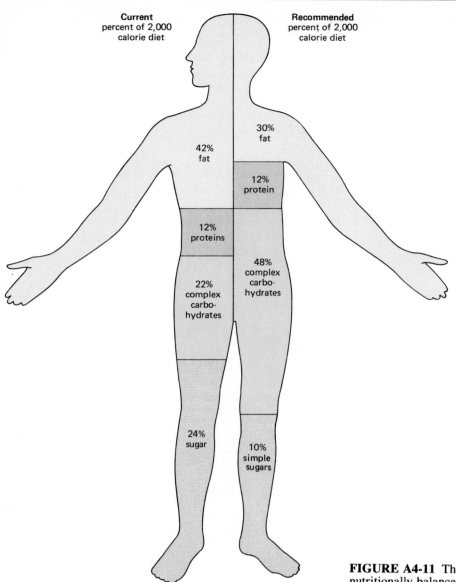

Current
percent of 2,000
calorie diet

Recommended
percent of 2,000
calorie diet

30%
fat

42%
fat

12%
protein

12%
proteins

48%
complex
carbo-
hydrates

22%
complex
carbo-
hydrates

24%
sugar

10%
simple
sugars

FIGURE A4-11 This figure contrasts a recommended, nutritionally balanced diet with a "typical" American diet.

etable. This food group also contains essential vitamins and minerals and the complex carbohydrates that supply energy.

- Protein: This group not only includes such traditional sources as eggs, fish, and meat, but also such vegetarian sources of protein as peanut butter, dried beans, lentils, and tofu. Two servings a day are usually considered adequate for an adult to supply the recommended 30 percent of your daily calories (Phoenix, 1989). Fish and poultry (without the skin) are lower in cholesterol and fats than red meat.

- Breads and cereals: Bread, cereals, and pasta are traditional foods from this group. Choose whole-grain breads, brown rice, and whole-wheat or spinach pastas for better nutrition. Hot

breakfast cereals like oatmeal are also good ways to get the three or four servings daily that you need from this group. This group supplies needed carbohydrates (as much as 60 percent of your calories should come from this group [Phoenix, 1988]). These foods are also high in fiber, which will reduce your risk of obesity, diabetes, CHD, cavities, periodontal disease, constipation, varicose veins, hemorrhoids, colon spasm, appendicitis, and large bowel cancer (Phoenix, 1988).

2. Cut down on sugar or its relatives — honey, sucrose, or corn syrup. Canned fruit, prepared breakfast cereals, and baked goods often contain surprisingly high amounts of sugar. Sugar provides high calories but low nutrition, thus displacing more important foods. It promotes tooth decay

and may be linked to hyperactivity, heart disease, and vitamin depletion — which means that it drains the vitamins stored in the body (Bruess and Richardson, 1989).

3. Avoid excessive salt, which can raise blood pressure levels. Read the labels to determine whether salt has been added to canned, frozen, and processed foods.

4. Watch your cholesterol intake. Fatty foods, especially fatty red meats, fried foods, dairy products, butter, and margarine, are often offenders. Fat is essential to your diet — about 10 percent of your caloric intake should be in the form of fat (Phoenix, 1989) — but saturated fats have highly undesirable side effects.

5. Be sure you drink enough water. Water carries food to cells, carries wastes away, regulates our body temperatures, and lubricates our joints. Our bodies are between 65 and 75 percent water. The recommended intake for an adult who is not engaged in strenuous work or in a hot environment is one-and-a-half quarts daily. It makes sense to pass up soft drinks, coffee, and tea, with their sugar and caffeine, in favor of a fruit or vegetable juice — or just plain water! Another argument against using a soft-drink as a snack or pick-me-up is that it linked with hypoglycemic symptoms — lack of energy and afternoon "blahs." The reason is that "when high concentrations of refined sugar are consumed without vegetables, complex carbohydrates, or proteins, the body produces a high amount of insulin, which moves the sugar into the cells for energy. The sugar is quickly used up, leaving the insulin but little sugar in the bloodstream. Consequently, the insulin, which would normally be working on the slower digested proteins, fats, and complex carbohydrates, causes hypoglycemic symptoms in the body" (Bruess and Richardson, 1989).

6. You should monitor your intake of caffeine. Caffeine, like other drugs, is addictive. Instant coffee contains about 65 mg per six ounces, while drip coffee may be as high as 180 mg. Soft-drinks containing caffeine range from 30 to 60 mg per twelve-ounce can. Caffeine doses of between 200 and 500 mg can produce "abnormally rapid heart, abnormal heart rhythms, increased blood pressure, birth defects, increased body temperature, and increased secretion of gastric acids leading to stomach problems" (Hoeger, 1989).

See Figure A4-12 for an overall guide to good eating.

Weight Management

Obesity is no favor to your body. Not only does each pound of fat give your heart a work-out that it doesn't need, it can also result in back problems. A paunchy abdomen pulls your lower spine forward. Excess body weight, even if it is well distributed, means increased pressure on the lumbar disks. ("Put Your Disk Problems Behind You," 1990). Excessive weight also reduces the body's ability to dissipate heat and increases strain on your joints and muscles. According to the 1988 Surgeon General's report on nutrition, "diseases of dietary excess and imbalance" contribute to coronary heart disease, stroke, atherosclerosis, diabetes, and cancer, which together accounted for more than two-thirds of all deaths in the United States" (Hoeger, 1989). (See Figure A4-13.)

Will Rogers reportedly once observed, "There are only two things that cause people to become overweight — chewing and swallowing; and the best exercise for losing weight is pushing yourself away from the table." A professional weight-management program may help you set up new eating habits and maintain them during the always-difficult adjustment period; but the role of will power cannot be overestimated, and it seems clear that exercise and diet must work together in controlling weight (Figure A4-14).

Literally hundreds of books are available on diet and nutrition. Avoid programs that aim primarily at weight loss. The goal here is lifestyle change, not a short-term change. Also avoid gimmicks.

> *Research . . . has shown that there is no such thing as spot reducing or losing "cellulite" from certain body parts. Cellulite is nothing but plain fat storage. . . . Other common fallacies regarding quick weight loss relate to the use of rubberized sweatsuits, steam baths, and mechanical vibrators. When an individual wears a sweatsuit or steps into a sauna, there is a significant amount of water (and not fat) loss. . . . As soon as you replace body fluids, the weight comes back quickly. Wearing rubberized sweatsuits not only increases the rate of body fluid loss, which is vital during prolonged exercise, but it also increases core temperature. Dehydration as a result of these methods leads to impaired cellular function and in extreme cases even death. Similarly, mechanical vibrators are worthless in a weight control program. Vibrating belts and turning rollers may feel good, but they require no effort whatsoever on the part of the muscles. Fat cannot be "shaken off"; it has to be burned off in muscle tissue (Hoeger, 1989).*

Bad eating habits are sometimes aggravated by personality traits like eating to relieve stress or boredom, for instance, or by such physical conditions as candy vending machines in the hallway, over-hurried lifestyles that lead to the consumption of convenience foods, and "social" eating. (See Figure A4-15.)

GUIDE TO GOOD EATING

Every day eat a wide variety of foods from the Four Food Groups in moderation.

You don't have to be a nutrition expert to eat for good health. The GUIDE TO GOOD EATING makes it easy. Even if you're watching your weight, looking for ways to cut back on fat or sodium, or trying to eat more fiber, this plan can work for you. Just follow the simple steps below.

Step 1—Eat foods from all Four Food Groups every day.

Foods from the Four Food Groups—Milk, Meat, Fruit-Vegetable, and Grain—can supply the more than 40 nutrients your body needs to stay healthy. Foods in each food group are good sources of different nutrients. That's why it's important to eat foods from all Four Food Groups every day.

Step 2—Include a wide variety of foods.

Foods within a food group are usually good sources of the same nutrients. But some foods are better sources of a particular nutrient than others. By eating different foods within each food group, you have a good chance of getting all the nutrients you need.

- Explore the dairy case. Try new milks, cheeses, and yogurts from the Milk Group.
- Experiment with new recipes for beef, chicken, fish, eggs, and dried beans from the Meat Group.
- Find creative ways to include foods from the Fruit-Vegetable Group. Add spinach, carrots, broccoli, mushrooms, and green pepper to your salads.
- Enjoy new tastes from the Grain Group. Try bagels, tortillas, or rye, pita, or cracked-wheat bread for sandwiches.

Step 3—Practice moderation.

By practicing moderation you can get the nutrients you need without getting too many calories or too much fat or sodium.

- Eat at least the recommended number of servings from each food group every day.
- Watch how many servings you have from the "Others" category.
- Eat foods in the serving sizes listed below.

Special Tips

If you are concerned about calories, fat, sodium, or fiber, choose foods from the Four Food Groups. Try the following:

To cut down on fat and calories:
- Begin by limiting high-fat foods from the "Others" category like salad dressings, mayonnaise, chips, cookies, cakes, and doughnuts.
- Use cooking methods that add little or no fat like baking, roasting, poaching, stir frying, steaming, and broiling.
- Choose skim, 1% or 2% milk; lowfat or nonfat yogurt; lowfat cottage cheese; and lowfat cheeses like part-skim mozzarella.
- Select leaner cuts of meat and trim off excess fat.

To limit sodium:
- Season food with herbs and spices instead of high-sodium items like salt, soy sauce, or steak sauce.
- Choose fresh rather than canned vegetables, fish, and meats.
- Look for prepared foods that say low- or reduced-sodium on the label.

To increase fiber:
- Eat fresh fruits and vegetables with their skins.
- Select whole grain breads, bran cereals, and brown rice.
- Include dried beans and peas.

No matter what your dietary goal, it all comes down to one simple rule of thumb: *Every day eat a wide variety of foods from the Four Food Groups in moderation.*

	Serving Size		Minimum Recommended Number of Servings*					Comments
			Children 1-10	Teenagers and Young Adults 11-24	Adults 25+	Pregnant Women	Breastfeeding Women	
Milk Group	1 cup / 1 cup / 1 oz / 1/2 cup / 1/2 cup	Milk / Yogurt / Cheese / Cottage cheese† / Ice cream, ice milk, frozen yogurt†	3	4	2	4	4	†Good sources of calcium such as milk, yogurt, and cheese are recommended daily. Cottage cheese, ice cream, ice milk, and frozen yogurt have about 1/4 to 1/3 the amount of calcium per serving as milk, yogurt, and cheese.
Meat Group	2-3 oz / 1 / 1/2 cup / 2 tbsp / 1/4 cup	Cooked, lean meat, fish, poultry / Egg‡ / Cooked, dried peas, dried beans‡ / Peanut butter‡ / Nuts, seeds‡	2	2	2	3	2	‡Eggs, dried beans, and peanut butter have about 1/2 the amount of protein per serving as meat.
Fruit-Vegetable Group	1/2 cup / 1/2 cup / 1 medium / 1/2 / 1/4 / 1/4 cup	Juice / Vegetable, fruit / Apple, banana, orange / Grapefruit / Cantaloupe / Dried fruit	4	4	4	4	4	Dark green, leafy, or orange vegetables and fruit are recommended 3 or 4 times a week for vitamin A. Good sources of vitamin C such as oranges, strawberries, tomatoes, potatoes, and green peppers are recommended daily.
Grain Group	1 slice / 1/2 / 1 oz / 1/2 cup / 1	Bread / English muffin, hamburger bun / Ready-to-eat cereal / Pasta, rice, grits, cooked cereal / Tortilla, roll, muffin	4	4	4	4	4	Whole grain, fortified, or enriched grain products are recommended.
Combination Foods	1 cup / 1 cup / 1/8 15" / 1	Soup / Macaroni and cheese, lasagna, stew, chili, casserole / Pizza / Sandwich, taco	These count as servings (or partial servings) from the food groups from which they are made.					Combination Foods supply the same nutrients as the foods they contain.
"Others" Category	1 oz / 2 / 1/16 9" / 1 tsp / 12 oz / 1 tsp / 1 tbsp	Potato chips, pretzels / Cookies / Layer cake / Sugar, jelly / Soft drink, beer / Margarine, butter / Salad dressing, mayonnaise	There is no recommended number of servings for foods in the "Others" category.					"Others" don't take the place of foods from the Four Food Groups in supplying nutrients. And they are often high in fat or calories.

*These servings provide the nutrients your body needs. They also supply about 1200 Calories. However, most people need more than 1200 Calories. If you do, add more servings.

FIGURE A4-12

GUIDE TO GOOD EATING

Every day eat a wide variety of foods from the Four Food Groups in moderation.

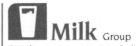**Milk** Group

Supplies many nutrients including:
- calcium
- protein
- riboflavin

2 servings for adults
3 servings for children
4 servings for teenagers, young adults, and pregnant or breastfeeding women

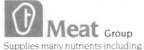**Meat** Group

Supplies many nutrients including:
- protein
- iron
- niacin
- thiamin

2 servings for all ages
3 servings for pregnant women

Fruit-Vegetable Group

Supplies many nutrients including:
- vitamin A
- vitamin C

4 servings for all ages

Grain Group

Supplies many nutrients including:
- carbohydrate
- iron
- thiamin
- niacin

4 servings for all ages

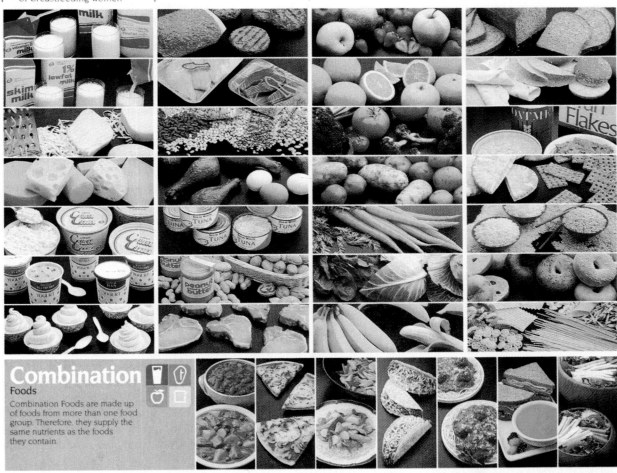

Combination
Foods

Combination Foods are made up of foods from more than one food group. Therefore, they supply the same nutrients as the foods they contain.

"Others"
Category

Foods in the "Others" category are often high in calories and/or low in nutrients. They don't take the place of foods from the Four Food Groups in supplying nutrients.

Condiments
Barbeque sauce
Catsup, mustard
Olives, pickles
Salt
Soy sauce

Chips and Related Products
Corn chips
Popcorn
Potato chips
Pretzels
Tortilla chips

Fats and Oils
Coffee whitener
Cream, sour cream
Gravy, cream sauce
Margarine, butter
Mayonnaise
Oil, lard, shortening
Salad dressing

Sweets
Brownies, cookies
Cakes, pies
Candy
Jelly, jam
Sugar, honey, syrup
Sweet rolls, doughnuts

Alcohol
Beer
Gin, vodka
Whiskey, rum
Wine

Other Beverages
Coffee, tea
Fruit-flavored drinks
Soft drinks

ISBN 1-55647-001-0

FIGURE A4-12 *continued*

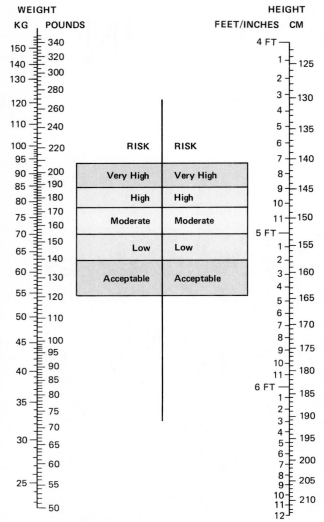

WEIGHT			HEIGHT	
KG	POUNDS		FEET/INCHES	CM

RISK   RISK

Very High	Very High
High	High
Moderate	Moderate
Low	Low
Acceptable	Acceptable

FIGURE A4-13 Are you overweight? To find out if your current level of fatness increases your chances of dying before your time, use the chart. Angle a pencil or the edge of a piece of paper from your weight (on the left) to your height (on the right). Read your risk where the pencil crosses the center line.

Stop Smoking

If a new drug were to suddenly be proposed by a company for acceptance by the Food and Drug Administration, and that drug was shown to contain some 3,000 toxic chemicals, would double the risk of a fatal heart attack, would make the risk of death from chronic obstructive lung disease six times greater among users, make the risk of dying from lung cancer ten times greater among users, and it was known that this new drug contributed to over 300,000 deaths a year in the U.S., there is little question that the drug would not approved for consumer use. Yet those devastating effects are clearly established for tobacco smokers today (Bruess and Richardson, 1989). No one says it better

than C. Everett Koop, former Surgeon General of the United States: "There is no serious debate about the hazards of cigarette smoking. It is the chief avoidable cause of death in this country. It is a 'disease' which each year is costing us billions of dollars in economic loss as well as much human suffering" (Bruess and Richardson, 1989). One study shows that the average age of smoking heart-attack victims is ten years less than that of nonsmokers (Phoenix, 1988). It is also a leading cause of lung cancer, emphysema, chronic bronchitis, and stroke.

But the decision to stop smoking is easy compared to actually quitting. Various commercial programs are available which report high success rates. Depending on your particular physiology and personality profile, one of these programs may be right for you; but they are expensive, and their success rates are not usually tested by scientific follow-ups.

A general help is sticking with your physical conditioning program. Aerobic exercise puts you in touch with your body's needs for a well-functioning cardiovascular system in a way that makes smoking lose some of its appeal.

Additional helps are getting rid of reminders like ashtrays and matches, avoiding the places where you usually smoke, such as parties or bars, changing your routine to avoid situations where you almost automatically light up — such as having a cigarette with coffee or after meals — and joining a support group. Substitute activities — playing with a pencil or chewing gum — sometimes provide the gratification that a cigarette used to supply.

Control Alcohol Consumption

Alcohol and other drugs can also work against your well-being. The Phoenix, Arizona Fire Department, which has a mandatory fitness program, offers the guidelines of no more than two drinks in any twenty-four hour period (Phoenix, 1989). Alcohol abuse can intensify your risk of heart disease, some kinds of cancer, liver and brain damage, ulcers, and gastritis. It is also a major factor in deaths from car accidents (Figure A4-16).

It is encouraging that, in our 1987 survey of Utah-Idaho EMTs, only 4 percent scored in the category that indicated high addictive potential when the national level of addiction is estimated at 30 percent by the designers of the test (Hawks, Hafen, and Karren, 1989).

To avoid alcohol abuse, avoid social situations that encourage excessive drinking. Never drive after drinking. If you find yourself drinking alone or drinking to escape, face up to these signs of alcohol dependence and get help through your physician or through Alcoholics Anonymous.

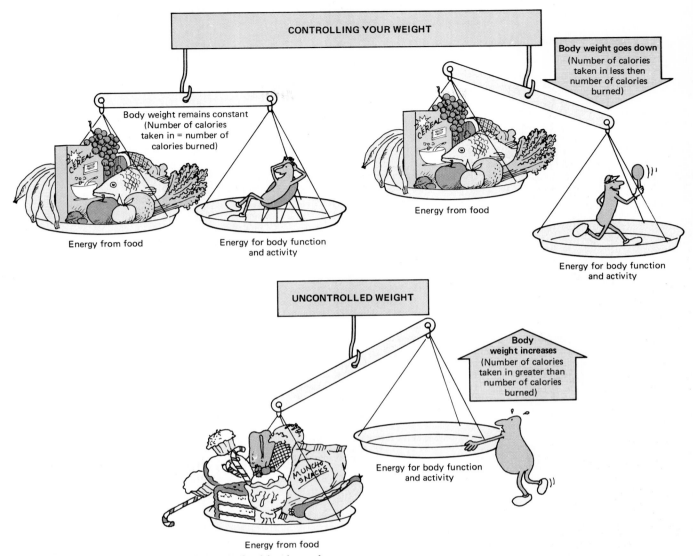

FIGURE A4-14 The relationship between food intake and calories burned.

Learn to Manage Stress

It is impossible, and not desirable, to avoid all stress, and probably some stress is actually necessary. However, prolonged and mismanaged stress can aggravate or cause many medical problems, among them fatigue, headaches, cramps, depression, heart disease, ulcers, and colitis. If you have a Type-A personality, you are at greater risk for heart disease, because stress-released hormones damage arteries. Individuals with Type-A personality typically speak and move rapidly, hold feelings in, have few interests outside work, are precise and numbers-oriented, find it difficult to relax, are excessively time-conscious, seek approval from others, are usually engaged in multiple tasks with impossible deadlines, and are continually hurried and overscheduled.

Another health risk stemming from your personality that can be controlled through stress management is your anger threshold. Hostility and anger may, according to current research, be the Type-A personality traits most responsible for increased heart disease. Our 1987 study of Utah-Idaho EMTs showed that 14 percent of the respondents fell into the safe zone, 53 percent were average, and an alarming 33 percent were in the high (or dangerous) category. According to the test's designers, the average score should be about seventeen for women and eighteen for men, and only 25 percent of the average respondents could be expected to score in the high zone. Our respondents' scores were about 18.5 for women and 18.6 for men (Hawks, Hafen, and Karren, 1989).

Smoking is a sure way to damage your health; it contributes to about one death in seven in the U.S. The main harmful effects come from nicotine, carbon monoxide, and tar. The first two contribute to heart disease, whereas tar causes lung disease and cancer.

Nonsmoker
— Cilia
Cells lining airways

Smoker
Smoke particles
Extra mucus produced

Nonsmoker
Bronchiole
Blood capillaries
Alveoli

Smoker
Coalesced alveoli

How smoking damages the lungs
Smoke particles irritate the lung airways, causing excess mucus production (top right). They also indirectly destroy the walls of the lungs' alveoli, which coalesce (above left and right). Both factors reduce lung efficiency. In addition, tar in tobacco smoke has a direct cancer-causing action.

FIGURE A4-15 How cigarette smoking damages the lungs.

FIGURE A4-16 Alcohol and society.

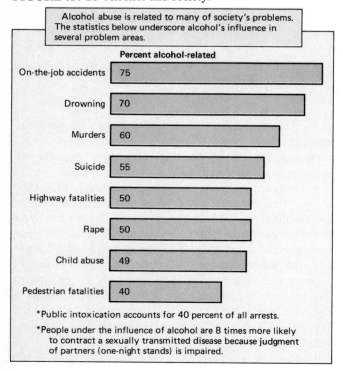

Alcohol abuse is related to many of society's problems. The statistics below underscore alcohol's influence in several problem areas.

Percent alcohol-related

On-the-job accidents	75
Drowning	70
Murders	60
Suicide	55
Highway fatalities	50
Rape	50
Child abuse	49
Pedestrian fatalities	40

*Public intoxication accounts for 40 percent of all arrests.

*People under the influence of alcohol are 8 times more likely to contract a sexually transmitted disease because judgment of partners (one-night stands) is impaired.

You probably already know that eating a balanced nutritional diet and getting exercise regularly are both excellent ways of controlling and managing stress. Here are some guidelines to help you manage stress effectively:

1. Be realistic. Plan your work to let you use your time and energy most effectively. Set practical goals and don't try to do too much. Evaluate your capabilities and achievements wisely. Give yourself credit for what you are achieving. If you are genuinely trying to do too much, reduce the burden rather than trying to increase your speed. Ask for help if the workload seems overwhelming. Learn to delegate and say no.

2. Manage change. Even a positive change in your life — like a marriage, the birth of a child, or moving to a new home — brings stress with it. Avoid making too many major changes too close together and build in adjustment periods.

3. Get another perspective on things to help you keep your own perspective. If you see a problem devel-

MANAGE STRESS

Pressures, demands and worries that make you feel tense are facts of life. The key is to keep them within manageable limits.

Some stress can be good, but too much can **INTERFERE** with your normal activities and contribute to **MANY MEDICAL PROBLEMS** — some serious. For example: fatigue, headaches, cramps, prolonged depression, heart disease, ulcers and colitis can result from stress.

Steps you can take to **PROTECT YOURSELF AGAINST STRESS**

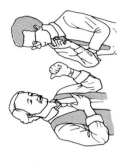

BE REALISTIC

Set practical goals — don't expect the impossible. Try not to tackle too much at one time.

LIMIT CHANGES

Avoid making too many major changes in your life at one time. Allow an adjustment period for each change.

TALK IT OVER

Discuss problems with the people involved, or with a close friend, before tensions build up.

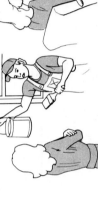

PLAN YOUR WORK

Organize your workload to use time and energy efficiently. Ask for help if workload seems overwhelming.

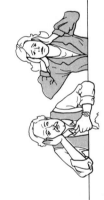

LEARN TO RELAX

Taking short breaks, weekend getaways, vacations, can help. Take a class in yoga or meditation. Doing something to relax every day is highly recommended. Regular exercise helps, too.

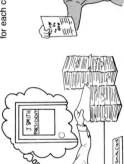

IMPROVE YOUR ENVIRONMENT

Rearrange your office, redecorate your apartment, etc. — little changes can help you feel in control and give you a lift.

SEEK PROFESSIONAL HELP

Don't ignore physical symptoms of stress. Consult your physician for treatment, advice or referral.

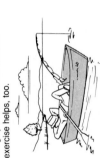
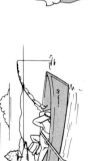

FIGURE A4-17

765

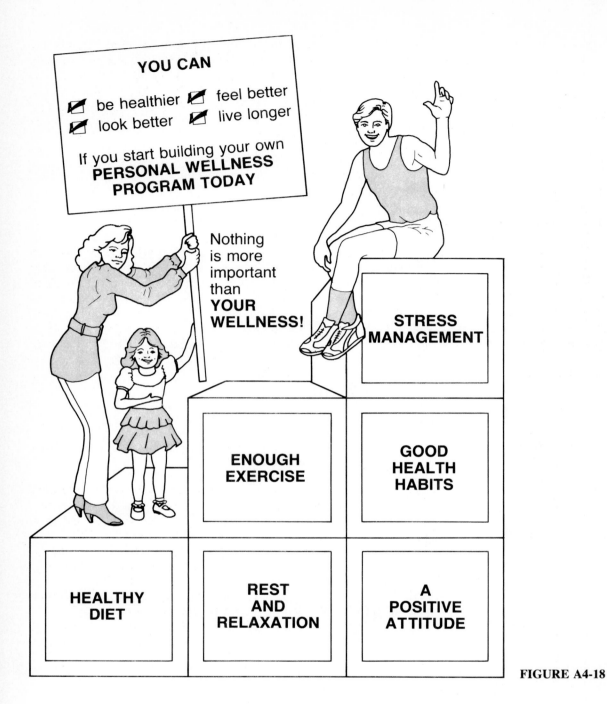

YOU CAN

☑ be healthier ☑ feel better
☑ look better   ☑ live longer

If you start building your own
**PERSONAL WELLNESS
PROGRAM TODAY**

Nothing is more important than **YOUR WELLNESS!**

STRESS MANAGEMENT

ENOUGH EXERCISE

GOOD HEALTH HABITS

HEALTHY DIET

REST AND RELAXATION

A POSITIVE ATTITUDE

FIGURE A4-18

oping at work, talk it over with the people involved. For personal difficulties, find a trusted friend or family member to whom you can "unload" who will not feel it necessary to burden you with advice. If you find that stress is prolonged or starting to cause emotional and physical symptoms, seek professional help from a counselor.

4. Build positive experiences into your life. Meditation or guided imagery that you can do for a few minutes every day will recharge your batteries. Plan time and give yourself permission to do pleasant things for yourself every day. You deserve the relaxation that comes from short breaks, weekend getaways, or vacations. Do not let the pressure of events intrude into this "reward" time for yourself. For many people, a physical conditioning program provides these needed pleasant experiences.

5. Improve your environment. Often when external events seem to weigh heavily upon you, small but deliberately chosen improvements that lift your spirits. Wash your car. Rearrange your office. Clean out your closet or desk. Cleanliness and order can boost your morale and cost nothing.

6. Learn to relax completely. Sometimes when you are keyed up, even falling sleep will not dissipate built-up tension. Being able to relax not only improves your rest but lets you deal quickly and effectively with tension during your work day. Again, many books are available on various relaxation techniques, but nearly all of them share a few basic principles: In a calm environment where you can sit comfortably, close your eyes and concentrate on breathing slowly and evenly. When the rhythm is established, concentrate on relaxing each muscle in your body. To still your mind, repeating a word or syllable as you breathe will reduce the number of distracting thoughts. Usually ten to twenty minutes of this exercise will yield good results. Some people can do a relaxation procedure on a bus. Others, just by establishing a breathing rhythm and concentrating on relaxing for a few seconds, can break a cycle of tension that is developing.

See Figure A4-17 for further tips on managing stress.

□ CONCLUSION

Whole books have been written on each of these aspects of a healthy lifestyle. Obviously, this chapter only touches the highlights. Much of wellness is listening to the messages from your own body and responding appropriately. Eating sensibly, getting enough exercise, taking reasonable precautions, and making a nutritious diet are not hard to do — and the rewards of working towards wellness pays rich personal as well as professional dividends.

□ BIBLIOGRAPHY

Breslow, Lester, and James E. Enstrom. "Persistence of Health Habits and Their Relationship to Mortality," *Preventative Medicine 9* (1980): 469–83.

Bruess, Clint E., and Glen E. Richardson. *Decisions for Health*. (2nd ed.). Dubuque, Iowa: William C. Brown Publishers, 1989.

City of Phoenix Fire Department. *Standing Operating Procedures*. 1988.

Elswick, Stephen A., et al. "Mandatory Physical Fitness: A Research Project for the National Fire Academy." *MIS Report 20* (August 1988).

Hawks, Steven R., Brent Q. Hafen, and Keith J. Karren. "How Does Your Health Rate?" *JEMS*, March 1989, pp. 46–51.

Healey, Tom. Personal communications.

Hoeger, Werner W. K. *Lifetime Physical Fitness and Wellness*. Englewood, Colorado: Morton Publishing Company, 1989.

Phoenix Fire Department Health/Fitness Manual. December 1988.

Pedrotti, Dean. "Heptavax: A Shot in the Arm for Health." *Firehouse*, November 1986, pp. 76–77.

"Put Your Disk Problems Behind You." *Prevention*, June 1990, 67–125.

Schatz, Mary Pulling. "Living with Your Lower Back." *Yoga Journal*, 1988.

☐ Glossary of Terms

A

Abandonment: a termination of an EMT-patient relationship by the EMT without consent of the patient and without care to the patient by qualified medical providers.

ABD dressings: one of many names for large, thick-layered, bulky pads used for quick application to stem profuse bleeding.

Abdominal aortic aneurysm: an aneurysm of the abdominal aorta, which is the continuation of the thoracic aorta.

Abdominal breather: a patient whose chest does not seem to move during respiration, but his abdomen does.

Abdominal cavity: the space bounded by the abdominal walls, the diaphragm, and the pelvis; contains most of the organs of digestion.

Abdominal evisceration: injuries in which abdominal organs are exposed.

Abdominal thrust: the Heimlich maneuver; the manual thrusts delivered to the abdominal region between the navel and xiphoid process to create pressure to help expel an airway obstruction.

Abdomino-pelvic cavity: the large body cavity below the diaphragm and above the pelvis.

Abduct: to draw away from the midline.

Abduction: the act of abducting; the state of being abducted.

Abortion: the premature expulsion from the uterus of the products of conception, the embryo, or of a nonviable fetus.

Abrasion: a scraped or scratched skin wound.

Abruptio placenta: premature separation of a normally implanted placenta from the uterine wall, usually with massive hemorrhage, occurring during the third trimester of pregnancy.

Abscess: a swollen, inflamed area of body tissue in which pus collects.

Absence attacks: a common name for petit mal seizures.

Absorption: passage of a substance through a membrane into blood.

Abstinence syndrome: a complex of signs and symptoms caused by nonuse of a substance to which the body has been habituated.

Acceleration-deceleration injury or accident: injury caused by the sudden acceleration and deceleration of the head as the brain is slapped back and forth by the skull and then rebounds.

Acetabulum: the cup-shaped cavity on the external surface of the innominate bone in which the rounded head of the femur fits.

Acetaminophen: pain reliever used as an aspirin substitute as it is less likely to cause gastric irritation.

Acetone: a colorless liquid found in small quantities in normal urine and in larger amounts in diabetic urine; a metabolic end product of the use of fat for routine energy needs.

Acidosis: an abnormal state of the body in which the pH falls below 7.35; excessive amounts of carbon dioxide (respiratory acidosis) and lactic and organic acids (metabolic acidosis) produce the acidotic state.

ACLS: see Advanced Cardiac Life Support.

Activated charcoal: powdered charcoal that has been treated to increase its powers of adsorption; used as a general-purpose antidote.

Acute: having rapid onset, severe symptoms, and a relatively short duration.

Acute abdomen: a term indicating the presence of some abdominal process that causes the sudden irritation of the peritoneum and intense pain.

Acute radiation syndrome: a progressive illness with predictable stages, but a wide variety of symptoms which may or may not occur after exposure to radiation.

Adam's apple: the projection on the anterior surface of the neck, formed by the thyroid cartilage of the larynx.

Addiction: the state of being strongly dependent upon some agent; drugs, tobacco, for example.

Adduction: the act of adducting; the movement of a part toward the midline of the body.

Adhesions: the growing together of normally separate tissues; the fibrous bands connecting such tissues.

Adipose tissue: fatty tissue.

Adrenal glands: the small gland on the superior aspect of the kidney; produces corticosteroids, catecholamines, and other hormones.

Adrenlin: the proprietary name for epinephrine.

Advanced cardiac life support (ACLS): the use of adjunctive equipment, cardiac monitoring, defi-brillation, intravenous lifeline, and drug infusion.

African sleeping sickness: tropical African disease, a form of trypanosomiasis, caused by some protozoa and spread by the bite of the tsetse fly, characterized by recurrent fever, drowsiness, often fatal.

Afterbirth: the placenta and membranes expelled after the birth of a child.

Agonal respirations: irregular gasping respirations, sometimes heard in dying patients.

Agoraphobia: "fear of the marketplace," a phobia which renders its victims terrified of leaving the safety of their own home.

AIDS: acquired immune deficiency syndrome; a fatal disease first noted in 1978 and caused by a virus. It is spread through direct contact with the blood, semen, or oral secretions of infected individuals.

AIDS-related complex: an AIDS-like illness that does not fit the rigid standards that the Center for Disease Control has established for diagnosing AIDS.

Airbags: installed in some vehicles, they are self-inflating on impact.

Air splints: a double-walled plastic tube that immobilizes a limb when sufficient air is blown into the space between the walls of the tube, to cause it to become almost rigid.

Airway: the route for passage of air and/or gases into and out of the lungs.

Alcoholic: pertaining to or containing alcohol; also a person who becomes habituated, dependent, or addicted to alcoholic consumption.

Alcoholism: addiction to alcohol; overuse that affects the individual's health and social functioning.

Alimentary canal or tract: the tubular passage that extends from mouth to anus and functions in digestion and absorption of food and elimination of residual waste.

Alkaline: having a pH greater than 7.0; in human physiology, having a pH greater than 7.35.

Alkalosis: a condition of an increase in base (alkaline).

Alpha particle: a positively charged nuclear particle consisting of two neutrons and two protons; ejected from the nucleus of a radioactive atom.

Alveolar pouch: terminal air sac of the lung.

Alveolus: a cavity; specifically, the socket

holding a tooth; or a terminal air sac of the lung.

Alzheimer's disease: associated with the elderly, but can affect younger people; causes confusion, emotional depression, irritability, and violence between lucid intervals.

Ambulance cots: adaptable cots carried in ambulances; there are three basic types.

Ambulatory: able to walk.

Amino acids: an organic acid in which one of the hydrogen atoms has been replaced by a molecular amine group, the chief component of protein.

Ammonia: an agent frequently used in pesticides, medications, and common household products.

Amnesia: loss of memory.

Amniotic fluid: the fluid surrounding the fetus in the uterus, contained in the amniotic sac.

Amniotic sac: a thick, transparent sac that holds the fetus suspended in the amniotic fluid.

Amputation: complete removal of an appendage.

Anaphylactic shock: an exaggerated allergic reaction with severe bronchospasm and vascular collapse, which may be rapidly fatal.

Anatomy: the structure of the body, or the study of body structure.

Anemia: the condition in which the blood is deficient in hemoglobin, red blood cells, or in total volume.

Anesthesia: a partial or complete loss of sensation with or without loss of consciousness; can result from drug administration or from injury or disease.

Anesthetic: without feeling.

Aneurysm: a permanent blood-filled dilation of a blood vessel resulting from disease or injury of the blood vessel wall.

Angina pectoris: a spasmodic pain in the chest, characterized by a sensation of severe constriction or pressure on the anterior chest; associated with insufficient blood supply to the heart; aggravated by exercise or tension and relieved by rest or medication.

Angiocath: the Deseret trade name for an intravenous cannula with a Teflon catheter over the metallic needle; has become a generic name for such a device.

Anorexia: loss of hunger or appetite.

Anoxia: without oxygen; a reduction of oxygen in body tissues below required physiology levels.

Antabase: trademark for a preparation of disulfiram, a drug used by alcoholics to assist in decreasing alcohol dependence; produces a breath odor similar to alcohol.

Antecubital space: the depression in the anterior region of the elbow.

Antepartum: before delivery.

Anterior: situated in front of, or in the forward part of; in anatomy, used in reference to the ventral or belly surface of the body.

Anterior chamber (of the eye): the space filled with aqueous humor between the cornea and the iris.

Anterior compartment syndrome: rapid swelling, increased tension, pain, and ischemic necrosis of the muscles of the anterior tibial compartment of the leg.

Antibodies: substances produced in the body in response to an antigen that destroys or inactivates the antigen.

Anticoagulants: a class of drugs that prevents clotting of blood.

Antidote: a substance used to counteract the effects of a drug or combat the effects of a poison.

Antihistamines: a drug that helps counteract the effects of allergic-type reactions.

Antiseptic: any preparation that prevents the growth of bacteria.

Anxiety: a feeling of apprehension, uncertainty, and fear.

Aorta: the largest artery in the body, originates at the left ventricle and terminates at the bifurcation of the iliac arteries.

Aortic semilunar valve: the valve at the outlet of the left ventricle into the aorta; prevents blood return to the heart from the aorta.

Apex: the peak, top or highest point.

Apgar scoring system: a method developed by Dr. Virginia Apgar for assessing the newborn infant at one minute of age by designating a score of 0, 1, or 2 for the following: A = appearance; P = pulse rate; G = grimace; A = activity; and R = respiration.

Aphonic: loss of voice.

Apical pulse: pulse taken from the apex of the heart; observed by placing the stethoscope under the left breast.

Apnea: absence of respiration.

Appendage: any subordinate organ or external part, for example, a leg, arm.

Appendicitis: inflammation of the vermiform appendix.

Aqueous humor: the limpid, water fluid that fills the space between the cornea and the lens of the eye.

Arachnoid: resembling a spider's web; the middle membrane of the three meninges that surround the brain and spinal cord.

Arcing injury: a burn caused when an electric current jumps from one surface to another.

Arrhythmia: disturbance of heart rate and rhythm; abnormal heart rhythm.

Arterial emboli: clots or other plugs brought by the blood from another artery and forced into a smaller one, thus obstructing the circulation.

Arterial pulse (pressure) points: points where an artery passes over a bony prominence or lies close to the skin; at these points the artery can be palpated and the arterial pulse taken.

Arterial system: all of the arteries considered together

Arteries: a blood vessel, consisting of three layers of tissue and smooth muscle, that carries blood away from the heart.

Arteriole: a small artery that at its distal end leads into a capillary.

Arteriosclerosis: a generic name for several conditions that cause the walls of the arteries to become thickened, hard, and inelastic.

Articulate: to unite to form a joint.

Artificial ventilation: movement of air into and out of the lungs by artificial means.

Aseptic: sterile; free of bacteria.

Asphyxia: suffocation; a condition characterized by hypercarbia and hypoxemia.

Aspiration: to inhale materials into the lungs.

Asthma: a condition marked by recurrent attacks of dyspnea with wheezing due to spasmodic construction of the bronchi, often as a response of allergens, or by mucous plugs in the bronchioles.

Asystole: lack of any electric or muscular activity in the heart; lack of a heartbeat.

Ataxic: failure of muscular coordination; often used to describe a staggering gait.

Atherosclerosis: a common form of arteriosclerosis caused by fat deposits in arterial walls.

Atria: either of the two upper chambers on each side of the heart that receive blood from the veins and in turn force it into the ventricles.

Atrial fibrillation: disorganized, ineffective quivering of the atria, causing an irregular, often rapid ventricular heart rate.

Atrial flutter: beating of the atria up to rates of 300 per minute note associated with equal beating of the ventricles.

Atrioventricular node: a cluster of specialized cells that retard the passage of the atrial stimulus toward the ventricles, allowing the atria to complete their contraction; located near the junction of the atrial septum with the ventricular septum, next to the septal leaflet of the tricuspid valve.

Auger: farm equipment, a boring tool.

Aura: a premonitory sensation of impending illness, usually used in connection with an epileptic attach.

Auricle: the external ear; ear flap; also atrium.

Auscultate: to listen.

Autoclave: an apparatus using steam under pressure for sterilization.

Autonomic discharge: a response from the autonomic nervous system which may stimulate any of the following: glands, cardiac muscle, smooth muscles.

Autonomic nervous system: part of the nervous system concerned with the regulation of bodily functions not controlled by conscious thought; composed of the sympathetic and parasympathetic systems.

Autopsy: the detailed examination of a body after death to determine cause of death.

AV node: atrioventricular node.

Avulsion: an injury that leaves a piece of

skin or other tissue either partially or completely torn away from the body.

Axilla: the armpit.

B

Back blows: sharp blows delivered with the EMT's hand over the patient's spine between the scapulae to relieve upper airway obstruction.

Backboard: *see* Spineboard.

Bacteria: sometimes called germs; a kind of microorganism; many bacteria cause disease.

Bactericide: an agent capable of killing bacteria.

"Bad trip": a drug episode resulting in a state of intense anxiety or panic.

Bag of waters: the amniotic sac and its contained amniotic fluid.

Bag-valve-mask: a portable artificial ventilation unit consisting of a face mask, one-way valve, and an inflatable bag; producing positive pressure ventilation.

Bandage: a material used to hold a dressing in place.

Bandage compress: a folded cloth or pad used for applying pressure to stop hemorrhage or as a wet dressing.

Barbiturates: a class of drugs that produce a calming, sedative effect.

Barotrauma: injury to the tissues of the body's air cavities from a failure to equalize internal pressure with changing ambient pressure.

Basic life support: maintenance of the ABCs (airway, breathing, and circulation) without adjunctive equipment.

Basilic vein: a large vein of the upper arm on the inner side of the biceps muscle.

Basilar skull: the base or basal part of the skull.

Basket stretcher: also called Stokes litter; shaped like a basket.

Battery: physical contact with a person's body or clothing without consent.

Battle's sign: a contusion on the mastoid process of either ear; sign of a basilar skull fracture.

Bends: pain in the limbs and abdomen occuring as a result of bubbles of nitrogen in the blood; caused by too rapid decompression; caisson disease; decompression sickness.

Beta particles: electrons, either positively charged (positron) or negatively charged (negatron), that are emitted during beta decay of a radionuclide.

Betadine: trademark for an antiseptic ointment containing povidone and iodine.

Biceps muscle: the large muscle of the front part of the arm that bends the forearm at the elbow; also, one of the hamstring muscles located on the back of the thigh that flexes and rotates the knee.

Bicuspid valve: one of the four heart valves, it lies between the left atrium and left ventricle of the heart.

Bilateral: on two or both sides.

Bile ducts: the tube which carries bile from the confluence of the hepatic and cystic ducts to the duodenum.

Biological death: present when irreversible brain damage has occurred, usually after 4-10 minutes of cardiac arrest.

Bipolar disorder: sometimes called manic-depressive disorder, causes a patient to swing to opposite sides of the spectrum.

Birth canal: the vagina and the lower part of the uterus.

Black eye: a discoloration of the skin or flesh around an eye, resulting from a sharp blow or contusion.

Bladder: an organ of the urinary system located in the pelvis just behind the pubic bone, which stores urine produced by the kidneys.

Blanket drag: *see* Drag.

Bleeder: in surgery, a small blood vessel that is bleeding profusely; also, a hemophiliac patient.

Bloated: distended with gas.

Blood clots: *see* Clot.

Blood pressure: the pressure exerted by the pulsatile flow of blood against the arterial walls.

Blood volume: the total amount of blood in the heart and blood vessels; represents 8 to 9 percent of body weight in kilograms.

Bloody show: the mucous and bloody discharge signaling the beginning of labor.

"Blue bloater": a patient with chronic bronchitis.

Blunt trauma: injury caused by impact of a blunt object, such as a rounded stone, in contrast to that caused by a sharp object such as a knife.

Botulism: food poisoning caused by *Clostridium botulinum* toxin.

Bounding pulse: unusually strong pulse.

Brachial artery: the artery of the arm that is the continuation of the axillary artery, that in turn branches at the elbow into the radial and ulnar arteries.

Brachial pulse: pulse produced by compressing the major artery of the upper arm; used to detect heart action and circulation in infants.

Bradycardia: abnormal condition where the heart rate is very slow, below 50 beats per minute.

Bradypnea: abnormal slowness of respiration, specifically a low respiratory frequency.

Brain: organ in the skull that controls all bodily functions and is the seat of consciousness.

Brain stem: the stem-like portion of the brain that connects the brain with the spinal cord; includes the pons, medulla, and mesencephalon.

Breech birth: the delivery during which the presenting part of the fetus is the buttocks or foot instead of the head.

Bronchi: the main branches of the trachea carrying air into various parts of the lung; also called bronchial tubes.

Bronchiolitis: a condition seen in children under 2 years of age characterized by dyspnea and wheezing, a viral infection often confused with asthma.

Bronchitis: inflammation of the bronchial tube.

Bronchospasm: severe constriction of the bronchial tree.

Bruise: an injury that does not break the skin but causes rupture of small underlying blood vessels with resulting tissue discoloration; a contusion.

Bruits: any abnormal sounds or murmurs heard on auscultation.

Bulky Dressing: thick, multi-layer dressing used to cover a large wound, control bleeding, and/or stabilize an impaled object.

Burn pads: one of many names for large, thick-layered, bulky pads used for quick application to stem profuse bleeding.

Burnout: a complex of signs and symptoms brought on by exhaustion from the stress of work.

Bursa (pl. Bursae): a fluid-filled sac that tends to lessen friction between movable parts of the body.

Butterfly strips: adhesive strips used to hold the edges of a wound together.

Buttocks: the prominence formed by the gluteal muscles on the posterior of both sides of the body.

C

Caesarean section (C-section): the delivery of a fetus by means of an incision into the uterus, usually through the abdominal wall.

Cafe coronary: common name for incident where people choke to death on a foreign object obstructing the upper airway.

Calamine: a powder consisting of zinc oxide and about .05 percent ferric oxide used in skin ointments.

Calcaneus: the largest tarsal bone, forming the prominence of the heel.

Calcium: a mineral substance necessary for life functioning; plays a vital role in heart contraction, nerve condition, and muscle contractions; cation with double valence.

Candida albicans: pathogen commonly part of the normal flora of the skin, mouth, and intestinal tract, but can cause a variety of infections.

Cannula(s): a word used to mean any of the kinds of tubes that can be inserted into one of the body cavities. A cannula may be used to draw fluids out or to give oxygen.

Canvas litter: lightweight, low cost, compact size, carrying device.

Capillaries: the very small blood vessels that carry blood to all parts of the body and the skin. Capillaries are a link between the ends of the arteries and the beginning of the beginning of the veins.

Capillary refill: a method of assessing the adequacy of circulation to the extremities. Gentle pressure is exerted on the nail bed until the underlying tissue whitens, then pressure is released, and the time for return of the pink color is observed.

Carbohydrate(s): a compound represented by the sugars, starches, and celluloses; contains carbon, hydrogen, and oxygen.

Carbon dioxide: CO_2; a colorless and odorless gas that neither supports combustion nor burns; a waste prod-uct of aerobic metabolism; in combination with water (H_2O)-, forms carbonic acid (H_2CO_3).

Carbon monoxide: CO; a colorless, odorless, and dangerous gas formed by the incomplete combustion of carbon; it combines four times as quickly with hemoglobin than oxygen; when in the presence of heme, replaces oxygen and reduces oxygen uptake in the lungs.

Carbonic acid: acid resulting from the mixture of carbon dioxide and water.

Cardiac arrest: the sudden cessation of cardiac function with no pulse, no blood pressure, unresponsiveness.

Cardiac asthma: a condition characterized by left heart failure and pulmonary edema with wheezing respirations; not related to bronchial asthma.

Cardiac compression: a technique of external heart massage to restore the pumping action of the heart.

Cardiac contusion: bruising of the heart.

Cardiac muscle: the heart muscle.

Cardiac standstill: the absence of cardiac contraction or electrical activity.

Cardiac tamponade: a condition in which the sac around the hearts fills with blood.

Cardiogenic shock: the inability of the heart to pump adequate amounts of blood to perfuse the vital organs.

Cardiopulmonary arrest: cessation of cardiac and respiratory activity.

Cardiopulmonary resuscitation (CPR): application of artificial ventilation and external cardiac compression in patients with cardiac arrest to pro-vide an adequate circulation to support life.

Cardiovascular system: pertaining to the heart and blood vessels.

Carotid artery: the principal artery of the neck, palpated easily on either side of the thyroid cartilage.

Carotid pulse: pulse taken at the ca-rotid artery.

Carpals: the eight small bones of the wrist.

Carpopedal: pertaining to or affecting the carpus and the foot.

Cartilage: a tough, elastic, connective tissue that covers opposite surfaces of movable joints and also forms parts of the skeleton, such as ear and nose.

Cataract: the partial or complete opacity of the crystalline lens of the eye or its capsule.

Catheter: a tube used for withdrawing or infusing fluids into various structures of the body.

Cat-scratch fever: a benign, subacute, re-gional lymphadenitis resulting from the scratch or bite of a cat or a scratch from a surface contaminated by a cat; it is marked by a primary papular eruption at the site of inoculation which may develop into a small ulcer.

Caudal: tail-like, at the tail.

Cavitation: formation of a partial vacuum, and susequent cavity, within a liquid. This describes the action of a high-velocity projectile on the human body, which is 60% water.

Cavity: a hollow or space, especially a space within a body or one of its organs.

Cellulitis: a spreading redness and swelling of the skin usually caused by infection.

Central nervous system: the portion of the nervous system consisting of the brain and spinal cord.

Cephalic vein: a large vein of the upper arm lying along the outer edge of the biceps muscle and emptying into the axillary vein.

Cerebellum: that portion of the brain behind and below the cortex, the general function of which is coordination of movement.

Cerebral cortex: the cells and fibers forming the convoluted layer of gray matter over the cerebral hemisphere of the brain.

Cerebral infarction: an ischemic condition of the brain, producing a persistent focal neurological deficit in the area of distribution of one of the cerebral arteries.

Cerebral thrombosis: thrombosis of a cerebral vessel, which may result in cerebral infarction.

Cerebrospinal fluid: fluid secreted by cells in cavities within the cerebrum. It circulates through the membranes that cover and protect the brain and spinal cord.

Cerebrovascular accident (CVA): sometimes called stroke or apoplexy; the sudden cessation of circulation to a region of the brain, due to thrombus, embolism, or hemorrhage.

Cerebrum: the portion of the brain controlling major function of the body, including movement, sensation, thinking, and emotions.

Cerumen: earwax.

Cervical collar: a device used to immobilize and support the neck.

Cervical spine: that portion of the spinal column consisting of the seven vertebrae that lie in the neck.

Cervical spondylosis: degenerative joint disease affecting the cervical vertebrae, intervertebral disks, and surrounding ligaments and connective tissue, sometimes with pain or paresthesia radiating down the arms as a result of pressure on the nerve roots.

Cervical vertebrae: the first seven vertebrae of the spinal column that lie in the neck.

Cervix: the lower portion, or neck, of the uterus.

CHEMTREC (Chemical Transportation Emergency Center): a division of Chemical Manufacturer's Association, available twenty-four hours a day toll free to answer questions involving hazardous materials.

Chest thrust: a series of manual thrusts to the chest to relieve upper airway obstruction.

Cheyne-Stokes breathing: breathing abnormality characterized by rhythmic waxing and waning of the depth of respiration, with regularly recurring periods of apnea; seen in association with central nervous system dysfunction.

Chief complaint: the problem for which a patient seeks help, stated in a word or short phrase.

Chlorhexidine: a topical anti-infective agent.

Chlorine: a greenish-yellow, incombustible, poisonous gas that is highly irritating to the respiratory organs.

Cholera: an acute, infectious, bacterial disease characterized by diarrhea, vomiting, cramps, collapse, and dehydration.

Cholesterol: a fatty substance found in animal tissue, egg yolks, and in various oils and fats; thought to contribute to arteriosclerosis.

Chronic: of long duration, or recurring over a period of time.

Chronic obstructive pulmonary disease (COPD): a term comprising chronic bronchitis, emphysema, and asthma; an illness that causes obstructive problems in the airways.

Cilia: the short, hairlike processes on the surface of the protozoans or of metazoan cells, which by their motion accomplish locomotion.

Circulatory overload: a condition of having too much fluid in the circulatory system.

Circulatory system: the body system consisting of the heart and blood vessels.

Circumduction: circular movement of a limb or eye.

Cirrhosis: chronic progressive fibrosis of the liver, often associated with heavy alcohol ingestion.

Clamping injury: usually involves a finger, or part of the hand, which has been strangled or stuck in a hole and cannot be readily extracted or has been extracted with damage.

Clavicle(s): the collarbone; attached to the uppermost part of the sternum at a right angle, and joins the scapular spine to form the point of the shoulder.

Clinical death: a term that refers to the lack of signs of life, when there is no pulse and no blood pressure; occurs immediately after the onset of cardiac arrest.

Clo units: the amount of clothing insulation needed to keep an average resting person comfortable at 21°C with air moving at 20 fpm and less than 50% relative humidity.

Clonic phase: pertaining to a spasm in which rigidity and relaxation succeed each other.

Closed-chest compression: external cardiac massage.

Closed wound: a wound in which the skin is not broken.

Clostridium perfringens: anaerobic bacteria that can cause food poisoning in cooked food held without proper refrigeration.

Clot: a semi-solidified mass, as of blood or lymph, also called a coagulum.

CO₂: the chemical formula for carbon dioxide.

Cocaine: powerful stimulant that induces an extreme state of euphoria.

Coccygeal spine: *see* Coccyx.

Coccyx: the lowest part of the backbone; composed of three to five small, fused vertebrae; also called the tailbone.

Colic: an intermittent painful intestinal cramp caused by strong peristaltic waves.

Colitis: inflammation of the colon.

Collagen: a general term referring to the structural tissues of the body other than bone; cartilage, membranes, tendons.

Collateral ligament(s): ligament located at the side of a joint, farthest from the center plane of motion.

Colloid: a fluid used for intravenous infusion.

Colostomy: An artificial opening into the colon.

Coma: state of unconsciousness from which the patient cannot be aroused, even by powerful stimulation.

Comatose: in a state of coma.

Combine: farm vehicle used for harvesting crops.

Come-a-long: a hand-operated winch of varying capacity (2-ton capacity is standard for ambulance equipment); used to effect forceful entry.

Compensatory shock: the first stage of shock.

Compound fracture(s): an open fracture; a fracture in which there is an open wound of the skin and soft tissues leading down to the location of the fracture.

Compress (compression dressing): a folded cloth or pad used for applying pressure to stop hemorrhage or as a wet dressing.

Compulsive drug use: preoccupation with the procurement and use of a drug.

Concussion: a jarring brain injury resulting from a head blow or fall.

Conduction: the transmission of a stimulus from one fiber to another within a muscle.

Condyle: rounded projection on a bone, may be covered by cartilage at the joining with another bone.

Condyloid joint: a joint where a rounded protuberance on a bone serves to form an articulation with another bone.

Congenital: referring to any condition that is present at birth.

Congestive heart failure (CHF): excessive blood or fluid in the lungs or body tissues caused by the failure of the ventricles to pump blood effectively.

Conjunctiva: the delicate membrane that lines the eyelids and covers the exposed surface of the eyeball.

Conjunctivitis: inflammation of the conjunctiva.

Connective tissue: the tissue that binds together and supports the various structures of the body.

Constipation: difficult, incomplete, or infrequent passage of stools; more common in less physically active older people.

Constrict: to make smaller by drawing together or by squeezing.

Contact burns: a burn caused by touching either a hot surface or a live electrical circuit.

Contamination: contact with an unsterile object or infective agent.

Contamination zone: the area in a hazardous materials emergency where the contamination is actually present.

Continuity: an unbroken, connected whole.

Contract: to draw together or to shorten.

Contraindicated: condition, sign, or symptom that makes a particular course of treatment or procedure inadvisable.

Control zone: the area surrounding or immediately adjacent to the contamination zone in a hazardous material emergency, the purpose of which is to prevent the spread of the contamination.

Contusions: a bruise; an injury which causes a hemorrhage into or beneath the skin, but does not break the skin.

Convection: the conveyance of heat in liquid or gaseous form by movement of heated particles (as when the warm air of a room ascends to the ceiling); the loss of body heat to the atmosphere when airs passes over the body.

Convex: rounded and somewhat elevated.

Coquille: a glass or lens shaped like a watch crystal; also a name for a similarly shaped extrication device.

Corn picker: farm equipment.

Cornea: the transparent structure covering the pupil.

Coronary artery: a blood vessel that supplies the myocardium.

Coronary artery disease: progressive narrowing and eventual obstruction of the coronary arteries by the atherosclerotic process.

Costal: pertaining to the ribs.

Costochondral: pertaining to a rib and its cartilaginous portion attached to the sternum.

Coumarin: an anticoagulant.

Coup-contrecoup: a type of head injury causing contusion or bruising of the brain.

CRAMS score: a trauma scoring system: Circulation; Respiration; Abdomen; Motor; and Speech; used to determine the probability of survival.

Cranial nerves: the twelve pairs of nerves connected directly with the brain.

Cranial skull: pertaining to the cranium.

Cranium: the portion of the skull enclosing the brain.

Cravat: a special type of bandage made from a large triangular piece of cloth and folded to form a band; used as a temporary dressing for a fracture or wound.

Crepitus: a grating sound heard and a sensation felt when the fractured ends of a bone rub together.

Crib: child's bed, or as a verb, to install cribbing.

Cribbing: a system of timbers or other supports used to prop up a vehicle or re-enforce a wall or embankment.

Cricoid cartilage: a firm ridge of cartilage that forms the lower part of the larynx.

Criminal abortion: an illegal attempt to produce an abortion, often under highly unsterile conditions, hazardous to the mother's life.

Crisis: any event that is seen as a crucial moment or turning point in the patient's life.

Critical burns: the most serious burns. Included are burns complicated by respiratory tract injury; third-degree burns involving critical areas or more than ten percent of the body surface; second-degree burns involving more than 20-25 percent of the body surface; and any otherwise moderate burn in an elderly or critically ill patient.

Critical incidence stress debriefing: A meeting of rescue workers after a stressful event to allow open discussion of their emotions and feelings.

Crossed-finger technique: method to open clenched jaw.

Croup: the general term for a group of viral infections that produce swelling of the larynx.

Crowing: a sound that occurs when the muscles around the larynx spasm.

Crowning: the stage of birth when the presenting part of the baby is visible at the vaginal orifice.

Crush points: two large objects coming together to cause a crushing action.

Cryotherapy: to treat with cold.

Crystalloid: a substance capable of crystallization that, in solution, may be diffused through animal membranes; does not contain protein molecules.

Culture: the cultivation of microorganisms, such as bacteria, for scientific study.

Cyanosis: blueness of the skin due to insufficient oxygen in the blood.

Cyst: a saclike structure containing fluid or semisolid matter.

Cystic fibrosis: a hereditary, chronic disease of the pancreas, lungs, etc. beginning in infancy in which there is an inability to digest foods and a difficulty in breathing.

Cystitis: inflammation of the urinary bladder.

Cytomegalovirus: one of a group of highly host-specific herpes viruses.

D

Deadspace: areas of the respiratory tract where gas exchange does not take place.

Decapitation: the removal of the head.

Decelerating aortic injury: a possible laceration of the aorta caused by a victim being hurled into an immovable object such as a dashboard.

Decompensation: failure of the heart to maintain sufficient circulation of the blood.

Decompression: removal of compression or pressure.

Decontamination: to remove foreign substance that could cause harm; frequently used to described removal of radioactive material from person, clothing, or area.

Decubitus position: the position assumed in lying down.

Defibrillation: application of an unsynchronized DC electrical shock to terminate ventricular fibrillation.

Dehydration: loss of water and electrolytes; excessive loss of body water.

Delirium: a mental disturbance marked by hallucinations, cerebral excitement, and physical restlessness, usually lasting only a short time.

Delirium tremens (DTs): a form of insanity, often temporary, caused by alcohol poisoning; characterized by sweating, tremor, great excitement, precordial pain, anxiety, and mental distress; occurs usually following heavy alcohol intake.

Demand-valve: an intermittent, positive pressure breathing unit used to assist or control ventilation; with a manual control, it is acceptable emergency equipment.

Dementia: a severe emotionally disturbed state, where the patient acts irrationally.

Deoxygenated: lacking in oxygen.

Department of Transportation (DOT): cabinet level department charged with overseeing nation's transportation regulations.

Depress: to decrease the force or activity.

Depressant: an agent that lowers functional activity, a sedative.

Depression: a mental state characterized by feelings of dejection, psychomotor retardation, insomnia, weight loss, often of delusional proportion.

Dermal: of or pertaining to the skin.

Dermatitis: inflammation of the skin.

Dermis: the inner layer of skin; contains the skin appendages, hair follicles, sweat glands, nerves, and blood vessels.

Dexedrine: trademark for preparations of dextroamphetamine sulfate.

Dextran: a water-soluble polysaccharide used as a synthetic plasma volume expander in infusions.

Diabetes: a general term referring to disorders characterized by excessive urine excretion, excessive thirst, and excessive hunger.

Diabetic: one who has diabetes; pertaining to diabetes.

Diabetic acidosis: a variety of metabolic acidosis produced by accumulation of ketone bodies resulting from uncontrolled diabetes mellitus.

Diabetic coma: result of an inadequate insulin supply that leads to unconsciousness, coma, and eventually death unless treated.

Diaphoresis: profuse perspiration.

Diaphragm: a large skeletal muscle which is a major component in the act of respiration and which separates the chest cavity from the abdominal cavity.

Diarrhea: a large number of bowel movements of abnormally liquid character.

Diastolic pressure: blood pressure measured when the heart is resting between beats, the lower of the two numbers in a blood pressure reading.

Digestion: the process or act of converting food into chemical substances that can be absorbed and assimilated.

Digestive system: the group of body organs that carries our digestion. Digestion is the process in the body in which food is broken down mechanically and chemically and is changed into forms that can enter the bloodstream and be used by the body.

Digitalis: a drug used in the treatment of congestive heart failure and certain atrial arrhythmias.

Dilate: to expand or enlarge.

Direct pressure: force applied directly on top of a wound to stop bleeding.

Direct transmission: the spread of disease by contact with an infected person, or by droplet spray from sneezing, coughing, or talking.

Dislocation: the state of being misaligned; the displacement of the ends of two bones at their joint so that the joint surfaces are no longer in proper contact.

Disoriented: the loss of proper bearings, or a state of mental confusion as to time, place, and identity.

Distal: farther from any point of reference; generally, the point of reference is the heart.

Distended: inflated or enlarged.

Distillation: separation of the more volatile parts of a substance from the less volatile by boiling and condensing the vapors into separate liquids.

Distress: physical or mental anguish or suffering.

Diuretic(s): a substance or drug used to decrease excess body fluid by increasing the secretion of urine by the kidney; often used in treatment of congestive heart failure.

Diverticulitis: inflammation of a diverticulum of the colon.

Diving reflex: a complex cardiovascular reflex resulting from submersion of the face or nose in water which constricts blood flow everywhere except to the brain.

Dorsal: of, toward, on, in, or near the back.

Dorsalis pedis artery: an artery located in the top back of the foot.

DOT: *see* Department of Transportation.

Drag: method of transportation utilizing various materials, e.g. sheet, blanket, or shirt to move a patient.

Draw-sheet: a method of transferring a patient from a bed to a stretcher, using the sheet on which he/she is lying as a hammock.

Dressing: protective covering for a wound, used to stop bleeding and to prevent contamination of the wound.

Drowning: death by suffocation after being submerged in liquid.

Drug abuse: the self-administration of a drug or drugs in a manner not in accord with approved medical or social patterns.

Drugs: any substance used as medicine.

Ductless glands: glands that have no external openings and that secrete internally one or more hormones.

Duodenum: first or most proximal portion of the small intestine, passing from the stomach to the jejunum.

Dura mater: the outermost and strongest of the three meninges.

Dysentery: severe inflammation of the mucous membrane of the large intestine, characterized by diarrhea, bloody stools, cramps, and fever.

Dysphagia: sensation of sticking or discomfort when swallowing.

Dyspnea: difficulty in breathing, with rapid, shallow respirations.

Dysrhythmias: disturbances in the cardiac rhythms.

E

Eardrum: a flexible membrane that forms most of the outer wall of the tympanic cavity and separates it from the external auditory canal; the tympanum.

Earwax: waxy substance secreted by the glands lining the passages of the external ear.

Ecchymosis: blood under the skin causing a black and blue mark, bruise.

Eclampsia: a toxic condition of pregnancy, causing convulsions and coma, associated with hypertension, edema, and proteinuria.

Ectopic pregnancy: a pregnancy in which the fetus is implanted elsewhere than in the uterus, e.g. in the fallopian tube or in the abdominal cavity; produces abdominal pain, bleeding.

Eczema: a superficial inflammatory process involving primarily the epidermis, characterized early by redness, itching, minute papules and vesicles, weeping, oozing, and crusting, and later by scaling, lichenification, and often pigmentation.

Edema: a condition in which fluid escapes into the body tissues from the vascular or lymphatic spaces and causes local or generalized swelling.

Edematous: swollen with fluid; having dropsy.

Egg: female reproductive cell; ovum.

Electrical-mechanical dissociation: the form of cardiac arrest in which the electrocardiogram displays an adequate heart rate and rhythm, but the heart is incapable of generating a palpable pulse and blood pressure in the circulation.

Electrocardiogram (ECG or EKG): a graphic tracing of the electrical currents generated by the process of depolarization and repolarization of the myocardial tissues.

Electrocution: death caused by passage of electrical current through the body.

Electrolyte: a substance whose molecules dissociate when put into solution.

Embolism: the sudden blocking of an artery or vein by a clot or foreign material which has been brought to the site of lodgement by the blood current.

Embolus: any foreign matter, as a blood clot or air bubble, carried in the bloodstream.

Embryo: in animals, the derivatives of the fertilized egg, that eventually become offspring, during their period of most rapid development; in man, from about two weeks after fertilization to the end of the seventh or eighth week.

Emergency blanket: a blanket used as a stretcher or for padding or protecting the patient.

Emesis: vomiting.

Emphysema: a chronic lung disease caused by distention of the alveoli and/or destruction of their walls; a pathological accumulation of air in tissues, or organs, as in subcutaneous emphysema.

EMS: Emergency Medical Services.

EMT: Emergency Medical Technician.

EMT-A: Emergency Medical Technician-Ambulance.

EMT-D: Emergency Medical Technician-Defibrillation.

Encephalitis: inflammation of the brain.

Endocarditis: infection of the valves of the lining of the heart.

Endocardium: the membrane lining the inside of the heart.

Endocrine glands: glands that produce hormones that regulate specific body functions.

Enema: a clyster or injection; a liquid injected into the rectum.

Endotracheal intubation: a method of intubation in which an endotracheal tube is placed through a patient's mouth or nose and directly through the larynx between the vocal cords into the trachea for the purpose of opening and maintaining an airway.

Enzyme: a protein substance capable of accelerating or producing by catalytic action some change in another substance for which it is often specific.

Epicardium: the layer of serous pericardium on the surface of the heart.

Epidermis: the outermost and nonvascular layer of the skin.

Epidural: located outside or above the dura, the outermost membrane that covers the brain.

Epidural hematoma: a hematoma outside the dura mater and under the skull.

Epigastric: relating to the epigastrium.

Epigastric region: the upper and middle regions of the abdomen within the costal angle.

Epiglottis: the lidlike cartilaginous structure overhanging the superior entrance to the larynx and serving to prevent food from entering the larynx and trachea while swallowing.

Epiglottitis: a bacterial infection occurring in children, marked by swelling of the epiglottis, high fever, pain on swallowing, and drooling; airway obstruction can result with great rapidity.

Epilepsy: a chronic brain disorder marked by paroxysmal attacks of brain dysfunction, usually associated with some alteration of consciousness, abnormal motor behavior, psychic or sensory disturbances; may be preceded by aura.

Epinephrine: adrenalin; hormone and drug that has powerful beta stimulating properties, used in the treatment of asthma, anaphylaxis, asystole, and fine ventricular fibrillation.

Equilibrium: balance.

Esophageal obturator airway: a device used to provide adequate airway by blocking off the esophageal opening with a cuffed obturator and providing ventilation through a series of side holes located at the level of the epiglottis.

Esophageal reflux: a burning pain under the sternum caused by gastric juices that reflux into the lower esophagus and attack its lining.

Esophageal varices: dilated veins in the wall of the esophagus that develop in patients with liver disease. If these enlarged veins rupture, subsequent bleeding can be fatal.

Esophagus: the portion of the digestive tract that lies between the pharynx and the stomach.

Estrogen: one of the classes of female sex hormones.

Etiology: the study of the factors that cause disease.

Eustachian tube: the tube leading from the back of the throat to the middle ear; serves to equalize pressure in the middle ear.

Evaporation: conversion of a liquid or solid to a gas.

Evert: to turn inside out, to turn outward.

Evisceration: internal organs exposed to the outside through a complete break in the abdominal wall.

Exhalation: the act of breathing out; expiration.

Expiration: breathing out; exhaling.

Extension: the act of straightening.

External auditory canal: the passage from the outer ear to the tympanic membrane.

External ear: all of the ear external to the tympanic membrane.

External maxillary artery: artery anterior to the angle of the mandible on the inner surface of the lower jaw that contributes much of the blood supply to the face.

Extremity: a limb; an arm or leg.

Extremity lift: transfer method using the arms and legs of the patient.

Extrication: disentanglement; freeing from entrapment.

Extrication back splint: transfer device used to immobilize the back.

Extrication collar: transfer device used to immobilize the head, neck, and spinal column.

F

Fallopian tubes: the bilateral tubes extending from the ovaries to the uterus.

False labor: ineffective pains which resemble labor pains, but which are not accompanied by effacement and dilatation of the cervix.

Falx: a sickle-shaped organ or structure; used as a general term in anatomical nomenclature to designate such a structure.

Fascia: a sheet or band of fibrous tissue; lies deep under the skin and acts as an anchor for muscle attachment.

Fats: adipose tissue; white or yellowish tissue that forms soft pads in the body and furnishes a reserve supply of energy.

Fatty acids: acids derived from fats; they contribute to a dangerous level of acidosis in uncontrolled diabetics.

Fecal: pertaining to feces.

Femoral artery: the principal artery of the thigh, a continuation of the iliac artery; supplies blood to the lower abdominal wall, the external genitalia, and the lower body extremities; pulse may be palpated in the groin area.

Femoral pulse: located approximately two fingerbreadths inferior to the midpoint line between the anterior superior iliac spine and the pubic symphysis.

Femur: the bone that extends from the pelvis to the knee; the longest and largest bone of the body; the thigh bone.

Fetal membranes: the double-walled bag of waters, or amniotic sac.

Fetal position: a position resembling that of the fetus in the uterus with the legs drawn up toward the abdomen.

Fetus: the unborn offspring in the postembryonic period after major structures have been outlined; in man from 7 to 8 weeks after fertilization until birth.

Fever: an elevation of body temperature beyond normal.

Fibers: threadlike strands.

Fibrillation: uncoordinated contractions of the myocardium resulting from independent individual muscle fiber activity.

Fibrin: fibrous protein material formed and utilized to produce a blood clot.

Fibula: the smaller of the two bones of the lower leg.

Filariasis: tropical disease caused by a parasitic worm transmitted by mosquitoes.

Finger sweep: technique to remove a foreign object from the oropharynx so that it does not reenter the airway.

Fireman's carry: a method whereby one EMT can carry a patient slung over the shoulder.

Fireman's drag: *see* Drag.

First-degree burns: mild, partial thickness burn, only involving the outer layer of skin.

Fisting: a practice common among homosexual men of forcing the clenched fist and forearm into the rectum.

Flaccid: a term meaning soft, limp, without any muscular tone.

Flail chest: a condition in which several ribs are broken, each in at least two places; or a sternal fracture or separation of the ribs from the sternum producing a free-floating segment of the chest wall that moves paradoxically on respiration.

Flail injuries: exhibiting abnormal or paradoxical mobility, as a flail joint or flail chest.

Flank: the part of the body below the ribs and above the ilium.

Flash burns: a burn caused when an extremity is close to an electrical flash or is struck by lightning.

Flash chamber: a chamber at the proximal end of an IV needle.

Flat lift: transport method lifting the patient so that he remains horizontal to the ground.

Flexion: the act of bending, or the condition of being bent.

Flexor: a muscle that flexes or bends a part of the body.

Fluid therapy: replacement of lost body fluids, as in dehydration following a severe burn.

Flutter pulse: repetitive, regular, and rapid beating of the heart.

Follicle: a deep, narrow pit in the skin containing the root of the hair; the duct of the sebaceous gland opens into the follicle.

Fontanelle: area in a baby's head where the skull bones have not yet completely grown together.

Foot drag: a single rescuer method of moving a patient by dragging him/her by the feet.

Forceps: two-pronged instrument for grasping, compressing, or pulling.

Foreign object: not normally a part of the body.

Foreskin: the fold of skin covering the glans penis.

Fourth-degree burn: in some areas, a burn that involves muscle and bone.

Fowler's position: the head of the patient is raised 18 to 20 inches above level, with the knees of the patient raised also.

Fracture: a break or rupture in a bone.
  avulsion: an indirect fracture caused by avulsion or pull of a ligament.
  comminuted: a fracture in which the bone is shattered, broken into small pieces.
  compression: a fracture produced by compression, e.g. vertebral fracture.
  depressed: a fracture of the skull in which a fragment is depressed.
  greenstick: an incomplete fracture, the bone is not broken all the way through; seen most often in children.
  impacted: a fracture in which the ends of the bone are jammed together.
  longitudinal: a break in a bone extending in a longitudinal direction.
  oblique: a fracture in which the break crosses the bone at an angle.
  spiral: a fracture in which the break line twists around and through the bone.
  transverse: a fracture in which the break line extends across the bone at right angle to the long axis.

Friction rubs: abnormal respiratory sound which resembles the sound of two pieces of leather rubbing together.

Frostbite: damage to the tissues as a result of prolonged exposure to extreme cold.

Full-thickness burn: a burn through all the layers of the skin into the subcutaneous tissues; a third-degree burn.

Fulminating: to occur suddenly with great intensity.

G

Gall bladder: the sac located just beneath the liver that concentrates and stores bile.

Gallstones: a small, hard concretion in the gallbladder or bile duct, composed chiefly of cholesterol crystals.

Gamma rays: an electromagnetic radiation emitted from radioactive substances analogous to x-rays.

Ganglia: a knot or mass; a group of nerve cell bodies located outside the central nervous system.

Gangrene: local tissue death as a result of an injury or inadequate blood supply.

Gastric distention: inflation of the stomach caused when excessive pressures are used during artificial ventilation or when several breaths are administered in rapid succession.

Gastritis: inflammation of the stomach.

Gastroenteritis: inflammation of the stomach and intestines.

Gastrointestinal tract: the digestive tract, including stomach, small intestine, large intestine, rectum, and anus.

Gauze: a light, open-meshed fabric of muslin or similar material.

Geiger counter: an instrument used to measure the level of radioactivity in the environment; designed to detect gamma radiation.

General purpose dressing: one of many names for large, thick-layered, bulky pads used for quick application to stem profuse bleeding.

Generalized: affecting many parts or all parts of the organism; not local.

Gene: biological unit contained within a chromosome which transmits specific physical hereditary characteristics.

Genital: pertaining to the reproductive organs.

Genitalia: the external sex organs.

Genitourinary system: the organs of reproduction, together with the organs concerned in production and excretion of urine.

Germs: any disease-causing organisms.

Gestation: the period of development of the young; pregnancy.

Giardia: a genus of flagellate protozoa found in the intestinal tract; it may cause a protracted intermittent diarrhea.

Glasgow Coma Scale: a method of quantifying a patient's state of consciousness.

Glaucoma: a disease that produces increased pressure within the eyeball; can lead to blindness.

Gliding joint: a type of synovial joint in which the opposed surfaces are flat or only slightly curved.

Globe: the eyeball.

Glucose: a simple sugar.

Glycogen: the form in which carbohydrates are stored in animal and human tissue.

Goiter: an enlargement of the thyroid gland, causing a swelling in the front part of the neck.

Gonad: an ovary or testis.

Good Samaritan laws: laws written to protect emergency care personnel which require a standard of care to be provided in good faith, to a level of training, and to the best of ability.

Gout: metabolic disease caused by excess uric acid in the blood, characterized by painful inflammation of such joints as the big toe.

Grafting: transplanting of tissue from one site to another.

Grain tanks: farm storage units

Grand mal seizures: severe epileptic seizure.

"Gray matter": the gray outer covering of the brain.

Greene body splint: a corset-type extrication device adjustable to patient's height with metal and straps.

Groin: the inguinal region; junction of the abdomen and the thigh.

Ground splint: asking the patient to keep his prone body very still as if it were splinted to the ground.

"Guarding": instinctive reaction to palpation of patient with abdominal pain.

Gurgling: a breathing sound indicating the presence of foreign matter in the airway.

H

Habituation: a situation in which a patient produces a tolerance to a drug and becomes psychologically dependent on the drug.

Hallucinations: a sensory perception not founded on objective reality; may involve smell, touch, taste, sight, and hearing.

Hand off: the act of transferring responsibility for a patient from one health care professional to another.

Hay baler: farm equipment.

Hazardous materials: a material that in any quantity poses a threat to life, health, or property.

Head-tilt/chin-lift maneuver: opening the airway by tilting the patient's head backward and lifting the chin forward, bringing the entire lower jaw with it.

Heart: a hollow muscular organ that receives the blood from the veins, sends it through the lungs to be oxygenated, then pumps it to the arteries.

Heart attack: a layman's term for a condition resulting from blockage of a coronary artery and subsequent death of part of the heart muscle; an acute myocardial infarction; a coronary.

Heart disease: abnormal condition of the heart or heart and circulation.

Heart failure: inability of the heart to maintain adequate circulation.

Heart muscle: *see* cardiac muscle.

Heat burns: *see* thermal burns.

Heat cramps: painful muscle cramps resulting from excessive loss of salt and water through sweating.

Heat exhaustion: prostration caused by excessive loss of water and salt through sweating; characterized by cold, clammy skin and a weak, rapid pulse.

Heat stroke: life-threatening condition caused by a disturbance in temperature regulation; characterized by extreme fever, hot and dry skin, delirium, or coma.

Heimlich maneuver: also known as manual thrust; a system developed by Heimlich to remove a foreign body from the airway.

Helium: a light, inert, colorless, elemental gas, preferred for inflation of balloons, etc. as it is nonflammable.

Hemangioma: a benign tumor made up of newly formed blood vessels.

Hematemesis: vomiting bright red blood.

Hematoma: localized collection of blood in the tissues as a result of injury or a broken blood vessel.

Hemiplegia: paralysis of one side of the body.

Hemodilution: an increase in the volume of blood plasma resulting in reduced concentration of red blood cells.

Hemoglobin: the oxygen-carrying pigment of the red blood cells; when it has absorbed oxygen in the lungs, it is bright red and called oxyhemoglobin; after it has given up its oxygen to the tissues, it is purple in color and is called reduced hemoglobin.

Hemophilia: an inherited blood disease occurring mostly in males, characterized by the inability of the blood to clot.

Hemoptysis: coughing up of bright red blood.

Hemorrhage: abnormally large amount of bleeding.

Hemorrhagic shock: a state of inadequate tissue perfusion due to blood loss.

Hemostat: an instrument for stopping hemorrhage by compressing the bleeding vessel; a type of clamp.

Hemothorax: an accumulation of blood in the chest cavity.

Hepatic: pertaining to the liver.

Hepatitis B: hepatitis caused by a virus that is spread through blood-to-blood contact (transfusion, needle stick), mucous membrane (saliva or sputum contact), or sexual contact. It is a serious disease with long-term side effects. Signs and symptoms are nausea, vomiting, fatigue, abdominal pain, and jaundice.

Hernia: the abnormal protrusion of any organ through an opening into another body cavity; most common in the inguinal hernia where a loop of intestine descends into the inguinal canal in the groin.

Herpes: a spreading, recurrent skin eruption caused by infection from the herpes virus.

Hetastarch: a colloid solution used as a volume expander for blood.

Hiatal hernia: occurs when part of the stomach bulges upward through the opening that allows the esophagus to pass through the diaphragm.

High-pressure regulators: one of two types of regulators attached to an oxygen cylinder, which can provide fifty psi to power a demand-valve type resuscitator or a suction device.

Hip: the joint where the femur articulates with the innominate bone.

History (patient): information about the patient's chief complaint, symptoms, data leading up to the acute episode, previous illnesses, family history, and surgical history.

Hormones: a substance secreted by an endocrine gland that has effects upon other glands or systems of the body.

Horse-collar technique: a cervical collar device made with a rolled-up blanket.

Host: the organism upon which or within which a parasite lives.

Humerus: the bone of the upper arm.

Hydration: the act of combining or causing to combine with water.

Hydrofluoric acid: a gaseous haloid acid, extremely poisonous and corrosive.

Hydrogen peroxide: a strongly disinfectant cleansing and bleaching liquid used in dilute solution in water, mainly as a wash or spray.

Hydrogen sulfide: an offensive and poisonous gas used as a chemical reagent.

Hydroplaning: a condition whereby the tires of a moving vehicle are lifted out of contact with a wet road surface, losing traction and directional control. With low pressure tires or worn tread it can occur at speeds as low as 25-35 mph.

Hymenoptera: an order of insects usually having two pairs of well developed membranous wings, as the bees, wasps, ants, etc.

Hyperflexion position: Flexion of a limb or part beyond the normal limit.

Hyperglycemia: abnormally increased concentration of sugar in the blood.

Hyperpnea: increased depth of respiration.

Hypertension: high blood pressure, usually in reference to a diatolis pressure greater than 90-95 mm Hg.

Hyperthermia: greatly increased body temperature.

Hypertonic phase: the phase that signals the end of the tonic phase of a seizure and is characterized by five to fifteen seconds of extreme muscular rigidity and hyperextension.

Hyperventilation: an increased rate and depth of breathing resulting in an abnormal lowering of arterial carbon dioxide, causing alkalosis.

Hypoglycemia: an abnormally diminished concentration of sugar in the blood; insulin shock.

Hyponatremia: too little sodium in the blood.

Hypopharynx: the lowest part of the pharynx leading to the larynx and esophagus.

Hypothermia: decreased body temperature.

Hypotension: abnormally low blood pressure.

Hypothyroidism: deficient function of the thyroid gland, characterized by low metabolism, lack of energy, thick skin, and intolerance to cold.

Hypovolemic shock: decreased amount of blood and fluids in the body.

Hypoxemia: a term that refers to inadequate oxygen in the blood; an arterial oxygen pressure of less than 60 torr.

Hypoxia: a low oxygen content in the blood; lack of oxygen in inspired air.

Hypoxic drive: patients with COPD lack the normal breathing reflex, and instead are driven to breathe by the lack of oxygen.

I

Ibuprofen: an anti-inflammatory.

ICU: intensive care unit.

Ileum: the distal portion of the small intestine, extending from the jejunum to the cecum.

Ilia: plural of ilium, the expansive superior portion of the hip bone.

Iliac crest: the highest point of the hipbone.

Immersion hypothermia: hypothermia brought on by placing or plunging the body into a cold liquid.

Immersion syndrome: the physiological changes that occur from the shock of sudden immersion in cold water.

Immunosuppressed: the artificial prevention or diminution of the immune response.

Impaction: state of being tightly wedged or firmly packed.

Impaled object: an object which has caused a puncture wound and which remains embedded in the wound.

Implantation: the insertion of an organ or tissue in a new site in the body.

Implied consent: in a true emergency where the patient is unconscious or disoriented and there is a significant risk of death, disability, or deterioration of condition, the law assumes that the patient would give his consent.

Incident command system: a management system designed to control, direct, and coordinate emergency response resources.

Incision: an open wound with smooth edges.

Incomplete abortion: an abortion in which some of the products of conception remain in the uterus.

Incontinence: inability to prevent the flow of urine or feces.

Incubator: a device that provides protection and temperature control for a newborn infant or a high-risk infant of any age.

Incus: Latin for anvil; named for its resemblance to an anvil, the middle bone of the middle ear; one of the three ossicles.

Indirect transmission: a means of transmitting a communicable disease through the use of a vector, such as food or water.

Induced abortion: an abortion that is performed in an authorized medical setting.

Inevitable abortion: vaginal bleeding, uterine contractions and cervical dilatation before term, where there is no possibility that the pregnancy will go to term.

Infarction: localized death of tissue resulting from the discontinuation of its blood supply.

Infection: an invasion of a body by disease-producing organisms.

Infectious: capable of being transmitted by infection.

Interior vena cava: one of the two largest veins in the body that empties venous blood into the right atrium receiving blood from the lower extremities and abdominal organs.

Infiltration: leakage of fluid into the interstitial compartment, usually as a result of improper cannulation of a vein, or by design, to render insensitive the area of surgical procedures, such as suturing.

Inflammation: a tissue reaction to disease, irritation, or infection, characterized by pain, heat, redness, and swelling.

Influenza: an acute viral infection involving the respiratory tract.

Informed consent: a patient has received, in terms that he understands, all of the information that would affect a reasonable person's decision to accept or refuse a treatment or procedure.

Infusion: induction by gravity of a therapeutic fluid other than blood into a vein.

Ingestion: intaking of food or other substances through the mouth.

Inguinal hernia: a rupture or separation of the abdominal wall so that a portion of the intestine projects into the groin area.

Inguinal ligaments: tough fibrous ligament that stretches between the lateral edge of the pubic symphysis and the anterior superior iliac spine.

Inhalation: the drawing of air or other gases into the lungs.

Inner ear: the labyrinth, containing the cochlea (the essential organs of hearing), the auditory nerve, and the semicircular canals that govern balance.

Innervate: the distribution or supply of nerves to a body part.

Innominate bones: one or two bones forming the pelvic girdle; made up of the fusion of the ilium, ischium, and pubis.

Inspiration: the breathing in of air into the lungs; inhalation.

Insulin: a hormone secreted by the islets of Langerhans in the pancreas; essential for the proper metabolism of blood sugar.

Insulin coma: another name for insulin shock.

Insulin reaction: another name for insulin shock.

Insulin shock: not a true form of shock; hypoglycemia caused by excessive insulin dosage, characterized by sweating, tremor, anxiety, unusual behavior, vertigo, and diplopia; may cause death of brain cells.

Integument: a covering or sheath; the skin.

Intercostal muscles: muscle between the ribs.

Intervertebral disc: the pad of fibrocartilage between the bodies of adjacent vertebrae.

Intestines: the portion of the alimentary canal extending from the pylorus to the anus.

Intoxication: the state of being affected by alcohol or another drug to the point of losing physical and mental control.

Intraabdominal: within the abdomen

Intramural hematoma: a hematoma within the walls of an organ.

Intrapleural space: a tiny space with negative pressure between the two layers of pleura.

Intrathoracic: within the thorax

Intravenous: within or into a vein.

Intravenous (IV) therapy: the administration of drugs, fluids, or blood directly into the circulatory system via a vein.

Intubation: the placement of a tube in the airway to improve ventilation.

Inverted: turned inside out or upside down.

Involuntary muscle: muscles that function without voluntary control; smooth (as opposed to skeletal) muscles.

Ionizing radiation: any radiation resulting when a stable, neutral atom is disrupted, releasing individual ions that bear either positive or negative charges.

Iris: colored portion of the eye surrounding the pupil.

Irregular pulse: one in which the beats occur at irregular intervals.

Irreversible shock: the final stage of shock.

Irrigation: cleansing by washing and rinsing with water or other fluids.

Irritable heart: neurocirculatory asthenia.

Ischemic: lacking oxygen.

Ischemic stroke: a stroke caused by an obstruction in circulation.

Ischium: either of the two lowermost portions of the hipbone.

Islets of Langerhans: clusters of cells in the pancreas that produce insulin.

Isotonic: having the same osmotic pressure as a reference solution; usually the intracellular fluid, or the red blood cell.

Isotope: any of two or more forms of an element of the same atomic number but having different atomic weights.

J

Jaundice: yellow color of the tissues seen in liver disease.

Jaw thrust maneuver: a procedure for opening the airway, wherein the jaw is lifted and pulled forward to keep the tongue from falling back into the airway.

Jejunum: that portion of the small intestine that extends from the duodenum to the ileum.

Joint: the juncture where two bones come in contact.

   ball-and-socket: a type of synovial joint in which a spheroidal surface on one bone (the ball) moves within a concavity (the socket) on the other bone, as in the hip bone.

   freely movable: a synovial joint, a special form of articulation permitting more or less free movement.

   hinge: a joint that allows angular movement.

   immovable: fibrous joint, one in which the components are connected by fibrous tissue.

   limited motion: a joint that cannot be moved through a full range of motion.

   pivot: a uniaxial joint in which one bone pivots within a bony or an osseoligamentous ring.

Joint capsule: a fibrous sac that, with its synovial lining, encloses a joint.

Jugular venous outflow: the flow of blood from the head, neck and face to the superior vena cava.

Jump kit: a closed container fitted with necessary portable equipment and supplies to be used in the emergency care of patients who are treated away from the ambulance.

K

Kaposi's sarcoma: a multifocal, metastasizing, malignant reticulosis with features resembling those of angiosarcoma, principally involving the skin.

Kendrick Extrication Device (KED): trade name for a commercial extrication device used in rescue work.

Kerlix: a type of self-adhering roller material.

Ketoacidosis: a condition arising in diabetics where their insulin dose is insufficient to their needs; fat is metabolized, instead of sugar, to ketones; characterized by excessive thirst, urination, vomiting, and hyperventilation of the Kussmaul type.

Ketone bodies: organic compounds, by-products of fat metabolism.

Ketosis: a condition characterized by an abnormally elevated concentration of ketone bodies in the body tissues and fluids; it is a complication of diabetes mellitus and starvation.

Kidneys: the paired organs located in the retroperitoneal cavities that filter blood and produce urine, also act as adjuncts to keep a proper acid-base balance.

Kidney stone: stones that pass from the kidney and into the ureter where they cause excruciating pain until they enter the bladder.

Killing zone: in a crisis situation, the area potentially exposed to hostile gunfire.

Kinetics: the science that deals with movements of parts of the body.

Kling: a type of self-adhering roller material.

Kussmaul respiration: a deep, rapid respiration characteristic of hyperglycemia, or diabetic coma, caused by acidosis and the necessity of the body to blow off carbon dioxide as a compensatory mechanism.

L

Labia: the lips, the folds of skin and mucous membranes that comprise the vulva.

Labor: the muscular contractions of the uterus designed to expel the fetus from the mother.

Labyrinthine system: a system of interconnecting canals or cavities, especially that constituting the internal ear.

Laceration: a wound made by tearing or cutting of body tissues.

Lacrimal gland: a small gland located in the upper outer angle of the orbit that secretes the tears.

Lactated Ringer's: a frequently used sterile intravenous solution containing sodium, potassium, calcium, and chloride ions in approximately isotonic concentrations; lactate is added as a buffer for acidotic conditions.

Lactic acid: an organic acid normally present in tissue and produced in carbohydrate matter by bacterial fermentation; one of the acids produced by anaerobic metabolism, contributing to the acidosis produced in cardiac arrest.

Ladder splint: a flexible splint consisting of two stout parallel wires and finer cross-wires; resembles a ladder.

Large intestines: the portion of the digestive tube that extends from the ileocecal valve to the anus. It is made up of the cecum, colon, and rectum.

Laryngeal edema: fluids invading the tissues of the larynx causing swelling.

Laryngectomy: the surgical removal of the larynx.

Laryngospasm: severe constriction of the larynx, often in response to allergy or noxious stimuli.

Larynx: the voice box.

Lasix: a medication used to rid the body of fluid.

Lateral: of or toward the side; away from the midline of the body.

Lateral immobilizer: a device that prevents sideward movements.

Lavage: a washing out of a hollow organ, such as the stomach.

Leaders: *See* Tendons.

Legionnaire's disease: an acute bronchopneumonia caused by bacteria.

Lens: the portion of the eye that focuses light rays onto the retina.

Lethargy: a lack of activity; drowsiness; indifference.

Leukemia: a disease of the blood-forming organs, characterized by proliferation of white blood cells and pathological changes in the bone marrow and other lymphoid tissue; cancer of the blood.

Librium: trade mark for preparations of chlordiazepoxide hydrochloride.

Ligament: tough band of fibrous tissues which connects bones to bones about a joint or supports any organ.

Light burns: burns resulting from concentrated sources of light, i.e. a welding torch or the sun.

Lipid: fat; any one of a group of fats that is insoluble in water but soluble in fat solvents.

Lipofuscin: any one of a class of fatty pigments formed by the solution of a pigment in fat.

Liquefy: to change to a liquid.

Litter: a type of stretcher for moving or carrying patients.

Liver: the large organ in the right upper quadrant of the abdomen that secretes bile, produces many essential proteins, detoxifies many substances, and store glycogen.

Lividity: redness caused by blood pooling in the dependent parts of the body that is seen 15 to 30 minutes after death.

Localized: confined to one spot or small area.

Locomotion: movement or the ability to move from one place to another.

Log roll: a method of rolling the body as a complete unit.

Long bones: a bone that has a longitudinal axis of considerable length consisting of a shaft and an extended portion at each end that is usually articular.

Lower extremity: the pelvis, legs, and feet.

LPM: abbreviation for liters per minute.

Lumbar spine: the lower part of the back formed by the lowest five non-fused vertebrae.

Lumbar vertebrae: vertebrae of the lumbar spine.

Lumbo-sacral: the area of the spine where the lumbar and sacrum meet.

Lumen: the cavity of tube-shaped organ such as blood vessel; the inside diameter of an artery.

Lung fields: referring to sections of the lung.

Lupus erythematosus: an inflammatory dermatitis.

Lymph: a straw-colored fluid that circulates in the lymphatic vessels and interstitial space.

Lymph nodes: any one of the round, oval, or bean-shaped bodies located along the course of the lymphatic vessels; producing lymphocytes and acting as filters for lymphatic system; when there is infection present, the lymph nodes in the area swell and are detected more easily in the neck and groin.

Lymphadenopathy: a disease of the lymph nodes.

Lymphatic system: an auxiliary part of the circulatory system, providing drainage for tissue fluid and returning it to the bloodstream.

Lymphatic vessels: the vessels through which lymph flows.

M

Macro-drip IV: a large-bore IV used for rapid fluid replacement by large drops of fluid.

Malaria: a parasitic disease causing intermittent chills and fever, spread by the bite of a previously infected anopheles mosquito.

Malignancy: a condition that is life-threatening, resistant to treatment, and severe; cancer.

Malleolus: the rounded projection on either side of the ankle joint.

Malleus: Latin for hammer; one of the three ossicles, or bones of the middle ear, named for its resemblance to a hammer.

Mandible: lower jawbone.

Manic-depressive disorder: marked by alternating periods of elation and depression.

"March" fracture: *see* Fatigue fracture.

Marijuana: a narcotic obtained from the dried leaves and flowers of the hemp plant.

Mastic: quickly-drying pasty cement.

Mastoid: a portion of the temporal bone that lies behind the ear, contains spongy bone tissue.

Mastoid cells: cells found in the large, spongy bone behind the ear.

Mastoiditis: inflammation of the mastoid, a bone located behind the ear.

Maxilla: the upper jawbone.

Maxillary bones: the two bones forming the upper jaw.

Maxillofacial: the lower half of the face.

Measles: acute viral disease with fever, bronchitis, and red blotchy rash.

Mechanical chest compression devices: "thumpers"; a compressor designed to imitate the appropriate manual techniques for chest compression.

Mechanical respirator: a mechanical device that delivers oxygen to a patient.

Mechanism of injury: factors involved in producing the injury.

Meconium: a dark green mucilaginous substance in the intestine of a full-term fetus, being a mixture of the secretions of the intestinal glands and some amniotic fluid.

Medalert tag: another name for medic alert identification system.

Mediastinal region: the space within the thorax that contains the heart, pericardium, large blood vessels, vagus nerve, trachea and esophagus; located between the left and right pleural spaces.

Medic Alert: identification system for patients with hidden medical condition

Medulla oblongata: the portion of the brain between the cerebellum and spinal cord that contains the centers for control of respiration, heart beat, and other major controls centers.

Melanin: the pigment that gives skin its color.

Meniere's disease: deafness, tinnitus, and vertigo resulting from nonsuppurative disease of the labyrinth.

Meninges: the three membranes covering the spinal cord and brain; the dura mater (external), arachnoid (middle), and pia mater (internal).

Meningitis: an inflammation of the meninges; characterized by a stiff neck, fever, and delirium.

Menopause: the point that marks the permanent cessation of menstrual activity.

Menstrual period: the time period of the menstrual flow; usually from three to seven days.

Menstruation: the normal periodic discharge of blood fluid from the uterus.

Metabolic acidosis: excessive amounts of lactic and other organic acids in the body.

Metabolic shock: shock caused by loss of body fluids with a change in biochemical equilibrium.

Metabolism: the conversion of food into energy and waste products.

Metacarpals: the five cylindrical bones of the hand extending from the wrist to the fingers.

Metatarsals: the five cylindrical bones of the foot extending from the ankles to the toes.

Metatarsus: the part of the foot between the tarsus and the toes, its skeleton being the five long bones extending from the tarsus to the phalanges.

Methedrine: trademark for preparations of methamphetamine hydrochloride.

Microcephaly: abnormal smallness of the head, usually associated with mental retardation.

Micro-drop IV: a small-bore IV used for children and maintenance of a lifeline.

Microflora: the plant life, visible only under the microscope, which is present in or characteristic of a special location.

Microorganisms: minute living organisms, usually microscopic.

Middle ear: the tympanic cavity and its ossicles.

Midline: the median line or plane of the body.

Migraine headache: an often familial symptom complex of periodic attacks of vascular headaches, usually temporal and unilateral in onset, commonly associated with irritability, nausea, vomiting, constipation, or diarrhea.

Military antishock trousers (MAST): an inflatable garment applied around the legs and abdomen, used in the treatment of shock.

Minor burns: any third-degree burns that involve less than 2 percent of the body surface or second-degree burns that involve less than 15 percent of the body surface.

Minor's consent: the right to consent is usually given to the parent or other person so close to the minor as to be treated as a parent.

Miscarriage: a lay term for the abortion or the premature expulsion of a nonliving fetus from the uterus.

Missed abortion: a situation in which the fetus has died at less than 20 weeks gestation and is retained in the uterus for at least two months thereafter.

Mitral valve: a valve located between the left atrium and left ventricle.

mmHg: millimeters of mercury.

Moderate burns: burns that are less serious than critical burns; included are third-degree burns that involve 2 to 10 percent of the body surface, excluding hands, feet, face, or genitalia; second degree burns that involve 15 to 25 percent of the body surface area; and first-degree burns that involve 50 to 70 percent of the body surface.

Mononucleosis: acute viral disease with fever, sore throat, and lymph node swelling.

Morphine: a narcotic analgesic used to relieve pain and anxiety; helpful in pulmonary edema because of its peripheral dilating effects.

Mortal: subject to death, destined to die.

Mouth to mask ventilation: The process of ventilating a patient by blowing through a mouthpiece connected to a face mask.

Mouth-to-mouth ventilation: the preferred emergency method of artificial ventilation when adjuncts are not available.

Mouth-to-nose ventilation: artificial ventilation in which the EMT's lips make a seal around the patient's nose as the EMT exhales into the patient's nose. The patient's mouth is kept closed, although sometimes the lips are spread apart during the exhalation by the patient.

Mucosa: any mucous membrane.

Mucous membrane: a membrane that lines many organs of the body and contains mucus-secreting glands.

Mucus: a viscid, slippery secretion that lubricates and protects various body structures.

Multiple births: the delivery of two or more babies during one episode of labor.

Multiple sclerosis: a disease in which there are patches of demyelination throughout the white matter of the central nervous system.

Multitrauma dressings: one of many names for large, thick-layered, bulky pads used for quick application to stem profuse bleeding.

Mummy board: a type of child-size restraining board.

Musculature: the muscular system of the body, or a part of the system.

Musculoskeletal system: all the collective bones, joints, muscles, and tendons of the body.

Myocardial infarction: the damaging or death of an area of heart muscle resulting from a reduction in the blood supply reaching that area.

Myocardium: heart muscle.

N

Narcotics: drugs used to depress the central nervous system, thereby relieving pain and producing sleep.

Nares: the external orifices of the nose; the nostrils.

Nasopharyngeal airway: an artificial airway positioned in the nasal cavity with the curvature of the airway following the nasal floor.

Nasopharynx: the upper part of the pharynx above the level of the palate.

National Association of EMTs: organization concerned primarily with maintaining and upgrading EMT knowledge and skills.

National Council of State EMS Training Coordinators: organization for communication between state EMS training coordinators.

National Registry of EMTS: organization involved in developing educational programs for national certification and maintaining a list of registered EMTs.

Nausea: an unpleasant sensation, vaguely referred to the epigastrium and abdomen, often culminating in vomiting.

Near-drowning: at least temporary survival after submersion in water.

Necrosis: a death of an area of tissue, usually caused by the cessation of blood supply.

Negligence: failure to perform an important or necessary technique or performing such a technique in a manner less than the accepted standard of care.

Nerve: a cordlike structure composed of a collection of fibers that convey impulses between a part of the central nervous system and some other region.
cranial: the twelve pairs of nerves connected with the brain.
spinal: the thirty-one pairs of nerves arising from the spinal cord.

Nervous system: the brain, spinal cord, and nerve branches fro the central, peripheral, and autonomic systems.
autonomic (involuntary): the portion of the nervous system concerned with regulation of the activity of cardiac muscle, smooth muscle, and glands.
cerebrospinal (voluntary): that portion of the nervous system consisting of the brain and spinal cord.

Neurogenic hyperventilation: a problem originating in the nervous system that causes rapid breathing and the giving off of excess carbon dioxide.

Neurogenic shock: shock caused by massive vasodilation and pooling of blood in the peripheral vessels to a degree that adequate perfusion cannot be maintained, resulting from loss of effective nervous control of blood vessels.

Neurological: of or relating to the branch of medical science dealing with the nervous system and its disorders.

Neurons: a nerve cell; the basic unit of the nervous system.
motor: an neuron possessing a motor function.
sensory: any neuron possessing a sensory function.

Neurotoxic: poisonous to nervous tissue.

Neurovascular: pertaining to both nervous and vascular elements; pertaining to the nerves that control the caliber of blood vessels.

Neutrons: particles of an atom that have no electrical charge.

Nitrogen: an element (N) making up about 80 percent of the atmosphere; present in the tissues of all plants and animals.

Nitroglycerine: drug used in the treatment of angina pectoris, usually taken under the tongue (sublingually).

Nonrebreathing masks: masks equipped with one-way valves that permit inhalation of oxygen from the reservoir bag and exhalation through the valve.

Norepinephrine: a hormone and drug used in the treatment of shock primarily for its alpha stimulating properties; causes vasoconstriction; trade name Levophed.

Normal saline (N.S): an intravenous solution containing 0.9 percent sodium chloride in water; used when volume replacement is desired.

Nosebleed: hemorrhage from the nose.

Nystagmus: continuous rolling movement of the eyeball.

O

O₂: symbol for oxygen.

Obstetric pack: a basic pack of equipment and supplies to be carried in an ambulance that is subject to emergency maternity call.

Obstructed airway: a blockage or obstruction in the airway which impairs respiration.

Obstructive airway disease: any disease which causes an obstructed airway.

Occipital lobe: the rear portion of each cerebral hemisphere of the brain, which receives messages from the optic nerve.

Occiput: the back of the skull.

Occlude: to close off or stop up; obstruct.

Occlusive dressing: a watertight dressing for a wound.

Ocular: pertaining to the eye.

One-rescuer cradle carry: method of movement where patient is carried in rescuer's arms, as one would a small child.

One-rescuer crutch: method of assisted, ambulatory movement where patient's arm is draped around the rescuer's neck for support and rescuer assists patient with an arm around patient's waist.

Open fracture: a fracture exposed to the exterior; an open wound lies over the fracture.

Open wound: a wound in which the affected tissues are exposed by an external opening.

Opiate: technically, one of several alkaloids derived from the opium poppy plant.

Opportunistic infections: infections capable of adapting to a tissue or host other than the normal one.

Opsite: a commercial, clear covering that is placed over an IV site.

Optic nerve: cranial nerve number two; the nerve that transmits visual impulses from the eye to the brain.

Oral airway: see nasopharyngeal airway.

Orbital fracture: fracture of the skull bone around the eye socket.

Orbits: the bony, pyramid-shaped cavities in the skull that hold the eyeballs.

Organic brain syndrome: neurological diseases that may cause disruptive or irrational behavior.

Oriented: the determination of one's position with respect to space and time.

Oropharyngeal airway: ventilatory adjunct placed in the patient's upper airway such that the distal curved part lies behind the base of the tongue and holds the tongue forward.

Oropharynx: area behind the base of the tongue between the soft palate and upper portion of the epiglottis.

Orthopedic: pertaining to the correction of deformities.

Oscilloscope: a display device with a screen for viewing an EKG or other physiologic data.

Ossicles: small bones; specifically, one of the three bones of the middle ear, malleus, incas, or stapes.

Osteoarthritis: a degenerative joint disease occurring chiefly in older persons, characterized by degeneration of the articular cartilage.

Osteoporosis: increased porosity of bone, loss of bone mass, resulting in fragility and weakness of the bones.

Ostomy: a general term referring to any operation in which an artificial opening is formed between two hollow organs or between one or more such viscera and the abdominal wall for discharge of intestinal contents or of urine.

Outer ear: *see* external ear.

Ovaries: the female gonad in which eggs and female hormones are produced.

Overdose: amount of medicine, drug, etc. in excess of that prescribed.

Ovulation: discharge of a mature ovum from the ovaries, occurring about every 28 days.

Ovum: egg.

Oxygen: a colorless, odorless, tasteless gas essential to life and comprising 21 percent of the atmosphere; chemical formula O₂.

Oxygenated: perfused with oxygen.

Oxygenation: to perfuse with oxygen.

Oxyhemoglobin: hemoglobin in its oxygenated state.

P

Pacemaker: a device generally implanted under a heavy muscle or fold of skin that maintains a regular cardiac rhythm and rate be delivering an electrical impulse through wires that are in direct contact with the heart.

Pacemaker cells: specialized heart cells which create a pulse, causing a wave of myocardial contractions.

Packstrap: A single-rescuer method of moving a patient by carrying the patient on rescuer's back with patient's arms draped over the rescuers shoulders.

Painful stimuli: any agent which stimulates pain.

Palate: roof of the mouth.

Palatine bones: the bones forming the roof of the mouth.

Pallor: a paleness of the skin.

Palmar: corresponding to the palm of the hand.

Palpate: to examine by feeling and pressing with the palms and fingers.

Palpation: the act of feeling with the hand for the purpose of determining the consistency of the part beneath, in physical diagnosis.

Pancreas: a large gland, 6 to 8 inches long, that secretes enzymes into the intestines for digestion of foods. It also manufactures insulin, which is secreted into the blood stream

Pancreatitis: an inflammation of the pancreas.

Paradoxical breathing: associated with flail chest, where a loose segment of chest wall moves in the opposite direction to the rest of the chest during respiratory movements.

Paradoxical undressing: a state of hypothermia wherein the body's thermal-regulating system becomes confused and while dangerously cold, the patient may undress because he thinks he is too warm.

Paralysis: loss or impairment of motor function of a part due to a lesion of the neural or muscular mechanism.

Paranoia: a mental disorder characterized by abnormal suspicions or other delusions, often of persecution or grandeur.

Paranoid schizophrenic: a psychotic state characterized by delusions of grandeur or persecution, often accompanied by hallucinations.

Paraplegia: the loss of both sensation and motion in the legs and lower parts of the body; most commonly due to damage of the spinal cord.

Parasitic: relating to an animal or vegetable organism that lives on or in another organism.

Parasympathetic nervous system: subdivision of the autonomic nervous system involved in control of involuntary, vegetative functions, mediated largely by the vagus nerve through the chemical acetylcholine.

Parathormone: hormone secreted by the parathyroid glands, important in regulating calcium in the body.

Parathyroid gland: small endocrine glands near or embedded in the thyroid gland that regulate blood calcium and phosphorus levels.

PARCER method: a study method standing for Preview, Ask, Read, Check, Evaluate, and Relate.

Paresthesia: an abnormal skin sensation, often of the pins-and-needles variety, indicating a disturbance in nerve function.

Pericardial tamponade: filling of the pericardial sac with fluid which limits the filling of the heart.

Parietal: pertaining to or forming any wall of an cavity.

Parkinson's disease: chronic, progressive nervous disease causing muscle tremors at rest, stiffness, and a rigid facial expression.

Partial neck breather: one who has had a tracheotomy, an incision into the windpipe.

Partial rebreathing mask: similar to the standard plastic face mask, but equipped with reservoir bags which permit the patient to rebreathe about one-third of his expired air.

Partial-thickness burns: a first or second-degree burns.

Patella: a small, flat bone that protects the knee joint; the kneecap.

Patent: open; unobstructed; obvious.

Pathogen: any disease producing microorganism or material.

Pathologic: indicative or cause by disease.

PCP: phencyclidine.

Pedal: pertaining to the foot or feet.

Pediatric: relating to children; medical practice devoted to the care of children up to age 15.

Pediatric Trauma Score: a cumulative trauma score which categorizes the physical condition of a child patient.

Pelvic cavity: the lowermost portion of the abdominal cavity containing the rectum, urinary bladder, and, in the female, the internal sex organs.

Pelvic girdle: the large, bony structure supporting the abdominal and pelvic organs, made up of the two innominate bones that arise in the area of the last nine vertebrae and sweep around to form a complete ring.

Penicillin: powerful antibiotic used in treatment of a wide variety of infections.

Penis: the male organ of urinary discharge and copulation.

Perfusion: the act of pouring through or into; the blood getting to the cells in order to exchange gases, nutrients, etc. with the cells.

Pericardial cavity: the space or sac formed by the two layers of the pericardium, and the inner visceral pericardium.

Pericardial sac: the double-layered sac holding the heart and the origins of the superior vena cava and pulmonary artery.

Pericardial space: the cavity between the two layers of the pericardium.

Pericardium: see Pericardial sac.

Perineum: the pelvic floor and associated structures occupying the pelvic outlet.

Periodontal disease: abnormal conditions dealing with the tissues that support the teeth.

Periosteum: the dense, fibrous tissue covering the bone.

Peripheral nervous system: the structures of the nervous system (especially nerve endings) that lie outside the brain and spinal cord.

Peripheral vascular resistance: the resistance to blood flow in the systemic circulation; depends on the degree of constriction or dilation of the small arteries, arterioles, venules, and veins making up the peripheral vascular system.

Peristalsis (peristaltic waves): the successive waves of muscular contraction and relaxation proceeding uniformly along a hollow tube, such as the esophagus or intestine; this motion propels the contents of the tube forward.

Peritoneal cavity: the abdominal cavity.

Peritoneum: the serous membrane lining the abdominal cavity.

Peritonitis: an inflammation of the peritoneum.

pH: a symbol used to indicate the acidity or alkalinity of a substance; the negative log of the concentration of hydrogen ions in a substance.

Phalanges: any bone of the finger or toe.

Pharyngeo-tracheal-lumen airway: a device used to manage and maintain an open airway.

Pharynx: the part of the alimentary canal between the cavity of the mouth and the esophagus; throat region.

Phencyclidine (PCP): "Angel dust," a very dangerous hallucinogen that can cause

arrhythmia, hypertension, hypotension, respiratory arrest, convulsions, coma, schizophrenia, paranoia, and amnesia.

Phenothiazine: a tranquilizer drug; also an anthelmintic.

Phlebitis: an inflammation of a vein manifested by tenderness, redness, and a slight edema along part of the length of the vein.

Phobia: an abnormal and persistent fear of a specific object or situation.

Phrenic nerve: the motor nerve of the diaphragm.

Physical dependence: habituation or use of a drug, or other maneuver, because of its physiologic support, and because of the undesirable effects of withdrawal.

Physiology: the study of body functions.

Pia mater: the innermost and most delicate of the three membranes covering the brain and spinal cord.

Piggyback carry: a one-man method of transport carrying the patient on one's back.

Pinch points: in farm equipment, where two objects meet to cause a pinching or pulling action.

"Pink puffers": an emphysema patient.

Pinna: the outer portion of the ear that leads to the ear canal.

Pituitary gland: the master gland of the body, located in the brain behind the eyes; influences the secretion of all other glands.

Placenta: a vascular organ attached to the uterine wall that supplies oxygen and nutrients to the fetus; also called the afterbirth.

Placenta previa: a delivery in which the placenta is the presenting part; may result in exsanguinating hemorrhage.

Plaque: any patch or flat area.

Plasma: the fluid portion of the blood, retains the clotting factors, but has no red or white cells.

Platelet: a small cellular element in the blood that assists in blood clotting.

Pleura: a continuous serous membrane that lines the outer surfaces of the lungs and the internal surface of the thoracic cavity.

Pleural cavities (space): the potential space between the parietal and visceral pleura.

Pleurisy: inflammation of the pleura.

Pneumatic antishock garment (PASG): an inflatable garment applied around the legs and abdomen, used in the treatment of shock.

Pneumocystis carinii pneumonia: a pulmonary disease of infants and debilitated persons in which white cellular detritus containing plasma cells appears in the lung tissue.

Pneumonia: an acute infectious disease of the lungs; causes an effusion.

Pneumothorax: an accumulation of air in the pleural cavity, usually entering after a wound or injury that causes a penetration of the chest wall or laceration of the lung.

Pocket masks: a device to aid in mouth-to-mouth resuscitation to prevent contact with the patient's mouth. It may be used with supplemental oxygen when fitted with an oxygen inlet.

Poison ivy: any of several American sumacs with grayish berries and pointed leaves in groups of three that can cause a rash if touched.

Poison oak: a shrubby western variety of poison ivy.

Poison sumac: a swamp shrub with greenish white flowers, grayish berries, and compound leaves of 7 to 13 leaflets that can cause a severe rash if touched.

Poliomyelitis: acute viral inflammation of the central nervous system characterized by fever, headache, sore throat, and stiffness of the neck and back; also called polio; infantile paralysis.

Polyuria: a condition of excessive urination.

Pons: a portion of tissue that connects the 2 halves of the brain.

Popliteal artery: the continuation of the femoral artery in the area behind the knee joint; used to auscultate pulse when taking a femoral blood pressure.

Positive pressure ventilators: ventilators capable of delivering large volumes of 100 percent oxygen, but with the drawback that they prevent the operator from feeling respiratory resistance as is the case with the use of a bag-valve-mask.

Posterior: situated in the back of or behind a surface.

Posterior tibial artery: the artery located posterior to the medial malleolus, supplies blood to the foot.

Postictal stupor: the third and final phase of a generalized seizure—the period of exhaustion and recovery following a convulsion. The patient's level of consciousness is depressed, and the airway may become obstructed by mucus, vomitus, or the relaxed pharyngeal muscles.

Potassium: a mineral substance necessary for the proper functioning of the heart and other tissues.

Power takeoff (PTO) shaft: the drive shaft that connects a tractor to farm implements.

Preeclampsia: the condition that precedes eclampsia, or toxemia of pregnancy, characterized by hypertension, edema, and seizures.

Premature: birth of a baby before the normal period of gestation (pregnancy) is over.

Prepartum hemorrhage: bleeding before birth of a baby, may be due to abruptio placenta, placenta previa, or ruptured uterus.

Pressure bandages: a bandage with which enough pressure is applied over a wound site to stop bleeding.

Pressure points: one of several places on the body where the blood flow of a given artery can be restricted by pressing the artery against an underlying bone.

Priapism: the persistent erection of the penis, especially when due to disease, injury, or excessive quantities of androgens.

Prickly heat: a cutaneous eruption accompanied by a prickling and itching sensation, caused by an inflammation of the sweat glands.

Primary survey: the process of finding and treating the most life-threatening emergencies first, dealing with breathing, heartbeat, and profuse bleeding.

Prinzmetal's angina: a variant of angina pectoris in which the attacks occur during rest.

Progesterone: ovarian hormone that prepares the uterus to receive the fertilized ovum.

Progressive shock: the second of the three stages of shock.

Prolapsed umbilical cord: a delivery in which the umbilical cord appears at the vaginal opening before the head of the infant.

Pronation: the act of assuming the prone position; placing or lying face downward; turning the hand palm down.

Proprioception: receiving stimuli within the tissues of the body, as within muscles and tendons.

Prostrate gland: a small gland that surrounds the male urethra where it emerges from the urinary bladder; it secretes a fluid that is part of the ejaculatory fluid.

Proteins: an essential nutrient, composed of amino acids in varying combinations.

Protocol: a precise and detailed plan for the emergency care given in a specific situation.

Protons: particles of an atom that have a positive electrical charge.

Pruritus: an itching that occurs as a symptom of some systemic change or illness.

psi: pounds per square inch.

Psychogenic shock: a shocklike condition due to excessive fear, joy, anger, or grief.

Psychological dependence: dependence of a drug, or other therapeutic maneuvers, because of its support to the patient's psyche, rather than to his physiologic function.

Pubic bones: the anterior inferior part of the hip bone on either side.

Pulmonary artery: the major artery leading from the right ventricle to the lungs.

Pulmonary circulation: the passage of blood from the right ventricle through the pulmonary artery and all of its branches and capillaries in the lungs, and then back to the left atrium through the pulmonary veins.

Pulmonary edema: condition of the lungs when the pulmonary vessels are filled with exudate and foam, usually secondary to left heart failure.

Pulmonary semilunar valve: one of the 4 heart valves (it lies between the right ventricle and the pulmonary artery).

Pulmonary valve: the valve between the right ventricle and the pulmonary artery.

Pulmonary vein: the veins that carry oxygenated blood from the lungs to the left atrium.

Pulse: the rhythmic expansion and contraction of an arterial wall caused by ventricular systole and diastole.

Pulse wave: the elevation of the pulse felt by the finger or shown graphically in a recording of pulse or pressure.

Puncture wounds: a result of any sharp object that pierced the skin.

Pupil: the small opening in the center of the iris.

Pupillary: pertaining to the pupil.

Purulent: a pussy condition; forming or containing pus.

Pus: fluid matter containing leukocytes and microorganisms.

Pyloric stenosis: an obstruction of the outlet of the stomach, a congenital abnormality characterized by excessive growth of the pyloric muscle.

Pyrogenic reactions: fever caused by foreign substance; in IV therapy, a fever caused by an IV contaminated with foreign protein.

Pyrogens: a fever producing substance.

R

Rabid: having or pertaining to rabies.

Rabies: viral disease of the CNS transmitted by the bite of an infected animal, invariably fatal unless treated before symptoms appear; also called hydrophobia from the supposed aversion of the victim to water.

Raccoon's sign: also called "coon's eyes;" bilateral symmetrical periorbital ecchymoses seen with skull fracture.

Radial artery: one of the major arteries of the forearm; the pulse is palpable at the base of the thumb.

Radial pulse: pulse taken where the radial artery crosses the distal end of the radius, that is, near the base of the thumb.

Radial styloid: part of the styloid processes, the bony prominences on the ends of the ulna and radius that form the socket for the wrist joint, the radial styloid being on the thumb side of the wrist.

Radiate: to diverge from a common center.

Radiation: the process of emitting energy in a particulate or wave form.

Radiation safety officer (RSO): an expert specially trained under government provisions to handle radioactive contamination.

Radine: a type of allergic reaction caused by specific chemicals.

Radioactive: emitting radioactivity; the spontaneous release of energy by particles that make up atoms.

Radius: the bone on the thumb side of the forearm.

Rads: a measure of the dose absorbed from ionizing radiation; equivalent to 100 ergs of energy per gram.

Rales: abnormal breath sounds produced by flow of air through alveoli and bronchioles constricted by spasm or filled by secretions.

Reactivity: normal contraction of the pupil in response to light aimed into the eye.

Receptor: a specialized area in a tissue that initiates a certain action upon specific stimulation.

Rectum: the distal portion of the large intestine.

Red blood cells: an erythrocyte; the cell that carries oxygen from alveoli to cell.

Reduce: to restore a part to its normal position.

Reeves Sleeve: corset-type extrication device.

Relative skin temperature: the quickest and most common type of temperature taken in the field; accomplished by touching the back of the hand to the patient's skin to monitor for abnormally high or low temperatures.

Renal: pertaining to the kidney.

Reoxygenate: to perfuse with oxygen after hypoxia.

Reproductive system: the organs in the male and female used in producing offspring.

Reservoir: the location where infecting organisms live and multiply.

Respiration: the act of breathing; the exchange of oxygen and carbon dioxide among the tissues, lungs, and atmosphere.

Respiratory: related to breathing or respiration.

Respiratory arrest: the cessation of breathing.

Respiratory depression: defined as breathing rate less than five per minute.

Respiratory system: a system of organs that controls the inspiration of oxygen and the expiration of carbon dioxide.

Responsive: acting or moving due to the application of a stimulus.

Retina: the lining of the back of the eye that receives visual images and transmits them via the optic nerve to the brain.

Retinal detachment: the sensory portion of the retina separates from the choroid.

Retinal vessels: the blood vessels of the retina.

Retraction: withdrawal of a body part, such as the testicles being withdrawn into the abdomen.

Retractions: the drawing in of the intercostal muscles above the clavicles; seen in respiratory arrest.

Rheumatic fever: infectious disease usually of children and young adults, characterized by intermittent fever, painful inflammation of the joints, and inflammation of the pericardium and heart valves.

Rhonchi: coarse rattling sounds somewhat like snoring, usually caused by secretions in the bronchial tubes.

Rib cage: the skeletal framework of the chest; composed of the sternum, the ribs, and the thoracic vertebrae.

Ribs: one of the 24 bones forming the thoracic cavity wall.
> **false:** the lower five ribs on either side which are not directly attached to the sternum.
> **floating:** the lower two ribs on either side which ordinarily do not have any ventral attachment.

true: the upper seven ribs on either side, which are connected to the sides of the sternum by their costal cartilages.

Rickettsia: parasite transmitted by the bite of infected ticks, lice, and fleas, causing Rocky Mountain spotted fever, Q fever, ricksettial pox, and typhus.

Rigor mortis: stiffening of a person's body and limbs shortly after death.

Rocky Mountain spotted fever: infectious ricksettial disease transmitted by tick bites, characterized by chills, fever, rash, headache, and pain in muscle and bone.

Roentgen: the international unit of x-ray or gamma radiation.

Roller bandage: a strip of rolled-up material used for bandages.

Rotation: the turning or movement of a body around its long axis.

Rules of Nines: a method of estimating the amount of skin surface burned.

Rupture: a tear or dissolution of continuity; a break of any organ or tissue.

Ruptured uterus: an uterine wall which rips open due to pressure.

S

Sacral spine: the lower part of the spine formed by five fused vertebrae.

Sacrum: part of the lower spine formed by five fused vertebrae.

Saddle joint: a joint having two saddle-shaped surfaces at right angles to each other.

Safe zone: the zone adjacent to the containment zone in a hazardous materials incident which is safe from contamination.

Sager splint: a traction splint with a padded arch support designed to fit into the patient's crotch on one end and an ankle harness on the other with an internal spring pulley-and-cable apparatus.

Salicylates: any salt of salicylic acid.

Saline: containing salt.

Salmonella: an organism related to that of typhoid fever which produces intestinal upsets.

Scald: burn or injury caused by hot liquid or steam.

Scapula: shoulder blade.

Scarring: the marking resulting from being scarred.

Scar tissue: the end product of a healed wound, usually whiter, tougher, and more gnarled than normal tissue.

SCBAs: self-contained breathing apparatus.

Schizophrenia: psychosis characterized by withdrawal from reality.

Sciatic nerve: a major collection of nerve fibers arising from the lumbosacral plexus and subserving most sensation of the lower extremity and motion of the leg and foot.

Sclera: the white, opaque, outer layer of the eyeball.

Scleroderma: chronic hardening and shrinking of the connective tissues of any part of the body.

Scoop stretcher: narrow stretcher that is first separated lengthwise, and then the two halves are slipped under the patient from each side; the halves are closed with locking brackets.

Scott air pack: a type of closed rescue breathing system suitable for use with radiation exposure.

Scrotum: a pouch of thickened skin hanging at the base of the penis, containing the testicles and their accessory ducts and glands.

Sebaceous gland: gland in the dermis which secretes an oily substance known as sebum.

Sebum: the secretion of the sebaceous gland; a thick, oily, semifluid substance composed of fat and epithelial debris from the cells of the skin.

Secondary survey: a head-to-toe evaluation of a patient to determine injuries.

Second-degree burns: burns in which the epidermis and a varying extent of the dermis are burned; there burns are characterized by blister formation.

Seizure: a sudden attack or recurrence of a disease; a convulsion; an attack of epilepsy.
> **febrile:** caused by high fever and most common in infants and children under four.
> **generalized:** affect the entire body; include both grand mal and petit mal seizures.
> **grand mal:** also known as major motor seizures, characterized by convulsions, always produce a loss of consciousness.
> **Jacksonian:** usually begin as convulsive movements in one part of the body, such as the foot, and subsequently spread.
> **myoclonic:** also called minor motor seizures, characterized by jerking activity of the limbs and trunk.
> **partial:** occur in a localized area of the brain.
> **petit mal:** also called absence attacks, do not involve convulsions, may be inherited, and almost always occur among young children.
> **psychomotor:** usually originate in the temporal lobe, typically in adults, and characterized by the repetition of inappropriate acts that may be mistaken for neurotic behavior.
> **status epilepticus:** the occurrence of two or more seizures without any period of complete consciousness between them.
> **unclassified:** includes all other kinds of seizures besides generalized, partial, and unilateral.
> **unilateral:** affect only one side of the body and one hemisphere of the brain.
> **withdrawal:** occur after dependency on a drug or alcohol when use ceases.

Self-contained breathing apparatus (SCAB): a complete unit for delivery of air to a rescuer who enters a contaminated area; contains a mask, controls, and air supply.

Senility: loss of mental faculties occurring as a result of the aging process.

Sensorium: a sensory nerve center.

Sepsis: the presence in the blood or other tissues of pathogenic microorganisms or their toxins.

Septic abortion: a serious uterine infection that commonly follows an illegal abortion.

Septic shock: a shock developing in the presence of, and as a result of, severe infection.

Septicemia: a systemic disease associated with the presence and persistence of pathogenic microorganisms or their toxins in the blood.

Septum: a dividing wall or partition, usually separating two cavities.

Serum: the liquid portion of the blood containing all of the dissolved constituents except those used for clotting.

Serum albumin: a natural colloid used as a volume expander for blood.

Shear points: in farm equipment, where two objects move close enough together to cause a cutting action.

Sheet drag: method of transport where a patient is moved by pulling the sheet on which he is laying.

Shirt drag: method of transport where a patient is moved by pulling on his clothing.

Shock: a state of inadequate tissue perfusion that may be a result of pump failure (cardiogenic shock), volume loss or sequestration (hypovolemic shock), vasodilation (neurogenic shock), or any combination of these.

Shoulder drag: method of transport where patient in a face up position is lifted under the shoulders and armpits and dragged head first with rescuer backing up.

Shoulder girdle: the encircling bony structure supporting the upper limbs; comprised of the scapulae, clavicles, and their central attachment.

Sickle cell anemia: a hereditary, genetically determined hemolytic anemia occurring in the black population; characterized by joint pain, acute attacks of abdominal pain, and recurrent embolic episodes.

Sigmoid: shaped like the letter "s" or the letter "c"; the sigmoid colon.

Sign: bodily evidence of disease found on physical examination.

Simple plastic face masks: *see* Pocket mask.

Sinusitis: inflammation of a sinus.

SKED: an extrication device used to stabilize a suspected neck or spinal injury victim.

Skeletal muscle: the most abundant muscle type; it allows movement and is mostly under voluntary control.

Skeleton: the hard, bony structure that forms the main support of the body.
appendicular: the bones of the limbs.
axial: the bones of the cranium, vertebral column, ribs, and sternum.

Skin: the outer integument of covering of the body, consisting of the dermis and the epidermis; the largest organ of the body; contains various sensory and regulatory mechanisms.

Sling: a triangular bandage applied around the neck to support an injured upper extremity; any wide or narrow material long enough to suspend an upper extremity by passing the material around the neck; used to support and protect an injury of the arm, shoulder, or clavicle.

Small intestine: the portion of the digestive tube between the stomach and the cecum, consisting of the duodenum, jejunum, and ileum.

Smooth muscle: a nonstriated muscle found in the walls of the internal organs and blood vessels; generally not under voluntary control.

Snapping rolls: high-speed farm equipment used for cutting.

Sniffing position: the position for endotracheal intubation with the neck flexed and the head extended.

Snoring: a breathing sound caused by partial obstruction of the upper airway by the base of the tongue.

Snowblindness: obscured vision caused by sunlight, reflected off snow.

Sodium chloride: NaCl, common table salt.

Soft palate: the soft, muscular tissue at the rear of the roof of the mouth.

Soft tissue: the nonbony and noncartilaginous tissue of the body.

Spasm: a sudden, violent, involuntary contraction of a muscle, or group of muscles, attended by pain and interference with function; a sudden but transitory constriction of a passage, canal, or orifice.

"Speed": amphetamines.

Sperm: the male reproductive cell.

Sphincter muscle: circular muscles that encircle a duct, tube, or opening in such a way that their contraction constricts the opening.

Sphygmomanometer: a device for measuring blood pressure.

Spinal column: the 33 bones (vertebrae) that enclose the spinal cord and protect it.

Spinal cord: the cord of nerve tissues extending from the brain down the length of the spine.

Spinal nerves: nerves coming out from the spinal cord.

Spine board: a device used primarily for transporting patients with suspected or actual spinal injuries.

Spleen: the largest lymphatic organ of the body; located in the left upper quadrant of the abdomen.

Splint: any support used to immobilize a fracture or to restrict movement of a part.

Spontaneous abortion: an abortion occurring naturally.

Spontaneous pneumothorax: a rupture of the lung parenchyma resulting in the accumulation of air in the pleural space without trauma.

Spores: the reproductive element of one of the lower organisms.

Spouse abuse: violent behavior between two people who are involved in an intimate relationship; either the man or the woman may be the abuser.

Sprains: a trauma to a joint causing injury to the ligaments.
first-degree (mild) sprain: characterized by pain with mild disability, some point tenderness, no abnormal motion, but frequently considerable swelling.
second-degree (moderate) sprain: sprain with pain, moderate disability, point tenderness, moderately abnormal motion, swelling, and hemorrhage.
third-degree (severe) sprain: sprain with pain, disability, loss of function, severely abnormal motion, and possible deformity, also tenderness, swelling, hemorrhage, and usually a torn ligament.

Sputum: expectorated matter, especially mucus or matter resulting from diseases of the air passages.

Stair-chair: a carrying device used to transverse stairs.

Stapes: Latin for stirrup; one of the three ossicles, or bones of the middle ear, named for its resemblance to a stirrup.

Staphylococcus: a bacteria that causes boils and other infections.

Status epilepticus: *see* Seizures.

Statute of limitations: a statutory time period during which a cause of action, such as a tort claim, must be legally commenced; failure to do so within the time period voids the claim.

Stereotyping: to give a fixed form to a person or situation.

Sterile: free from living organisms, such as bacteria.

Sternal rub: a maneuver used to test the patient's responsiveness by rubbing the patient's sternum with the rescuer's knuckles.

Sternocleidomastoid muscles: muscles on either side of the neck that allow movement of the head.

Sternum: the long, flat bone located in the midline in the anterior part of the thoracic cage; articulates above with the clavicles and along the sides with the cartilages of the first seven ribs.

Steroids: a group name for compounds that contain a hydrogenated cyclopentophenanthrene-ring system; substances include progesterone, adrenocortical hormones, and the gonadal hormones.

Stethoscope: instrument used in the determination of blood pressure and in the detection of heart, breath, and bowel sounds.

Stimulants: any agent that increases the level of bodily activity.

Stimuli: anything that causes or changes an activity in an organism.

Stokes litter: a wire basket stretcher used in rescue work.

Stoma: a small opening, especially an artificially created opening such as made by tracheostomy.

Stomach: the part of the digestive tract between the esophagus (food pipe) and the duodenum. The stomach churns food and starts the process of digestion.

Stool: the fecal discharge from the bowels.

Stored energy: in farm equipment, hazards

that remain after machinery has been shut down.

Straddle injury: an injury that usually occurs to the genital area from an object between the legs.

Strain: a muscle pull; a stretched or torn muscle.

Strangling injury: an injury in which an object constricts an extremity and cuts off circulation.

Street drugs: drugs acquired "on the street" by addicts from pushers or other addicts, not prescribed by a physician.

Striated muscle: muscle that has characteristic stripes, or striations, under the microscope; voluntary, skeletal muscle.

Stridor: harsh, high-pitched respiratory sound associated with severe upper airway obstruction, such as laryngeal edema.

Stroke: cerebrovascular accident.

Stroke volume: the amount of blood pumped forward by the heart each time the ventricles contract.

Strychnine: an extremely poisonous alkaloid.

Styloid processes: bony prominences at the ends of the radius and ulna that form the socket for the wrist joint.

Subarachnoid space: between the arachnoid (middle layer) and the pia mater (innermost layer) of the brain.

Subcutaneous connective tissue: a layer of fatty tissue just below the skin.

Subcutaneous emphysema: a condition in which trauma to the lung or airway results in the escape of air into body tissues, especially the chest wall, neck, and face; a crackling sensation will be felt on palpation of the skin.

Subdiaphragmatic abdominal thrust: *see* Heimlich maneuver.

Subdural: beneath the dura and outside the brain.

Subdural hematoma: a collection of blood or clot between the dura mater and the arachnoid usually caused by a laceration or rupture of a menin-geal blood vessel.

Subdural space: between the dura mater (outermost layer) and the arachnoid (middle layer) of the brain.

Subjective interview: a part of the secondary survey that uses the patient and bystanders as sources of information by having them answer specific questions.

Substernal notch: the point where the ribs meet the sternum.

Sucking chest wound: open pneumothorax.

Suction unit: equipment for clearing blood, vomitus, and other liquids from the airway.

Sudden infant death syndrome (SIDS): crib death; death of an infant after the first few weeks of life where the cause cannot be established by careful autopsy.

Suffocation: the act of having one's breathing blocked; suffering from lack of oxygen.

Suicide: self-inflicted death.

Sulphur dioxide: a colorless nonflammable gas having a strong, suffocating odor.

Sunstroke: form of heatstroke due to prolonged sun exposure.

Superficial: on the surface; opposite of deep.

Superior vena cava: one of the two largest veins in the body that empty venous blood into the right atrium; it receives blood from the upper extremities, head, and neck.

Supination: turning the forearm so that the palm faces upward.

Supine hypotensive syndrome: a pregnancy complication where a pregnant patient lying supine has a mask created by the uterus, fetus, and placenta compressing her inferior vena cava.

Suprapubic: the lower central abdominal region, above the pubis.

Swathe: a cravat tied around the body to decrease movement of a part.

Sweat gland: a gland that secretes water and electrolytes through the skin.

Symmetry: correspondence of opposite parts in size, shape, and position.

Sympathetic nervous system: a part of the autonomic nervous system that causes blood vessels to constrict, stimulates sweating, increases the heart rate, causes the sphincter muscles to constrict, and prepares the body to respond to stress.

Symptom: a subjective sensation or awareness of disturbance of bodily function.

Syncope: fainting.

Synovial fluid: a clear, viscid fluid that lubricates joints; secreted by the synovial membrane.

Synovial membrane: a membrane that lines the inside of the joint and secretes a fluid that lubricates the joint.

Synovium: the lining membrane of a joint cavity.

Syphilis: contagious disease spread venereally or congenitally that, untreated, runs its course over many years.

Syrup of Ipecac: preparation of the dried root of a shrub found in Brazil and other parts of South America that can cause vomiting.

Systemic: refers to anything that affects the body as a whole.

Systemic circulation: the passage of blood from the left ventricle through the aorta and all of its branches and capillaries and back to the right atrium through the venules, veins, and venae cavae.

Systolic: the highest peak pressure exerted on the arterial walls during ventricular contraction.

T

Tachycardia: abnormally rapid heart rate, over 100 beats per minute.

Tachypnea: excessively rapid rate of respiration, over 25 per minute in adults.

Talk-down technique: soothing and supportive communication with a person

high on drugs or alcohol in an effort to get them to relax.

Talus: the highest of the tarsal bones and the one which articulates with the tibia and fibula to form the ankle joint; the ankle bone.

Tarsal bones: the seven bones of the ankle.

Tarsus: the region of the articulation between the foot and the leg.

Telemetry: the measurement of diagnostic signs by electrical instruments and the transmission of them, especially by radio, to a distant place for recording; used for EKG signals.

Temporal artery: the artery located on either side of the face that supplies the scalp; it can be palpated just anterior to the ear at the temporomandibular joint.

Temporal bones: a pair of compound bones forming the sides of the skull.

Temporal lobe: a region of the cerebral hemisphere below and lateral to the frontal and occipital lobes; contains the control center for speech.

Temporomandibular joint: the joint formed by the articulation between the mandible and the cranium, just in front of the ear.

Ten-code system: a radio communications system which utilizes commonly used numbers to communicate EMS phrases.

Tendon: a tough band of dense, fibrous, connective tissue that attaches muscles to bone and other parts.

  tendon of insertion: the tendon connecting a muscle's point of action to the bone.

  tendon of origin: a tendon lying at the base of a muscle and attaching it to a bone.

Tension of pneumothorax: situation in which air enters the pleural space through a one-way valve defect in the lung, causing progressive increase in intrapleural pressure, with lung collapse and impairment of circulation.

Tentorium: an anatomical part resembling a tent or a covering.

Testis (pl. testes): the male reproductive gland that produces spermatozoa.

Tetanus: an infectious disease caused by an exotoxin of a bacteria, Clostridium tetani, that is usually introduced through a wound, characterized by extreme body rigidity and spasms, trismus, or opisthotonos, of voluntary body muscles.

Therapy regulators: regulator to be used in oxygen therapy, it has a control to adjust the flow rate.

Thermal burns: burns caused by heat; the most common type of burn.

Third-degree burns: burns that extend through the dermis and into or beyond the subcutaneous fat.

Thoracic region: the area pertaining to or affecting the chest.

Thoracic spine: the 12 vertebrae that attach to the 12 ribs; the upper part of the back.

Thoracic vertebrae: the 12 vertebrae that lie between the cervical vertebrae and the lumbar vertebrae.

Thorax: the part of the body between the neck and the diaphragm, encased by the ribs.

Thorazine: trade mark for preparations of chlorpromazine hydrochloride.

Thready pulse: a pulse that is weak or scarcely audible, characteristic of a person in shock.

Threatened abortion: bleeding and cramps during pregnancy which may go on to complete abortion or may subside, allowing the pregnancy to go to term.

Threshold: point at which an effect is produced.

Thrombophlebitis: a condition in which inflammation of a vein leads to the formation of a clot in the vein.

Thrombus: a blood clot which forms inside a blood vessel.

"Thumpers": mechanical chest compression device.

Thymus gland: a ductless, gland-like body situated in the anterior mediastinal cavity, which reaches its maximum development during the early years of childhood and then undergoes involution.

Thyroid cartilage: a firm prominence of cartilage that forms the upper part of the larynx; the Adam's apple.

Thyroid gland: a ductless endocrine gland lying in front of the trachea; produces hormones involved in metabolism regulation.

Thyroxin: hormone secreted by the thyroid gland.

Tibia: the larger of the two bones in the leg; the shin bone.

Tidal air: the air in the tidal volume; *see* tidal volume.

Tidal volume: the amount of air inhaled or exhaled during any level of activity; the volume of one breath at rest approximates 500 milliliters.

Tine test: a test for tuberculosis.

TKO: abbreviation for "to keep open."

Tolerance: the state of enduring, or of less susceptibility to the effects of a drug or poison after repeated doses.

Tonic phase: first stage of a convulsive seizure where the patient's body can become rigid for up to 30 seconds per episode.

Tonsil: either of two small, lymph tissue organs at the back of the throat.

Tonsil suction tips: large-bore tips that fasten onto suction tubing used to suction the pharynx.

Torsion: twisting.

Torso: the trunk of the body.

Tort claim: a civil court action to determine whether the rights of an individual have been violated.

Tourniquet: constrictive device used on the extremities to impede venous blood return to the heart or obstruct arterial blood flow to the extremity.

Toxemia: a condition wherein the blood contains poisonous products manufactured by body cells or microorganisms.

Toxemia of pregnancy: a condition sometimes occurring during the second half of pregnancy manifested by symptoms of eclampsia.

Toxins: poisons.

Trachea: the cartilaginous tube extending from the larynx to its division into the primary bronchi; windpipe.

Tracheostomy tube: a surgical opening made through the anterior neck, entering into the trachea.

Traction: pulling or exerting force to straighten the alignment of a part of the body.

Traction splint: a splint designed to apply tension to fractured bones and hold them in alignment while they heal.

Tracts: groups of nerve fibers within the brain or spinal cord.

Transection: a tranverse cut.

Transfusion: an injection of blood, saline solution, or other liquid into a vein.

Transient ischemic attack (TIA): a recurrent episode of neurologic deficit, often a warning sign of an impending stroke.

Transverse: across from side to side.

Trapezius muscles: originates at occipital bone, ligamentum nuchae, spinous processes of seventh cervical and all thoracic vertebrae; rotates scapula to raise shoulder in abduction of arm, draws scapula backward.

Trauma: surgical definition, physical injury; psychiatric definition, emotional distress relation to a specific incident.

Trauma packs: one of many names for large, thick-layered bulky pads used for quick application to stem profuse bleeding.

Trauma score: a quick appraisal system based on assigned numbers for respiratory rate and effort, capillary refill time, blood pressure, and the Glasgow coma scale, which can be helpful in indicating the condition of a trauma victim.

Trendelenberg position: the stock position, achieved by elevating the foot of the long spine board.

Triage: a system used for sorting patients to determine the order in which they will receive medical attention.

Triangular bandage: a piece of cloth cut in the shape of a right-angled triangular; used as a sling, or folded for a cravat bandage.

Trichinosis: disease caused by the trichina organism found in raw pork.

Tricuspid: the atrioventricular valve between the right atrium and right ventricle.

Tuberculosis: an infectious disease caused by the tubercle bacillus, affecting primarily the lungs, but can affect other organs. Spread by coughing or sneezing.

Tumor: a new growth of tissue in which the multiplication of cells is uncontrolled and progressive.

Turbinates: shaped like a top, a turbinate bone.

Tympanic membrane: the eardrum.

Type A personality: a hard driving, competitive, often hostile individual.

Typhoid: resembling typhus; any of a group of related anthropod-borne infectious diseases caused by species of Rickettsia and marked by malaise, severe headache, sustained high fever, and a macular or maculopapular eruption which appears from the third to the seventh day.

U

Ulcer: an open lesion of the skin or mucous membrane.

Ulna: the larger bone of the forearm, on the side opposite that of the thumb.

Ulnar artery: a major artery of the forearm; pulse is palpable on the medial wrist at the base of the fifth finger.

Ulnar styloid: part of the styloid processes, the bony prominences on the ends of the ulna and radius that form the socket for the wrist joint, the ulnar styloid being on the little finger side of the wrist.

Ultrasound: a high-frequency sound used to obtain images for medical diagnostic purposes.

Ultraviolet light burns: burns resulting from the rays of the sun.

Umbilical cord: the flexible, cordlike structure connecting the fetus at the navel with the placenta and containing two umbilical arteries and one vein that nourish the fetus and remove its waste.

Umbilical hernia: rupture of the viscera at the navel.

Umbilicus: the navel.

Universal dressing: a large (9 × 36 inches) dressing of multilayered material that can be used open, folded, or rolled to cover most wounds, to pad splints, or to form a cervical collar.

Upper extremity: that part of the skeleton consisting of the shoulder girdle, the arm, and the hand.

Uremia: a toxic condition caused by waste products of metabolism accumulating in the blood as a result of failure of kidney function.

Ureter: either of the tubes that convey urine from the kidneys to the bladder.

Urethra: the canal that leads urine from the bladder to the urethral orifice.

Urinary bladder: see Bladder.

Urinary system: the organs that control the discharge of certain waste materials filtered from the blood and excreted as urine.

Uterine inversion: turning inside out of the uterus.

Uterus: the muscular organ that hold and nourishes the fetus, opening into the vagina through the cervix; the womb.

V

Vacutainer: a commercial container for blood samples.

Vagina: genital canal in the female extending from the uterus to the vulva; the birth canal.

Vagus nerve: the 10th cranial nerve, chief mediator of the parasympathetic system.

Valium: a drug used as a tranquilizer and muscle relaxant.

Valvular heart disease: pertaining to diseases that cause damage to the heart valves.

Varices: plural of varix, an enlarged and tortuous vein, artery, or lymphatic vessel.

Vascular: relating to, or containing blood vessels.

Vasoconstriction: the diminution of the caliber of vessels, especially constriction of arterioles leading to decreased blood flow to a part.

Vasodilation: dilation of a vessel, especially dilation of arterioles leading to increased blood flow to a part.

Vasomotor center: the area that controls dilation and constriction of the blood vessels.

Vein: any blood vessel that carries blood from the tissues to the heart.

Venae cava: the two largest veins of the body returning blood to the right atrium.

Venacaval: pertaining to the venae cava.

Venipuncture: a surgical puncture of a vein for any purpose.

Venomous: containing poison secreted by animals and deposited in bite wounds.

Venous blood: unoxygenated blood, containing hemoglobin in the reduced state.

Ventilation: supplying air to the lungs.

Ventral: referring to the abdomen; directed toward or situated on the belly surface; opposite of dorsal.

Ventral cavity: composed of the thoracic cavity and the abdomino-pelvic cavity.

Ventricles: the thick-walled, muscular chambers in the heart that receive blood from the atrium and force blood into the arteries; also any small cavities; cerebral chambers containing cerebrospinal fluid.

Ventricular failure: absent ventricular contractions.

Ventricular fibrillation: a rapid, tremulous, and ineffectual contraction of the cardiac myofibils, producing no cardiac output; cardiac arrest.

Ventricular standstill: asystole; no muscular contraction of the ventricles.

Venules: very small veins.

Vernix caseosa: the white, cheesy deposit covering the skin of the newborn.

Vertebra (pl. vertebrae): any one of the 33 bones of the spinal column.

Vertebral arch: the posterior projection of each vertebra through which the spinal cord passes.

Vertigo: dizziness; an illusion of movement; sensation as if the external world were revolving around the patient.
central: vertigo due to some disease of the central nervous system.
labyrinthine: a form associated with the labyrinth of the ear.

Vial of Life Program: an emergency medical information system, similar to Medic Alert, which uses a small bottle or vial kept in the refrigerator which contains patient's medical information; sign or card near front entrance tell EMTs that the vial is present.

Virus: the specific agent of a type of infectious disease; specifically, a group of microbes that can pass through fine fibers that bacteria cannot pass through.

Viscera: internal organs, usually referring to the abdominal organs.

Vital signs: in basic EMT-level care, pulse rate and character, breathing rate and character, blood pressure, and relative skin temperature.

Vitreous body: the transparent substance that fills the part of the eyeball between the lens and the retina.

Vitreous humor: the fluid behind the lens of the eye.

Vocal cords: either of two pairs of folds of mucous membrane in the larynx that project into the cavity of the larynx; activated by the passing of air over the folds, causing vibration; source of the voice sound.

Voice box: the larynx.

Voluntary muscle: muscle under direct voluntary control of the brain, which can be contracted or relaxed at will; skeletal muscle.

Voluntary nervous system: that functional part of the nervous system which influences the activity of voluntary muscles and movements throughout the body.

Waterchill: a method of heat loss where water conducts heat away from the body 240 times more quickly than in air.

Wernicke-Korsakoff syndrome: organic brain disorder caused by thiamin defi-ciency stemming from chronic alcohol consumption.

Wharton's jelly: the soft, jelly-like homogeneous intercellular substance of the umbilical cord.

Wheal: a raised area on the skin resulting from an allergic reaction.

Wheezes: whistling respiratory sounds.

White blood cells: also called leukocytes and WBCs. Blood cells involved with destroying microorganisms and producing antibodies to fight off infection.

White matter: the inner mass of cerebral tissue; it has interconnecting nerve fibers intermixed with small sections of "gray matter" that form the control centers of nerve cells.

Windchill: the relationship of wind velocity and temperature in determining the effect on a living organism.

Windpipe: the trachea.

Withdrawal: physical or psychological removal of oneself from a situation.

Wound: a bodily injury caused by physical means, with disruption of the normal continuity of structures.

Wrap points: in farm equipment, an aggressive component moving in a circular motion.

X

Xiphoid process: one of three components of the sternum; the narrow, cartilaginous lower tip of the sternum.

Y

Yawning: a deep, involuntary inspiration with the mouth open, often accompanied by the act of stretching.

Yeast: a general term including single-celled usually rounded fungi that produce by budding.

Yoke: a connecting structure; a depression or ridge connecting two structures.

Z

Zinc oxide: a very fine, odorless, amorphous, white or yellowish white powder used topically as an astringent and protectant.

Zone: *see* specific zones, e.g. Safety zone.

Zygote: the cell resulting from union of a male and a female gameta, until it divides; the fertilized ovum.

□ INDEX

A

Abandonment, 11
Abbreviations, 21
"ABCs," 86, 124
Abdomen
 acute, 423-46
 anatomy, *29*, 326
 assessment, 74-75
  of children, 458
 bloated, 74
 closed wound (internal), 326-28
 cramps
  abortion, 499
  food poisoning, 353
  heat cramps, 554-55
 distended, 74
 edematous, 74
 evisceration, 329, *330*
 examination procedures, 424
 gastrointestinal tract, 36
 guarding, 75, 424
 injury, 326-30, *327*
  from auto accident, 180
  emergency care of, 329-30
  fetal position, 328
  from projectiles, 193
  signs and symptoms, *328*
 internal bleeding, 326
 open wound, 326
 pain, 423-24
  as complication in pregnancy, 498
 quadrants, 28, *29*
Abdominal aortic aneurysm, 426-27
Abdominal cavity, 26, 36, 326, *327*
Abdominal thrusts, 96
Abdominal walls, 326
Abortion, 499
 spontaneous, 499
Abrasions, 187-88, 196-97
Abruptio placenta, 501
Abscess, 46
"Absence attacks," 431
Abstinence syndrome, 357
Abuse
 child, 13, 471-74, *472*
 of elderly, 483
 spouse, 601-7
Acceleration-deceleration contusion, 259
Achilles tendon, *30*
Acidosis, 416
Acquired immunodeficiency syndrome. *See* AIDS
Activated charcoal, 346-47
Acute Myocardial Infarction (AMI), 399, 402-3
Adam's apple, 34
Adolescents, 452
 examination of, 455-56
 injury or illness. *See* Children (pediatric emergencies)

Adrenal gland, *38*
Advanced airway management, 707-18
Advanced cardiac life support, 133
Age, and heart attack, 396
Agonal respirations, 61
Agoraphobia, 594
AIDS, 441-46
 CPR, 139, 446
 destruction of virus, 447
 signs and symptoms, 444
 transmission, 443-44
 universal precautions, 444-46
Air bags, 186, 660
Air embolism, 574
Airway, 80
 adjuncts, 104-7
 advanced airway management, 707-18
  endotracheal intubation, 708-12
  esophageal gastric tube, 715-16
  esophageal obturator airway, 712-15
  pharyngeo-tracheal-lumen airway, 716-18
  transillumination (lighted stylet) intubation, 709-12
 anatomy, *95*
 assessment, 53-54
 obstruction, 94-101
  children, 100-101, 462-63
  cross-finger technique, 86-88
  emergency care, 94-101
  head injury, 253
  removal of, 94-101
  shock, *165*
  signs and symptoms, 97
  snoring, 85
Alcohol. *See also* Alcoholism
 abuse, disorders of, *355*
 controlling consumption, 764
 emergencies, *359*
 emergency treatment, 357-58
 violent patient, 365
Alcoholism, 355
 acute intoxication, 362
 addiction, 357
 crisis management, 364-65
 delirium tremens (DTs), 360, 362
 emergencies, *359*
 hypoglycemia, 362
 hypothermia, 362, 365
 insulin shock similarity, 362
 withdrawal syndrome, 362
Alimentary canal, 29
Alimentary tract, 36
Alkali, eye injury from, 294
Alkalosis, 392-93
Allergic reactions
 IV, 731
 venom, 380
Allergies
 shock, 161, 164-66, *165*, 169

All-terrain vehicle (ATV) accidents, 188
Alveolar collapse, oxygen concentration and, 119
Alveolar pouches, 34
Alveoli, 34
Alzheimer's disease, 483
Ambulance
 accidents, 675
 air, 693-96
 colors and markings, 675
 cots, 618, 633-34
 CPR, 136-37
 driving, 675-84
  bad weather, 678-79
  escorts, 684
  hazards, 678-82
  laws, 675-77
  mistakes common, 677
  safety, 675-77
 equipment, 684-86
  checklist, 684-86
 loading of stretcher, *634*
 maintenance, 686-88
  carbon monoxide in, 688-89
  daily inspection, *687*
  winter, 688
 run, phases of, 689-93, *692*
 types, *676*
 warning devices, 683-84
American Heart Association (AHA), 3, 86, 88, 94
American Red Cross, 2
American Trauma Society, 16
Ammonia, 343
Amniotic fluid, 485
Amputation, 201-3
 partial amputation, 201-3
Anatomical planes, 19, *20*
Anatomical regions, 19-21
Anatomical terminology, 18-19
Anatomy, generally, 17-47
 topographic, *22*
Aneurysm, 409
 abdominal aortic, 426-27
Angina pectoris, 397-98
Angular-impact collisions, 187
Ankle, 26
 assessment, 76-77
 dislocation, 227
 fracture, 244-46, *248*
 pulse in, 77
Anoxia, 80
 cardiac arrest, 83
 shock, 157-58
Anterior abdominal surface area, 28
Anticipatory phase of disaster, 644
Anticoagulants, 84
Anxiety, 594
Aorta, 34
Aortic semilunar valve, 33, 34

Apgar scoring, 496-97
Aphonic, 95
Apnea, 60
Apoplexy. *See* Stroke (apoplexy, cerebrovascular accident)
Appendicitis, 423
Appendicular skeleton, 25
Appendix, *37*
  secondary survey, 75
Arachnoid tissue, 42
Arms
  chest pains, 399
  collarbone fracture, 237, *238*
  elbow fracture, 238
  fracture, 238-40
  heart disease assessment, 399
  injury assessment, 77-78
  neurological survey, 255
Arterial pulse points, 34-35
Arteriosclerosis, 395
Artery(ies), 34, 122
  arterial hemorrhage, 142-44
  brachial, 147, 150
  carotid, *125*
  coronary, 395-96
  femoral, 150
  obstruction of, 395-96
Artificial ventilation, 79-103
  ambulance equipment, 684-86
  anatomy associated with, 80
  bag-valve-mask, 86, 117-18, 138
  children, 88, 91, 119
  CPR, *125*, 138
  demand-valve resuscitator, *118*, 118
  gunshot wounds, 207-9
  head-tilt/chin-lift, 90, *125*
  laryngectomy, 91
  lightning-strike victims, 527
  masks, 112-18
  mouth-to-mouth, 89-91, *90*
  mouth-to-nose, *90*, 91
  mouth-to-stoma, 91-92
  nasopharyngeal, *106*
  newborn baby, 506-7
  oropharyngeal, 105-6, *106*
  pocket mask, 115-16, *116*
  positive-pressure resuscitator, 119
  rescue breathing, 89-94
Asphyxia
  drowning deaths, 570
  traumatic, *313*, 319
Aspiration
  drowning, 570
  poisoning, 348-51
Aspirin poisoning, 343
Assessment. *See* Patient assessment
Asthma, 102
  acute, 388-89
  bronchospasm, 388
  children, 388, 465
  dyspnea, 83
  status asthmaticus, 388-89
  wheezing, 388
Asthmatic attack, acute, 388-89
Atherosclerosis, 395-96, *396*
  cardiac arrest from, 123
Atria, 31
ATV accidents, 188
"Aura," 435
Automated defibrillation, 737-42
Automatic Implantable Cardioverter Defibrillators (AICDs), 744
Automobile accidents
  access, 660-63
  emergency medical care, 663-67

extrication from, 663-67
kinetics of trauma in, 179-86
  ejection, 185
  head-on impact, 179-82, *183*
  lateral impact, 184-85
  rear impact, 182
  restraints and, 185-86
  rotational impact, 185
pregnancy and, 508
reporting of, 656
scene of, 656-57
traffic control, 657-58
ventilation of victims, 94
Avulsion, 199
Axial skeleton, 22-24

B
Babies (Infants). *See also* Children (pediatric emergencies); Pregnancy
  artificial ventilation, 506-7
  back blows, *101*
  brachial pulse on, 135
  cardiorespiratory emergencies, 461-67
  chest thrust, 100
  CPR, 133-36, *134*
  delivery, 485
  examination of, 454
  eye damage from oxygen, 119
  labor complications, 497-506
  newborn, 496-97, 506-7
    apgar scoring, 496-97
    meconium passage, 507
  premature, 506
  stillborn, 507
  Sudden Infant Death Syndrome (SIDS), 468-71
  vital signs, 457-58
Back
  assessment, 75
  blows, *100*
Backboards, 207, *619*, 622, 669-70
  difficulties, 670-71
  extrication equipment, 669-70
Bacteria, 440
Bag-valve-mask breathing apparatus, 86
Ball-and-socket joint, 25
Ballistics, 191
Bandage, bandaging, 212-19
  air splint, 151, *233*
  chest, *323*
  collarbone fracture, *237*
  compress, 214
  evisceration, *330*
  gauze pads, 215
  pressure, 219
  rib fracture, *320*
  roller, 215, *216*
  sanitary napkins, 213
  slings, *219*, 219
  triangular, 215
Baptism, of stillborn babies, 507
Barotrauma, 575-76
"Barrel chest," 84
Barton, Clara, 2
Basic life support, 79-103
  assessment, 86
  CPR, 120-39
  termination of, 137
Basket stretcher, *619*, 624, *625*
Battery, 12
Battle's sign, 255, 256-57
Bee stings, 379-80
Bends (decompression sickness), 574-75
Biceps, *30*

Bicuspid valve, 34
Bile ducts, 423
Biological death, 83
Bipolar disorder, 594-95
Birth canal, 486
Bites, 199-201, 370-84
  insect, 375-79
  snakes, 371-75
Black eye, 296
Black widow spider, 376
Bladder, 26
  injury, 331
Blanket, emergency, 623-24
Blanket drag, 615
Blanket lift, *625*
Blast injuries, 193-94
Bleeding (hemorrhaging), 140-55
  abdominal, 154
  abortion, 499
  arterial, 142-44
  assessment, 54-55, 141-42
  capillary, 144
  characteristics, *144*
  control of, 140-55
    direct pressure, 147-50
    elevation, 147
    tourniquet, 152
  cryotherapy, 152
  internal, 152-54
    after delivery, 504
    ectopic pregnancy, 499-501
    extremity, 154
    signs and symptoms, 152-53
  labor, 502-3
  lacerations, 146
  MAST, 151
  nosebleeds, 154-55, *155*
  oxygen deprivations, 141
  premature babies, 506
  pressure points, 147
  shock treatment, 154
  skull fracture, 258
  throat, 306
  vaginal, 499, 501, 502
  venous, 144
Blood
  backup, IV, 731
  cells
    radiation exposure, 541
    red, 141
    white, 141
  clot, 408-09
  congestive heart failure, 399
  in ears, 254-55
  head injury, 254
  oxygenation, 157
  physiology, 31-34, 720
  pressure
    children, 467
    cuff, 54, 58
    diastolic, 61
    head injury, 254
    heatstroke, 552
    hypothermia, 557
    internal bleeding, 152
    MAST, 151
    and pulse, 54-55, 58-60
    shock, 158-59, 164
    systolic, 61, 166
    technique, *62*, 62-63
  shock, 141
  transfusion, 720, 732
  vessels, 34, 141
    anatomy, 34

cardiovascular system, 141
  injury, 144
  shock, 159
  wounds, closed, 196
"Blue bloater," 386
Blueness (cyanosis), 55, 64
Blunt trauma, 203, 311
Body fluids, 720
"Body packers," overdose due to, 365
Body regulators. *See* Endocrine system
Bones. *See* Skeletal system
Brachialis muscle, *30*
Brachial pulse, 54, 135
Bradycardia, 736
Bradypnea, 60-61
Brain
  anatomy, *40*, 42
  central nervous system, 42
  cerebellum, 42, *252*
  cerebrum, 42, 251, *252*
  concussion, 259
  contusion, 259-62
  corpus callosum, *40*
  damage
    contusion, 259-62
    heatstroke, 549
    hematoma, 261-62
    insulin shock, 417
    stroke, 408
  fainting, 161
  injury
    acceleration-deceleration, 259
    assessment, 253-58
    coup-contrecoup, *261*
    epidural hematoma, *261*, 262
    impaled objects, 262
    patient history, 252-53
    physiology of, 252
    puncture wound, 262
    subdural hematoma, *261*, 261-62
  medulla, 252
  pons, *40*
  skull fracture, 258
  tissue
    bruise, 259
    laceration, 262
    swelling, 261
  trauma, *260*
Breastbone. *See* Sternum
Breathing apparatus, bag-valve-mask, 86
Breathing (respiration), 36, 80
  abdominal breather, 60
  agonal, 61
  apnea, 60
  assessment, 54, *61*
  chest injury, 311
  Cheyne-Stokes, 60, 369
  children, 91, 135, 457
  depth, 60
  emergencies, 384-93
  establishing breathlessness, *125*
  expiration (exhalation), 36
  head injury, 254
  heatstroke, 552
  hyperventilation, 392-93
  inspiration (inhalation), 36
  nasal passages, 34
  newborn babies, 506-7
  paradoxical, 315, *316*
  rate, 254
  rescue, 89-94
  shortness of breath. *See* Dyspnea
  spinal cord injury, 268
  symmetry of, 86

Breath odor, 71-72
Breech birth, 504-5
Bronchi, 34
  asthma, 388
  bronchiolitis, 462
Bronchial tubes. *See* Bronchi
Bronchioles
  asthma, 388
  emphysema, 385
Bronchiolitis, 462
Bronchitis, chronic, 102, 385-87
Bronchospasm, 85
Brown recluse spider, 376-77
Bruises, 23, 196
  coup-contrecoup, 259
  head injury, 259-62
Bullet wounds, kinetics of, 191-93
"Burn-out" syndrome, 588-91
  critical incident stress debriefing (CISD)
    to deal with, 591-92
Burns, 507-9
  chemical, 522-25
    ammonia, 524-25
    hydrofluoric acid, 524
  children, 516
  classification, 512-14
  contact, 511
  degrees, 512, *514*
    first degree, 511
    second degree, 512
    third degree, 512
  depth, *514*
  elderly, 516
  electrical, 525-28
    emergency care, 526-27
  emergency treatment, 516-18, 520,
    523-25, 528-29
  and eyes, 524
  inhalation injuries, 519-20
    emergency care, 520
  from "laying the bike down," 188
  lightning, 527-28
  patient transportation, 528-29
  radiant, 521-22
  rule of nines, 514, *515*
  scald, 507-9, 522
  severity, 514-15
    critical, 514-15, *516*
    minor, 515
    moderate, 514-15
  thermal, 515, 521
Buttocks, 45

C
"Cafe coronary," 95
Calcaneus, 26
Capillaries, 34
  bleeding, 144
Car accidents. *See* Automobile accidents
Carbohydrates, 36
Carbon dioxide, 31, 81
Carbon monoxide poisoning, 349-50
Cardiac arrest, 123
  children, 133, 466
  hypothermia, 563
  steps preceding CPR, 124-26, *125*
Cardiac asthma, 389
Cardiac compression, 121
  CPR, *136*
  mistakes, 133
  newborn baby, 507
Cardiac contusion, *318*
Cardiac emergencies, 394-406, *404*

Cardiac injuries, *318*
Cardiac risk factors, 396-97
Cardiac tamponade, 317-19
Cardiopulmonary arrest, 123
  oxygen delivery for, 112
Cardiopulmonary Resuscitation (CPR), 3,
  123
  changeover sequence, 132
  children, 133-36, *134*, 507
  complications, 133
  disease transmission from, 139
  electrical shock, 528
  interruptions of, 130
  mechanical, 138
  mistakes, 133
  "one-man," 126-30, *127*
  patient transportation, 136-37
  preceding steps, 124-26
  psychological considerations, 138
  retraining for, 137
  signs of successful, 132
  Sudden Infant Death Syndrome, 133
  "two-man," 130-32, *131*
Cardiovascular disease, in firefighters, 756
Cardiovascular system, 31
  disease, 395-96
  shock, 158-59
Carotid pulse, 54, 122, *126*, 135, 166
Carpals, 26
Car seats, 186
Catheters, 107
Cavitation from projectile, 192
Cavities, *28*
  abdomino-pelvic, 28
  body, 28
  chest, *311*
  pelvic, 28
  thoracic, 28
Central nervous system. *See* Nervous system
Cerebellum, 42, 251
Cerebral cortex, 42
Cerebrospinal fluid, 42, 254-55
Cerebrovascular accident (CVA). *See* Stroke
  (apoplexy, cerebrovascular accident)
Cerebrum, 42, 251
Cervical collar, 54, 57
Cervical spine, 53-54
  injury
    facial trauma and, 301
    signs of, 86
    surveying for, 72
Cervical vertebrae, 24
Cervix, *39*
Cesarean section, 502
Chain of evidence, 13
Chair-lift, 626, 631
Chair litter carry method of transfer, *631*,
  631-33
Chest, 80
  anatomy, 311
  assessment, 73-74
  blunt trauma, 311
  compression injury, 319
  emergency care, *313*, 314-15
  flail chest, *315-16*, 315-16
  heart contusions, 317
  injury, 311-24, 328
    from auto accident, 180-81, 185
    from projectiles, 193
  lung contusions, 316-17
  pain, heart attack related, *401*
  palpating, 85-86
  signs and symptoms, 311-14, *312-14*
  thrust, airway obstruction, 100

Cheyne-Stokes respiration, 60, 369
Chief complaint, 58
Childbirth, generally, 484-509. *See also* Pregnancy
Children (pediatric emergencies), 452-76
  alertness assessment, 454
  artificial ventilation, *101*, 119
  assessment, 454-56
  burns, 510-29
  cardiorespiratory emergencies, 461-67
    asthma, 465
    bronchiolitis, 465-66
    cardiac arrest, 466
    convulsions, 466-67
    croup, 463-64
    epiglottitis, 464
    shock, 467
    SIDS, 468-71
  carotid pulse on, 135
  child abuse, 13, 471-74, *472*
  CPR, 133-36
  dehydration, 458
  differences from adults, 453
  examination of, 454-56
  history, 456-57
  neurological assessment, 458-59
  parents, 453-54
  pediatric coma score, 459
  poisoning, 345
  psychological emergencies, 584-85
  PTS score, 459-60
  reassurance, 456
  transport, 474-76
  trauma, 459-60
  vital signs, 457-58
Chlorine gas, 343
Cholesterol, 396-97
Chronic bronchitis, 102, 385-87
Chronic Obstructive Pulmonary Disease (COPD), 36, 60, 385-89
Circulation
  assessment, 54-55
    after fracture, *230*
  child/infant CPR, 135
  pulmonary, 31, *121*
  systemic, 31, *121*
Circulatory system, 31-34, *32-33*, 141
  overload, 731
  shock, 161
Clamping injury, *206*, 206
Clavicles, 24, 80
  fracture, 237
Clinical death, 83
Clot, 408-9
Clothes drag method of transfer, 614
Clothing
  body temperature, 547
  frostbite, 565
  protective, 654
Cocaine, 368-69
Coccygeal spine, *266*
Coccyx, 24
Code of Ethics, 14-15
Cold, protecting IV solutions from, 731
Cold injuries. *See* Frostbite; Hypothermia
Colicky pain, 424
Collarbone (clavicle), 25
  fracture, 237
Collisions. *See* Vehicular accidents
Colon, *37*
Colostomy, 75
Coma
  diabetic, 61, 415-17
  hypothermia, 563

Communicable diseases, 440-41
  transmission, 440
Communications, 697-706
  control center, 700
  disasters, 648
  dispatch, 701-2
    medical control cards, *703*
  information gathering, 701-2
  IV therapy, 732
  radio equipment, 702-4
  radio terms, 699
  relaying information to physician, 699-700
  special needs, 584-87
  times, 699
Communications system, 698-99
Compression, 410
Concussion, 259
Conduction and convection, 548
Condyles, 26
Congestive heart failure. *See under* Heart
Conjunctiva, objects in, 290
Consciousness
  assessment of, 55, 65
  levels
    children, 459
    head injury, 255-56
    shock, 163
  neurological examination, 65-68
Consent
  implied, 12
  informed, 12
  minor's, 12
Constipation, 428
Contact lenses, 297-98
  extended use of, 293, 297
Contamination. *See also* Hazardous materials emergencies
  open wounds, 196
  radiation, 540-45
Contractions, 487
  timing, 490
Contusion, 196, 259-62, 316-17
Convulsions
  alcohol/drug abuse, 358
  children, 466-67
  heatstroke, 552
COPD, 36, 60, 385-89
Coral snake, 375
Corset-type extrication devices, 671
Costal, 28
Costochondral separation, 133
Coughing
  asthma, 388
  chronic bronchitis, 385-87
  coughing blood, 392
  croup, 85
  dyspnea, 384
  emphysema, 387
  respiratory assessment, 84
CPR. *See* Cardiopulmonary Resuscitation (CPR)
Cranial nerves, 22, 42
Cranium, 22
Crime scene management, 600-601
Crime victims, 13
Crisis intervention, 593-611
Critical incident stress debriefing (CISD), 591-92
Crossed-finger technique, 86-88
Croup, 85
Crowing, 85
Crowning, 486
Cryotherapy, 152

CUPS procedure, 66
Cyanosis (blueness), 55, 64
Cystitis, 423

D
Deaf, communicating with the, 586
Death
  alcoholism, 355
  asthma, 389
  biological, 83
  burns, 509
  "cafe coronary," 95
  carbon monoxide poisoning, 350
  childbirth, 507
  children, 476
  clinical, 83
  drowning, 569-70
  and dying, 609-11
  heart attack, 395
  heatstroke, 552
  hypothermia, 563
  insulin shock, 417
  lightning, 527-28
  radiation, 541
  shock, 157
  SIDS, 468-71
  from trauma, 66
Decompensation, 387
Decompression sickness, 574-75
Decontamination, radiation, 544-45
Defibrillation, 138
  automated, 737-42
  Automatic Implantable Cardioverter Defibrillators (AICDs), 744
  EMT-D prehospital defibrillation, 733-44
  maintenance checklist, 742
  manual, 737, 742-43
  precautions, 744
  troubleshooting, 742-43
Dehydration
  children, 458
  diabetic coma, 416
  and fever, 458
  shock, 158
Delirium tremens (DTs), 362
Deltoid muscles, *30*
Dementia in elderly, 483
Depression
  crisis, 594-95
  geriatric, 481
Dermatitis, 352
Diabetes
  and burns, 516
  causes, 415
  coma, 415-17
  diabetic emergencies, 414-21
  hyperglycemia, 415
  hypoglycemia (insulin shock), 415, 417-21
Diabetic coma, 61, 415-17
Diaphoresis. *See* Sweating (disphoresis, perspiring)
Diaphragm, 80, *311*
Diarrhea, 428
Diastolic pressure, 61
Digestive system, 36-38, *37*
Digitalis, 84
Dilation of pupils, 254
Disasters, 643-52
  communications, 648
  disaster assistance, 644
  management of, 649-50
  planning for, 644-47

prewarning, 647-48
reactions to, 648-49
stress on personnel, 651-52
Disentanglement, 667-70
farm equipment, 340
Dislocations, 25, *198*, 225-27
ankle, 227
elbow, 226
hip, 227
knee, 227
shoulder, 226
wrist, 226-27
Dispatch, 701-2
medical control cards, *703*
Dissipation of energy, 191
Distal pulse, 77
Diverticulitis, 423
Diving emergencies, 572-76
Diving reflex, mammalian, 571
Dizziness, 437
Dog bites, 199-201
Drag on bullet, 191
Draw-sheet, *620*, 626-29
Dressings, 212-19
amputation, 202
and bandages, 212-19
human bites, 201
occlusive, 215
pressure, 219
sucking chest wound, *323*
Drowning and near drowning, 569-72
emergency care, 571-72
Drug(s)
abuse, 355, 356
signs and symptoms, 358
addiction, 357
cocaine, 358
compulsive use, 357
crisis management, 364-65
emergency consequences of abuse, 356
emergency treatment, 357-58
hallucinogens, 356
heatstroke, 550
hyperventilation, 365
hypothermia, 557
inhalants, 356
narcotics, 357
overdose procedures, 365-67
phencyclidine (PCP), 358, 368
"physical dependence," 357
psychological dependence, 357
talk-down technique, 367-68
tolerance, 357
violent patients, 365
withdrawal, 355
Drug-related injuries, reporting
requirements, 13
Drug toxicity in elderly, 483
Ductless glands. *See* Endocrine system
Duodenum, 36
Dura mater, 42
Dying patient, 609-11
legal requirements and, 13-14
Dyspnea, 60-61, 83-84, 384
congestive heart failure, 84
COPD, 385
emphysema, 385
and heart disease, 84
and myocardial infarction, 84
and pulmonary embolism, 84, 391

E
Ear(s)
anatomy, *46*, 46

cerebrospinal fluid, 254
drum, 46
earwax, 46
foreign objects in, 305-6
injury, 305-6, *306*
inner, 46
middle, 46
outer, 46
Ecchymosis, 196
Eclampsia, 430, 499
Ectopic pregnancy, 499-501
Edema. *See* Swelling (edema)
Ejection from vehicle, 185, 187
Elbow
dislocation, 226
fracture, 238
Elderly
burns, 516
geriatric emergencies, 477-88
hypothermia, 482, 563
Embolism
air, 574
cerebral, *409*
pulmonary, 102-3, 389-91
childbirth, 391, 504
dyspnea, 391
hyperventilation, 392
Embolus (wandering clot), 409
air, 730
plastic, 730
pulmonary, in elderly, 482
Embryo, 38
Emergency blanket, *619*, 623-24
Emergency Childbirth Record, sample
form, *498*
Emergency medical dispatcher, 49
Emergency medical services, 2-3
symbol, *4*
Emergency medical system (EMS), 3-4
Emergency medical technician(s) (EMTs),
2-7. *See also* Lifestyle of EMTs, healthy
burnout, 588-92
code of ethics, 14-15
D - defibrillation, 733-44
disaster response, 644-47
education, 6
functions, 7-10
initial role, 5
legal problems associated with, 10-14
levels of training, 5
oath of, 15
stress, 587-88, 651-52
Emotional stress, 757-61
Emphysema, 102, 385-87
subcutaneous, 322-23
traumatic, *313*
EMS Incident Report, sample form, *706*
Endocrine system, *38*, 38-39
Endotracheal intubation, 708-12
Endotracheal tube, 118
Energy
dissipation of, 191
effect of, 179
Entrance wounds, 207
Enzymes, 36
Epidural, 251
Epigastric, 28
Epiglottis, 34, 81
airway closure, 95
Epiglottitis, 95
Epilepsy, 430
seizures, 429-38
Esophageal gastric tube airway, 715-16
Esophageal obturator airway, 118, 712-15

Esophageal reflux (heartburn), 427-28
Esophageal varices, 426
Esophagus, 81
Ethnicity, patient responses and, 10
Eustachian tube, 46
Evacuation, disaster, 647-48
Evaporation, heat loss, 549
Evidence, chain of, 13
Exit wounds, 207
Extremities, injuries to, 193
Extremity lift, 629-31
Extrication, 653-73
access to patient, 660-63
ambulance equipment for, 654-55
basic principles of, 655
chemical hazards, 657
disentanglement, 667-70
farm equipment, 340
electrical hazards, 657
extrication device, *669*
rope-sling, 671
stabilizing patient, 663-67,
668-69
tools, 654-55
traffic control, 657-58
transfer, *669*, 669-71
underground, 671-72
vehicle stabilization, 659
water, 671
Extruded eyeball, 295-96
Eye(s)
anatomy, 45-46
anterior chamber, 45
aqueous humor, 45
assessment, 290
black, 296
burns, 296, 524
cataract, 46
chemical burns, 293-94, 524
conjunctiva, 45
conjunctivitis, 45
contact lenses, 297-98
cornea, 45, 296
diagnostic significance of, 70
emergency care of, 296
extruded eyeball, 295-96
foreign objects in, 290-91, *291*
globe, 290, 293
and head injury, 256
impaled objects, 295
injuries, 71, 119, 289-98
iris, 45
lens, 45
lids, injury to, 291-93, *292*
movements, 256
optic nerve, 46
orbits, 290
injury to, *293*
pupils, 290
assessment, 70
central nervous system emergencies,
256
constriction, 254
dilation, 254
head injuries, 254, 256
heatstroke, 552
hypothermia, 557
neurological examination, 256
skull fracture, 258
retina, 45
detachment, 296
sclera (whites), 45
vitreous body, 45
vitreous humor, 45

F

Face, 16
  assessment, 70
  burns, 515-16
  injury, 299-311
    from auto accident, 181
    emergency care of, 300-301
Face-masks, pocket, 92-94
Facial bones, *303*
Fainting, 437-38
  in elderly, 482
  shock, 161, 164
Fallopian tubes, 39
Falls
  by elderly, 482-83
  kinetics of trauma from, 179, 188-89
Farm injuries, 334-41
  causes, 334-36
  emergency care, 336, 340
  special seriousness, 334
Farm machinery, 337-39
  combines, 337-39
  corn pickers, 339
  grain tanks and augers, 339
  hay balers, 339
  operational controls, 339
  power takeoff shafts, 337
  shutdown of equipment, 339-40
  snapping rolls, 339
Feces, blood in, 75
Federal Communications Commission (FCC), 699
Feet-first fall, 189
Felonies, reporting requirements, 13
Femoral artery, *150*, 150
Femur, 26
  fracture, 242-44
  traction splint, 243
Ferno K.E.D. (Kendrick Extrication Device), 276
Fetal membranes, 485
Fetus, 39
Fever
  children, 458
  heatstroke, 550
Fibrillation, ventricular, 122, 735-36
Fibula, 26
Fingers
  clamping injury, 206
  fracture, 240-41, *241*
Finger sweeps, 98
Fire ant bite, 378
Firefighters, cardiovascular disease in, 756
Fireman's carry method of transfer, *615-16*, 615
First responders, interacting with, 5-6
Fitness program for EMTs, 748-56
Flat lift carry, 627-29, *629*
Flat stretcher (folding emergency stretcher), 621
Flu symptoms, carbon monoxide poisoning and, 349
Folding stair chair, 626
Follicle, 44
Food
  anaphylactic shock, 161
  poisoning, 353
  tube (esophagus), 81
Foot (feet), 26
  assessment, 76-77, *77*
  burns, 516
  distal pulse, 77
  fracture, 244-46
Force, defined, 177-78

Fractures, 227-35
  ankle, 244-46, 248
  arm, 238-40, *240*
  assessment after, *230*
  assessment for, 222-23
  classification, *228*
  closed (simple), *228*
  collarbone, 237
  comminuted, 229
  compression, 229, 319
  depressed, 229
  elbow, 238, *239*
  emergency care of, 230-32
  fatigue, 229
  femur, *243*
  fibula, 244
  finger, 240-41, *241*
  foot, 244-46, *248*
  forearm, 238-40, *240*
  greenstick, 229
  hand, 240-41
  hip, 242
  humerus, 238, *239*
  impacted, 229
  and internal bleeding, 152
  jaw, 303-4
  kneecap, 244, *246*
  leg, 242-48
  longitudinal, 227
  "march fractures," 229
  mechanisms of injury, 229
  oblique, 227
  open (compound), *228*
  patella (kneecap), 244, *246*
  pelvis, *241*, 241-42
  penis, 331-32
  ribs, 319-20
  scapula, 237-38
  and shock treatment, 168
  signs and symptoms, *229*
  skull, 258
  spiral, 227-29
  thigh, 242-44
  tibia, *231*, 244
  toe, 244-46
  traction splint, 243, *245*
  transverse, 227
  types, 227-29
  wrist, 240
Frontalis muscle, *30*
Frostbite, 565-67, *566*
  assessment, 565
  emergency care, 565-67

G

Gallbladder, 36, *37*
Ganglia, 42
Gangrene
  bandaging, 214
  frostbite, 565
Gas from silos, 337
Gastric distention, *94*, 94
Gastrocnemius muscles, *30*
Gastroenteritis, 423
Gastrointestinal tract, 36
Gauze compresses, 213-14
Geiger counter, 543
Genes, 39
Genitalia, 39
  burns, 516
  injury, 326
    female, 332
    male, 331-32
  pelvic assessment, 75

Genitourinary system. *See* Reproductive system; Urinary system
Geriatric emergencies, 477-88
  assessment, 480-81
  signs and symptoms, 478
Glands
  ductless, 38-39
  sebaceous, 44
  sweat, 44
Glasgow Coma Scale, 66, *67*
Glaucoma, 296
Gluteus maximus, *30*
Glycogen, 39
Gonads, 39
Good Samaritan laws, 11
Grand mal seizures, 431, *434*
Gunshot wound, 207-9
Gurgling, 85
Gynecological emergencies. *See* Pregnancy

H

Hallucinations, 362
  hallucinogenic drugs, 356
Hand
  burns, 516
  clamping injury, *206*, 206
  fracture, 240-41
Hazardous materials emergencies, 530-45
  general procedures for handling, 532-40
    HazMat protective suits, *538*
    plan implementation, 535
    preincident planning, 535
  identifications, 532, *533-34*
  nine step decon, *536*
  radiation emergencies, 540
    emergency procedures, 542-44
    personal decontamination, 544-45
    vehicle decontamination, 545
  zones, 535-40
Head-first fall, 189
Head injury, 249-64
  assessment, 253-58
  from auto accident, 182, 185
  from bullet, 192
  closed, 262-63
  emergency care, 263-64
  neurological assessment, 255-58
  open, 262-63
  puncture wound, 262
  signs and symptoms, *253*, 259
  skull fracture, 258
  vital signs, 254
  water rescue, 572
Head-on collisions
  automobile, 179-82
  motorcycle, 187
Head tilt/chin lift, 52, *88*, 88
Health risks for EMTs, 747-48
Heart
  anatomy, 31, 121-22, *122*, 395, 734-35
  angina pectoris, 397-98
    distinguished from MI, *399*
  aorta, transection, 320-21
  attack (myocardial infarction), 122, *400*, 402-3
    and chest pains, *401*
    distinguished from angina pectoris, *399*
    dyspnea, 402
    risk factors, 396-97
    signs and symptoms, *400*
  blood flow, 402
  congestive heart failure, 399
  causes of, 403-4
  dyspnea, 404

noisy lung sounds, 356
  signs and symptoms, 404
  tachycardia, 358
  wheezing, 404
contusions, 317
coronary artery diseases, 121, 395-96
  disease, 397-98
  and burns, 516
  risk factors, *397*
heartburn, 427-28
injuries, 317-19, *318*
  from auto accident, 180-81
  flail chest and, 315
muscle, 31, 123
oxygen, lack of, 123
pericardial tamponade, *313*, 317-19
rate, newborn babies, 497, 507
traumatic asphyxia, *313*, 319
valves, damage to, 395
Heart attack, 122, 482
Heat cramps, 549, 554-56, *558*
Heat exhaustion, 549, 553-54, *558-59*
  different from heatstroke, 554
Heat loss, 547-48, 549
  newborn babies, 496
Heat regulation, 547-48
Heatstroke (sunstroke), 549-53, *559*
Heimlich maneuver, 97
Helmet removal, *287-88*
Hematoma, 196
  epidural, 262
  subdural, 261-62
Hemoglobin, 34
Hemophiliacs, 144
Hemopneumothorax, 193
Hemoptysis, 102-3
Hemorrhage. *See also* Bleeding
  (hemorrhaging)
  abdominal injury, 326-27
  abortion, 499
  arterial, 142-43
  body control of, 142
  capillaries, 144
  cerebral, 409-10
  childbirth, 502-3
  ectopic pregnancy, 500-501
  effects of, 142
  from facial injury, 302
  grades of, 63-64
  internal, 152, *154*
  labor, 502-3
  MAST, 151
  open wounds, 199
  prepartum, 502-3
  and shock, 150
  stages of, 142, *143*
  stroke, 409-10
  tourniquet, 151
  vein, 144
Hemorrhagic shock, 159-60, 161, 164
Hemothorax
  chest injury, 312, 321
  CPR, 130
Hepatitis B, *442*
Hernia (rupture), 38, 329-30
  inguinal, 38
  umbilical, 38
Hip(s), 26
  dislocation, 227
  fracture, 242
  traction splint, 243
History taking, 68-69
Hostility in patients, 598-601
Humerus, 25
Hydrofluoric acid, 524

Hyperflexion position, 182
Hyperglycemia, 415-17
Hyperpnea, 61
Hyperthermia, 549
Hyperventilation, 61, 103, 392-93
  for head-injured patient, 263
  neurogenic, 61
Hypoglycemia (insulin shock), 362, 415, 417-21
  alcoholism, 362
Hyponatremia, 570
Hypothalamus, *40*
Hypothermia, 556-67
  CPR, 560-62
  elderly, 482, 563
  emergency care, 559-62
  immersion, 563-65
  levels of, 557-59
  signs and symptoms, *561*
  stages, *560*
Hypovolemic shock, 366
Hypoxemia, 66
Hypoxia, 100

I
Ileostomy, 75
Ileum, 36
Ilia, 26
Immobilization. *See* Moving patients
Immune system, 440
Impact phase of disaster, 644
Impaled object, generally, 209-10
Implied consent, 12
Incident command system, 644
Incisions, 197-98
Incontinence, 259
Incus, 46
Industrial rescue, 340-41
Infants. *See* Babies (Infants)
Infection-control measures, 196
Infection from human bites, 201
Infectious disease control, 439-51
  transmission, 440
Inferior vena cava, 31
Infiltration, 731
Inflammation, clamping injury and, 206
Information transmittal. *See* Reporting information
Informed consent, 12
Infusion, 720
Inhalation injury, 519-20
Injury. *See also* Kinetics of trauma
  among EMTs, 747
  mechanism of, 177
Insect bites, 375-79
  anaphylactic shock, 161
Insect stings, 379-80
  anaphylactic shock, 161, 380
Insulin, 39
  shock, 362, 415, 417-21
International Red Cross, 2
Intervertebral disc, 24
Intestines, 26, 36
Intrapleura space, 36
Intrathoracic pressure, 123
Intravenous (IV) therapy, 719-32
  blood transfusions, 732
  communications, 732
  complications, 730-32
  discontinuation, 732
  patient assessment, 728, *729*
  procedure, 723-27
  set-up, 720-23
Intubation, transillumination (lighted stylet), 709-12

Ipecac, 346
Islets of Langerhans, 39

J
Jaw
  fracture, 303-4
  injury, *303*
  lower (mandible), 301
  thrust maneuver, 85, 88-89
  upper (maxilla), 301
Jejunum, 36
Jellyfish, *382*
Joints
  ball-and-socket, 25
  condyloid, 28
  elbow, 27
  gliding, 27-28
  hinge, 26
  immovable, *27*, 225
  knee, 27
  movable, *27*, 225
  movements, 26-28, 225
  pivot, 27
  rotation, 26
  saddle, 28
Jump kit, 50

K
Kenrick extrication device (KED), 626, 667
Ketoacidosis, 415-17
Kidneys, 38
  diabetes, 415
  injury, 331
  stones, 423
  urinary system, *38*
Kinetic energy formula, 177, 190
Kinetics of trauma, 176-94
  automobile accidents, 179-86
    ejection, 185
    head-on impact, 179-82, *183*
    lateral impact, 184-85
    rear impact, 182
    restraints and, 185-86
    rotational impact, 185
  blast injuries, 193-94
  falls, 179, 188-89
  motorcycle accidents, 186-88
  penetrating trauma, 189-93
    bullet wounds, 191-93
    low velocity, 190
    medium and high velocity, 191-92
    shotgun wounds, 192
  recreation vehicles accidents, 188
  velocity-mass interaction, 177-79
Knee(s), 26
  dislocation, 227
Kneecap (patella), 26
  fracture, 244

L
Labor (childbirth). *See also* Pregnancy
  ambulance equipment, 491
  complications of delivery, 504-6
  emergency delivery, 490-96
  stages, 486, *489-90*
  transporting, 487
Lacerations, 22, 198
  bleeding from, 146
  brain, 262
  descending aorta, *313*
  face, *198*
  lung, 322-23
  penis, 331
  scalp, *198*

Lactated Ringer's solution, 720
Lap belts, 186
Laryngectomy, 94-95
Laryngospasm, 368
Larynx (voice box), 34
   deviation of, 72
   respiration, 80
Lateral-impact collisions, 184-85
Lateral recumbent position, 17, *19*
Lattissimus muscle, *30*
Law
   ambulance driving, 675-77
   child abuse reporting, 474
   Good Samaritan legislation, 11
   malpractice insurance, 14
   reporting, 704-6
"Laying the bike down" (evasive action), 187-88
Leg(s), 26
   assessment, 76-77
   fracture, 242-48
   heat cramps, 554-56
   injury assessment, 76-77
Legal requirements, dying patient and, 13-14
Lifestyle of EMTs, healthy, 745-69
   alcohol consumption, 764
   cancer prevention, 753
   controllable health factors, 754
   disease prevention, 756-57
   emotional stress, 757-61
   fitness program, 748-56
   health risks for EMTs, 747-48
   nutrition, 756
   smoking, 764
   stress management, 765-69
   weight management, 761-64
   wellness and, 746-47
Lifting of patients, 624-26
Ligament(s), 221
   collateral, 221
   injury, 221
Lightning, 527-28
Liver
   alcohol abuse, *355*
   laceration from CPR, 130
   secondary survey of, 75
Log-roll maneuver, 55, *56*
"Look, Listen, Feel, Smell" approach to secondary survey, 69-70
Lumbar vertebrae, 24
Lung(s), 34-36, 80
   bronchial obstruction, *386*
   bronchial tubes, 34
   chest injury, 311-17
   contusions, 316-17
   emphysema, 385
   fractured ribs, 319-20
   injury from auto accident, 180-81
   intrapleural space, 36
   laceration of, 314
   nasal passages, 34
   pleura, 36
   respiratory system, 34-36
Lung fields, 85
Lyme disease (Lyme borreliosis), 379
Lymphatic system, 31

M
Macro drip IV, 721-22
Malleus, 46
Malpractice insurance, 14
Mammalian diving reflex, 571
Mandible, 24

Manic-depressive disorder, 594-95
Manure storage ponds, injuries at, 337
Marijuana, 356
Marine animals, *382*
Mask, oxygen, 112, 114-18
Masseter muscle, *30*
MAST (Military Anti-Shock Trousers). *See* Pneumatic antishock garment (PASG)
Mastoid cells, 46
Mastoiditis, 46
Maxillary bones, 24
Mechanical chest compression devices, 138
Mechanism of injury, 177. *See also* Kinetics of trauma
   spinal cord injury, 268
Meconium passage, 507
Medic Alert tags, 64-65
Medical terminology, 19-21
Medulla oblongata, 42, 251
Membrane(s)
   brain, *251*
   fetal, 485
   meninges, 42
   synovial, 31
Meninges, 42
Meningitis, *442*, 467-68
Metacarpals, 26
Metatarsals, 26
Micro drip IV, *721*
Military Anti-Shock Trousers (MAST). *See* Pneumatic antishock garment (PASG)
Minor's consent, 12
Miscarriage, 499
Modified Jaw Thrust, 52
Mononucleosis, *442*
Motor vehicle accidents. *See* Vehicular accidents
Mouth
   human bites, 201
   injury, *302*
   jaw fracture, *303*, 303-4
Mouth-to-mask ventilation, 92-94
Mouth-to-mouth ventilation, 89-91, *90*
Mouth-to-nose ventilation, *90*, 91
Mouth-to-stoma ventilation, 91-92
Movement terminology. *See* Moving patients
Moving patients, 613-36
   disentanglement, 667
   equipment, 618-24
   extrication. *See* Extrication
   guidelines, 616-17
   IV therapy, 727-28
   lifting, 624-26
   lifts and carries, 626-33
   special concerns, 634-36
   types of moves, 614-15
   when to move, 513-14
Mucosa, 113, 519
"Mules," overdose due to, 365
Multiple casualty incidents. *See* Disasters
Muscles, 28-31, *30*
   cardiac, 28, 31
   fibers, 28
   injury, 223-25
   skeletal (voluntary), 28-29, 221
   smooth (involuntary), 29, 31, 221
   tone, newborn babies, 497
Musculoskeletal injuries, 196, 220-35
   anatomy, 221-22
   assessment, 222-23
   causes, 222
Myocardial infarction, 122, 482
Myocardium, 31, 123

N
Narcotics, 357
Nasal cannula, 112-14
Nasal passages, 34
Nasopharyngeal airway, 86, *106*, 106-7
National Association for Search and Rescue, 16
National Association of Emergency Medical Technicians (NAEMT), 14-15
National Council of State EMT Training Coordinators and EMS Clearinghouse, 15-16
National Registry of Emergency Medical Technicians, 15
Nausea
   heatstroke, 552
   poisoning, 344
Neck
   injury, *308-9*
      from auto accident, 182, 185
   physical examination, 72
   secondary survey of, 72
Negligence, 11
Nerve(s)
   anatomy, *40*
   brachial, *41*
   cranial, 22, 42
   femoral, *41*
   heart, of the, *41*
   sciatic, *41*
   spinal, 22, 42
   vagus, 43
Nervous system, 39-43, *40-41*, 250-51
   assessment after fracture, *230*
   autonomic, 41, *43*, 43
   central, 22, 42
      Wernicke-Korsakoff Syndrome, 362
   cerebrospinal
      and lightning strike, 527
   head injury, 250-51, 255-58
   neurons, 39
   parasympathetic, 43
   peripheral, 41
   and shock, 161
   sympathetic, 43
   voluntary, 41
Neurogenic hyperventilation, 61
Neurological examination
   assessment, 65-68
   children, 458-59
   head injury, 255-58
   sample record, 67
Newborn. *See under* Babies (Infants)
Nose
   bleeds, 154-55, *155*, 305
   cerebrospinal fluid, 254
   foreign objects in, 305
   fracture, 305
   human bites, 201
   injury, 305
Nutrition for EMTs, 756

O
Oath, EMT, 15
Oblique muscles, *30*
Obstetrics. *See* Pregnancy
Occipital lobe, 42
Occlusion, 396
Occlusive dressing, 215
Opium, 356
Oral airway, 86
Orbicularis muscles, *30*
Oropharyngeal airway, 105-6, *106*
Ossicles, 46

Ovaries, 39
Ovum, 39
Oxygen
  administration of, 110-12
    asthmatic attack, 388
    for children, 463-64
    child respiratory illness, 463-64
    and CPR, 138
    drowning, 574
    masks, 112, 114-18
    newborn babies, 497
    poisoning, 350
    premature babies, 506
  anoxia (lack of), 80
    cardiac arrest, 83
    shock, 157-58
  blood flow, 31
  blood vessels, 31-34
  cardiovascular system, 31-34
  circulatory system, 31
  cylinders, 109
  equipment, 107-19
  hypoxemia, 66
  medical hazards of, 119
  respiratory system, 34
Oxyhemoglobin, 34

P
Packaging, 613
PAIN, 69
Palate, 24
Palatine bones, 24
Palmar surface method of burn
  measurement, 514
Pancreas, 36
Pancreatitis, 360
Paralysis
  assessment of, 77
  contusions, 261
  musculoskeletal injury, 230
  spinal injury, 77
Paranoia, 597-98
Parathormone, 39
Parathyroid, 39
Paresthesia, 230
Partial neck breather, 92
Past medical history, 68-69
Patella, 26
  fracture, 244
Patient assessment, 47-78
  airway, 53-54
  bleeding, 54-55
  blood pressure, 61-63
  breathing, 54
  cervical spine, 53-54
  chief complaint, 58
  disability, 55-57
  establishing rapport, 50-51
  history, 68-69
  neuro exam, 65-68
  pediatric, 454-56
  primary survey, 52-69
  pulse, 58-60
  pyramid, 51
  reporting, 704
  respiration, 60-61
  routine, 49
  secondary survey, 69-78
  temperature, 64
  trauma, 66-68
  visual, 84
  vital signs, 58-64
Pectoralis muscles, *30*

Pediatric emergencies. *See* Children
  (pediatric emergencies)
Pelvis, 26
  fracture, *241*, 241-42
  injury, 75, 185
  pelvic cavity, 26, *327*
  pelvic girdle, 26
Penetrating injuries, 207-11
  kinetics of, 189-93
    bullet wounds, 191-93
    low velocity, 190
    medium and high velocity, 191-92
    shotgun wounds, 192
Penis, 39
  injury, 331-32
  persistent erection of (priapism), 75
Perfusion, 157
Pericardial space, 31, 121
Pericardial tamponade, *313*, 317-19
Pericardium, 31
Peristalsis, 36
Peritoneum, 326
Peritonitis, 75, 360
Perspiration. *See* Sweating (disphoresis,
  perspiring)
Phalanges, 26
Pharyngeo-tracheal-lumen (PTL) airway,
  716-18
Pharynx, 34
  injury, *306-7*
Phencyclidine (PCP), 358, 368
Phlebitis, 727, 730
Phobia, 594
Physical examination. *See also* Patient
  assessment
  adolescents, 455-56
  anxiety during, 48
  children, 454-56
Physician, relaying information to, 699-700
Physiology, generally, 17-47
Pia mater, 42
Piggyback carry, 615
Pineal body, *38*
"Pink puffers," 385
Pituitary body, *38*
Pit viper snakes, 374-75
Placenta (afterbirth), 485
  abruptio, 501-2
  previa, 501
Pleura, 36, 81
Pneumatic antishock garment (PASG), 151,
  172-75, *174*, 209, 227
  pericardial tamponade and, 319
Pneumonia, 102, 389, 482
Pneumothorax, 193
  chest injury, *312*, 322
  CPR, 130
  dyspnea, 311
  respiratory assessment, 311
  shock, 311
  spontaneous, *312*, 322
  tension pneumothorax, 193, *312*,
    321-22
Pocket face-masks, 92-94
Poison(s), poisoning, 342-53
  absorbed, 343, 351
  assessment, 344
  corrosive, 351
  food, 353
  ingested, 343-48
    children, 345
    emergency care, 345-48
    examination, 344
    history taking, 343-44

poisonous plants, 351-53
  signs and symptoms, 344
  vomiting, 346-47
inhaled, 343, 348-51
  carbon monoxide, 349-50
  emergency care, 350-51
  signs and symptoms, 348-49
injection, 343
ivy, *352*, 352
oak, *352*, 352
plants, 351-53
poison centers, 344-45
sea animals, 380-83
skin color, 344
snake venom, 372-73
sumac, *352*, 352
Pole stretcher, *619*, 621
Polyuria, 415
Pons, *40*, 42
Portuguese Man-of-War, *382*
Position(s), anatomical, 18-19
Positive-pressure ventilators, 119
Postimpact phase of disaster, 644
Power takeoff shafts (farm equipment), 337
Preeclampsia, 499
Prefixes, 19-21
Pregnancy
  anatomy, *485*
  complications, 497-506
    abruptio placenta, 501-2
    placenta previa, 501
    prepartum hemorrhage, 502-3
    prolapsed umbilical cord, 503-4
    ruptured uterus, 502
    spontaneous abortion, 499
    toxemia, 498-99
  ectopic, 423, 499-501
  emergency delivery, 490-96
  labor (childbirth), 485, *489-90*
    complications, 504-6
    multiple births, 506
  newborn assessment, 496-97
  newborn care, 496-97
  normal, 485
  trauma, 507-9
Preimpact phase of disaster, 644
Premature birth, 506
Pressure points, 147
Priapism, 75, 257
Primary phase blast injury, 193
Primary survey, 52-69
Prinzmetal's angina, 397
Profile of bullet, 191
Projectile injuries, kinetics of, 189-93
Prolapsed cord, 503-4
Prone position, 18, *19*
Protective clothing, 654
Pruritis, 362
Psychogenic shock, 161, 164
Psychological emergencies, 577-92
  bystander responses, 580
  communicating in, 583-84
    blind, 586-87
    deaf, *586*, 586
    developmentally disabled, 587
    geriatric, 584
    non-English-speaking, 587
    pediatric, 584-85
  disasters, 648-49
  family responses, 580
  general principles of, 578
  management of, 581-83
  patient assessment, 580-81
  patient responses, 579-80

Psychological Emergencies (*cont.*)
  physical disorders resembling, 581
  signs and symptoms, *579*
Psychomotor seizures, 431
Pubic bone, 75
Pulmonary artery, 34
Pulmonary circulation, 31, *121*
Pulmonary disease, chronic obstructive, 36, 60, 385-87
Pulmonary edema, 391-92
  congestive heart failure, 391-92
Pulmonary embolism, 102-3, 389-91
  childbirth, 391, 504
  dyspnea, 391
  hyperventilation, 392
Pulmonary embolus in elderly, 482
Pulmonary semilunar valve, 34
Pulmonary veins, 34
Pulse
  apical, 59
  and blood pressure, 54-55, 58-60
  bounding, 58
  brachial, 54, 135
  carotid, 54, 122, *126*, 135, 166
  children, 457
  distal, 77
  evaluating, *54*
  femoral, 54, 122
  heat exhaustion, 554
  heatstroke, 552
  hypothermia, 557
  irregular, 58
  normal, 58
  radial, 54, 122, 166
  shock symptoms, 163-64, 166
  thready, 58
  wave, 724
Pulse points, arterial, 34-35
Punctures, 198-99
Pupils. *See under* Eye(s)
Pyrogenic reaction, 730

Q
Quadrants, 28, *29*

R
Rabies, 200
Raccoon's sign ("raccoon's eyes"), 255, 258
Radiation, heat loss, 547-48
Radiation emergencies, 540-45
Radio, emergency use of. *See* Communications
Radius, 25
Rads, 541
Rales
  children, 462
  respiratory emergencies, 85
Rape, 607-9
Rape trauma syndrome, 607-9
Rattlesnakes, 371-75
Rear-impact collisions, 182
Recoil phase of disaster, 644
Record keeping, 704-6
Rectum, 26
Rectus muscles, *30*
Report, writing, 78-79
Reporting information, 68, 704-6
Reporting requirements, 13
Repositioning patient, 613
Reproductive organs, *39*
Reproductive system, *39*
  injury, 331-32
Rescue. *See* Extrication
Respiration. *See* Breathing (respiration)

Respiratory emergencies, 384-93. *See also* Breathing (respiration)
Respiratory system, *35*
  anatomy, 34-36, 82
  arrest, 83
  assessment, 84-85
  auscultation, 73, 84
  difficulties, 384-93
    children, 91, 461-67
  distress signs, 84, *85*
  head injury, 254
  injury, from burns, 519-20
  palpating exam, 85-86
  rate, children, 457
Restraints, vehicular, 185-86
Reye's syndrome, 468
Rhonchi, 85
Rib(s), 25
  cage, 31
  false, 25
  floating, 25
  fracture, *320*, *327*
  true, 25
Rickettsial infection, 161
Rings, clamping injury, 206
Roentgens, 541
Rollover, vehicular, 185
Rope-sling extrication, 671
Rotational-impact collisions, 185
"Rule of Nines, the," 511
Rupture. *See also* Hernia (rupture)
  uterus, 502

S
Sacrum, 24
Salt, heat cramps, 555-56
SAMPLE, 68
Sartorius muscle, *30*
Scalp
  injury, 254, 258
  secondary survey of, 72
Scapula (shoulder blade), 25
Scoop stretcher, 618-21, *621*
Scorpion, 377-78
Scrotum, injury, 332
Seat carry method of transfer, 629
Secondary phase blast injury, 193
Secondary survey, 69-78
Seizures, 430-37
  assessment, 435
  aura, 435
  children, *433*
  emergency care, *432-33*, 435-37
  phases, 435
  status epilepticus, 431
  types of, 431-35
    atonic, *433*
    febrile, 431
    grand mal, 431, *434*, *436*
    infantile spasms, *433*
    Jacksonian, 442
    myoclonic, *433*
    petit mal (absence attacks), 431
    psychomotor, *433*
    simple partial, *432*
    withdrawal, 431
Semitendinosus muscle, *30*
Septicemia, 468
Septic shock, 102, 160-61, 164
Septum, 31
Serratus muscles, *30*
Sexual assault, 607-9
  genital injuries from, 332
Sheet drag, 614-15

Shirt drag, 614
Shock, 156-75
  anaphylactic, 161, 164-66, *165*, 169
  assessment, 166-67
  from burns, 516
  cardiogenic, 161, 164
  causes of, 158-59
  children, 166, 467
  dark-skinned patients, *167*
  in elderly, 482
  electrical, 525-28
  fluid volume, 160
  gunshot wounds, 209
  hemorrhagic, 159-60, 161, 164
  hypovolemic, 366
  "irreversible shock," 162
  management, 167-72
  neurogenic, 161
  from pelvic injury, 242
  physiology of, 157-58
  pregnant women, 168
  prevention, *172*, 172
  psychogenic (fainting), 161, 164
  septic, 102, 160-61, 164
  severity factors, 159
  signs and symptoms, 162-66, *163*
  and skin color, 166
  and skin temperature, 166
  stages of, 161-62
    compensatory, 161
    progressive, 161-62
  thigh fracture, 243
  traumatic, 158
  treatment, 167-72
  vasovagal. *See* Shock, neurogenic
  wound. *See* Shock, hemorrhagic
Shoes, removing, 76
Shotgun wounds, kinetics of, 192
Shoulder(s)
  blade, 25
  dislocation, 226
  girdle, 25
Shoulder belts, 186
Sigmoid, 28
Silo injuries, 337
Skeletal system, 21-28, *23*, *222*
Skin
  anatomy, *44*, 44-45
  assessment, 64
  burns, 514
  color
    newborn babies, 496
    poisoning, 344
    shock, *167*
  dermis, 44
  epidermis, 44
  frostbite, 565-67
  hair, *44*
  during heart attack, 400
  heat exhaustion, 554
  heatstroke, 554
  melanin (pigmentation), 44
  sebaceous glands, 44
  subcutaneous connective tissue, 44
  subcutaneous emphysema, 322
  sweat glands, 44
Skull, 22-24
  basilar, 250-51
  cranial, 250
  facial, 251
  fracture, 258
  injury to, 258
Sling and swathe, *234*
Smoking, 764
Snakebite, 371-75

emergency care, 373-75
kit, 374
signs and symptoms, 372-74
Snakes, 371
Snake venom, 372-73
Snoring, upper airway obstruction, 85
Snowmobile accidents, 188
SOAP reporting method, 705
Sodium chloride, 44
Soft tissue injury, 195-204. *See also*
  Wounds
Soleus muscle, *30*
Spasm, 85
Sperm, 39
Sphygmomanometer, 58, *61*
  technique, 62-63
Spinal column, 22, 24
Spinal cord, 22, 42, 266-67
  divisions of, 40
  and head injury, 255
  injury. *See* Spinal injury
  tracts, 42
Spinal injury, 266-88
  assessment, 268
  cervical, 86, 301
  emergency care for, *272*, 272-85
  and extrication, 669-71, *672*
  extrication collar, 273-76
  head injury, 255
  helmet removal, *287-88*, 287-88
  mechanisms of injury, *267*, 267-68
  patient transfer, 276-85
  signs and symptoms, 268, *271*
  water rescue, 572
Spinal nerves, 22, 42
Spineboard
  automobile accidents, 669-71
  CPR, 128
  patient transfer, 276-85, 669-71
Spleen, *29*
Splenius muscle, *30*
Splint(s), 232-35
  air, 151, *233*
  dislocations, 232
  extrication equipment, 655
  fixation, 233
  improvised, 232-33
  MAST, 151
  PASG, 151
  pillow, *235*
  self-splint, 232
  sling and swathe, 234
  traction, 243, *245*
  wrist fracture, *240*
Spouse abuse, 601-7
Sprains, *198*, 223-25
  emergency care (RICE), 224
Stab wounds, 207
Stairchair, *620*, 626
Standard routines, 48
Stapes, 46
Status asthmaticus, 388-89, *390*
Status epilepticus, 431
Stem words, 20
Sternum, 25
  and CPR, 130
Stethoscope, 58, *61*
Stingrays, *382*
Stings, 379-80
Stokes litter, 624
Stoma, 72, 91-92
Stomach, secondary survey of, 75
Strains, *198*, 225
Strangling injury, 206
Stress

disasters, 651-52
emotional, 757-61
response of EMT to, 587-88
Stress management, 765-69
Stretchers
  patient transfer, 633-34
  types, 619-22
Stridor, 85
Stroke (apoplexy, cerebrovascular accident),
  408-13
  causes, 408-10
    compression, 410
    embolus, 409
    hemorrhage, 409-10
    thrombus, 408
  coma, 408
  consciousness level, 410-11
  emergency care, 412-13
  risk factors, 408
  signs and symptoms, 410-12
  speech problem, 411
Strychnine, 348
Styloid processes, 25
Subarachnoid space, 42
Subdural space, 42, 251
Sucking chest wound, *323*, 323-24
Suction equipment, *107*, 107
Sudden Infant Death Syndrome (SIDS),
  468-71
Suffixes, 19-21
Suffocation, oxygen masks and, 112
Suicide, 595-97
Sunstroke, 549-53, *559*
Superior vena cava, 31
Supine hypotensive syndrome, 487-90
Supine position, 18, *19*
Suprapubic, 28
Sweating (disphoresis, perspiring)
  body temperature, 549-50
  heat exhaustion, 553-54
  heatstroke, 549-52
  shock, 163
Swelling (edema)
  burns, 516
  and closed wounds, 196
  and congestive heart failure, 404
Syncope in elderly, 482
Synovial fluid, 31
Synovial membrane, 31
Syrup of ipecac, 346
Systemic circulation, 31, *121*
Systemic condition, 53
Systolic pressure, 54

T

Tachycardia, 735-36
Tachypnea, 61
Talus, 26
Tarsal bones, 26
Temperature
  body
    adjustment, 547
    assessment, 64
    children, 458
    heat exhaustion, 64, 554
    heat loss, 547-49
    heatstroke, 64, 553
    normal, 64
    oral, 64
    technique, 64
  skin, 64
Temporal bones, 24
Temporalis muscle, *30*
Temporal lobe, 42
Tendons, 28, 221

injury to, 221
of insertion, 221
of origin, 221
Tension pneumothorax, 193, *312*, 321-22
Terminology, 48
Tertiary phase blast injury, 193-94
Testicle, rupture of, 332
Thighs, 26
Thoracic vertebrae, 24
Thorax. *See* Chest
Three-man carry method of transfer, 631
Three-man log roll method of transfer, 280
Thorat (pharynx), 34
  injury, *306-7*, 306-9
Thrombophlebitis, 391
Thrombus (clot), 408
Thymus gland, *38*
Thyroid gland, *38*, 39
Thyroxin, 39
Tibia, 26
Tibialis anterior muscle, *30*
Ticks, 378-79
Tidal volume, 114
Tissue, injuries to soft, 195-204
Toe fracture, 244-46
Tongue
  facial injury and, 301
  upper airway obstruction and, *81*
Tooth (teeth), face injury and, 301
Tort, 11-12
Tourniquet, 151
Toxemia, 430, 498-99
Toxicity of oxygen, 119
Toxins from poisonous plants, 352, *353*
Trachea (windpipe), 34, 81
  deviation of, 72
Tracheostomy tube, 92
Tractor (farm equipment), 334-36
Trajectory of projectile, 191
Transection, 320-21
Transfer techniques. *See also* Moving
  patients
  spinal injury, 276-85
Transient ischemic attacks (TIAs), 408
Transillumination (lighted stylet) intubation,
  709-12
Transport, 78. *See also* Moving patients;
  Packaging
Trauma
  assessment, 66-68
  blunt, 203, 311
  geriatric, 481-82
  kinetics of. *See* Kinetics of trauma
  pregnancy, 507-9
  scale, 66, *67*
  traumatic shock, 158
Triage, 636-42
  conduct of, 640-42
  log, 642
  tags, 638-40
  three-level systems, 638
Triceps muscle, *30*
Tricuspid value, 31
Tuberculosis, *442*
Two-rescuer immobilization, 281

U

Ulcer and internal bleeding, 152
Ulna, 25
Umbilical cord, 485
  around neck, 505
  prolapsed, 503-4
Unconsciousness, 437-38
  AMI and, 402
  CPR, 123

Unconsciousness (*cont.*)
  hypothermia, 563
  spinal cord injury, 268
"Universal body-substance isolation," 446
Ureters, 38
Urinary bladder, 38
Urinary system, *38*
  injury, 331
Urine, blood in, 75
Uterine inversion, 504
Uterus, 39
  pregnancy, 485
  rupture of, 502

V
Vagina, 39
Vasodilation, 103
Vehicular accidents. *See also* Automobile accidents
  blunt trauma from, 331
  kinetics of trauma from, 179-88
    motorcycle, 186-88
    recreation vehicles, 188
Veins, 34
Ventilation
  of car accident victims, 94
  mouth-to-mask, 92-94

Ventilators, positive-pressure, 119
Ventricles, 31
Ventricular fibrillation, 122, 735-36
Ventricular tachycardia, 735-36
Vernix caseosa, 492
Vertebrae (anatomy), *24*, 24-25
Vertigo, 437
Vial of Life program, 65
Victims of crime, 13
Violent patients, 598-601
Viruses, 440
Visual assessment, 84
Vital signs, 58
Vocal cords, 34
Vomiting
  gastrointestinal complaint, 427
  poisons, 346-47

W
Waterchill, 548
Water emergencies, 568-76
  barotraum, 575-76
  bends, 574-75
  diving, 572-76
  drowning, 569-72
Weight management, 761-64
Wellness, health and, 746-47

Wernicke-Korsakoff syndrome, 360
Wheezing
  children, 462
  respiratory emergencies, 85
Windchill, 548, *549*
Windpipe, 34, 81
Wounds
  abrasions, 196-97
  avulsions, 199
  bites, 199-201, *200*
  care of, *203*, 203-4
  clamping injury, *206*, 206
  classification, *197*
  closed, 196
  entrance, 207
  exit, 207
  gunshot, 207-9
  impaled objects, 209-10
  incisions, 197-98
  lacerations, 198
  open, 196-204
  punctures, 198-99, 262
  stab, 207
  traumatic amputations, *201*, 201-3

X
Xiphoid process, 97